Advances in Food Authenticity Testing

Advances in Food Authenticity Testing

Edited by

Gerard Downey
Teagasc Food Research Centre
Dublin, Republic of Ireland

ELSEVIER

AMSTERDAM • BOSTON • CAMBRIDGE • HEIDELBERG
LONDON • NEW YORK • OXFORD • PARIS • SAN DIEGO
SAN FRANCISCO • SINGAPORE • SYDNEY • TOKYO
Woodhead Publishing is an imprint of Elsevier

WP
WOODHEAD PUBLISHING

Woodhead Publishing is an imprint of Elsevier
The Officers' Mess Business Centre, Royston Road, Duxford, CB22 4QH, United Kingdom
50 Hampshire Street, 5th Floor, Cambridge, MA 02139, United States
The Boulevard, Langford Lane, Kidlington, OX5 1GB, United Kingdom

Library of Congress Cataloging-in-Publication Data
A catalog record for this book is available from the Library of Congress

British Library Cataloguing-in-Publication Data
A catalogue record for this book is available from the British Library

ISBN: 978-0-08-100220-9

Publisher: Nikki Levy
Acquisition Editor: Rob Sykes
Editorial Project Manager: Karen Miller
Production Project Manager: Debbie Clark
Designer: Greg Harris

Typeset by TNQ Books and Journals

Contents

List of Contributors

O. Abbas Walloon Agricultural Research Centre (CRA-W), Gembloux, Belgium

G.A. Abernethy Fonterra Research & Development Centre, Palmerston North, New Zealand

J. Amaral University of Porto, Porto, Portugal

I. Amin Universiti Putra Malaysia, Serdang, Selangor, Malaysia

M.L. Ashour Ain Shams University, Cairo, Egypt

V. Baeten Walloon Agricultural Research Centre (CRA-W), Gembloux, Belgium

J.G. Bendall Fonterra Research & Development Centre, Palmerston North, New Zealand

L. Bontempo Research and Innovation Centre, Trentino, Italy

T. Brendel Eurofins Medigenomix GmbH, Ebersberg, Germany

S. Broeders Scientific Institute of Public Health, Brussels, Belgium

T. Cajka University of California, Davis, Davis, CA, United States

F. Camin Research and Innovation Centre, Trentino, Italy

S. Circi University of Rome, Rome, Italy

D. Cozzolino Central Queensland University, Rockhampton, Queensland, Australia

A. Dankowska Poznań University of Economics and Business, Poznań, Poland

D. Deforce Ghent University, Ghent, Belgium

M. De Loose Institute for Agricultural and Fisheries Research (ILVO), Merelbeke, Belgium

S.R. Delwiche USDA, Agricultural Research Service, Beltsville, MD, United States

G. Downey Teagasc Food Research Centre, Dublin, Republic of Ireland

L. Dugo Università Campus Bio-Medico of Rome, Rome, Italy

T. Dymerski Gdansk University of Technology, Gdańsk, Poland

S.H. El-Ahmady Ain Shams University, Cairo, Egypt

M. Espiñeira ANFACO-CECOPESCA, Vigo, Spain

C. Fanali Università Campus Bio-Medico of Rome, Rome, Italy

O. Fiehn University of California, Davis, Davis, CA, United States

M.-A. Fraiture Scientific Institute of Public Health, Brussels, Belgium

M.M. Giusti College of Food Agriculture and Environmental Sciences, The Ohio State University, OH, United States

P. Herman Scientific Institute of Public Health, Brussels, Belgium

S.E. Holroyd Fonterra Research & Development Centre, Palmerston North, New Zealand

D.W. Lachenmeier Chemisches und Veterinäruntersuchungsamt (CVUA) Karlsruhe, Karlsruhe, Germany

F. Lago ANFACO-CECOPESCA, Vigo, Spain

K.H. Laursen University of Copenhagen, Copenhagen, Denmark

E. Maestri University of Parma, Parma, Italy

I. Mafra University of Porto, Porto, Portugal

L. Mannina Sapienza University of Rome, Rome, Italy

N. Marmiroli University of Parma, Parma, Italy

M.J. Martelo-Vidal University of Santiago de Compostela, Lugo, Spain

L. Meira University of Porto, Porto, Portugal

L. Mondello Università Campus Bio-Medico of Rome, Rome, Italy

M. Muilwijk Wageningen University and Research Centre, Wageningen, The Netherlands

W.F. Nader Eurofins Global Control GmbH, Hamburg, Germany

J. Namieśnik Gdansk University of Technology, Gdańsk, Poland

T. Nur Azira International Islamic University Malaysia, Kuala Lumpur, Malaysia

M.B.P.P. Oliveira University of Porto, Porto, Portugal

P. Oliveri University of Genova, Genova, Italy

V.A. Parvathy ICAR-Indian Institute of Spices Research, Kozhikode, Kerala, India

A.M. Pustjens Wageningen University and Research Centre, Wageningen, The Netherlands

K. Riddellova ALS Czech Republic s.r.o., Prague, Czech Republic

P. Rinke SGF International E.V., Nieder-Olm, Germany

L.E. Rodriguez-Saona College of Food Agriculture and Environmental Sciences, The Ohio State University, OH, United States

N.H. Roosens Scientific Institute of Public Health, Brussels, Belgium

A. Roßmann Isolab GmbH Laboratory for Stable Isotopes, Schweitenkirchen, Germany

B. Sasikumar ICAR-Indian Institute of Spices Research, Kozhikode, Kerala, India

R. Schubbert Eurofins Medigenomix GmbH, Ebersberg, Germany

T.E. Sheeja ICAR-Indian Institute of Spices Research, Kozhikode, Kerala, India

M. Shotts College of Food Agriculture and Environmental Sciences, The Ohio State University, OH, United States

M.R. Showalter University of California, Davis, Davis, CA, United States

R. Simonetti University of Genova, Genova, Italy

M. Śliwińska Gdansk University of Technology, Gdańsk, Poland

A.P. Sobolev National Research Council, Rome, Italy

V.P. Swetha ICAR-Indian Institute of Spices Research, Kozhikode, Kerala, India

I. Taverniers Institute for Agricultural and Fisheries Research (ILVO), Merelbeke, Belgium

F. Ulberth European Commission, Geel, Belgium

S.M. van Ruth Wageningen University and Research Centre, Wageningen, The Netherlands

M. Vázquez University of Santiago de Compostela, Lugo, Spain

W. Wardencki Gdansk University of Technology, Gdańsk, Poland

Y. Weesepoel Wageningen University and Research Centre, Wageningen, The Netherlands

P. Wiśniewska Gdansk University of Technology, Gdańsk, Poland

Introduction

1

G. Downey
Teagasc Food Research Centre, Dublin, Republic of Ireland

Food security is a primeval concern and people have developed systems of agricultural production, safe storage, processing, and transportation in order to satisfy their food requirement needs. Since the industrial revolution and the accelerated accumulation of scientific knowledge in the last two centuries, major inroads have been made in addressing the problems around providing sufficient food for earth's population, although about 793 million people globally were estimated to be undernourished in 2015 (FAO, 2015). For those living in the developed regions of the world, food insufficiency is not generally of relevance although societal problems concerning equitable food distribution are a current reality. However, issues around the safety and quality of the food supply are foremost in the minds of consumers and regulatory authorities in these countries. Food safety is of course paramount for the food industry and regulatory industries given the increased amount of dietary energy now consumed in the form of processed foods by the populations of developed countries (Monteiro et al., 2013) and the increasing complexity and length of food distribution and supply chains. However, consumer sensitivity to the possibility that their food may not be what it claims to be is generally assumed to be increasing.

A significant reason for this is sensitivity perhaps lies in the print and broadcast media's greater coverage of food scandals involving false labeling. Detailed descriptions of and investigations into recent scandals such as the presence of Sudan-1 dye in a wide range of foodstuffs in the United Kingdom in 2005, the detection of melamine in milk sourced in China in 2008, and the more recent horsemeat scandal uncovered in Ireland in 2013 have all been covered extensively in the public arena and have doubtlessly contributed to public concern. The melamine scandal in particular has been responsible for heightened awareness because this adulteration also had a significant food safety dimension due to the toxic effects of this compound, especially in babies and young children. Indeed, it is partly in response to this particularly egregious adulteration that consumers now increasingly treat food adulteration as a potential food safety issue with all the attention that this implies.

Regulatory agencies around the world are now devoting more resources to this problem not least because many of the adulterations, eg, those involving illicit alcohol, can involve revenue losses to the state. Operation OPSON is a multicountry (currently 47 states) joint cooperation between Europol and INTERPOL, which also includes public authorities and private companies. Operated through annual, targeted exercises, the most recent (OPSON IV) was conducted between December 2014 and January 2015 and, in this short period, OPSON seized more than 2500 tons of illicit and counterfeit food including mozzarella cheese, strawberries, eggs, cooking oil, and dried fruit (Europol, 2015). This type of cross-border organization is a recognition of the increasing globalization of trade in food and especially food ingredients and the extended nature of food supply chains.

Within Europe, food fraud has been a long-standing subject of research and concern. The European Commission funded a number of research projects through its Framework Programmes 3–7 covering the period 1994 until now. These projects have ranged from collaborative research activities such as FAIM (1994–97) and TRACE (2005–10) to actions focused on specific analytical techniques (Food analysis using isotopic techniques, 1996–98) or authenticity issues (FATAUTHENTICATION; Authentication of fats and fat products used in food and feed, 2010–12). Recognizing the need for greater communication between states regarding intelligence around potential adulteration incidents, the Commission formed the Food Fraud Network (FFN) in 2015. This pan-European body is designed specifically to detect and prevent violations of food chain rules across borders and to collect information that is needed (in accordance with applicable national rules) to further refer a case to investigation or prosecution.

To support these regulatory and commercial initiatives, research scientists have devoted considerable resources to the development of analytical techniques to identify foods or food ingredients that are in breach of labeling requirements and may consequently be adulterated. A quick and rather crude search of the Web of Science using the search terms "food authentic*" and "food adulteration" revealed that 334 research articles with one or the other of these terms in the publication title had appeared in the decade between 2006 and 2016. Given that many publications will have more specific titles, it may not be unreasonable to conclude that the total number of such outputs may be 5 or even 10 times this number. Given this evidence of a flourishing research community focusing on analytical problems related to food adulteration, it was considered timely to gather together the most up-to-date information on the techniques and their use in specific application types in this book.

In Part 1, the focus is on advances in methods for food authenticity testing. This collection of 11 chapters contains contributions from experts in fields as diverse as differential scanning calorimetry to mass spectrometry and DNA fingerprinting. All of these authors have contributed information on the latest developments in these methods and the chapters will be invaluable to anyone practicing in the field or considering adding new techniques to their analytical repertoire.

Part 2 contains reports on advances in authenticity testing of a range of food types. These four chapters cover strategies for confirming the geographic origin of foods and testing for authenticity in meat, fish, and cereals.

Part 3 comprises 10 chapters, each of which deals with specific food products or analytical tools to support authenticity testing. Among the former are chapters dealing with adulteration testing methods for dairy products, cereals and cereal products, alcoholic beverages, and fruit and fruit juice products. Of increasing interest is the food supplement sector of the food industry, and one chapter focuses on the methods being currently applied to detect offenses in this industry segment. Last, but not least, is a chapter on the most appropriate chemometric tools suitable for and that are being used to tackle authenticity and adulteration practices.

I trust that you will find the book useful and profitable.

Gerard Downey
Dublin, February 2016

References

Europol, 2015. https://www.europol.europa.eu/content/record-seizures-fake-food-and-drink-interpol-europol-operation (accessed 04.03.16.).

FAO, 2015. The State of Food Insecurity in the World 2015. http://www.fao.org/hunger/key-messages/en/ (accessed 04.03.16.).

Monteiro, C.A., Moubarac, J.-C., Cannon, G., Ng, S.W., Popkin, B., November 2013. Ultra-processed products are becoming dominant in the global food system. Obesity Reviews 14 (Suppl. 2), 21–28. http://dx.doi.org/10.1111/obr.12107.

Part One

Advances in Methods for Food Authenticity Testing

Advances in DNA Fingerprinting for Food Authenticity Testing

2

W.F. Nader[1], *T. Brendel*[2], *R. Schubbert*[2]
[1]Eurofins Global Control GmbH, Hamburg, Germany; [2]Eurofins Medigenomix GmbH, Ebersberg, Germany

Chapter Outline

2.1 Introduction

For the last two decades, analysis of DNA in food has become a routine procedure to detect genetically modified organisms, allergens, pathogens, and adulterations in food. Many cases of food fraud have been uncovered by DNA testing, for example, undeclared horse meat in beef products (FSA, 2013), *Pinus armandii* in Chinese pine nuts (Nader et al., 2013), persipan declared as marzipan (Brüning et al., 2011), and overfished species like yellowfin (*Thunnus albacares*) or bigeye tuna (*Thunnus obesus*) in canned tuna declared as skipjack (*Katsuwonus pelamis*) (Chuang et al., 2012). The horse meat scandal stunned the food industry and trade in the European Union (EU) in 2013. Adulteration of pine nuts by the species *P. armandii* (Chinese white pine) affects food safety, since these latter cause significant and long-lasting taste disturbances (Pine mouth syndrome).

The authenticity testing mentioned herein is based on the detection of species-specific DNA sequences. Animal species are commonly differentiated based on sequences of mitochondrial genes, which code for the subunit I of cytochrome c oxidase. Plant species can be distinguished by differences of the intergenic spacer regions in the plastid chloroplast DNA or the internal transcribed spacer (ITS) region of the nuclear ribosomal cistron (18S-5.8S-26S) (Nader et al., 2013).

Certain specialty foods like basmati rice and Angus beef require authenticity testing beyond the species level because crop varieties and breeds of livestock have to be identified and distinguished. Basmati and its adulterants, ordinary long-grain rice varieties, belong to the same species *Oryza sativa*. Angus cattle are a premium breed of *Bos taurus*, and meat from ordinary cattle can frequently be found declared as genuine Angus beef.

Traceability is a major requirement of EU food legislation (Regulation (EC) No 178/2002) and is particularly strict for meat products (Regulation (EC) No 1760/2000; Commission Implementing Regulation (EU) No 931/2011). Controlling this traceability requires the differentiation of individual animals, which can be achieved by DNA analysis as well (Vázquez et al., 2004).

Individual animals, breeds of livestock, and crop varieties cannot be identified based on the genetic elements commonly used for species differentiation (see previous discussion) because these DNA sequences are stable and well established within a species. For testing at this level, DNA sequences are required with a high degree of polymorphism, which changes frequently within generations. Genetic elements, which meet these requirements, are highly polymorphic mini- and microsatellites and single nucleotide mutations, the so-called single nucleotide polymorphisms (SNPs). These three groups of genetic elements provide the markers for DNA fingerprinting capable of analysis at the level of individuals, breeds, and varieties.

DNA fingerprinting used to identify human individuals was first applied by Sir Alec Jeffreys as a forensic tool to solve an immigration case in 1985 and later the Enderby murder in 1986 (Jobling and Gill, 2004). The original method applied by Jeffreys was based on polymorphisms of minisatellites and was later replaced by genotyping of microsatellites, also called simple sequence repeats (SSRs). SSR typing has revolutionized forensics since then and has now even become a major tool to solve decades-old cold cases.

Genotyping based on SNPs utilizes differences of single nucleotides and is widely used for breeding of plants and animals and for the identification and paternity testing of cattle (Heaton et al., 2002).

This chapter will describe in detail scientific and technological aspects of DNA fingerprinting and two applications of SSR genotyping in food, ie, authenticity testing of high-value rice varieties and traceability checks on pork meat. Legal and economic aspects will be discussed with regard to the DNA analysis of basmati and jasmine rice.

2.2 Scientific Background of DNA Fingerprinting and Its Applications

2.2.1 *Mini- and Microsatellites*

Minisatellites are often referred to as variable number of tandem repeats (VNTRs) and microsatellites as short tandem repeats (STRs) or SSRs. The names mini- or microsatellites are historically derived from the behavior of certain fractions of DNA in the cesium chloride density gradient during ultracentrifugation. These fractions form satellites, strong and localized bands above or below the main band.

VNTRs and SSRs are tandem repeats of short repeat units. The size of the repeat unit is the main feature to classify a tandem repeat as a mini- or microsatellite. It is generally accepted that repeat units of microsatellites contain less than 9 base pairs (Richard et al., 2008).

Tandem repeats occur in virtually all prokaryotic and eukaryotic genomes. The most simple repeat structures consist of mononucleotide repeats, homopolymers of poly(AT) and poly(GC) tracts, which were first observed in a very basic eukaryotic life form, the myxomycete *Physarum polycephalum* (Nader et al., 1985, 1986).

Mini- and microsatellites occur frequently in eukaryotes. About 253,000 (90 per - megabase) microsatellites have been detected in the human genome (Richard et al., 2008), and according to Sonah et al. (2011) the rice genome contains over 135,000 SSRs with a frequency of about 360 per megabase.

Lengths of mini- and microsatellites can be highly variable, and mutations lead to the gain or loss of one or more repeats. Short microsatellites tend to expand while longer ones tend to contract. The variability of microsatellites depends on the length and structure of the tandem repeat and the location in the genome. The mutation rates are estimated at between 10^{-2} and 10^{-6} per locus and generation in the human genome (Eckert and Hile, 2009). In contrast, the average mutation rate for nucleotide conversions generating SNPs is much lower and estimated to be $\sim 2.3 \times 10^{-8}$ per nucleotide site. However, these might occur all over the genome and consequently are at least as frequent as changes in SSRs with 175 mutations at single nucleotide sites per diploid genome per generation (Nachman and Crowell, 2000).

Replication slippage is generally thought to be the main pathway causing the high mutation rates of tandem repeats (Ellegren, 2004). Slippage involves the transient dissociation of the replicating DNA strands and, during reassociation, loops might form on the template or nascent strands due to the tandem repeat structure. Loops on the nascent strand lead to an increase of the repeat length and on the template strand to a decrease. In most cases, the mismatch repair system corrects these changes, but in a small unrepaired fraction these mutations are manifested (Levinson and Gutman, 1987).

Mini- and microsatellites are often considered to be nonfunctional "junk" DNA. However, recent studies on variations of tandem repeats within functional genes of the yeast *Saccharomyces cerevisiae* reveal that these change the capability of the cells to adhere and form biofilms and thus contribute to the fast adaptation of these microorganisms to changing environments (Verstrepen et al., 2005). Hypervariable repeats located within developmental genes of the dog genome supposedly permit the fast evolution of the limb and skull morphology of these animals (Fondon and Garner, 2004). Mini- and microsatellites might therefore significantly contribute to the genetic variability of organisms and may possibly be a driving force in evolution.

Mini- and microsatellites are highly polymorphic, and therefore these elements are used extensively in applied genomics. Their role in modern forensics has already been described herein but there are numerous other applications. Microsatellite typing was used for the identification of laboratory and industrial strains of the yeast *S. cerevisiae* and pathogenic *Candida* strains (Lunel et al., 1998). It was furthermore applied to investigate the origin of domestic horses (Vilà et al., 2001) and French wine grapes (Bower et al., 1999). Microsatellites play an important role in marker-assisted plant and animal breeding (Phuc et al., 2005; Gupta et al., 2001). In biological conservation, analysis of microsatellites became an important tool with which to determine the genetic diversity of populations and to prevent inbreeding of populations in captivity in reintroduction projects (Nader et al., 1999). Applications for the control of food authenticity and traceability will be discussed in detail later.

2.2.2 Single Nucleotide Polymorphism

DNA fingerprinting can be also performed on the basis of SNPs. This method has substituted SSR typing in many applications (Gupta et al., 2001). SNPs occur at single base pair positions in the genome, at which two different alleles exist in the individuals of a population or among different crop varieties. The abundance of the least frequent allele should be 1% or greater (Guerra and Yu, 2010). SSRs and SNPs are referred to as second- and third-generation markers, respectively (Gupta et al., 2001). Advantages of SNPs over SSRs include their higher abundance within genomes; in any genome, one SNP can be found in every 100 to 300 base pairs while SSRs occur less frequently by one to two orders of magnitude. The human genome reveals one microsatellite in every 10,000 base pairs and the rice genome reveals one in every 3000 base pairs (see previous mention). SNPs are also more homogenously distributed over the genome than are SSRs; they are also more stable due to their lower mutation rate (see previous mention). Due to these characteristics, SNPs are the markers of choice for genotyping of human and animal diseases, in personalized medicine (for example, in pharmacogenomics), genome-wide association studies and marker-assisted breeding of animals and plants (Gupta et al., 2001; Feltus et al., 2004).

One advantage of SSRs over SNPs is their polyallelic nature. For each SNP, four different alleles should occur, but in most cases only two alleles have been observed at a specific locus in the genome of a population. By analyzing only a small panel of SSR markers, crop varieties can be detected and differentiated in food. Similarly, meat can be traced back to individual animals or parents. The high abundance of SNPs largely offsets this disadvantage of only two alleles being present, and numerous SNPs can be analyzed simultaneously, for example, by applying multiarray DNA biochip technologies (see following discussion).

In contrast to SSRs, SNPs have not yet been established as routine markers for food analysis, and potential applications are still at the stage of fundamental research (Spaniolas et al., 2014).

Another alternative to SSR markers are insertions/deletions (InDels). In the rice genome, for example, 400,000 InDels have been mapped, many of these being polymorphic and therefore suitable for DNA fingerprinting (Steele et al., 2008). The cause of most of these insertions or deletions is unknown, but many of them have been created through the transposition of transposons and retroelements.

2.3 The Methodology of DNA Fingerprinting

2.3.1 First-Generation Markers: RFLP, ISSR, and RAPD

First applications of DNA fingerprinting were based on markers derived from restriction fragment length polymorphisms (RFLPs), inter simple sequence repeats (ISSRs), and randomly amplified polymorphic DNA (RAPD). These markers are considered as first generation.

RFLPs can be caused by all possible mutations including InDels, contractions and expansions of VNTRs and SSRs, and exchanges of single nucleotides. Therefore, RFLP analysis can also be used for SSR genotyping. Nader et al. (1999) applied RFLP typing to analyze the genetic diversity of the scarlet macaw (*Ara macao*) in Costa Rica. The method involves the isolation of DNA from the biological material and its digestion with restriction endonucleases to generate restriction fragments. The fragments are then separated by electrophoresis on agarose or polyacrylamide gels followed by Southern blotting. DNA bound to the membrane is hybridized with labeled probes consisting of repeats that are typical for microsatellites, eg, $(CAC)_5$ or $(GGAT)_4$. DNA hybrids are then visualized by labeling of the probes, for example, by the enzymatic cleavage of colorogenic substrates or radioactive isotopes. Band patterns are evaluated manually or by computer programs to differentiate individuals and determine parental relationships among them.

Inter simple sequence repeat−polymerase chain reaction (ISSR−PCR) has been used for testing genetic diversity (Kantety et al., 1995), cultivar identification (Charters et al., 1996), molecular mapping (Ratnaparkhe et al., 1998), seed authenticity testing (Kumar et al., 2001), and various other applications. In a study combining ISSR-PCR and fingerprinting with SSR markers, Nagaraju et al. (2002) evaluated the genetic relationships in traditional and evolved basmati and in semidwarf non-basmati rice varieties. ISSR analysis is based on the PCR amplification of the regions between adjacent and inversely orientated SSRs. These have to be close enough to allow efficient amplification. Inversions, insertions, deletions, and mutational events of microsatellites at multiple loci in the genome yield differences in the band pattern. It is not suited to differentiate between individuals in a population that show no or only few differences in their ISSR band patterns, whereas closely related subspecies and species reveal specific banding profiles or fingerprints. For the primer design, DNA sequences are selected that represent tandem repeats typically found in microsatellites.

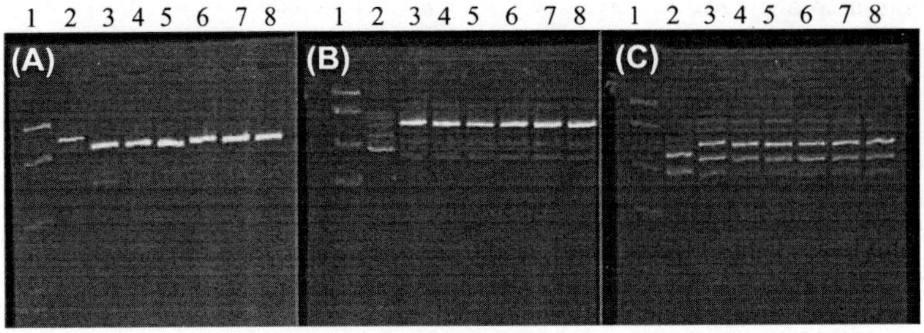

Figure 2.1 Analysis of basmati rice varieties by inter simple sequence repeat-polymerase chain reaction (ISSR-PCR). Amplification in the PCR reactions was performed with primers AGAGAGAGAGAGAGAGYT (agarose gel a), CACACACACACACACAG (gel b) and GAGAGAGAGAGAGAGAT (gel c). After amplification, amplicons were separated on agarose gels and visualized by staining with ethidium bromide. Lane 1 on the agarose gels contains the molecular weight marker FastRuler (*Life Technologies, Inc., Foster City, CA, USA*; fragment lengths: 1500, 850, 400, 200, and 50 base pairs). Amplicons of the following basmati varieties were separated on the other lanes of gels (A to C): Pusa Basmati-1 (lane 2), Taraori (HBC-19) (lane 3), Basmati 2000 (lanes 4 and 7), Basmati 515 (lanes 5 and 8) and Super Basmati (lane 6).

PCR amplicons are separated by gel electrophoresis and can then be visualized by staining with intercalating fluorescent dyes like ethidium bromide. Alternatively, one might use primers that are labeled by, eg, radioactivity or by conjugation with digoxigenin. Fig. 2.1A–C show results of an ISSR analysis of five different varieties of basmati rice and three different primers. These results will be discussed later in the context of basmati authenticity testing.

RAPD analysis is a special type of PCR involving short primers with arbitrary nucleotide sequences of generally 10 bases, which randomly bind to various regions in the genome. Amplified fragments are analyzed by agarose gel electrophoresis, and polymorphisms are identified on the basis of banding patterns resulting after staining with ethidium bromide.

Due to the rapid development of modern technologies for DNA analysis over the last two decades, RFLP, RAPD, and ISSR markers have lost their importance for DNA fingerprinting. They are still useful in certain cases in which there is no or only a little available information about DNA sequences of the targeted genome, for example, if genomes of rare or exotic organisms have to be analyzed. In food analysis, DNA fingerprinting based on ISSR markers has been applied to trace and differentiate wild coffee harvested in Ethiopian rain forests (Zeltz et al., 2005).

2.3.2 Second-Generation Markers: SSRs

Modern DNA fingerprinting methods based on SSR markers comprise the direct amplification of the microsatellite loci by the PCR with primers hybridizing to the flanking sequences of these multiple repeats. The amplified alleles of different repeat lengths are then analyzed by gel or capillary electrophoresis. DNA sequence data for the design of primers fitting a large variety of different SSRs have become available due to various whole-genome sequencing projects and to the development of cost-effective high-throughput sequencing methods (Di Bella et al., 2013). Genomes of important crop and livestock such as rice (International Rice Genome Sequencing Project, 2005), wheat (Brenchley et al., 2012), cattle (Zimin et al., 2009), and swine (Archibald et al., 2010) have been sequenced and Websites like Gramene (www.gramene.org) hold SSR and SNP allelic data for these organisms.

In 2000 Bligh published her pioneering work on the differentiation of basmati from non-basmati rice varieties by SSR genotyping, and her method became a standard procedure for basmati authenticity testing (Nader et al., 2013). Like other self-pollinators, rice varieties are also particularly suited for DNA fingerprinting considering that they are, in most cases, homozygous pure lines that reveal only one allele per marker.

The method is capable of analyzing even complex mixtures in a reliable and quantitative manner, and the following example of the analysis of a rice sample obtained from a customer and declared as basmati describes the procedure in more detail.

DNA extracted from the sample and purified over silica membrane spin columns served as a template for the PCR amplification of 10 standard SSR markers, published by the UK Food Standards Agency (FSA) in 2004: RM1, RM44, RM55, RM171, RM201, RM202, RM223, RM229, RM241, and RM348. The markers belong to a panel of 50 SSR loci that are published on the Gramene Website together with primer sequences suited for their PCR amplification (Gramene, 2015). These SSRs were found to be highly polymorphic and are therefore used by the Generation Challenge Program for rice diversity analysis. Primers for amplification of the SSR markers RM1, RM201, RM202, and RM171 were labeled at the 5′-end with the fluorescent dye FAM (6-carboxylfluorescein), markers RM223, RM229, and RM241 were labeled with JOE (6-carboxy-4,5-dichloro-2,7-dimethoxy-fluorescein), and markers RM348, RM44, and RM55 with TAMRA (carboxy-tetramethyl-rhodamine).

After amplification, PCR products marked with different fluorescent dyes were combined into four mixtures: (1) RM202 and RM348; (2) RM1, RM223, and RM44; (3) RM201 and RM229; and (4) RM171, RM241, and RM55. Polynucleotides in each mixture were separated on an ABI 3130XL Genetic Analyzer with POP4 polymers on 36-cm capillary arrays (Life Technologies, Foster City, CA, USA) in the presence of ILS 600 internal size standards (Promega Inc, Madison, WI, USA). Fluorescent signals were quantified by laser-induced fluorescence and, due to the different labeling, alleles from three different SSR markers could be analyzed simultaneously during each chromatographic run. Chromatograms of the 10 markers are shown in Fig. 2.2.

Stutter peaks are observed for all markers with the exception of RM348. These are caused by replication slippage, which is also considered to be the main pathway causing the high mutation rates of tandem repeats in VNTRs and SSRs (see previous discussion). Stutter peaks represent minor amplification products, differing from the main amplicon by multiples of the length of the repeat unit (Ellegren, 2004). In contrast to SSR mutations in vivo, which lead to both extension and contraction of

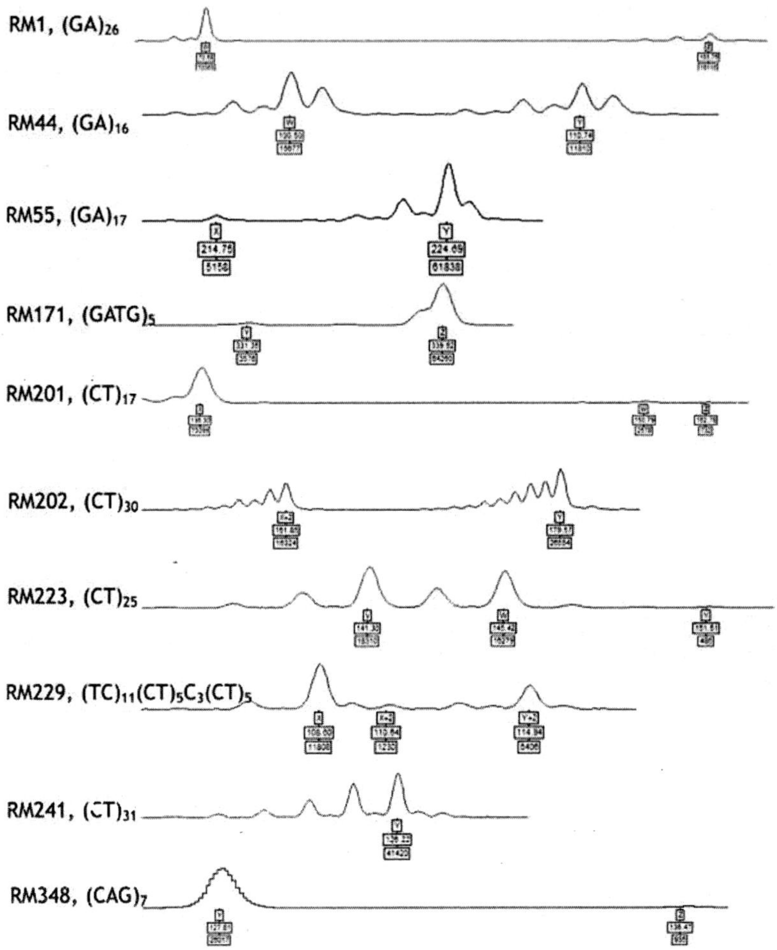

Figure 2.2 Separation of amplified alleles of simple sequence repeat markers in a rice sample by capillary electrophoresis. Allele type (W, X, Y, and Z), size of fragment (in base pairs), and intensity of fluorescent signals are indicated in the boxes under each allele peak. Details are described in the text.

the microsatellite locus, stutter peaks generally appear in PCR as products that are shorter than the size of the corresponding SSR allele. Strong stuttering is observed with markers RM1, RM44, RM55, RM201, RM223, and RM241, which are characterized by simple dinucleotide repeat structures $(GA)_n/(CT)_n$, whereas this effect is less pronounced in the markers with more complex repeat structures, RM171 [$(GATG)_5$] and RM229 [$(TC)_{11}(CT)_5C_3(CT)_5$], and absent in RM348 [$(CAG)_7$].

In order to compensate for this stutter effect, only the peak of each allele with the highest fluorescence intensity is evaluated. Fragment sizes and peak areas are analyzed with the GeneScan/Genotyper or GeneMapper software and results are then transferred into an Excel sheet for further calculations (Table 2.1).

Table 2.1 Combinatorial Approach to Identify and Quantify Rice Varieties in a Mixture by Simple Sequence Repeat (SSR) Fingerprinting Evaluation of Data From Fig. 2.2

		RM1		RM44		RM55		RM171		RM201		RM202		RM223		RM229		RM241		RM348	
1	Pusa Basmati-1	W		Y		Y		Z		X		Y		W		X		Y		Y	
2	Pusa 1121	W		Y		X		Y		X		Y		W		X		Y		Y	
3	Pusa 1509	W		Y		X		Z		X		Y		W		Y+2		Y		Y	
4	Sugandha	Z		W		Y		Z		X		X+2		V		Y+2		Y		Y	
5	Analytical results	W	65%	Y	61%	Y	92%	Z	92%	X	95%	Y	67%	W	61%	X	61%	Y	100%	Y	96%
6		Z	35%	W	39%	X	8%	Y	8%	W	4%	X+2	33%	V	38%	Y+2	34%	–	0%	Z	4%
7		–	0%	–	0%	–	0%	–	0%	Z	1%	–	0%	Y	1%	X+2	5%	–	0%	–	0%
Hypothesis 1: Mixture of Pusa Basmati-1, Sugandha, and Pusa 1121																					
8	Step 1: 57%	W	8%	Y	4%	Y	35%	Z	35%	X	38%	Y	10%	W	4%	X	4%	Y	43%	Y	39%
9	Pusa Basmati-1	Z	35%	W	39%	X	8%	Y	8%	W	4%	X+2	33%	V	38%	Y+2	34%	–	0%	Z	4%
10	subtracted	–	0%	–	0%	–	0%	–	0%	Z	1%	–	0%	Y	1%	X+2	5%	–	0%	–	0%
11	Step 2: 34%	W	8%	Y	4%	Y	1%	Z	1%	X	4%	Y	10%	W	4%	X	4%	Y	9%	Y	5%
12	Sugandha subtracted	Z	1%	W	5%	X	8%	Y	8%	W	4%	X+2	0%	V	4%	Y+2	0%	–	0%	Z	4%
13		–	0%	–	0%	–	0%	–	0%	Z	1%	–	0%	Y	1%	X+2	5%	–	0%	–	0%
14	Step 3: 4%	W	4%	Y	0%	Y	1%	Z	1%	X	0%	Y	6%	W	0%	X	0%	Y	5%	Y	1%
15	Pusa 1121 subtracted	Z	1%	W	5%	X	4%	Y	4%	W	4%	X+2	0%	V	4%	Y+2	0%	–	0%	Z	4%
16		–	0%	–	0%	–	0%	–	0%	Z	1%	–	0%	Y	1%	X+2	5%	–	0%	–	0%

Continued

Table 2.1 Combinatorial Approach to Identify and Quantify Rice Varieties in a Mixture by Simple Sequence Repeat (SSR) Fingerprinting Evaluation of Data From Fig. 2.2—cont'd

		RM1		RM44		RM55		RM171		RM201		RM202		RM223		RM229		RM241		RM348	
Hypothesis 2: Mixture of Pusa Basmati-1, Sugandha, and Pusa 1509																					
17	Step 1: 57%	W	8%	Y	4%	Y	35%	Z	35%	X	38%	Y	10%	W	4%	X	4%	Y	43%	Y	39%
18	Pusa Basmati-1	Z	35%	W	39%	X	8%	Y	8%	W	4%	X+2	33%	V	38%	Y+2	34%	–	0%	Z	4%
19	subtracted	–	0%	–	0%	–	0%	–	0%	Z	1%	–	0%	Y	1%	X+2	5%	–	0%	–	0%
20	Step 2: 30%	W	8%	Y	4%	Y	5%	Z	5%	X	8%	Y	10%	W	4%	X	4%	Y	13%	Y	9%
21	Sugandha subtracted	Z	5%	W	9%	X	8%	Y	8%	W	4%	X+2	3%	V	8%	Y+2	4%	–	0%	Z	4%
22		–	0%	–	0%	–	0%	–	0%	Z	1%	–	0%	Y	1%	X+2	5%	–	0%	–	0%
23	Step 3: 4%	W	4%	Y	0%	Y	5%	Z	1%	X	4%	Y	6%	W	0%	X	4%	Y	9%	Y	5%
24	Pusa 1509 subtracted	Z	5%	W	9%	X	4%	Y	8%	W	4%	X+2	3%	V	8%	Y+2	0%	–	0%	Z	4%
25		–	0%	–	0%	–	0%	–	0%	Z	1%	–	0%	Y	1%	X+2	5%	–	0%	–	0%

Fluorescence emission intensity directly correlates to the number of copies generated by PCR, permitting a quantitative analysis of each allele in relation to the whole allele mixture found for each SSR marker.

Shorter alleles of SSR markers are amplified more efficiently than the longer ones during PCR. Therefore, correction factors have to be applied on the fluorescent intensities to compensate for the allelic imbalance caused by the PCR reaction and to avoid longer SSR alleles being underestimated in relation to shorter ones.

Table 2.1 summarizes in rows 5–7 the quantitative results of the SSR typing illustrated by the chromatograms in Fig. 2.2 for each allele and after applying the corresponding correction factors. The letters V to Z characterize the alleles of each of the 10 microsatellite markers with V being the shortest and Z the longest tandem repeat (FSA, 2004). In a combinatorial approach, different hypotheses are generated to explain the allelic pattern determined for the sample by putative mixtures of rice varieties. For the present case, the allelic pattern can be explained by a mixture of the varieties Pusa Basmati-1, Pusa 1121, and the non-basmati variety Sugandha (hypothesis 1) or Pusa Basmati-1 with Sugandha and Pusa 1509 (hypothesis 2).

The allele patterns of these varieties have been determined from reference materials obtained from official sources and from trade (Nader et al., 2013, 2014) and are summarized in rows 1–4. These varieties are furthermore listed in Table 2.2. Initially, the dominant variety in the mixture is identified; this is Pusa Basmati-1 and would fit both hypotheses at a concentration of 57%. The percentage expresses the relative DNA content of the variety in the mixture in relation to the total rice DNA detected (see further comments following). Consequently, 57% are subtracted from all alleles that belong to Pusa Basmati-1. Residual alleles are listed in rows 8–10 for hypothesis 1 and 17–19 for hypothesis 2.

In a second step, the concentration of Sugandha is estimated at 34% to fit hypothesis 1 and 30% to fit hypothesis 2. These fractions are then subtracted from all alleles that belong to Sugandha and that are left over from the first evaluation step. Residual alleles are summarized in rows 11–13 for hypothesis 1 and in rows 17–19 for hypothesis 2. Finally, the concentrations of Pusa 1121 and 1509 are estimated at 4% for both hypotheses, and these fractions are subtracted from the alleles left over from step 2. Residual alleles are listed in rows 14–16 for hypothesis 1 and 23–25 for hypothesis 2. The residual allele patterns can be attributed to two different rice varieties, which cannot be identified due to the lack of reference materials. In addition to 57% Pusa Basmati-1, the sample therefore either contains 34% Sugandha, 4% Pusa 1121, and 4% of unidentified nonbasmati varieties or 30% Sugandha, 4% Pusa 1509, and 9% unidentified. For ISO 17025 accreditation, the test was fully validated by addressing precision, accuracy, linearity, and sensitivity (Nader et al., 2013). The analytical uncertainty U depends on the complexity of the mixture and might vary between $U = \pm 3\%$ (absolute) for samples with one major variety >95% and $U = \pm 6\%$ (absolute) for complex mixtures such as in the example described previously. In a quantitative proficiency test of the FSA (2006) involving 11 independent laboratories, an uncertainty of ±6% was determined, which corresponds to the result obtained by the authors (Nader et al., 2013).

Table 2.2 DNA Fingerprints of Various Rice Varieties Based on the Analysis of 10 Standard Simple Sequence Repeat (SSR) Markers

Variety	Origin	RM1	RM44	RM55	RM171	RM201	RM202	RM223	RM229	RM241	RM348	*fgr*
Traditional Basmati Varieties												
Taraori (HBC-19, Karnal local)	India	W	Y	X	Y	X	Y	W	Y	Y	Z	+/+
Basmati 386	India	W	Y	X	Y	X	Y	W	Y	Y	Z	+/+
Kernel (Basmati Pakistan)	Pakistan	W	Y	X	Y	X	Y	W	Y	Y	Z	+/+
Basmati 370	Pak./In.	W	X	Z	Y	X	Y	W	Y	Z	Z	+/+
Type 3 (Dehradun)	India	W	X	Z	Y	X	Y	W	Y	Z	Z	+/+
Ranbir Basmati (IET 11348)	India	W−1	X+1	Z	Y	X	Y	Y	Y	Z+2	Z	+/+
Evolved Basmati Varieties												
Super Basmati	Pakistan	W	X	X	Z	X	Y	W	Y	Z	Z	+/+
Basmati 385	Pakistan	Y	Y	Z	Y	X	X	W	Y	Z	Z	+/+
Basmati 198	Pakistan	Y	X	Z	Y	X	X	W	Y	Z	Z	+/+
D-98*	Pakistan	Y	X+2	Z	Y	X	X	W−2	Y	Y−2	Z	+/+
Pusa Basmati-1 (IET 10364)	India	W	Y	Y	Z	X	Y	W	X	Y	Y	+/+
Kasturi (IET 8580)	India	W	W	Y	Z	X	Y	V	Y	Z	Y	+/+

Punjab Basmati (IET 8580)	India	Y+2/Z+5	X+1	Z+3/Z	Y	X	X	Y	Y	X−4/Z	Z	+/+
Haryana Basmati IET 10367)	India	Z	W	Y	Z	X	X	Y	X	Y	Y/Z	+/+
Mahi Sugandha (IET 12601)	India	Y	W	Y	Z	Z	X	X	X	Z	Z	+/+
Basmati 2000	Pakistan	W	X	X	Z	X	Y	W	Y	Z	Z	y
Basmati 515	Pakistan	W	X	X	Z	X	Y	W	Y	Z	Z	+/+
Pusa 1121 (IET, 18004)	India	W	Y	X	Y	X	Y	W	X	Y	Y	+/+
Pusa 1509 (IET 21960)	India	W	Y	X	Z	X	Y	W	Y+2	Y	Y	+/+
Indian and Pakistani Nonbasmati Varieties Frequently Observed as Adulterants												
Superfine	Pakistan	Z	W	Y	Z	Z	Y−4	V	Y	Y	Y	+/+
Sugandha	India	Z	W	Y	Z	X	X+2/Y	V	Y+2	Y	Y	+/+
Sherbati	India	W	W	Y	W	Z	Y	Z	X	X	Y	−/−
Parmal	India	Z	W	Y	Z	Z	X	Y	X	Y	Y	−/−
Pak 386	Pakistan	Y	W	Y	Z	Z	Y	X	Y	Y	Y	−/−
IRRI-9	IRRI	Y+2	W	Y	Z	Z/W	X	Y	X+2	Y−4	Y	−/−
KS-282	Pakistan	W/Y+2/Z	W	Y	Z	Z	Y	Y	X	Y−4	Y	−/−
Supri	Pakistan	Z+2	W	Y	W	W	Y+4	Z	X	Y−2	Y	−/−
Other Rice Varieties of Importance												
Hom Mali (KMDL 105/ RD15)	Thailand	Z+5	W+2	Z+2	Z	W	Y	V	X	Y−2	Y	+/+
Phka Romeat, Rumdeng, Rumduol	Cambodia	Z+5	W+2	Z+2	Z	W	Y	V	X	Y−2	Y	+/+

Continued

Table 2.2 DNA Fingerprints of Various Rice Varieties Based on the Analysis of 10 Standard Simple Sequence Repeat (SSR) Markers—cont'd

Variety	Origin	RM1	RM44	RM55	RM171	RM201	RM202	RM223	RM229	RM241	RM348	*fgr*
Pathumtani 1	Thailand	Z+5	W	Y	Z+4	W	Y+4	V	X	Y	Y	+/+
Sen Kra Oub	Cambodia	W+6	W+2	Y	Z	W	X	W−12	Y+2	Y	Y	+/+
Vietnamese Jasmine rice	Vietnam	Y	W+2	Y	Z	W	Y	V	X	Y	Y	+/+
Paw San	Myanmar	W+10	Y−2	Z	X−3	W	Y+2	W−2	Y+2	Y	Y	−/−
Arborio Risotto rice	Italy	W+8	X	Z+2	X−3	X	Y−8	X	Z−2	Y−8	Z	−/−
Carnaroli Risotto rice	Italy	W+8	X	Z+2	X−3	X+2	Y−8	X	Z−2	Y−8	Z	−/−
Baldo Risotto rice	Italy	Y−8	Y	Z	X−3	X	Y−8	Z−4	Z−2	Y+6	Z	−/−
Vialone Nero Risotto rice	Italy	W+10	X	Z	X−3	X	Y−8	X	Z−2	Y−6	Z	−/−
Bomba Paella rice	Spain	W+12	X	Z+4	Z	X	Y−8	Y	Y+4	Y−2	Z	−/−

Note: DNA fingerprints were established by the authors based on reference materials obtained from authorities and traders. Each letter V to Z represents a DNA fragment of a distinct length (FSA, 2004). For several varieties more than one allele is observed for some markers and these are listed separated by a slash.

* According to a statement of the Pakistani Trade Development Authority, the variety D98 is the same as PK-198, which is an approved basmati variety. However, DNA fingerprints between the two varieties differ significantly.

The method determines the relative amount of DNA of each variety in relation to the total rice DNA in the mixture. Because DNA contents of rice kernels might vary depending on the processing stage and the variety, the results do not necessarily reflect the weight proportions of each type of rice. Brown rice with bran and germ contains more DNA than white milled rice, which primarily consists of the starch body. Furthermore, the DNA content might vary among rice varieties. In the validation study for the ISO 17025 accreditation process, which was mentioned before, DNA contents were determined for different rice samples (Brendel and Schubbert, unpublished results) and ranged between 17 ± 2 for white milled jasmine rice over 140 ± 67 for white milled to 296 ± 82 µg/g for brown basmati rice. Results are average values of six independent DNA extractions. However, the relative DNA amounts of rice varieties reflect quite well the weight proportions, because in practice mainly mixtures have to be analyzed, which consist of rice of one common processing stage (paddy, brown, milled, or parboiled rice) and of varieties that are related to each other and do not significantly differ in their DNA contents.

This was shown during routine preshipment inspections of basmati rice in Pakistan by analyzing basmati authenticity with the DNA fingerprinting method in comparison with the visual testing performed traditionally in this country. The latter method is based on morphological differences between kernels of different varieties, which are manually selected from the sample (Nader et al., 2014). Separated grains are then weighed to determine the relative content of each variety. Samples of 59 individual lots were analyzed with both methods in parallel. Contents of the variety Super Basmati determined by visual testing were in a range between 93.3% and 99% (w/w). The average difference of these results to the contents determined by DNA fingerprinting (DNA/DNA) was $1.39 \pm 1.18\%$ with a maximum deviation of 5.7%. These results indicate that both the relative DNA content and the relative weight do not differ significantly.

As an alternative to capillary electrophoresis, amplified SSR alleles can be separated by agarose or slab gel (polyacrylamide) electrophoresis. However, a study by Vemireddy et al. (2007) on authenticity testing of basmati rice revealed that capillary electrophoresis is essential for this kind of application due to its higher reproducibility and lower analytical uncertainty with regard to the quantification of SSR alleles in a mixture of various rice varieties.

InDel markers are longer than the relatively short SSRs and were introduced for basmati authenticity testing by Steele et al. (2008) as an alternative to microsatellite markers. Due to their length, InDels can be analyzed on agarose gels making this technology more cost effective and suitable for smaller laboratories without special equipment like DNA sequencers.

Another technology possibly suited for laboratories without special equipment such as DNA sequencers is a lab-on-a-chip method developed by Agilent Technologies, Inc., Santa Clara, CA, USA (Garrett and Clarke, 2007). PCR amplified SSRs or InDels are separated by capillary gel electrophoresis on a chip in the presence of intercalating fluorescent dye ethidium bromide.

2.3.3 Third-Generation Markers: SNPs

Mini- and microsatellite typing uses the analysis of length differences of the repeats by electrophoresis. In contrast, genotyping at SNP loci is based on the selective detection of the differences in one base pair and distinguishes the single base mismatch from the perfect match. New techniques have been developed for SNP analysis like oligonucleotide arrays on DNA chips and matrix-assisted laser desorption/ionization mass spectrometry (MALDI-TOF MS) detection systems (for a review, see Gupta et al., 2001). For genotyping of individual humans, animals, and crop varieties only plus/minus assays are required and these can be automated. Many thousand SNP loci can be analyzed simultaneously on a DNA chip, making SNP typing a powerful tool for genome mapping and detecting even minor differences between individuals and populations.

For food, quantitative analytical systems are required since most often foodstuff contains materials from different individual animals or plant varieties. Quantitative SNP analysis is feasible with the MassARRAY iPLEX Platform, a MALDI-TOF MS technology (Gabriel et al., 2009). Real-time-PCR can be used for quantitative SNP analysis as well, eg, with two allele-specific TaqMan probes containing distinct fluorescent dyes. The KASP genotyping technology (Kompetitive Allele Specific PCR) is routinely used in plant breeding and is a cost-efficient alternative to chip-based SNP-typing systems in applications that require small to moderate numbers of markers (Semagn et al., 2013). The method is also suitable for quantitative SNP analysis by using two allele-specific primers conjugated with different fluorescent dyes, HEX (hexachloro-6-carboxy-fluorescein) and FAM (6-carboxy-fluorescein). Fluorescence emission intensities of each dye are measured by an end point fluorescent reading and are directly correlated to the number of templates of each SNP allele in the sample. The ratio of the fluorescence intensities of both dyes therefore corresponds to the ratio of both SNP alleles.

2.4 DNA Fingerprinting for Authenticity Testing of Rice Varieties

Rice is not only the most important staple food globally but it is also characterized by an extraordinary varietal diversity. The International Rice Information System (IRIS; www.iris.irri.org) recognizes around 5000 released varieties and the gene bank collection of the International Rice Research Institute, IRRI, holds more than 117,000 types of rice (Nader et al., 2014). Garris et al. (2005) analyzed 234 rice accessions representing the geographic range of *O. sativa* by SSR genotyping and sequence analysis of chloroplast DNA and classified the five subspecies *indica*, *aus*, *aromatic*, *temperate japonica*, and *tropical japonica*.

Rice varieties differ in many characteristics such as adaptation to different climates and soils, tolerance to salt and drought, resistance to pests, and shape. The chemical composition, morphology, and structure of the starch body are quite variable as well, affecting the cooking characteristics, taste, and texture of rice. A large variety of traditional rice dishes are found worldwide, for example, risotto, paella, sushi, and biryani, and their diversity is mainly due to these aforementioned differences. Sushi, rice cakes, rice crackers, and rice paper for spring rolls are made from sticky *japonica* rice varieties. Biryani requires nonsticky, fluffy cooking rice varieties. Paella rice varieties are characterized by their high-absorption capacity for the associated broth, and cooked risotto rice by its creamy consistency. Special rice varieties best suited to prepare these dishes have been evolved by breeding and are traded as prime quality and at a higher price than varieties that mainly serve as staple food. Examples are the aromatic jasmine and basmati rice varieties, Arborio and Carnaroli risotto rice, Bomba paella rice, and Koshihikari sushi rice.

2.4.1 Case Study: Basmati Rice

Adulteration of high-value varieties with cheaper rice was first reported in literature for basmati rice. Basmati (the Hindi word for aroma) rice is indigenous to the Indian subcontinent and is characterized by its aroma and special cooking characteristics. The major aroma compound is 2-acetyl-1-pyrroline, which gives the rice its distinct popcorn flavor. Many other aromatic compounds have been found that contribute to the special flavor of basmati and that supposedly cause the differences in smell and taste observed between basmati and jasmine rice (Bryant and McClung, 2009). Basmati is furthermore characterized by its lengthwise excessive elongation during cooking and the soft and fluffy texture of the cooked rice.

Purity and quality of basmati rice has been traditionally tested in the countries of origin by chemical and visual methods. Experienced experts can visually distinguish basmati and nonbasmati rice varieties due to morphological differences of the milled kernels (Nader et al., 2014; see previous Section 2.3.2). Amylose content, alkaline spread, and gel length are chemical properties that characterize the typical cooking behavior of basmati and that can be tested by rather simple methods (Masoumias et al., 2013). Over recent decades, basmati has developed from a primarily ethnic food to one of the most important types of rice on the EU market. Due to its lower yields in the field, basmati rice is more expensive than other rice varieties that are mainly used as staple food. Depending on the harvests in Pakistan and India, prices can be twice as high as for normal long-grain indica rice. Consequently, basmati rice is frequently adulterated with cheaper nonbasmati varieties.

Based on the DNA fingerprinting method of Bligh (2000) which was described earlier, the Food Standards Agency (2004) examined 363 samples sold as basmati rice across the United Kingdom for authenticity and reported that 17% of samples contained more than 20% of nonbasmati and 9% were adulterated at levels in excess of 60%. As a consequence of these adulterations, the British Retail Consortium, Rice Association and the British Rice Millers Association released a Code of Practice on basmati rice in 2005, which became a legal standard in the United Kingdom and was also adopted as a general trade standard by the Grain and Feed Trade Association and the private sector in other EU member states.

The Code of Practice was developed in consultation with Indian and Pakistani rice exporters (All India Rice Exporters Association, AIREA; and the Rice Exporters Association of Pakistan, REAP) and defines 15 rice varieties as basmati. In the United Kingdom the code has been enforced as a legal standard by food control authorities and has since then led to a steady improvement of basmati authenticity (Nader et al., 2013).

Recently the French rice association, the Syndicat de la Rizerie Français (2015), published its own code of practice, which includes four new basmati varieties in addition to the 15 listed in the UK Code of Practice.

Basmati rice has been furthermore tested at the retail level by consumer organizations in France, Germany, and Switzerland (Union Fédérale des Consommateurs Que Choisir, 2009; Stiftung Warentest, 2010; Saldo, 2010) based on SSR analysis. The test by the German Stiftung Warentest revealed that 5 out of 31 samples did not comply with the UK Code of Practice and two of these did not even contain basmati rice but rather 100% of a nonaromatic rice without the fragrance gene *frg* (see later discussion).

Article 6 of the UK Code of Practice defines the DNA fingerprinting method published by the Food Standards Agency in 2004 as the standard procedure for authenticity testing. This method is based on the 10 standard SSR markers described in detail under Section 2.2 of this chapter. Table 2.2 reveals the allelic patterns of various rice varieties for these markers and the presence or absence of the fragrance gene *fgr*, a specific 8 base pair deletion in the gene *BADH2*, which codes for the enzyme betaine aldehyde dehydrogenase and supposedly causes the typical aroma of basmati and jasmine rice because of a lack of this enzyme (Bradbury et al., 2005). A quantitative screening test for basmati has been developed on the basis of this InDel marker, and the absence of the deletion indicates the presence of nonbasmati varieties (Bucher et al., 2014). However, as can be seen from Table 2.2, screening of the fragrant gene is not sufficient to test for basmati authenticity because numerous other rice varieties are also aromatic and homozygous for the *fgr* gene. These are not considered as basmati due to their different origin and cooking characteristics. Examples are the aromatic nonbasmati varieties Superfine from Pakistan and Sugandha from India, which would pass the screening as genuine basmati.

Of the 15 rice varieties listed as genuine basmati rice by the UK Code of Practice, seven are considered traditional varieties (Table 2.2). Taraori (HBC-19), Kernel (Basmati Pakistan) and Basmati 386 on one hand and Basmati 370 and Type 3 (Dehradun) on the other cannot be distinguished by genotyping with the 10 standard SSR markers because they are genetically closely related. They were collected from the same landraces by different institutions but were notified under different names. The Rice Research Station in Kala Shah Kaku in Pakistan notified Kernel Basmati and Basmati 370, the Haryana Agriculture University Taraori (HBC-19), the Punjab Agriculture University Basmati 217 and 386, and the Nagina Rice Research Station in Uttar Pradesh Type 3 (All Indian Rice Exporters Association, 2016).

The variety Ranbir was selected from the cultivar Basmati 370 and reported by the Sher-e-Kashmir University in Jammu (Siddiq et al., 2012). The DNA fingerprint obtained from a Ranbir reference material obtained by the Food Standards Agency

(2004) is different from Basmati 370 (Table 2.2) but all samples obtained so far as Ranbir by Eurofins revealed the same allelic pattern as Basmati 370 and Type 3. This indicates that the source of such reference materials is not always reliable even if these are official sources. The genotype of Ranbir as published by the FSA (2004) should be revised accordingly.

Due to the low yield of landrace basmati varieties, only Taraori, Type 3, and Ranbir are cultivated at significant quantities in India, whereas in Pakistan traditional varieties are no longer in use. By crossing basmati landraces with high-yield indica long-grain rice varieties, new varieties were developed of which the varieties Pusa 1121, Pusa 1509, Pusa Basmati-1, Super Basmati, and Basmati 515 play the most significant role in agriculture in India and Pakistan today. The most important basmati varieties cultivated in India are Pusa 1121 and 1509, which are exported on a large scale to the Middle East, Iran, and the United States. Pusa 1121 is also grown in Pakistan under the name Kainat 1121. Pusa 1121 and 1509 were reported in 2008 and 2013 as basmati and are characterized by their extraordinary kernel length and elongation during cooking. Because these varieties were reported after 2005, they are not listed as genuine basmati in the UK Code of Practice but are in the new French Code of Practice. Efforts to recognize Pusa 1121 in the UK as basmati failed due to the argument that an evolved variety only qualifies as basmati if at least one of the parents is a traditional basmati. Pusa 1121 is a sister line of Pusa Basmati-1, and evolved basmati varieties are the parents (Siddiq et al., 2012).

The French Code of Practice also includes the new Pakistani varieties Basmati 2000 and 515, which were evolved from Super Basmati and which cannot be distinguished from their ancestor by DNA fingerprinting using the 10 standard SSR markers (Table 2.2). The exact breeding history of these lines remains unclear. Based on ISSR- and RAPD-PCR analysis, no significant differences could be found between these lines and Super Basmati, whereas the genetic distance to Indian Taraori and Pusa Basmati-1 is quite obvious (Fig. 2.1). DNA fingerprinting with an extended panel of SSR markers revealed differences between Basmati 515, Basmati 2000, and Super Basmati but also a pronounced genetic diversity in the variety Super Basmati, which is probably due to the degeneration of the seed materials used in Pakistani agriculture and which complicates its differentiation from Basmati 515 and 2000. DNA fingerprinting of single kernels in samples of Super Basmati frequently reveals a diversity of alleles for the markers RM118, RM152, RM212, RM224, and RM252 (Gramene, 2015) with six different alleles observed for the marker RM252 (Nader et al., unpublished results). In contrast only one unique DNA fingerprint with one allele per SSR is observed with the 10 standard markers, defined by the FSA (2004; Table 2.2). This is probably due to differences in mutation rates of microsatellites (see previous mention under Section 2.2.1), which might be lower for the 10 standard markers than for the markers tested additionally.

DNA fingerprinting is furthermore applied to control basmati imports for compliance with EU customs legislation. According to Commission Implementing Regulation (EU) No 706/2014, husked brown cargo rice of nine basmati varieties qualifies for a zero rate of import duty. These include all landraces and the evolved varieties Pusa Basmati-1 and Super Basmati (Table 2.2). For tax exemption, only one variety is allowed per consignment and admixtures of contrasting varieties (basmati and nonbasmati) are tolerated up to 5% (w/w) (Commission Regulation (EU) No 272/2010).

In contrast to EU customs legislation, both the UK and French Code of Practice tolerate mixtures of various basmati rice varieties and nonbasmati admixtures up to 7% (w/w). Analytical methods to control compliance with these codes therefore have to be able to identify and quantify various rice varieties even in complex mixtures; this can be achieved with the procedure described in detail in Section 2.2.

Currently 23 varieties are officially approved in India as basmati (All Indian Rice Exporters Association, 2016) and 9 in Pakistan. Of these 14 have been notified after the publication of the UK Code of Practice on Basmati Rice in 2005. Thus a revision of the current basmati definition in the EU and the adaptation of the DNA fingerprinting method to the rice breeding practice in the source countries seems necessary. Several of the new varieties cannot be distinguished from the older varieties based on DNA fingerprinting with the 10 standard SSR markers (see above). Examples are the varieties CSR 30 (Yamini) and Pusa Basmati-6 (Pusa 1401), which resemble Taraori Basmati and Pusa Basmati-1.

2.4.2 Case Study: Jasmine Rice

Theoretically, the DNA fingerprinting method can be applied to identify and quantify all rice varieties as long as reference materials are available to establish the corresponding genotype. Jasmine rice comprises aromatic varieties that are cultivated in Thailand, Cambodia, Laos, and South Vietnam and are imported into the EU in large quantities. In Thailand, jasmine rice is traded under the name Hom Mali (Thai words for fragrant jasmine) and comprises the two varieties Khao Dawk Mali 105 (KDML 105) and Kor Kho 15 (RD15), which are genetically identical with regard to the 10 standard SSR markers. Varieties Phka Rumduol, Phka Rumdeng, and Phka Romeat are traded in Cambodia as Phka Malis, which means "fragrant flower." They are genetically identical to Hom Mali with regard to the 10 standard SSR markers and the additional markers RM72, RM212, RM252, RM348, RM440, and RM525, but differences are reported for the markers RM152 in the case of Phka Rumdeng and RM263 for Phka Rumduol (CARDI, 2013). Varieties of Hom Mali and Phka Malis are photosensitive, can only be grown during the rainy season and harvested once per year. They are genetically closely related to each other and were probably derived from one single landrace.

The photo-insensitive varieties Pathumthani 1 and Sen Kra Oub have probably evolved from these landrace varieties by breeding and can be cultivated and harvested throughout the entire year. They can be readily distinguished from each other and from Hom Mali and Phka Malis by DNA fingerprinting based on the 10 standard SSR markers (Table 2.2).

In the EU, the term "jasmine rice" (Riz Jasmine) is defined in the French Code of Practice as fragrant rice from Thailand or Cambodia. "Riz Jasmine Thaï" must contain a minimum of 92% (w/w) Hom Mali or 80% (w/w) Pathumthani. In contrast only Hom Mali and Phka Malis varieties are called "jasmine rice" in Thailand and Cambodia.

2.4.3 Further Candidates for Rice DNA Authenticity Testing

DNA fingerprinting based on the 10 standard markers can be also applied for authenticity testing of risotto rice; distinct allele patterns were derived for the varieties Arborio, Carnaroli, Baldo, and Vialone Nano (Table 2.2).

Bomba paella rice is characterized by its high absorption capacity for the cooking broth and is grown traditionally in Southern Spain. Wankhade et al. reported in 2010 that Bomba cultivars from four different regions in Spain were highly polymorphic with regard to six out of 10 SSR markers. A different set of markers was used by these authors than in the study reported in Table 2.1 with only RM171 in common. The genotype for Bomba in Table 2.2 therefore represents only one cultivar and further studies are necessary to characterize this genetically diverse variety in more detail for authenticity testing. The genetic diversity of Bomba is supposedly caused by the high level of heterozygosity of this variety.

DNA fingerprinting is also the method of choice to give new or so far unknown rice varieties with specific characteristics an identity and to market these as specialties at a higher price. As an example, the aromatic variety Paw San from Myanmar is widely unknown outside this country. It significantly differs from basmati and jasmine rice with some unique features in particular related to cooking characteristics, which might create a new market and export opportunities for Myanmar. A reference material of this rice was obtained from the trade and its DNA fingerprint is listed in Table 2.2. In contrast to jasmine and basmati rice, Paw San does not contain the fragrance gene *frg*, which is characterized by an eight–base pair deletion in the *BADH2* gene (see previous mention). Instead, Myint et al. (2012) detected a three–base pair insertion in this gene in eight of 18 different accessions of Paw San, obtained from different sources and regions in Myanmar. Similar to the eight–base pair deletion of *frg*, this insertion might cause the inactivation of the betaine aldehyde dehydrogenase and therefore the typical aroma of the rice.

2.5 Meat Traceability

In the light of the bovine spongiform encephalopathy (BSE) crisis, the EU imposed a compulsory traceability and labeling system for fresh beef and veal (Regulation (EC) No. 1760/2000). The system imposed full traceability of the meat back to individual animals. Traceability can be verified by fingerprinting (Vázquez et al., 2004) of DNA extracted from meat and from samples obtained from individual animals prior to slaughtering. Practical systems, integrated into the ear tags every animal has to wear according to Regulation (EC) No. 1760/2000, have been developed to sample and conserve DNA from the animals.

In addition, regulation (EU) No. 1169/2011 imposes stricter labeling rules for unprocessed meats from swine, sheep, goat, and poultry while Commission Implementing Regulation (EU) No 1337/2013 requires food business operators to establish a traceability system that provides the link between the meat and the animal or group of animals from which it has been obtained. DNA fingerprinting would actually be the method of choice for the verification of these legally imposed traceability systems. However, experience after the implementation of beef traceability in 2000 has shown that the industry is quite reluctant to establish such voluntary verification systems.

Notwithstanding this, some companies are setting up universal DNA-based traceability systems to support certain claims made on their products and to distinguish themselves from the competition. Claims can be on a certain geographic origin or a distinct quality due to a special breed. For swine, such a system is under development at the laboratory of the authors (Brendel and Schubbert, unpublished results) to verify that pork labeled as a Berkshire or Gloucester Old Spot sired breed contains only meat that is sired by particular Berkshire or Gloucester boars used on distinct farms.

In principle, such traceability systems can be based on two concepts. A direct link between animals and meat products can be made by matching the DNA fingerprints. For this approach, DNA of all animals in the herd would require analysis and fingerprints would be kept in a data base, but this is costly. Alternatively, DNA fingerprints may only be established for the breeding animals and meat samples can then be traced back to specific breeds by paternity testing.

The latter "proof of descent" concept is cost efficient and was tested by Eurofins in a feasibility study. DNA was extracted from bristles of breeding boars (Berkshire and Gloucester Old Spot) and fingerprints were established based on 11 tetrameric (repeat units of four base pairs) SSR markers with a commercially available kit (Animaltype Pig, Biotype Diagnostic GmbH, Dresden, Germany; Caratti et al., 2010). In a blind study, meats of different origins were then analyzed with the same marker panel, and DNA profiles were compared with the fingerprints of the breeding animals. Using the panel of tetrameric SSR markers, it was possible to unambiguously trace specific meat samples back to a sire.

2.6 Future Trends

Until now the most prominent example of the application of DNA fingerprinting in food authenticity testing is that of basmati rice due to a strong industry and retail interest to ensure the reputation of this specialty as a premium product. The method became the main pillar for the Code of Practice on basmati rice, which has developed to a trade standard far beyond the United Kingdom.

Similar success stories can therefore be expected for other premium foods, when industry and trade have a strong commercial interests to safeguard the reputation of such products. Such interests might concern other rice varieties like premium sushi, jasmine, risotto, or paella rice, but also special cocoas or coffees that are sold at premium prices. Arriba cocoa is a highly aromatic variety from Ecuador, and there are strong indications of adulterations with bulk cocoa. Methods to distinguish the premium Arriba varieties have been recently developed and are based on sequence differences in the chloroplast DNA (Hermann et al., 2014) or DNA fingerprinting with SSR markers (Hermann et al., 2015).

The legislators in the EU have obliged business operators handling meat to impose traceability and to provide a direct link between their product and the individual animal or animal herd; this was first done for cattle in 2000 and since 2013 also for goats, sheep, swine, and poultry. Under current legislation, this link only has to be provided by documentation and does not require a parallel analytical system that allows its verification. So far there are not many examples of industry and the retail sectors establishing such verification systems voluntarily. But consumer trust was severely affected by the horse meat scandal, and this might encourage business operators to establish such verification systems to protect their brands. DNA fingerprinting is the most elegant and straightforward approach to provide the direct link between the final product and the individual animal or animal herd.

Costs involved in the establishment of such systems are often overestimated. Not every animal has to be tested, and it is sufficient to keep backup samples of tissues, like hair, of each slaughtered animal and to control traceability by spot-checking meat. Alternatively, databases containing DNA fingerprints of the sires can be established and meat checked randomly by paternity testing, as discussed under Section 2.5.

The horse meat scandal concerned processed food for which exact labeling concerning the origin of the animals is not required by EU legislation and which may contain meat of different animals. As was shown for DNA fingerprinting of basmati rice, the quantitative analysis of several varieties is feasible in a mixture. Also, in processed meat, the differentiation and quantification of different animals should be possible in order to verify traceability claims made by business operators and to confirm the origin of these meats in a more efficient manner.

References

AIREA, 2016. Notified Varieties of Basmati Rice. All Indian Rice Exporters Association, New Delhi. Available from: http://www.airea.net/page/8/varieties (accessed 26.05.16.).

Archibald, A.l., Bolund, L., Churcher, C., Fredholm, M., Groenen, M.A.M., Harlizius, B., Lee, K.-T., Milan, D., Rogers, J., Rothschild, M.F., Uenishi, H., Wang, J., Schook, L.B., The Swine Genome Sequencing Consortium, 2010. Pig genome sequence – analysis and publication strategy. BMC Genomics 11, 438.

Bligh, H.F.J., 2000. Detection of adulteration of basmati rice with non-premium long-grain rice. International Journal of Food Science and Technology 35, 257–265.

Bowers, J., Boursiquot, J.-M., This, P., Chu, K., Johansson, H., Meredith, C., 1999. Historical genetics: the parentage of Chardonnay, Gamay, and other wine grapes of northeastern France. Science 285, 1562–1565.

Bradbury, L.M.T., Fitzgerald, T.L., Henry, R.J., Jin, Q.S., Waters, D.L.E., 2005. The gene for fragrance in rice. Plant Biotechnology 3 (3), 363–370.

Brenchley, R., Spannagl, M., Pfeifer, M., Barker, G.L.A., D'Amore, R., Allen, A.M., McKenzie, N., Kramer, M., Kerhornou, A., Bolser, D., Kay, S., Waite, D., Trick, D., Bancroft, I., Gu, Y., Huo, N., Luo, M.C., Sehgal, S., Kianian, S., Gill, B., Anderson, O., Kersey, P., Dvorak, J., McCombie, R., Hall, A., Mayer, K.F.X., Edwards, K.J., Bevan, M.W., Hall, N., 2012. Analysis of the bread wheat genome using whole genome shotgun sequencing. Nature 491 (7426), 705–710.

BRC, BRMA and the Rice Association, 2005. Code of Practice on Basmati Rice of the British Retail Consortium, British Rice Millers Association and the Rice Association. London.

Brüning, P., Haase, I., Matissek, R., Fischer, M., 2011. Marzipan: polymerase chain reaction-driven methods for authenticity control. Journal of Agricultural and Food Chemistry 59 (22), 11910–11917.

Bryant, R.J., McClung, A.M., 2011. Volatile profiles of aromatic and non-aromatic rice cultivars using SPME/GC–MS. Food Chemistry 124, 501–513.

Bucher, T.B., Fridez, F., Köppel, R., 2014. Duplex real-time PCR for the determination of non-basmati rice in basmati rice (*Oryza sativa*). European Food Research and Technology 238 (3), 417–423.

Caratti, S., Rossi, L., Sona, B., Origlia, S., Viara, S., Martano, G., et al., 2010. Analysis of 11 tetrameric STRs in wild boars for forensic purposes. Forensic Science International: Genetics 4 (5), 339–342.

CARDI, 2013. Aromatic Authenticity to Jasmine Rice Type and Fragrance Genes Analysis. Cambodian Agricultural Research and Development Institute, Phnom Penh. Available from: http://www.cardi.org.kh/index.php?page=detail&ctype=article&id=212&lg=en (accessed 04.06.15.).

Charters, Y.M., Robertson, A., Wilkinson, M.J., Ramsay, G., 1996. PCR analysis of oilseed rape cultivars (*Brassica napus* L. *ssp. oleifera*) using 5′-anchored simple sequence repeat (SSR) primers. Theoretical and Applied Genetics 92, 442–447.

Chuang, P.-S., Chen, M.-I., Shiao, J.-C., 2012. Identification of tuna species by a real-time polymerase chain reaction technique. Food Chemistry 133, 1055–1061.

Commission Implementing Regulation (EU) No 931/2011 of 19 September 2011 on the Traceability Requirements Set by Regulation (EC) No 178/2002 of the European Parliament and of the Council for Food of Animal Origin, OJ L242, 20.9.2011, pp. 2–3.

Commission Implementing Regulation (EU) No 706/2014 of 25 June 2014 Amending Regulation (EC) No 972/2006 as Regards the Import Duty Applicable to Basmati Rice, OJ L186, 26.6.2014, pp. 54–55.

Commission Implementing Regulation (EU) No 1337/2013 of 13 December 2013 Laying Down Rules for the Application of Regulation (EU) No 1169/2011 of the European Parliament and of the Council as Regards the Indication of the Country of Origin or Place of Provenance for Fresh, Chilled and Frozen Meat of Swine, Sheep, Goats and Poultry, OJ L335, 14.12.2013, pp. 19–22.

Commission Regulation (EU) No 272/2010 of 30 March 2010 Amending Regulation (EC) No 972/2006 Laying Down Special Rules for Imports of Basmati Rice and a Transitional Control System for Determining Their Origin. OJ L84, 31.3.2010, pp. 23–24.

Di Bella, J.M., Bao, Y., Gloor, G.B., Burton, J.P., Reid, G., 2013. High throughput sequencing methods and analysis for microbiome research. Journal of Microbiological Methods 95, 401–414.

Eckert, K.A., Hile, S.E., 2009. Every microsatellite is different: 'Intrinsic DNA features dictate mutagenesis of common microsatellites present in the human genome. Molecular Carcinogenesis 48 (4), 379–388.

Ellegren, H., 2004. Microsatellites: simple sequences with complex evolution. Nature Reviews Genetics 5, 435–445.

Feltus, F.A., Wan, J., Schulze, S.R., Estill, J.C., Jiang, N., Paterson, A., 2004. An SNP Resource for rice genetics and breeding based on subspecies indica and japonica genome alignments. Genome Research 14, 1812–1819.

Fondon, J.W., Garner, H.R., 2004. Molecular origins of rapid and continuous morphological evolution. Proceedings of the National Academy of Sciences of the United States of America 101, 18058–18063.

FSA, 2004. Survey on Basmati Rice, Food Surveillance Information: Sheet 47/04 of the Food Standards Agency (London).

FSA, 2006. Report on the Ring Trial of the Quantitative Determination of Non-basmati Rice Varieties in a Mixture With Basmati Rice Varieties of the Food Standards Agency, London.

FSA, 2013. Report of the Investigation by the Food Standards Agency into Incidents of Adulteration of Comminuted Beef Products With Horse Meat and DNA of the Food Standards Agency, London.

Gabriel, S., Ziaugra, L., Tabba, D., 2009. SNP genotyping using the Sequenom MassARRAY iPLEX platform. Current Protocols in Human Genetics 60, 2.12.1–2.12.18.

Garrett, G., Clarke, M.-A., 2007. Use of the Agilent 2100 Bioanalyzer for Basmati Rice Authenticity Testing. Agilent Technologies, Inc., Santa Clara, CA, USA.

Guerra, R., Yu, Z., 2006. Single nucleotide polymorphisms and their applications. In: Zhang, W., Shmulevich, I. (Eds.), Computational and Statistical Approaches to Genomics. Springer, Heidelberg, pp. 311–349.

Garris, A., Tai, T.T., Coburn, J., Kresovich, S., McCouch, S., 2005. Genetic structure and diversity in *Oryza sativa* L. Genetics 169, 1631–1638.

Gupta, P.K., Roy, J.K., Prasad, M., 2001. Single nucleotide polymorphisms: a new paradigm for molecular marker technology and DNA polymorphism detection with emphasis on their use in plants. Current Science. India 80 (4), 524–535.

Gramene, 2015. SSR Primers From McCouch et al. (2002). Available from: http://archive.gramene.org/markers/microsat/ssr.html (accessed 07.07.15.).

Heaton, M.P., Harhay, G.P., Bennett, G.L., Stone, R.T., Grosse, W.M., Casas, E., Keele, J.W., Smith, T.P., Chitko-McKown, C.G., Laegreid, W.W., 2002. Selection and use of SNP markers for animal identification and paternity analysis in U.S. beef cattle. Mammalian Genome 13 (5), 272–281.

Herrmann, L., Haase, I., Blauhut, M., Barz, N., Fischer, M., 2014. DNA-based differentiation of the Ecuadorian cocoa types CCN-51and Arriba based on sequence differences in the chloroplast genome. Journal of Agricultural and Food Chemistry 62, 12118–12127.

Herrmann, L., Felbinger, C., Haase, I., Rudolph, B., Fischer, M., 2015. Food fingerprinting: characterization of the Ecuadorean type CCN-51 of *Theobroma cacao* L. using microsatellite markers. Journal of Agricultural and Food Chemistry 63, 4539–4544.

International Rice Genome Sequencing Project, 2015. The map-based sequence of the rice genome. Nature 436, 793–800.

Jeffreys, A.J., Brookfield, J.F., Semeonoff, R., 1985. Positive identification of an immigration test-case using human DNA fingerprints. Nature 317 (6040), 818–819.

Jobling, M.A., Gill, P., 2004. Encoded evidence: DNA in forensic analysis. Nature Reviews Genetics 5 (10), 739–751.

Kantety, R.V., Zeng, X., Bennetzen, J.L., Zehr, B.E., 1995. Assessment of genetic diversity in dent and popcorn (*Zea mays* L.) inbred lines using inter-simple repeat (ISSR) amplification. Molecular Breeding 1, 365–373.

Kumar, L.D., Kathirvel, M., Rao, G.V., Nagaraju, J., 2001. DNA profiling of disputed chilli samples (*Capsicum annum*) using ISSR-PCR and FISSR-PCR marker assays. Science International 116, 63–68.

Levinson, G., Gutman, G.A., 1987. High frequencies of short frameshifts in poly-CA/TG tandem repeats borne by bacteriophage M13 in *Escherichia coli* K-12. Nucleic Acids Research 15, 5323–5338.

Lunel, F.V., Licciardello, L., Stefani, S., Verbrugh, H.A., Melchers, W., Meis, G.M., Scherer, S., Van Belkum, A., 1998. Lack of consistent short sequence repeat polymorphisms in genetically homologous colonizing and invasive *Candida albicans* strains. Journal of Bacteriology 180, 3771–3778.

Masoumiasl, A., Amiri-Fahliani, R., Khoshroo, A.R., 2013. Some local and commercial rice (*Oryza sativa* L.) varieties - comparison for aroma and other qualitative properties. International Journal of Agriculture and Crop Sciences 5 (19), 2184–2189.

Myint, K.M., Courtois, B., Risterucci, A.-M., Frouin, J., Soe, K., Thet, K.M., Vanavichit, A., Glaszmann, J.-C., 2012. Specific patterns of genetic diversity among aromatic rice varieties in Myanmar. Rice 5, 20.

Nachman, M.W., Crowell, S.L., 2000. Estimate of the mutation rate per nucleotide in humans. Genetics 156, 297–304.

Nader, W.F., Edlind, T.D., Huettermann, A., Sauer, H.W., 1985. Cloning of *Physarum* actin sequences in an exonuclease-deficient bacterial host. Proceedings of the National Academy of Sciences of the United States of America 82 (9), 2698–2702.

Nader, W.F., Isenberg, G., Sauer, H.W., 1986. Structure of *Physarum* actin gene locus ardA: a nonpalindromic sequence causes inviability of phage lambda and recA-independent deletions. Gene 48 (1), 133–144.

Nader, W.F., Werner, D., Wink, M., 1999. Genetic diversity of scarlet macaws (*Ara macao*) in a breeding project and in the wild in Costa Rica. Biological Conservation 87, 269–272.

Nader, W.F., Brendel, T., Schubbert, R., 2013. DNA-analysis: enhancing the control of food authenticity through emerging technologies. Agro Food Industry Hi Tech 24 (1), 42–46.

Nader, W.F., Grote, A.K., Cuevas Montilla, E., 2014. Impacts of food safety and authenticity issues on the rice trade. In: Sontag, J. (Ed.), Rice Processing – The Comprehensive Guide to Global Technology and Innovative Products. Erling Verlag, Clenze, pp. 159–176.

Nagaraju, J., Kathirvel, M., Ramesh Kumar, R., Siddiq, E.A., Hasnain, S.E., 2002. Genetic analysis of traditional and evolved basmati and non-basmati rice varieties by using fluorescence-based ISSR-PCR and SSR markers. Proceedings of the National Academy of Sciences of the United States of America 99 (9), 5836–5841.

Phuc, N.V., Lang, N.T., Buu, B.C., 2005. STS and microsatellite marker-assisted selection for bacterial blight resistance in rice, *Oryza sativa* L. Omonrice 13, 18–25.

Ratnaparkhe, M.B., Tekeoglu, M., Muehlbauer, F.J., 1998. Inter-simple-sequence-repeat (ISSR) polymorphisms are useful for finding markers associated with disease resistance gene clusters. Theoretical and Applied Genetics 97, 515–519.

Regulation (EC) No 178/2002 of the European Parliament and of the Council of 28 January 2002 Laying Down the General Principles and Requirements of Food Law, Establishing the European Food SafetyAuthority and Laying Down Procedures in Matters of Food Safety, OJ L31, 1.2.2002, pp. 1–24.

Regulation (EC) No 1760/2000 of the European Parliament and of the Council of 17 July 2000 Establishing a System for the Identification and Registration of Bovine Animals and Regarding the Labelling of Beef and Beef Products and Repealing Council Regulation (EC) No 820/97, OJ L204, 11.8.2000, pp. 1–11.

Regulation (EU) No 1169/2011 of the European Parliament and of the Council of 25 October 2011 on the Provision of Food Information to Consumers, Amending Regulations (EC) No 1924/2006 and (EC) No 1925/2006 of the European Parliament and of the Council, and Repealing Commission Directive 87/250/EEC, Council Directive 90/496/EEC, Commission Directive 1999/10/EC, Directive 2000/13/EC of the European Parliament and of the Council, Commission Directives 2002/67/EC and 2008/5/EC and Commission Regulation (EC) No 608/2004, OJ L304, 22.11.2011, pp. 18–63.

Richard, G.F., Kerrest, A., Dujon, B., 2008. Comparative genomics and molecular dynamics of DNA repeats in eukaryotes. Microbiology and Molecular Biology Reviews 72 (4), 686–727.

Saldo, 2010. Nicht jeder Basmati Reis ist ein Genuß. Available from: https://www.saldo.ch/tests/tests/detail/d/nicht-jeder-basmati-reis-ist-ein-genuss/ (accessed 04.06.15.).

Semagn, K., Babu, R., Hearne, S., Olsen, M., 2013. Single nucleotide polymorphism genotyping using Kompetitive Allele Specific PCR (KASP): overview of the technology and its application in crop improvement. Molecular Breeding 33 (1), 1–14.

Siddiq, E.A., Vemireddy, L.R., Nagaraju, J., 2012. Basmati rices: genetics, breeding and trade. Agriculture Research 1 (1), 25–36.

Sonah, H., Deshmukh, R.K., Sharma, A., Singh, V.P., Gupta, D.K., Gacche, R.J., Rana, J.C., Singh, N.K., Sharma, T.R., 2011. Genome-wide distribution and organization of microsatellites in plants: an Insight into marker development in *Brachyp*odium. PLoS One 6 (6), e21298.

Spaniolas, S., Bazakos, C., Tucker, G.A., Bennett, M.J., 2014. Comparison of SNP-based detection assays for food analysis: coffee authentication. Journal of AOAC International 97 (4), 1114–1120.

Steele, K., Ogden, R., McEwing, R., Briggs, H., Gorham, J., 2008. InDel markers distinguish basmatis from other fragrant rice varieties. Field Crops Research 105, 81–87.

Stiftung Warentest, 2010. 'Duftreis ist selten dufte', *Stiftung Warentest*, Berlin. Test 8, 20–27.

Syndicat de la Rizerie Français, 2015. Code des Usages relatif au riz destiné à la consummation humaine, Paris.

Union Fédérale des Consommateurs Que Choisir, 2009. 'Riz parfumés – L'authenticité en question'. Que Choisir, Paris 471, 50–55.

Vázquez, J.F., Pérez, T., Ureña, F., Gudín, E., Albornoz, J., Domínguez, A., 2004. Practical application of DNA fingerprinting to trace beef. Journal of Food Protection 67 (5), 972–979.

Vemireddy, L.R., Archak, S., Nagaraju, J., 2007. Capillary electrophoresis is essential for microsatellite marker based detection and quantification of adulteration of basmati rice (*Oryza sativa*). Journal of Agricultural and Food Chemistry 55, 8112–8117.

Verstrepen, K.J., Jansen, A., Lewitter, F., Fink, G.R., 2005. Intragenic tandem repeats generate functional variability. Nature Genetics 37, 986–990.

Vilà, C., Leonard, J.A., Götherström, A., Marklund, S., Sandberg, K., Lidén, K., Wayne, R.K., Ellegren, H., 2001. Widespread origin of domestic horse lineages. Science 291, 474–477.

Wankhade, S.D., Cornejo, M.J., Mateu-Andres, I., 2010. Microsatellite marker-based genetic variability in Spanish rice cultivars and landraces. Spanish Journal of Agricultural Research 8 (4), 995–1004.

Zeltz, P., Schneider, S., Volkmann, J., Willmund, R., 2005. Traceability of wild-growing coffee from Ethiopian rainforest by genetic fingerprinting. Deutsche Lebensmittel-Rundschau 101 (3), 89–92.

Zimin, A.V., Delcher, A.L., Florea, L., Kelley, D.R., Schatz, M.C., Puiu, D., Hanrahan, F., Pertea, G., Van Tassell, C.P., Sonstegard, T.S., Marçais, G., Roberts, M., Subramanian, P., Yorke, J.A., Salzberg, S.L., 2009. A whole-genome assembly of the domestic cow, Bos Taurus. Genome Biology 10, R42.

Advances in Ultraviolet and Visible Light Spectroscopy for Food Authenticity Testing

3

M.J. Martelo-Vidal, M. Vázquez
University of Santiago de Compostela, Lugo, Spain

Chapter Outline

3.1 Introduction

The presence on retail markets of food adulteration and fraud such as substitutions of cheaper or inferior food products is evident. The current demand for high-quality products provides an opportunity for fraudsters based on the fact that the consumer cannot identify fraud in ingredients or processes (Wlasiuk et al., 2015; Wu and Sun, 2013).

Thus, it is of utmost importance to protect the reputation of quality foodstuffs and minimize malpractices that may undermine their position in the marketplace. Regulatory authorities, food processing companies and importers, as well as consumers are increasingly interested in control activities, traceability, and labeling of products (Wójcicki et al., 2015; Wu and Sun, 2013). They need rapid and specific analytical methods to enable food authentication and compliance with European Union (EU) rules on food labeling, presentation of products, and protection of public health (Nunes, 2014; Aparicio et al., 2013; Cozzolino, 2014; Morsy and Sun, 2013).

Food producers should provide food descriptions and information that can enable confirmation of foodstuff authenticity through verification of label descriptions. These descriptions may include aspects such as the identity of products and ingredients, region of origin and/or species, and variety of ingredients (Arvanitoyannis, 2008; Biancolillo et al., 2014).

Ultraviolet—visible (UV—VIS) spectroscopy is one of the most common laboratory techniques for food analysis. It is a useful tool for both quantitative and qualitative analyse. There are many different spectral methods, each of which is appropriate for a large range of analytical problems; these include molecular or atomic spectroscopy depending on the chemical species to be analyzed, different types of interaction of radiation with matter (absorption, reflection, emission, or diffraction), and different spectral regions to be used in analyses (Penner, 2010; Lourenco et al., 2012; Kumirska et al., 2010). In the past, UV—VIS analysis was used only for color measurement or simple determination of chemical concentrations using filter photometers (Liauw, Baylor, and O'Rourke, 2010).

The electromagnetic spectrum includes a wide range of radiation that varies according to wavelength or frequency and energy (Fig. 3.1); ultraviolet (UV) and visible (VIS) radiation is a very small region. Other regions included in the electromagnetic spectrum are near infrared (NIR), mid and far infrared (MIR and FIR), and X-rays (Owen, 2000). Absorption of radiation in the UV—VIS region results in changes in electron distributions (Dufour, 2009; Skoog et al., 2008, 2013).

Measurement of the absorption of UV—VIS absorption has many applications in the quantitative determination of organic and inorganic molecules as well as to determine the functional groups on molecules (Skoog et al., 2008). Furthermore, the attractiveness of UV—VIS spectroscopy is due to the availability of good

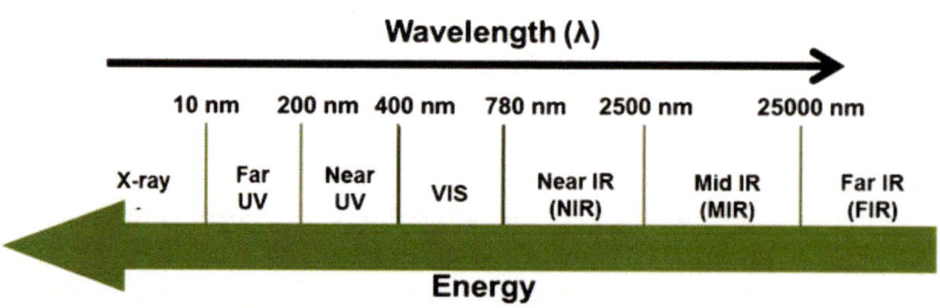

Figure 3.1 Electromagnetic spectrum according to major wavelength ranges.

instrumentation, ease of use, accuracy, precision, and speed of the method (Sánchez Rojas and Bosch Ojeda, 2009; Snyder et al., 2014).

Absorptions in the UV−VIS zone arise due to electronic and vibrational excitations (Gauglitz and Moore, 2014; Skoog et al., 2013; Hof, 2005). Electrons are excited by absorption of energy and this absorption can be related to the concentration of absorbing molecules (Van Maarschalkerweerd and Husted, 2015).

The UV spectrum ranges from 190 to 400 nm while the VIS region extends from 400 to 780 nm (Gauglitz and Moore, 2014). All organic compounds contain electrons susceptible to excitation to higher levels as a result of absorbed electronic radiation (Skoog et al., 2008). Spectral data therefore reflects the molecular composition of foods. Spectroscopy in the visible wavelength range directly provides color information, and such wavelengths are used to quantify pigments in samples (Alamprese et al., 2013).

3.2 Fundamentals of Ultraviolet and Visible Light Spectroscopy in Food Analysis

In spectroscopy, when incident light interacts with samples, many diverse outcomes are possible: the incident light (I_0) may be reflected (I_R), scattered (I_S), absorbed (I_A), or transmitted (I_T) (Fig. 3.2). The amount of radiation passing through the sample is measured and compared to a reference sample in order to determine concentration of one or more specific analytes. Such radiation is attenuated by the sample (light absorbed); thus absorption spectroscopy measures the amount of light absorbed by the sample. Absorbance is the measure most used for quantitative and qualitative analyse in chemistry, biology, and agriculture applications (Penner, 2010; Skoog et al., 2013). According to Beer's law, absorbance is proportional to concentration of analyte (c), to path length (b), and to absorptivity constant (a). Absorbance is dimensionless, and, furthermore, the absorptivity constant must have units that eliminate units of b and c (Eq. (3.1)).

$$A = a \cdot b \cdot c = \varepsilon \cdot b \cdot c \tag{3.1}$$

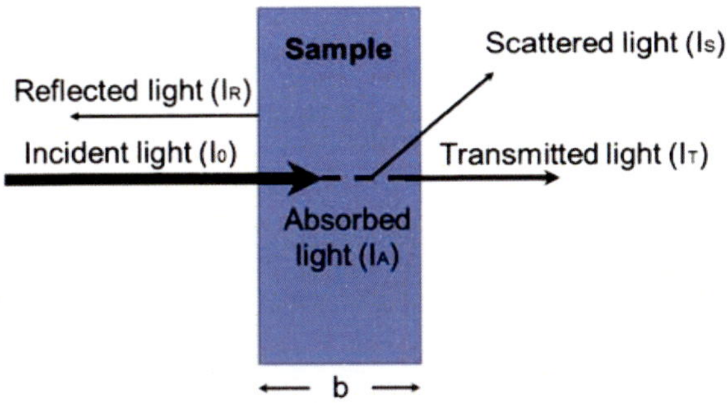

Figure 3.2 Energy of incident light when interacting with samples.

When concentration is expressed as moles per liter (mol L^{-1}) and path length in centimeters (cm), the absorptivity constant is the molar absorptivity (ε) with L mol^{-1} cm^{-1} as units (Skoog et al., 2013; Hollas, 2004).

Transmittance (T) expresses the relationship between light incident and transmitted (ratio of I_T and I_0), and the intensity of light decreases from I_0 to I_T (Penner, 2010; Skoog et al., 2013; Lourenco et al., 2012). Thus, transmittance is defined as the quantity of incident light that it is transmitted by the sample (Eq. (3.2)). Often this is expressed as a percentage (%T):

$$T = \frac{I_T}{I_0} \tag{3.2}$$

The relationship between absorbance and transmittance of a sample is defined as the negative logarithm of transmittance (Eq. (3.3)). When absorption of a sample increases, transmittance decreases (Liauw et al., 2010):

$$A = -\log T = -\log \frac{I_T}{I_0} = \log \frac{I_0}{I_T} \tag{3.3}$$

Reflectance is defined as the fraction of incident energy reflected by the surface (Eq. (3.4)):

$$R = \frac{I_R}{I_0} \tag{3.4}$$

Absorbance may be obtained from reflectance (R) from Eq. (3.5):

$$A = \log \frac{1}{R} \tag{3.5}$$

Absorption of UV–VIS radiation at appropriate wavelengths causes electronic transitions between orbitals. Therefore absorbances due to vibrational and rotational levels of orbitals are overlaid on those arising from electronic levels, providing absorption spectra with wide bands (Lourenco et al., 2012; Hof, 2005).

Signals provided by UV–VIS spectrophotometers may be associated with pigments or with the results of chemical reactions between analytes such as colorimetric methods used for the analysis of proteins. UV–VIS spectra have continuous absorption bands arising from a combination of overlapping peaks caused by superimposition of vibrational and rotational transitions of two or more components of a sample (Kumirska et al., 2010; Liauw et al., 2010). The main parameters that characterize a spectral band are the location of the maximum and its intensity.

Chromophores are characteristic structures in a molecule that absorb UV–VIS radiation. They have multiple bonds such as C=C or C=O and are comprised of heteroatoms and transition metals (Dufour, 2009; Buglass, 2011; Kumirska et al., 2010).

Table 3.1 Relationship of Wavelengths to Absorbed and Observed Colors in UV−VIS Spectroscopy

Wavelength (nm)	Absorbed Color	Transmitted Color (Observed)
<380	Ultraviolet	Colorless
380−420	Violet	Yellow-green
420−440	Violet-blue	Yellow
440−470	Blue	Orange
470−500	Blue-green	Red
500−520	Green	Purple
520−550	Yellow-green	Violet
550−580	Yellow	Violet-blue
580−620	Orange	Blue
620−680	Red	Blue-green
680−780	Purple	Green
>780	Near infrared	Colorless

Molecules such as carotenoids and chlorophylls with double-conjugated bonds (Penner, 2010; Dufour, 2009) absorb in the VIS spectral range; this spectral zone is perceived by human eye as color (Ruiz-Altisent et al., 2010) with violet at the short wavelength ending with red at high wavelengths (Table 3.1). The human eye cannot detect any color in the UV zone (190−400 nm). Absorptions in this spectral zone are caused by peptide bonds in proteins and aromatic amino acids of proteins and vitamins. Compounds with isolated double, triple, and peptide bonds and molecules with aromatic and carbonyl groups have maximum absorbance in the UV region.

Measurements observed UV−VIS spectroscopy can be classified on the basis of the physical state of the sample phase, eg, liquid (homogeneous samples, liquid in a flowing sample, and immiscible samples), solid (powders, chunks, and surfaces), and gaseous. Sometimes raw samples are inappropriate for analysis because of their complex nature or size. Therefore, sample preparation and representative sampling are required prior to analysis (Cullum and Vo-Dinh, 2005). Moreover, pretreatment of spectral data measured and the development of chemometric models to obtain useful information from spectra have helped to exploit the advantages of UV−VIS spectral data.

In spite of the fact that assignment of specific absorptions observed in UV−VIS spectra is complicated by the presence of overlapping bands, UV−VIS spectroscopy can provide information about food component absorptions that, combined with chemometric data treatments, make it an excellent technique for quantification and classification of foodstuffs (Tan et al., 2015).

Chemometrics uses mathematical and statistical methods to analyze spectral data from chemical systems such as foods, extracting relevant information to determine or quantify components (Blanco and Maspoch, 2007; Lourenco et al., 2012). It is very important to consider factors that can affect the position and intensity of absorbance such as temperature, concentration of sample, pH of solution, presence of impurities or bubbles in solution, and solvents used. These should be controlled before and during analysis to obtain high-precision measurements and avoid baseline shifts by performing all spectral analyses under the same conditions.

Any solvent used should be completely transparent to avoid modification of analyte absorbance. Furthermore, the concentration of a sample can affect the measured intensity with high concentrations possibly causing changes in the shape or position of characteristic bands. Changes in temperature can also displace absorption bands while absorptivity can be affected by physicochemical changes of the sample (Penner, 2010; Skoog et al., 2013; Owen, 2000).

Simple mathematical pretreatments can help to correct all these possible deviations while use of chemometric techniques can also help to extract useful information contained in the spectra (Karoui and Dufour, 2008).

Usually, absorbance mode measurements are used on liquid samples, transmittance mode on solid and liquid samples, and reflectance mode used on solid samples such as powders or opaque liquids (Liauw et al., 2010; Gauglitz and Moore, 2014).

The principal radiation sources used in UV—VIS spectroscopy are deuterium and tungsten/halogen lamps. Instruments used in all techniques of UV—VIS spectroscopy have similar components, including a radiation source, radiation detectors, and sample cells (Penner, 2010).

When there is only one absorbing species in a sample and no baseline offset, Beer's law is useful to determine analyte concentration in a sample, but when there are more absorbing species, chemometric tools are useful. The main tools used to extract information from sample spectra are:

1. For quantification: Partial least squares (PLS) regression, principal component analysis (PCA), principal component regression (PCR), and multiple linear regression (MLR).
2. For classification: Linear discriminant analysis (LDA), soft independent modeling of class analogy (SIMCA), or support vector machine (SVM) classification.

Moreover, data pretreatments are often required to enhance the important information contained in spectral data, eg, normalization, mean-centering, smoothing, or derivatives (Lourenco et al., 2012; Liauw et al., 2010).

Multiplicative scatter correction (MSC) is perhaps the most commonly deployed normalization method, used to compensate for baseline shifts and multiplicative effects. Standard normal variate (SNV) is used to eliminate multiplicative effects while first and second derivatives calculated using the Savitzky—Golay algorithm are often used to eliminate baseline offsets and resolve (partially or entirely) overlapping peaks (Rinnan et al., 2009; Cozzolino et al., 2011; Lourenco et al., 2012).

To perform a successful UV—VIS spectral analysis (Nicolaï et al., 2007; Cozzolino et al., 2011; Blanco and Maspoch, 2007; Blanco and Alcalá, 2009) and get good prediction results on new samples, all experiments must begin by selecting a good, representative set of calibration samples. Samples used for model development must be similar to those likely to be encountered in future analysis. Moreover, it is best to include the widest possible variability and the greatest number of samples possible to develop calibration models. A number of pretreatment and modeling methods should be examined to obtain the most accurate mathematical models for both quantification and classification. Critically, models obtained must be validated by application to new, unknown samples.

Hyperspectral imaging is a technique related to UV—VIS spectroscopy. It is a new UV—VIS spectral technique capable of performing analysis in real time and, critically, collecting spectral and spatial data from foodstuffs in one step. This technique does not involve contact directly with materials being analyzed (Pu et al., 2015). Hyperspectral imaging uses traditional spectroscopy and traditional digital imaging. It is useful for a large range of foodstuffs, homogenized or not. It has been reported to be useful for determining pH, color, chemical composition, and contaminations using either reflectance or transmittance measurement modes (Kamruzzaman et al., 2015).

Its main uses are in vegetables, fruits, meats, and fish to determine intrinsic and extrinsic characteristics of food products (Dai et al., 2014). Principal uses of hyperspectral imaging involve the VIS and NIR spectral ranges. Data collected using hyperspectral systems consist in a three-dimensional data array with two spatial and one spectral dimension. Samples are illuminated with light from a tungsten-halogen or LED source. Reflected light enters an objective lens in the hyperspectral camera and is separated into individual wavelengths by diffraction and measured (Gowen et al., 2007; Kamruzzaman et al., 2015). Each pixel in a hyperspectral image contains the spectral data of a specific position in the sample, and the resulting complete spectrum is like a fingerprint that can be used to determine, for example, food composition (ElMasry et al., 2012). The principal advantage of this technique is the possibility of obtaining spatial information potentially describing the physical distribution of chemical compounds in a sample by one measurement (ElMasry and Sun, 2010).

Nowadays the main research focuses on (1) UV—VIS spectroscopy combined with other spectral ranges such as NIR and MIR spectroscopy, (2) using different pretreatments to remove unwanted spectral variations, and (3) using chemometric tools to obtain robust models from multivariate spectral (and spatial) data.

3.3 Application of UV—VIS Spectroscopy for Authentication of Foodstuffs

For many years UV—VIS spectroscopy has been the cheapest and most used spectroscopic tool for quantification of macro- and microcomponents in foods, eg, carbohydrates, amino acids, proteins, sugars, vitamins, polyphenols, or minerals. Moreover, lipid oxidation, levels of pigmentation in foods, and characterization of foodstuffs have also been determined (Lourenco et al., 2012; Karoui and Dufour, 2008).

Nowadays studies concerning authenticity for UV—VIS spectroscopy are very scarce (Reidet al., 2006) but use of these spectral zones is increasing as a result of advances in spectrophotometer design and construction, spectral data processing, and available chemometric tools. Progress in the availability and performance of mathematical models to determine multicomponents or quality parameters of foodstuffs facilitates advances in authentication of foodstuffs (Martelo-Vidal and Vázquez, 2014a; Rohman and Man, 2011; Nunes, 2014).

There are European systems and several EU regulations in existence to protect and facilitate development of foodstuffs. These systems stimulate quality foodstuff production and protect such products from fraud such as the use of mixtures or imitations. They also help to detect specific characteristics of products by correct identification (Reid et al., 2006; Primrose et al., 2010).

Nowadays several methods are available to confirm the authenticity of foodstuffs, eg, chromatography, mass spectrometry, polymerase chain reaction, microscopy, electronic spin resonance, electronic nose or tongue, or enzymatic analysis (Morsy and Sun, 2013; Reid et al., 2006; Wlasiuk et al., 2015). However, their principal disadvantages are that they are slow and expensive techniques (equipment and reagents), need trained staff, have high maintenance costs, and require sophisticated infrastructure and even complete laboratories (Souto et al., 2010; Acevedo et al., 2007). UV−VIS spectroscopy can also be used to monitor and supervise processes (Lourenco et al., 2012).

Tables 3.2 and 3.3 show some examples of qualitative and quantitative applications of foodstuffs using UV−VIS spectroscopy.

3.3.1 Authentication of Geographical Origin

Protected designation of origin (PDO) is the name of a geographical region or specific area that is recognized by official rules to produce certain foods with special characteristics related to location. The PDO regulation covers agricultural products and foodstuffs that are produced, processed, and prepared in a given geographical area using recognized know-how in this specific zone. Therefore, it is very important for food producers and regulatory institutions to determine and quantify the specific quality parameters of such products to avoid fraud and to confirm their geographical origin.

Thus, the use of UV−VIS spectroscopy for confirming geographical origin or to classify foods, and consequently determine food authenticity, potentially represents a simple and low-cost technique for use in ordinary laboratories. A large number of classification and characterization studies of vegetables and fruits, juices, olive oils, alcoholic beverages, honeys, or coffee using PDO labels use spectroscopy in UV−VIS zone alone or combined with NIR and MIR spectroscopy.

Dried *sclerotium* of mushroom *Wolfiporia extensa* from three different geographical origins of southwestern China was discriminated using UV absorbance spectroscopy (range of 190−450 nm) and chemometric tools. Smoothing was applied such as pretreatment of spectral data. Moreover, partial least squares discriminant analysis (PLS-DA) and hierarchical cluster analysis (HCA) were used to discriminate by origin. High correct classification percentages (95%) were obtained using PLS-DA analysis (Li et al., 2014). Differentiation and classification of *La Mancha* red and white PDO wines was performed using UV and VIS spectroscopy in the wavelength range 300−800 nm. SIMCA was used as a classification method, and a correct classification

Table 3.2 Examples of Food Classification Using UV–VIS Spectroscopy Only or Combined with NIR and MIR Spectroscopy

Food	Spectral Region	Pretreatment	Method	References
Craft beer	210–400 nm	1ª and 2ª derivative, smoothing	SIMCA	Biancolillo et al. (2014)
		De-trending	PLS-DA	
		SNV, MSC	MSC	
Brazilian, Argentinean and Sri Lankan black tea, Brazilian and Argentinean green tea	180–800 nm	No pretreatment	SPA-LDA, KNN, CART, SIMCA, PLS-DA, and PCA-LDA	Diniz et al. (2016)
Belgian beers	450–800 nm	No pretreatment	LDA	Mignani et al. (2013)
Lager beers from different factories	320–800 nm	SNV	LDA	Vera et al. (2011)
		1ª derivative		
Canned lager beer Chinese	240–400 nm	1ª derivative	LDA	Tan et al. (2015)
	380–700 nm	2ª derivative		
Fresh Atlantic salmon fillet stored under different atmospheres	400–1100 nm	SNV	PCA	Sone et al. (2012)
			PLS	
Fresh and frozen-thawed pork meat	400–1000 nm	No pretreatment	LS-SVM	Pu et al. (2014)

Continued

Table 3.2 Continued

Food	Spectral Region	Pretreatment	Method	References
Rice wines	325–1075 nm	SNV Smoothing	PLS	Liu et al. (2008)
Italian red wines	340–740 nm	SNV 2^a derivative	LDA	Casale et al. (2010)
Australian red wines	400–4000 cm^{-1}	SNV 2^a derivative	LDA SIMCA	Riovanto et al. (2011)
Decaffeinated and caffeinated coffee	225–352 nm	No pretreatment	SIMCA LDA	Souto et al. (2010)
Different brands and fake tequilas	250–500 nm	Centered Smoothing	SVM LDA PCA	Contreras et al. (2010)

Table 3.3 Examples of Quantification of Components and Quality Parameters of Foods Using UV–VIS Spectroscopy only or Combined with NIR and MIR Spectroscopy

Food	Spectral Region	Component	Pre-treatment	Method	Reference
Belgian beers	450–800 nm	Ethanol	No pretreatment	PLS	Mignani et al. (2013)
Fish fillets of grass carp	400–1000 nm	Total volatile basic nitrogen (TVB-N)	No pretreatment	LS-SVM	Cheng et al. (2014)
Pork meat	400–1000 nm	pH and thawing loss percentage	No pretreatment	LS-SVM	Pu et al. (2014)
Pork meat	400–800 nm 400–1100 nm	Intramuscular fat, pH, color, drip lost	1^a and 2^a derivative SNV De-Trending	MPLS	Savenije et al. (2006)
Rice wine	300–1000 nm	Alcohol, total sugar content, pH	Smoothing	PLS	Ouyang et al. (2016)
Red wine from PDO Valdeorras	200–800 nm	Phenolic compounds	No pretreatment	PLS	Figueiredo-Gonzalez et al. (2013)
Red wine from Galician PDO	190–2500 nm	Phenolic compounds	SNV, MSC, 1ª and 2ª derivative, smoothing, de-trending, normalize, centered and scaled, baseline	PLC PCR	Martelo-Vidal and Vázquez (2014b)
White egg	200–860 nm	Yolk contamination	No pretreatment	LV-SVM	Yao et al. (2014)
Algal oil	453–1026 nm	Docosahexaenoic acid and eicosapentaenoic acid	Smoothing, MSC, SNV, 1ª and 2ª derivative	PCR PLS	Wu and He (2014)
Ewe's milk	300–1710 nm	pH, density, nonfat in dry matter, fat, protein, lactose, ash and freezing point	Normalization, 1ª derivative	PLSR	Mouazen et al. (2009)

rate of wines from the same PDO was around 90% (Urbano et al., 2006). Moreover, UV–VIS spectroscopy (190–780 nm) was applied to classify Galician white wines from PDO regions *Rías Baixas, Ribeira Sacra, Ribeiro, Valdeorras*, and *Monterrei* (Martelo-Vidal and Vázquez, 2014e) and to discriminate Galician white wines from subzones inside the PDO *Rías Baixas* area (Martelo-Vidal et al., 2013). Different data pretreatments and regions of spectra were used to develop LDA, SVM, SIMCA, and artificial neural network (ANN) models. All PDOs and subzones inside PDO *Rías Baixas* assayed were 100% correctly classified using different ranges of spectra. Furthermore, red wines from *Ribeira Sacra* and *Rías Baixas* were classified by PDO using UV–VIS and NIR spectroscopy. LDA and SVM models using raw spectral data and centered spectral data were developed. LDA models without pretreatment provided the best classification (100% correct classification) (Martelo-Vidal and Vázquez, 2014a). UV spectral data were used to classify Argentinean white wines (from Mendoza, San Juan, and Rio Negro) produced by *Sauvignon blanc* grape. Models obtained using LDA and PLS-DA provided 100% correct classification of wines (Azcarate et al., 2013b). Furthermore, VIS spectroscopy, in range of 495–700 nm, and chemometric models (LDA and PLS-DA) were used on Spanish PDO olive oils (*Andalusia, La Rioja*, and *Catalonia*) to classify them on the basis of geographical origin, obtaining correct classification values of 92.5% (Pizarro et al., 2013).

Confirming the geographical origin of products with UV–VIS spectroscopy can confirm authenticity of foodstuffs in a few minutes, protecting production areas, economic value of products, and consumers.

3.3.2 Authentication of Variety or Species

Other possible adulterations relate to varieties or species of ingredients used in foodstuffs. Consumers are not familiar with morphological, chemical, and taxonomical characteristics of diverse foods. For these reasons, bad practices and adulterations are possible by substitution of species or varieties or by producing mixtures involving varieties or species of lower commercial value. UV–VIS spectral data alone or combined with other spectral zones can also be useful to classify foods on the basis of variety or species used in food elaboration, thereby confirming authenticity.

Varieties of olive oil, grapes for wine, fish, seafood, and meats are suitable for authentication. Different adulterations of canned products of Atlantic blue crabmeat (*Callinectes sapidus*) with blue swimmer crabmeat (*Portunus pelagicus*) (Gayo and Hale, 2007) were determined.

On the other hand, in several foodstuffs such as wines or olive oils, varietal composition is fixed by production rules (Casale et al., 2007). White wines from Galician PDO (*Rías Baixas, Ribeira Sacra, Ribeiro, Valdeorras*, and *Monterrei*) were classified by grape variety using spectral data in UV, VIS, and NIR zones (Martelo-Vidal and Vázquez, 2014d). Sometimes the compositional differences between varieties are based on harvest or geographical conditions (microclimate, soil, or topography). For the authentication of varieties, it can be interesting to quantify and detect differences in composition, growing, and process. These differences can involve the content and quality of sterols, colorants, fatty acids, volatile compounds, or polyphenols that can be characteristic of one or several varieties (Gad et al., 2013a; Sarbu et al., 2012).

The polyphenols of red wines such as *trans*-resveratrol, quercetin, catechin, malvin, epicatechin, oenin, and syringic acid were determined in Galician red wines using UV−VIS and NIR spectroscopy and chemometric tools (PCR and PLS). Residual predictive deviation (RPD) was used to evaluate the prediction capacity of the models obtained. Calibrations of polyphenols provided values of RPD higher than 1.4 (1.50 for *trans*-resveratrol, 1.54 for quercetin, 3.24 for quercetin, 1.50 for malvin, 1.98 for epicatechin, 3 for oenin, and 1.74 for syringic acid). They were recommended for prediction of polyphenol composition (Martelo-Vidal and Vázquez, 2014b). In another study, four subspecies of kiwi (*Actinidia chinensis*: Hayward, Haenam, Bidan, and Daeheung) and three of pomelo (*Citrus maxima*: Kao Paen, Thong Dee, and Tha Knoi) were analyzed using UV−VIS spectral data to perform classifications according to species and subspecies. One hundred percent correct classification was obtained for all subspecies (Sarbu et al., 2012). Furthermore, flavonoids such as kaempferol, quercetin, and myricetin were analyzed using UV spectral data and chemometric tools (least squares support vector machine; LS-SVM) in Laurel (*Laurus nobilis*), St. John's wort (*Hypericum perforatum*), and green tea. LS-SVM models provided determination coefficients (r^2) of 0.9992 (kaempferol), 0.9996 (quercetin), and 0.9992 (myricetin) (Sohrabi and Darabi, 2016).

3.3.3 Purity or Quality Determination

Sometimes foods are adulterated with other substances such as water or sugar added to juices and colorants added to olive oils or meats. Other adulterations involve mixtures with lower-quality meats, fish, or juices. Incorrect declarations of vintages in wines and incorrect or absent labeling of hydrogenated oils on bakery products are also frauds (Boggia et al., 2013; Aroca-Santos et al., 2015; Alamprese et al., 2013; Da Costa Filho, 2014). Identification and quantification of adulterants in olive oils of the *Picual* variety were performed with UV−VIS spectroscopy and ANNs. These adulterants were analyzed in mixtures of *Picual* extra virgin olive adulterated with refined oils from olives, orujo olive oil, sunflower oil, and corn oil (Aroca-Santos et al., 2015).

Spectral data covering different ranges (UV−VIS, NIR, MIR, and UV−VIS−NIR−MIR) were used to detect different levels of adulterations of bovine minced beef with turkey meat. UV−VIS spectral data and LDA modeling provided 100% correct classification when levels of adulteration were highest. Moreover, when PLS models were used on UV−VIS spectra, the following values were obtained: r^2, 0.815−0.963; RMSECV, 6.70−9.12; and RMSEP, 8.61−21.51. Better models were obtained using UV−VIS−NIR−MIR spectra (r^2, 0.951−0.994; RMSECV, 2.58−5.90; and RMSEP 5.33−10.15; Alamprese et al., 2013).

Other applications include quantification of acid value, as an indicator of free fatty acids of edible oils by UV–VIS spectroscopy, analyzing the effect of heating edible corn, sunflower, rapeseed, peanut, soybean, and sesame oils on acid value to provide information on quality and degree of refining. PLS models used provided r^2 values of 0.991–0.998 and RMSEPs of 0.0230–0.0794 (Zhang et al., 2015). Moreover, VIS spectroscopy combined with NIR data was applied to Saudi honeys adulterated with different concentrations of glucose syrup to predict the quantity of glucose concentration in such honey mixtures (Mouazen and Al Walaan, 2014).

3.3.4 Discrimination of Fresh from Cold-Stored and Frozen-Thawed Products

Mainly in the fish and meat processing industry, product quality depends on raw materials and their freshness. In food collection and distribution, it is important to preserve the integrity of the cold chain to avoid contamination by microbial growth and loss of quality nutrients, which can affect organoleptic characteristics and product integrity (Pu et al., 2014; Uddin et al., 2005; Zhu et al., 2013; Cheng et al., 2015). VIS combined with NIR hyperspectral imaging was applied to classify fresh and frozen-thawed pork *Longissimus dorsi* muscles using PLS-DA (Ma et al., 2015), to discriminate between fresh and frozen-thawed fillets of West African Goatfish (*Pseudupeneus prayensis*) (100% and 98.5%, respectively, of correct classification accuracy) (Ottavian et al., 2014), or to discriminate fresh or frozen-thawed swordfish cutlets (*Xiphias gladius* L.) (100% and 96.7%, respectively, of correct classification) (Fasolato et al., 2012).

3.4 Suitable Foodstuffs for Testing Using Ultraviolet and Visible Light Spectroscopy Analysis

Spectral analysis can supply results in real time and may be used to determine a wide range of parameters in foodstuffs in an environmentally friendly manner (Gonzalez-Caballero et al., 2010).

In analysis using spectral data and chemometric models, calibrations are performed using multivariate calibration methods. Accuracy of quantification models is evaluated by correlation and determination coefficients (r and r^2), root mean square errors of calibration, prediction or cross-validation (RMSEC, RMSECP, or RMSECV), standard errors of calibration, cross-validation or prediction (SEC, SECV or SEP), or residual prediction deviations (RPD).

In classification models, values for the percentage correct classification are commonly used (Lourenco et al., 2012; Cozzolino et al., 2011; Nicolaï et al., 2007). Moreover, PCA is normally performed prior to calibration as a data-reduction method, to detect patterns and distribution of samples within the dataset, and to detect outliers (Martelo-Vidal et al., 2013). It is important to state that PCA is not a modeling method and that evidence of separate clustering of, for example, meat of different species in a PCA scores plot does not constitute development of a predictive model.

In the following section, reports of food groups for which UV–VIS spectroscopy was applied, either alone or in combination with other spectroscopic techniques, are summarized.

3.4.1 Oils

One of the main applications of UV–VIS spectroscopy is its use to analyze vegetable oils. Olive oil is the main oil studied. Commercialization of olive oil has significantly increased in recent years due to its nutritional value ascribed to its content of polyunsaturated fatty acids (PUFAs) and antioxidants (Jacomelli et al., 2010; Casale et al., 2012; Fernandes et al., 2013). The major reported frauds affecting oils are failure to declare the presence of mixtures of different quality oils or different species of olives, adulterations with hydrogenated oils or other vegetable fats, and incorrect declaration of geographical origin.

Absorbance spectra (400–715 nm) of extra virgin olive oils from PDO *Riviera Ligure* (Italy) were successfully used to verify geographic origin (Casale et al., 2007). These authors reported 100% correct classification and 89.10% of correct prediction of models to determine the origin of extra virgin olive oils into PDO from *Riviera Ligure*. These authors claimed that UV–VIS spectral data alone or combined with data from an electronic nose were useful to confirm the geographical origin of virgin olive oils and consequently their authenticity with regard to this property.

UV–VIS spectral data alone and combined with NIR and MIR were used to verify PDO *Chianti Classico* olive oils from the Tuscany region of Italy; these authors reported classification models (SIMCA and unequal class models), which could discriminate olive oil from this Tuscany region from other Italian olive oils produced using the same olive varieties. One hundred percent correct classification was obtained with SIMCA models using UV–VIS–NIR–MIR and 97.5% using UV–VIS spectral data alone (Casale et al., 2012).

Moreover, UV–VIS spectral data were used to predict contents of oleic and linoleic acids and to classify Italian olive oils (Casale et al., 2012). Spectra were collected in absorbance mode pretreated using normalization and first-derivative calculation. Results showed that UV–VIS spectral data alone produced models to classify oils by geographical origin using SIMCA with a 97.5% correct classification rate. PLS models developed to predict concentrations of oleic and linoleic acids using UV–VIS spectra were not useful because, in the UV–VIS region, there are no characteristic absorptions by these fatty acids. Calibrations performed in UV–VIS–NIR–MIR spectral data provided RMSECV values from 0.107 to 0.801 and RMESP from 0.447 to 0.687 for oleic acid and RMSECV from 0.043 to 0.315 and RMSEP from 0.153 to 0.352 for linoleic acids.

A similar analysis was performed using UV–VIS and NIR spectroscopy and an electronic tongue and nose (Oliveri et al., 2011). Pretreatments in this case were not used in order to reduce the time of analysis. Models built for the PDO *Chianti Classico* oil using NIR and UV–VIS data showed good classification rates; in all cases, correct classification was higher than 95%, providing very satisfactory models to confirm the geographic origin of olive oils.

Moreover, a study performed to classify Spanish virgin olive oils with regard to PDO using UV–VIS spectral data as fingerprints combined with LDA and PLS-DA obtained 100% correct classifications (Pizarro et al., 2013).

On the other hand, UV spectral data coupled with partial least squares regression (PLSR) analysis was used to detect extra virgin olive oil and palm oil in blended vegetable edible oils (Jiang et al., 2015). Good results for prediction of contents of extra virgin olive oils ($r^2 = 0.981$ and RMSEP = 0.271) and adulterants (like palm oils) ($r^2 = 0.981$ and RMSEP 0.082) in blends of extra virgin olive oils plus sunflower oils and extra virgin olive oils ($r^2 = 1.000$ and RMSEP = 0.001) and also adulterants (like palm oils) ($r^2 = 1.000$ and RMSEP = 0.001) in blends of extra virgin olive oils plus soybean oils were obtained.

UV–VIS spectral data were used to determine carotenoids (lutein and β-carotenes) and chlorophylls (pheophytin-a and pheophytin-b) of extra virgin olive oils as representative oil pigments. Results showed that UV–VIS spectral data were analytically oriented to the chromophores, extracting quantitative information for the most important pigments in extra virgin olive oils. Models performed using UV–VIS spectral deconvolution provided values of r^2 around 0.96 and 0.85. Therefore these models could provide reliable concentration of the pigments assayed (Domenici et al., 2014).

The application of UV–VIS spectroscopy to determine acid value in edible oils (Zhang et al., 2015) has been reported. PLS and PCR models were developed with best values of $r^2 = 0.9893$ and RMSEC = 0.051 for PLS calibrations and $r^2 = 0.9911$ and RMSEP = 0.0459 for PLS predictions.

Combining VIS and NIR spectral data, it was possible to determine docosahexaenoic acid (DHA) and eicosapentaenoic acid (EPA) in algal oil using different data pretreatments (smoothing, SNV, MSC, first and second derivatives) and PLS models (Wu and He, 2014). Accuracy and predictive abilities of the established PLSR models provided values of $r^2 = 0.995$ and RMSEC = 0.476 for calibrations and $r^2 = 0.951$ and RMSECV = 1.451 for DHA predictions. Values of r^2 equal to 0.997 and RMSEC equal to 0.021 were obtained for EPA calibrations; r^2 was 0.921 and RMSECV was 0.108 for EPA predictions. These authors concluded that these spectral data were suitable for rapid analysis of EPA and DHA in algal oils and that these techniques could be used to rapidly measure polyunsaturated fatty acids, thus facilitating checks on the labeling of algal oil foods.

3.4.2 Spices and Tea

Tea is the most consumed beverage in the world (Lucio-Gutiérrez et al., 2012). The principal importance of tea is due to its health benefits, contributing to minimize blood sugar and pressure, promote digestion, provide amino acids and vitamins, regulate body temperature, and promote antioxidant activity associated with polyphenols (Marchese et al., 2014; Palacios-Morillo et al., 2013). Moreover, in China it is used as a remedy to treat diabetes mellitus (Cai et al., 2013). There are many varieties of tea with multiple patterns of phenolic compounds. Some varieties are processed, and they can differ substantially from each other.

UV–VIS spectroscopy, alone or combined with NIR and MIR spectroscopy, has been used to determine quality and to classify varieties of tea, aromatic herbs, and culinary spices. It has been used to quantify the content of antioxidant or other different components to determine authenticity.

UV–VIS combined with NIR spectroscopy was used to discriminate between five green tea varieties, using an unsupervised method to explore the dataset and a supervised method to discriminate (Wang et al., 2015). These authors used PCA as the unsupervised method and random forest (RF) as the supervised procedures. Good classification results using UV–VIS and NIR spectroscopy jointly were obtained, producing an overall correct classification rate of 96%.

UV–VIS absorbance spectral data combined with pattern recognition methods were applied to differentiate three tea varieties (black, green, and Pu'er). Classification methods used were SVM, ANNs, and LDA. Results of this research provided models combining PCA scores and a multilayer perceptron ANN to produce 100% correct classification. Moreover, LDA models provided sensitivity values of 93.2–100% and 96.7–100% for specificity (Palacios-Morillo et al., 2013).

Total catechins of green tea from Ethiopia and Sri Lanka were quantified and characterized using UV–VIS spectral data in absorbance mode. Beer's law and standard solutions were used to develop the models. Optical properties of catechins in the solvents such as water, methanol, ethanol, and acetonitrile were calculated. Limits of detection were in the range 3.1×10^{-2} to 1.6×10^{-1} gm/L and reproducibilities had RSD values lower than 2%. After method validation, values of $17.14 \pm 0.01\%$ of catechins in Ethiopian green tea leaves and $7.17 \pm 0.12\%$ of catechins in Sri Lanka tea leaves were obtained (Atomssa and Gholap, 2015).

Adulterated culinary spices were determined using UV–VIS spectroscopy in absorbance mode (Di Anibalet al., 2014). K-nearest neighbors (KNN) and PLS-DA were used as multivariate analysis methods to discriminate adulterated from nonadulterated culinary spices. The results provided by models supplied very good classifications, 89–100% for PLS-DA and 83–92% using KNN.

3.4.3 Mushrooms

Principal adulterations regarding mushrooms could be an incorrect declaration of species, incorrect declaration of geographical origin or process, no declaration of genetic modifications, adulterations by addition of water, or incorrect declarations of nutraceutical and functional properties.

The fungus *Wolfiporia extensa* is used in functional foods, nutraceutical and medicinal, and was analyzed to discriminate between different source geographical origins (Li et al., 2014). Wild *W. extensa* from three different growing locations of Yunnan (Chuxiong, Honghe, Pu'er; all from southwestern China) was analyzed. UV absorbance spectra without any pretreatment were used and subject to PLS-DA and HCA, obtaining good classification by growing place of mushroom (95% correct classification). The models fitted very well to their geographical origins based on low contents of polar constituents. All samples used were discriminated accurately by geographical origin. Therefore this technique is simple, low cost, and effective, and has significant advantages for discrimination purposes from other species of fungi.

Combined VIS and NIR reflectance spectra were applied to discriminate between different production origins of the black-brown mushroom *Auricularia auricular* (Liu and He, 2011). This variety of mushroom has a high content of carbohydrates, proteins, minerals, and polysaccharides with consequent claimed high benefits for health. Therefore the quality parameters are very important and there is a relationship with the geographical origin. The authors used back propagation artificial neural networks (BP-ANNs) and LV-SVM. Data preprocessing involved smoothing and second derivative followed by SNV. The results showed excellent accuracy with 98.30% correct recognition by the BP-ANN model and 96.70% by the LS-SVM model.

The same spectral regions and BP-ANNs were used to discriminate between three different varieties of fragrant mushrooms (Yang and He, 2008). In this case, the authors used absorbance spectra; pretreatment of data involved smoothing and MSC. Correct classification rates of up to 91% were obtained. The authors concluded that these methods can discriminate fragrance mushrooms with commercial importance from others with lower value or toxic contents.

Another application of spectral data is to determine fungus contamination on foodstuffs. VIS and NIR spectroscopies were used in reflectance mode to detect fungal infections on citrus fruit by detecting initial decay symptoms induced by the fungus (Lorente et al., 2015). The use of VIS and NIR spectral data jointly provided good results with 95.07% correct classification accuracy using PCA and MLR. The authors concluded that further research is needed to establish accurate models for detection of fungal contamination.

3.4.4 Meat

Quality parameters of meat are related to appearance, preservation methods, addition of adulterants, or different classifications according to geographical origin or species. Several studies have been performed using spectral data to determine meat quality parameters and consequently to determine authenticity. Some of these parameters have included Warner-Bratzler force, pH, sensory attributes, color, volatile basic nitrogen, fat, and microbial contaminations.

Recently, research about reflectance and hyperspectral imaging has shown advantages for meat spectral analysis. Some models to predict pH, color (L^*, a^*, and b^* parameters), intramuscular fat, and shear force on intact pork samples were obtained using VIS and NIR spectroscopy (Balage et al., 2015). These authors used reflectance spectra and PLSR models; preprocessing steps applied were MSC and first derivative. Predictive models for pH and color parameters had higher accuracy than other previously reported studies, but the authors concluded that further investigations are required to obtain robust models.

The potential use of VIS and NIR hyperspectral imaging to obtain classifications of fresh and frozen-thawed (one or twice) pork meat has been studied (Pu et al., 2015). Good probabilistic neural network (PNN) classification models using all spectral data were obtained, with correct classification rates of 100% and 97.7% being reported in classification and validation, respectively. However, hyperspectral imaging data are characterized by high dimensionality and colinearity so the authors selected specific wavelengths to improve these calibrations. Good classification models were obtained using six wavelengths only. The average classification accuracy of a PNN model using these optimum wavelengths combined with gray-level-gradient co-occurrence matrix (OW-GLGCM) was the highest (92.02%), followed by optimum wavelengths combined with gray-level co-occurrence matrix (OW-GLCM) (91.29%), optimum wavelengths combined with histogram statistics (OW-HS) (91.29%), and optimum wavelengths alone (OW) (86.36%). The authors concluded that the use of PNN models developed using both spectral and textural data was better than those obtained using single-spectra extraction, improving the correct classification rate of fresh and frozen-thawed pork meat.

VIS and NIR hyperspectral imaging spectra were used to detect adulteration of mince beef meat with horse meat using PLS regression (Kamruzzaman et al., 2015). Results were very good to predict adulteration, providing $r^2 = 0.990$ and SEC = 1.14% for calibration; $r^2 = 0.990$ and SECV = 1.56% for cross-validation; and $r^2 = 0.980$ and SEP = 2.23% for prediction models using all spectral data without pretreatment. When only four specific wavelengths were used, $r^2 = 0.980$ and SEP = 2.20% was obtained.

Other authors used UV–VIS, NIR, and MIR spectroscopy separately and in combination to detect bovine meat adulterations with turkey meat (Alamprese et al., 2013). Spectra were collected in diffuse reflectance mode, and both SNV and first derivative were used as spectral pretreatments. Results provided by these authors stated that LDA of UV–VIS spectra produced models with only low percentages of average correct classification (78.6%) but 88.3% and 84.8% of average correct classifications using NIR and MIR spectral ranges, respectively. The authors determined that better models were obtained using NIR and MIR spectra when they evaluated all spectral regions jointly (UV–VIS–NIR–MIR).

3.4.5 *Fish and Seafood*

Fish is one of the main sources of nutrients with positive effects on human health but it is a product with a short shelf life. New techniques of preservation and storage have been developed in recent years that allow for a longer shelf life of fish products. Producers and consumers have a greater interest in quality parameters, the positive nutritional effects of fish products, their textural properties, and safety.

For these reasons, it is necessary to look for new techniques to detect adulterations and to determine chemical composition and contaminants to ensure quality and authenticity of fish products.

The main authenticity issues relating to fish and seafood consist of incorrect claims regarding the origin of fish, incorrect labeling with regard to fish species, and incorrect labeling for frozen and fresh seafood. There are few studies related to UV–VIS spectral data in this application field but several do use the VIS spectral range in combination with NIR and MIR ranges.

The use of VIS and NIR hyperspectral imaging in reflectance mode to rapidly discriminate fresh from cooled and frozen-thawed fillets of carp was studied (Cheng et al., 2015). These authors used SIMCA, PLS-DA, LS-SVM, and PNN models to perform different classifications; for data pretreatments, they used MSC, SNV, first and second derivatives. Results of these studies showed PNN to produce the best classification model using first derivative pretreatment with 94.3% correct classification. The authors concluded, however, that all models performed were useful to discriminate fresh from cooled or frozen-thawed fish.

Hyperspectral imaging was also used to determine the freshness of rainbow trout using different data pretreatments and PLS-DA (Khojastehnazhand et al., 2014). Results showed that VIS and NIR hyperspectral imaging was useful when PLS-DA was applied coupled with smoothing, second derivative and MSC or SNV, providing 100% correct classification of fillets of different freshness levels. VIS−NIR hyperspectral imaging was used to determine freshness of salmon stored under different packing atmospheres, producing 88.30% correct classification when authors used SNV as a pretreatment of spectral data (Sone et al., 2012).

The use of VIS and NIR spectroscopy, hyperspectral imaging, and computer vision on fish and fish products was reviewed recently (He et al., 2015). It was concluded that these spectral imaging techniques provide a fast and nondestructive technique with which to classify fish and fish products as well as determine their quality.

In addition, VIS and NIR spectral data were used to detect and quantify adulterations in crabmeat (Gayo and Hale, 2007). Results of this research provided models with a high coefficient of determination (0.984) and low standard errors (5.64) using all spectral data. Models were improved when only one part of the spectrum was used (400−1700 nm), providing values of 0.987 and 5.17 for determination coefficient and standard error, respectively. Therefore, results demonstrated that VIS combined with NIR spectra can be used to discriminate and to quantify species of adulterated crabmeat.

3.4.6 Rice

Rice is one of the most produced and consumed cereals worldwide. It has advantages for human health related to its high-fiber content, vitamins, and other bioactive molecules such as phenolic compounds (Bordiga et al., 2014; Liu et al., 2014). UV−VIS spectral data is a powerful tool to determine composition or classify rice according to geographical origin. Hyperspectral imaging was also reported to be effective in rice authentication studies. Likely frauds could be the use of different rice variety to that declared on label, incorrect geographical origin claims, or substitutions of good-quality grains by poor.

VIS and NIR spectral data were used to classify rice wines according to their ages using BP neural networks in transmittance mode (Liu et al., 2008). In this case, authors used SNV and smoothing to reduce noise in the data and PLS to select important variables. Rice wines were 1, 3, or 5 years old. The discrimination rate was 96.67%, showing that VIS and NIR spectral data processed by BP-ANN are suitable to discriminate rice wines from different vintages and thereby prevent fraud arising from mislabeling of rice wine age. Moreover, Chinese rice wines from the "Pagoda" brand "Shaoxing" (vintage 2000–2005) were classified by vintage year using VIS and NIR spectral data. Bottles of wine rice were scanned in transmission mode. Discriminant analysis of data using raw spectral data provided percentages of correct classification from 92.9% for 2000 and 2001 vintage to 100% for 2002, 2003, 2004, and 2005 vintages (Yu et al., 2007).

3.4.7 Juices

Frauds involving fruit juice include adulteration with water, sugars, acids, or addition of other juices or of lower quality.

With authenticity objectives, UV–VIS spectral data were used in absorbance mode to obtain a rapid and cheaper method to determine possible frauds in juices (Boggia et al., 2013). PCA results provided useful information with two principal components accounting for 96.8% of total variance in this study and producing a good separation of different juices. The authors concluded that rapid and cheap analysis using UV–VIS spectral data is useful as a screening technique to detect adulterations on juices.

Kiwi and grapefruit are tasty, rich in polyphenols, and vitamins. UV–VIS spectroscopy was used to classify and obtain spectral fingerprints of different varieties of these fruits (Sarbu et al., 2012). In this case, the authors prepared different extracts of kiwi and pomelo, which were mixed with methanol in proportions of 1:10. Spectral data were measured in absorbance mode. Normalized and first-derivative steps were used as pretreatments of data. Major absorptions of both fruit types appeared in the UV spectral range. These authors combined PCA and LDA to develop predictive models, and their results showed that kiwi and pomelo were correctly classified—100%. They concluded that the models can be used to classify kiwi and grapefruit.

3.4.8 Wine and Vine

Wine is extensively consumed around the world. It has a high commercial value. The geographical origin and composition of wine are very important with regard to its quality. The constantly increasing demands by markets and the internationalization of trade mean that this industry has to increase both productivity and quality levels. Adulterations and frauds have been reported in wine such as incorrect labeling of grape species, adding water or other liquids (eg, juices, volatile compounds, oils), presence of contaminants arising from manipulation or poor practices, incorrect declarations of alcohol contents, inappropriate sugar additions to increase alcoholic grade, and incorrect declaration of geographical origin (Martelo-Vidal et al., 2013).

European rules were developed to ensure correct labeling of wine geographic origin monitoring cultivation, varieties used, process conditions, and localization of production. There are a number of techniques that can determine these parameters, but they are very expensive and time-consuming. For this reason, new techniques to detect adulterations and ensure authenticity using rapid and low-cost methods were investigated. The main spectral research on wines and grapes was performed using NIR and MIR spectroscopy in combination with chemometric tools (Cozzolino et al., 2008;

Bellincontro et al., 2011; Ferrer-Gallego et al., 2013). As mentioned earlier, UV−VIS spectral data sometimes combined with those spectra, comply with the characteristics and advantages mentioned given that, in the UV−VIS spectral zone, polyphenols and benzoic (235−305 nm), hydroxycinnamic compounds (227−245 nm and 310−332 nm and 350−390 nm), anthocyans (267−275 nm), flavonols (250−270 nm) and other wine compounds absorb (Azcarate et al., 2013a; Uríčková and Sádecká, 2015). Therefore authenticity of wines could be confirmed by measuring differences in composition (polyphenols, organic acid, tannins, or colorant composition) or by determining grape maturation.

The discrimination of wines from different zones is an issue of authenticity, considering that wines from a PDO could be adulterated using external grapes (eg, differences based on quality composition of grapes, topography, or special production and cultural activities). UV−VIS spectral data combined with chemometric tools were used to classify wines produced with *Sauvignon blanc* grapes from Argentina (Azcarate et al., 2013b) using LDA and PLS-DA. *Sauvignon blanc* wine samples from three different places in Argentina (Mendoza, San Juan, and Rio Negro) were analyzed. Results obtained with both classification models provided 100% correct classification of wines. Although the models were good, these authors concluded that some factors could limit method accuracy such as the number of samples analyzed or similarity of wines produced in areas which were very close together. They used the same techniques to classify wines produced from the *torrontés* grapes from Mendoza, San Juan, and Rio Negro zones of Argentina (Azcarate et al., 2013a). In this case, they used more wine samples and results provided 100% correct classification. They concluded that these models can be used to classify wines elaborated with *torrontés* grapes from different provinces of Argentina.

UV−VIS spectral data were used to quantify two types of tannins in South African red wines with PLS models (Aleixandre-Tudo et al., 2015). Models of calibration provided 0.890 of correlation coefficient and RMSEP of 0.160 for methylcellulose-precipitable tannins, a correlation coefficient of 0.930 and RMSEP of 0.080 for bovine serum albumin tannins. Similar analysis was performed on Australian wines using MLR and UV spectra, and results were similar with correlation coefficient of 0.920 and SECV of 0.200 g/L for methylcellulose-precipitable tannins (Dambergs et al., 2012). These results suggest that UV and VIS spectral data are suitable to detect tannins on wines, and thus could be used to determine the authenticity of wines. As commented previously, determining the geographical production zones is important to ensure authenticity of wine.

UV−VIS spectral data collected in transmittance mode were used to classify Chilean red wines from different zones of the Casablanca valley (Saavedra et al., 2011). Chemometric tools used by authors were LDA, PLS-DA, and SIMCA with data centered and scaled. Samples showed characteristic bands around 475−545 nm and exhibited differences between samples with different anthocyanin contents. Results provided by the authors showed 100% correct classification of wines using LDA and SIMCA.

UV−VIS spectral data were also used to classify Spanish wines (Acevedo et al., 2007). The authors performed several experiments with all spectra selected to compare different methods of classification. Moreover, they performed other classifications using only a set of selected wavelengths. On first experiments with all spectra, the authors reported good classification results for SVM with 96.53% and 97.89% average correct classification in the case of white and red wines from different PDO regions. Some PDOs were correctly classified with SVM obtaining 100% correct classification (Penedés and Rioja white wines and La Mancha, Penedés, Rioja, and Toro red wines).

UV–VIS spectra were also used to classify wines from Spanish PDO Castilla la Mancha using as criteria zones of PDO, aging process, and grape variety. Classification models were obtained using SIMCA (Urbano et al., 2006) with the authors reporting 90% average correct classification of white wines by zones of PDO and 80% average correct classification of red wines by zones of PDO. Classification of wines according to grape variety and aging was greater than 75% of average correct classification. Therefore, they concluded that SIMCA combined with UV and VIS spectral zones were useful for screening wines from Castilla la Mancha PDO, obtaining results in less than 10 min. UV spectral data were useful to discriminate wines from the same PDO. In the range of 300–400 nm, esters from hydroxycynamic compounds absorbed. When both spectral ranges (UV and VIS) were used jointly, they were reported to provide information about classification according to aging process. Therefore, vegetable secondary metabolism results in phenolic compositions in wines that may be useful to discriminate them according to vintage. Differences in this secondary metabolism are due to grape varieties, topography of soils, grape culture activities, and wine production conditions.

VIS and NIR hyperspectral imaging have been studied to discriminate between grape varieties from Australia (Cabernet Sauvignon, Merlot, Shiraz, and Semillon) (Lacar et al., 2001). Both raw and derivative spectral data were analyzed using an ANOVA one-way test. F-tests were used to compare mean of varieties and each block assayed to test for equal reflectance between vine varieties. The Tukey post hoc test was used to perform multiple pairwise mean comparisons to further determine which means differed from another. Spectral data in the ranges 720–740, 550, and 600 nm showed differences due to different varieties of grape. Cabernet Sauvignon and Semillon showed the most differences in the VIS region. The authors concluded that chlorophyll content, structure of leaf, and water content were responsible for significant differences. Results showed that Cabernet Sauvignon was the most different from 512 to 580 nm. They concluded that wavelengths with the most discrimination power were 512, 580, 611, 649, 690, and 763 nm.

3.4.9 Beer

Beer is probably the oldest beverage. Brewing influences beer composition and fermentation of components. They are generally starches from cereals such as barley, wheat, maize, or rice (Cetó et al., 2013). Thus monitoring parameters on process and final product are very important to guarantee quality, safety, consumer confidence, and authenticity. Color, pH, alcoholic content, yeast used, hop variety, organoleptic characteristics, or country of production are important characteristics of quality and authenticity to be determined on beer.

Absorptions of beer on bands 250–300 nm and 300–350 nm were relating to iso and alpha acids, vitamins of group B, and phenolic compounds (aromatic groups and multiple bonds conjugated). Absorptions of beer in the VIS zone relate to yellow-green pigments such as riboflavin and flavonols. Moreover, 400–430 nm and 490–560 nm absorptions correspond to red and brown colors, principally in ale beers (Tan et al., 2015; Vera et al., 2011; Biancolillo et al., 2014).

The main adulterations of beers could be inappropriate additions of sugars, incorrect declarations of origin, no declarations of use of genetically modified cereals, and incorrect declarations of alcoholic strength.

Diffuse light absorption spectroscopy in VIS and NIR spectral ranges were used to predict alcoholic content of golden ale, lager, and weiss beers from several countries (Mignani et al., 2012a, 2013). Normalized and first-derivative spectral data and LDA (with VIS) and PLS (with NIR) models were developed (Mignani et al., 2012a). Misclassification rates for LDA models were about 11% in calibration and 13% in cross-validation. The authors concluded that this spectral method is useful to determine alcohol contents using NIR spectra and classification using VIS data, but neither is useful to discriminate Belgian beers from others (Mignani et al., 2013).

On the other hand, other authors used similar spectral ranges to monitor quality parameters in craft beers (Giovenzana et al., 2014). They used a portable device measuring from 400 to 980 nm (VIS and NIR spectra) to determine pH and SSC. The quantitative analysis was performed to classify beers according to optical properties. They used PLS models after smoothing and second-derivative spectral pretreatments were applied. Changes in spectra of different beers in the 500–600 nm range were observed. The best model quantified SSC and pH of one type of craft beer (Lambrate type) with a determination coefficient of 0.890 and 0.14 of RMSECV for SSC and determination coefficient of 0.890 and 0.1 of RMSECV, respectively.

Other authors used only UV–VIS spectral data to classify beers. Sometimes companies make products of the same brand in different places, thus geographical origin of products could affect the final product. Classification of beers according to brand, production location, and type is useful to confirm authenticity and quality of beers.

UV–VIS spectral data combined with MS e-nose and an MIR optical tongue was used to classify selected beer brands (Vera et al., 2011; Tan et al., 2015; Biancolillo et al., 2014). Results exhibited correct classification rates ranging from 16.7% to 100% when only UV–VIS spectral data were used. But in this case, classification rates improved when data were analyzed jointly, obtaining correct classification rates from 66.70% to 100%.

UV–VIS spectroscopy was used to discriminate Chinese beer of different brands (Tan et al., 2015). On spectral inspections, these authors observed a strong band at 250–300 nm and a weak band at 300–350 nm. These absorptions were related to polyphenolic acids and vitamin B; LDA models produced correct classification rates of 78.5% to 86.7%.

Different spectral zones (NIR, MIR, VIS, and UV) were used separately to characterize Italian beers (Biancolillo et al., 2014). Results showed that UV and VIS zones were the best for classification. PLS-DA models provided 77.8% correct classification while SIMCA analysis provided 92.9%.

The UV zone alone was used to classify Trappist and non-Trappist beers (Weeranantanaphan and Downey, 2010). PLS-DA provided 100% classification of Rochefort type of Trappist samples and 94.4% classification of non-Rochefort types. Discrimination of Trappist and non-Trappist beers was achieved with 95.7% and 95.8% correct classification rates, respectively, after applying SNV to spectra. With SIMCA models, correct classification rates for Rochefort and non-Rochefort beers were 75% and 94.4%, respectively.

3.4.10 Miscellaneous

UV−VIS spectra have also been used to address authenticity issues in a variety of different foodstuffs as follows: (1) to classify species of coffee (Souto et al., 2010; Dias et al., 2013; Belay et al., 2008); (2) to identify adulterated tequilas (Contreras et al., 2010); (3) to classify Scotch whisky by origin (Mignani et al., 2012b); and (4) to obtain quality models of thyme using UV spectral data (Gad et al., 2013b).

3.5 Case Study: Wine Authentication

In this case study, rapid methods based on UV−VIS−NIR spectroscopy were developed for analysis of Galician wines (Northwest Spain). UV−VIS−NIR spectroscopy in wine was applied to analyze grapes and wine composition, obtaining quality information to verify the authenticity and origin of white and red wines.

Authenticity was established by UV−VIS−NIR spectra as fingerprints for the PDO studied (Rías Baixas, Ribeiro, Monterrei, Ribeira Sacra, and Valdeorras) for white and red wines (vintages 2009, 2010, and 2011). Moreover, a rapid analysis of the composition for ethanol, glucose, glycerol, organic acids, and phenolic compounds of wines based on UV−VIS−NIR spectra was also obtained.

It was also possible to identify the subzone within a PDO and the wine composition regarding grape varieties used in its production (Martelo-Vidal and Vázquez, 2014a,b,c,d,e, 2015; Martelo-Vidal et al., 2013).

In the just-mentioned studies, all samples were measured in transmittance mode from 190 to 2500 nm at 2 nm intervals using a quartz cell with a 1 mm path length. Different pretreatments were evaluated to minimize, reduce, and remove undesirable noise. Fig. 3.3 shows UV−VIS spectra of white and red wines from the Galician PDO.

In raw spectral data (Fig. 3.3A), there are several differences between red and white wines; these are more pronounced in the second-derivative spectra (Fig. 3.3B). These spectral differences were observed from 202 to 230 nm in the UV, related principally

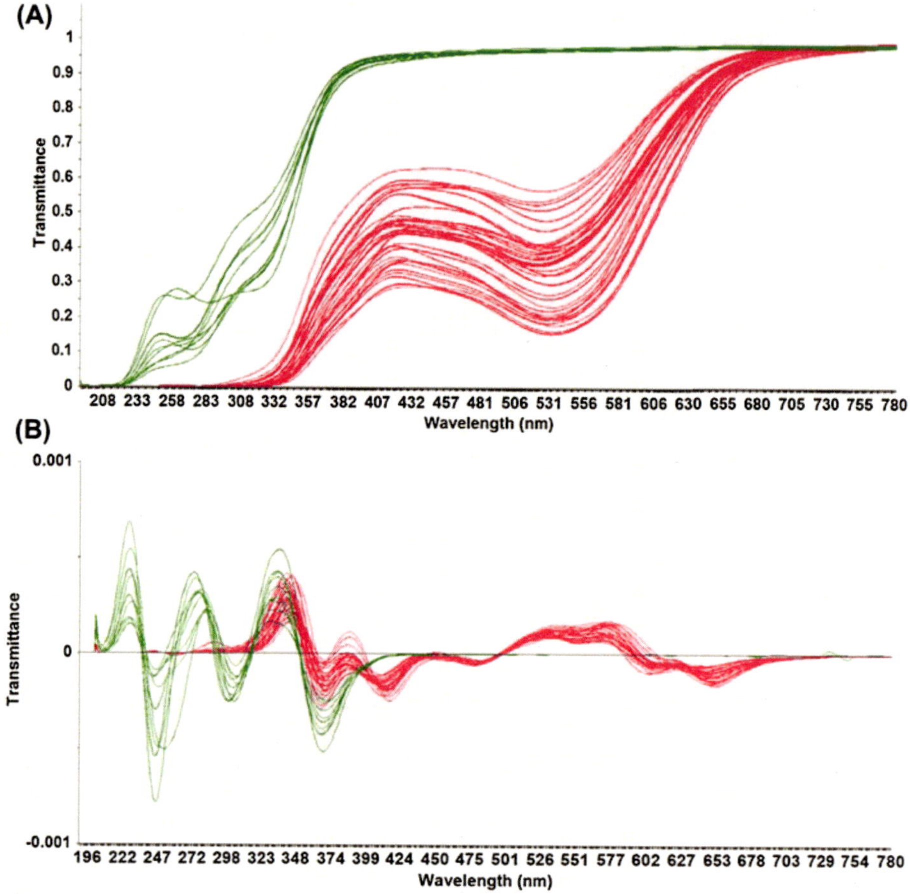

Figure 3.3 Spectral data of red (*pink color*) and white (*green color*) Galician wines, (A) raw spectra and (B) second-derivative spectra.

to carboxyl groups of organic acids, and 230–350 nm and 310–332 nm, which are principal absorptions of benzene ring compounds such as hydroxycinnamic acids and other phenolic compounds.

There were absorptions of benzoic acids around 230–300 nm. Absorptions at wavelengths from 250 to 270 nm are related to flavonols; catechin absorptions were around 280 nm. Principal absorptions of red wines were in the VIS spectral range. Absorptions around 420 nm were related to anthocyanins and tannins (yellow components), and absorptions around 500 and 525 nm were related to free anthocyanins and combinations with tannins (red components). Absorptions around 610–650 nm were related to free anthocyanins or combinations of tannins and anthocyanins (principally blue colors in young red wines) (Ribéreau-Gayon et al., 2000; Uríčková and Sádecká, 2015).

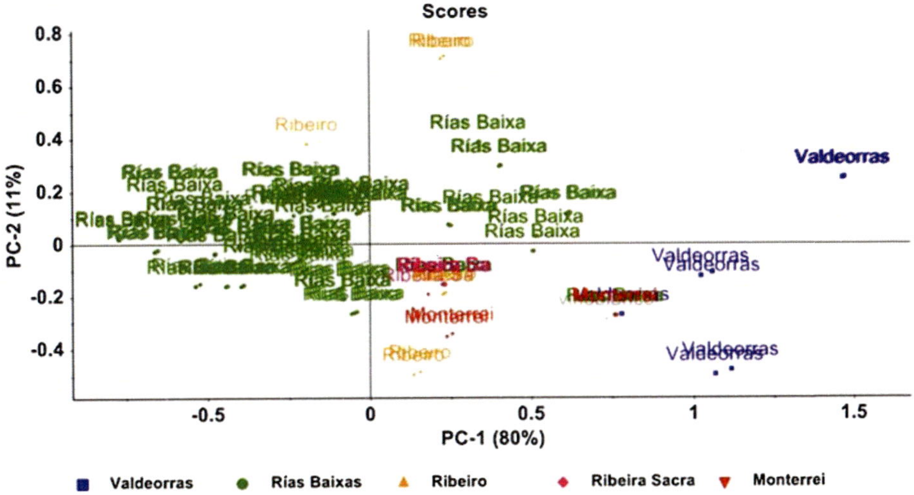

Figure 3.4 PCA score plot of raw data of Galician white wines.

PCA analysis was performed to detect patterns and outliers among samples. For example, a PCA score plot explaining 91% of total variance explained by PCs 1 and 2 can be seen in Fig. 3.4.

There is a clear trend to separation of samples by PDO. The principal cause of this separation could be the grape variety or climatological conditions. Rías Baixas PDO are localized in a coastal climate and grapes used in wines are mainly the *albariño* grape variety. Valdeorras wines were localized in a continental climate and grapes principally used are of the *godello* variety. On the other hand, Ribeiro, Monterrei, and Ribeira Sacra are localized in continental climate. They are shown slightly overlapped in Fig. 3.4.

Results of ANN, LDA, SIMCA, and SVM models using UV–VIS–NIR spectroscopy (using all spectra and fragments of them) to classify monovarietal Galician white wines showed a good fit. In these cases, white wines were from PDO Rías Baixas, Ribeira Sacra, Monterrei, Valdeorras, and Ribeiro. Furthermore, the feasibility of classifying wines by grape variety (albariño, treixadura, palomino, and godello varieties) and to classify wines from subzones of PDO Rías Baixas were also studied.

Results of the models showed that most of the monovarietal white wines were correctly classified in the corresponding PDO using ANN, LDA, SVM, and SIMCA using different regions of the combined UV–VIS–NIR spectrum. Classifications using ANN show that wines from PDO Valdeorras, Ribeira Sacra, and Monterrei were the best classified, obtaining 100% correct classification. On the other hand, the worst-classified white wines were PDO Rías Baixas with only 30% correct classification.

The results for white wines using ANN according to the subzones of PDO Rías Baixas provided a correct classification of 100% for wines from subzones Rosal and Ribeira do Ulla, while wines from Condado were classified correctly at a level of

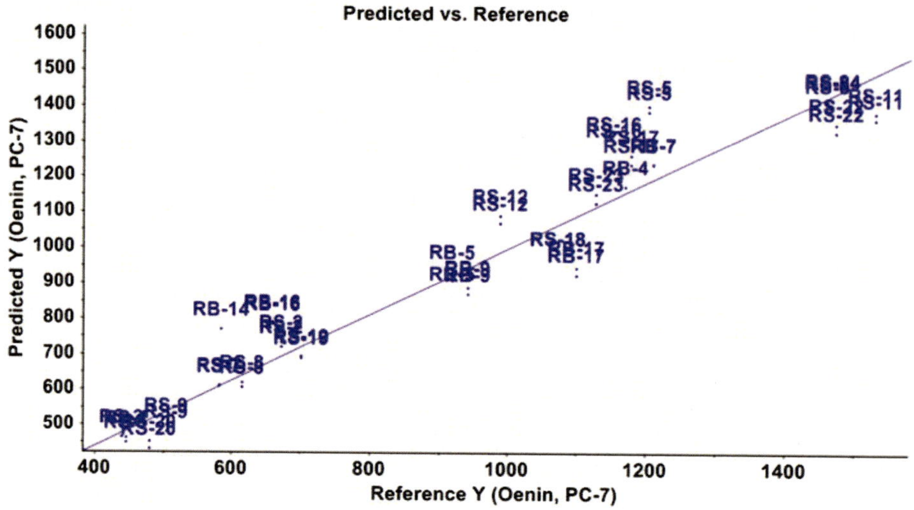

Figure 3.5 Prediction and real values of oenin (mg/L) in red wines.

93.33% and a corresponding value of 76.67% for Salnés wines (Martelo-Vidal and Vázquez, 2014e).

Classifications performed with LDA provided 86.0% correct classifications in UV–VIS–NIR zone, followed by 81.7% in VIS-NIR and 80.6% in VIS-only spectral regions. The model using SIMCA provided 100% correct classification for the wines of subzone Condado using the whole spectrum, NIR, and VIS-NIR regions. Furthermore, the rate of correct classification was 100% for subzone Rosal in UV region and 100% for subzones Ribeiras de Ulla and Salnés in UV–VIS region (Martelo-Vidal et al., 2013). Classifications of white wines according to grape variety provided a 100% correct classification using ANN (Martelo-Vidal and Vázquez, 2014d).

Polyphenolic profiles can be used for authentication of PDO wines. Therefore quantification of polyphenolic profiles in red wines using UV–VIS–NIR spectral data was performed using different sets of data (all red wines of study, only wines from PDO Rías Baixas, only wines from PDO Ribeira Sacra, and only wines made from grapes of mencía variety) using PCR and PLS models. With PCR, good prediction models for phenolic composition for all wines studied were not obtained. Good predictions were only obtained for *trans*-resveratrol and quercetin for Rías Baixas red wines and for quercetin, oenin, and syringic acid for Ribeira Sacra red wines. Results were improved using PLS calibrations. For all wines studied together, calibration models provided good models for oenin and catechin. Polyphenolic composition of Rías Baixas red wines was well predicted with all models. For Ribeira Sacra red wines, good models were obtained to predict quercetin, epicatechin, oenin, and syringic acid.

For wines of the Mencía variety, the best models were obtained for prediction of catechin, malvin, oenin, and syringic acid (Martelo-Vidal and Vázquez, 2014b). For example, Fig. 3.5 shows the relationship of predicted and real values obtained for oenin phenolic compound. Good agreement for all wines studied was obtained.

Classification of Galician red wines from PDO Rías Baixas and Ribeira Sacra using UV–VIS–NIR spectral data and different spectral regions provided good classification models. Classification with LDA provided 100% correct classification with different combinations of pretreatments and with data not pretreated (Martelo-Vidal and Vázquez, 2014a).

Results obtained from these case studies carried out with different varietal white wines from PDO Rías Baixas, Ribeira Sacra, Valdeorras, Monterrei, and Ribeiro and with red wines from PDO Rías Baixas and Ribeira Sacra showed the feasibility of using UV–VIS spectral data, alone or combined with NIR, and with classification and quantification chemometric tools as a rapid technique for wine analysis and wine authentication.

References

Acevedo, F.J., Jiménez, J., Maldonado, S., Domínguez, E., Narváez, A., 2007. Classification of wines produced in specific regions by UV-visible spectroscopy combined with support vector machines. Journal of Agricultural and Food Chemistry 55 (17), 6842–6849.

Alamprese, C., Casale, M., Sinelli, N., Lanteri, S., Casiraghi, E., 2013. Detection of minced beef adulteration with turkey meat by UV-vis, NIR and MIR spectroscopy. LWT – Food Science and Technology 53 (1), 225–232.

Aleixandre-Tudo, J.L., Nieuwoudt, H., Aleixandre, J.L., Du Toit, W.J., 2015. Robust ultraviolet–visible (UV–Vis) partial least-squares (PLS) models for tannin quantification in red wine. Journal of Agricultural and Food Chemistry 63 (4), 1088–1098.

Aparicio, R., Morales, M.T., Aparicio-Ruiz, R., Tena, N., Garcia-Gonzalez, D.L., 2013. Authenticity of olive oil: mapping and comparing official methods and promising alternatives. Food Research International 54 (2), 2025–2038.

Aroca-Santos, R., Cancilla, J.C., Matute, G., Torrecilla, J.S., 2015. Identifying and quantifying adulterants in extra virgin olive oil of the picual varietal by absorption spectroscopy and nonlinear modeling. Journal of Agricultural and Food Chemistry 63 (23), 5646–5652.

Arvanitoyannis, I.S., 2008. "Trends in Food Authentication", Modern Techniques for Food Authentication. Elsevier Science Publication, Amsterdam, pp. 617–643.

Atomssa, T., Gholap, A., 2015. Characterization and determination of catechins in green tea leaves using UV-visible spectrometer. Journal of Engineering and Technology Research 7 (1), 22–31.

Azcarate, S.M., Cantarelli, M.A., Marchevsky, E.J., Camiña, J.M., 2013a. Evaluation of geographic origin of Torrontés wines by chemometrics. Journal of Food Research 2 (5), 48.

Azcarate, S.M., Cantarelli, M.Á., Pellerano, R.G., Marchevsky, E.J., Camiña, J.M., 2013b. Classification of Argentinean Sauvignon blanc wines by UV spectroscopy and chemometric methods. Journal of Food Science 78 (3), C432–C436.

Balage, J.M., da Luz e Silva, S., Gomide, C.A., Bonin, M.d.N., Figueira, A.C., 2015. Predicting pork quality using Vis/NIR spectroscopy. Meat Science 108, 37–43.

Belay, A., Ture, K., Redi, M., Asfaw, A., 2008. Measurement of caffeine in coffee beans with UV/vis spectrometer. Food Chemistry 108 (1), 310–315.

Bellincontro, A., Cozzolino, D., Mencarelli, F., 2011. Application of NIR-AOTF spectroscopy to monitor aleatico grape dehydration for passito wine production. American Journal of Enology and Viticulture 62 (2), 256–260.

Biancolillo, A., Bucci, R., Magrì, A.L., Magrì, A.D., Marini, F., 2014. Data-fusion for multiplatform characterization of an italian craft beer aimed at its authentication. Analytica Chimica Acta 820, 23–31.

Blanco, M., Alcalá, M., 2009. Multivariate calibration for quantitative analysis. In: Sun, D. (Ed.), Near Infrared Spectroscopy for Food Quality Analysis and Control, first ed. Academy Press – Elsevier, Inc., USA, pp. 51–82.

Blanco, M., Maspoch, S., 2007. Calibración multivariable. In: Blanco, M., Cerdá, V. (Eds.), Temas avanzados de quimiometría: Advanced Topics in Chemometrics. Edicions UIB, pp. 233–280.

Boggia, R., Casolino, M.C., Hysenaj, V., Oliveri, P., Zunin, P., 2013. A screening method based on UV–Visible spectroscopy and multivariate analysis to assess addition of filler juices and water to pomegranate juices. Food Chemistry 140 (4), 735–741.

Bordiga, M., Gomez-Alonso, S., Locatelli, M., Travaglia, F., Coïsson, J.D., Hermosin-Gutierrez, I., Arlorio, M., 2014. Phenolics characterization and antioxidant activity of six different pigmented *Oryza sativa* L. cultivars grown in Piedmont (Italy). Food Research International 65 (Part B), 282–290.

Buglass, A.J., 2011. Handbook of Alcoholic Beverages: Technical, Analytical and Nutritional Aspects. John Wiley and Sons.

Cai, W., Xie, L., Chen, Y., Zhang, H., 2013. Purification, characterization and anticoagulant activity of the polysaccharides from green tea. Carbohydrate Polymers 92 (2), 1086–1090.

Casale, M., Armanino, C., Casolino, C., Forina, M., 2007. Combining information from headspace mass spectrometry and visible spectroscopy in the classification of the Ligurian olive oils. Analytica Chimica Acta 589 (1), 89–95.

Casale, M., Oliveri, P., Armanino, C., Lanteri, S., Forina, M., 2010. NIR and UV-vis spectroscopy, artificial nose and tongue: comparison of four fingerprinting techniques for the characterisation of Italian red wines. Analytica Chimica Acta 668 (2), 143–148.

Casale, M., Oliveri, P., Casolino, C., Sinelli, N., Zunin, P., Armanino, C., Forina, M., Lanteri, S., 2012. Characterisation of PDO olive oil Chianti Classico by non-selective (UV-visible, NIR and MIR spectroscopy) and selective (fatty acid composition) analytical techniques. Analytica Chimica Acta 712, 56–63.

Cetó, X., Gutiérrez-Capitán, M., Calvo, D., Del Valle, M., 2013. Beer classification by means of a potentiometric electronic tongue. Food Chemistry 141 (3), 2533–2540.

Cheng, J., Sun, D., Zeng, X., Pu, H., 2014. Non-destructive and rapid determination of TVB-N content for freshness evaluation of grass carp (*Ctenopharyngodon idella*) by hyperspectral imaging. Innovative Food Science and Emerging Technologies 21, 179–187.

Cheng, J., Sun, D., Pu, H., Chen, X., Liu, Y., Zhang, H., Li, J., 2015. Integration of classifiers analysis and hyperspectral imaging for rapid discrimination of fresh from cold-stored and frozen-thawed fish fillets. Journal of Food Engineering 161, 33–39.

Contreras, U., Barbosa-García, O., Pichardo-Molina, J.L., Ramos-Ortíz, G., Maldonado, J.L., Meneses-Nava, M.A., Ornelas-Soto, N.E., López-de-Alba, P.L., 2010. Screening method for identification of adulterate and fake tequilas by using UV–VIS spectroscopy and chemometrics. Food Research International 43 (10), 2356–2362.

Cozzolino, D., Cynkar, W.U., Dambergs, R.G., Mercurio, M.D., Smith, P.A., 2008. Measurement of condensed tannins and dry matter in red grape homogenates using near infrared spectroscopy and partial least squares. Journal of Agricultural and Food Chemistry 56 (17), 7631–7636.

Cozzolino, D., Cynkar, W.U., Shah, N., Smith, P., 2011. Multivariate data analysis applied to spectroscopy: potential application to juice and fruit quality. Food Research International 44 (7), 1888–1896.

Cozzolino, D., 2014. An overview of the use of infrared spectroscopy and chemometrics in authenticity and traceability of cereals. Food Research International 60, 262–265.

Cullum, B.M., Vo-Dinh, T., 2005. Sample collection and preparation of liquid and solids. In: Handbook of Spectroscopy. Wiley-VCH Verlag GmbH and Co. KGaA, pp. 17–35.

Da Costa Filho, P.A., 2014. Developing a rapid and sensitive method for determination of trans-fatty acids in edible oils using middle-infrared spectroscopy. Food Chemistry 158, 1–7.

Dai, Q., Sun, D., Cheng, J., Pu, H., Zeng, X., Xiong, Z., 2014. Recent advances in de-noising methods and their applications in hyperspectral image processing for the food industry. Comprehensive Reviews in Food Science and Food Safety 13 (6), 1207–1218.

Dambergs, R.G., Mercurio, M.D., Kassara, S., Cozzolino, D., Smith, P.A., 2012. Rapid measurement of methyl cellulose precipitable tannins using ultraviolet spectroscopy with chemometrics: application to red wine and inter-laboratory calibration transfer. Applied Spectroscopy 66 (6), 656–664.

Di Anibal, C., Susana Rodriguez, M., Albertengo, L., 2014. UV-visible spectroscopy and multivariate classification as a screening tool to identify adulteration of culinary spices with Sudan I and blends of Sudan I plus IV dyes. Food Analytical Methods 7 (5), 1090–1096.

Dias, R.C.E., Alves, S.T., Benassi, M.D.T., 2013. Spectrophotometric method for quantification of kahweol in coffee. Journal of Food Composition and Analysis 31 (1), 137–143.

Diniz, P.H.G.D., Barbosa, M.F., de Melo Milanez, K.D.T., Pistonesi, M.F., de Araújo, M.C.U., 2016. Using UV–Vis spectroscopy for simultaneous geographical and varietal classification of tea infusions simulating a home-made tea cup. Food Chemistry 192, 374–379.

Domenici, V., Ancora, D., Cifelli, M., Serani, A., Veracini, C.A., Zandomeneghi, M., 2014. Extraction of pigment information from near-UV vis absorption spectra of extra virgin olive oils. Journal of Agricultural and Food Chemistry 62 (38), 9317–9325.

Dufour, E., 2009. Principles of infrared spectroscopy. In: Sun, D. (Ed.), Near Infrared Spectroscopy for Food Quality Analysis and Control, first ed. Academy Press – Elsevier, Inc., USA, pp. 1–27.

ElMasry, G., Sun, D., 2010. Principles of hyperspectral imaging technology. Hyperspectral Imaging for Food Quality Analysis and Control 3–43.

ElMasry, G., Sun, D., Allen, P., 2012. Near-infrared hyperspectral imaging for predicting colour, pH and tenderness of fresh beef. Journal of Food Engineering 110 (1), 127–140.

Fasolato, L., Balzan, S., Riovanto, R., Berzaghi, P., Mirisola, M., Ferlito, J.C., Serva, L., Benozzo, F., Passera, R., Tepedino, V., Novelli, E., 2012. Comparison of visible and near-infrared reflectance spectroscopy to authenticate fresh and frozen-thawed swordfish (*Xiphias gladius* L). Journal of Aquatic Food Product Technology 21 (5), 493–507.

Fernandes, J.K., Umebara, T., Lenzi, M.K., da Silva Alves, E.T., 2013. Image analysis for composition monitoring. Commercial blends of olive and soybean oil. Acta Scientiarum - Technology 35 (2), 317–324.

Ferrer-Gallego, R., Miguel Hernandez-Hierro, J., Rivas-Gonzalo, J.C., Teresa Escribano-Bailon, M., 2013. A comparative study to distinguish the vineyard of origin by NIRS using entire grapes, skins and seeds. Journal of the Science of Food and Agriculture 93 (4), 967–972.

Figueiredo-Gonzalez, M., Cancho-Grande, B., Simal-Gandara, J., 2013. Garnacha Tintorera-based sweet wines: chromatic properties and global phenolic composition by means of UV-Vis spectrophotometry. Food Chemistry 140 (1–2), 217–224.

Gad, H.A., El-Ahmady, S.H., Abou-Shoer, M.I., Al-Azizi, M.M., 2013a. Application of chemometrics in authentication of herbal medicines: a review. Phytochemical Analysis 24 (1), 1–24.

Gad, H.A., El-Ahmady, S.H., Abou-Shoer, M.I., Al-Azizi, M.M., 2013b. A modern approach to the authentication and quality assessment of thyme using UV spectroscopy and chemometric analysis. Phytochemical Analysis 24 (6), 520–526.

Gauglitz, G., Moore, D.S., 2014. Handbook of Spectroscopy, 4 Volume Set. John Wiley and Sons.

Gayo, J., Hale, S.A., 2007. Detection and quantification of species authenticity and adulteration in crabmeat using visible and near-infrared spectroscopy. Journal of Agricultural and Food Chemistry 55 (3), 585–592.

Giovenzana, V., Beghi, R., Guidetti, R., 2014. Rapid evaluation of craft beer quality during fermentation process by vis/NIR spectroscopy. Journal of Food Engineering 142, 80–86.

Gonzalez-Caballero, V., Sanchez, M., Lopez, M., Perez-Marin, D., 2010. First steps towards the development of a non-destructive technique for the quality control of wine grapes during on-vine ripening and on arrival at the winery. Journal of Food Engineering 101 (2), 158–165.

Gowen, A.A., O'Donnell, C.P., Cullen, P.J., Downey, G., Frias, J.M., 2007. Hyperspectral imaging – an emerging process analytical tool for food quality and safety control. Trends in Food Science and Technology 18 (12), 590–598.

He, H., Wu, D., Sun, D., 2015. Nondestuuctive spectroscopic and imaging techniques for quality evaluation and assessment of fish and fish products. Critical Reviews in Food Science and Nutrition 55 (6), 864–886.

Hof, M., 2005. Basics of optical spectroscopy. In: Handbook of Spectroscopy. Wiley-VCH Verlag GmbH and Co. KGaA, pp. 37–47.

Hollas, J.M., 2004. Modern Spectroscopy. John Wiley and Sons.

Jacomelli, M., Pitozzi, V., Zaid, M., Larrosa, M., Tonini, G., Martini, A., Urbani, S., Taticchi, A., Servili, M., Dolara, P., 2010. Dietary extra-virgin olive oil rich in phenolic antioxidants and the aging process: long-term effects in the rat. The Journal of Nutritional Biochemistry 21 (4), 290–296.

Jiang, L., Zheng, H., Lu, H., 2015. Application of UV spectrometry and chemometric models for detecting olive oil-vegetable oil blends adulteration. Journal of Food Science and Technology-mysore 52 (1), 479–485.

Kamruzzaman, M., Makino, Y., Oshita, S., 2015. Non-invasive analytical technology for the detection of contamination, adulteration, and authenticity of meat, poultry, and fish: a review. Analytica Chimica Acta 853, 19–29.

Karoui, R., Dufour, E., 2008. Spectroscopic technique: fluorescence and ultraviolet-visible (UV-Vis) spectroscopy. In: Sun, D.W. (Ed.), Modern Techniques for Food Authentication. Elsevier, Burlington, London, San Diego, New York, pp. 201–246.

Khojastehnazhand, M., Khoshtaghaza, M.H., Mojaradi, B., Rezaei, M., Goodarzi, M., Saeys, W., 2014. Comparison of visible–near infrared and short wave infrared hyperspectral imaging for the evaluation of rainbow trout freshness. Food Research International 56, 25–34.

Kumirska, J., Czerwicka, M., Kaczynski, Z., Bychowska, A., Brzozowski, K., Thoeming, J., Stepnowski, P., 2010. Application of spectroscopic methods for structural analysis of chitin and chitosan. Marine Drugs 8 (5), 1567–1636.

Lacar, F., Lewis, M., Grierson, I., 2001. Use of hyperspectral reflectance for discrimination between grape varieties. In: Geoscience and Remote Sensing Symposium, 2001. IGARSS'01. IEEE 2001 International IEEE, p. 2878.

Li, Y., Zhang, J., Zhao, Y., Li, Z., Li, T., Wang, Y., 2014. Characteristic fingerprint based on low polar constituents for discrimination of *Wolfiporia extensa* according to geographical origin using UV spectroscopy and chemometrics methods. Journal of Analytical Methods in Chemistry 2014, 519424.

Liauw, M.A., Baylor, L.C., O'Rourke, P.E., 2010. UV-visible spectroscopy for on-line analysis. In: Process Analytical Technology. John Wiley and Sons, Ltd, pp. 81–106.

Liu, F., He, Y., 2011. Discrimination of producing areas of *Auricularia auricula* using visible/near infrared spectroscopy. Food and Bioprocess Technology 4 (3), 387–394.

Liu, F., Cao, F., Wang, L., He, Y., 2008. Discrimination of rice wine age using visible and near infrared spectroscopy combined with BP neural network. In: Image and Signal Processing, 2008. CISP'08. Congress on IEEE, p. 267.

Liu, C., Liu, W., Lu, X., Chen, W., Yang, J., Zheng, L., 2014. Nondestructive determination of transgenic Bacillus thuringiensis rice seeds (*Oryza sativa* L.) using multispectral imaging and chemometric methods. Food Chemistry 153.

Lorente, D., Escandell-Montero, P., Cubero, S., Gómez-Sanchis, J., Blasco, J., 2015. Visible–NIR reflectance spectroscopy and manifold learning methods applied to the detection of fungal infections on citrus fruit. Journal of Food Engineering 163, 17–24.

Lourenco, N.D., Lopes, J.A., Almeida, C.F., Sarraguca, M.C., Pinheiro, H.M., 2012. Bioreactor monitoring with spectroscopy and chemometrics: a review. Analytical and Bioanalytical Chemistry 404 (4), 1211–1237.

Lucio-Gutiérrez, J.R., Coello, J., Maspoch, S., 2012. Enhanced chromatographic fingerprinting of herb materials by multi-wavelength selection and chemometrics. Analytica Chimica Acta 710, 40–49.

Ma, J., Pu, H., Sun, D., Gao, W., Qu, J., Ma, K., 2015. Application of Vis–NIR hyperspectral imaging in classification between fresh and frozen-thawed pork Longissimus Dorsi muscles. International Journal of Refrigeration 50, 10–18.

Marchese, A., Coppo, E., Sobolev, A.P., Rossi, D., Mannina, L., Daglia, M., 2014. Influence of in vitro simulated gastroduodenal digestion on the antibacterial activity, metabolic profiling and polyphenols content of green tea (Camellia sinensis). Food Research International 63 (Part B), 182–191.

Martelo-Vidal, M.J., Vázquez, M., 2014a. Classification of red wines from controlled designation of origin by ultraviolet-visible and near-infrared spectral analysis. Ciencia e Tecnica Vitivinicola 29 (1), 35–43.

Martelo-Vidal, M.J., Vázquez, M., 2014b. Determination of polyphenolic compounds of red wines by UV-VIS-NIR spectroscopy and chemometrics tools. Food Chemistry 158, 28–34.

Martelo-Vidal, M.J., Vázquez, M., 2014c. Evaluation of ultraviolet, visible, and near infrared spectroscopy for the analysis of wine compounds. Czech Journal of Food Sciences 32 (1), 37–47.

Martelo-Vidal, M.J., Vázquez, M., 2014d. Rapid authentication of white wines. Part 2: classification by grape variety. Agro Food Industry Hi-tech 25 (6), 20–22.

Martelo-Vidal, M.J., Vázquez, M., 2014e. Rapid authentication of white wines. Part 1: classification by designation of origin. Agro Food Industry Hi-Tech 25 (5), 44–48.

Martelo-Vidal, M.J., Vázquez, M., 2015. Application of artificial neural networks coupled to UV-VIS-NIR spectroscopy for the rapid quantification of wine compounds in aqueous mixtures. CYTA – Journal of Food 13 (1), 32–39.

Martelo-Vidal, M.J., Domínguez-Agis, F., Vázquez, M., 2013. Ultraviolet/visible/near-infrared spectral analysis and chemometric tools for the discrimination of wines between subzones inside a controlled designation of origin: a case study of Rías Baixas. Australian Journal of Grape and Wine Research 19 (1), 62–67.

Mignani, A., Ciaccheri, L., Mencaglia, A., Ottevaere, H., Baca, E.E.S., Thienpont, H., 2012a. Optical measurements and pattern recognition techniques for autheticating top-fermented and bottom-fermented beers and predicting the alcoholic strength. In: Sensors, 2012. IEEE, p. 1.

Mignani, A.G., Ciaccheri, L., Gordillo, B., Mencaglia, A.A., González-Miret, M.L., Heredia, F.J., Culshaw, B., 2012b. Identifying the production region of single-malt Scotch whiskies using optical spectroscopy and pattern recognition techniques. Sensors and Actuators B: Chemical 171–172, 458–462.

Mignani, A.G., Ciaccheri, L., Mencaglia, A.A., Ottevaere, H., Báca, E.E.S., Thienpont, H., 2013. Optical measurements and pattern-recognition techniques for identifying the characteristics of beer and distinguishing Belgian beers. Sensors and Actuators B: Chemical 179, 140–149.

Morsy, N., Sun, D., 2013. Robust linear and non-linear models of NIR spectroscopy for detection and quantification of adulterants in fresh and frozen-thawed minced beef. Meat Science 93 (2), 292–302.

Mouazen, A., Al Walaan, N., 2014. Glucose adulteration in Saudi honey with visible and near infrared spectroscopy. International Journal of Food Properties 17 (10), 2263–2274.

Mouazen, A.M., Dridi, S., Rouissi, H., De Baerdemaeker, J., Ramon, H., 2009. Prediction of selected ewe's milk properties and differentiating between pasture and box feeding using visible and near infrared spectroscopy. Biosystems Engineering 104 (3), 353–361.

Nicolaï, B.M., Beullens, K., Bobelyn, E., Peirs, A., Saeys, W., Theron, K.I., Lammertyn, J., 2007. Nondestructive measurement of fruit and vegetable quality by means of NIR spectroscopy: a review. Postharvest Biology and Technology 46 (2), 99–118.

Nunes, C.A., 2014. Vibrational spectroscopy and chemometrics to assess authenticity, adulteration and intrinsic quality parameters of edible oils and fats. Food Research International 60, 255–261.

Oliveri, P., Casale, M., Casolino, M.C., Baldo, M.A., Grifi, F.N., Forina, M., 2011. Comparison between classical and innovative class-modelling techniques for the characterisation of a PDO olive oil. Analytical and Bioanalytical Chemistry 399 (6), 2105–2113.

Ottavian, M., Fasolato, L., Serva, L., Facco, P., Barolo, M., 2014. Data fusion for food authentication: fresh/frozen–thawed discrimination in West African Goatfish (*Pseudupeneus prayensis*) fillets. Food and Bioprocess Technology 7 (4), 1025–1036.

Ouyang, Q., Zhao, J., Pan, W., Chen, Q., 2016. Real-time monitoring of process parameters in rice wine fermentation by a portable spectral analytical system combined with multivariate analysis. Food Chemistry 190, 135–141.

Owen, T., 2000. Fundamentals of UV-visible Spectroscopy: A Primer. Agilent Technologies.

Palacios-Morillo, A., Alcázar, Á., de Pablos, F., Jurado, J.M., 2013. Differentiation of tea varieties using UV–Vis spectra and pattern recognition techniques. Spectrochimica Acta Part A: Molecular and Biomolecular Spectroscopy 103, 79–83.

Penner, M.H., 2010. Basic principles of spectroscopy. In: Food Analysis. Springer, pp. 375–385.

Pizarro, C., Rodríguez-Tecedor, S., Pérez-del-Notario, N., Esteban-Díez, I., González-Sáiz, J.M., 2013. Classification of Spanish extra virgin olive oils by data fusion of visible spectroscopic fingerprints and chemical descriptors. Food Chemistry 138 (2–3), 915–922.

Primrose, S., Woolfe, M., Rollinson, S., 2010. Food forensics: methods for determining the authenticity of foodstuffs. Trends in Food Science and Technology 21 (12), 582–590.

Pu, H., Sun, D., Ma, J., Liu, D., Cheng, J., 2014. Using wavelet textural features of visible and near infrared hyperspectral image to differentiate between fresh and frozen–thawed pork. Food and Bioprocess Technology 7 (11), 3088–3099.

Pu, H., Sun, D., Ma, J., Cheng, J., 2015. Classification of fresh and frozen-thawed pork muscles using visible and near infrared hyperspectral imaging and textural analysis. Meat Science 99, 81–88.

Reid, L.M., O'Donnell, C.P., Downey, G., 2006. Recent technological advances for the determination of food authenticity. Trends in Food Science and Technology 17 (7), 344–353.

Ribéreau-Gayon, P., Glories, Y., Maujean, A., Dubourdieu, D., 2000. Handbook of enology. The Chemistry of Wine and Stabilisation and Treatments 2.

Rinnan, A., Nørgaard, L., van den Berg, F., Thygesen, J., Bro, R., Engelsen, S.B., 2009. Data pre-procesing. In: Sun, D. (Ed.), Near Infrared Spectroscopy for Food Quality Analysis and Control, first ed. Academy Press – Elsevier, Inc., USA, pp. 27–50.

Riovanto, R., Cynkar, W.U., Berzaghi, P., Cozzolino, D., 2011. Discrimination between Shiraz wines from different Australian regions: the role of spectroscopy and chemometrics. Journal of Agricultural and Food Chemistry 59 (18), 10356–10360.

Rohman, A., Man, Y.B.C., 2011. Analysis of chicken fat as adulterant in cod liver oil using Fourier transform infrared (FTIR) spectroscopy and chemometrics. Cyta – Journal of Food 9 (3), 187–191.

Ruiz-Altisent, M., Ruiz-Garcia, L., Moreda, G., Lu, R., Hernandez-Sanchez, N., Correa, E., Diezma, B., Nicolaï, B., García-Ramos, J., 2010. Sensors for product characterization and quality of specialty crops – a review. Computers and Electronics in Agriculture 74 (2), 176–194.

Saavedra, J., Fuentealba, C., Yanez, L., Bravo, M., Quiroz, W., Lukacsy, G., Carot, J.M., 2011. Chemometric approaches for the zoning of Pinot Noir wines from the Casablanca valley, Chile. Food Chemistry 127 (4), 1842–1847.

Sánchez Rojas, F., Bosch Ojeda, C., 2009. Recent development in derivative ultraviolet/visible absorption spectrophotometry: 2004–2008: a review. Analytica Chimica Acta 635 (1), 22–44.

Sarbu, C., Nascu-Briciu, R.D., Kot-Wasik, A., Gorinstein, S., Wasik, A., Namiesnik, J., 2012. Classification and fingerprinting of kiwi and pomelo fruits by multivariate analysis of chromatographic and spectroscopic data. Food Chemistry 130 (4), 994–1002.

Savenije, B., Geesink, G.H., Van Der Palen, J.G.P., Hemke, G., Hopkins, D., Ouali, A., 2006. Prediction of pork quality using visible/near-infrared reflectance spectroscopy. Meat Science 73 (1), 181–187.

Skoog, D.A., Crouch, S.R., Holler, F.J., 2008. Principios de analisis instrumental (Principles of Instrumental Analysis). Cengage Learning Editores.

Skoog, D., West, D., Holler, F., Crouch, S., 2013. Fundamentals of Analytical Chemistry. Cengage Learning.

Snyder, A.B., Sweeney, C.F., Rodriguez-Saona, L.E., Giusti, M.M., 2014. Rapid authentication of concord juice concentration in a grape juice blend using Fourier-transform infrared spectroscopy and chemometric analysis. Food Chemistry 147, 295–301.

Sohrabi, M., Darabi, G., 2016. The application of continuous wavelet transform and least squares support vector machine for the simultaneous quantitative spectrophotometric determination of Myricetin, Kaempferol and Quercetin as flavonoids in pharmaceutical plants. Spectrochimica Acta. Part A, Molecular and Biomolecular Spectroscopy 152, 443–452.

Sone, I., Olsen, R.L., Sivertsen, A.H., Eilertsen, G., Heia, K., 2012. Classification of fresh Atlantic salmon (*Salmo salar* L.) fillets stored under different atmospheres by hyperspectral imaging. Journal of Food Engineering 109 (3), 482–489.

Souto, U.T.C.P., Pontes, M.J.C., Silva, E.C., Galvão, R.K.H., Araújo, M.C.U., Sanches, F.A.C., Cunha, F.A.S., Oliveira, M.S.R., 2010. UV–Vis spectrometric classification of coffees by SPA–LDA. Food Chemistry 119 (1), 368–371.

Tan, J., Li, R., Jiang, Z., 2015. Chemometric classification of Chinese lager beers according to manufacturer based on data fusion of fluorescence, UV and visible spectroscopies. Food Chemistry 184, 30–36.

Uddin, M., Okazaki, E., Turza, S., Yumiko, Y., Tanaka, M., Fukuda, Y., 2005. Non-destructive visible/NIR spectroscopy for differentiation of fresh and frozen-thawed fish. Journal of Food Science 70 (8), c506–c510.

Urbano, M., de Castro, M., Perez, P., Garcia-Olmo, J., Gomez-Nieto, M., 2006. Ultraviolet-visible spectroscopy and pattern recognition methods for differentiation and classification of wines. Food Chemistry 97 (1), 166–175.

Uríčková, V., Sádecká, J., 2015. Determination of geographical origin of alcoholic beverages using ultraviolet, visible and infrared spectroscopy: a review. Spectrochimica Acta Part A: Molecular and Biomolecular Spectroscopy 148, 131–137.

Van Maarschalkerweerd, M., Husted, S., 2015. Recent developments in fast spectroscopy for plant mineral analysis. Frontiers in Plant Science 6, 169.

Vera, L., Aceña, L., Guasch, J., Boqué, R., Mestres, M., Busto, O., 2011. Discrimination and sensory description of beers through data fusion. Talanta 87, 136–142.

Wang, X., Huang, J., Fan, W., Lu, H., 2015. Identification of green tea varieties and fast quantification of total polyphenols by near-infrared spectroscopy and ultraviolet-visible spectroscopy with chemometric algorithms. Analytical Methods 7 (2), 787–792.

Weeranantanaphan, J., Downey, G., 2010. Identity confirmation of a branded, fermented cereal product by UV spectroscopy: a feasibility study involving a Trappist beer. Journal of the Institute of Brewing 116 (1), 56–61.

Wlasiuk, P., Martyna, A., Zadora, G., 2015. A likelihood ratio model for the determination of the geographical origin of olive oil. Analytica Chimica Acta 853, 187–199.

Wójcicki, K., Khmelinskii, I., Sikorski, M., Caponio, F., Paradiso, V.M., Summo, C., Pasqualone, A., Sikorska, E., 2015. Spectroscopic techniques and chemometrics in analysis of blends of extra virgin with refined and mild deodorized olive oils. European Journal of Lipid Science and Technology 117 (1), 92–102.

Wu, D., He, Y., 2014. Potential of spectroscopic techniques and chemometric analysis for rapid measurement of docosahexaenoic acid and eicosapentaenoic acid in algal oil. Food Chemistry 158, 93–100.

Wu, D., Sun, D., 2013. Advanced applications of hyperspectral imaging technology for food quality and safety analysis and assessment: a review — Part I: fundamentals. Innovative Food Science and Emerging Technologies 19, 1–14.

Yang, H., He, Y., 2008. Design and implement of variety discriminator of fragrant mushrooms based on Vis/NIR spectroscopy and BP-ANN. In: Automation and Logistics, 2008. ICAL 2008. IEEE International Conference on IEEE, p. 2727.

Yao, L., Zhou, W., Wang, T., Liu, M., Yu, C., 2014. Quantification of egg yolk contamination in egg white using UV/Vis spectroscopy: prediction model development and analysis. Food Control 43, 88–97.

Yu, H.Y., Ying, B., Sun, T., Niu, X.Y., Pan, X.X., 2007. Vintage year determination of bottled Chinese rice wine by VIS-NIR spectroscopy. Journal of Food Science 72 (3), E125–E129.

Zhang, W., Li, N., Feng, Y., Su, S., Li, T., Liang, B., 2015. A unique quantitative method of acid value of edible oils and studying the impact of heating on edible oils by UV–Vis spectrometry. Food Chemistry 185, 326–332.

Zhu, F., Zhang, D., He, Y., Liu, F., Sun, D., 2013. Application of visible and near infrared hyperspectral imaging to differentiate between fresh and frozen-thawed fish fillets. Food and Bioprocess Technology 6 (10), 2931–2937.

Advances in Infrared Spectroscopy for Food Authenticity Testing

4

L.E. Rodriguez-Saona, M.M. Giusti, M. Shotts
College of Food Agriculture and Environmental Sciences, The Ohio State University, OH, United States

Chapter Outline

4.1 Introduction

Counterfeiting is a worldwide and growing concern that is estimated to be worth \$250 billion (Chaudhry and Zimmerman, 2013), representing an annual cost to the global food industry of \$49 billion in counterfeited products (Perks, 2007).

Economically motivated adulteration and contamination of foods is estimated to cost the US industry $10 to $15 billion per year with up to 10% of food products in retail stores having some degree of adulteration (Grocery Manufacturing Association, 2015). Currently, only about 1% of imported foods are randomly inspected by federal agencies primarily due to limited resources and time-consuming protocols required for testing (Johnson, 2014).

Vibrational spectroscopy is the collective term used to describe two analytical techniques: infrared (IR) and Raman spectroscopy. These techniques measure molecular vibrations either by the absorption of light quanta (IR) or the inelastic scattering of photons (Raman); either method generates spectral signature profiles ("fingerprints") that are reproducible and distinct for different raw materials as well as adulterants and chemical contaminants. Vibrational spectroscopy can provide rapid and cost-effective techniques required for effective surveillance of our food supply to deter acts of economic adulteration, counterfeiting, or vandalism (Ellis et al., 2015). Advances in supervised pattern recognition techniques have provided the capability for targeted and nontargeted screening of tampered ingredients using these spectral profiles, thus enabling real-time and field-based measurements to control the raw material stream. The development of portable and handheld optical systems for chemical identification has incorporated the analytical precision of spectroscopy to field applications with spectral resolution equivalent to bench-top instruments (Sorak et al., 2012).

Sensor technologies are directed at improving efficiency, throughput, and reliability of critical processes, such as monitoring incoming raw materials. Implementation of rapid testing by industry and regulatory agencies would help to streamline food safety and quality assurance and prevent the growing danger to consumers from adulterated or substituted products as evidenced by recent incidents involving melamine in milk-derived products, Sudan 3 in turmeric powder, or peanut-tainted cumin seeds.

This chapter will present the current state of the research on authentication applications for high-value raw materials (fats, extra virgin olive oil, milk, and fruit juices among others) susceptible to economically motivated tampering. Our primary focus will be on near- and mid-infrared (MIR) spectroscopies due to their wide versatility and application in the food industry. We will also present Raman spectroscopy as a closely related vibrational spectroscopy technique that offers potential for food application because of its ease of use, high specificity, nondestructive and structure-probing characteristics, minimal sample preparation, ability to collect data through packaging, and suitability for use in aqueous systems (Ozaki, 1998; Li and Church, 2014).

4.2 Vibrational Spectroscopy as a Screening Method

Vibrational spectroscopy techniques are based on the oscillations of atoms in molecules, generating information about the molecular vibrational energy transitions that are related to molecular conformation, structure, intermolecular interaction(s), and chemical bonding (Li and Church, 2014). In IR spectroscopy, samples are exposed to a source of thermal radiation (1500–2000 K) in the infrared region of the electromagnetic spectrum (13,000–40 cm^{-1}) and radiation is absorbed by the sample, changing the molecular dipole moment, resulting in a spectrum showing distinct frequencies corresponding to the vibrational frequencies of the bonds in the sample. In contrast, the Raman effect is an inelastic light-scattering phenomenon that depends on a change in the shape of the electron distribution in the molecule (polarizability) during the particular mode of vibration (Li and Church, 2014).

Vibrational spectroscopic techniques have significant potential in the field of food authentication, as they provide resolution of unique chemical information allowing rapid monitoring of subtle compositional changes to help detect potential ingredient tampering. The complex spectrum reflects the total biochemical composition, with bands arising from bond vibrations from food constituents with known assignment in many cases. The complementary nature of IR and Raman information provides versatility to the analyst in identifying the technique best suited for screening adulteration because the spectra are a unique reflection of the molecular structure of the matrix. Virtually every organic compound will absorb IR radiation, and the intensity of the signal is associated with the concentration of the compound allowing for identification and quantitative analysis of materials; this capability has made infrared spectroscopy a workhorse for food applications. On the other hand, the Raman effect is weak and sample fluorescence has been a major limiting factor for food applications, but recent advances in laser technology using excitation wavelengths in the NIR range combined with sensitive detectors are showing great promise in the food and agricultural fields.

4.2.1 Fundamentals of Infrared Spectroscopy

IR spectroscopy is based on the interaction of IR radiation (heat) with bonds in a chemical structure; thus, a portion of the radiation is absorbed by molecular bonds of the sample matter resulting in light being absent or attenuated at certain frequencies in reflectance of transmission spectra (Colthup et al., 1990). IR spectra are commonly divided into three regions: far-IR (40–400 cm^{-1}), MIR (400–4000 cm^{-1}), and NIR (4000–14,000 cm^{-1}). Absorption of infrared radiation by a molecule causes a shift in the dipole moment as a result of molecular vibrations, stretching and contracting of bonds, and bending or twisting of bonds. Because of this specificity, conserved atomic arrangements (known as "functional groups") can be identified in any sample, despite the slightly different vibrational modes associated with the unique connectivity and environment of each molecule (Maurer et al., 2012). When functional groups are excited by incident radiation, they can move from the lowest vibrational state ($\nu = 0$) to the first excited energy state ($\nu = 1$). The radiation frequency that causes this energy transition is equal to the initial vibratory frequency of the bond and is known as the fundamental absorption (Colthup et al., 1990). Absorptions of this type are most commonly associated with the MIR region. Molecules that interact with the higher intensity light of the NIR region are capable of further energetic transitions ($\nu = 2$ or 3); these transitions are referred to as overtones (Colthup et al., 1990). The IR region's sensitivity to changes in structure and conditions make it well suited for analysis of components in a complex matrix (Griffiths and de Haseth, 2006).

MIR and NIR regions are most useful for food authentication applications because of their unique fingerprinting capabilities and have been extensively covered in the literature. No significant role on food authenticity has been played by far-IR and for that reason, we will not discuss it in this chapter.

4.2.2 Mid-Infrared Spectroscopy

MIR is well suited for a variety of qualitative and quantitative applications because absorption bands in the spectrum are related to the vibrational modes of specific functional groups (Fig. 4.1), and their band position and intensity are correlated with the energy of the bond and its concentration in the matrix (Li-Chan et al., 2010). A portion of the MIR region, between 650 and 1500 cm^{-1}, is known as the fingerprint region because it contains a complex series of absorptions arising from multiple bonds deforming simultaneously producing a unique spectral pattern allowing the identification of similar substances (Günzler and Gremlich, 2002).

4.2.2.1 Instrumentation

MIR spectrometers have been commercially available since the 1940s relying on prisms to act as dispersive elements, but by the mid-1950s diffraction gratings were introduced into dispersive machines. Conventional dispersive IR systems separate the incident infrared radiation into its component wavelengths for analysis at the

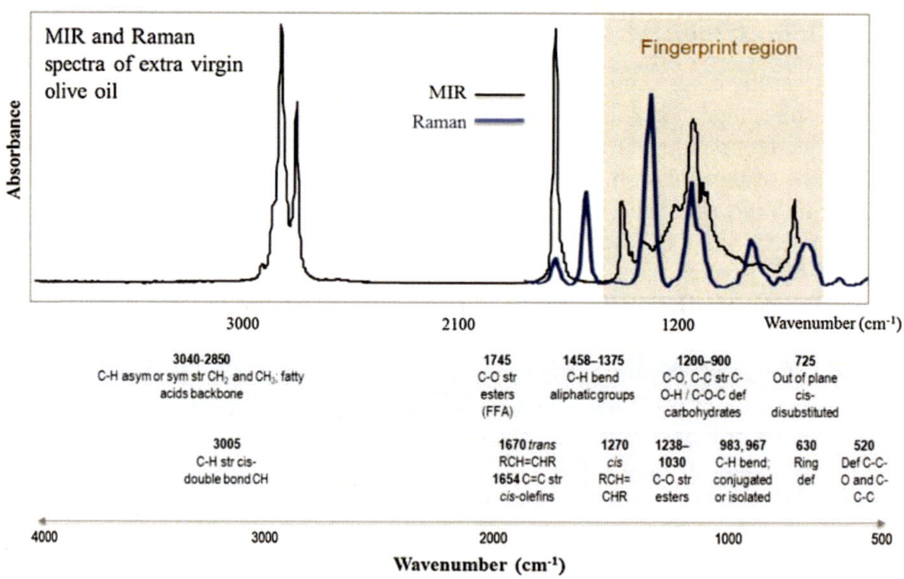

Figure 4.1 Representative mid-infrared (MIR) and Raman spectra of extra virgin olive oil and their corresponding functional group band assignments. Shaded area (650–1500 cm^{-1}) highlights the fingerprint region.

detector. A major advance in the field of MIR spectroscopy was the development of Fourier transform infrared spectroscopy (FT-IR), employing an interferometer and exploiting the well-established mathematical process of Fourier transformation. FT-IR dramatically improved the quality of IR spectra and minimized the time required to obtain data. FT-IR allows for measuring all of the IR frequencies simultaneously, using an optical device called an interferometer. The interferometer produces a unique signal that has all of the infrared frequencies "encoded" into it resulting in extremely fast measurements ($\sim$1 s) rather than the several minutes often required by in dispersive units. A common FT-IR spectrometer (Fig. 4.2) consists of infrared energy emitted from a glowing blackbody source, an interferometer, a sample compartment, a detector, an amplifier, an A/D convertor, and a computer. Interferometers employ a beam splitter that transmits 50% of the light and reflects the remaining part. The reflected light hits a fixed mirror while the transmitted part of the beam is directed to a movable mirror.

The light returning from the two mirrors is recombined at the beam splitter, with the two beams having a difference in path length. The resulting signal is called an interferogram, which has the unique property that every data point (a function of the moving mirror position) contains information about every infrared frequency that comes from the source. The interferogram signal is a function of the change in optical path length from the moving mirror and is then Fourier transformed to obtain a frequency domain, which is deconvolved to yield a spectrum.

FT-IR systems have been widely used in food analysis with advantages such as faster data collection speeds because of simultaneous detection of all frequencies in one scan, increased energy throughput over a monochromator producing a much higher signal-to-noise ratio than dispersive systems, reduced scan time without loss of resolution, superior wavelength resolution, and superior wavelength accuracy obtained through the use of an internal laser to maintain wavelength calibration, as

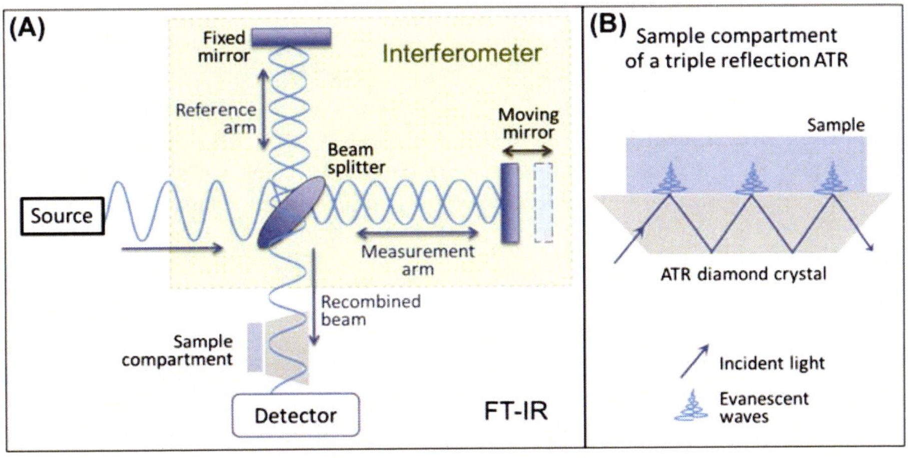

Figure 4.2 Schematic diagram of a Fourier transform infrared spectrometer (FT-IR) (A) and details of the Michelson interferometer, and the attenuated total reflectance (ATR) accessory (B).

opposed to the external calibration required by dispersive systems (Griffiths and Haseth, 1986).

4.2.2.2 Sampling Modes

The traditional method of analysis for IR spectrometers is transmittance of IR radiation done by placing the sample directly into the path of the IR beam (with the help of sample holder) and scanning. Liquids and pastes are generally the easiest samples to run using a demountable liquid cell or a sealed cell, but solid samples (with the exception of thin films) require sample preparation that includes making a pellet (typically potassium bromide, KBr) or a mull that are time consuming and can be destructive. However, transmission analysis sets forth a variety of sampling issues for complex matrices that have plagued MIR methods (Griffiths and de Haseth, 2006). Drawbacks of the use of the transmission model include the effort in preventing bubble formation in the liquid cells, difficulty in cleaning these cells, and the complexity and labor involved in making good KBr pellets.

The advent of attenuated total reflectance (ATR) has overcome many of these issues (Li-Chan et al., 2010) by improving the versatility of IR systems, allowing IR spectra to be obtained from the surface of a material (Günzler and Gremlich, 2002). The ATR accessory is placed between the beam splitter and the detector in the signal path; it consists of a high refractive index crystal that directly contacts the sample. The IR beam enters the crystal at a predetermined angle, reaches the interface of the crystal and the sample, and is completely reflected back into the crystal (Fig. 4.2). At the point of reflection, an evanescent wave is produced that penetrates the sample and is absorbed (Günzler and Gremlich, 2002). Although this wave minimally penetrates the sample (1−4 μm for MIR), multiple bounce ATR devices allow for many contact points between the sample and the IR beam, resulting in absorption by the sample at each point of reflection. A wide variety of high-refractive index materials have been used for ATR including zinc selenide (ZnSe), germanium, AMTIR, and diamond. Each of these has unique properties and must be matched to the sample in question, most commonly in order to assure that the refractive index of the crystal is much higher than that of the sample. If the refractive index of the sample is close to or greater than that of the crystal, internal reflectance will not occur. The only other requirement for ATR sampling is that the sample comes into direct contact with the crystal; in some cases this may require the application of pressure to the sample by using pressure clamps. ATR sampling accessories now include temperature and environmentally controlled units that allow for a great deal of control during data collection.

4.2.3 Near-Infrared Spectroscopy

NIR spectroscopy is a well-established branch of spectroscopy that measures chemical bonds on the basis of overtones and combination bands of specific functional groups (Fig. 4.3). NIR spectroscopy follows the theory of anharmonic oscillation in which energy levels are not equally spaced, potentially resulting in transitions between energy states that are greater than one (Blanco and Villarroya, 2002).

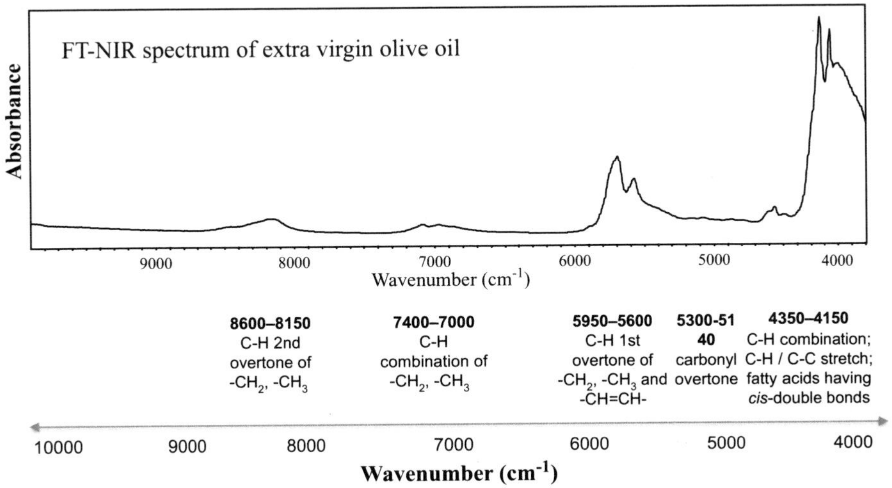

Figure 4.3 Representative near-infrared (NIR) spectrum of extra virgin olive oil and its corresponding functional group band assignments.

Although NIR bands are one or two orders of magnitude lower in intensity than corresponding bands in the MIR region, a consequence is that the NIR region enables direct analysis of samples that are highly absorbing and strongly light scattering without dilution or extensive sample preparation, provides deeper light penetration into a sample (>10 mm) and allows direct measurement of samples contained in glass or plastic containers (Rodriguez-Saona et al., 2001). However, in comparison to the well-separated, distinctly identifiable bands of MIR, the overlapping bands in the NIR region do not allow for determination of structure from spectra alone (Ismail et al., 1999). By contrast, NIR excels at determination of major components in complex matrices allowing for quantitative determination of proteins (primarily N—H bonds), lipids (C—H), and carbohydrates (O—H) (Li-Chan et al., 2010).

Unlike MIR, the higher-energy NIR radiation can be used to directly analyze solids with diffuse reflectance spectroscopy. In this technique, a small amount of incident radiation penetrates the solid surface of a sample and is reflected several times before exiting and being captured by a suitably located detector (Ismail et al., 1999). More IR radiation is absorbed as a result of the multiple reflections, allowing for the analysis of solid, minimally prepared samples (Günzler and Heise, 2000). As opposed to MIR instrumentation relying mainly on the interferometer, NIR offers several options depending on the application and location of the test (in-line, at-line, or in the laboratory). A review of NIR instrumentation is available in the book by Ciurczak and Igne (2015) and includes the rugged filter-based instruments, rugged and fast acousto-optic tunable filter (AOTF) instruments, grating instruments that are still the workhorses of the analytical laboratory, Fourier transform—NIR instruments offering extremely fast data acquisition and highest spectral resolution, and the virtually instantaneous and rugged photodiode array instruments (Ciurczak and Igne, 2015). These properties have led to the development of NIR methods for process monitoring and quality assurance in a variety of food applications (Rodriguez-Otero and Hermida, 1996; Gonzaga and Pasquini, 2006; Woodcock et al., 2008; Du et al., 2012).

4.2.4 Raman Spectroscopy

Raman spectroscopy is another vibrational technique that provides information about the vibrations of the molecules contained within the Raman shift spectrum of scattered intensity (Fig. 4.1). We direct the reader to excellent material on the fundamentals (Reichenbächer and Popp, 2012; Siebert and Hildebrandt, 2008) and food applications (Yang and Ying, 2011; Li and Church, 2014) of Raman spectroscopy.

Raman and infrared spectroscopy are based on the vibrational transitions occurring in the ground electronic state of molecules. Raman scattering arises from the changes in the polarizability or shape of the electron distribution in the molecule as it vibrates; in contrast, infrared absorption requires a change of the intrinsic dipole moment with the molecular vibration. Thus, IR and Raman spectroscopies are complementary techniques (Fig. 4.1) since transitions allowed in Raman may be forbidden in IR or vice versa. An IR signal is strongest in asymmetric polar moieties, whereas Raman is strong for symmetric, electron-rich moieties. For example, O—H stretching modes of water and alcohols have strong absorption in the infrared region but produce relatively weak Raman signals (Reichenbächer and Popp, 2012; Ali et al., 2013) making Raman ideal for measurements of solutions.

For every 10 million photons that are incident on a sample, only one of those will be Raman scattered. Using an excitation wavelength in the UV and visible range enhances the Raman signal, but the trade-off is fluorescence that can completely overwhelm the Raman signal. For many years, Raman spectroscopy was considered to be of very limited use in food science because of drawbacks such as fluorescence, photodecomposition, and wave number calibration problems together with the difficulty of obtaining high-resolution spectra (Baeten and Aparicio, 2000). New-generation Raman spectrometers are equipped with a longer excitation wavelength (NIR, 1064 nm) that eliminates the fluorescence limitation but results in diminished Raman signal intensity. In order to address this signal limitation, InGaAs array detectors are available. Also, surface-enhanced Raman spectroscopy (SERS) phenomena can be exploited (Craig et al., 2013) by using metallic nanostructures (typically gold and silver) to enhance, by an order of 10^8-10^{14}, the Raman signal of sample molecules that are in a certain proximity to the metal surface due to the large electromagnetic field induced by localized surface plasmon resonance (Zhang et al., 2005), resulting in limits of detection (LODs) of SERS applications in ppb or even at single-molecule level.

4.3 Chemometrics in Vibrational Spectroscopy

The development of IR methods has been aided by increases in computing power, and specifically the application of chemometric tools that can extract information from large spectral data sets. Advances in vibrational spectroscopy instrumentation and multivariate statistical analysis techniques (chemometrics) have shown potential for analysis of complex multispectral information for the discrimination, classification, and identification of biological systems. Infrared spectra contain many overlapping bands, preventing data interpretation by simple visual inspection. Multivariate data generated from an IR experiment consist of the results of observations of many different frequencies for each sample, and each variable may be regarded as constituting a different dimension, such that if there are *n* variables (IR bands) each object may be said to reside at a unique position in an abstract entity referred to as n-dimensional hyperspace. This hyperspace, though difficult to visualize, uses multivariate analysis for simplification or dimensionality reduction (Ellis and Goodacre, 2006).

Classification techniques can be divided into unsupervised (when samples are classified without any prior knowledge of groups contained in the data set, ie, the category membership of samples) and supervised (in which prior knowledge is required). Supervised classification models are developed on a training set of samples with known categories, and then the model performance is evaluated by comparing the classification predictions to the true categories of a set of entirely separate validation samples (Roggo et al., 2007). Table 4.1 summarizes the main chemometric methods used for qualitative and quantitative analysis. We will further describe here some of the methods most commonly used.

Among unsupervised methods, principal component analysis (PCA) is often used to reveal sample patterns and groupings. PCA attempts to reduce a large data set to a smaller number of orthogonal variables, or principal components (PCs), that retain

Table 4.1 Description of Common Chemometric Methods and the Type of Discriminant Analysis Associated With Each

Multivariate Analysis	Description
Classification – Unsupervised Analyses	
Hierarchical Clustering Analysis (HCA)	Successive partitions of the data set resulting in a cluster sequence that can be represented with a dendrogram to visualize the obtained structure of clustering. Ward's algorithm of minimum variance is very popular and highly efficient in computing distances between all possible pairs of clusters.
Principal Component Analysis (PCA)	Reduces the number of variables (scores) and transforms the original measurement variables into new, uncorrelated variables (loadings), used to assess the similarities or differences between classes. Interrelationships among different variables and sample patterns and groupings can be studied.
Classification – Supervised Analyses	
k-nearest neighbors (k-NN)	Nonparametric classification method based on a local metric related to similarities among samples. The shortest Euclidean distance is used to assign the class membership. The optimal K value is selected usually by means of cross-validation, and the K giving the lowest classification error is the optimal one.

Continued

Table 4.1 Description of Common Chemometric Methods and the Type of Discriminant Analysis Associated With Each—cont'd

Multivariate Analysis	Description
Soft independent modeling by class analogy (SIMCA)	Each class is independently modeled by PCA, explaining the major sources of variance with fewer variables. For each class, an acceptance boundary is defined based on the maximum residuals of the samples from that group. Each class is modeled by a number of PCs assessed by cross-validation. An unknown sample is assigned to the class with the smallest residual variance during the prediction.
Partial Least Squares Discriminant Analysis (PLS-DA)	Approach that maximizes the covariance between the independent variables X (ie, spectra) and the corresponding dependent variable Y (ie, groups) of highly multidimensional data. Permits the prediction of Y based on a reduced number of factors (latent variables). The main advantage is the handling of highly collinear and noisy data. Provides a visual interpretation of complex data sets illustrating the separation between different groups.
Linear Discriminant Analysis (LDA)	Parametric and PCA-based method that finds the optimal linear combination of the original variables. The transformed observations are called discriminant functions that maximize variance between groups and minimize variance within groups. LDA selects the directions that achieve a maximum separation among the different classes using Euclidean distance to classify unknown samples.
Support vector machine (SVM)	Nonlinear pattern recognition method based on finding the widest margin of separation between classes. Using a mapping function (kernel function), SVM can deal with complex classification problems that are not linear in the initial dimension but may be at high dimensional spaces. The kernel function algorithm embodies the principle of structural risk minimization and offers potential for self-adjustment and self-learning.
Supervised locally linear embedding (SLLE)	Nonlinear dimensionality reduction method based on the assumption that each data point and its neighbors lie on a locally linear patch of the manifold. SLLE uses the known class label information to calculate the Euclidean distance. Classification is accomplished by the nearest centroid algorithm. The method computes a centroid (mean) for each class and compares the profile of a new sample to each of these class centroids. The new sample is assigned to the class with the nearest centroid.

Table 4.1 Description of Common Chemometric Methods and the Type of Discriminant Analysis Associated With Each—cont'd

Multivariate Analysis	Description
Classification and Quantitative Supervised Analyses	
Artificial Neural Networks (ANN)	Nonlinear computational methods inspired by the functioning of human brain. Black-box that receives multiple inputs (X, ie, spectral intensities) and produces multiple outputs (Y, chemical value). ANN poses characteristics such as adaptivity, noise (data), and fault (neurons and connections lost) tolerance. The modeling (training) process obtains output values from the input layer of neurons. The training error decreases with the increasing number of training iterations and reaches an asymptotic value. The network might learn a relevant part of noise with the systematic information. Validation procedures are applied by using an external data set to obtain the optimal number of iterations.
Quantitative Supervised Analyses	
Principal component regression (PCR)	Spectral data are treated with a PCA and then a multiple linear regression is performed on the scores as predictive variables. PCA suppresses the spectral colinearity but there is no guarantee that the computed principal components are correlated to the studied property.
Partial Least Squares Regression (PLSR)	Regressions are computed with least squares algorithms. The goal is to establish a linear link between the spectral data X and the reference values Y. This technique models both X and Y in order to find the variables in X matrix that best describe the Y matrix. PLSR can be enhanced using orthogonal signal corrections (OSC). PLSR has the PCR advantages without the drawbacks by selecting latent variables according to the covariance matrix between data and investigated parameter.

the major variance of the original variables (Kemsley, 1996). Each sample is assigned a score on each of these principal components, and graphical representation of these scores can be used to uncover relationships or clustering within a data set (Karoui and De Baerdemaeker, 2007). Graphical display (Fig. 4.4) is helpful in finding outliers or misclassified samples, revealing characteristics that can be hidden in the original data. Most common methods for supervised classification of vibrational spectroscopy include soft independent modeling of class analogy and partial least squares discriminant analysis.

Soft Independent Modeling of Class Analogy (SIMCA) is a pattern recognition method based on PCA that reduces the dimensionality of multivariate data to permit

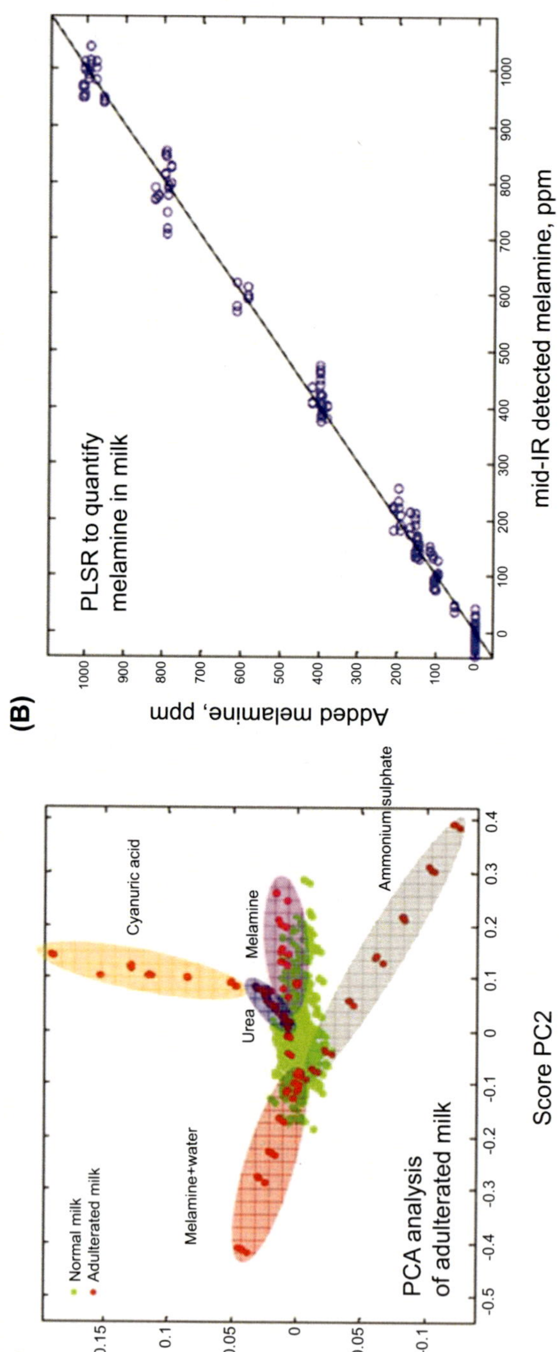

Figure 4.4 (A) Unsupervised classification analysis (PCA) of milk powders contaminated with melamine and related N-containing agents and (B) quantitative analyses (PLSR) of melamine concentration in milk samples by MIR spectroscopy.
Modified from FOSS Analytical. 2009. Food Protein Workshop: Developing a Toolbox of Analytical Solutions to Address Adulteration. Possibilities of FTIR and NIR for the Detection of Adulteration in Food and Feed. Maryland USP Meeting Center, USP Headquarters, Rockville. June 17, 2009 6a. Breakout Session A.

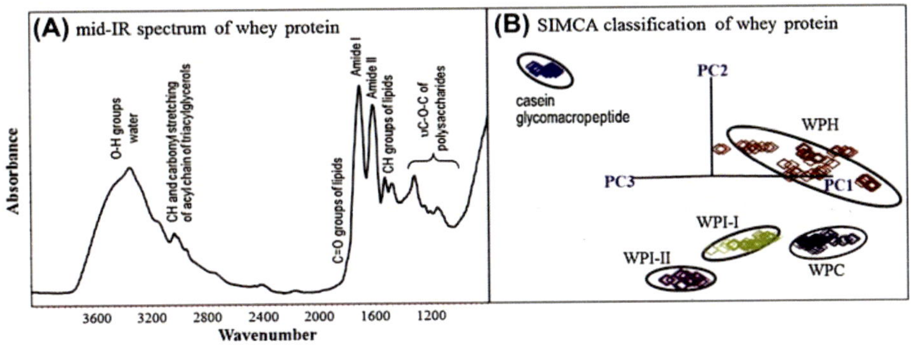

Figure 4.5 (A) Mid-infrared (MIR) spectrum of whey protein concentrate and (B) soft independent modeling of class analogy (SIMCA) classification of whey protein powders. Modified from Wang, T., Tan, S.Y., Mutilangi, W., Aykas, D.P., Rodriguez-Saona, L.E., 2015. Authentication of whey protein powders by portable mid-infrared spectrometers combined with pattern recognition analysis. Journal of Food Science 80 (10), C2111–C2116.

investigation of any systematic variation present in the samples (Wold et al., 1983; De Maesschalck et al., 1999; Lavine, 2000). The analysis generates a classification model that differentiates samples based on their group identification. A probability boundary of 95% confidence level is defined for each class based on the maximum residuals of the calibration samples from that group (Fig. 4.5). Each class is modeled by a number of PCs assessed by cross-validation. SIMCA is particularly useful when analyzing data sets with many classes. Comparison of loadings and scores plots supports investigations in terms of the relationship between important variables that can be specific to the group of interest.

Partial Least Squares Discriminant Analysis (PLS-DA) is a classification algorithm that combines the properties of PLS regression with discriminant analysis (Ballabio and Consonni, 2013). PLS-DA optimizes separation between different groups of samples that is accomplished by linking two data matrices X (ie, spectra) and Y (ie, groups) and maximizing the covariance between the independent and dependent variable of highly multidimensional data by finding a linear subspace of the explanatory variables. This new subspace permits the prediction of the Y variable based on a reduced number of factors (PLS latent variables) (Gromski et al., 2015).

PLS-DA handles highly collinear and noisy data and provides several statistics (loading weights and regression coefficients) that can be used to identify the most important variables associated with the classification. This technique provides a visual interpretation of complex data sets illustrating the separation between different groups. The advantage of PLS-DA is that the main sources of variability in the data set are modeled by the so-called latent variables (LVs), therefore, in the associated scores and loadings, making easy the visualization and understanding of data structure and relations in the data set (Chen et al., 2015). The model constructed with the training data set can be used to assign unknown samples to a previously defined class based on its measured spectrum. PLS-DA uses the appropriate number of LVs, that is, linear combinations of the original variables, to maximize the discrimination between the classes. The number of LVs can be optimized by the criterion of lowest prediction error in cross-validation (Chen et al., 2015).

Partial Least Squares Regression (PLSR) is a multivariate method that analyzes data that are strongly collinear (correlated), noisy, and multidimensional (X-variables) (Wold et al., 2001). PLSR combines the features of PCA and multiple linear regression to compress a large number of variables into a few latent variables (PLS factors) by attempting to explain the maximum variance in both the spectra and reference data sets in the form of a linear equation (Karoui and De Baerdemaeker, 2007). The selection of reference data and spectral regions plays an important role in the creation of PLSR quantification models (Fig. 4.4). It is particularly useful when the number of independent variables (wavelengths) is much larger than that of dependent variables (reference value).

A very important advantage of PLSR is that it takes the error into account both in the concentration measured by the reference method and the spectra collected by infrared spectrometers. It does not assume that the concentrations used as reference numbers are error-free since the potential for error in sample preparation, dilutions, weighing, etc. can be significant (Brereton, 2000). Thus, PLSR is becoming a standard tool for modeling correlated relationships between multivariate measurements (Dejong, 1993). The robustness of a model is determined by the variance included in the model and the number of samples—in both cases, higher levels will yield a more robust model. Calibration models may be internally validated using full cross-validation (CV) and externally validated with an independent validation set, eg, using approximately 25% of the samples to validate the prediction performance of the models.

4.4 Screening Capabilities of Vibrational Spectroscopy to Detect Adulteration in Foods

New and challenging risks have emerged as food supply chains have become increasingly global and complex (GMA, 2010; Jackson, 2009). One of the risks gaining attention from industry, governments, and standards-setting organizations is fraud conducted for economic gain by food producers, manufacturers, processors, distributors, or retailers. Food fraud is the deliberate substitution, addition, tampering, or misrepresentation of food, food ingredients, or food packaging, or false or misleading statements made about a product for economic gain (Spink, 2011). Adulteration criminals engineer fraudulent ingredients specifically to evade existing quality assurance (QA) and quality control (QC) systems implemented by purchasers, including GMP testing and hazard analysis and critical control points (HACCP) plans (Moore et al., 2012). Consequently, only the criminal knows how the food ingredient has been manipulated but generally lacks the expertise to assess whether such a manipulation poses any toxicological or hygienic risks to the purchaser or the consumer (Moore et al., 2012). Counterfeiters target high-value products, including those with a strong brand name, resulting in potentially serious counterfeit with ingredients unlikely to have been subjected to the rigorous quality control normally applied to food products.

Moore et al. (2012) summarized results from the US Pharmacopeial Convention's Food Chemicals Codex, including 1000 records with analytical methods collected from 677 references showing that olive oil, milk, honey, and saffron were the most common targets for adulteration reported in scholarly journals. Potentially harmful issues identified include spices diluted with lead chromate and lead tetraoxide, substitution of Chinese star anise with toxic Japanese star anise, and melamine adulteration of high-protein-content foods (Table 4.2).

The risk of international incidents is becoming greater as more major manufacturing companies adopt strategies of global branding, or extend brand names across product ranges. Due to the global nature of the food supply, adulteration continues to be an area of concern for regulatory agencies, the food industry, and consumers. Although there is a wide range of food products and risks, food ingredients and additives present a unique risk because they are used in so many food products throughout the supply chain (Moore et al., 2012). The development and validation of new and increasingly sophisticated techniques for the authentication and analysis of foods and their implementation as part of quality control programs and risk-management systems will

Table 4.2 Top Ingredients in Scholarly Records Data Set Associated With Fraud and Economically Motivated Adulteration From 1980 to 2010

Ingredient	Total Number of Records of Adulteration	Percentage of Total Record
Olive oil	167	16
Milk	143	14
Honey	71	7
Saffron (*Crocus sativus* L.)	57	5
Orange juice	43	4
Coffee	34	3
Apple juice	20	2
Grape wine (*Vitis vinifera*)	16	2
Maple syrup	16	2
Vanilla extract	16	2

Adapted from Moore, J.C., Spink, J., Lipp, M., 2012. Development and application of a database of food ingredient fraud and economically motivated adulteration from 1980 to 2010. Journal of Food Science 77 (4), R118–R126.

enable enhanced surveillance of the food supply to prevent economically motivated food fraud.

Economically motivated adulteration can have serious consequences for public health. In 1981, street vendors in Spain sold colza oil (lubricant for machinery) to customers as "olive oil" (NY Times, 1987). The toxic compounds derived during the refinement process of colza oil caused toxic oil syndrome, a musculoskeletal disease that killed over 600 people in Spain (WHO, 2004). In 2008, milk and infant formula were adulterated with melamine resulting in $18 billion in fines, recalls, and reparations, and physical harm with 300,000 people becoming ill, more than 50,000 infant hospitalizations and six infant deaths (Guan, 2009). By July 2010, Chinese authorities were still reporting seizures from melamine-contaminated dairy products as the result of illegal reuse of material from the 2008 adulterations (Guan, 2010).

Rapid and cost-effective techniques are required for effective surveillance of our food supply to avoid toxic contamination and acts of economic adulteration, counterfeiting, terror, vandalism, or poor manufacturing practices. Analytical methods for determining whether a raw material is adulterated or contaminated are time consuming and labor intensive. An ideal sensor would be capable of detecting and identifying multiple contaminants in real or near-real time, operate in an autonomous, unattended fashion for an extended period of time, would not require frequent maintenance, would have a low overall life cycle cost and low false alarm rates (Kalasinsky et al., 2007). Vibrational spectroscopy-based detection can address a number of limitations of more conventional strategies and may become an optimal threat detection and identification system technology (Ellis et al., 2012). Vibrational spectroscopy (NIR, MIR, and Raman) in combination with supervised pattern recognition techniques offer reproducible, rapid (<1 min), and nondestructive screening of large volumes of food products, can be automated, and reduce the need for solvents and toxic reagents associated with wet chemical methods and traditional analysis. Infrared spectroscopy may differentiate minor target components in the food matrix (Rodriguez-Saona and Allendorf, 2011). Furthermore, real-time capabilities of this technology may be improved through complementary portable NIR, IR, and Raman analysis. In the following section, we present some reports describing the use of vibrational spectroscopy for authentication (Table 4.3) and adulteration (Table 4.4) of foods.

4.4.1 Monitoring Authenticity and Adulteration of Milk Products

MIR and NIR have been used to determine the typical spectral profiles of milk and dairy products to use as a tool for monitoring the authenticity of these commodities (Table 4.3). Milk adulteration (Table 4.4) by addition of water, neutralizers, salt, sugar, high solid contents, whey, or hydrogen peroxide (Kartheek et al., 2011) is done either for financial gain or lack of proper hygienic conditions of processing, storing, transportation, and marketing and could bring economic problems and health concerns. NIR spectroscopy combined with a modified support vector machine has shown success for quantifying whey, starch, and sucrose adulterants in milk powder (Borin et al.,

Table 4.3 Vibrational Spectroscopy Combined With Multivariate Analysis to Authenticate Various Foods

Sample	Materials Used	Type	Method	Multivariate Analysis	(%) Correct Classification	References
Fruits and Fruit Products						
Coffee	Arabica ($n = 60$), Robusta ($n = 54$)	VA	NIR	PCA-LDA	87 (lyophilized); 95 (beverage)	Downey and Boussion (1996)
	Arabica ($n = 29$), Robusta ($n = 27$)	VA	MIR, NIR	PCA-FDA	100	Downey et al. (1997)
	Freeze-dried Arabica ($n = 29$) Robusta ($n = 23$)	VA	MIR DRIFT	PCA-LDA	98	Briandet et al. (1996a,b)
Concord grape juice	Grapes (4 varieties, 17 lots)	AU	MIR ATR 3-Reflect	SIMCA	100	Snyder et al. (2014)
Pomegranate juice	Grape juice (2–14% v/v)	AU	MIR	SIMCA	98	Vardin et al. (2008)
Apple juice	Authentic ($n = 224$), adulterated with sugar solutions ($n = 480$)	AU	MIR ATR	k-NN, PLS dummy variable	82–97	Kelly and Downey (2005)
Mango juice	Sucrose solutions ($n = 165$)	AU	MIR ATR	PLS-DA	100	Jha and Gunasekaran (2010)
Multiple juices	Cranberry, Concord grape, blueberry, plum apple	AU	MIR ATR 3-Reflect	SIMCA	100	He et al. (2007)
Orange juice	Orange pulp wash, grapefruit juice and sugar/acid mix	AU	NIR reflectance	PCA-FDA	94 at >50 g/kg	Twomey et al. (1995)

Continued

Table 4.3 Vibrational Spectroscopy Combined With Multivariate Analysis to Authenticate Various Foods—cont'd

Sample	Materials Used	Type	Method	Multivariate Analysis	(%) Correct Classification	References
Strawberry	Jams, wide range of commercial fruit types ($n = 36$)	VA	MIR DRIFT & HATR	PCA/PLS -DA	91–98 (PLSDA)	Defernez and Wilson (1995)
Raspberry	Purees, raspberry, apple, blackcurrant, blackberry, plum, cherry, apricot, grape ($n = 692$)	VA	MIR	PLS dummy variable	94	Holland et al. (1998)
	Blackberry, plum, apple, strawberry, blackcurrant, apricot, cherry ($n = 911$)	VA	MIR ATR	PLS dummy variable	95	Kemsley et al. (1996)
Wine	Riesling ($n = 144$) and Chardonnay ($n = 125$)	VA	Vis-NIR	DPLS	100 (Riesling) 97 (Chardonnay)	Cozzolino et al. (2003)
	Rias Baixas ($n = 19$) and Ribeira Sacra ($n = 20$)	DO	Vis-NIR	SVM and LDA	100 (LDA)	Martelo-Vidal and Vazquez (2014)
Oils						
Camellia oil	Pure ($n = 166$) and nonpure ($n = 17$)	AU	FT-NIR transflectance	HCA, PCA-DA, RBFNN	98	Li et al. (2012)
Extra virgin olive oil	Hazelnut, sunflower, corn, corn germ, soybean ($n = 30$)	AU	MIR transmittance	LDA	100	Lerma-Garcia et al. (2010)

	Greece, Italy, Portugal, Spain ($n = 60$)	VA	MIR ATR	PLS-DA, GA-LDA	96–100	Tapp et al. (2003)
	16 other vegetable oils ($n = 150$)	AU	MIR ATR	LDA, ANN	100 (LDA)	Marigheto et al. (1998)
	Refined olive oils	AU	MIR ATR	PCA-DA	75–99	Lai et al. (1994)
	Canola, walnut, sunflower, soybean, peanut, corn, sesame oils	AU	MIR ATR	PCA-DA	100 at >20 mg/L	Tay et al. (2002)
	Peanut oil ($n = 192$)	AU	MIR ATR	LDA	88.3%	Vasconcelos et al. (2015)
Hazelnut oil	Extra virgin olive oil	AU	MIR ATR	PLS-DA	20	Ozen and Mauer (2002)
Shacha Inchi oil	Corn, canola, flax, cottonseed, sunflower, high oleic sunflower and olive ($n = 21$)	AU	MIR ATR 3-Reflect	SIMCA, PLS	94–100	Maurer et al. (2012)
Honey and Milk Products						
Honey	Artisanal Irish honey ($n = 580$)	AU	MIR	SIMCA	92	Kelly et al. (2006)
	Unifloral ($n = 11$) and polyfloral ($n = 411$) types	BO	MIR ATR	PCA-LDA	92–100	Ruoff et al. (2006)
	Unifloral ($n = 8$) and polyfloral ($n = 364$) types	BO	FT-NIR	PCA-LDA	94–100	Ruoff et al. (2006)
	Unifloral ($n = 130$)	BO	MIR ATR	PCA-SVM	98.6	Lenhardt et al. (2014)

Continued

Table 4.3 Vibrational Spectroscopy Combined With Multivariate Analysis to Authenticate Various Foods—cont'd

Sample	Materials Used	Type	Method	Multivariate Analysis	(%) Correct Classification	References
Milk	Water, whey, hydrogen peroxide, urea, and synthetic milk	AU	MIR ATR	SIMCA	100 at >3% v/v	Santos et al. (2013)
	Water and whey ($n = 90$, 1–97% v/v)	AU	NIR reflectance	SIMCA, PLS-DA	87–97 at >11%	Kasemsumran et al. (2007)
	Melamine, urea, ammonium nitrate ($n = 813$)	AU	NIR transflectance	Non-linear methods	89–97	Zhang et al. (2014)
	Urea, melamine, tetracycline, and glucose (0.01–0.3 g/L)	AU	(2D) IR correlation spectroscopy	PLS-DA	92.5	Yang et al. (2013)
	Melamine	AU	NIR	LS-SVM, PLS-DA	100 at >1 ppm	Lu et al. (2009)
Organic bovine butter	Conventional bovine butter	AU	MIR ATR	SIMCA	100	Pujolras et al. (2015)
Whey protein	Whey protein concentrate, isolate and hydrolyzate powders ($n = 30$)	AU	MIR ATR	SIMCA	95	Wang et al. (2015)

ATR, Attenuated total reflectance; *AU*, authentication; *BO*, botanical origin; *DO*, designation of origin; *DPLS*, discriminant partial least squares; *DRIFT*, diffuse reflection; *FDA*, functional data analysis; *FT*, Fourier transform; *GA-LDA*, genetic algorithm linear discriminant analysis; *HATR*, horizontal ATR accessory; *MIR*, middle infrared spectroscopy; *NIR*, Fourier transform near infrared spectroscopy; *RBFNN*, radial basis function neural network; *VA*, varietal authentication; *Vis-NIR*, visible near infrared spectroscopy. Abbreviations used under multivariate analysis (ANN, k-NN, LDA, PCA, PLS-DA, SIMCA, SVM) are defined in Table 4.1.

Table 4.4 Vibrational Spectroscopy Combined With Multivariate Analysis to Determine Presence of Specific Adulterants in Various Foods

Sample	Type of Adulterant	Method	Multivariate Analysis	LOD (%)	References
Fruit and Fruit Products					
Apple juice	Sugar solutions, HFCS	NIR	PLSR	9.5 (HFCS)–18.5 (sugar mix)	León et al. (2005)
	Authentic ($n = 224$), adulterated with sugar solutions ($n = 480$)	MIR ATR	PLSR	10	Kelly and Downey (2005)
Coffee	Arabica, Robusta blends ($n = 18$)	MIR	PLSR	1.2	Briandet et al. (1996a,b)
Concord grape juice	Niagara, red grape and white grape blends ($n = 64$)	MIR ATR	PLSR	5	Snyder et al. (2014)
Raspberry purees	Apple, strawberry, plum and sugar solutions ($n = 112$)	MIR ATR	PLSR	20	Kemsley et al. (1996)
Strawberry fruit	Apple, plum, sugar solutions, red grape and rhubarb	MIR	PLSR	10	Holland et al. (1998)
Oils					
Hazelnut oil	Sunflower oils (2–10% v/v)	MIR ATR	PLSR	2	Ozen and Mauer (2002)

Continued

Table 4.4 Vibrational Spectroscopy Combined With Multivariate Analysis to Determine Presence of Specific Adulterants in Various Foods—cont'd

Sample	Type of Adulterant	Method	Multivariate Analysis	LOD (%)	References
Extra virgin olive oil	Sunflower oil ($n = 138$)	Vis-NIR	PLSR	SEP: 0.8	Downey et al. (2006)
	High oleic sunflower, pomace olive, high linoleic sunflower, canola and hazelnut oils ($n = 94$)	MIR ATR	PLSR	SEP: 1 (Canola)-20 (Hazelnut)	Maggio et al. (2010)
	peanut oil ($n = 192$)	MIR ATR	PCR, PLSR	0.5 v/v	Vasconcelos et al. (2015)
	Soybean, sunflower, corn, walnut and hazelnut oil ($n = 525$)	NIR transmittance	PLSR	0.6–1.3 v/v	Christy et al. (2004)
	Sunflower, soybean, sesame, corn oils	MIR transmittance	A_{3006}/A_{2925}	6 (sun, soy), 9 (corn, sesame)	Vlachos et al. (2006)
	Binary blends of corn, sunflower, rapeseed and cottonseed oils	MIR HATR	PLSR	SEP: 1.4; LOD 5%	Gurdeniz and Ozen (2009)
	Palm oils (1–50% w/w)	MIR ATR multiple bounce	PLSR, PCR	0.29 (PLSR); 0.37 (PCR)	Rohman and Che Man (2010)
	Refined olive and walnut oils ($n = 44$; 0–22% w/w)	MIR ATR 10 reflections	PLSR	SEP: 1.3	Lai et al. (1995)

	Soybean, sunflower, corn. canola, hazelnut, high oleic safflower, peanut, palm and refined olive oils	FT-NIR transmittance	PLS1	SECV: 0.9 (high linoleic acid), 2.2 (high oleic acid), 1 (palm olein), 3.7 (refined olive)	Azizian et al. (2015)
Milk Products					
Butter	Beef fat	MIR ATR	PLS	2.4	Nurrulhidayah et al. (2013a)
	Chicken fat	ATR 12 Reflection	PLS	4.3	Nurrulhidayah et al. (2013b)
Milk	Melamine in infant formula	MIR ATR DRIFT, NIR	PLSR	1 ppm	Mauer et al. (2009)
	Melamine in milk	MIR, NIR	Non-linear regression	0.76 ± 0.11 ppm	Balabin and Smirnov (2011)
		MIR ATR	PLSR	2.5 ppm, LOQ 15 ppm	Jawaid et al. (2013)

ATR, Attenuated total reflectance; *DRIFT*, diffuse reflection; *FT*, Fourier transform; *HATR*, horizontal ATR accessory; *HFCS*, high-fructose corn syrup; *LS-SVM*, least squares support vector machines; *LOD*, limit of detection; *LOQ*, limit of quantitation; *MIR*, middle infrared spectroscopy; *NIR*, near infrared spectroscopy; *SECV*, standard error of cross-validation; *SEP*, standard error of prediction; *v/v*, volume/volume. Abbreviations used under multivariate analysis (PCA, PCR, PLSR) are defined in Table 4.1.

2006) and addition of aqueous solutions of dextrin or starch containing pseudoproteins (melamine, urea, or ammonium nitrate) to liquid cow milk (Zhang et al., 2014), but only at levels of adulteration greater than 5% (Alves da Rocha et al., 2015).

The fingerprinting characteristics of MIR spectra allowed for detecting whey, urea, and hydrogen peroxide in liquid milk, exhibiting well-separated clusters between control and adulterated milk samples, clustering samples according to the type of adulterant used in the milk-spiking process (Santos et al., 2013). Whey protein added to milk as an inexpensive protein source is difficult to detect due to structural similarities to other milk proteins. Mendenhall and Brown (1991) examined 135 nonfat dry milk samples containing various concentrations of WPC (1.3–33% w/w) and reported a strong correlation ($r^2 > 0.99$) between the actual concentrations and predicted values by MIR combined with PLSR; a detection limit was identified as 5.6% w/w whey protein concentrate. Similarly, FT-Raman spectroscopy using a 1064-nm beam from a Nd:YAG laser and combined with PLS-DA correctly classified 100% of adulterated milk powder samples by the addition of whey (1–40% w/w) (Almeida et al., 2011).

Van der Ven et al. (2002) showed that MIR spectra correlated to various functional properties of whey and casein hydrolysates, and Wang et al. (2015) characterized whey protein powders (WPC, WPI, and WPH) based on their unique infrared profile associated with functional group vibrations in the 1800–900 cm^{-1} wavenumber range (Fig. 4.5). Pattern recognition analysis (SIMCA) showed well-separated clustering among the powder samples (Fig. 4.5) whose orientation in the 3D space, defined by using the first 3 PCs, correlated with whey protein type. Furthermore, the WPI clusters were separated depending on the source of whey (acid or sweet), while samples of casein glycomacropeptide (GMP) were distinguished from the whey protein powders (Wang et al., 2015). Efforts have also been directed to predict whey protein fractions such as α-lactalbumin and β-lactoglobulin using MIR spectra; however, the authors indicated that the results might not be accurate when variation of genetic levels was involved (De Marchi et al., 2010; Rutten et al., 2011).

Melamine, an industrial chemical, was intentionally added to foods to boost apparent protein content; however, it forms extremely insoluble crystals (Perdigao and Champness, 2006) in animal kidneys, leading to acute renal failure. These contamination incidents (2007, 2008) prompted the US Food and Drug Administration (FDA) and other regulatory agencies to develop analytical tools to monitor food ingredients for melamine and cyanuric acid. FDA broadened its domestic and import sampling and testing of dairy ingredients and products from Chinese sources and warned consumers about certain products with possible melamine contamination (Jackson, 2009). NIR spectroscopy has been reported as a rapid method for detecting melamine in milk powder with detection limits of 75–100 ppm (Foss, 2009). The technique has shown potential as a tool for screening adulteration in milk (Fig. 4.4) with unspecific adulteration detection levels at 250–500 ppm (Foss, 2009). In addition, IR spectroscopy has been reported as a rapid method for detecting pure melamine in milk powder with detection limits <1 ppm (Balabin and Smirnov, 2011; Lu et al., 2009; Mauer et al., 2009). Jawaid et al. (2013) reported LOD and LOQ of 2.5 ppm and 15 ppm, respectively, for the detection of melamine in both freeze-dried and powdered milk using an ATR-MIR technique. Although these authors report detection limits of 1 ppm, caution would be advised because these calibrations were done by serial dilutions of the contaminant (melamine) in powders that can result in the introduction of artifacts (nonrandom variations such as moisture changes and irregular distribution of the contaminant, among others) and they would not likely resemble samples in a processing plant. Furthermore, there is no information on loadings weights and the models were not validated with an independent sample set to demonstrate the reliability of the methods. Finally, surface-enhanced Raman scattering using gold nanoparticles has also shown promise for detection melamine in liquid milk displaying good linearity ($R^2 = 0.99$) in the concentration range of 0.31−5.0 mg/L in milk with a limit of detection of 0.17 mg/L and requiring a 30-min extraction procedure (Giovannozzi et al., 2014).

The potential of a Klarite SERS-active substrate to detect added melamine content in various food matrices gave LOD of SERS of 0.033 μg/mL, lower than that of HPLC (1 μg/mL) and showed a unique peak at 682 cm^{-1} assigned to the in-plane deformation of the triazine ring in melamine molecules (Lin et al., 2008). Mecker et al. (2012) detected melamine content in a wide variety of solid matrices, including milk powder, infant formula, lactose, povidone, whey protein, wheat bran, and wheat gluten, using a portable Raman spectrometer employing AuNPs agglomerates. These authors reported LODs ranging from 100 to 200 μg/L depending on the sample matrix. Betz et al. (2012) determined the potential for detecting melamine in infant formula by SERS on low-cost surfaces of Cu tape and coin, reporting detection to the 5 ppb level. A strong peak between 676 and 690 cm^{-1} was used to identify melamine contamination.

4.4.2 Monitoring Authenticity and Adulteration of Fruits and Fruit Juices

Authentication of fruit juices (Table 4.3) is a major challenge for an industry that is fast growing and expanding. Traditional methods to monitor authenticity such as HPLC, GC, or sensory methods are time consuming and require well-trained personnel. Giusti et al. (2011) summarized the applications of infrared and chemometrics for monitoring the authenticity of fruit juices. Infrared technology showed potential in detection of foreign materials, differentiation of different juice commodities, or even to evaluate geographical origin of a juice.

Adulteration of fruit juice (Table 4.4) by dilution with water, addition of sugars (cane and beet sucrose, invert or medium invert syrup, high-fructose corn syrup, and hydrolyzed inulin syrup), pulp wash solids, or a less-expensive fruit juice is a problem because the price of sugar and syrups is significantly cheaper than the juice itself. Detecting adulteration in juices is challenging because the similarity in compositional profiles of commercial sweeteners available and the natural variation in authentic samples, including differences in species, maturity, climate, growing regions, seasons, processing, and storage conditions (Kelly and Downey, 2005). An ATR-IR sampling approach combined with k-nearest neighbors and discriminant PLS using a sample set of 224 authentic apple juices and 480 adulterated (partially inverted cane syrup, beet sucrose, high-fructose corn syrup, and a synthetic solution of fructose, glucose, and sucrose at levels ranging from 10% to 40% w/w) gave a correct classification rate of 82–96% depending on the adulterant type and level of adulteration (Kelly and Downey, 2005). Similar results were reported using NIR transflectance spectroscopy and discriminant PLS with accuracy rates of 91–100% for adulterated apple juice (León et al., 2005). Both ATR-IR and NIR methods were considered to show promise as a rapid-screening technique for the detection of a broad range of potential adulterants in apple juice.

Pomegranate juice is in high demand and short supply, leading to incentives to extend limited supplies by addition of other juices, sugars, and small amounts of deeply colored fruit juices such as blackcurrant or aronia juice to imitate the color (Zhang et al., 2009). Zhang et al. (2009) surveyed 45 commercial juices from 23 different manufacturers purchased at local grocery stores and reported that only ~35% qualified as authentic pomegranate juice. Due to the high demand for and short supply of pomegranate juice, adulteration is typically carried out to extend limited supplies by addition of cheaper juices or to mask the astringent taste and uncharacteristically pale color of low-quality juice. ATR spectroscopy and chemometric techniques detected adulteration of pomegranate juice concentrate with grape juice concentrate (2–14% v/v) using the 1780–1685 cm^{-1} region, which corresponds to C=O stretching (Vardin et al., 2008).

He et al. (2007) reported that the phenolic compounds provided signature-like spectral information improving the classification modeling power over the whole juice or sugar-rich fraction models allowing for the differentiation of juices with different origins. The ATR technique assisted by a simple fractionation and chemometrics provided a promising analytical method for the assurance of juice quality and authenticity (He et al., 2007). Similar to pomegranate juice, there is an increased market demand for Concord grape products spurred by positive health-benefit news, resulting in higher prices for Concord concentrate. However, grapes of other varieties have vastly different prices, making juice manufacturers vulnerable to fraudulent behavior from suppliers and competitors. A simple solid-phase extraction step, targeted at isolating the phenolic fraction, provided signature-like spectral information allowing prediction of the content of Concord grape juice in a grape juice blend at levels >5% w/w using attenuated total reflectance infrared spectroscopy and chemometrics (Snyder et al., 2014).

4.4.3 Monitoring Authenticity and Adulteration of Oils and Fats

An important field of application of vibrational spectroscopy has been the detection of adulteration in vegetable oils, especially extra virgin olive oil (EVOO). A review by Nunes (2014) summarizes the applications of vibrational spectroscopy and chemometrics to assess authenticity and adulteration of edible oils and fats. We will further discuss the efforts on applications of vibrational spectroscopy for authentication (Table 4.3) and detection of adulteration (Table 4.4) of EVOO and cocoa butter.

4.4.3.1 Extra Virgin Olive Oil

A report issued by the UC Davis Olive Center in 2010 showed that 69% of imported olive oils labeled as "extra virgin" failed to meet the international standard for EVOO (Frankel et al., 2011). The high price of extra virgin olive oil and its reputation as a healthy and delectable oil makes it a preferred target for fraudsters. Adulteration may take place by deliberate mislabeling of less expensive olive oil categories or by the addition of less-expensive edible oils to virgin olive oil for the purpose of financial gain (Aparicio et al., 2013).

NIR spectroscopy has been evaluated for quantification of adulterants in EVOO (Table 4.4). Authentication of virgin olive oil by geographical origin using NIR and pattern recognition analysis (ANNs and PLS-DA) showed promising results in spite of the similarity of cultivar compositions between different denominations of origin (Bertran, 2000; Galtier et al., 2007). NIR combined with SIMCA successfully classified EVOO from eastern Mediterranean countries on the basis of their geographical origin and discriminated between authentic EVOO and oils adulterated with sunflower oil at levels as low as 1% w/w (Downey et al., 2002).

The ability of NIR and discriminant analysis to identify adulteration of extra virgin olive oil was reported by Wesley et al. (1996), predicting adulteration by sunflower oil, rapeseed oil, and soybean oil in 90% of the cases; PLS regression could predict levels of adulteration with a standard error of performance of ±2.8%. Christy et al. (2004) developed an NIR procedure for the classification and quantification of the adulteration of pure olive oil by soybean, sunflower, corn, walnut, and hazelnut oils predicting the adulterants in olive oil with error limits ranging from 0.6% (corn) to 1.3% (sunflower) w/w. Furthermore, their PCA models classified unknown adulterated olive oil mixtures with almost 100% certainty (Christy et al., 2004). More recently, Azizian et al. (2015) described a rapid Fourier transform near infrared (FT-NIR) spectroscopic procedure combined with PLSR to screen for the authenticity of EVOOs and to determine the kind and amount of an adulterant in EVOO based on the relative intensities of two unique carbonyl overtone absorptions attributed to volatile (5280 cm^{-1}) and nonvolatile (5180 cm^{-1}) components.

The fingerprinting characteristics of MIR have shown promise for the authentication (Table 4.3) and quantitation of adulteration (Table 4.4) of pure olive oils. Lai et al. (1995) estimated the level of adulteration of olive oil by refined olive oil (SEP 0.9% w/w) and walnut oil (SEP 0.7% w/w) using MIR equipped with an ATR accessory and coupled with PLS regression. Vlachos et al. (2006) used a transmittance MIR approach to determine extra virgin olive oil adulteration with lower-priced vegetable oils (sunflower, soybean, sesame, corn oils) by monitoring the band shift observed at 3009 cm^{-1} assigned to the C—H stretching vibration of the *cis*-double bond. Internal reflection MIR spectroscopy and chemometrics were used by de la Mata et al. (2012) to distinguish between various blends of olive oils, while Bendini et al. (2007) investigated the capability to discriminate virgin olive oils based on geographic origin. Other MIR studies have included authentication of EVOO (Gurdeniz and Ozen, 2009; Lerma-Garcia et al., 2010; Rohman et al., 2014) and the determination of sunflower oils (Küpper et al., 2001; Tay et al., 2002), soybean and sunflower oils

(Oussama et al., 2012), hazelnut oil (Groselj et al., 2008), and palm oil (Rohman and Che Man, 2010) as adulterants in extra virgin olive oil. Finally, Sun et al. (2015) evaluated the application of FT-IR and supervised locally linear embedding (SLLE) methods on a total of 300 oil samples including 40 EVOO, 5 pure camellia oil, 5 soybean oils, 5 sunflower oils, 5 corn oils, and 240 mixed oil samples adulterated at levels ranging from 1% to 90% w/w. Results from the nearest centroid classification with SLLE models showed misclassification rates of 3.42%, while PCA was inadequate in detecting adulteration because of severe overlapping among the different types of oil samples (Sun et al., 2015).

Yang and Irudayaraj (2001) compared NIR, MIR, and FT-Raman (1064-nm laser) spectroscopic techniques to quantify the amount of olive pomace oil adulteration in extra virgin olive oil reporting that all techniques gave high correlation ($R^2 > 0.99$), but Raman had a lower standard error of prediction of 1.7% w/w for validation samples than NIR and MIR models (SEP of 3.3% w/w).

4.4.3.2 Cocoa Butter

According to the European Chocolate Directive (2000/36/EC), the addition of up to 5% of vegetable fats other than cocoa butter, the so-called cocoa butter equivalents, is allowed in chocolate products. The permitted fats are palm oil, illipe, sal, shea, kokum gurgi, and mango kernel. MIR spectroscopy has been used for the rapid identification of pure cocoa butter and of their mixtures with other vegetable fats (Goodacre and Anklam, 2001). Samples consisted of pure cocoa butter from various geographical origins, cocoa butter equivalents, and mixtures of cocoa butter with cocoa butter equivalents at various concentrations (5–20% w/w). Classification models based on canonical variate analysis (CVA) were able to distinguish between cocoa butter mixed with cocoa butter equivalents at the 10% and 20% w/w levels. MIR showed great potential as a rapid-screening method for detection of cocoa butter adulteration, however, a single global model based on PLS was not able to accurately predict the level of addition (Goodacre and Anklam, 2001).

ATR-IR spectroscopy and PLS regression detected the presence of lard (0–15% w/w) in chocolate formulations with a standard error of cross-validation of 1.3% w/w and CV of 5.2% w/w (Che Man et al., 2005). Maurer and Rodriguez-Saona (2013) reported the application of ATR-MIR spectroscopy in combination with multivariate analysis (SIMCA and PLSR) as a screening tool for assuring the quality of incoming raw materials. SIMCA classified cocoa butters in distinct clusters due to the stretching vibrations of the ester (–C=O) linkage (1660–1720 cm^{-1}), but group patterns were not associated with melting characteristics. In addition, regression models ($R^2 > 0.93$) were developed for the prediction of melting characteristics and levels of major fatty acids and triacylglycerols (Maurer and Rodriguez-Saona, 2013). Fig. 4.6A shows the SIMCA clustering by using ATR MIR spectra for pure cocoa butter and some potential adulterants, displaying the spectral similarities of palm oil and lard with cocoa butter while coconut oil, cottonseed oil, and mainly mineral oil showed marked differences in spectral profile (unpublished data). Furthermore, Fig. 4.6B shows that SIMCA pattern recognition analysis successfully discriminated between pure cocoa butter and the adulterated samples at levels above 1% w/w (unpublished data).

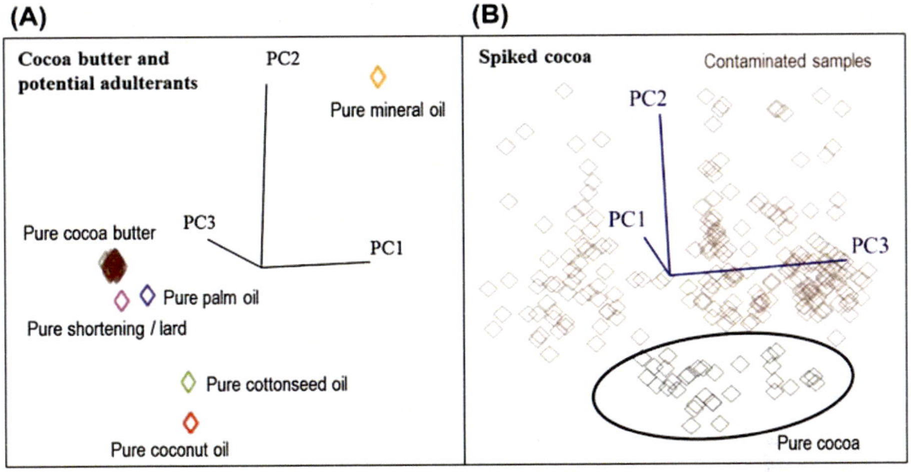

Figure 4.6 (A) Soft independent analysis of class analogy (SIMCA) projection plot for the first three principal components for classification of pure cocoa butter and pure adulterants including palm oil, lard, cottonseed oil, coconut oil, and mineral oil and (B) spiked cocoa butter with adulterants at levels ranging from 1% to 10% w/w (unpublished data).

4.4.4 Unintentional Contaminants

Vibrational spectroscopy has also shown potential for the detection of food contaminants and we will focus this review on research pertaining to detection of mycotoxins, acrylamide, and pesticides in food matrices. Mycotoxins account annually for millions of dollars in losses worldwide, in condemned agricultural products and in animal and human health (CAST, 2003). The surveillance of mycotoxin contamination of human foods by low-tech and simple methods could have a significant effect on public health in low-income countries, leading to improved economic sustainability of the industry, enhanced food safety efforts, and enhanced international trade efforts (Murphy et al., 2006). A review by McMullin et al. (2015) summarizes the advancements in IR-spectroscopic approaches for the determination of fungal-derived contaminations in food crops.

4.4.4.1 Mycotoxins

Most publications focus on NIR spectroscopy because it offers higher-sampling fields, depth of penetration, and opportunities for online sorting capabilities. Berardo et al. (2005) reported the feasibility of quantifying the mold infection and metabolites produced in maize grain and flours by *Fusarium verticillioides* using NIRS. Among mycotoxins, NIR detection of deoxynivalenol (DON) from *Fusarium*-damaged wheat kernels and ground wheat has been most researched (Pettersson and Aberg, 2003; De Girolamo et al., 2009; Siuda et al., 2008; Bolduan et al., 2009; Beyer et al., 2006; Dvoracek et al., 2012). FT-NIR was used for the qualitative and quantitative prediction of DON in 262 wheat samples (143 durum and 119 common) derived from 32 different varieties naturally infected by *Fusarium graminearum* or *Fusarium culmorum*. The method gave a standard error of calibration of 386 μg/kg and $r^2 = 0.7$ and resulted in 69% correct classification rate using a threshold of 300 μg/kg; however, the model failed with samples around their set DON threshold (De Girolamo, 2009). To improve the robustness of the method, De Girolamo et al. (2014) used a linear discriminant analysis (LDA) approach on 500 samples of naturally contaminated durum wheat (<50 to 16,000 μg/kg) and successfully discriminated highly contaminated wheat samples with overall classification and false compliance rates of 90% and 5%, respectively, using a cutoff of 1400 μg/kg fulfilling the requirement of the European official guidelines for screening methods.

Fernandez-Ibañez et al. (2009) evaluated the application of NIR spectroscopy and PLS-DA for rapid detection of Aflatoxin B1 in maize and barley as an analytical quality assessment tool. The most significant bands related to fungal infection were around 870–1200 nm, corresponding to NH in most amino acids and aromatic rings and structures in cell wall components (ie, phenolics) that might be interpreted as deteriorative alterations of kernels. Delwiche and Hareland (2004) identified bands ~1200 nm as the best wavelengths to use in a spectral difference model to discriminate deoxynivalenol in wheat kernels. FT-NIR spectra allowed for detecting aflatoxin in maize ($r^2 = 0.82$; SECV = 0.2) and barley ($r^2 = 0.84$; SECV = 0.18) and gave 100% correct classification for detecting aflatoxin presence at 20 ppb level using an external set of cereals (Fernandez-Ibañez et al., 2009). Their findings were better than those reported by Pearson et al. (2001) that, working in a range of 550–1700 nm, obtained more than 95% of simple corn kernels correctly classified when AFB1 content was high (>100 ppb) or low (<10 ppb); however, classification accuracy was reduced to 25% in the range between 10 and 100 ppb. Other research has reported that NIR spectroscopy could accurately predict the percentage of *F. verticillioides* infection in maize kernels and the content of ergosterol and fumosin B1 in meals (Berardo et al., 2005).

Interferometer-based instruments in the MIR range have also been evaluated for detection of mycotoxins taking advantage of their excellent signal-to-noise ratio and high spectral resolution. Fig. 4.7 shows the unique ATR MIR spectral fingerprints of mycotoxins (aflatoxin) and the ability of SIMCA to discriminate spiked peanuts at levels >1 ppm (unpublished data).

Kos et al. (2002, 2003, 2004) described the successful application of MIR spectroscopy with ATR for the detection of fungal contamination (ergosterol and deoxynivalenol; DON) in corn. Sieving of samples (100–250 μm sieve) increased repeatability of DON concentration determinations by ATR MIR spectroscopy in corn, classifying correctly 100% of the time as opposed to 79% for unsieved samples and was identified as a necessary step for increasing toxin determination accuracy (Kos et al., 2007).

4.4.4.2 Acrylamide

Another important food contaminant is acrylamide. In 2002, significant amounts of acrylamide were detected in some foods processed at high temperatures, notably in potato products, cereal foods, and coffee. Acrylamide is a known animal carcinogen

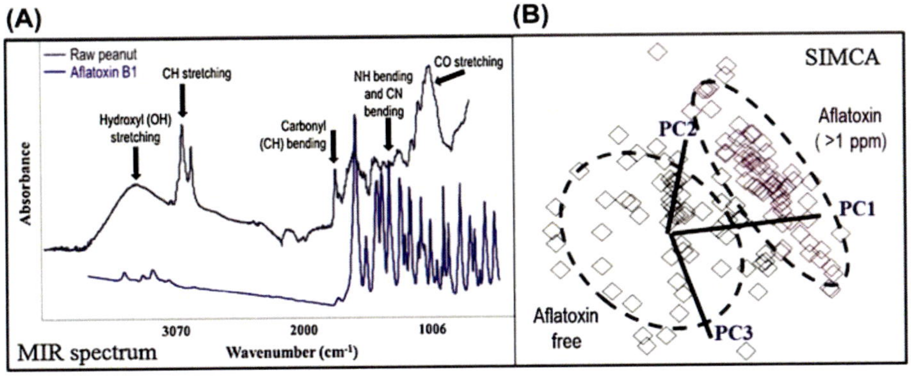

Figure 4.7 (A) Mid-infrared (MIR) spectrum of a raw peanut with the Aflatoxin B1 spectra overlaid showing the sensitivity of the fingerprint region, and (B) SIMCA class projection discriminating aflatoxin-free peanuts from peanuts containing higher than 1 ppm aflatoxin levels (unpublished data).

and human neurotoxicant, and is classified as a "probable carcinogen to humans." Since the discovery of acrylamide in foods, the American Cancer Society, the FDA, and many other organizations have recognized the need for further research on this topic (American Cancer Society, 2015). The food industry is modifying processing operations to limit acrylamide formation as consumer concerns increase as a result of new scientific evidence or federal/state regulations. However, there is a need to develop simple, low-cost method(s) to be used for routine monitoring of acrylamide in food as current analytical methods are highly sophisticated, time consuming, and labor intensive. Proposition 65, or the Safe Drinking Water and Toxic Enforcement Act of 1986, is a state law that requires businesses in California to warn citizens of significant exposures to chemicals that can potentially cause cancer or reproductive harm. Businesses can either reformulate products to lower exposures below the level deemed significant by the state or they can warn citizens of the exposures by labeling their products or posting a warning sign. Since 1990, acrylamide has been listed under Proposition 65 and both the California Attorney General and private interest groups have filed lawsuits against a number of US food manufacturers and restaurant chains, alleging that food sold by these companies contains acrylamide without warning. Since its adoption, Proposition 65 has been criticized by the food industry because of its potential impact on food labeling (Posnick, 2007).

Analysis of acrylamide in food requires the development and validation of analytical methods for screening and quantification of acrylamide and their implementation in quality control programs and risk management systems by food producers and authorities. NIR spectral analysis focused on a starch band at 1934 nm that correlated with predetermined quantities of acrylamide ($R^2 = 0.95$, prediction error of 257 ppb). The authors concluded that NIR spectral models were accurate enough for screening of acrylamide contents in processed potato chips, giving a good indirect representation of acrylamide (Segtnan et al., 2006). Evaluation of the feasibility of using online monitoring of acrylamide in chips using NIR gave a model with a $R^2 = 0.83$

and prediction error of 266 ppb (Pedreschi et al., 2010). NIR research on screening acrylamide in potato chips had focused on evaluating a single cultivar of potato tuber (Saturna) and palm oil (as frying medium) with no other ingredients and manipulating frying conditions (time and temperature) to generate varying levels of acrylamide ranging from 40 to 2987 μg/kg (Pedreschi et al., 2010; Segtnan et al., 2006). Ayvaz and Rodriguez-Saona (2015) showed that handheld and portable infrared spectrometers gave good linear correlation between the predicted acrylamide levels and actual acrylamide concentrations measured by LC-MS/MS ($rPred > 0.90$ and $SEP < 100$ μg/kg) allowing for simple and rapid screening of acrylamide in potato chips.

4.4.4.3 Pesticides

A field in which Raman spectroscopy has shown great potential is the detection of pesticides in foods. A review by Craig et al. (2013) provides an overview of the applications of SERS in monitoring food contaminants and adulteration. Current standard routine analyses for trace pesticides are based on chromatography techniques (Vongsvivut et al., 2010). Vongsvivut et al. (2010) reported a highly sensitive SERS technique for detection of organophosphorus pesticides in the ppm range using silver colloids (AgNPs). A portable Raman instrument was used to quantify the content of tricyclazole in paddy rice by SERS using the ratio of the signal at 424 cm^{-1} to the strong pyridine peak at 1035 cm^{-1} of giving a coefficient of correlation (R^2) of 0.995 and LOD of 0.002 mg/L. More interestingly, portable Raman devices have been used successfully for the detection of the organophosphate and organothiophosphate pesticides on apple skins (Xu et al., 2014).

4.5 The Future of Vibrational Spectroscopy in Food Authentication: Portable and Handheld Technology

Optical technology is rapidly developing and instruments are already available commercially as portable, handheld, and microdevices (Ellis and Goodacre, 2006) that can be used when it is not practical or economical to use the more sophisticated and costly instruments used in research laboratories. An excellent review article by Ellis et al. (2015) summarizes the developments in portable and handheld and/or remote sensor devices that are positioned for on/at-line analysis at points of vulnerability along complex food supply networks. Advantages of these sensor devices include low cost, small size, compactness, robustness, high throughput, and ease of operation for *in-field* routine analysis. Miniaturization of vibrational spectrometers into commercially available portable and handheld IR and Raman spectrometers (Table 4.5) has occurred within the last few years, partly driven by developments in microelectromechanical systems (Sorak et al., 2012).

The development of handheld and portable optical systems (Fig. 4.8) for chemical identification has incorporated the analytical precision of spectroscopy to field

Table 4.5 Commercially Available Portable and Handheld Vibrational Spectrometers

Company	Product Name	Spectral Range (per cm)	Weight (kg)	Size (cm)	Specifications
MIR					
Acroptix	FTIR-Rocket	1700–5000 or 830–4000	1.2	18 × 16 × 8	Mercury-cadmium-telluride detector
Agilent	4500	650–4500	6.8	22 × 29 × 19	Triple reflection ATR
	4300	650–4500	2.2	10 × 19 × 35	Handheld, DGTS detector
	4100 Exoscan	650–4500	3.2	17.1 × 11.9 × 22.4	Handheld, ATR, diffuse
	Cary 630	650–4000	3.6	15 × 20 × 20	ATR
Pyreos	MIR	909–1818	0.23	4.5 × 2.5 × 1	OEM interferometer or ATR
Thermo Fisher	Gemini Analyzer	650–4000	1.9	25.6 × 14.6 × 6.1	FT-IR: ATR diamond crystal, single bounce
	TruDefender	650–4500	1.3	5.3 × 19.6 × 11.2	Handheld, ATR diamond crystal
NIR					
ARCoptix	FT-NIR Rocket	3800–11,000	1.2	18 × 16 × 8	InGaAs, PDA
Avantes	AvaSpec-UV/VIS/NIR	200–1100	3.5	18.5 × 14.5 × 18.5	Dual channel broad band Channel 1: UV/VIS with replaceable slit Channel 2: NIR with replaceable slit
	AvaSpec-Mini	220–1100	0.174	9.5 × 6.8 × 2	Grating/filter
BWTEK	I-Spec nano	4500–7700	0.5	12 × 6 × 3	Diffuse reflectance
Brimrose	Luminar 5030	4300–9000	n/a	n/a	Acousto-optic tunable filter – NIR, diffuse reflection
JDSU	MicroNIR pro	6000–11,000	0.06	4.5 × 4.4	128 pixel InGaAs, PDA

Continued

Table 4.5 Commercially Available Portable and Handheld Vibrational Spectrometers—cont'd

Company	Product Name	Spectral Range (per cm)	Weight (kg)	Size (cm)	Specifications
Ocean Optics	NIRQuest 512–2.5	900–2500	1.18	18.2 × 11 × 4.7	Grating/filter
	Flame-NIR	950–1700	0.265	8.89 × 6.35 × 3.19	InGaAs detector
	Ventana-VIS-NIR	430–1100	0.9	17 × 11 × 5	Fluorescence
	STS-NIR	650–1100	0.068	4 × 4.2 × 2.4	ELIS1024 detector
Scentronic	SentroID	5800–11,000	1.1	23 × 8 × 4.2	OEM System
StellarNet	Dwarf–Star	900–1700	0.07	5 × 3 × 2	InGaAs detector, PDA
Thermo Fisher	Phazir	4100–6250	1.8	26.6 × 25.1 × 10.9	MEMS Chip

Company	Product Name	Spectral Range (per cm)	Laser (nm)	Weight (kg)	Size (cm)	Specifications
Raman						
Agiltron	PinPointer	200–3000	532, 785	1.36	21.4 × 10.8 × 6.3	
Airsense Analytics	LS-ID	250–2875	785	0.4	13 × 7 × 4	CCD array detectors
Bruker	BRAVO	300–3200	785, 1064	1.5	27 × 15.6 × 6.2	Duo LASER™ excitation, laser class 1M
BWTEK	NanoRam	176–2900	785	1.2	22 × 10 × 5	TE cooled linear CCD array
	Tactic ID	176–2900	785	0.9	19 × 10 × 5	Linear CCD array
Chemring Detection	THOR-1064	160–2200	1064	1.5	22.9 × 11.5 × 5.1	CCD array detectors

Metrohm	Mira M-1	400–2300	785	0.54	12.5 × 8.5 × 3.9	Orbital Raster Scan
	Mira M-2	400–2300	1064	0.82	14.4 × 9.3 × 6.4	
Ocean Optics	ID Raman Mini	400–2300	785	0.33	9.1 × 7.1 × 3.8	NIR-enhanced CCD array
Rigaku	Progeny	200–2500	1064	1.6	29.9 × 8.1 × 7.4	512 pixels, TE cooled InGaAs
Sciaps	Inspector 300	175–2875	785	1.7	19 × 17.5 × 4.3	CCD array
	Inspector 500	100–2500	1030	2.7	20 × 17.5 × 4.3	Type III-IV semiconductor array
Snowy Range	CBEx	400–2300	785	0.33	9.1 × 7.1 × 3.8	Orbital Raster Scan
	CBEx 1064	400–2300	1064	0.77	11.3 × 7.9 × 5.7	
StellarNet	HR-TEC	200–2200	785	0.4	2.5 × 7.6 × 12.7	CCD array detectors
	SR-TEC-IG	400–3500	1064	0.4	2.5 × 7.6 × 12.7	InGaAs detector
Thermo Fisher	First Defender RM	250–2875	785	0.82	4.4 × 19.3 × 10.7	CCD array detectors
	First Defender RMX	250–2875	785	0.92	19.6 × 11.4 × 6.1	
	TruNarc	250–2875	785	0.505	16.3 × 10.4 × 5.1	
	TruScan GP	250–2875	785	0.9	20.8 × 10.7 × 4.3	
	TruScan RM	250–2875	785	0.9	20.8 × 10.7 × 4.3	
	Gemini Analyzer	250–2875	785	1.9	25.6 × 14.6 × 6.1	Raman
TSI	ASSURX	250–2350	785	1.9	23.1 × 10.1 × 22.2	CCD detector
Wasatch Photonics	NOVA	200–2500	785	0.82	16.2 × 13.2 × 3.7	Volume phase holographic grating

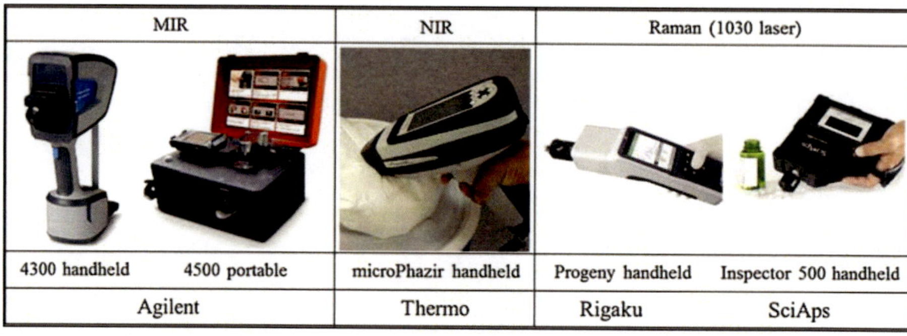

Figure 4.8 Examples of commercially available portable and handheld vibrational spectrometers.

applications with spectral resolution equivalent to bench-top instruments. Thus, the unique spectrum associated with functional groups allows for the chemically based discrimination of biological systems and produces complex biochemical fingerprints that are distinct and reproducible for different materials. Raman spectroscopy is positioning as an attractive fingerprinting technique for various applications including pharmaceuticals, petrochemicals, and law enforcement (Volodin et al., 2014). Advantages of Raman spectroscopy include portable and ruggedized instrumentation for field deployment (Fig. 4.8), little or no sample preparation requirement, noncontact and nondestructive capabilities, and the relatively weak Raman response of water, allowing measurement of aqueous solutions. Furthermore, new generations of handheld and portable Raman spectrometers are equipped with longer excitation wavelength (NIR, 1030 nm) and InGaAs array detectors that eliminate potential fluorescence limitations.

Our research group has shown the utility and efficacy of portable and handheld infrared for a range of food applications, showing that the technology provides simple, rapid, robust, and sensitive on-site analysis of quality parameters and in situ authentication of food products. The sensor technologies are directed at improving efficiency, throughput, and reliability of critical processes, such as monitoring incoming raw materials. In order for the technique to become a routine screening tool, research needs to resolve limits of sensitivity of the method, generate a library of major threat agents and evaluation of powerful multivariate classification methods. Portable and handheld spectroscopy has already demonstrated its potential to move from the confines of the relatively stable and controlled laboratory environment and out into the potentially more challenging and dynamic environs of the food supply chain (Ellis et al., 2015).

ATR, Attenuated total reflectance; *CCD*, charged couple device; *DGTS*, deuterated triglycine sulfate; *DRIFT*, diffuse reflection; *ELIS-1024*, 2.8V sensor features sample and hold capability, selectable resolution, and advanced power management; *HATR*, horizontal ATR accessory; *InGaAs*, indium gallium arsenide; *Laser class 1M*, safe for all conditions, except when passed through magnifying optics; *MEMS*, microelectromechanical systems; *OEM*, original equipment manufacturer; *PDA*, photodiode array; *TE*, thermoelectrically; *UV/VIS*, ultraviolet—visible spectroscopy.

Sources of Further Information

More information about the principles and applications of infrared vibrational spectroscopy can be found:

1. Ciurczak, E.W., Igne, B., 2015. Pharmaceutical and Medical Applications of Near-Infrared Spectroscopy, second ed. CRC Press, Boca Raton, Taylor and Francis Group.
2. Ellis, D.I., Muhamadali, H., Haughey, SA, Elliott, C.T., Goodacre, R., 2015. Point-and-shoot: rapid quantitative detection methods for on-site food fraud analysis – moving out of the laboratory and into the food supply chain. Analytical Methods 7, 9401–9414.
3. Giusti, M.M., Atnip, A., Sweeney, C., Rodriguez-Saona, L.E., 2011. Rapid Authentication of Fruit Juices by Infrared Spectroscopic Techniques. In: Ebeler, S.E., Takeoka, G.R. Winterhalter, P. (Eds.).Progress in authentication of food and wine. Washington, D.C. Am. Chem. Soc., Div. Agric. Food Chem. pp. 275–299.
4. Li-Chan, E.C.Y., Chalmers, J.M., Griffiths, P.R., 2010. Applications of Vibrational Spectroscopy to Food Science. Eds. John Wiley and Sons, Chichester, UK.
5. Rodriguez-Saona, L.E., Allendorf, M.E., 2011. Use of FT-IR for rapid authentication and detection of adulteration of food. Annual Review of Food Science and Technology. 2, 467–483.

References

Ali, S.M., Bonnier, F., Lambkin, H., Flynn, K., McDonagh, V., Healy, C., Lee, T.C., Lyng, F.M., Byrne, H.J., 2013. A comparison of Raman, FTIR and ATR-FTIR micro spectroscopy for imaging human skin tissue sections. Analytical Methods 5 (9), 2281–2291.

Almeida, M.R., Oliveira, S., Stephani, R., de Oliveira, L.F.C., 2011. Fourier-transform Raman analysis of milk powder: a potential method for rapid quality screening. Journal of Raman Spectroscopy 42 (7), 1548–1552.

Alves da Rocha, R., Paiva, I.M., Anjos, V., Furtado, M.A., Bell, M.J., 2015. Quantification of whey in fluid milk using confocal Raman microscopy and artificial neural network. Journal of Dairy Science 98 (6), 3559–3567.

American Cancer Society, 2015. Acrylamide and Cancer Risk. [Online] Available at: http://www.cancer.org/cancer/cancercauses/othercarcinogens/athome/acrylamide.

Aparicio, R., Hardwood, J., 2013. Technological aspects. Springer, US. In: Handbook of Olive Oil: Analysis and Properties. Springer Science Business Media, New York.

Ayvaz, H., Rodriguez-Saona, L.E., 2015. Application of handheld and portable spectrometers for screening acrylamide content in commercial potato chips. Food Chemistry 174, p154–162.

Azizian, H., Mossoba, M.M., Fardin-Kia, A.R., Delmonte, P., Karunathilaka, S.R., Kramer, J.K., 2015. Novel, rapid identification, and quantification of adulterants in extra virgin olive oil using near-infrared spectroscopy and chemometrics. Lipids 50 (7), 705–718.

Baeten, V., Aparicio, R., 2000. Edible oils and fats authentication by Fourier transform Raman spectrometry. Biotechnologie, Agronomie, Societe et Environnement 4 (4), 196–203.

Balabin, R.M., Smirnov, S.V., 2011. Melamine detection by mid-and near-infrared (MIR/NIR) spectroscopy: a quick and sensitive method for dairy products analysis including liquid milk, infant formula, and milk powder. Talanta 85 (1), 562–568.

Ballabio, D., Consonni, V., 2013. Classification tools in chemistry. Part 1: linear models. PLS-DA. Analytical Methods 5, 3790–3798.

Bendini, A., Cerretani, L., Virgilio, F.D., Belloni, P., Lercker, G., Toschi, T.G., 2007. In-process monitoring in industrial olive mill by means of FT-NIR. European Journal of Lipid Science and Technology 109, 498–504.

Berardo, N., Pisacane, V., Battilani, P., Scandolara, A., Pietri, A., Marocco, A., 2005. Rapid detection of kernel rots and mycotoxins in maize by near-infrared reflectance spectroscopy. Journal of Agricultural and Food Chemistry 53 (21), 8128–8134.

Bertran, E., Blanco, M., Coello, J., Iturriaga, H., Maspoch, S., Montoliu, I., 2000. Near infrared spectrometry and pattern recognition as screening methods for the authentication of virgin olive oils of very close geographical origins. JNIRS 8, 45–52.

Betz, J.F., Cheng, Y., Rubloff, G.W., 2012. Direct SERS detection of contaminants in a complex mixture: rapid, single step screening for melamine in liquid infant formula. Analyst 137 (4), 826–828.

Beyer, M., Klix, M.B., Klink, H., Verreet, J.A., 2006. Quantifying the effects of previous crop, tillage, cultivar and triazole fungicides on the deoxynivalenol content of wheat grain-a review. Journal of Plant Diseases and Protection 241–246.

Blanco, M., Villarroya, I., 2002. NIR spectroscopy: a rapid-response analytical tool. Trends in Analytical Chemistry 21, 240–250.

Bolduan, C., Miedaner, T., Schipprack, W., Dhillon, B.S., Melchinger, A.E., 2009. Genetic variation for resistance to ear rots and mycotoxins contamination in early European maize inbred lines. Crop Science 49, 2019–2028.

Borin, A., Ferrão, M.F., Mello, C., Maretto, D.A., Poppi, R.J., 2006. Least-squares support vector machines and near infrared spectroscopy for quantification of common adulterants in powdered milk. Analytica Chimica Acta 579 (1), 25–32.

Brereton, R.G., 2000. Introduction to multivariate calibration in analytical chemistry. Analyst 125, 2125–2154.

Briandet, R., Kemsley, E.K., Wilson, R.H., 1996a. Approaches to adulteration detection in instant coffees using infrared spectroscopy and chemometrics. Journal of the Science of Food and Agriculture 71, 359–366.

Briandet, R., Kemsley, E.K., Wilson, R.H., 1996b. Discrimination of *Arabica* and *Robusta* in instant coffee by Fourier transform infrared spectroscopy and chemometrics. Journal of Agricultural and Food Chemistry 44, 170–174.

Chaudhry, P., Zimmerman, A., 2013. The global growth of counterfeit trade. In: Protecting Your Intellectual Property Rights. Springer, New York, pp. 7–31.

Che Man, Y.B., Syahariza, Z.A., Mirghani, M.E.S., et al., 2005. Analysis of potential lard adulteration in chocolate and chocolate products using Fourier transform infrared spectroscopy. Food Chemistry 90, 815–819.

Chen, H., Lin, Z., Mo, L., Wu, T., Tan, C., 2015. Near-infrared spectroscopy as a diagnostic tool for distinguishing between normal and malignant colorectal tissues. BioMed Research International 7. Article ID 472197.

Christy, A.A., Kasemsumran, S., Du, Y., Ozaki, Y., 2004. The detection and quantification of adulteration in olive oil by near-infrared spectroscopy and chemometrics. Analytical Sciences 20, 935–940.

Ciurczak, E.W., Igne, B., 2015. Pharmaceutical and Medical Applications of Near-infrared Spectroscopy, second ed. CRC Press Taylor and Francis Group, Boca Raton.

Colthup, N.B., Daly, L.H., Wiberley, S.E., 1990. Vibrational and rotational spectra. In: Introduction to Infrared and Raman Spectroscopy. Academic Press, Inc, UK, pp. 1–73. Edition: Elsevier Inc.

Council for Agricultural Science and Technology (CAST), 2003. Mycotoxins: risks in plant, animal, and human systems. Task Force Reports (139), 136–142.

Cozzolino, D., Smyth, H., Gishen, M., 2003. Feasibility study on the use of visible and near-infrared spectroscopy together with chemometrics to discriminate between commercial white wines of different varietal origins. Journal of Agricultural and Food Chemistry 51, 7703–7708.

Craig, A.P., Franca, A.S., Irudayaraj, J., 2013. Surface-enhanced Raman spectroscopy applied to food safety. Annual Review of Food Science and Technology 4, 369–380.

De Girolamo, A., Cervellieri, S., Visconti, A., Pascale, M., 2014. Rapid analysis of deoxynivalenol in durum wheat by FT-NIR spectroscopy. Toxins 6 (11), 3129–3143.

De Girolamo, A., Lippolis, V., Nordkvist, E., Visconti, A., 2009. Rapid and non-invasive analysis of deoxynivalenol in durum and common wheat by Fourier-transform near infrared (FT-NIR) spectroscopy. Food Additives and Contaminants: Part A 26, 907–917.

de la Mata, P., Dominguez-Vidal, A., Bosque-Sendra, J.M., Ruiz-Medina, A., Cuadros-Rodríguez, L., Ayora-Cañada, M.J., 2012. Olive oil assessment in edible oil blends by means of ATR-FTIR and chemometrics. Food Control 23 (2), 449–455.

De Maesschalck, R., Candolfi, A., Masart, D.L., Heuerding, S., 1999. Decision criteria for soft independent modeling of class analogy applied to near infrared data. Chemometrics and Intelligent Laboratory Systems 47, 65–77.

De Marchi, M., Bonfatti, V., Cecchinato, A., Di Martino, G., Carnier, P., 2010. Prediction of protein composition of individual cow milk using mid-infrared spectroscopy. Italian Journal of Animal Science 8 (2s), 399–401.

Defernez, M., Wilson, R.H., 1995. Mid-infrared spectroscopy and chemometrics for determining the type of fruit used in jam. Journal of the Science of Food and Agriculture 67, 461–467.

Dejong, S., 1993. PLS fits closer than PCR. Journal of Chemometrics 7, 551–557.

Delwiche, S.R., Hareland, G.A., 2004. Detection of scab-damaged hard red spring wheat kernels by near infrared reflectance. Cereal Chemistry 81, 643–649.

Downey, G., Boussion, J., 1996. Authentication of coffee bean variety by near-infrared reflectance spectroscopy of dried extract. Journal of the Science of Food and Agriculture 71, 41–49.

Downey, G., Kelly, J.D., 2006. Food Authentication Using Infrared Spectroscopic Methods Project RMIS No. 4907.

Downey, G., Briandet, R., Wilson, R.H., Kemsley, E.K., 1997. Near- and mid- infrared spectroscopies in food authentication: coffee varietal identification. Journal of Agricultural and Food Chemistry 45 (11), 4357–4361.

Downey, G., McIntire, P., Davies, A.Y., 2002. Detecting and quantifying sunflower oil adulteration in extra virgin olive oils from the eastern mediterranean by visible and near-infrared spectroscopy. Journal of Agricultural and Food Chemistry 50, 5520–5525.

Du, R., Lai, K., Xiao, Z., Shen, Y., Wang, X., Huang, Y., 2012. Evaluation of the quality of deep frying oils with Fourier transform near-infrared and mid-infrared spectroscopy. Journal of Food Science 77 (2), C261–C266.

Dvoracek, V., Prohaskova, A., Chrpova, J., Stockova, L., 2012. Near infrared spectroscopy for deoxynivalenol content estimation in intact wheat grain. Plant, Soil and Environment 58, 196–203.

Ellis, D.I., Goodacre, R., 2006. Metabolic fingerprinting in disease diagnosis: biomedical applications of infrared and Raman spectroscopy. Analyst 131 (8), 875–885.

Ellis, D.I., Brewster, V.L., Dunn, W.B., Allwood, J.W., Golovanov, A.P., Goodacre, R., 2012. Fingerprinting food: current technologies for the detection of food adulteration and contamination. Chemical Society Reviews 41 (17), 5706–5727.

Ellis, D.I., Muhamadali, H., Haughey, S.A., Elliott, C.T., Goodacre, R., 2015. Point-and-Shoot: rapid quantitative detection methods for on-site food fraud analysis – moving out of the laboratory and into the food supply chain. Analytical Methods 7, 9401–9414.

Fernandez-Ibañez, V., Soldado, A., Martinez- Fernandez, A., Roza Delgado, B., 2009. Application of near infrared spectroscopy for rapid detection of aflatoxin B1 in maize and Barely as analytical quality assessment. Food Chemistry 113, 629–634.

FOSS Analytical, 2009. Food Protein Workshop: Developing a Toolbox of Analytical Solutions to Address Adulteration. Possibilities of FTIR and NIR for the Detection of Adulteration in Food and Feed. Maryland USP Meeting Center, USP Headquarters, Rockville. June 17, 2009 6a. Breakout Session A.

Frankel, E.N., Mailer, R.J., Wang, S.C., Shoemaker, C.F., Guinard, J.X., Flynn, J.D., Sturzenberger, N.D., 2011. Evaluation of Extra-Virgin Olive Oil Sold in California. UC Davis Olive Center at Robert Mondavi Institute. http://olivecenter.ucdavis.edu/research/files/report041211finalreduced.pdf.

Galtier, O., Dupuy, N., Le Dreau, Y., Ollivier, D., Pinatel, C., Kister, J., Artaud, J., 2007. Geographic origins and compositions of virgin oils determinated by chemometric analysis of NIR spectra. Analytica Chimica Acta 595, 136–144.

Giovannozzi, A.M., Rolle, F., Sega, M., Abete, M.C., Marchis, D., Rossi, A.M., 2014. Rapid and sensitive detection of melamine in milk with gold nanoparticles by Surface Enhanced Raman Scattering. Food Chemistry 159, 250–256.

Giusti, M.M., Atnip, A., Sweeney, C., Rodriguez-Saona, L.E., 2011. Rapid authentication of fruit juices by infrared spectroscopic techniques. In: Ebeler, S.E., Takeoka, G.R., Winterhalter, P. (Eds.), Progress in Authentication of Food and Wine. ACS, Washington, DC, pp. 275–299.

Gonzaga, F.B., Pasquini, C., 2006. A new method for determination of the oxidative stability of edible oils at frying temperatures using near infrared emission spectroscopy. Analytica Chimica Acta 570, 129–135.

Goodacre, R., Anklam, E., 2001. Fourier transform infrared spectroscopy and chemometrics as a tool for the rapid detection of other vegetables fats mixed in cocoa butter. Journal of the American Oil Chemists' Society 78 (10), 993–1000.

Griffiths, P.R., de Haseth, J.A., 1986. Fourier transform infrared spectroscopy, Vol. 83. In: Chemical Analysis – a Series of Monographs of Analytical Chemistry and Its Applications. J. Wiley Sons, Chichester, New York, Brisbane, Toronto, Singapore.

Griffiths, P.R., de Haseth, J.A., 2006. Introduction to vibrational spectroscopy. Fourier Transform Infrared Spectrometry, second ed. John Wiley & Sons, Inc, New Jersey, Hoboken, pp. 1–18.

Grocery Manufacturers Association (GMA) and A.T. Kearney Research. 2015. URL (http://www.atkearney.com/index.php/News-media/economic-adulteration-and-counterfeiting-of-global-food-and-consumer-product.html).

Grocery Manufacturers Association (GMA). 2010. Available from: http://www.gmaonline.org/downloads/research-and-reports/consumerproductfraud.pdf.

Gromski, P.S., Muhamadali, H., Ellis, D.I., Xu, Y., Correa, E., Turner, M.L., Goodacre, R., 2015. A tutorial review: metabolomics and partial least squares-discriminant analysis—a marriage of convenience or a shotgun wedding. Analytica Chimica Acta 879, 10–23.

Groselj, N., Vracko, M., Pierna, J.A.F., Baeten, V., Novic, M., 2008. The use of FT-MIR spectroscopy and counter-propagation artificial neural networks for tracing the adulteration of olive oil. Acta Chimica Slovenica 55, 935–941.

Guan, G., Zhang, Z., Han, M.Y., 2010. A simple, reliable and sensitive colorimetric visualization of melamine in milk by unmodified gold nanoparticles. Analyst 135, 1070–1075.

Guan, N., Fan, Q., Ding, J., Zhao, Y., Lu, J., Ai, Y., Guobin, X., Sainan, Z., Chen, Y., Jiang, L., Miao, J., Zhang, H., Zhao, D., Liu, X., Yao, Y., 2009. Melamine-contaminated powdered formula and urolithiasis in young children. New England Journal of Medicine 360, 1067–1074.

Günzler, H., Gremlich, H.U., 2002. IR Spectroscopy. An Introduction. Wiley-VCH, Weinheim, Germany vol. 34 (15), 374.

Günzler, H., Gremlich, H., Blümich, M.J., 2002. Spectrometers. Wiley-vch. IR Spectroscopy: An Introduction. Federal Republic of Germany: Wiley-VCH, Weinheim, pp. 1–7, 37–91.

Günzler, H., Heise, H.M., 2000. IR Spectroscopy. Wiley-VCH, New York, ISBN 3527288961.

Gurdeniz, G., Ozen, B., 2009. Detection of adulteration of extra-virgin olive oil by chemometric analysis of mid-infrared spectral data. Food Chemistry 116 (2), 519–525.

He, J., Rodriguez-Saona, L.E., Giusti, M.M., 2007. Midinfrared spectroscopy for juice authentication- rapid differentiation of commercial juices. Journal of Agricultural and Food Chemistry 55, 4443–4452.

Holland, J.K., Kemsley, E.K., Wilson, R.H., 1998. Use of Fourier transform infrared spectroscopy and partial least squares regression for the detection of adulteration of strawberry purees. Journal of the Science of Food and Agriculture 76, 263–269.

Ismail, A.A., Nicodemo, A., Sedman, J., van de Voort, F., Holzbaur, I.E., 1999. Infrared spectroscopy of lipids: principles and applications. In: Hamilton, R.J., Cast, J. (Eds.), Spectral Properties of Lipids. CRC Press, Boca Raton, FL, pp. 235–269.

Jackson, L.S., 2009. Chemical food safety issues in the United States: past, present, and future. Journal of Agricultural and Food Chemistry 57 (18), 8161–8170.

Jawaid, S., Talpur, F.N., Sherazi, S.T.H., Nizamani, S.M., Khaskheli, A.A., 2013. Rapid detection of melamine adulteration in dairy milk by SB-ATR–Fourier transform infrared spectroscopy. Food Chemistry 141 (3), 3066–3071.

Jha, S.N., Gunasekaran, S., 2010. Authentication of sweetness of mango juice using Fourier transform infrared-attenuated total reflection spectroscopy. Journal of Food Engineering 101 (3), 337–342.

Johnson, R., 2014. The Federal Food Safety System: A Primer. Congressional Research Service.

Kalasinsky, K., Hadfield, T., Shea, A., Kalasinky, V., Nelson, M., Neiss, J., Drauch, A., Vanni, G., Treado, P., 2007. Raman chemical imaging spectroscopy reagentless detection and identification of pathogens: signature development and evaluation. Analytical Chemistry 79, 2658–2673.

Karoui, R., De Baerdemaeker, J., 2007. A review of the analytical methods coupled with chemometrics tools for the determination of the quality and identity of dairy products. Food Chemistry 102, 621–640.

Kartheek, M., Smith, A.A., Muthu, A.K., Manavalan, R., 2011. Determination of adulterants in food: a review. Journal of Chemical and Pharmaceutical Research 3 (2), 629–636.

Kasemsumran, S., Thanapase, W., Kiatsoonthon, A., 2007. Feasibility of near-infrared spectroscopy to detect and to quantify adulterants in cow milk. Analytical Science 23 (7), 907–910.

Kelly, J.D., Petisco, C., Downey, G., 2006. Potential of near infrared transflectance spectroscopy to detect adulteration of irish honey by beet invert syrup and high fructose corn syrup. JNIRS 14 (2), 39.

Kelly, J.F., Downey, G., 2005. Detection of sugar adulterants in apple juice using Fourier transform infrared spectroscopy and chemometrics. Journal of Agricultural and Food Chemistry 53 (9), 3281–3286.

Kemsley, E.K., Holland, J.K., Defernez, M., Wilson, R.H., 1996. Detection of adulteration of raspberry purees using infrared spectroscopy and chemometrics. Journal of Agricultural and Food Chemistry 44 (12), 3864–3870.

Kemsley, E.K., 1996. Discriminant analysis of high-dimensional data: a comparison of principal components analysis and partial least squares data reduction methods. Chemometrics and Intelligent Laboratory Systems 33, 47–61.

Kos, G., Krska, R., Lohninger, H., Griffiths, P.R., 2004. A comparative study of mid-infrared diffuse reflection (DR) and attenuated total reflection (ATR) spectroscopy for the detection of fungal infection on RWA2-corn. Analytical and Bioanalytical Chemistry 378, 159–166.

Kos, G., Lohninger, H., Krska, R., 2003. Development of a method for the determination of Fusarium fungi on corn using mid-infrared spectroscopy with attenuated total reflection and chemometrics. Analytical Chemistry 75 (5), 1211–1217.

Kos, G., Lohninger, H., Krska, R., 2002. Fourier transform mid-infrared spectroscopy with attenuated total reflection (FT-IR/ATR) as a tool for the detection of Fusarium on maize. Vibrational Spectroscopy 29, 115–119.

Kos, G., Lohninger, H., Mizaikoff, B., Krska, R., 2007. Optimisation of a sample preparation procedure for the screening of fungal infection and assessment of deoxynivalenol content in maize using mid-infrared attenuated total reflection spectroscopy. Food Additives & Contaminants 24, 721–729.

Küpper, L., Heise, H.M., Lampen, P., Davies, A.N., McIntyre, P., 2001. Authentication and quantification of extra virgin olive oils by attenuated total reflectance infrared spectroscopy using silver halide fiber probes and partial least-squares calibration. Applied Spectroscopy 55 (5), 563–570.

Lai, Y.W., Kemsley, E.K., Wilson, R.H., 1994. Potential of Fourier transform infrared spectroscopy for the authentication of vegetable oils. Journal of Agricultural and Food Chemistry 42 (5), 1154–1159.

Lai, Y.W., Kemsley, E.K., Wilson, R.H., 1995. Quantitative analysis of potential adulterants of extra virgin olive oil using infrared spectroscopy. Food Chemistry 53 (1), 95–98.

Lavine, B.K., 2000. Clustering and classification of analytical data. In: Meyers, R.A. (Ed.), Encyclopedia of Analytical Chemistry. John Wiley and Sons, New York, NY, pp. 1–21.

Lenhardt, L., Zeković, I., Dramićanin, T., Tešić, Ž., Milojković-Opsenica, D., Dramićanin, M.D., 2014. Authentication of the botanical origin of unifloral honey by infrared spectroscopy coupled with support vector machine algorithm. Physica Scripta (T162), 014042.

León, L., Kelly, J.D., Downey, G., 2005. Detection of apple juice adulteration using near-infrared transflectance spectroscopy. Applied Spectroscopy 59 (5), 593–599.

Lerma-García, M.J., Ramis-Ramos, G., Herrero-Martínez, J.M., Simó-Alfonso, E.F., 2010. Authentication of extra virgin olive oils by Fourier-transform infrared spectroscopy. Food Chemistry 118, 78–83.

Li, S., Zhu, X., Zhang, J., Li, G., Su, D., Shan, Y., 2012. Authentication of pure camellia oil by using near infrared spectroscopy and pattern recognition techniques. Journal of Food Science 77 (4), C374–C380.

Li, Y.S., Church, J.S., 2014. Raman spectroscopy in the analysis of food and pharmaceutical nanomaterials. Journal of Food and Drug Analysis 22 (1), 29–48.

Li-Chan, E., Chalmers, J.M., Griffiths, P.R., 2010. Application of Vibrational Spectroscopy for the Study of Heat-induced Changes in Food Components. Wiley, West Sussex, United Kingdom, pp. 213–228. John Wiley & Sons Ltd.

Lin, M., He, L., Awika, J., Yang, L., Ledoux, D.R., Li, H.A., Mustapha, A., 2008. Detection of melamine in gluten, chicken feed, and processed foods using surface enhanced Raman spectroscopy and HPLC. Journal of Food Science 73 (8), T129–T134.

Lu, C., Xiang, B., Hao, G., Xu, J., Wang, Z., Chen, C., 2009. Rapid detection of melamine in milk powder by near infrared spectroscopy. JNIRS 17 (2), 59.

Maggio, R.M., Cerretani, L., Chiavaro, E., Kaufman, T.S., Bendini, A., 2010. A novel chemometric strategy for the estimation of extra virgin olive oil adulteration with edible oils. Food Control 21, 890–895.

Marigheto, N.A., Kemsley, E.K., Defernez, M., Wilson, R.H., 1998. A comparison of mid-infrared and Raman spectroscopies for the authentication of edible oils. JAOCS 75 (8), 987–992.

Martelo-Vidal, M.J., Vazquez, M., 2014. Evaluation of ultraviolet, visible, and near infrared spectroscopy for the analysis of wine compounds. Czech Journal of Food Sciences 32, 37.

Mauer, L.J., Chernyshova, A.A., Hiatt, A., Deering, A., Davis, R., 2009. Melamine detection in infant formula powder using near- and mid-infrared spectroscopy. Journal of Agricultural and Food Chemistry 57 (10), 3974–3980.

Maurer, N.E., Rodriguez-Saona, L.E., 2013. Rapid assessment of quality parameters in cocoa butter using ATR-MIR spectroscopy and multivariate analysis. JAOCS 90 (4), 475–481.

Maurer, N.E., Hatta-Sakoda, B., Pascual-Chagman, G., Rodriguez-Saona, L.E., 2012. Characterization and authentication of a novel vegetable source of Omega-3 fatty acids, Sacha Inchi (*Plukenetia volubilis* L.) oil. Food Chemistry 134, 1173–1180.

McMullin, D., Mizaikoff, B., Krska, R., 2015. Advancements in IR spectroscopic approaches for the determination of fungal derived contaminations in food crops. Analytical and Bioanalytical Chemistry 407 (3), 653–660.

Mecker, L.C., Tyner, K.M., Kauffman, J.F., Arzhantsev, S., Mans, D.J., Gryniewicz-Ruzicka, C.M., 2012. Selective melamine detection in multiple sample matrices with a portable Raman instrument using surface enhanced Raman spectroscopy-active gold nanoparticles. Analytica Chimica Acta 733, 48–55.

Mendenhall, I.V., Brown, R.J., 1991. Fourier transform infrared determination of whey powder in nonfat dry milk. Journal of Dairy Science 74, 2896–2900.

Moore, J.C., Spink, J., Lipp, M., 2012. Development and application of a database of food ingredient fraud and economically motivated adulteration from 1980 to 2010. Journal of Food Science 77 (4), R118–R126.

Nunes, C.A., 2014. Vibrational spectroscopy and chemometrics to assess authenticity, adulteration and intrinsic quality parameters of edible oils and fats. Food Research International 60, 255–261.

Nurrulhidayah, A.F., Che Man, Y.B., Rohman, A., Amin, I., Shuhaimi, M., Khatib, A., 2013a. Authentication analysis of butter from beef fat using Fourier Transform Infrared (FTIR) spectroscopy coupled with chemometrics. International Food Research Journal 20 (3), 383–1388.

Nurrulhidayah, A.F., Rohman, A., Amin, I., Shuhaimi, M., Khatib, A., 2013b. Analysis of chicken fat as adulterant in butter using Fourier transform infrared spectroscopy and chemometrics. Grasas Y Aceites 64 (4), 349–355.

NY Times: New York Times, 1987. A Long Trial in Spain on Fatal Tainted Food. The New York Times Company, New York City, New York. August 2, 1987. Available from: http://www.nytimes.com/1987/08/02/world/a-long-trial-in-spain-on-fatal-tainted-food.html.

Oussama, A., Elabadi, F., Platikanov, S., Kzaiber, F., Tauler, R., 2012. Detection of olive oil adulteration using FT-IR spectroscopy and PLS with variable importance of projections (VIP) scores. Journal of the American Chemical Society 89 (10), 1807–1812.

Ozaki, Y., 1998. Raman spectroscopy. In: Mossoba, M. (Ed.), Spectral Methods in Food Analysis: Instrumentation and Applications. Marcel Dekker, Inc, New York, pp. 427–462.

Ozen, B.F., Mauer, L.J., 2002. Detection of hazelnut oil adulteration using FT-IR spectroscopy. Journal of Agricultural and Food Chemistry 50, 3898–3901.

Pearson, T.C., Wicklow, D.T., Maghirang, E.B., Xie, F., Dowell, F.E., 2001. Detecting aflatoxin in single corn kernels by transmittance and reflectance spectroscopy. Transactions of the American Society of Agricultural Engineers 44 (5), 1247–1254.

Pedreschi, F., Segtanan, V.H., Knutsen, S.H., 2010. On-line monitoring of fat, dry matter and acrylamide contents in potato chips using near infrared reflectance and visual reflectance imaging. Food Chemistry 121, 616–620.

Perdigao, L.M., Champness, N.R., 2006. Surface self-assembly of the cyanuric acid-melamine hydrogen bonded network. Chemical communications 1, 538–540.

Perks, B., 2007. Fighting Food Fraud With Science. Chemistry World Magazine. Royal Society of Chemistry (accessed 01.16.). http://www.rsc.org/images/FightingFoodFraudWithScience_tcm18-98167.pdf.

Pettersson, H., Åberg, L., 2003. Near infrared spectroscopy for determination of mycotoxins in cereals. Food Control 14 (4), 229–232.

Posnick, R., 2007. June/July 2007 Ask the Regulators: Acrylamide, Furan, and the FDA. Reproduced from Food Safety Magazine by the Target Group. http://www.fda.gov/Food/FoodborneIllnessContaminants/ChemicalContaminants/ucm194482.htm.

Pujolras, M.P., Ayvaz, H., Shotts, M.L., Pittman Jr., R.A., Herringshaw, S., Rodriguez-Saona, L.E., 2015. Portable infrared spectrometer to characterize and differentiate between organic and conventional bovine butter. Journal of the American Oil Chemists' Society 92 (2), 75–184.

Reichenbächer, M., Popp, J., 2012. Vibrational spectroscopy. In: Reichenbächer, M., Popp, J. (Eds.), Challenges in Molecular Structure Determination. Springer–Verlag, Berlin Heidelberg, pp. 63–143.

Rodriguez-Otero, J.L., Hermida, M., 1996. Analysis of fermented milk products by near infrared reflectance spectroscopy. Journal of Association Official Analytical Chemists International 79, 817–821.

Rodriguez-Saona, L.E., Allendorf, M.E., 2011. Use of FTIR for rapid authentication and detection of adulteration of food. Annual Review of Food Science and Technology 2, 467–483.

Rodriguez-Saona, L.E., Fry, F.S., McLaughlin, M.A., Calvey, E.M., 2001. Rapid analysis of sugars in fruit juices by FT-NIR spectroscopy. Carbohydrate Research 366, 63–74.

Roggo, Y., Chalus, P., Maurer, L., Lema-Martinez, C., Edmond, A., Jent, N., 2007. A review of near infrared spectrsopcy and chemometrics in pharmaceutical technologies. Journal of Pharmaceutical and Biomedical Analysis 44, 683–700.

Rohman, A., Che Man, Y.B., 2010. Fourier transform infrared (FTIR) spectroscopy for analysis of extra virgin olive oil adulterated with palm oil. Food Research International 43 (3), 886–892.

Rohman, A., Setyaningrum, D.L., Riyanto, S., 2014. FTIR spectroscopy combined with partial least square for analysis of red fruit oil in ternary mixture system. International Journal of Spectroscopy 2014, 1–5.

Ruoff, K., Luginbühl, W., Künzli, R., Iglesias, M.T., Bogdanov, S., Bosset, J.O., von der Ohe, K., von der Ohe, W., Amadò, R., 2006. Authentication of the botanical and geographical origin of honey by mid-infrared spectroscopy. Journal of Agricultural and Food Chemistry 54 (18), 6873–6880.

Rutten, M.J.M., Bovenhuis, H., Heck, J.M.L., van Arendonk, J.A.M., 2011. Predicting bovine milk protein composition based on Fourier transform infrared spectra. Journal of Dairy Science 94, 5683–5690.

Santos, P.M., Pereira-Filho, E.R., Rodriguez-Saona, L.E., 2013. Application of hand-held and portable infrared spectrometers in bovine milk analysis. Journal of Agricultural and Food Chemistry 61 (6), 1205–1211.

Segtnan, V.H., Kita, A., Mielnik, M., Jørgensen, K., Knutsen, S.H., 2006. Screening of acrylamide contents in potato crisps using process variable settings and near-infrared spectroscopy. Molecular Nutrition & Food Research 50 (9), 811–817.

Siebert, F., Hildebrandt, P., 2008. Theory of infrared absorption and Raman spectroscopy. Ch. 2. In: Vibrational Spectroscopy in Life Science. WILEY-VCH Verlag GmbH & Co. KGaA, Weinheim.

Siuda, R., Balcerowska, G., Kupcewicz, B., Lenc, L., 2008. A modified approach to evaluation of DON content in scab damaged ground wheat by use of diffuse reflectance spectroscopy. Food Analytical Methods 1, 283–292.

Snyder, A.B., Sweeney, C.F., Rodriguez-Saona, L.E., Giusti, M.M., 2014. Rapid authentication of Concord juice concentration in a grape juice blend using Fourier-transform infrared spectroscopy and chemometric analysis. Food Chemistry 147, 295–301.

Sorak, D., Herberholz, L., Iwascek, S., Altinpinar, S., Pfeifer, F., Siesler, H.W., 2012. New developments and applications of handheld Raman, mid-infrared, and near-infrared spectrometers. Applied Spectroscopy 47 (2), 83–115.

Spink, J., 2011. The challenge of intellectual property enforcement for agriculture technology transfers, additives, raw materials, and finished goods against product fraud and counterfeiters. Journal of Intellectual Property Rights 16 (3), 183–193.

Sun, X., Zhang, L., Li, P., Xu, B., Ma, F., Zhang, Q., Zhang, W., 2015. Fatty acid profiles based adulteration detection for flaxseed oil by gas chromatography mass spectrometry. Food Science and Technology 63, 430–436.

Tapp, H., Defernez, M., Kemsley, E.K., 2003. FTIR spectroscopy and multivariate analysis can distinguish the geographic origin of extra virgin olive oils. Journal of Agricultural and Food Chemistry 51 (21), 6110–6115.

Tay, A., Singh, R.K., Krishnan, S.S., Gore, J.P., 2002. Authentication of olive oil adulterated with vegetable oils using Fourier transform infrared spectroscopy. Food Science and Technology 35, 99–103.

Twomey, M., Downey, G., McNulty, P., 1995. The potential of NIR spectroscopy for the detection of the adulteration of Orange juice. Journal of the Science of Food and Agriculture 67, 77–84.

Van der Ven, C., Gruppen, H., de Bont, D.B.A., Voragen, A.G.J., 2002. Optimisation of the angiotensin converting enzyme inhibition by whey protein hydrolysates using response surface methodology. International Dairy Journal 12 (10), 813–820.

Vardin, H., Tay, A., Ozen, B., Mauer, L., 2008. Authentication of pomegranate juice concentrate using FTIR spectroscopy and chemometrics. Food Chemistry 108 (2), 742–748.

Vasconcelos, M., Coelho, L., Barros, A., Martins de Almeida, J.M.M., 2015. Study of adulteration of extra virgin olive oil with peanut oil using FTIR spectroscopy and chemometrics. Cogent Food & Agriculture (1), 1018695.

Vlachos, N., Skopelitis, Y., Psaroudaki, M., Konstantinidou, V., Chatzilazarou, A., Tegou, E., 2006. Applications of Fourier transform-infrared spectroscopy to edible oils. Analytica Chimica Acta 74, 459–465.

Volodin, V.A., Marin, D.V., Sachkov, V.A., Gorokhov, E.B., Rinnert, H., Vergnat, M., 2014. Applying an improved phonon confinement model to the analysis of Raman spectra of germanium nanocrystals. Journal of Experimental and Theoretical Physics 118 (1), 65–71.

Vongsvivut, J., Robertson, E.G., Menaughton, D., 2010. Surface-enhanced Raman spectroscopic analysis of fonofos pesticide adsorbed on silver and gold nanoparticles. Journal of Raman Spectroscopy 41, 1137–1148.

Wang, T., Tan, S.Y., Mutilangi, W., Aykas, D.P., Rodriguez-Saona, L.E., 2015. Authentication of whey protein powders by portable mid-infrared spectrometers combined with pattern recognition analysis. Journal of Food Science 80 (10), C2111–C2116.

Wesley, I., Pacheco, F., McGill, A., 1996. Identification of adulterants in olive oils. Journal of the American Oil Chemists' Society 73 (4), 515–518.

Wold, S., Sjöström, M., Eriksson, L., 2001. PLS-regression: a basic tool of chemometrics. Chemometrics and Intelligent Laboratory Systems 58 (10), 109–130.

Wold, S., Martens, H., Wold, H., 1983. The Multivariate Calibration Problem in Chemistry Solved by the PLS Method. Springer, Berlin Heidelberg, pp. 286–293.

Woodcock, T., Fagan, C., O'Donnell, C.P., Downey, G., 2008. Application of near and mid-infrared spectroscopy to determine cheese quality and authenticity. Food and Bioprocess Technology 1 (2), 117–129.

World Health Organization (WHO), 2004. In: Terracini, B. (Ed.), Toxic Oil Syndrome Ten Years of Progress. World Health Organization, Geneva, Switzerland, pp. 5–35. Available from: http://www.euro.who.int/__data/assets/pdf_file/0005/98447/E84423.pdf.

Xu, M.L., Liu, J.B., Lu, J., 2014. Determination and control of pesticide residues in beverages: a review of extraction techniques, chromatography, and rapid detection methods. Applied Spectroscopy Reviews 49 (2), 97–120.

Yang, H., Irudayaraj, J., 2001. Comparison of near-infrared, Fourier transform-infrared, and Fourier transform-Raman methods for determining olive pomace oil adulteration in extra virgin olive oil. Journal of the American Oil Chemists' Society 78 (9), 889–895.

Yang, R., Liu, R., Xu, K., Yang, Y., 2013. Discrimination of adulterated milk based on two-dimensional correlation spectroscopy (2D-COS) combined with kernel orthogonal projection to latent structure (K-OPLS). Applied Spectroscopy 67 (12), 1363–1367.

Yang, D., Ying, Y., 2011. Applications of Raman spectroscopy in agricultural products and food analysis: a review. Applied Spectroscopy Reviews 46, 539–560.

Zhang, L.G., Zhang, X., Ni, L.J., Xue, Z.B., Gu, X., Huang, S.X., 2014. Rapid identification of adulterated cow milk by non-linear pattern recognition methods based on near infrared spectroscopy. Food Chemistry 145, 342–348.

Zhang, X., Young, M.A., Lyandres, O., Van Duyne, R.P., 2005. Rapid detection of an anthrax biomarker by surface-enhanced Raman spectroscopy. Journal of the American Chemical Society 127, 4484–4489.

Zhang, Y., Wang, D., Lee, R., Henning, S.M., Heber, D., 2009. Absence of pomegranate ellagitannins in the majority of commercial pomegranate extracts: implication for standardization and quality control. Food Chemistry 57, 7395–7400.

Advances in Fluorescence Emission Spectroscopy for Food Authenticity Testing

5

A. Dankowska
Poznań University of Economics and Business, Poznań, Poland

Chapter Outline

5.1 Introduction

Food authenticity is a very important issue for consumers, producers, and distributors. Accurate labeling is important to help consumers select appropriate types of product to fulfill their demands and to avoid some ingredients in the case of people who do not consume specific products in their diet owing to health, religious, or ethical reasons. Authentication methods applied to food can be classified according to different criteria. Separation techniques, such as gas chromatography, focus on the existence or absence of certain chemical compounds in the adulterated sample. Physical techniques are based on a combination of measurements, eg, light absorbance at different frequencies or over the whole spectrum. Fluorescence is one of the physical techniques that have been investigated for food authentication. The potential of fluorescence spectroscopy for monitoring food products has increased over the past few years with the widespread application of chemometric tools together with technical and optical developments in equipment. Fluorescence spectroscopy is a rapid, sensitive, and nondestructive analytical technique that can be used to record fingerprints of food products. The potential of fluorescence techniques (conventional excitation-emission matrix and synchronous fluorescence spectroscopy) for food authenticity testing is unquestionable, especially when it is combined with powerful multivariate analysis tools such as principal component analysis, parallel factor analysis, and factorial discriminant analysis.

Fluorescence is the emission of light by a fluorophore, which is a compound that absorbs energy in the form of light at a specific wavelength and radiates energy in the form of emitted light at a longer wavelength (Guilbault, 1999). Fluorescence spectroscopy offers several inherent advantages for the characterization of food products compared with other spectrophotometric techniques. The principal advantages of fluorescence spectroscopy are rapidity and sensitivity as the method is around 100 to 1000 times more sensitive than other spectrophotometric techniques (Strasburg and Ludescher, 1995). Fluorescence spectroscopy is able to determine various properties of foods with very little or any use of chemicals and the avoidance of time-consuming sample preparation (Andersen and Mortensen, 2008).

5.1.1 Principles of Fluorescence

There are several types of fluorescence measurements that are usually carried out in food analysis:

- Emission spectrum—obtained by recording emission intensity as a function of the emission wavelength λem.
- Excitation spectrum—obtained when λex is scanned while observation is conducted at a fixed λem.
- Total excitation-emission matrix luminescence spectroscopy (EEM)—a three-dimensional landscape is obtained when a set of emission spectra is recorded at different values of λex (this enables one to obtain more information on the fluorescent species present in the sample).
- Synchronous fluorescence spectroscopy (SFS)—values of λex and λem are scanned simultaneously while maintaining a constant wavelength interval ($\Delta\lambda$) between λex and λem (spectral overlap can be overcome and selectivity can be enhanced) (Guilbault, 1999).

This last technique provides some important advantages, such as spectral simplification, bandwidth narrowing, reduced scattering interference, and improved resolution. SFS is efficient in increasing analytical selectivity yet it maintains the fluorimetric high sensitivity. SFS has become an attractive alternative for the simultaneous determination of complex samples containing multiple compounds. Synchronous fluorescence techniques can be further divided into (Li et al., 2010):

- Conventional synchronous fluorescence spectroscopy known as constant-wavelength SFS (CWSFS), in which a constant wavelength difference is maintained between the excitation and emission monochromators.

- Constant-energy SFS (CESFS)—the excitation and the emission monochromators are synchronized so that a constant energy difference is maintained between two monochromators. Considerable improvements in selectivity of the analysis of polycyclic aromatic hydrocarbon (PAH) mixtures were made with this technique.
- Variable-angle SFS (VASFS)—the fluorescence measurement is carried out through the simultaneous scanning of the excitation and the emission monochromators at different rates. This technique is known for its flexibility as well as high selectivity.
- Matrix isopotential SFS (MISFS) —it is possible to make use of a cut in the total fluorescence spectrum. The cut can be obtained by joining points of equal intensity to produce an isopotential trajectory.

Recently, a combination of synchronous fluorescence spectrometry with other techniques and chemometrics has been developed in order to overcome spectral overlapping problems in multicomponent samples. First among these is the derivative technique, which is an excellent way of band narrowing and signal enhancing for minor spectral features. A combination of the derivative technique and SFS approaches provides synergistic effects for better resolution and selectivity. Secondly, we can consider the low-temperature technique, which has shown excellent band-narrowing features. A combination of the low-temperature technique and SFS provides better resolution than traditional fluorescence methods. Finally, chemometrics is one of the modern approaches to improve applicability of analytical methods (Li et al., 2010).

Fluorescence spectra can by acquired using different measurement geometries (Fig. 5.1). Right-angle geometry is used for diluted samples while front-face

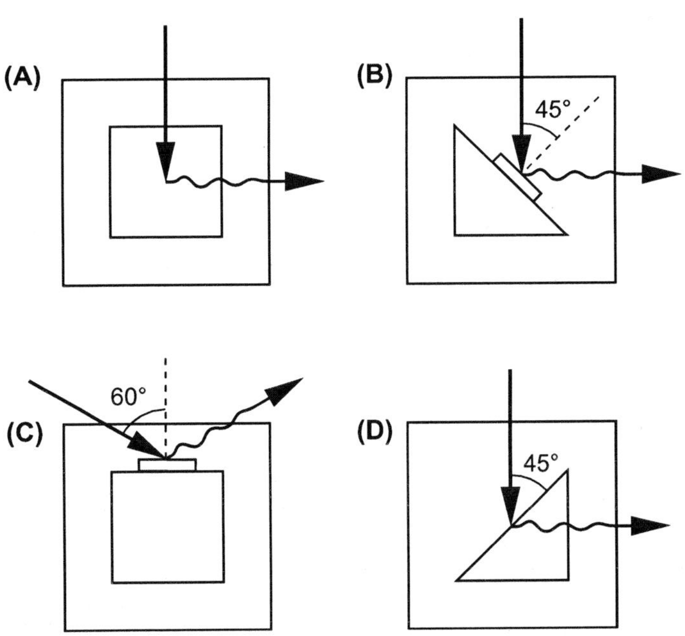

Figure 5.1 (A) Right-angle geometry, (B) front-face geometry (45°), (C) front-face geometry (60°), and (D) 45° angle geometry with a triangular cell.

fluorescence spectroscopy is deployed for bulk liquid or solid samples. Applicability of conventional right-angle fluorescence is limited by spectral overlap; the inner-filter effect, scattered light, and reflected light can also limit the spectroscopy under certain conditions, eg, high concentrations of the fluorescent species. To avoid these problems, the method of front-face fluorescence spectroscopy is used for bulk liquid and solid samples (Li et al., 2010).

Spectra obtained with right-angle geometry are used for further analysis with no pretreatment. Samples analyzed with this geometry must be diluted, and concentration of the analyzed product is fixed. Front-face fluorescence spectra are normalized by the reduction of the area under each spectrum to the value of one to minimize scattering effects and delete differences between spectra due to different amounts of sample. A first or second derivative algorithm is sometimes used to enhance differences between spectra and resolve overlapping bands (Bertrand and Scotter, 1992; Sikorska, 2008). Patra and Mishra (2002) proposed the use of a reversed triangle cuvette to resolve overlapping bands.

Besides factors related to the nature of the food sample as well as fluorophore concentration, the molecular environment of the inherent fluorophores will influence the fluorescence signal, eg, scatter, quenching, concentration, and molecular environment. Scattering and reflection of the incident light have a substantial effect on fluorescence measurements both with respect to the optical depth of sampling and the fluorescence signal obtained. Raman scatter is related to vibrational states of the bulk substances in the sample and reflects a constant energy loss. Raman scatter can in many cases be neglected because of its weak contribution to the fluorescence signal. Alternatively, corrections of the fluorescence signal can be performed either by subtracting the pure solvent or background scatter contribution or by specifically addressing the scatter in the modeling of the fluorescence data. Fluorescence quenching refers to any process that decreases the fluorescence intensity of a sample—a deactivation of the excited molecule by molecular interactions. Moreover, fluorescence intensity depends on the concentration, the molar absorptivity, and the quantum yield of a fluorophore. Fluorescence intensity is approximately linearly proportional to the concentration of the fluorophore in solutions with optical density values below 0.05 AU. Additionally, the polarity of the local environment of a fluorophore influences emission characteristics, especially in the case of polar fluorophores. In more polar environments, fluorophores relax to a lower vibrational energy state, resulting in emission at longer wavelengths (Christensen et al., 2006).

5.2 What Adulterations Can Fluorescence Emission Spectroscopy Be Used to Detect?

Food contains a wide range of naturally occurring fluorescent compounds that are important for its nutritional, compositional and technological quality; they include alkaloids, aromatic amino acids, coumarins, flavonoids, nucleic acids, porphyrins, mycotoxins, vitamins, and cofactors (Christensen et al., 2006; Karoui and Blecker, 2011). Moreover, fluorescent compounds are sensitive at the molecular level to changes that occur during food processing, handling, or storage; for that reason, fluorescence methods are useful for qualitative and/or quantitative detection of food adulteration. Fluorescence techniques are used for authentication of different food products, in particular for detection of quality changes in products, determination of the level of lipid oxidation in foods such as fish and meat (Aubourg, 1999; Wold and Mielnik, 2000; Wold et al., 2002), as well as classification of the botanical and/or geographical origins of products or product brands. Besides confirmation of food authenticity, fluorescence spectroscopy is used for monitoring various types of bioprocesses, eg, yeast or bacterial cultivations (Grote et al., 2014) or classification of food raw materials originating from different feeding systems (Hammami et al., 2010, 2013).

Fluorophores can be divided into two main classes: intrinsic and extrinsic. Intrinsic fluorophores are those that occur naturally. They include aromatic amino acids (tryptophan, tyrosine, and phenylalanine in proteins), vitamin A and B2, reduced nicotinamide adenine dinucleotide (NADH), derivatives of pyridoxal and chlorophyll, some nucleotides, and numerous other compounds that can be found at low or very low concentration in food. Extrinsic fluorophores are added to the sample to provide fluorescence when none exists or to change the spectral properties of the sample (Karoui et al., 2003). An overview of fluorophores in different food systems is presented in Table 5.1 (Karoui and Blecker, 2011).

Fluorophore concentration depends on botanical and geographical origin, production process, storage condition, and freshness of the product. Therefore, fluorimetry can be widely applied to food authentication, in particular, for the following:

1. Detection of adulteration
   a. Adulteration of the process. It is common that a commodity commands a premium price because it is prepared by a specific process, eg, orange juice obtained by squeezing the fruit, hence pulp wash is not permitted in pure orange juice.
   b. Adulteration of species or variety. It involves mixing authentic products with a similar but less expensive alternative, eg, orange juice adulterated with apple juice or olive oil blended with another oil.
   c. Adulteration of geographical origin. Products from one region may be of considerably greater value than similar products from other areas.
   d. Adulteration of brand. Selling a product as a more expensive brand; commonly this concerns manufactured products more than commodities (eg, whisky).
2. Freshness detection. Substitution of a fresh product with an expired one, mislabeling food with prolonged expiry date, or selling frozen products as fresh are examples of fraudulent practices that might be potentially harmful to consumers' health.
3. Grading and categorization. Selling products of cheaper grade as more expensive ones is a fraudulent practice. This type of food mislabeling, whilst not necessarily unsafe, deceives the consumer as to the nature of the product being purchased. Fig. 5.2 presents examples of synchronous fluorescence spectra (at wavelength intervals equal to 10 and 80 nm) obtained for food authentication: different food products, different edible oils, different grades of olive oils, fresh and expired olive oils, and cocoa butter adulterated with cocoa butter equivalent (CBE) (Table 5.2).

Table 5.1 Overview of Fluorescence in Different Food Systems

Fluorophore	Products								
	Dairy Products	Honey	Meat	Alcohols	Fish	Egg	Edible Oils	Cereal	Sugar
Amino acids and nucleic acids		✓		✓	✓			✓	
Caramel				✓					
Collagen	✓								
Chlorophyll				✓			✓		
Ferulic acid								✓	
Maillard products						✓			✓
NADH					✓				✓
FAD	✓		✓				✓		
Oxidation products			✓				✓		
Polyphenols		✓		✓			✓		✓
Retinol	✓								
Riboflavin	✓			✓				✓	
Tocopherols							✓		

FAD, flavin adenine dinucleotide; *NADH*, reduced nicotinamide adenine dinucleotide.
Christensen, J., Nørgaard, L., Bro, R., Engelsen, S.B., 2006. Multivariate autofluorescence of intact food systems. Chemical Reviews 106 (6), 1979–1994; Sádecká, J., Tóthová, J., 2007. Fluorescence spectroscopy and chemometrics in the food classification – a review. Czech Journal of Food Science 25 (4), 159–173; Karoui, R, Blecker, C., 2011. Fluorescence spectroscopy measurement for quality assessment of food systems—a review. Food Bioprocess Technology 4 (3), 364–386.

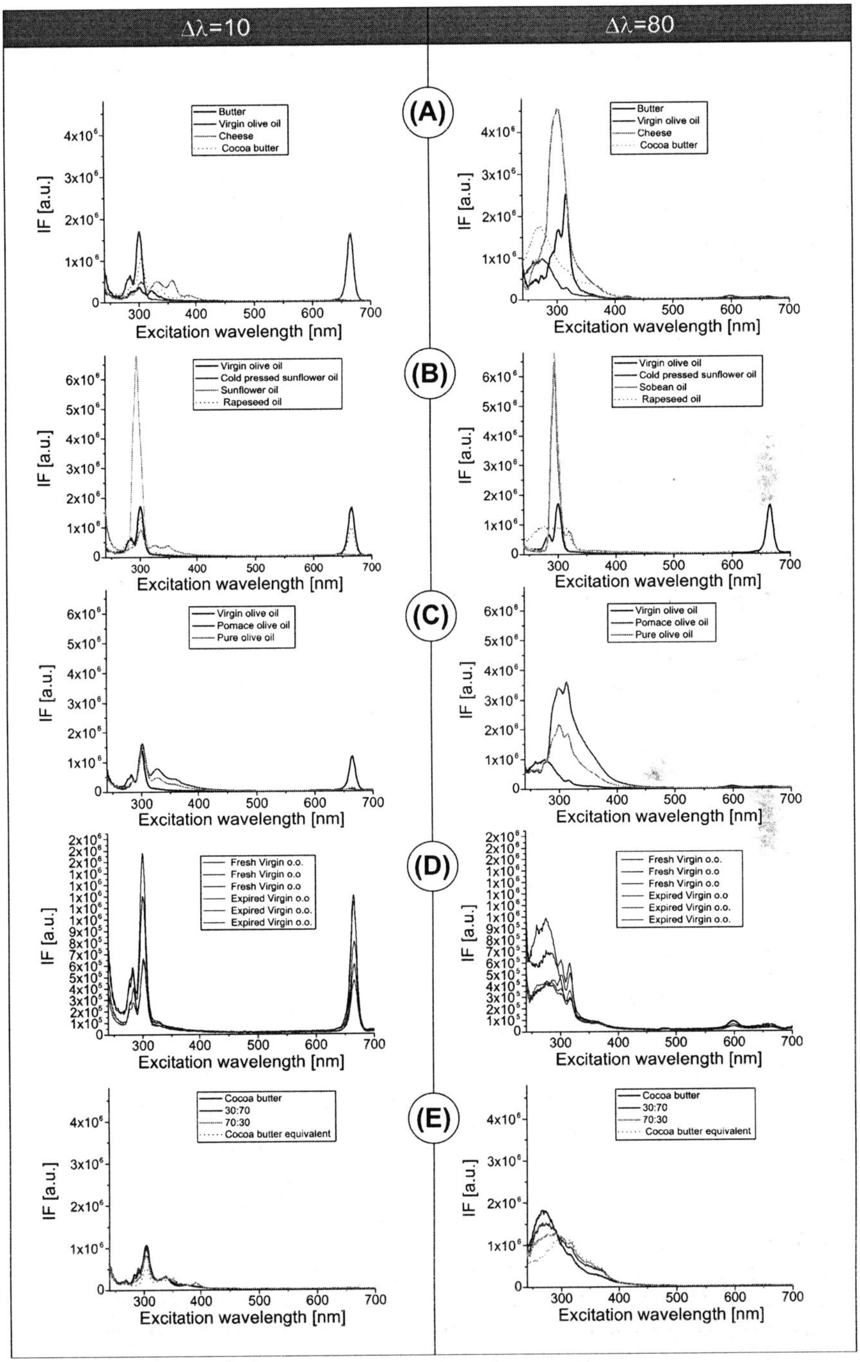

Figure 5.2 Examples of synchronous fluorescence spectra obtained at $\Delta\lambda$: (A) different food products, (B) different edible oils, (C) different grades of olive oil, (D) fresh and expired olive oil, and (E) cocoa butter adulterated with cocoa butter equivalent (CBE).

Table 5.2 Fluorescence and Multivariate Analysis Techniques for Food Authentication (a) Adulteration, (b) Detection of Food Freshness, and (c) Food Grading and Categorization

Food Sample	Fluorescence Technique	Fluorophore	Multivariate Analysis Technique	References
(a) Food Adulteration (Different Process, Botanical or Geographical Origin, Brand)				
Beer	TLS, 3D-SFS	Amino acids, vitamins polyphenols	None	Insińska-Rak et al. (2007)
Brandy	EEM	Caramel, phenolic compounds	PARAFAC-PLS	Markechová et al. (2014)
Butter	SFS	Polyphenols, tocochromanoles, chlorophylls	SPA, LOD, MLR, LDA	Dankowska et al. (2014)
Cheese	SFS	Polyphenols, tocochromanoles, chlorophylls	SPA, LOD, MLD, MLR, PCA, LDA	Dankowska et al. (2015)
Honey	RA- 3D-SFS	Phenolic compounds	None	Sergiel et al. (2014)
Honey	FF-SFS	Phenolic compounds	PCA, PLS-DA	Lenhardt et al. (2014)
Honey	3DFS	Aromatic amino acids, phenolic compounds	PCA, PLS, BP-ANN	Chen et al. (2014)
Honey	FF-ES, FF-ExS	Aromatic amino and nucleic acids, HMF, furosine, polyphenols	PCA, FDA	Karoui et al. (2007a)
Milk (with melamine)	ES	Triton X-114 excitation at 235 nm	LOD, regression analysis	Nascimento et al. (2015)
Milk fat, butter	2D and 3D FF-FS	Fatty acids, tryptophan, tocopherol, riboflavin	PCA	Ntakatsane et al. (2013)
Olive oil	RA-EEM, RA-SFS	Fatty acids, oxidative products	PCA, HCA	Poulli et al. (2005)

Olive oil	TSFS, SFS	Polyphenols, tocochromanoles, chlorophylls	PLS	Poulli et al. (2006)
Olive oil	SFS	Polyphenols, tocochromanoles, chlorophylls	SPA, PCA, LDA, MLR,LOD	Dankowska et al. (2013a)
Olive oil	SFS	Polyphenols, tocochromanoles, chlorophylls	LOD, MLR	Dankowska et al. (2009)
Olive oil	RA-EEM	Conjugated hydroperoxides, vitamin E, chlorophylls	PCA, PARAFAC, LDA, PLSR	Guimet et al. (2005)
Orange juice	3D-FF-FS	Flavonoids and phenolic compounds	ICA, MLR	Ammari et al. (2015)
Spices	SFS	Sudan I dye	PLS-DA	Di Anibal et al. (2015)
Virgin olive oil	TSFS	Polyphenols, tocopherols, tocotrienols, chlorophylls	PLS	Poulli et al. (2007)
Virgin olive oil/ hazelnut	ES	Pigments and tocopherols, hydrolysis products	Regression analysis, ANOVA	Sayago et al. (2004)
Walnut oil	ES	Fatty acid oxidation products, tocopherols, carotenoids, chlorophyll	SIMCA, PLS	Li et al. (2015)
Wine	FF-EEM	Polyphenols, vitamins and amino acids	PARAFAC	Airado-Rodriguez et al. (2011)
Wine spirits	TSFS	Caramel	LOQ, LOD, precision, repeatability, and recovery	Sádecká and Tóthová (2010)
Olive oil	TSFS, SFS	Oxidation products	PCR, PLS	Wójcicki et al. (2015)
(b) Food Freshness				
Apples	FF	Chlorophyll	Regression analysis	De Ell et al. (1996)
Beer	RA-EMM	Aromatic amino acids, riboflavin	PCA, kNN, LDA	Sikorska et al. (2006)

Continued

Table 5.2 Fluorescence and Multivariate Analysis Techniques for Food Authentication (a) Adulteration, (b) Detection of Food Freshness, and (c) Food Grading and Categorization—cont'd

Food Sample	Fluorescence Technique	Fluorophore	Multivariate Analysis Technique	References
Cakes	FF-FS	Vitamin A, oxidation products, lumichrome	PCA	Botoso et al. (2013)
Eggs	FF (22.5°)	Tryptophan, vitamin A, conjugated linoleic acid (CLA)	PCA, FDA	Karoui et al. (2006b,c)
Extra virgin olive oil	ExS	Phenolic compounds, vitamin E, hydroperoxides	PLS	Cheikhousman et al. (2004, 2005)
Olive oil	TLS, SFS	Tocopherols, chlorophyll, phenolic compounds	Regression analysis, PCA	Sikorska et al. (2008a)
Meat	FF-FS	Oxidation products	Multivariate regression	Wold et al. (2002)
Rapeseed oils	FS	Tocopherols	PLS	Mas et al. (2004)
Meat	FF-EMM (180°)	Amino acids, lipid oxidation products	PCA, PLS, PARAFAC	Moller et al. (2003)
(c) Grading and Categorization				
Brandy	SFS	Tyrosine, tryptophan, ferulic, *p*-coumaric, caffeic acids, chlorophyll, lignin, scopoletin, umbelliferon, 4-methylumbelliferon, gallic, vanillic and syringic acids, tryptophol, tyrosol, lignin	PCA, HCA, LDA	Píš et al. (2011)
Cereal flour	FF-SFS	Tryptophan, ferulic acid, *p*-hydroxycinnamic acids such as coumaric and caffeic acid, riboflavin lutein and xanthophyll	PCA, cluster analysis, PLS-DA	Zeković et al. (2012)

Fish fillets	FF (56°)	Tryptophan, NADH	PCA, FDA	Karoui et al. (2006e)
Hard cheeses	ES	Aromatic amino acids, tryptophan, CLA, phenolic compounds, aromatic acids, polycyclic aromatic hydrocarbons	PCA	Karoui et al. (2005)
Olive oil	SFS	Polyphenols, tocopherols, tocotrienols, chlorophylls	SPA, PCA, LDA, MLR, LOD	Dankowska et al. (2013b)
Olive oil	RA-EEM	Tocopherols, oxidation products	NMF, LDA, PLSR PARAFAC,	Guimet et al. (2006)
Olive oil	RA-EEM	Chlorophylls, vitamin E, oxidation products	PCA, PARAFAC	Guimet et al. (2004a)
Olive oil	RA-EEM	Chlorophylls, vitamin E, oxidation products	CA	Guimet et al. (2004b)
Sheep milk	FF-FS	Vitamin A, CLA, phenolic compounds	FDA, PCA	Hammami et al. (2010)
Soft cheese	FF (56°)	Tryptophan, casein, lipid oxidation products, vitamin A	PCA, CCSWA	Karoui et al. (2006a)
Vegetable oils	RA-SFS, TSFS	Tocopherols, polyphenols, chlorophylls,	kNN, LDA	Sikorska et al. (2005)
Olive oil	SEEM	Chlorophylls, tocopherols, phenols, riboflavin	PCA, PLS	Dupuy et al. (2005)
Wine	FF (56°)	Stilbenes, anthocyanins, flavanols, tannins, proteins	PCA, FDA	Dufour et al. (2006)

3D-SFS, three-dimensional synchronous fluorescence spectroscopy; *3DFS*, three-dimensional fluorescence spectroscopy; *CA*, cluster analysis; *CCSWA*, common components and specific weights analysis; *DA*, discriminant analysis; *EEM*, excitation emission matrix fluorescence spectra; *EFS*, emission fluorescence spectroscopy; *FDA*, factorial discriminant analysis; *FF*, front face; *FS*, fluorescence spectroscopy; *ExS*, fluorescence excitation spectra; *HCA*, hierarchical cluster analysis; *ICA*, independent components analysis; *kNN*, k-nearest neighbors; *LDA*, linear discriminant analysis; *LOD*, limit of detection; *LOQ*, limit of determination; NADH, reduced nicotinamide adenine dinucleotide; *PARAFAC*, parallel factor analysis; *PCA*, principal component analysis; *PLS*, partial least squares; *RA*, right angle; *SEEM*, synchronous excitation-emission fluorescence spectra; *SFS*, synchronous fluorescence spectroscopy; *SIMCA*, soft independent modeling by class analogy; *TLS*, total luminescence spectra; *TSFS*, total synchronous fluorescence spectroscopy.

5.3 Applications of Fluorescence Emission Spectroscopy for Food Authentication – Examples

5.3.1 Edible Oils and Fats

Edible oils contain different fluorophores such as tocopherols, chlorophylls, and polyphenols depending on the botanical origin of the oil as well as the technology applied in their extraction. Refining processes decrease the vitamin E and chlorophyll contents, so refined oils are more susceptible to oxidation processes, and oxidative changes in fatty acids are reflected in their emission fluorescence spectra. A wide peak is found between 400 and 500 nm for excitation at 365 nm (Kyriakidis and Skarkalis, 2000).

Many studies regarding vegetable oils on fluorescence spectroscopy analysis are reported in the literature. Sikorska et al. (2005) applied total luminescence and SFS to characterize and differentiate edible oils, including soybean, sunflower, rapeseed, peanut, olive, grape-seed, linseed, and corn oils. Bands attributed to tocopherols, chlorophylls, and unidentified fluorescent components were detected in SFS spectra. Both fluorescence methods provided a very good discrimination between oil classes with a low classification error. Guimet et al. (2006) studied the capabilities of nonnegative matrix factorization (NMF) used together with linear discriminant analysis (LDA) for discriminating between the different types of oils by means of excitation-emission fluorescence spectroscopy. The main advantage of NMF with respect to discriminant multiway partial least squares regression (PLSR) is that basic functions are more interpretable than PLS loadings because they are positive and correspond to parts of the spectra that are more easily related to the fluorescent compounds of the oils.

Most papers on the use of fluorescence spectra for analysis of edible oils concern the problem of extra virgin olive oil authenticity. Extra virgin olive oil is highly valued because it is traditionally pressed and does not undergo the refining process. For this reason, this category of olive oil is the most expensive and is sometimes adulterated with olive-pomace oil and refined olive oil or pure olive oil (a blend of refined olive oil with extra virgin olive oil) or even with seed oils.

Guimet et al. (2005) developed a fast screening method based on excitation-emission fluorescence (EEM) spectra for detecting adulteration with olive-pomace oil at 5% level in extra virgin olive oil. EEM spectra were used by the same author for differentiation between virgin and pure olive oils. It was established that oxidation products contribute most to the separation between the two oil categories. The ranges studied were $\lambda ex = 300-400$ nm, $\lambda em = 400-695$ nm with $\lambda ex = 300-400$ nm, and $\lambda em = 400-600$ nm. Unfold principal component analysis (U-PCA) and parallel factor analysis (PARAFAC) were applied to analyze the types of olive oils. The three-component PARAFAC model was found to be the most interpretable and enabled a good distinction between the two groups of olive oils. Moreover, it was shown that differentiation between virgin and pure olive oils is better when the chlorophyll fluorescence region is not included in the models (Guimet et al., 2004a).

Poulli et al. compared SFS spectra with EEM spectra measured for edible and lampante olive oils (olive oils unfit for human consumption). SFS showed a reduced spectral complexity and high amplification of fluorescence bands; a wavelength interval $\Delta\lambda$ of 80 nm provided the best differentiation between olive oil samples. According to the findings, virgin olive oil showed one low-intensity band at 370 nm while lampante virgin olive oil showed medium-intensity bands at 385 and 450 nm. Maximum differentiation between oil samples was found in the spectral range 429–545 nm, originating from oleic acid (Poulli et al., 2005).

Dankowska et al. (2013b) examined the potential of SFS for the classification of olive oils. Spectra were measured in the region 240–700 nm with wavelength intervals of 10, 30, 60, and 80 nm. For the first time, the successive projection algorithm (SPA) was applied for the determination of representative wavelengths in fluorescence spectra. SPA is an approach suitable for selecting effective wavelength variables from spectra; it has been compared to the genetic algorithm, which is a popular method for variable selection in multivariate calibration, and the results proved to be in favor of SPA (Araújo et al., 2001). Classification errors of the LDA analysis were in the range 0.9–6.4% for measurements collected at all wavelength intervals. The best classification accuracy was obtained for synchronous fluorescence intensities acquired for a wavelength interval of 10 nm.

SFS was also applied for the detection of extra virgin olive oil adulteration by olive oil (Dankowska and Małecka, 2009). Olive oils are blends of refined and virgin oils and must possess free acidity of no more than 1% and conform to standards within their category (IOC, 2015). Synchronous fluorescence spectra were collected in the region 240–700 nm at wavelength intervals of 10, 30, 60, and 80 nm. Results showed that the ability to detect olive oil in extra virgin olive oil was better using a wavelength interval of 60 or 80 nm than one of 10 or 30 nm. According to the data acquired at 60 and 80 nm wavelength intervals, the lowest detection limits of adulteration were 8.9% and 8.4% at the wavelengths 350 and 302 nm, respectively.

Poulli et al. (2007) applied total synchronous fluorescence (TSFS) for the detection of virgin olive adulteration with olive-pomace, corn, sunflower, soybean, rapeseed, and walnut oils. TSFS spectra were acquired by varying the excitation wavelength over the region 250–720 nm and the wavelength interval from 20 to 120 nm. Adulterants could be discriminated from virgin olive oil using a wavelength interval of 20 nm and excitation wavelength region 315–400, 315–392, 315–375, 315–365, 315–375, and 315–360 for olive-pomace, corn, sunflower, soybean, rapeseed, and walnut oils, respectively. PLSR was used to quantify adulteration and enabled detection of olive-pomace, corn, sunflower, soybean, rapeseed, and walnut oil in virgin olive oil at levels of 2.6%, 3.8%, 4.3%, 4.2%, 3.6%, and 13.8% (w/w), respectively. The problem of extra virgin olive oil adulteration with sunflower oil was analyzed by Poulli et al. (2006) using TSFS spectra measured at wavelength intervals of 20 and 80 nm followed by PLSR analysis. This technique was reported to detect sunflower oil in virgin olive oil at levels down to 3.4% (w/v) using an 80-nm wavelength interval.

Sayago et al. (2004) applied the measurement of emission fluorescence spectroscopy followed by multivariate analysis to assess the genuineness of olive oil in admixtures with hazelnut oils. The authors examined seven virgin olive oil samples of different European varieties, as well as virgin hazelnut oils from roasted hazelnuts and their corresponding refined oils obtained on laboratory scale and their mixtures.

The amount of hazelnut oil added to olive oil ranged from 5% to 30%. Fluorescence emission spectra of oil samples and admixtures in the region 300–800 nm were collected at 350-nm excitation wavelength. Raw spectral data were subjected to mathematical treatment by calculation of the first derivative, selection of the maximum values, and application of one-way ANOVA to assess the most prominent variables in the discrimination process. Linear discriminant analysis applied to each admixture separately and to the whole set of samples allowed 100% correct classification in the calibration set.

A few papers have been published in recent years on the use of fluorescence in vegetable oils other than olive oil. Li et al. (2015) compared the potential of Fourier transform infrared (FTIR) and fluorescence spectroscopy, combined with soft independent modeling of class analogies (SIMCA) and PLS, in detecting the authenticity of walnut oil and the adulteration amounts of soybean oil in walnut oil. The classification error of soybean oil adulterated with walnut oil as measured by fluorescence spectroscopy was below 5% (w/w) while the classification limit of soybean oil in walnut oil with a SIMCA model of FTIR spectra was 10% (w/w). Fluorescence spectroscopy was more applicable than FTIR in the adulteration detection of walnut oil.

Fluorescence spectroscopy was also applied for the authentication of fats of animal origin. Dankowska et al. (2014) applied SFS with multivariate data analysis for the determination of butter adulteration. Butter fats, palm oil, and coconut fat oils exhibit differences in fluorescence spectra caused by the different content of tocopherols, tocotrienols, and chlorophylls; these differences make it possible to distinguish between butter fat and palm and coconut oils (Ntakatsane et al., 2013). Synchronous fluorescence spectra were collected in the range 240–700 nm with wavelength intervals of 10, 30, 60, and 80 nm. The lowest detection limit of adulteration of butter fat with palm and coconut oils of 5.5% (w/w) was obtained for measurements acquired at a 60-nm wavelength interval and an excitation wavelength of 313 nm. Highest prediction accuracy of multiple linear regression (MLR) models was in the case of fluorescence intensities measured at the 60-nm wavelength interval with errors of classification and prediction equal to 3.8% and 3.9% (Dankowska et al., 2014).

5.3.2 Dairy Products and Eggs

Dairy products contain many fluorophores such as aromatic amino acids, nucleic acids, tryptophan residues of proteins, riboflavin, vitamin A, conjugated linoleic acid (CLA), and PAHs (Karoui and Blecker, 2011). Tryptophan residues in proteins are excited at 290 nm with maximum emission at about 345 nm, while emission fluorescence in the 305–450 nm region allows analysis of fluorescent Maillard-reaction products (maximum emission at 440 nm (Karoui et al., 2007b). Riboflavin has a strong and broad fluorescence emission peak in the region of 525–531 nm (excitation wavelength 380 nm). In ultraviolet light, riboflavin is degraded into two fluorescent products: lumichrome and lumiflavin (Andersen and Mortensen, 2008; Karoui et al., 2007b). Excitation spectra of vitamin A recorded between 250 and 350 nm with the emission wavelength set at 410 nm provide information on the development of protein–fat globule interactions during milk coagulation. The shape of the vitamin A excitation spectrum has been correlated with the physical state of triglycerides in the fat globule (Karoui et al., 2007b). Since these products differ in their manufacturing processes, geographic locations, animal feed, and breeds as well as the conditions of milk production, it is apparent that their structures at the molecular level and, as a consequence, their intrinsic fluorophores are different. Fluorescence enables the classification of cheese according to geographical origin (Karoui et al., 2004), milk preparation (raw milk or milk from a thermized milk process) (Karoui et al., 2005), and season of production, manufacturing processes, or sampling zones (Karoui et al., 2007b).

Front-face fluorescence spectroscopy in combination with a mid-infrared (MIR) spectroscopy was used to discriminate between Emmental cheeses originating from different European countries. The first 20 principal components of the PCA were extracted from each data set (MIR and fluorescence spectra), pooled (concatenated) into a single matrix, and analyzed by factorial discriminant. Correct classifications for 89% of the calibration spectra and 76.7% of the validation spectra were recorded (Karoui et al., 2004).

Moreover, Karoui et al. (2005) examined the potential of MIR and intrinsic fluorescence spectroscopies in determining geographical origins of different hard cheeses. As a result, 80% and 100% correct classification rates were obtained by applying factorial discriminant analysis (FDA) to the MIR and fluorescence spectra, respectively.

Karoui et al. (2007b) examined 15 traditional and stabilized retail soft cheeses with different manufacturing processes using front-face fluorescence spectroscopy. The spectral patterns yielded information on protein structure, protein—protein and protein—fat globule interactions, and the degree of degradation of riboflavin at molecular level. Fluorescence spectroscopy allowed for identification of cheeses by their manufacturing processes and sampling zones (Karoui et al., 2007b).

Dankowska et al. (2015) evaluated the potential of synchronous fluorescence spectroscopy followed by chemometric analysis (SPA) combined with MLR and LDA for the detection of cheese adulteration with plant oils. Cheese is made from milk; therefore, the only fat it contains is milk fat. Cheese-like products are obtained by total or partial substitution of milk fat by significantly cheaper plant oils. Results obtained have shown that fat contained in cheese and cheese-like products exhibits significant differences in fluorescent intensities. Lowest detection limits of adulteration of cheese fat with cheese-like product fat, namely 3.0% and 4.4% (w/w), were obtained by measurements acquired at higher (60 and 80 nm) than lower wavelength intervals (10 and 30 nm). MLR models for fluorescence intensities obtained at the wavelength interval of 60 nm enabled the prediction of the addition of plant oils with error of calibration and prediction equal to 1.5% and 1.7% (Dankowska et al., 2015).

Fluorimetric procedures were proposed for melamine determination in milk. Zhang et al. (2012) have exploited quenching of the fluorescence of quantum dots by melamine, ie, the inner-filter effect caused by Au nanoparticles on the fluorescence of CdTe. The detection limit was estimated at 0.8 mg/L (95% confidence level). Results for different milk samples agreed with those obtained by high-performance liquid chromatography (Nascimento et al., 2015).

Fluorescence spectroscopy is also a promising approach for determining egg freshness. In the study 79 fresh white-shelled eggs came directly from the producer. The eggs were stored in daylight at room temperature for up to 29 days. The fluorescence emission spectra of tryptophan residues (excitation: 290 nm; emission: 305–430 nm) of proteins and the excitation spectra of vitamin A (emission: 410 nm; excitation: 270–350 nm) were recorded directly on egg yolk samples. The first five principal components of the PCA extracted from each data set (tryptophan and vitamin A fluorescence spectra) were pooled into a single matrix and analyzed by FDA. Correct classifications were obtained for 97.5% of the calibration and 96.3.1% of the validation spectra. The intensity at 672 nm of a fresh egg is stronger than that of an old one (Karoui et al., 2006b).

5.3.3 Meat, Fish, and Meat and Fish Products

Meat authenticity has many aspects for consumers such as species, geographical origin, meat cuts, breed, wild or farmed meat, organic or conventional meat, fresh or frozen-thawed meat, and freshness. Fluorophores in meat include collagen and NADH, protein fluorescence, and suggestions for some fluorescent oxidation compounds were also reported (Swatland, 2000, 2001). Meat tissue at this excitation wavelength gives only weak fluorescence signals whereas fat, bone, cartilage, and connective tissue give a stronger fluorescence emission signal (Egelandsdal et al., 2002). Fluorescence emission spectra assigned to fluorescent oxidation products were found to correlate with lipid oxidation and rancidity of meat. Tryptophan fluorescence (excitation 290 nm) was correlated with the texture of meat emulsions and sausages and meat tenderness. Autofluorescence images reflecting collagen fluorescence were used for evaluating lipid oxidation in chicken meat. Veberg et al. (2006) studied the formation of the fluorescent compounds in meat undergoing lipid oxidation. A PARAFAC decomposition of the recorded fluorescence landscapes revealed the presence of five fluorophores, of which tryptophan was assigned as the dominant one. The remaining four components were suggested to arise from salting and fatty acid oxidation products (Veberg et al., 2006).

Front-face autofluorescence of meat products was measured in an attempt to measure and predict lipid oxidation. Three sample sets were studied: turkey meat with added aldehydes, raw and heat-treated turkey meat, and meat loaf at different process steps. In the experiment semiquantitative amounts of volatile compounds were found by correcting peak intensities from the integrator against the peak of the internal standard. Multivariate regression was used to correlate spectral data with sensorially assessed rancidity or volatile profiles. Results verified that the increase in fluorescence during storage originated from aldehydes reacting with the meat matrix. Fluorescence spectroscopy modeled sensorially assessed rancidity with the same accuracy as direct measurement of volatile compounds ($R = 0.9$). RMSECV (root mean square error of cross validation) values obtained for acidic odor and flavor were in the range from 0.48 to 0.64. Errors for rancid odor and flavor were higher and were in the range from 0.58 to 1.05 (Wold et al., 2002).

Fish authenticity has similar issues to those of meat, including species, geographical origin, wild or farm-raised fish, organic or conventional fish, fresh or frozen-thawed fish, and freshness. Important fluorophores of fish muscle include aromatic amino acids and nucleic acids (excitation 250 nm, emission 280–480 nm), tryptophan residues in proteins (excitation 290 nm, emission 305–400 nm), and NADH (excitation 336 nm, emission 360–600 nm) (Kamruzzaman et al., 2015). During freezing, storage, and thawing, fish muscle may undergo protein denaturation and lipid oxidation. Fluorescence spectrometry was used to measure lipid oxidation products during frozen fish storage (Aubourg, 1999; Duflos et al., 2002). Aromatic amino acids and nucleic acid fluorescence emission spectra as well as tryptophan and NADH fluorescence spectra recorded on cod, mackerel, salmon, and whiting fillets were reported to be fingerprints that allowed the evaluation of fish freshness. Percentages of correct classification reached 100%, 92%, 83%, and 92% at various times of storage, 1, 5, 8, and 13 days, respectively. According to the authors, the technique based on the intrinsic fluorescence of fish muscle might be adapted for online monitoring of fish freshness (Dufour et al., 2003).

NADH emission spectra (excitation 340 nm) of fresh fish showed a maximum at 455 nm, while frozen-thawed fish was characterized by a maximum at 379 nm (Karoui et al., 2006d).

5.3.4 Honey

Honey is a remarkable natural mixture including a large number of complicated fluorescent compounds mainly aromatic in nature. The presence of fluorophores (aromatic amino acids, vitamins, cofactors, and phenolic compounds) in honey makes fluorescence spectroscopy a valuable technique with which to determine the botanical origin of honey (Sádecká and Tóthová, 2007).

Lenhardt et al. (2014) showed that single synchronous fluorescence spectra of different honeys differ significantly. Synchronous fluorescence spectra of three monofloral (linden, sunflower, and acacia), polyfloral (meadow mix), and fake (fake acacia and linden) honey types (109 samples) were collected in an excitation range of 240–500 nm for synchronous wavelength intervals of 30–300 nm. Both principal component and partial least squares discriminant analyses were performed on this data set. Mean cross-validated classification error of 0.2% was found for a model accounting only for monofloral samples and 4.8% for a model including both the monofloral and polyfloral groups (Lenhardt et al., 2014).

According to Sergiel et al. (2014), right-angle geometry three-dimensional synchronous fluorescence spectroscopy (3D-SFS) is able to differentiate and classify different honey types, including acacia, buckwheat, heather, linden, multiflower, and rape honeys. The fraction of phenolic compounds was initially isolated and preconcentrated from samples analyzed by means of polymeric reversed phase Strata X solid phase extraction (SPE).

Karoui et al. (2007a) used front-face fluorescence spectroscopy as a tool for the classification of honey samples ($n = 62$) according to their botanical origins. Honey fluorescence spectra from seven floral origins, namely, acacia, alpine rose, chestnut, rape, honeydew, alpine polyfloral, and lowland polyfloral were scanned after excitation at 250 nm (emission: 280–480 nm), 290 nm (emission: 305–500 nm), 373 nm (emission: 380–600 nm), and emission set at 450 nm (excitation: 290–440 nm). Correct classification rates of 100% and 90% were observed for the calibration and the validation samples, respectively. Ruoff et al. (2006) studied fluorescence spectra of 371 honey samples originating from Switzerland, Germany, Italy, Spain, France, Slovenia, and Denmark. Excitation spectra (220−400 nm) were recorded with emission measured at 420 nm. Samples were classified according to their geographical origin by chemometric tools with the error rates of the discriminant models ranging from 0.1% to 7.5%. The samples could also be correctly classified by LDA according to their geographical origin except for one Swiss sample classified as of German provenance (Ruoff et al., 2006).

Spectra of fake honey samples showed pronounced differences from those of genuine honey, according to Chen et al. (2014) who used a three-dimensional fluorescence spectroscopy technique followed by multivariate analysis. Data of 3D spectra were compressed using characteristic extraction and PCA. Then, PLS and back propagation neural network (BP-ANN) algorithms were used for modeling. The results showed that BP-ANN model was superior to PLS models, and the optimum prediction results were obtained as follow: root mean square error of prediction (RMSEP) = 0.0235 and $R = 0.9787$ in the prediction set. The study demonstrated that the 3D fluorescence spectroscopy technique combined with multivariate calibration has potential for rapid, nondestructive, and accurate quantitative analysis in honey adulteration. Ghosh et al. (2005) measured front-face fluorescence spectra to monitor adulteration of honey with cane sugar syrup. Using an excitation wavelength of 340 nm, pure honey samples were characterized by a maximum located at 510 nm, ascribed to flavins, while cane sugar syrup adulterated samples exhibited a maximum located around 430 nm. By applying FDA to the data sets, classification rates of 100% and 90% were observed for the calibration and validation samples, respectively.

5.3.5 Fruits, Vegetables, and Juices

Fluorescence spectroscopy is considered to have potential for assessing mealiness in apples since a good correlation was obtained between mealiness and fluorescence spectra (Moshou et al., 2005). In the study, it is observed that the fluorescence values decreased with mealiness level for the Jonagold and Cox apples. Based on the fluorescence curves, different fluorescence parameters could be defined. The slope of the fluorescence curve at the origin and normalized fluorescence have proven to be reliable parameters in classifying apples according to their mealiness level for both cultivars. The achieved classification performance was around 85%.

Chlorophyll fluorescence has been suggested as a tool for evaluating changes in apples during maturation, the quality of apple juice during processing, and the ripening of papaya fruit (Bron et al., 2004). Regarding apple quality, a neural networks analysis achieved an accuracy of 95% using a test material classified by an expert as "bad" and "good" apples. Seiden et al. measured fluorescence emission spectra obtained that were evaluated to classify the juices according to variety and to relate measurements to the maturity of apples. Emission values were recorded in the interval of 275−560 nm and excitation wavelengths of 315 and 265 nm were chosen, as they yielded the richest spectra. The obtained spectra were analyzed by PCA. On the first loading vector the areas around (ex/em) 315/440 nm and 265/350 nm have the highest loadings, while for the second loading vector the area from 330 to 370 nm (ex 265 nm) has high loadings. PLS was used to develop models between the most significant spectral principal components and soluble solids, titratable acidity, time of picking, and variety. The measured value for soluble solids (in percent sucrose) was plotted against the value predicted by the PLS model based on the fluorescence spectra with the root mean square error of cross-validation RMSECV around 0.5%. Moreover, by developing a SIMCA model on one-half of the samples, it was possible to classify correctly the remaining half of the samples as either Jonagold or Elstar (Seiden et al., 1996).

Ammari et al. (2015) studied the adulteration of orange juice by grapefruit juice by 3D-front-face fluorescence spectroscopy followed by independent components analysis (ICA) and by classical methods such as free radical scavenging activity and total flavonoid content. The results clearly indicated that frauds resulting from the addition of grapefruit juice to orange juice could be detected in this sample set at least at levels as low as 1%.

5.3.6 Alcohols

Fluorophore profiles of alcoholic drinks differ significantly depending on the kind of alcohol, geographical origin, processing, and aging. Phenolic acids, stilbenes, anthocyanins, flavanols, and tannins are the best-known fluorescent molecules in wines with the nature and amounts of these molecules differing from one grape variety to another. Wine processing and aging also affect phenolic compounds. Regarding vitamins, it can be stated that vitamin C is present in fresh must and decreases during the fermentation process. Vitamin A (retinol) is present in wine in very small amounts. The principal forms of riboflavin are flavin-mononucleotide (FMN) and flavin-adenine-dinucleotide (FAD). Free riboflavin is also present in raw and processed fruits and fermented beverages. FAD, and sometimes FMN, is present together with free riboflavin in significant amounts in beer, while free riboflavin is the only form of riboflavin present in significant amounts in wine (Andre-Lacueva et al., 1998). In beers, there are three groups of fluorescent components: amino acids, vitamins, and phenolics. The measurement of their concentrations provides a new approach to evaluation of product quality. In the study of Apperson et al. (2002), fluorescence signals for beer samples were stated to have originated from aromatic amino acids, NADH, riboflavin, and vitamin B6. Fluorescence spectroscopy enabled the detection of differences in beer composition, eg, the content of riboflavin and vitamin B6. Concentrations of beer components depend on the type of beer, brewing conditions, and the raw materials used (Insińska-Rak et al., 2007).

Dufour et al. (2006) examined the ability of emission and excitation spectra to distinguish between typical and nontypical Beaujolais wines by applying FDA to the principal components of the PCA performed on the excitation fluorescence data or emission fluorescence data. Two groups were created for the wines under investigation, ie, typical wines and others. Correct classification rates of 95% and 87% were obtained for the emission fluorescence data set and the excitation fluorescence data set, respectively.

PARAFAC in combination with front-face fluorescence spectroscopy was applied in the evaluation of wine samples according to their appellation and aging condition. Excitation-emission matrices (EEMs) were obtained from front-face fluorescence measurements of untreated wine samples of 245–345 and 300–500 nm for excitation and emission, respectively. Interpretation of PARAFAC-score values enabled discrimination and clustering of wine samples belonging to different appellations. When plotting the scores of second PARAFAC component against the third, a good separation between Rioja and Ribera del Guadiana samples was achieved. In addition, the effect of aging was studied using the same methodology. An improved discrimination between Rioja and non-Rioja samples for Crianza and Reserva wines compared to young wines was found (Airado-Rodrıguez et al., 2011).

Sádecká and Tóthová (2010) carried out research aimed at distinguishing between brandies aged in oak casks and nonaged, caramel-colored mixed wine spirits, with the subsequent determination of caramel in the latter. SFS was shown to differentiate caramel from oakwood extract. Oakwood extract showed a band at 280 nm while caramel has a characteristic band at 387 nm. Based on this, caramel quantity in nonaged mixed wine spirits was calculated from fluorescence intensity measured at 387 nm. The calibration curve was linear over the range from 5 to 56 mg/L, and the limit of determination reported was 5 mg/L (Sádecká and Tóthová, 2010).

Brandy is rich in phenolic acids due to its production from grapes and maturation in wooden barrels. Phenolic acids play a significant role in defining the sensory characteristics of wine and brandy and, therefore, are often analyzed in alcoholic beverages. Synchronous fluorescence spectra of mixtures containing phenolic acids (gallic, vanillic, syringic, and ferulic) and scopoletin have been used for the determination of these compounds by PLS regression. The leave-one-out cross-validation method was used to select the optimum number of five PLS components. The PLS model captured 100% of variance in the spectral block, and it accounted for 99.34% of variance in the concentration block. The performance of the model was evaluated by means of root mean square error of cross-validation, root mean square error of prediction, and coefficient of determination. The PLS results were found to be in good agreement with those obtained by the HPLC method RMSECV of PLS models acquired for gallic acid, vanillic acid, syringic acid, ferulic acid, and scopoletin and equaled: 0.01659, 0.00243, 0.00118, 0.00213, and 0.00019 (mg/L), respectively (Žiak et al., 2014).

Markechová et al. (2014) combined excitation emission matrix fluorescence with PARAFAC and PLS regression to determine the content of mixed wine spirits in adulterated brandy samples. Excitation emission matrix fluorescence spectra were measured in the emission wavelength range of 485–580 nm and in the excitation wavelength range of 363–475 nm. The model created using PARAFAC–PLS was able to predict the mixed wine spirits level in adulterated brandy with a very low RMSEP of 1.9% and a square of the correlation (R2) between reference contents and the predicted values of 0.995.

Synchronous fluorescence spectroscopy in combination with multivariate data analysis has been introduced for the characterization and classification of brandy and wine distillates. Synchronous fluorescence spectra were recorded from 220 to 700 nm with constant difference between excitation and emission wavelengths (10–100 nm) followed by a classification of samples using PCA, hierarchical cluster analysis (HCA) and LDA. Using PCA, 99.5% of brandy and wine distillate samples were clustered correctly. HCA showed that brandy and wine distillate samples created two clusters. LDA performed on selected wavelengths provided 99.2% correct classification of these two sample types (Píš et al., 2011).

5.3.7 Cereals and Cereal Products

In cereals and cereal-related products, the most intense fluorescence band is due to tryptophan emission, the second band originates from ferulic acid, and the third one is due to the presence of riboflavin with interference of lutein and xanthophyll emissions. Additional fluorescence emission is observed in spectra of rice samples at an excitation wavelength of about 480 nm (Zeković et al., 2012). Ferulic acid and riboflavin spectra have been reported to be capable of accurately monitoring wheat flour refinement and milling efficiency. Flour aleurone due to fluorescence properties of ferulic acid has a good potential for online monitoring of mill performance. Aleurone fluorescence was strongly related to the refinement of reduction flours for all of the common Canadian wheat classes examined (Symons and Dexter, 1992, 1993).

These results have recently been confirmed by Karoui et al. (2006d) where tryptophan fluorescence spectra of 59 samples (complete Kamut, semicomplete Kamut, soft wheat flours, pasta and semolinas manufactured from complete Kamut, semicomplete Kamut, and hard wheat flours) were scanned after excitation at 290 nm. Statistical analysis performed on the flour spectra clearly differentiated varieties of wheat flours as well as pasta samples manufactured from different wheat flours. The best discrimination was obtained from tryptophan spectra recorded on semolinas since the four groups were well discriminated. Correct classification of 61.9% was obtained for pasta spectra. A better classification was obtained for flour and semolina spectra since correct classification amounted to 86.7% and 87.9%, respectively.

Cereal flours could be discriminated and classified using data obtained with front-face synchronous fluorescence measurements. Discrimination and classification were possible for low synchronous intervals of 20 nm or less, and the best results were achieved with a combination of synchronous fluorescence measurements using 7 and 20 nm synchronous intervals. The difference between the SF spectra of different flours can be clearly observed from three emission band centers and intensities (Zeković et al., 2012). Zandomeneghi (1999) used front-face fluorescence spectroscopy (excitation 275 nm; emission 280−575 nm) to differentiate between different cereal flours (ie, rice, wheat, maize). The strong differences between the four species appeared to be sufficient for a clear recognition of the species considered. A quantitative index based on the intensity data appeared to be a possible parameter in discriminating between cereal species or cultivars. In another study, fluorescence spectroscopy was used to classify wheat flours and rye flours (Ram et al., 2004). Front-face fluorescence spectra were assessed to differentiate between red and white wheat kernels. Emission spectra (370−570 nm) were recorded after excitation at 350 nm, and a clear difference was observed between the two group samples. The data were analyzed by PLS and neutral networks analyses. Classification accuracies were 85% for the calibration and 72% for the validation samples.

5.3.8 Sugar and Confectionary

Fluorescence analyses of sugar and sugar solutions are all based on measuring impurities in the sugar since saccharose itself does not possess the ability to fluoresce. The main fluorophores of sugar are Millard products, polyphenolic compounds, tyrosine, and tryptophan. Fluorescence signals dominated by the aromatic amino acids were used for the classification of sugars according to their production site and for the prediction of several quality and process parameters. A sample set of 47 raw sugar samples representing a varied selection was analyzed. The spectral profiles of the fluorophores were estimated with the three-way decomposition model PARAFA, and PLS calibration models were built from the unfolded fluorescence data set. Three principal fluorophores were found in raw sugar, and one of them was characterized as an ultraviolet color precursor that participates in color development during storage. The other two fluorophores fluoresce in the visible wavelength area and were potential colorants. Since all the resolved fluorophores correlate to color, they could be used as indicator substances in further studies of the color development in cane sugar processing. The lowest root mean square error of cross-validation for prediction of color using PLS equaled 1622 (ICUSA units). It has been demonstrated that chemometric methods applied to multiwavelength fluorescence data can determine the chemical characteristics of fluorophores in raw cane sugar without any knowledge of their exact chemical structure (Baunsgaard et al., 2000a).

In combination with multivariate statistical analyses, fluorescence spectroscopy has proved to be a promising screening method for predicting quality parameters in beet sugar samples (Munck et al., 1998). In one study, it was reported possible to classify white sugar samples (Nørgaard, 1995). Another study of beet sugar samples utilized the three-dimensional structure of the fluorescence excitation-emission landscapes to resolve spectral excitation and emission profiles of fluorophores present in the sugar with a multiway chemometric model, PARAFAC (Bro, 1999). Four fluorescent components were found to capture all chemical variation in the fluorescence data of 268 sugar samples. Concentrations of the four components estimated from the sugar samples could be correlated with several quality and process parameters, and they were characterized as potential indicator substances of the chemistry of the sugar process, which was confirmed by the use of HPLC analysis (Baunsgaard et al., 2000b; Karoui and Blecker, 2011).

5.4 Future Trends

Quantitative analysis of food adulterants is an important health and economic issue and it needs to be fast and simple. Miniaturization and automation are the most significant future trends in fluorescence spectroscopy. These developments will reduce analysis time, improve accuracy and precision, and reduce the volume of reagents.

Moreover, many studies have demonstrated the potential use of hyperspectral imaging for authentication purposes. The requirement of real-time monitoring of food products has encouraged the development of nondestructive measurement systems.

Hyperspectral imaging is a rapid, reagentless, nondestructive analytical technique that integrates traditional spectroscopic and imaging techniques into one system to obtain both spectral and spatial information from an object; such information cannot be achieved with either digital imaging or conventional spectroscopic techniques. The main advantage of a hyperspectral imaging system is its ability to incorporate both spectroscopic and imaging techniques to directly and simultaneously assess different components and determine the spatial distribution of such components in the products under test (Kamruzzaman et al., 2015). Fluorescence sensors will need to measure directly on the process line and the need for online measurements arises. The use of fiber optics for the connection between the spectrometer and the sensing device may be the future.

Another issue is searching for ways to reduce the time needed for the calibration stage including the development of calibration equations. Minimizing or eliminating the sample preparation step is highly desirable in food analysis. Kalivas et al. (2014) reported the application of a newly developed pure component Tikhonov regularization (PCTR) process that does not require a laboratory or reference analysis method, hence is a greener calibration approach. The PCTR method requires an analyte pure component spectrum and nonanalyte spectra. Results are shown to be better than those obtained using ridge regression against reference calibration samples. Flexibility of PCTR allows the use of reference samples and combination with other instrumental methods and food products.

Moreover, it is important to improve quantitative analysis and search for alternative solutions. For concentrated samples with saturating absorption, a derived absorbance plot seems to correlate well with observed synchronous fluorescence spectra. Advanced statistical analysis must be applied for simultaneous extraction of the pure components from SF spectra of dilute mixtures of the fluorophores. It was shown that the MCR—ALS can be used for the simultaneous extraction of the pure synchronous profile at various wavelength offsets from the TSFS data set of the dilute aqueous mixtures of fluorophores (Kumar and Kumar, 2012).

Finally, another current trend is toward data fusion, eg, fluorescence combined with ultraviolet and visible. Tan et al. (2015) showed that fluorescence, UV and visible spectroscopies provide complementary information and revealed that data fusion can improve the discrimination performance. Fluorescence spectroscopy has high sensitivity and selectivity, but only a small proportion of compounds exhibit fluorescence. UV—visible spectroscopy has limited applications because of its relatively low sensitivity and spectral overlap; many organic compounds can absorb UV or visible light. Thus, they may complement each other on certain occasions, for example, when used as detectors for liquid chromatography. Compared with individual spectroscopy, data fusion often shows improved discrimination ability. Fusion of fluorescence, UV, and visible spectroscopic data is promising for food authentication and is worth further investigation. Moreover, the fusion of fluorescence and infrared techniques enables better understanding of structural modifications at the molecular level for a given product. The joint analysis of data sets may allow a very efficient management of all the spectroscopic information collected, contributing to a better understanding of the main structural modifications affecting proteins and lipids during food processing.

Other improvements include the use of quantum dots (Zhang et al., 2012; Tang et al., 2013). Recent research has shown that, with the use of quantum dots, a simple, reliable, fast, and environmentally friendly procedure can be developed, eg, for melamine determination in adulterated milk by exploiting, for the first time, the fluorescence quenching of Triton X-114 (Nascimento et al., 2015).

References

Airado-Rodríguez, D., Durán-Merás, I., Galeano-Díaz, T., Wold, J.P., 2011. Front-face fluorescence spectroscopy: a new tool for control in the wine industry. Journal of Food Composition and Analysis 24 (2), 257–264.

Ammari, F., Redjdal, L., Rutledge, D.N., 2015. Detection of orange juice frauds using front-face fluorescence spectroscopy and independent components analysis. Food Chemistry 168, 211–217.

Andersen, C.M., Mortensen, G., 2008. Fluorescence spectroscopy: a rapid tool for analyzing dairy products. Journal of Agricultural and Food Chemistry 56 (3), 720–729.

Andres-Lacueva, C., Mattivi, E., Tonon, D., 1998. Determination of riboflavin, flavin mononucleotide and flavin–adenine dinucleotide in wine and other beverages by high-performance liquid chromatography with fluorescence detection. Journal of Chromatography A 823 (1–2), 355–363.

Apperson, K., Leiper, K.A., McKeown, I.P., Birch, D.J.S., 2002. Beer fluorescence and the isolation, characterisation and silica adsorption of haze-active beer proteins. Journal of the Institute of Brewing 108 (2), 193–199.

Araújo, M.C.U., Saldanha, T.C.B., Galvão, R.K.H., Yoneyama, T., Chame, H.C., Visani, V., 2001. The successive projections algorithm for variable selection inspectroscopic multicomponent analysis. Chemometrics and Intelligent Laboratory Systems 57, 65–73.

Aubourg, S.P., 1999. Recent advances in assessment of marine lipid oxidation by using fluorescence. Review. Journal of the American Oil Chemists' Society 76 (4), 409–419.

Baunsgaard, D., Nørgaard, L., Godshall, M.A., 2000a. Fluorescence of raw cane sugars evaluated by chemometrics. Journal of Agricultural and Food Chemistry 48 (10), 4955–4962.

Baunsgaard, D., Andersson, C.A., Arndal, A., Munck, L., 2000b. Multiway chemometrics for mathematical separation of fluorescent colorants and colour precursors from spectrofluorometry of beet sugar and beet sugar thick juice as validated by HPLC analysis. Food Chemistry 70 (1), 113–121.

Bertrand, D., Scotter, C.N.G., 1992. Application of multivariate analyses to NIR spectra of gelatinized starch. Applied Spectroscopy 46 (2), 1420–1425.

Botosoa, E.P., Chèné, C., Karoui, R., 2013. Use of front face fluorescence for monitoring lipid oxidation during ageing of cakes. Food Chemistry 141 (2), 1130–1139.

Bro, R., 1999. Exploratory study of sugar production using fluorescence spectroscopy and multi-way analysis. Chemometrics and Intelligent Laboratory Systems 46 (2), 133–147.

Bron, I.U., Ribeiro, R.V., Azzolini, M., Jacomino, A.P., Machado, E.C., 2004. Chlorophyll fluorescence as a tool to evaluate the ripening of 'Golden' papaya fruit. Postharvest Biology and Technology 33 (2), 163–173.

Cheikhousman, R., Zude, M., Jouan-Rimbaud Bouveresse, D., Rutledge, D.N., Birlouez-Aragon, I., 2004. Fluorescence spectroscopy for monitoring extra virgin olive oil deterioration upon heating. Czech Journal of Food Sciences 22, 147–150.

Cheikhousman, R., Zude, M., Bouveresse, D.J.-R., Léger, C.L., Rutledge, D.N., Birlouez-Aragon, I., 2005. Fluorescence spectroscopy for monitoring deterioration of extra virgin olive oil during heating. Analytical and Bioanalytical Chemistry 382 (6), 1438–1443.

Chen, Q., Qi, S., Li, H., Han, X., Ouyang, Q., Zhao, J., 2014. Determination of rice syrup adulterant concentration in honey using three-dimensional fluorescence spectra and multivariate calibrations. Spectrochimica Acta Part A: Molecular and Biomolecular Spectroscopy 131, 177–182.

Christensen, J., Nørgaard, L., Bro, R., Engelsen, S.B., 2006. Multivariate autofluorescence of intact food systems. Chemical Reviews 106 (6), 1979–1994.

Dankowska, A., Małecka, M., 2009. Application of synchronous fluorescence spectroscopy for determination of extra virgin olive oil adulteration. European Journal of Lipid Science and Technology 111 (12), 1233–1239.

Dankowska, A., Małecka, M., Kowalewski, W., 2013a. Utilization of synchronous fluorescence spectroscopy to detect adulteration of olive oil. Żywność Nauka Technologia Jakość 87 (2), 106–115 (in Polish).

Dankowska, A., Małecka, M., Kowalewski, W., 2013b. Discrimination of edible olive oils by means of synchronous fluorescence spectroscopy with multivariate data analysis. Grasas Y Aceites 64 (4), 425–431.

Dankowska, A., Małecka, M., Kowalewski, W., 2014. Application of synchronous fluorescence spectroscopy with multivariate data analysis for determination of butter adulteration. International Journal of Food Science and Technology 49 (12), 2628–2634.

Dankowska, A., Małecka, M., Kowalewski, W., 2015. Detection of plant oil addition to cheese by synchronous fluorescence spectroscopy. Dairy Science and Technology 95 (4), 413–424.

De Ell, J.R., Prange, R.K., Murr, D.P., 1996. Chlorophyll fluorescence of delicious apples at harvest as a potential predictor of superficial scald development during storage. Postharvest Biology and Technology 9 (1), 1–6.

Di Anibal, C.V., Rodríguez, M.S., Albertengo, L., 2015. Synchronous fluorescence and multivariate classification analysis as a screening tool for determining Sudan I dye in culinary spices. Application of synchronous fluorescence spectroscopy for determination of extra virgin olive oil adulteration. Food Control 56, 18–23.

Duflos, G., Le Fur, B., Mulak, V., Becel, P., Malle, P., 2002. Comparison of methods of differentiating between fresh and frozen-thawed fish or fillets. Journal of the Science of Food and Agriculture 82, 1341–1345.

Dufour, E., Frencia, J.P., Kane, E., 2003. Development of a rapid method based on front-face fluorescence spectroscopy for the monitoring of fish freshness. Food Research International 36 (5), 415–423.

Dufour, E., Letort, A., Laguet, A., Lebecque, A., Serra, J.N., 2006. Investigation of variety, typicality and vintage of French and German wines using front-face fluorescence spectroscopy. Analytica Chimica Acta 563 (1–2), 292–299.

Dupuy, N., Le Dréau, Y., Ollivier, D., Artaud, J., Pinaltel, C., Jacky Kister, J., 2005. Origin of French virgin olive oil registered designation of origins predicted by chemometric analysis of synchronous excitation-emission fluorescence spectra. Journal of Agricultural and Food Chemistry 53 (24), 9361–9368.

Egelandsdal, B., Wold, J.P., Sponnich, A., Neegard, S., Hildrum, K.I., 2002. On attempts to measure the tenderness of Longissimus Dorsi muscles using fluorescence emission spectra. Meat Science 60 (2), 187–202.

Ghosh, N., Verma, Y., Majudmer, S.K., Gupta, P.K., 2005. A fluorescence spectroscopic study of honey and cane sugar syrup. Food Science and Technology Research 11 (1), 59–62.

Grote, B., Zense, T., Hitzmann, B., 2014. 2D-fluorescence and multivariate data analysis for monitoring of sourdough fermentation process. Food Control 38, 8–18.

Guilbault, G.G., 1999. Practical Fluorescence. Marcel Dekker, New York, pp. 378–380.

Guimet, F., Ferré, J., Boqué, R., Rius, X., 2004a. Application of unfold principal component analysis and parallel factor analysis to the exploratory analysis of olive oils by means of excitation-emission matrix fluorescence spectroscopy. Analytica Chimica Acta 515 (1), 75–85.

Guimet, F., Boqué, R., Ferré, J., 2004b. Cluster analysis applied to the exploratory analysis of commercial spanish olive oils by means of excitation-emission fluorescence spectroscopy. Journal of Agricultural and Food Chemistry 52 (22), 6673–6679.

Guimet, F., Ferré, J., Boqué, R., 2005. Rapid detection of olive-pomace oil adulteration in extra virgin olive oils from the protected denomination of origin "Siurana" using excitation-emission fluorescence spectroscopy and three-way methods of analysis. Analytica Chimica Acta 544 (1–2), 143–152.

Guimet, F., Boqué, R., Ferre, J., 2006. Application of non-negative matrix factorization combined with Fisher's linear discriminant analysis for classification of olive oil excitation-emission fluorescence spectra. Chemometric and Intelligent Laboratory Systems 81 (4), 94–106.

Hammami, M., Rouissi, H., Salah, N., Selmi, H., Al-Otaibi, M., Blecker, C., Karoui, R., 2010. Fluorescence spectroscopy coupled with factorial discriminant analysis technique to identify sheep milk from different feeding systems. Food Chemistry 122 (4), 1344–1350.

Hammami, M., Dridi, S., Zaïdi, F., Maâmouri, O., Rouissi, H., Blecker, C., Karoui, R., 2013. Use of front-face fluorescence spectroscopy to differentiate sheep milks from different genotypes and feeding systems. International Journal of Food Properties 16 (6), 1322–1338.

Insińska-Rak, M., Sikorska, E., Czerwińska, I., Kruzińska, A., Nowacka, G., Sikorski, M., 2007. Fluorescence spectroscopy for analysis of beer. Polish Journal of Food and Nutrition Sciences 57 (4), 239–243.

IOC, 2015. Trade Standard Applying to Olive Oil and Pomace-oil. COI/T.15/NC No 3/Rev. 8.

Kalivas, J.H., Georgiou, C.A., Moira, M., Tsafaras, I., Petrakis, E.A., Mousdis, G.A., 2014. Food adulteration analysis without laboratory prepared or determined reference food adulterant values. Food Chemistry 148, 289–293.

Kamruzzaman, M., Makino, Y., Oshita, S., 2015. Non-invasive analytical technology for the detection of contamination, adulteration, and authenticity of meat, poultry, and fish: a review. Analytica Chimica Acta 853 (1), 19–29.

Karoui, R., Blecker, C., 2011. Fluorescence spectroscopy measurement for quality assessment of food systems—a review. Food Bioprocess Technology 4 (3), 364–386.

Karoui, R., Mazerolles, G., Dufour, E., 2003. Spectroscopic techniques coupled with chemometric tools for structure and texture determinations in dairy products. International Dairy Journal 3 (4), 607–620.

Karoui, R., Dufour, E., Pillonel, L., Schaller, E., Picque, D., Cattenoz, T., Bosset, J.O., 2004. Determining the geographic origin of Emmental cheeses produced during winter and summer using a technique based on the concatenation of MIR and fluorescence spectroscopic data. European Food Research and Technology 219 (2), 184–189.

Karoui, R., Bosset, J.O., Mazerolles, G., Kulmyrzaev, A., Dufour, E., 2005. Monitoring the geographic origin of both experimental French Jura hard cheeses and Swiss Gruyère and L'Etivaz PDO cheeses using mid-infrared and fluorescence spectroscopies: a preliminary investigation. International Dairy Journal 15 (3), 275–286.

Karoui, R., Dufour, E., De Baerdemaeker, J., 2006a. Common components and specific weights analysis: a tool for monitoring the molecular structure of semi-hard cheese throughout ripening. Analytica Chimica Acta 572 (1), 125–133.

Karoui, R., Kemps, B., Bamelis, F., De Ketelaere, B., Merten, K., Schoonheydt, R., Decuypere, E., De Baerdemaeker, J., 2006b. Development of a rapid method based on front-face fluorescence spectroscopy for the monitoring of egg freshness: 2—evolution of egg yolk. European Food Research and Technology 223 (2), 180–188.

Karoui, R., Kemps, B., Bamelis, F., De Ketelaere, B., Mertens, K., Schoonheydt, R., et al., 2006c. Development of a rapid method based on front face fluorescence spectroscopy for the monitoring of egg freshness: 1—Evolution of thick and thin albumens. European Food Research and Technology 223 (3), 303–312.

Karoui, R., Cartaud, G., Dufour, E., 2006d. Front-face fluorescence spectroscopy as a rapid and non-destructive tool for differentiating various cereal products: a preliminary investigation. Journal of Agricultural and Food Chemistry 54 (2), 2027–2034.

Karoui, R., Thomas, E., Dufour, E., 2006e. Utilisation of a rapid technique based on front-face fluorescence spectroscopy for differentiating between fresh and frozen—thawed fish fillets. Food Research International 39 (3), 349–355.

Karoui, R., Dufour, E., Bosset, J.O., De Baerdemaeker, J., 2007a. The use of front face fluorescence spectroscopy to classify the botanical origin of honey samples produced in Switzerland. Food Chemistry 101 (1), 314–323.

Karoui, R., Dufour, E., Schoonheydt, R., De Baerdemaeker, J., 2007b. Characterization of soft cheese by front face fluorescence spectroscopy coupled with chemometric tools: effect of the manufacturing process and sampling zone. Food Chemistry 100 (2), 632–642.

Kumar, K., Kumar, M.A., 2012. Application of 'multivariate curve resolution alternating least square (MCR—ALS)' analysis to extract pure component synchronous fluorescence spectra at various wavelength offsets from total synchronous fluorescence spectroscopy (TSFS) data set of dilute aqueous solutions of fluorophores. Chemometrics and Intelligent Laboratory Systems 116, 78–86.

Kyriakidis, N.B., Skarkalis, P., 2000. Fluorescence spectra measurement of olive oil and other vegetable oils. Journal of American Oil Chemists' Society 83 (6), 1435–1439.

Lenhardt, L., Zeković, I., Dramićanin, T., Dramićanin, M.D., Bro, R., 2014. D'etermination of the botanical origin of honey by front-face synchronous fluorescence spectroscopy. Applied Spectroscopy 68 (5), 557–563.

Li, Y.-Q., Li, X.-Y., Falih Shindi, A.A., Zou, Z.-X., Liu, Q., Lin, L.-R., Li, N., 2010. Synchronous fluorescence spectroscopy and its applications in clinical analysis and food safety evaluation' chapter. Reviews in Fluorescence 2010, 95–117.

Li, B., Wang, H., Zhao, Q., Ouyang, J., Wu, Y., 2015. Rapid detection of authenticity and adulteration of walnut oil by FTIR and fluorescence spectroscopy: a comparative study. Food Chemistry 181 (15), 25–30.

Markechová, D., Májek, P., Sádecká, J., 2014. Fluorescence spectroscopy and multivariate methods for the determination of brandy adulteration with mixed wine spirit. Food Chemistry 159 (15), 193–199.

Mas, P.A., Rimbaud Bouveresse, D.J.R., Birlouez-Aragon, I., 2004. Fluorescence spectroscopy for monitoring rapeseed oil upon heating. Czech Journal of Food Science 22, 127–129.

Moller, J.K.S., Parolari, G., Gabba, L., Christensen, J., Skibsted, L.H., 2003. Monitoring chemical changes of dry-cured parma ham during processing by surface autofluorescence spectroscopy. Journal of Agricultural and Food Chemistry 51 (5), 1224–1230.

Moshou, D., Wahlen, S., Strasser, R., Schenk, A., De Baerdemaeker, J., Ramon, H., 2005. Chlorophyll fluorescence as a tool for online quality sorting of apples. Biosystems Engineering 91 (2), 163–172.

Munck, L., Nørgaard, L., Engelsen, S.B., Bro, R., Andersson, C.A., 1998. Chemometrics in food science—a demonstration of the feasibility of a highly exploratory, inductive evaluation strategy of fundamental scientific significance. Chemometrics and Intelligent Laboratory Systems 44 (1–2), 31–60.

Nascimento, C.F., Rocha, D.L., Rocha, F.R.P., 2015. A fast and environmental friendly analytical procedure for determination of melamine in milk exploiting fluorescence quenching. Food Chemistry 169, 314–319.

Norgaard, L., 1995. A multivariate chemometric approach to fluorescence spectroscopy. Talanta 42 (9), 1305–1324.

Ntakatsane, M., Liu, X.M., Zhou, P., 2013. Short Communication: rapid detection of milk fat adulteration with vegetable oil by fluorescence spectroscopy. Journal of Dairy Science 96 (4), 2130–2136.

Patra, D., Mishra, A.K., 2002. Recent developments in multi-component synchronous fluorescence scan analysis. TrAC Trends in Analytical Chemistry 21 (12), 787–798.

Píš, Ľ., Májek, P., Sádecká, J., 2011. Synchronous fluorescence spectroscopy for differentiating between brandies and wine distillates. Acta Chimica Slovaca 4 (1), 47–58.

Poulli, K.I., Mousdis, G.A., Georgiou, C.A., 2005. Classification of edible and lampante virgin olive oil based on synchronous fluorescence and total luminescence spectroscopy. Analytica Chimica Acta 542 (2), 151–156.

Poulli, K.I., Mousdis, G.A., Georgiou, C.A., 2006. Synchronous fluorescence spectroscopy for quantitative determination of virgin olive oil adulteration with sunflower oil. Analytical and Bioanalytical Chemistry 386 (5), 1571–1575.

Poulli, K.I., Mousdis, G.A., Georgiou, C.A., 2007. Rapid synchronous fluorescence method for virgin olive oil adulteration assessment. Food Chemistry 105 (1), 369–375.

Ram, M.S., Seitz, L.M., Dowell, F.E., 2004. Natural fluorescence of red and white wheat kernels. Cereal Chemistry 81 (2), 244–248.

Ruoff, K., Luginbuhl, W., Kunzli, R., Bogdanov, S., Bosset, J., Von der Ohe, K., Von der Ohe, W., Amado, R., 2006. Authentication of the botanical and geographical origin of honey by front face fluorescence spectroscopy. Journal of Agricultural and Food Chemistry 54 (18), 6858–6866.

Sádecká, J., Tóthová, J., 2007. Fluorescence spectroscopy and chemometrics in the food classification – a review. Czech Journal of Food Science 25 (4), 159–173.

Sádecká, J., Tóthová, J., 2010. Determination of caramel in non-aged mixed wine spirits by synchronous fluorescence spectroscopy. European Food Research and Technology 230 (5), 797–802.

Sayago, A., Moralesn, M.T., Aparcio, R., 2004. Detection of hazelnut oil in virgin olive oil by spectrofluorimetric method. European Food Research and Technology 218 (5), 480–483.

Seiden, P., Bro, R., Poll, L., Munck, L.J., 1996. Exploring fluorescence spectra of apple juice and their connection to quality parameters by chemometrics. Journal of Agriculture and Food Chemistry 44 (10), 3202–3205.

Sergiel, I., Pohl, P., Biesaga, M., Mironczyk, A., 2014. Suitability of three-dimensional synchronous fluorescence spectroscopy for fingerprint analysis of honey samples with reference to their phenolic profiles. Food Chemistry 145, 319–326.

Sikorska, E., Górecki, T., Khmelinskii, I.V., Sikorki, M., Kozioł, J., 2005. Classification of edible oils using synchronous scanning fluorescence spectroscopy. Food Chemistry 89 (2), 217–225.

Sikorska, E., Górecki, T., Khmelinskii, I.V., Sikorski, M., De Keukeleire, D., 2006. Monitoring beer during storage by fluorescence spectroscopy. Food Chemistry 96 (4), 632–639.
Sikorska, E., Khmelinskii, I.V., Sikorski, M., Caponio, F., Bilancia, M.T., Pasqualone, A., Gomes, T., 2008. Fluorescence spectroscopy in monitoring of extra virgin olive oil during storage. International Journal of Food Science and Technology 43 (1), 52–61.
Sikorska, E., 2008. Fluorescence Methods in Food. Poznań University of Economics Press.
Strasburg, G.M., Ludescher, R.D., 1995. Theory and applications of fluorescence spectroscopy in food research. Trends in Food Science and Technology 6 (3), 69–75.
Swatland, H.J., 2000. Connective and adipose tissue detection by simultaneous fluorescence and reflectance measurements with an on-line meat probe. Food Research International 33 (9), 749–757.
Swatland, H.J., 2001. A note on the stereological anatomy of four probe sites in beef carcasses. Food Research International 34 (9), 633–637.
Symons, S.J., Dexter, J.E., 1993. Relationship of flour aleurone fluorescence to flour refinement for some Canadian hard common wheat classes. Cereal Chemistry 70 (1), 90–95.
Symons, S.J., Dexter, J.E., 1992. Estimation of milling efficiency: prediction of flour refinement by the measurement of pericarp fluorescence. Cereal Chemistry 69 (2), 137–141.
Tan, J., Li, R., Jiang, Z.T., 2015. Chemometric classification of Chinese lager beers according to manufacturer based on data fusion of fluorescence, UV and visible spectroscopies. Food Chemistry 184, 30–36.
Tang, G., Du, L., Su, X., 2013. Detection of melamine based on the fluorescence resonance energy transfer between CdTe QDs and Rhodamine B. Food Chemistry 141 (4), 4060–4065.
Veberg, A., Vogt, G., Wold, J.P., 2006. Fluorescence in aldehyde model systems related to lipid oxidation. LWT – Food Science and Technology 39 (5), 562–568.
Wójcicki, K., Khmelinskii, I., Sikorski, M., Caponio, F., Paradiso, V.M., Summo, C., Pasqualone, A., Sikorska, E., 2015. Spectroscopic techniques and chemometrics in analysis of blends of extra virgin with refined and mild deodorized olive oils. European Journal of Lipid Science and Technology 117 (1), 92–102.
Wold, J.P., Mielnik, M., 2000. Nondestructive assessment of lipid oxidation in minced poultry meat by autofluorescence spectroscopy. Journal of Food Science 65 (1), 87–95.
Wold, J.P., Mielnik, M., Pettersen, M.K., Aaby, K., Baardreth, P., 2002. Rapid assessment of rancidity in complex meat products by front face fluorescence spectroscopy. Journal of Food Science 67 (6), 2397–2404.
Zandomeneghi, M., 1999. Fluorescence of cereal flours. Journal of Agricultural and Food Chemistry 47 (3), 878–882.
Zeković, I., Lenhardt, L., Dramićanin, T., Dramićanin, M., 2012. Classification of intact cereal flours by front-face synchronous fluorescence spectroscopy. Food Analytical Methods 5 (5), 1205–1213.
Zhang, M., Cao, X., Li, H., Guan, F., Guo, J., Shen, F., 2012. Sensitive fluorescent detection of melamine in raw milk based on the inner filter effect of Au nanoparticles on the fluorescence of CdTe quantum dots. Food Chemistry 135 (3), 1894–1900.
Žiak, Ľ., Sádecká, J., Májek, P., Hroboňová, K., 2014. Simultaneous determination of phenolic acids and scopoletin in brandies using synchronous fluorescence spectrometry coupled with partial least squares. Food Analytical Methods 7 (3), 563–570.

Advances in Nuclear Magnetic Resonance Spectroscopy for Food Authenticity Testing

6

A.P. Sobolev[1], *S. Circi*[2], *L. Mannina*[3]
[1]National Research Council, Rome, Italy; [2]University of Rome, Rome, Italy; [3]Sapienza University of Rome, Rome, Italy

Chapter Outline

6.1 Introduction

Any foodstuff is a complex matrix including many compounds, ranging widely in concentration, with different chemical structures and physicochemical properties, which originate from biological raw material and/or are produced during treatment, storage, etc. Therefore an exhaustive food characterization, important to assure its quality and authenticity, usually needs different and complementary analytical techniques to be used. Nuclear magnetic resonance (NMR) spectroscopy is not only a robust quantitative analytical technique, it also has proper tools for identification of compounds even in the absence of standards. One of the main advantages of NMR is that it does not require complicated sample preparation or separation of components prior to the actual analysis, and the determination of very different chemical species can be performed in a single experiment.

Some NMR methodologies, for instance, low-field NMR relaxometry and magnetic resonance imaging (MRI), are completely noninvasive and produce plenty of information regarding the texture of the sample, water distribution, and molecular dynamics, all of which can be important in determining product authenticity. High-resolution NMR simultaneously brings "high-throughput" spectroscopic/structural information on a wide range of metabolites with high analytical precision, giving a foodstuff metabolic fingerprint, which is important to assure its quality, genuineness, geographical origin, etc.

In this chapter some important aspects of NMR methodologies are reported together with relevant examples of NMR applications in authenticity confirmation.

6.2 Nuclear Magnetic Resonance Methodologies in Food Analysis

The discovery of NMR phenomenon gave birth to a variety of methodologies based on it to investigate the structure, chemical composition, and molecular dynamics of solids, liquids, and semisolid matrices. Most of these methodologies have found application in food science and therefore have potential in food authenticity testing. Principal NMR methodologies such as solid-state NMR, liquid-state NMR, and MRI require specific instrumentation and different approaches to sample preparation, data acquisition, and processing, and provide different kinds of information. A brief description of the most important NMR methodologies suitable for food authentication is given next.

Low-field ^1H NMR relaxometry (Hills, 2006) is an important tool used to investigate the proton relaxation behavior of the most abundant components of intact foodstuffs. In particular, by detecting proton signals predominantly contributed by H_2O contained in foodstuffs, information on water compartmentation, diffusion, and movement can be obtained. Some of the advantages of this technique are that it is noninvasive, does not require any pretreatment of the sample and has the potential for through-package analysis. Once developed, standard protocols based on the rapid and simple measurements can be easily transferred to quality control applications.

According to the literature, various foodstuffs such as banana (Raffo et al., 2005), kiwifruits (Capitani et al., 2010), mozzarella cheese (Gianferri et al., 2007), and meat (Brown et al., 2000) have been investigated by means of low-field NMR providing important information on food texture and ripening status. The feasibility of using NMR relaxometry to check the authenticity of food was demonstrated in the case of honey (Ribeiro et al., 2014), vegetable oil (Zhang et al., 2013), and milk adulterations (Santos et al., 2016).

High-resolution magic angle spinning (HRMAS) NMR spectroscopy is a reliable tool used to study intrinsically inhomogeneous matrices that include solid and liquid components such as in the case of animal tissues and many types of foodstuffs. Rapid spinning of the sample, typically at 4–6 kHz, at the magic angle (54.74 degrees with respect to the magnetic field direction) provides a reduction of line-broadening effects typical for solids caused by sample heterogeneity and residual anisotropic interactions.

It produces highly resolved NMR spectra of low molecular weight components and offers the almost unique opportunity of analyzing samples without any pretreatment. Within the same experiment it is possible to identify polar and nonpolar metabolites simultaneously and therefore to characterize the whole metabolic content of a specific intact tissue. Application of the HR-MAS technique to characterize the metabolic composition of intact food samples was reviewed by Valentini et al. (2011). A study by Corsaro et al. (2015) gives an interesting example of HR-MAS application for authentication of four different foodstuffs [cherry tomato of Pachino, the protected geographical indication (PGI) Interdonato lemon of Messina, several protected designation of origin (PDO) extra virgin olive oils from Sicily, and red garlic of Nubia] typical of the Mediterranean diet.

Correlations observed between the isotope ratio of deuterium to hydrogen ($^2H/^1H$) of methyl and methylene groups of ethanol in wine and its geographic origin are the basis of the ^2H Site-Specific Natural Isotopic Fractionation (SNIF) NMR method for wine authentication (Martin and Martin, 1983; Ogrinc et al., 2003). Confirmation of the geographical origin of wine using SNIF NMR was approved by the European Union in 1990 (EC Reg. 2676/90). Another example of an SNIF-NMR application was reported by Cotte et al. (2007) to characterize and control the authenticity of honey. Relative deuterium concentration and specific deuterium-site locations have also been determined in other alcoholic beverages, fruit juices, aromas and perfumes, fats and oils, milk, and drugs (Rossman, 2001).

Liquid-state high-field NMR has been extensively used in foodstuffs analysis (Mannina et al., 2012). One of the most important characteristics of this technique is its high throughput because of the high resolution of NMR spectra that permits the direct qualitative and quantitative analysis of complex mixtures without physical separation of the corresponding components. This characteristic makes liquid-state NMR one of the most attractive and suitable techniques for the direct analysis of liquid foods (beverages, oils, etc.) and even for solid foods, although a minimal manipulation to extract metabolites is necessary.

Both targeted and untargeted approaches to the analysis can be used. In the case of a specific component to be analyzed, a selective extraction can be also performed before the NMR analysis to concentrate the selected component and avoid interference from other compounds. Several general untargeted approaches such as metabolic profiling, metabolic fingerprinting, and metabolomics developed for the analysis of metabolites in biological samples using liquid-state NMR or diverse analytical methods have been successfully applied for food analysis. Metabolic profiling consists in identification and quantification of a number of selected metabolites belonging to various classes of compounds in a given sample often without a separation procedure. Metabolic fingerprinting is used when classification of samples without recognition of individual specific metabolites is sufficient; in this case the NMR spectrum can be considered as a fingerprint of the foodstuff and all the NMR resonances are measured without any identification. Metabolomics (Fiehn, 2002) is the most comprehensive approach aimed at identification and quantification of all metabolites present in a given sample.

Selected examples of all the approaches applied for food authenticity testing involving NMR spectroscopy are reported next.

6.3 Sample Preparation for Nuclear Magnetic Resonance Analysis

The different NMR methodologies require specific procedures for sample preparation, although some common aspects have to be considered. Proper sampling is a crucial point of any analytical protocol. As previously underlined, a foodstuff is a complex matrix in which the distribution of metabolites can be heterogeneous. If it is necessary to analyze just a piece of sample because it is impossible to put the foodstuff as a whole into the instrument (the most common case), it is important to perform the sampling in a correct way. For instance, one can choose to take different parts of the foodstuff to have a "representative" sample to analyze.

In addition, conservation requires suitable care to preserve the quality and composition of foodstuffs. In fact, some operations such as harvesting for vegetables and slaughtering of animals can be followed by enzymatic action and other degradation processes. Freezing in liquid nitrogen followed by storage in the dark at low temperature are the most common procedures used to avoid chemical or enzymatic degradation.

In the cases of low-field ^{1}H NMR relaxometry, HR-MAS NMR, and MRI, samples can be analyzed as is, without any pretreatment. In liquid-state NMR, as reported by Fukusaky and Kobayashi (2005), "the optimum preparation protocol should be developed on a case-by case basis...depending on the foodstuff, on the characteristics of target metabolites, the number of metabolites being examined and their respective quantities."

If an untargeted analysis is required, a sample can be analyzed as is (liquid foodstuffs) or after a pretreatment or a suitable extraction (liquid and solid samples) step. Olive oils, vinegars, wines, and fruit juices are often analyzed without any treatment, whereas dilution of a viscous liquid such as honey is recommended.

In the case of solid foodstuffs, after sample homogenization and/or disruption, an extraction with a suitable solvent has to be performed both for vegetal samples (Kaiser et al., 2009; Kim and Verpoorte, 2010) and for animal tissues (Lin et al., 2007; Wu et al., 2008). The combination of methanol/H_2O/chloroform in different proportions is often used since it allows the analyst to extract both hydrophobic and hydrophilic compounds. It has been used in the case of maize (Piccioni et al., 2009) and lettuce (Sobolev et al., 2005) as well as in animal-derived foodstuffs such as sea bass (Mannina et al., 2008) and meat (Jung et al., 2010).

In the case of targeted NMR analysis, the choice of extraction solvent to isolate selected metabolites is a crucial decision. Acetic acid/H_2O is used for extracting specific target compounds such as polyphenols (McDougall et al., 2008). Chloroform/ethyl acetate/2-butanol mixture is used to extract aromatic compounds (Khatib et al., 2006). Solid phase extraction (SPE) has also been suggested for isolation of compounds of interest, eliminating interference from high molecular weight compounds (Beretta et al., 2008). In the case of blueberry, SPE has facilitated a reduction in sugar content and enabled NMR characterization of anthocyanins, a group not easily identifiable in aqueous solution (Capitani et al., 2014).

Another important aspect to be considered is the necessity to obtain reproducible NMR spectra without undesirable variations between samples. This aspect is particularly important when critical information is derived from a comparison between spectra such as, for instance, in the case of fruit varieties, development, type of farming, etc.

To have reproducible and comparable spectra, it is extremely important to control pH and temperature: these have to be maintained constant within a set of experiments. In particular, variation of pH causes changes in the chemical shift of NMR signals of compounds with acidic or basic functional groups (organic acids, amino acids, etc.). Therefore the use of suitable buffered solution in proper concentration or the addition of small volumes of acid or basic solutions are often recommended.

6.4 Spectral Assignment and Quantitative Analysis

Most foodstuffs are complex mixtures and their NMR analysis can be challenging because they are generally constituted of a myriad distinct compounds (saccharides, polysaccharides, lipids, peptides, amino acids, etc.), which are present in a large range of concentrations. The corresponding ^{1}H NMR spectra of foodstuffs are highly complex because of the presence of numerous, often multiplet, resonances. Excellent reviews relevant to the NMR-based structural assignment of compounds present in mixtures are available in the literature (Novoa-Carballal et al., 2011; McKenzie et al., 2011).

As with any other analytical method, each individual compound in a mixture can be identified by its characteristic signals in an NMR spectrum after comparison with the NMR spectrum of the pure compound (database matching approach). One of the main limitations of this approach is that an exhaustive database should be available, otherwise it would require an enormous number of compounds to be synthesized or isolated from natural sources. Another limitation is the variation of NMR spectral parameters (chemical shifts, relaxation times, etc.) that can occur when the compound is analyzed in a mixture, as opposed to alone in solution. These variations arise because of interactions with other molecules or, more simply, because of changes in experimental conditions (eg, concentration, ionic strength, pH, temperature, solvent, etc.). In this case, it is clear that some chemical shift values can be different from the values found in a library database, thereby precluding unambiguous identification.

Along with database matching, another complementary approach for identification of metabolites present in food samples relies on specific NMR experiments that enable signal editing to reveal correlations between different signals present in NMR spectra (NMR elucidation approach).

Frequently used signal editing approaches consist in removing NMR signals caused by either low (diffusion filters) or high molecular weight compounds (relaxation spin–spin or T_2 filters). Widely used correlation experiments produce 2D maps (or even nD maps, $n > 2$) with the cross-correlations between the proton signals of the same molecule (^{1}H–^{1}H COSY, ^{1}H–^{1}H TOCSY, ^{1}H–^{1}H NOESY) or between ^{1}H and ^{13}C NMR signals (2D HSQC for directly bound H—C or 2D HMBC for long-range correlations between protons and carbons generally two or three bonds away).

Finally, it is also useful to confirm assignments by directly adding to the investigated sample an appropriate amount of a pure chemical standard, once its presence has been inferred or at least suspected. Overall, considering the high level of complexity of food samples, the highest information content can only be reached by combining all of these approaches.

Apart from qualitative and structural information, robust quantitative data can be obtained from NMR spectra. As a quantitative method, ^{1}H NMR is unbiased versus all classes of organic compounds because of the proportionality of an NMR signal integral only to the number of equivalent protons and the molar concentration of the corresponding compound(s) independent of its structure or physicochemical properties. Taking into account that each NMR spectrum is a sum of single scans repeated periodically, the recycling time (the time interval between consecutive scans) has to be sufficiently long (at least five times the longitudinal relaxation time (T_1) of the slowest relaxing nuclei) to assure the complete relaxation of all nuclei in mixture components and internal standard molecules.

6.5 Adulterations Detected by Nuclear Magnetic Resonance Spectroscopy

Food adulteration has been practiced for a long time and has become more sophisticated recently. Foods having high sensory and nutritional value such as olive oils, milk, fish, etc. are the most prone to adulteration. Determination of food authenticity and detection of adulteration have become an important question in quality control and safety of food.

Common adulteration practices and frauds consist in:

- undeclared mixing of high-quality expensive products with cheaper ones;
- addition of components that are not permitted;
- geographical origin or variety not conforming to that declared.

6.5.1 Tomatoes

^{1}H NMR spectroscopy has been applied to the study of tomato fruit metabolite profiles since the beginning of the 21st century (Sobolev et al., 2003; Le Gall et al., 2003). The assignment of NMR spectra (up to 45 different metabolites have been identified) provided a foundation for further studies in which the influence of different factors (ripening stage, cultivar/genetic background, cultivation method, etc.) on the metabolite profile have been investigated. All these studies can be considered as a useful background for the authenticity testing of tomato fruits. Some promising results have been already obtained in this specific field, for example, the comparison of metabolic profiles of conventionally and organically grown tomatoes (Hohmann et al., 2014). Two different tomato cultivars and four different producers were tested. The most important differences in metabolite profiles were attributed to the effect of cultivars, whereas the differences between organic and conventional fruits were less pronounced. Two different linear discriminant analysis (LDA) models were built to discriminate organic and conventional tomatoes. The first one included all variables and only the tomatoes from one of the producers as a calibration (training) set. In the validation performed using tomatoes from different producers, merely 72.2% of group identities were predicted correctly. The second LDA model included only variables from selected spectral regions and tomatoes from all the producers for calibration. Validation performed using a limited number of independent samples revealed only 1 out of 18 samples misclassified. Taking into account that the number of variables in both LDA models was comparable or even higher than the number of samples, there was a high possibility of overfitting. It is not clear why a drastically different bucket width was used to generate variables for two LDA analyses and how this arbitrary choice could influence the entire feasibility of statistical approach.

Another example of an authenticity testing approach is tomato analysis by HR-MAS NMR of tomato pulp tissue reported by Corsaro et al. (2015). Sicilian PGI cherry tomato of Pachino is one of the food products most subject to fraud. Its metabolite profile has been compared with those from other cherry tomato fruits of dubious provenance (non-Pachino) including two coming directly from China. Sugars, gamma-aminobutyric acid, glutamic acid, trigonelline, tryptophan, and tyrosine concentration turned out to be higher in Pachino cherry tomatoes whereas that of alanine, guanosine, and methanol was higher in non-Pachino ones. Principal components analysis (PCA) applied to 14 Pachino and 14 non-Pachino tomatoes showed that PC1 (accounting for 31% of variability) was able to separate two groups of cherry tomatoes except for one sample.

6.5.2 Honey

NMR spectroscopy can make an important contribution to the authenticity testing of honey. One of the main adulteration issues encountered in honey is the presence of exogenous sugar, either from deliberate addition to honey of a cheaper sugar source or from the use of sugar for bee feeding during the production season (which is prohibited). Different NMR methodologies [such as SNIF-NMR (Cotte et al., 2007), low-field ^{1}H NMR relaxometry (Ribeiro et al., 2014), and high-resolution NMR (Bertelli et al., 2010; Spiteri et al., 2015)] have been proposed to reveal these types of adulteration.

SNIF-NMR measurement is performed on ethanol obtained from fermentation of the honey and extracted by distillation. The isotopic composition of ethanol indicates the nature of the sugars from which it is derived. According to Cotte et al. (2007), the use of SNIF-NMR was limited by a minimum detection level as high as 20% w/w or above depending on the botanical origin of honey and the type of syrup.

Low-field ^{1}H NMR relaxometry applied directly to honey samples spiked with up to 80% of high-fructose syrup was able to reveal adulteration as low as 10% w/w (Ribeiro et al., 2014). This method relies on measurement of the T_2 relaxation time of water present in the sample. Biexponential T_2 relaxation curves were observed, indicating the occurrence of two water populations and their T_2 relaxation times were significantly affected by concentration of adulterants in pure honey, decreasing at higher fructose syrup concentrations.

Unlike SNIF-NMR and low-field ^{1}H NMR relaxometry, high-resolution NMR of honey solutions or extracts deals not only with bulk components of the honey matrix (principal sugars, water) but also with minor components (minor sugars, organic acids, amino acids, etc.) that can be excellent markers of adulteration. In the specific case of exogenous sugar addition, signals of some minor components of a sugar fraction (di- and oligosaccharides) are present only in the adulterated honey spectrum or at least are of greater intensity in adulterated samples (Bertelli et al., 2010). Sugar syrup concentrations as low as 10% w/w can be detected (Fig. 6.1).

In a bulk screening study, 518 reference honey spectra have been compared to 205 commercial samples using independent components analysis. Several unidentified signals, correlated to low levels of minor sugars and/or unusually high concentrations of organic acids, have been hypothesized to be a marker of sugar syrup addition. It is noteworthy that, according to statistical analysis, a significant number of the commercial samples appeared as outliers with respect to authentic samples; that is, most probably these commercial honeys have been adulterated with exogenous sugars (Spiteri et al., 2015).

High-resolution NMR spectroscopy has been extensively used for verification of botanical origin of monofloral honeys, commodities that are also frequently subjected to adulteration. Using this methodology, a number of studies dedicated to discovery of biomarkers linked to botanical origin have been undertaken (Donarski et al., 2010; Schievano et al., 2012, 2013; Spiteri et al., 2015). For example, kynurenic acid has been found to be a biomarker of sweet chestnut honey, whereas α-isophorone and 2,5-dihydroxyphenylacetic acid have been confirmed as markers of strawberry-tree honey (Donarski et al., 2010). Extraction and NMR characterization of hydrophobic metabolites from honeys of different botanical origins, that is, chestnut, linden, orange, acacia, eucalyptus, honeydew, and polyfloral honeys, has been proposed by Schievano et al. (2012, 2013). This approach is focused on retaining the aroma compounds and those hydrophobic substances that vary the most in honeys from various botanical origins, whereas ubiquitous and less specific carbohydrates are eliminated from the analysis. In fact, for each monofloral honey under study, two or more specific marker compounds were identified including chrysin and pinocembrin for acacia honey or 8-hydroxylinalool and caffeine for orange honey. Along with other analytical methods, high-resolution NMR has contributed to the qualitative and quantitative characterization of Manuka honey, a food that shows a very particular antimicrobial activity (Le Gresley et al., 2012; Spiteri et al., 2015). Because of mixing or mislabeling of Manuka honey with other honeys similar in color, or pollen morphology such as kanuka, rewarewa, or honeydew, the authenticity of commercial Manuka product is an important issue. The presence of relatively high levels of methylglyoxal and dihydroxyacetone, which can be efficiently quantified by ^{1}H NMR, is a good marker of authentic Manuka honey (Spiteri et al., 2015).

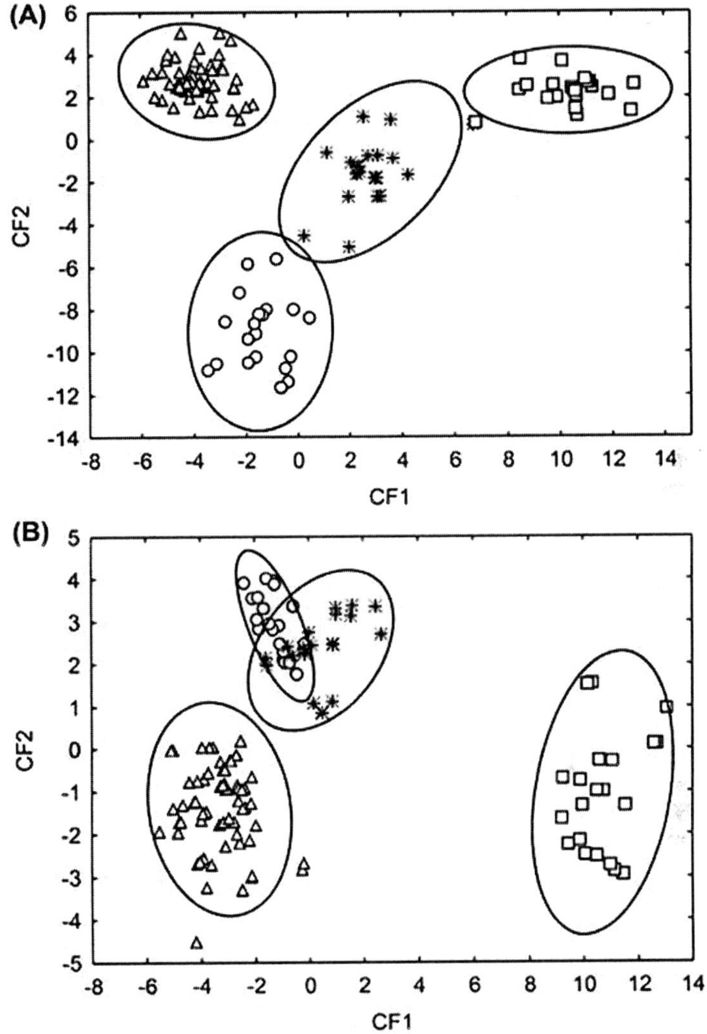

Figure 6.1 (A) Score plot of the first two canonical functions for the data set obtained from 1D ^{1}H NMR spectra of adulterated honey in dimethyl sulfoxide (DMSO-d_6). (B) Score plot of the first two canonical functions for the data set obtained from 2D $^{1}H-^{13}C$ HMBC (Heteronuclear Multiple Bond Correlation) NMR of the same honey samples: 10% adulterated honeys (○), 20% adulterated honeys (*), 40% adulterated chestnut honeys (□), authentic honeys (Δ). Reproduced with permission from Bertelli, D., Lolli, M., Papotti, G., Bortolotti, L., Serra, G., Plessi, M., 2010. Detection of honey adulteration by sugar syrups using one-dimensional and two-dimensional high-resolution nuclear magnetic resonance. Journal of Agricultural and Food Chemistry 58, 8495–8501. Copyright (2010) American Chemical Society.

6.5.3 Wine

An analytical method suitable for wine authenticity testing must be capable of answering questions concerning the discrimination of grape varieties, wine geographical origin, and vintage year.

A targeted approach based on high-resolution NMR has been useful in determining some specific markers of grape varieties [like shikimic acid (Godelmann et al., 2013)], or wine technology [caftaric acid as an indicator of the oxidation levels that a wine has undergone (Godelmann et al., 2013)]. Proline is the most abundant amino acid in wine and therefore appears to be a marker for ripeness (Lopez-Rituerto et al., 2009). Polyphenols extracted from wine and analyzed by ^{1}H NMR are a good marker for variety, geographical origin, and vintage of Greek wines (Anastasiadi et al., 2009).

Another typical adulteration of wine, addition of sugars before fermentation, can be revealed by SNIF-NMR usually in combination with isotope-ratio mass spectrometry to detect all possible sources of exogenous sugars (mostly from beet and cane) (Ogrinc et al., 2003).

Besides targeted analysis, the untargeted NMR approach to wine authenticity testing has been applied in conjunction with advanced multivariate statistical analysis (Godelmann et al., 2013). All latent factors important for wine identity such as grape variety, origin, vintage, and technology are coded in multivariate metabolite patterns in the whole NMR spectra rather than in single spectral markers. Among wine polyphenols, anthocyanins are mainly responsible for the color of red wines and their addition to increase color [by blending the wine with another one (Rossissimo) very rich in anthocyanins or by the addition of anthocyanins extracted from black rice] can be considered an adulteration. ^{1}H NMR in conjunction with proper statistical analysis was applied to discriminate the provenance of added anthocyanins (from black rise or Rossissimo wine) in unextracted samples of five different types of wines (a white wine, a rosé wine, and three red wines) (Ferrari et al., 2011). The data were subjected to three different classification methods: partial least squares discriminant analysis (PLS-DA), interval PLS-DA, and wavelet iterative linear modeling approach-discriminant version. The classification method based on wavelet-based variables selection was the best; it permitted an efficiency in validation greater than 95% to be reached.

6.5.4 Vinegar

In the case of vinegar, the most relevant frauds concern both balsamic and traditional balsamic vinegars. This special vinegar, which is produced by a well-established process, can be the subject of falsification of the aging process and addition of sugar and must (Consonni et al., 2008). Very interesting results were obtained using NMR methodology in the study of these vinegars. Examination of the ^{1}H NMR spectrum (Consonni and Gatti, 2004; Caligiani et al., 2007) has facilitated assessment of the aging process of both traditional balsamic vinegar of Modena and balsamic vinegar of Modena (Consonni and Gatti, 2004) and to differentiate traditional balsamic vinegars from their balsamic counterparts (Caligiani et al., 2007). Ethanol, acetic acid, malic acid, glucose, and 5-hydroxymethyl-2-furfural can be considered to be markers of the aging processes: sugars and 5-hydroxymethyl-2-furfural levels largely increase because of water loss and degradation reactions whereas the level of acetate and ethanol decreases. Traditional balsamic vinegars contain high levels of glucose, fructose, 5-hydroxymethyl-2-furfural, and 2,3-butanediol, whereas balsamic vinegars are characterized by high levels of acetic and lactic acid, acetoin, and ethanol.

Brazilian vinegars (56 samples) from different raw materials (honey, orange, pineapple, rice, wine, apple, and alcohol/agrin vinegars) have been characterized and well discriminated using NMR and statistical analyses including PCA, hierarchical cluster analysis (HCA), k-nearest neighbor (KNN), soft independent modeling by class analogy (SIMCA) and PLS-DA (Boffo et al., 2009). The KNN, SIMCA, and PLS-DA methods were used to build predictive models for classification of vinegar type wine, apple, and alcohol/agrin. A 100% correct classification of all samples (27 samples—22 as training set) was obtained. Validated models were used to predict the class of 21 commercial samples, which were correctly classified. Application of PCA and HCA methods resulted in the natural clustering of the samples according to the raw material used. In particular, the PCA score plot, reported in Fig. 6.2, shows a clear grouping of vinegar samples according to their origin. The first principal component, PC1, describes 18.5% of total variance,

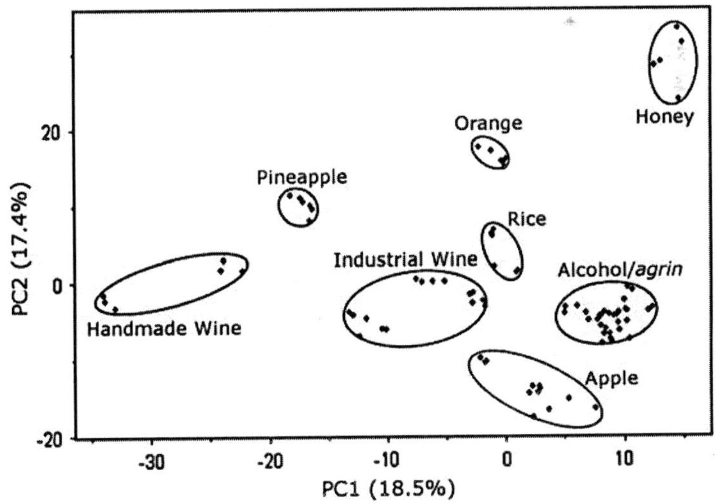

Figure 6.2 PCA score plot (PC1 and PC2) showing the vinegar groupings according the raw material used for the production.
Reprinted from Boffo, E.F., Tavares, L.A., Ferreira, M.M.C., Ferreira, A.G., 2009. Classification of Brazilian vinegars according to their ^{1}H NMR spectra by pattern recognition analysis. LWT – Food Science and Technology 42, 1455–1460. Copyright (2009), with permission from Elsevier.

whereas the second component, PC2, describes 17.4%; the two PCs together express 35.9% of the total variability.

Every type of vinegar contains specific markers. For instance, wine vinegars are characterized by a high concentration of ethyl acetate, glycerol, methanol, and tartaric acid, while glycerol and ethyl acetate signals are not detectable in alcohol/agrin vinegars. Apple vinegars are rich in alanine while pineapple vinegar has a high content of tartaric acid. Orange and rice vinegars both have a high content of lactic acid.

6.5.5 Olive Oils

NMR spectroscopy can make an important contribution to testing olive oil authenticity and quality and confirming the geographical origin of a sample (Mannina and Sobolev, 2011). An important aspect of this methodology is that it allows the sample to be analyzed without any chemical manipulation. In the case of olive oil, sometimes called "yellow gold" on account of its nutritional and sensory properties, one of the main adulterations is the addition of low-grade oils of different botanical origin such as seed oil or refined olive oils.

The assignment of ^{1}H, ^{13}C, and ^{31}P NMR spectra of oils of different origin (Sacchi et al., 1996; Fauhl et al., 2000; Vlahov, 1999; Spyros and Dais, 2009) in terms of major and minor compounds can be considered the fundamental background for olive oil authenticity testing by NMR.

The ^{13}C NMR approach has been useful for a variety of purposes since it allows detection of acyl positional distribution in the glycerol moiety (Sacchi et al., 1997; Shaw et al., 1997; Mannina et al., 1999). Two groups of resonances are observed in the carbonyl region of the ^{13}C NMR spectrum of an olive oil, one group being caused by fatty chains in position *sn*-2 of the glycerol moiety and the other being caused by fatty acids in position *sn*-1,3. This information can be useful to determine some fraudulent practices, such as the chemical esterification of glycerol to lower the acidity of an oil. For instance, the presence of a palmitic residue in position *sn*-2 of the glycerol moiety is a clear indication of adulteration since palmitic chains are preferentially present in position *sn*-1,3.

^{31}P NMR spectroscopy together with multivariate statistical analysis has allowed the detection (down to 5% w/w) of extra virgin olive oil adulteration with lampante olive oil and refined olive oil (Fragaki et al., 2005).

^{1}H NMR methodology has been used both to detect the fraudulent addition of low-quality oils and to confirm the geographical origin of olive oils. This methodology allows the detection of both major (triglycerides) and minor (squalene, β-sitosterol, terpenes, aldehydes, etc.) compounds.

A fraud very difficult to detect is the addition of low-quality hazelnut oils (for instance, those produced from rotten hazelnuts) to olive oils since these two types of oils have a similar chemical composition. To deal with this problem, different ^{1}H NMR protocols based on the statistical analysis of selected ^{1}H signals (fatty chains and triacylglycerides or fatty chains and squalene, and β-sitosterol) have been proposed (Mannina et al., 2009; Fauhl et al., 2000) allowing the detection of hazelnut oil down to 10% (Fig. 6.3).

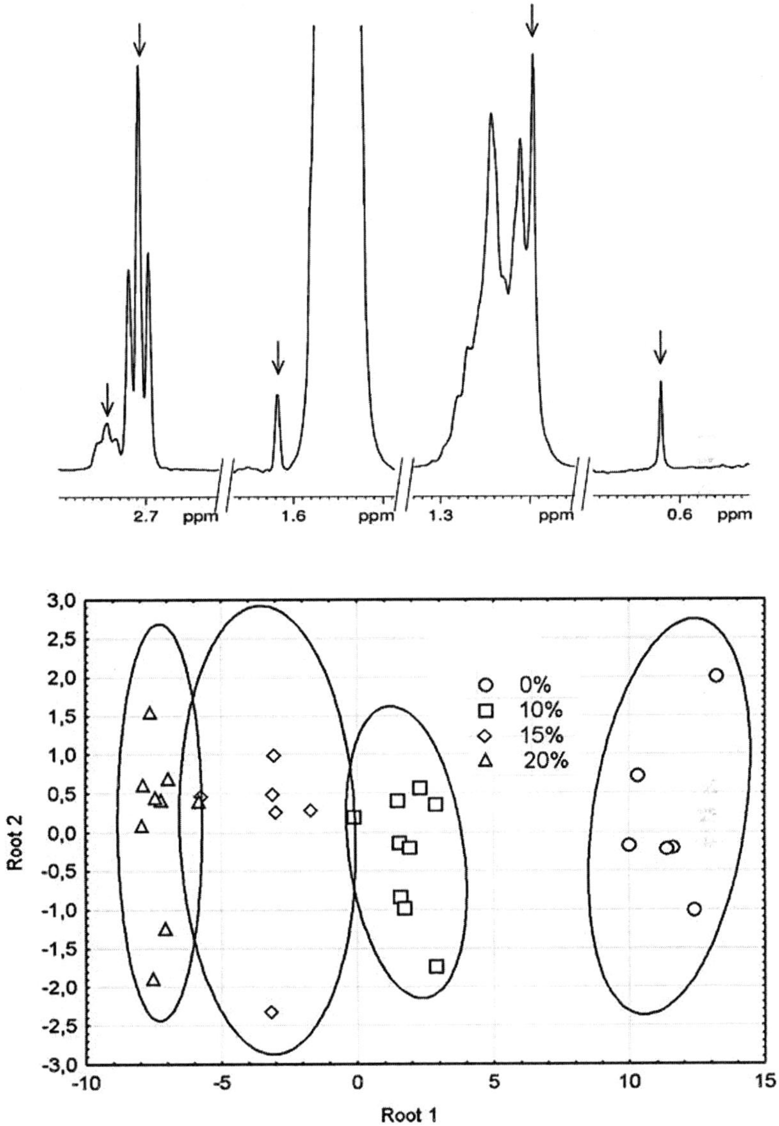

Figure 6.3 LDA applied to the intensity of five ^{1}H NMR resonances (*labeled with arrows*) in 600 MHz ^{1}H spectra of different samples of olive oils and hazelnut–olive oil mixtures. Percentages (v/v) of hazelnut oil in olive oil: 0% (○), 10% (□), 15% (◇), and 20% (Δ) Adapted from Mannina, L., D'Imperio, M., Capitani, D., Rezzi, S., Guillou, C., Mavromoustakos, T., Molero Vilchez, M.D., Fernández, A.H., Thomas, F., Aparicio, R., 2009. ^{1}H NMR-based protocol for the detection of adulterations of refined olive oil with refined hazelnut oil. Journal of Agricultural and Food Chemistry 57, 11550–11556.

Another important issue is confirmation of the geographical origin of extra virgin olive oils. High-resolution NMR together with a suitable statistical approach constitutes a powerful tool for the geographical characterization of olive oils on international (Mediterranean countries), national, regional, and PDO scales (Mannina and Sobolev, 2011; Alonso-Salces et al., 2010; Longobardi et al., 2012). Robust databases and statistical models have been created producing unique capabilities with which to define the geographical origin of olive oils. A significant example involves the NMR-based models created to define and confirm the declared geographical origin of olive oil samples from Liguria, an Italian region. PLS-DA and SIMCA have been used as modeling techniques resulting in a good classification, and the "class" olive oils from Liguria have been well defined with respect to other olive oils coming from the Mediterranean area (896 samples from Italy, Spain, France, Greece, and Turkey) during three consecutive harvest years (2005, 2006, and 2007) (Mannina et al., 2010). The results of PLS-DA and SIMCA are reported in Table 6.1.

This study highlights some important general aspects. The variability of some compounds in the three harvests can be caused by different factors such as the different climatic conditions, for instance, hot summer in 2005 and 2006 and/or rainy autumn in 2005.

Table 6.1 Classification Accuracy (PLS-DA), Sensitivity, and Specificity (SIMCA) for Ligurian Olive Oils

	Global Model	2004/ 2005	2005/ 2006	2006/ 2007
PLS-DA				
Classification accuracy (modeling)	89.3%	88.7%	92.4%	86.8%
Classification accuracy (cross-validation)	84.4%	88.7%	91.1%	86.8%
Classification accuracy (test set)	84.1%	34.7%	79.2%	54.6%
SIMCA				
Sensitivity (model)	84.3%	96.8%	93.7%	94.0%
Specificity (model)	70.6%	87.0%	78.7%	78.5%
Sensitivity (cross-validation)	83.6%	82.3%	81.0%	85.1%
Specificity (cross-validation)	72.0%	89.1%	79.8%	80.8%
Sensitivity (test)	92.8%	0.0%	14.6%	41.5%
Specificity (test)	70.6%	100.0%	93.5%	90.2%

PLS-DA, Partial least squares discriminant analysis; *SIMCA*, soft independent modeling of class analogy.
Reprinted from Mannina, L., Marini, F., Gobbino, M., Sobolev, A.P., Capitani, D., 2010. NMR and chemometrics in tracing European olive oils: the case study of Ligurian samples. Talanta 80, 2141–2148. Copyright (2010), with permission from Elsevier.

However, Ligurian olive oils are always characterized by a high amount of terpenes and a low amount of saturated fatty chains. Therefore the NMR and chemometric approach extended to a relevant number of samples representative of the Mediterranean production could be useful not only to discriminate a specific PDO with respect to the others but also to define sensory and quality markers specific to the PDO product.

6.5.6 Meat

In the case of meat, the most common adulterations are undeclared mixing of meat from different species and mixing of expensive meat cuts with cheaper ones. NMR methodologies have given some interesting results in meat authentication, species identification within meat products, and determination of geographical origin.

Adulteration of pure beef muscle tissue with offal (beef liver or kidney) was investigated using NMR methodology and suitable data elaboration including PCA, PLS, and PLS-DA (Al-Jowder et al., 2001). PCA applied to a data set (97 samples) consisting of pure samples of muscle tissue and offal has shown three groupings corresponding to beef muscle, kidney, and liver species, 90% of the information being within the first two PCs. Quantitative analysis of muscle/offal mixtures was carried out using PLS calibration and internal cross-validation. The predicted amounts of added kidney and added liver versus the actual concentrations of adulterants have shown correlation coefficient values of 0.990 and 0.986, respectively, and a standard error of prediction of 3.51% w/w and 3.93% w/w, respectively. PLS-DA applied to discriminate between three beef cuts, namely, brisket, neck, and silverside, obtained a success rate of 97% using a model dimensionality of 18 scores.

A simple screening protocol based on 60 MHz ^{1}H NMR measurements was used to distinguish beef from horse meat using their different triglyceride signatures (Jakes et al., 2015). In particular, the integrated olefinic and bis-allylic peak areas were used in a naïve Bayes classification model, whereas the olefinic, bis-allylic, and terminal CH_3 regions were used as input in PCA. Applying the model to 107 extracts prepared from new, completely independent samples resulted in all but one being correctly authenticated.

Another important aspect is the control of beef geographical origin. According to European Regulations, beef must be labeled according to its geographical origin. NMR coupled to pattern recognition techniques has given very interesting results in addressing this particular analytical issue (Jung et al., 2010). Significant differences between raw beef samples obtained from New Zealand, Australia, the United States, and Korea have been demonstrated using an NMR−chemometric-based approach (Fig. 6.4).

^{1}H time domain nuclear magnetic resonance (^{1}H TD-NMR) has been proposed to obtain information on meat quality. A correlation between T_2 relaxation times of pork M. *Longissimus dorsi* and the values of 14 technological parameters commonly used to assess pork meat quality was reported (Brown et al., 2000). The parameters used to measure water-holding capacity of meat, that is, drip loss and filter paper press, are those better correlated to the NMR signal of pork meat giving correlation coefficients of 0.74 and 0.71.

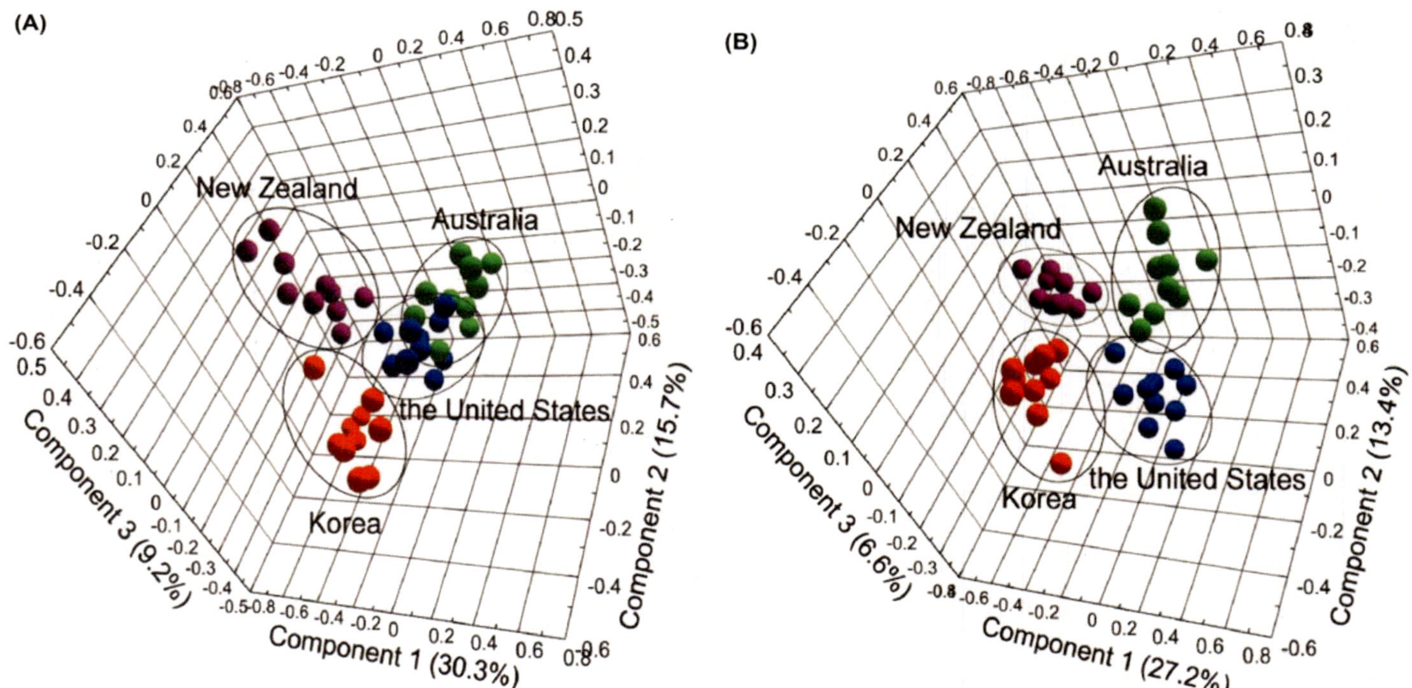

Figure 6.4 PCA (A) and OPLS-DA (Orthogonal Partial Least Squares Discriminant Analysis) (B) 3D score plots derived from the ^{1}H NMR spectra of beef sirloin (or chuck) extracts obtained from Australia, Korea, New Zealand, and the United States.

Reproduced with permission from Jung, Y., Lee, J., Kwon, J., Lee, K.S., Ryu, D.H., Hwang, G.S., 2010. Discrimination of the geographical origin of beef by ^{1}H NMR-based metabolomics. Journal of Agricultural and Food Chemistry 58 (19), 10458–10466. Copyright (2010) American Chemical Society.

6.5.7 Milk

Milk, a fundamental dietary constituent, is one of the seven top foods subjected to adulteration. Typical commercial frauds involve mixing milks from different animal species, addition of water, addition of exogenous compounds (salts, sugars, and melamine, for example), and neutralization to mask acidity.

^{1}H TD-NMR has been proposed as a rapid method to identify and quantify milk adulteration such as addition of whey, tap water, synthetic milk, synthetic urine, urea, and hydrogen peroxide (Santos et al., 2016). Milk samples were spiked with known levels of whey, urea, hydrogen peroxide, synthetic urine, and synthetic milk. A total of 78 milk samples was analyzed. T_2 relaxation times turned out to be significantly different between authentic and adulterated samples and correlated with the level of adulteration. Regression models to estimate the level of adulteration in milk samples were obtained either with the full ^{1}H TD-NMR dataset (multivariate approach) or only T_2 values (univariate approach) with standard errors of prediction of 2.34% and 3.79% v/v, respectively. SIMCA and KNN classification models were also developed to classify control and adulterated milk samples based on the level of adulteration. The results obtained with both models showed a similar and quite satisfactorily predictability, with sensitivity and specificity ranging from 0.66 (control sample) to 1.00 (adulterated sample).

Low-field NMR methodology has also been used to discriminate fresh from aged milks stored at 30°C for 96 h. Relaxation time signals T_1 and T_2 were measured to analyze synthetically the combination and mobility of water molecules whereas T_{21}, T_{22} proton density values obtained by T_2 inversion allow the change of bound water and free water to be observed. The result shows that the total moisture in fresh milk decreases first and then increases during the process of metamorphism since the free water decreases, and the bound water first decreases and then increases (Liu et al., 2014).

^{1}H NMR methodology (400 MHz NMR and 700 MHz HR-MAS NMR) has been used to quantify melamine, a very toxic contaminant, and to distinguish between melamine-contaminated and melamine-free infant formulas (Lachenmeier et al., 2009). NMR spectra can provide quantification of the melamine concentrations by integration of the signal of the NH_2 groups at about 5.93 ppm. The results show that NMR can be used for screening purposes at levels down to the lower mg/kg range. For contaminated Chinese infant formulas or candy, identical results were obtained when comparing NMR with solid phase extraction liquid chromatography tandem mass spectrometry.

^{1}H and ^{13}C NMR have made an important contribution to the authenticity of milk products, offering the possibility of identifying the species of animal from which the milk originated. Examination of fatty acid composition using ^{13}C NMR (Andreotti et al., 2000, 2002) has allowed discrimination between milks of different animal species (cow, buffalo, etc.). Brescia et al. (2004) have reported a comparison between cow and buffalo milk collected in different breeding areas in Apulia, a region of Southern Italy, based on their different triglyceride contents determined by ^{1}H NMR. Multivariate statistical analyses (PCA, HCA, and DA) applied on NMR data permitted buffalo and cow milks to be distinguished. In particular, DA applied on the first three PCs using the species of the animals from which samples were collected as classes for assignment has shown a highly satisfactory recognition ability of the two classes since all samples were correctly classified. The prediction ability of the model obtained after splitting the data set into a training and test set has shown 97% of the training set samples and 94.5% of the test set samples assigned correctly.

NMR together with isotope-ratio mass spectrometry in combination with chemometric methods (PCA and DA) were proposed as a tool to confirm the geographical origin of 39 milk samples (Sacco et al., 2009). Cow milk samples from different areas of Southern Italy (Apulia and Basilicata) and Central–Eastern Europe have been analyzed. The comparison between ^{1}H NMR spectra of the aqueous extracts of Southern Italy and foreign milk samples showed differences in amino acids content and a higher sugar content in foreign milk with respect to milk from Southern Italy. This could be caused by different feeding regimes of animals. The classification ability and the prediction ability were shown by DA to be 95% and 90%, respectively, using samples of known geographical origin for assignment.

6.5.8 Coffee

In the case of roasted coffee, the main commercial fraud is the addition of less expensive *Coffea canephora* var. Robusta to the higher quality *Coffea arabica* species when coffee is labeled as "100% Arabica." A German standard method (DIN 10779, 1999), which is laborious and time consuming, is based on the quantification of 16-*O*-methylcafestol (16-OMC) in roasted coffee beans to detect *C. canephora* in blends. NMR studies of lipophilic extracts of authentic roasted and green coffees have confirmed the presence of specific markers for Robusta, namely, 16-OMC and for Arabica, kahweol (Monakhova et al., 2015). Quantitative determination of esterified 16-OMC directly in coffee extracts has allowed the detection of Robusta in Arabica in coffee blends (Monakhova et al., 2015; Schievano et al., 2014). To evaluate the accuracy of the proposed method, the quantities of 16-OMC found by NMR were compared to those determined by the DIN method. The detection limit has been estimated by Monakhova et al. (2015) using experimental blends with different ratios of Arabica and Robusta authentic samples. It can be clearly seen that the presence of 16-OMC in the ^{1}H spectrum can be identified beginning from 2% to 3% w/w of Robusta. The relative 16-OMC integrals ranged from 0.055 for 2% to 0.270 for 7% w/w of Robusta in blends (percentage compared with tetramethylsilane (TMS) integrals). The authors propose for routine analysis a threshold value of the relative 16-OMC integral as 0.075. This means that coffee samples declared as 100% Arabica, for which the relative integral of 16-OMC signal exceeds 0.075, should be considered as suspicious and will require other investigations (reference HPLC analysis, DIN 10779, 1999).

^{13}C NMR spectroscopy coupled with PCA and OPLS-DA has also been applied to distinguish species and origin of green coffee bean samples of Arabica from Brazil, Colombia, Guatemala, and Tanzania, and Robusta from Indonesia and Vietnam (Wei et al., 2012). The levels of 14 metabolites in the classification models were found to be significantly different, including sucrose, caffeine, chlorogenic acid, choline, amino acids, organic acids, and trigonelline. The quality of the proposed OPLS models turned out to be high giving proper Rx^2 and Q^2 values. (Rx^2 is defined as the proportion of variance in the data explained by the model and indicates goodness of fit. Q^2 is defined as the proportion of variance in the data predictable by the model and indicates predictability.)

^1H NMR together with PCA followed by LDA was also applied to quality and authenticity control of 98 instant spray-dried coffees obtained from three different producers (Charlton et al., 2002): 99% of the samples have been correctly attributed to their manufacturer. Blind testing of the PCA model with an additional 36 samples of instant coffee (different sources including coffees produced by the same three manufacturers) resulted in a 100% success rate in identifying the samples from the three manufacturers. The authors underline that it is only possible to identify the manufacturer of a coffee if the samples from that manufacturer are employed in the building of the original model.

6.6 Future Trends

NMR methodologies have already shown significant potential in food analysis and authenticity testing. The versatility of NMR and the possibility to employ either targeted or untargeted approaches enable the analyst to develop a suitable protocol for any specific problem. Despite these advantages, important challenges still remain. Because of high capital and maintenance costs of NMR equipment, as well as the necessity for highly qualified operating personnel, high-resolution NMR is still too expensive for day-to-day application. To reduce the cost per single measurement and make NMR more accessible, the complete automation of NMR analysis is in progress. Spectral processing, peak assignment, and statistical analysis of NMR data are still too laborious and sometimes constitute a bottleneck in the entire analysis. Fortunately, the constant development of software suitable for assignment and quantification of metabolites in food matrices should significantly help and encourage the application of NMR. The creation and development of interactive databases containing NMR data for foodstuffs together with the standardization of successful analytical protocols are also important requirements to facilitate greater NMR application in the field of authenticity testing.

References

Al-Jowder, O., Casuscelli, F., Defernez, M., Kemsley, E.K., Wilson, R.H., Colquhoun, I.J., 2001. High resolution NMR studies of meat composition and authenticity. In: Webb, G.A., Belton, P.S., Gil, A.M., Delgadillo, I. (Eds.), Magnetic Resonance in Food Science: A View to the Future. Royal Society of Chemistry, Cambrige, UK, pp. 232–238.

Alonso-Salces, R.M., Moreno-Rojas, J.M., Holland, M.V., Reniero, F., Guillou, C., Héberger, K., 2010. Virgin olive oil authentication by multivariate analyses of ^1H NMR fingerprints and $d^{13}C$ and d^2H Data. Journal of Agriculture and Food Chemistry 58, 5586–5596.

Anastasiadi, M., Zira, A., Magiatis, P., Haroutounian, S.A., Skaltsounis, A.L., Mikros, E., 2009. ^{1}H NMR-based metabonomics for the classification of Greek wines according to variety, region, and vintage. Comparison with HPLC data. Journal of Agriculture and Food Chemistry 57, 11067−11074.

Andreotti, G., Lamanna, R., Trivellone, E., Motta, A., 2002. ^{13}C NMR spectra of TAG: an easy way to distinguish milks from different animal species. Journal of the American Oil Chemists' Society 79, 123−127.

Andreotti, G., Trivellone, E., Lamanna, R., Di Luccia, A., Motta, A., 2000. Milk identification of different species: ^{13}C NMR spectroscopy of triacylglycerols from cows and buffaloes' milks. Journal of Dairy Science 83, 2432−2437.

Beretta, G., Caneva, E., Regazzoni, L., Bakhtyari, N.G., Facino, R.M., 2008. A solid-phase extraction procedure coupled to ^{1}H NMR, with chemometric analysis, to seek reliable markers of the botanical origin of honey. Analytica Chimica Acta 620, 176−182.

Bertelli, D., Lolli, M., Papotti, G., Bortolotti, L., Serra, G., Plessi, M., 2010. Detection of honey adulteration by sugar syrups using one-dimensional and two-dimensional high-resolution nuclear magnetic resonance. Journal of Agriculture and Food Chemistry 58, 8495−8501.

Brescia, M.A., Mazzilli, V., Sgaramella, A., Ghelli, S., Fanizzi, F.P., Sacco, A., 2004. ^{1}H NMR characterization of milk lipids: a comparison between cow and buffalo milk. Journal of the American Oil Chemists' Society 81, 431−436.

Boffo, E.F., Tavares, L.A., Ferreira, M.M.C., Ferreira, A.G., 2009. Classification of Brazilian vinegars according to their ^{1}H NMR spectra by pattern recognition analysis. LWT − Food Science and Technology 42, 1455−1460.

Brown, R.J.S., Capozzi, F., Cavani, C., Cremonini, M.A., Petracci, M., Placucci, G., 2000. Relationships between ^{1}H NMR relaxation data and some technological parameters of meat: a chemometric approach. Journal of Magnetic Resonance 147, 89−94.

Caligiani, A., Acquotti, D., Palla, G., Bocchi, V., 2007. Identification and quantification of the main organic components of vinegars by high resolution ^{1}H NMR spectroscopy. Analytica Chimica Acta 585, 110−119.

Capitani, D., Mannina, L., Proietti, N., Sobolev, A.P., Tomassini, A., Miccheli, A., Di Cocco, M.E., Capuani, G., De Salvador, R., Delfini, M., 2010. Monitoring of metabolic profiling and water status of Hayward kiwifruits by nuclear magnetic resonance. Talanta 82, 1826−1838.

Capitani, D., Sobolev, A.P., Delfini, M., Vista, S., Antiochia, R., Proietti, N., Bubici, S., Ferrante, G., Carradori, S., De Salvador, F.R., Mannina, L., 2014. NMR methodologies in the analysis of blueberries. Electrophoresis 35, 1615−1626.

Charlton, A.J., Farrington, W.H.H., Brereton, P., 2002. Application of ^{1}H NMR and multivariate statistics for screening complex mixtures: quality control and authenticity of instant coffee. Journal of Agricultural and Food Chemistry 50, 3098−3103.

Consonni, R., Cagliani, L.R., Benevelli, F., Spraul, M., Humpfer, E., Stocchero, M., 2008. NMR and chemometric methods: a powerful combination for characterization of balsamic and traditional balsamic vinegar of Modena. Analytica Chimica Acta 611, 31−40.

Consonni, R., Gatti, A., 2004. ^{1}H NMR studies on Italian balsamic and traditional balsamic vinegars. Journal of Agricultural and Food Chemistry 52, 3446−3450.

Corsaro, C., Mallamace, D., Vasi, S., Ferrantelli, V., Dugo, G., Cicero, N., 2015. ^{1}H HR-MAS NMR spectroscopy and the metabolite determination of typical foods in Mediterranean diet. Journal of Analytical Methods in Chemistry 2015, 175696.

Cotte, J.F., Casabianca, H., Lhéritier, J., Perrucchietti, C., Sanglar, C., Waton, H., Grenier-Loustalot, M.F., 2007. Study and validity of ^{13}C stable carbon isotopic ratio analysis by mass spectrometry and ^{2}H site-specific natural isotopic fractionation by nuclear magnetic resonance isotopic measurements to characterize and control the authenticity of honey. Analytica Chimica Acta 582, 125–136.

DIN 10779, 1999. Bestimmung des Gehaltes an 16-Methyl-O-cafestol in Röstkaffe. HPLC Verfahren, Berlin, Germany.

Donarski, J.A., Jones, S.A., Harrison, M., Driffield, M., Charlton, A.J., 2010. Identification of botanical biomarkers found in Corsican honey. Food Chemistry 118, 987–994.

Fauhl, C., Reniero, F., Guillou, C., 2000. ^{1}H NMR as a tool for the analysis of mixtures of virgin olive oil with oils of different botanical origin. Magnetic Resonance in Chemistry 38, 436–443.

Ferrari, E., Foca, G., Vignali, M., Tassi, L., Ulrici, A., 2011. Adulteration of the anthocyanin content of red wines: perspectives for authentication by Fourier transform-near infrared and ^{1}H NMR spectroscopies. Analytica Chimica Acta 701, 139–151.

Fiehn, O., 2002. Metabolomics – the link between genotypes and phenotypes. Plant Molecular Biology 48, 155–171.

Fragaki, G., Spyros, A., Siragakis, G., Salivaras, E., Dais, P., 2005. Detection of extra virgin olive oil adulteration with lampante olive oil and refined olive oil using NMR spectroscopy and multivariate statistical analysis. Journal of Agricultural and Food Chemistry 53, 2810–2816.

Fukusaki, E., Kobayashi, A., 2005. Plant metabolomics: potential for practical operation. Journal of Bioscience and Bioengineering 100, 347–354.

Gianferri, R., D'Aiuto, V., Curini, R., Delfini, M., Brosio, E., 2007. Proton NMR transverse relaxation measurements to study water dynamic states and age-related changes in Mozzarella di Bufala Campana cheese. Food Chemistry 105, 720–726.

Godelmann, R., Fang, F., Humpfer, E., SchÜtz, B., Bansbach, M., SchÄfer, H., Spraul, M., 2013. Targeted and nontargeted wine analysis by ^{1}H NMR spectroscopy combined with multivariate statistical analysis. Differentiation of important parameters: grape variety, geographical origin, year of vintage. Journal of Agricultural and Food Chemistry 61, 5610–5619.

Le Gall, G., Colquhoun, I.J., Davis, A.L., Collins, G.J., Verhoeyen, M.E., 2003. Metabolite profiling of tomato (*Lycopersicon esculentum*) using ^{1}H NMR spectroscopy as a tool to detect potential unintended effects following a genetic modification. Journal of Agricultural and Food Chemistry 51, 2447–2456.

Le Gresley, A., Kenny, J., Cassar, C., Kelly, A., Sinclair, A., Fielder, M.D., 2012. The application of high resolution diffusion NMR to the analysis of manuka honey. Food Chemistry 135, 2879–2886.

Hills, B.P., 2006. Applications of Low Field NMR to Food Science in: Annual Reports on NMR Spectroscopy. Academic Press, Oxford, UK.

Hohmann, M., Christoph, N., Wachter, H., Holzgrabe, U., 2014. ^{1}H NMR profiling as an approach to differentiate conventionally and organically grown tomatoes. Journal of Agricultural and Food Chemistry 62, 8530–8540.

Jakes, W., Gerdova, A., Defernez, M., Watson, A.D., McCallum, C., Limer, E., Colquhoun, I.J., Williamson, D.C., Kemsley, E.K., 2015. Authentication of beef versus horse meat using 60 MHz ^{1}H NMR spectroscopy. Food Chemistry 175, 1–9.

Jung, Y., Lee, J., Kwon, J., Lee, K.S., Ryu, D.H., Hwang, G.S., 2010. Discrimination of the geographical origin of beef by ^{1}H NMR-based metabolomics. Journal of Agricultural and Food Chemistry 58 (19), 10458–10466.

Kaiser, K.A., Barding Jr., G.A., Larive, C.K., 2009. A comparison of metabolite extraction strategies for ^{1}H NMR-based metabolic profiling using mature leaf tissue from the model plant *Arabidopsis thaliana*. Magnetic Resonance in Chemistry 47, S147–S156.

Kim, H.K., Verpoorte, R., 2010. Sample preparation for plant metabolomics. Phytochemical Analysis 21, 4–13.

Khatib, A., Wilson, E.G., Kim, H.K., Lefeber, A.W.M., Erkelens, C., Choi, Y.H., Verpoorte, R., 2006. Application of two-dimensional J-resolved nuclear magnetic resonance spectroscopy to differentiation of beer. Analytica Chimica Acta 559, 264–270.

Lachenmeier, D.W., Humpfer, E., Fang, F., Schutz, B., Dvortsak, P., Sproll, C., Spraul, M., 2009. NMR-spectroscopy for nontargeted screening and simultaneous quantification of health-relevant compounds in foods: the example of melamine. Journal of Agricultural and Food Chemistry 57, 7194–7199.

Lin, C.Y., Wu, H., Tjeerdema, R.S., Viant, M.R., 2007. Evaluation of metabolite extraction strategies from tissue samples using NMR metabolomics. Metabolomics 3, 55–67.

Liu, Y., Cao, J., Zhang, H., He, Y., Xu, X., 2014. Nuclear magnetic resonance rapidly testing method on the moisture content of fresh milk. Journal of Chemical and Pharmaceutical Research 6 (1), 254–258.

Longobardi, F., Ventrella, A., Napoli, C., Humpfer, E., Schütz, B., Schäfer, H., Kontominas, M.G., Sacco, A., 2012. Classification of olive oils according to geographical origin by using ^{1}H NMR fingerprinting combined with multivariate analysis. Food Chemistry 130, 177–183.

Lopez-Rituerto, E., Cabredo, S., Lopez, M., Avenoza, A., Busto, J.H., Peregrina, J.M., 2009. A thorough study on the use of quantitative ^{1}H NMR in Rioja red wine fermentation process. Journal of Agricultural and Food Chemistry 57, 2112–2118.

Mannina, L., D'Imperio, M., Capitani, D., Rezzi, S., Guillou, C., Mavromoustakos, T., Molero Vilchez, M.D., Fernández, A.H., Thomas, F., Aparicio, R., 2009. ^{1}H NMR-based protocol for the detection of adulterations of refined olive oil with refined hazelnut oil. Journal of Agricultural and Food Chemistry 57, 11550–11556.

Mannina, L., Luchinat, C., Emanuele, M.C., Segre, A., 1999. Acyl positional distribution of glycerol tri-esters in vegetable oils: a ^{13}C NMR study. Chemistry and Physics of Lipids 103, 47–55.

Mannina, L., Marini, F., Gobbino, M., Sobolev, A.P., Capitani, D., 2010. NMR and chemometrics in tracing European olive oils: the case study of Ligurian samples. Talanta 80, 2141–2148.

Mannina, L., Sobolev, A.P., 2011. High resolution NMR characterization of olive oils in terms of quality, authenticity, and geographical origin. Magnetic Resonance in Chemistry 49, S3–S11.

Mannina, L., Sobolev, A.P., Capitani, D., Iaffaldano, N., Rosato, M.P., Ragni, P., Reale, A., Sorrentino, E., D'Amico, I., Coppola, R., 2008. NMR metabolic profiling of organic and aqueous sea bass extracts: implications in the discrimination of wild and cultured sea bass. Talanta 77, 433–444.

Mannina, L., Sobolev, A.P., Viel, S., 2012. Liquid state ^{1}H high field NMR in food analysis. Progress in Nuclear Magnetic Resonance Spectroscopy 66, 1–39.

Martin, G.J., Martin, M.L., 1983. Determination of specific isotopic fractionation by natural abundance deuterium NMR – application to the detection of wine chaptalization. Journal de Chimie Physique et de Physico-Chimie Biologique 80, 293–297.

McDougall, G., Martinussen, I., Stewart, D., 2008. Towards fruitful metabolomics: high throughput analyses of polyphenol composition in berries using direct infusion mass spectrometry. Journal of Chromatography B: Biomedical Sciences and Applications 871, 362–369.

McKenzie, J.S., Donarski, J.A., Wilson, J.C., Charlton, A.J., 2011. Analysis of complex mixtures using high-resolution nuclear magnetic resonance spectroscopy and chemometrics. Progress in Nuclear Magnetic Resonance Spectroscopy 59, 336–359.

Monakhova, Y.B., Ruge, W., Kuballa, T., Ilse, M., Winkelmann, O., Diehl, B., Thomas, F., Lachenmeier, D.W., 2015. Rapid approach to identify the presence of *Arabica* and *Robusta* species in coffee using ^{1}H NMR spectroscopy. Food Chemistry 182, 178–184.

Novoa-Carballal, R., Fernandez-Megia, E., Jimenez, C., Riguera, R., 2011. NMR methods for unravelling the spectra of complex mixtures. Natural Product Reports 28, 78–98.

Ogrinc, N., Košir, I.J., Spangenberg, J.E., Kidrič, J., 2003. The application of NMR and MS methods for detection of adulteration of wine, fruit juices, and olive oil. A review. Analytical and Bioanalytical Chemistry 376, 424–430.

Piccioni, F., Capitani, D., Zolla, L., Mannina, L., 2009. NMR metabolic profiling of transgenic maize with the *CryIA(b)* gene. Journal of Agricultural and Food Chemistry 57, 6041–6049.

EC Regulation No 2676/90, September 17, 1990. Official Journal of the European Communities (L 272), 64.

Raffo, A., Gianferri, R., Barbieri, R., Brosio, E., 2005. Ripening of banana fruit monitored by water relaxation and diffusion ^{1}H NMR measurements. Food Chemistry 89, 149–158.

Ribeiro, R.O.R., Mársico, E.T., Carneiro, C.S., Monteiro, M.L.G., Conte Júnior, C., Jesus, C.S., 2014. Detection of honey adulteration of high fructose corn syrup by low field nuclear magnetic resonance (LF ^{1}H NMR). Journal of Food Engineering 135, 39–43.

Rossmann, A., 2001. Determination of stable isotope ratios in food analysis. Food Reviews International 17, 347–381.

Sacchi, R., Patumi, M., Fontanazza, G., Barone, P., Fiordiponti, P., Mannina, L., Rossi, L., Segre, A.L., 1996. A high field ^{1}H magnetic resonance study of the minor components in virgin olive oils. Journal of the American Oil Chemists' Society 73, 747–758.

Sacchi, R., Addeo, F., Paolillo, L., 1997. ^{1}H and ^{13}C NMR of virgin olive oil. An overview. Magnetic Resonance in Chemistry 35, S133–S145.

Sacco, D., Brescia, M.A., Sgaramella, A., Casiello, G., Buccolieri, A., Ogrinc, N., Sacco, A., 2009. Discrimination between Southern Italy and foreign milk samples using spectroscopic and analytical data. Food Chemistry 114, 1559–1563.

Santos, P.M., Pereira-Filho, E.R., Colnago, L.A., 2016. Detection and quantification of milk adulteration using time domain nuclear magnetic resonance (TD-NMR). Microchemical Journal 124, 15–19.

Schievano, E., Morelato, E., Facchin, C., Mammi, S., 2013. Characterization of markers of botanical origin and other compounds extracted from unifloral honeys. Journal of Agricultural and Food Chemistry 61, 1747–1755.

Schievano, E., Stocchero, M., Morelato, E., Facchin, C., Mammi, S., 2012. An NMR-based metabolomic approach to identify the botanical origin of honey. Metabolomics 8, 679–690.

Schievano, E., Finotello, C., De Angelis, E., Mammi, S., Navarini, L., 2014. Rapid authentication of coffee blends and quantification of 16-O-methylcafestol in roasted coffee beans by Nuclear Magnetic Resonance. Journal of Agricultural and Food Chemistry 62, 12309–12314.

Shaw, A.D., di Camillo, A., Vlahov, G., Jones, A., Bianchi, G., Rowland, J., Kell, D.B., 1997. Discrimination of the variety and region of origin of extra virgin olive oils using ^{13}C NMR and multivariate calibration with variable reduction. Analytica Chimica Acta 348, 357–374.

Sobolev, A.P., Brosio, E., Gianferri, R., Segre, A.L., 2005. Metabolic profile of lettuce leaves by high-field NMR spectra. Magnetic Resonance in Chemistry 43, 625–638.

Sobolev, A.P., Segre, A.L., Lamanna, R., 2003. Proton high-field NMR study of tomato juice. Magnetic Resonance in Chemistry 41, 237–245.

Spyros, A., Dais, P., 2009. ^{31}P NMR spectroscopy in food analysis. Progress in Nuclear Magnetic Resonance Spectroscopy 54, 195–207.

Spiteri, M., Jamin, E., Thomas, F., Rebours, A., Lees, M., Rogers, K.M., Rutledge, D.N., 2015. Fast and global authenticity screening of honey using ^{1}H-NMR profiling. Food Chemistry 189, 60–66.

Valentini, M., Ritota, M., Cafiero, C., Cozzolino, S., Leita, L., Sequi, P., 2011. The HRMAS-NMR tool in foodstuff characterisation. Magnetic Resonance in Chemistry 49 (1), S121–S125.

Vlahov, G., 1999. Application of NMR to the study of olive oils. Progress in Nuclear Magnetic Resonance Spectroscopy 35, 341–357.

Wei, F., Furihata, K., Koda, M., Hu, F., Kato, R., Miyakawa, T., et al., 2012. ^{13}C NMR-based metabolomics for the classification of green coffee beans according to variety and origin. Journal of Agricultural and Food Chemistry 60, 10118–10125.

Wu, H., Southam, A.D., Hines, A., Viant, M.R., 2008. High-throughput tissue extraction protocol for NMR and MS-based metabolomics. Analytical Biochemistry 372, 204–212.

Zhang, Q., Saleh, A.S.M., Shen, Q., 2013. Discrimination of edible vegetable oil adulteration with used frying oil by low field nuclear magnetic resonance. Food and Bioprocess Technology 6, 2562–2570.

Advances in Mass Spectrometry for Food Authenticity Testing: An Omics Perspective

7

T. Cajka[1], *M.R. Showalter*[1], *K. Riddellova*[2], *O. Fiehn*[1]
[1]University of California, Davis, Davis, CA, United States; [2]ALS Czech Republic s.r.o., Prague, Czech Republic

Chapter Outline

7.1 Introduction

In recent years, there has been an increasing interest in issues related to food, diet, and nutrition among consumers. The globalization of food markets suggests that consumers may encounter diverse foods, and therefore may have questions about the origin and safety of the food they eat. Recent food scares such as bovine spongiform encephalopathy and avian flu outbreaks or the adulteration of milk with melamine have led to media and public attention regarding the origin of food and the more general concept of food authenticity. In general, *food authenticity* refers to whether a food purchased by a consumer matches its description. *Food fraud* is committed when food is deliberately placed on the market, mainly for financial gain, with the intention of deceiving the consumer (Carcea et al., 2009).

A wide range of methods has been developed for food authenticity testing and detection of adulteration. Many of these methods are based on simple assays using various physicochemical and biochemical measurements or morphological features (eg, pollen analysis for botanical origin of honey). In the last few years, advances in mass spectrometry (MS) have led to the development of novel methods applicable in food authenticity and adulteration areas in either an untargeted manner or by targeting specific compounds. These omics-based methods are moving toward maximum collection of information (features, markers) on sample composition in comparison to previous approaches that focused on a single or limited number of markers (Cevallos-Cevallos et al., 2009; Riedl et al., 2015; Ibanez et al., 2013; Wishart, 2008; Pischetsrieder and Baeuerlein, 2009; Cunsolo et al., 2014).

7.2 Process of Using Mass Spectrometry in the Analysis of Food

Foods are complex matrices containing hundreds to thousands of volatile, semivolatile, and nonvolatile compounds. Therefore, in most cases, extraction procedures are needed to isolate a subset of components and/or to remove some components that would otherwise interfere with the detection process.

As Fig. 7.1 shows, several MS-based approaches exist for the analysis of food. In general, these techniques can be divided into (1) direct MS techniques in which

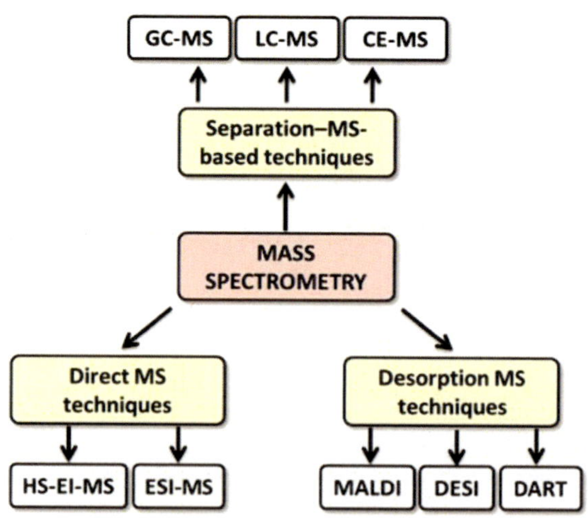

Figure 7.1 Analytical workflow for mass spectrometry in the analysis of food.

isolated compounds or sample extracts are immediately introduced into the ion source of a mass spectrometer, (2) desorption techniques in which compounds are desorbed using UV laser, high temperature, or solvent spraying prior to ionization, and (3) techniques involving a pre-separation step such as gas chromatography (GC), liquid chromatography (LC), or capillary electrophoresis prior to ionization and MS detection.

7.2.1 Direct MS Techniques

In headspace-MS (HS-MS), volatile compounds are extracted from the headspace above the sample. Headspace methods include static headspace, dynamic headspace (purge and trap), and solid-phase microextraction (SPME). After desorption in a hot GC injection port, the volatiles are immediately introduced via a short microbore capillary into the ion source of a mass spectrometer [usually a single quadrupole or time-of-flight (TOF) MS] where they are fragmented using electron ionization (EI) at 70 eV. These fragments are recorded as the abundance of each ion of different mass-to-charge ratios (*m/z*) and intensities of particular fragments (*m/z*) are subsequently submitted to statistical analysis. This technique is capable of analyzing samples in very short times (<5 min) and with minimal sample preparation (Vera et al., 2011; Vaclavik et al., 2014a).

For direct infusion MS, the most common method used for ionization is electrospray ionization (ESI). ESI-MS fingerprinting can be adapted to analyze polar and lipophilic extracts in both positive and negative ion modes. The sample or extract can be introduced using an LC-MS running solvent as a plug flow in a short (2–3 min) LC run or introduced continuously using nanoinfusion devices (eg, chip-based NanoMate). ESI-MS fingerprint data can be generated using both unit resolution and high-resolution MS instruments such as TOF [mass resolving power 10,000–50,000 full width at half maximum (FWHM), mass accuracy <1–5 ppm] and orbital ion trap (mass resolving power 50,000–240,000 FWHM, mass accuracy <1 ppm). With an analysis cycle time of 3–5 min per sample, ESI-MS fingerprinting can be considered as an ideal choice for high-throughput analysis (Draper et al., 2013; Han et al., 2012).

7.2.2 Desorption MS Techniques

In addition to direct MS methods, desorption MS techniques can be used for fingerprinting or profiling. Among them, matrix-assisted laser desorption/ionization (MALDI) and ambient MS techniques such as desorption electrospray ionization (DESI) and direct analysis in real time (DART) represent the most promising techniques (Vaclavik et al., 2014a). MALDI-MS enables detection of analytes varying in molecular weight and rapid examination of small quantities of complex samples. Although MALDI is largely used in biological studies to characterize large molecules, it has also been applied to the ionization of intermediate and low-molecular-weight compounds (<500 Da) (Wolfender et al., 2015). Ion suppression and matrix interferences can be reduced with the use of modified matrices and adapted experimental protocols. Ambient desorption ionization techniques, such as DESI and DART, have advantages compared to conventional desorption ionization techniques, including the ability to directly examine samples in the open atmosphere with high sample throughput (<1 min per single analysis). Additionally, only minimal or even no sample preparation is required for this method (Cody et al., 2005; Takats et al., 2004).

7.2.3 Chromatographic and Electrokinetic Separation–MS-Based Techniques

7.2.3.1 Liquid Chromatography-Mass Spectrometry

Several LC configurations have been described for the analysis of complex food mixtures. Currently, reversed-phase LC (RPLC) followed by hydrophilic interaction chromatography (HILIC) and normal-phase LC (NPLC) are the most frequently used LC-based separation techniques (Wolfender et al., 2015; Gika et al., 2014).

Improvements in chromatographic performance have been achieved by the introduction of ultrahigh-performance LC (UHPLC). Because current UHPLC systems are capable of operations at high back pressures (up to 1200–1500 bar), columns with sub-2-μm particles can be operated at high mobile-phase flow rates without loss of resolution (Fekete et al., 2014). Chromatographic resolution similar to that with sub-2-μm totally porous particles at comparable or even higher speeds without high back pressure can also be achieved with fused-core technology utilizing 2.6–2.8-μm particles with a 0.35–0.5-μm porous shell fused to a solid core (Guillarme et al., 2010).

Choice of ionization mode in LC-MS plays a major role in the profile that will be obtained. Ionization efficiency can be enhanced by using mobile-phase modifiers leading to the formation of a different type of molecular species. For LC-MS, ESI is the most commonly used method of ionization while atmospheric-pressure chemical ionization (APCI) is preferred for more specific applications such as the analysis of triacylglycerols (Cajka and Fiehn, 2014).

Most untargeted MS-based omics analyses rely on a mass spectrometer permitting full mass spectral acquisition, usually in high-resolution mode. TOF-based mass spectrometers, such as single TOF and quadrupole/time-of-flight (QTOF) and orbital ion trap-based MS (single orbital ion trap, quadrupole/orbital ion trap) are most commonly used in untargeted omics studies. Current high-resolution MS instruments used in omics research are available with a broad range of mass resolving power (10,000–450,000 FWHM) and mass accuracy typically better than 1–5 ppm (Wolfender et al., 2015; Holcapek et al., 2012).

For targeted analysis, triple quadrupole (QqQ) and quadrupole/linear ion trap (QLIT) represent the most popular and frequently used mass spectrometers. Both QqQ and QLIT are routinely operated via selected reaction monitoring and/or multiple reaction monitoring (MRM). In addition, QLIT enables MS^3 functionality together with QqQ fragmentation patterns, thus proving the more useful information needed for structural information. Current QqQ and QLIT instruments are capable of very low dwell times (1–5 ms). Therefore, when using an optimized MRM workflow, up to several hundreds of MRM transitions can be accommodated within a single LC-MS run (Holcapek et al., 2012; Cajka and Fiehn, 2016).

7.2.3.2 Gas Chromatography-Mass Spectrometry

Gas chromatography-mass spectrometry (GC-MS) techniques have historically enabled both the separation and identification of low-molecular-weight compounds in complex food samples. Capillary GC has very high peak capacity compared to HPLC or even UHPLC. In addition, EI affords spectral patterns that can be easily searched against established databases because the ionization energy is fixed at 70 eV (Wolfender et al., 2015).

However, the compounds must be sufficiently volatile; thus GC is restricted to the analysis of low-molecular-weight analytes, typically below 1000 Da. Direct GC-MS analysis is possible for organic volatiles isolated using, for example, headspace or SPME. Direct GC-MS can be also used for analysis of medium-polar and nonpolar analytes (Vaclavik et al., 2014a). A derivatization step is required for analysis of polar analytes to increase their volatility and thermal stability. Numerous derivatization reactions can be used to mask polar functional groups (alkylation, silylation, and acylation). Among these derivatizations, a two-step procedure involving the combination of methoximation and trimethylsilylation has successfully enabled the analysis of a wide range of polar analytes by GC-MS (Dettmer et al., 2007).

EI is the preferred ionization technique in GC-MS because of its highly reproducible mass fragmentation and the possibility of interinstrument, library-based searching for the identification of analytes (Wolfender et al., 2015). Because EI fragmentation can be too extensive, the use of soft ionization techniques such as chemical ionization (CI) can enhance detection of molecular ion-based species. Recently, APCI as a commercial ionization source for GC-MS became available. APCI overcomes some common disadvantages of EI and CI and is complementary to both ion sources through its use of a more universal and soft ionization process. APCI sources reduce fragmentation, allowing the molecular ion species to be more easily observed (Wachsmuth et al., 2015; Li et al., 2015).

Most of the GC-MS-based untargeted methods rely on a mass spectrometer capable of full mass spectral acquisition. Unit mass resolution TOF and single quadrupole mass spectrometers dominate in untargeted metabolomics studies (Dettmer et al., 2007). The most frequently used unit-resolution TOF instrument from LECO features a unique deconvolution software algorithm together with high acquisition speeds of up to 500 spectra/s fully compatible with fast GC and comprehensive two-dimensional gas chromatography (GC×GC). High-resolution GC-MS instruments are available such as high-resolution/accurate mass TOF analyzers (mass resolving power 5000−12,500 FWHM) but these provide only moderate acquisition speeds (20−50 spectra/s). Very recently, high-speed high-resolution/accurate mass TOF mass analyzers permitting high acquisition speeds (up to 200 spectra/s) as well as high mass resolving power (50,000 FWHM) have become available (Cajka, 2013). GC-Q/orbital ion trap-based MS capable of a mass resolving power of up to 120,000 FWHM has recently been introduced. However, when running this instrument with the highest acquisition speed available (18 spectra/s), the mass resolving power is reduced to 12,500 FWHM (https://www.thermoscientific.com/content/dam/tfs/ATG/CMD/cmd-documents/bro/spec/ms/gcms/PS-10458-GC-MS-Q-Exactive-Orbitrap-PS10458-EN.pdf). High-resolution tandem

MS/MS has also been enabled on a GC-Q/HRTOFMS instrument with an EI/CI ion source, permitting the selection of precursor ions and monitoring of product ions through the entire mass range with high mass accuracy (Cajka, 2013).

7.2.3.3 Capillary Electrophoresis-Mass Spectrometry

Capillary electrophoresis-mass spectrometry (CE-MS) is applicable to charged analytes such as nucleic acids, amino acids, carboxylic acids, sugar phosphates, charged lipids, or peptides (Hirayama et al., 2014; Ramautar et al., 2012). These charged analytes migrate through a capillary initiated by an electric field between the electrodes and are separated based on their electrophoretic mobility. Practically, if two charged analytes have the same size, the analyte with the greater charge will move faster; or if two analytes have the same charge, the smaller analyte will move faster because of reduced friction (Bjerrum, 2015). ESI is the most commonly used ionization method in CE-MS-based omics analysis and various types of MS have been coupled to CE, including full mass spectra acquisition analyzers such as TOF, QTOF, orbital ion trap, or single quadrupole, QqQ and QLIT operated in selected ion monitoring/MRM mode for targeted analysis (Hirayama et al., 2014).

7.3 Mass Spectrometry-Based Approaches for Food Authenticity Testing and Adulteration Detection

MS-based methods for food authenticity testing and adulteration detection can be divided into targeted and untargeted methods. Targeted methods for food authenticity testing and adulteration detection focus mainly on components such as Sudan dyes (Rebane et al., 2010), pharmaceuticals (Vaclavik et al., 2014b), or melamine (Rovina and Siddiquee, 2015).

Untargeted MS-based omics disciplines such as metabolomics and lipidomics target small molecules, typically below 1000–2000 Da, while peptidomics and proteomics focus on much larger molecules (up to ~500,000 Da) (Herrero et al., 2012). In the latter case, the analysis of high-molecular-weight intact proteins or peptides is feasible because multiply charged species are formed during electrospray ionization, which reduces the *m/z* ratio and thus effectively extends the mass range of mass spectrometers (Parker et al., 2009).

As we discuss in further sections, untargeted MS-based omics methods, which are primarily focused on detection of widest possible pattern of components, can be transformed after method optimization and validation of suitable biomarker(s) to a targeted method for monitoring only a few specific analytes (Cajka and Fiehn, 2016). This significantly simplifies data processing.

Reliability of MS-based omics approaches for food authenticity depends in part on the number of samples used. As Fig. 7.2 shows, only a few samples are needed to evaluate the application potential of a particular method. During this step, various parameters such as analyte coverage, instrument sensitivity, and robustness are assessed.

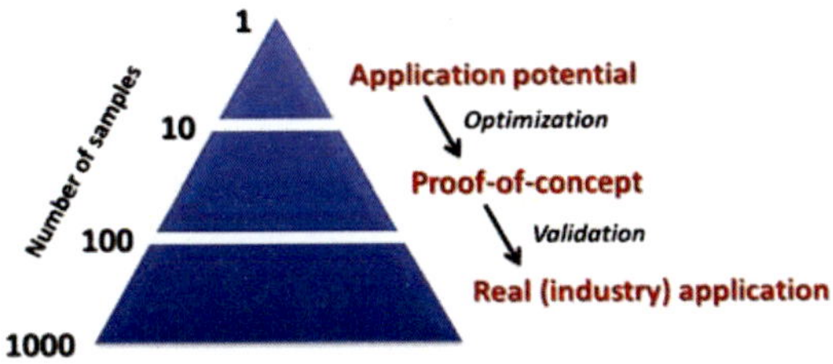

Figure 7.2 Steps in omics-based untargeted to targeted workflow related to number of samples required.

The next step is analysis of a large series of samples to create a statistical model permitting sample classification or discrimination based on sample origin (proof-of-concept). Ideally, potential biomarkers are further validated using a much larger set of samples with high biological variability to establish a targeted method and confirm that the method is suitable for use in a food control laboratory or industry.

As finding unique biomarkers is not always feasible, sample classification can also be based upon the entire pattern of features (Riedl et al., 2015). This requires the use of multivariate data analysis to establish a statistical model for case—control comparison. To this end, supervised pattern recognition techniques such as partial least squares discriminant analysis (PLS-DA), orthogonal projections to latent structures modeling discriminant analysis (OPLS-DA), linear discriminant analysis (LDA), soft independent modeling of class analogy (SIMCA), support vector machines (SVMs), or artificial neural networks (ANNs) are frequently used (Berrueta et al., 2007).

Current practice also involves a validation step to demonstrate the model is able to perform classification of unknown samples. Typically, this is done by observing how successful the model is at classifying samples of known origin once the data set is split into (1) a training set and (2) a testing set. *Recognition ability* represents the percentage of samples in the training set successfully classified while *prediction ability* is a percentage of samples in the test set correctly classified using the model developed during the training step. Sensitivity and specificity are also calculated. *Sensitivity* is the percentage of objects belonging to a given class that are correctly identified by the model while *specificity* is the percentage of objects foreign to the modeled class that are correctly classified as foreign (Berrueta et al., 2007; Gonzalez-Arjona et al., 1999).

The validation procedure can be performed using (1) leave-one-out cross-validation, (2) *k*-fold cross-validation or, preferably, using (3) external validation (Berrueta et al., 2007). However, these statistical models cannot take into account all biological variability of samples and the final sample classification in the untargeted workflow will always have some probability of incorrect classification. This is analogous to targeted analysis in which concentration along with the uncertainty of the measurement is reported.

Another problem encountered with untargeted fingerprinting and profiling methods is that of batch effects. Batch effects arise from analyzing unknown samples whose authenticity is to be determined at later times than samples used to build the statistical model (training set). Therefore batch effects must always be taken into account in spite of performing frequently used analytical normalization techniques, such as scaling by the total ion current (De Livera et al., 2015). Use of quality control samples with a composition similar to analyzed samples is highly recommended to check for batch effects and/or for further raw data normalization (Cajka and Fiehn, 2016).

Furthermore, the features obtained when analyzing the training (calibration) set must match exactly the features for new "unknown" samples. This can be a problem and is most often encountered with separation-MS-based methods and is caused by retention time shifts between different batches when processing hundreds of features. These challenges highlight the value of transforming an untargeted approach to a targeted method in which only the most important features are extracted from the data set during data processing (Cajka and Fiehn, 2016). On the contrary, preprocessing of direct MS and desorption MS datasets is greatly simplified because peak finding and feature alignments are unnecessary. Data processing of these MS methods can be simplified even further if a low-resolution, unit-mass spectrometer is used because features are binned according to mass (*m*/*z*) separated by one unit (Draper et al., 2013). In any case, processing raw data files represents a very critical step in the overall workflow and should be streamlined as much as possible to avoid potential biases.

Table 7.1 highlights different levels of difficulty when implementing food authenticity and fraud detection methods. Targeted methods, because of their specificity, are relatively straightforward. On the other hand, the use of untargeted methods for authenticity of one specific product and differentiation of botanical/animal or

Table 7.1 Difficulties Associated With Implementation of Food Authenticity and Fraud Detection Methods

Implementation	Aim	Example
Easy	Detection of adulterant (target analysis)	Detection of melamine in milk (Vaclavik et al., 2010)
Easy	Detection of species-specific peptides (target analysis)	Detection of horse and pork in highly processed food (von Bargen et al., 2014)
Easy–medium	Detection of species-specific metabolites (target analysis)	Detection of extra virgin olive oil adulteration with hazelnut oil (Calvano et al., 2012)
Medium	Authenticity of one product collected over a season (untargeted analysis)	Distinguishing a group of Rochefort 6, 8, 10 beers from other specialty beers (Cajka et al., 2010b)
Medium	Authenticity based on botanical origin (untargeted analysis)	Differentiation of unifloral honeys (Ampuero et al., 2004)
High	Authenticity based on geographical origin (untargeted analysis)	Distinguishing olive oils labeled "Liguria" (protected designation of origin) from other olive oils (Cajka et al., 2010a)

geographical origin of a sample is more difficult because a large number of authentic samples are needed to establish a reliable statistical model to differentiate these samples. In addition, variability associated with year, season, and composition of raw materials (or feed) represents another challenge in studies focused on food authenticity based on botanical/animal/geographical origin (Hrbek et al., 2014; Cajka et al., 2009, 2010a). An important question that should always be addressed is whether samples used for food authenticity studies are *really* authentic. It is not unusual that some studies have built statistical models based on samples from the retail market with (a priori) expected but not guaranteed authenticity. In the following sections, we will discuss current untargeted MS-based omics methods and their application to food authenticity and food fraud detection.

7.3.1 Proteomics and Peptidomics

MS is a workhorse in proteomics and peptidomics research. Currently, bottom-up and top-down approaches are the two fundamental strategies employed for protein/peptide identification and characterization. Fig. 7.3 shows a general workflow in proteomics analysis including (A) bottom-up, (B) bottom-up shotgun, and (C) top-down approaches (Herrero et al., 2012).

In bottom-up approaches, proteins are converted into peptides using enzymes such as trypsin and the resulting peptides are analyzed using MS or MS/MS. Preseparation of proteins using two-dimensional gel electrophoresis (2-DE) or differential in-gel electrophoresis followed by in-gel digestion of spot(s) is usually used in combination with soft ionization techniques such as MALDI (Fig. 7.3A). Alternatively, in-solution digestion of an entire protein mixture or in-gel digestion of bands obtained using sodium dodecyl sulfate/polyacrylamide gel electrophoresis can be used followed by separation of a peptide mixture using, for instance, UHPLC, nanoflow LC, or CE. Soft ionization techniques such as ESI are usually used followed by MS or MS/MS detection (Fig. 7.3B). Conversely, a top-down approach (Fig. 7.3C) works without protein digestion and the intact proteins are directly analyzed in a mass spectrometer forming characteristic fragments (Herrero et al., 2012).

For food authenticity and fraud detection, bottom-up approaches are usually used for matrices such as fish, shellfish, meat, milk, and cheese. Reviewing original papers focused on food authenticity, most of them focused on application potential or proof-of-concept. Although a limited number of samples were used for analysis, proteomics and peptidomics seem to be highly specific. Species-specific peptides from analyzed proteins in an untargeted workflow were consequently used for targeted analysis using LC-MS/MS in many cases.

7.3.1.1 Meat and Meat Products

Labeling of meat is important because it supports consumer choice based on moral, religious, ethical, dietary, or health factors. This problem became even more visible in 2013 following the discovery of horse meat in a frozen beef burger in Ireland; this led to the exposure of pan-European food fraud in an incident now known as

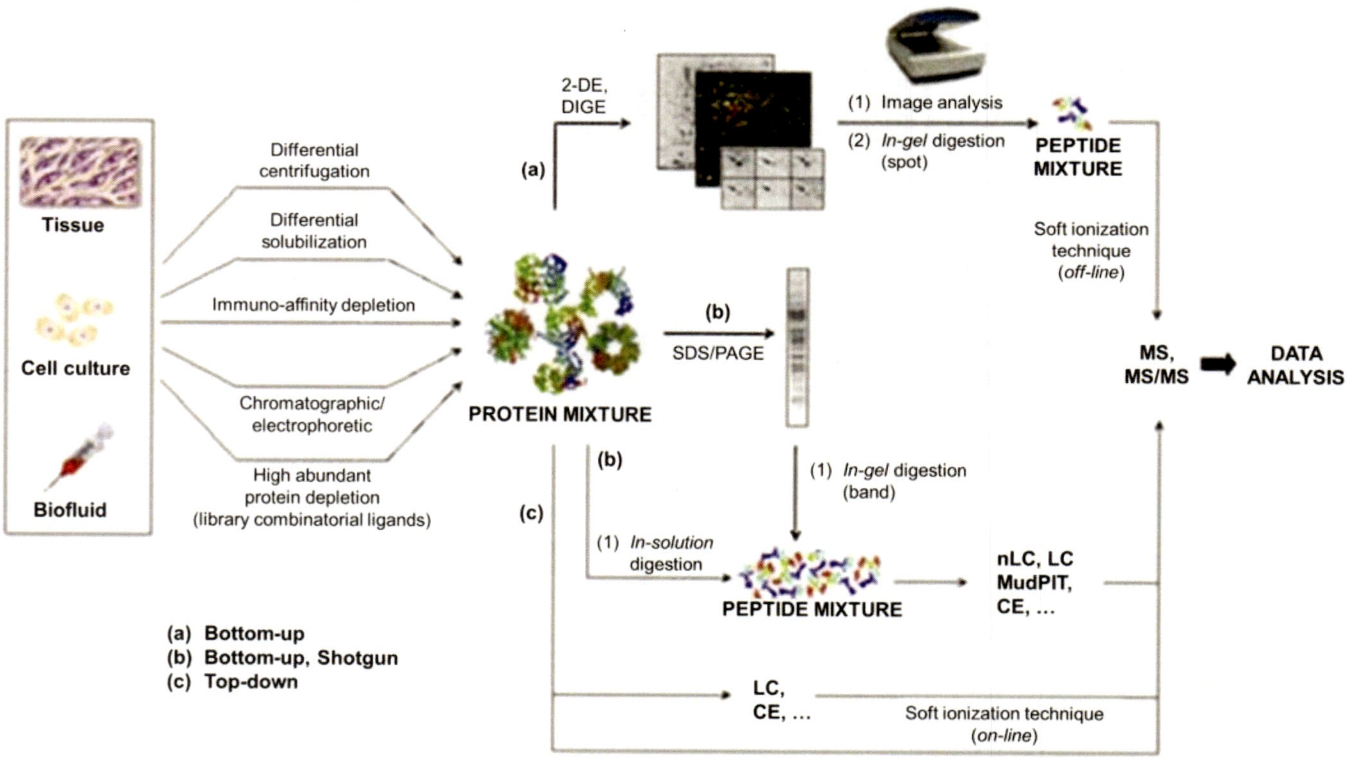

Figure 7.3 Scheme of MS-based proteomics strategies. *2-DE*, Two-dimensional gel electrophoresis; *DIGE*, differential in-gel electrophoresis; *SDS/PAGE*, sodium dodecyl sulfate/polyacrylamide gel electrophoresis; *LC*, liquid chromatography; *CE*, capillary electrophoresis; *nLC*, nanoliquid chromatography; *MudPIT*, multidimensional protein identification technology.
Reproduced from Herrero, M., Simo, C., Garcia-Canas, V., Ibanez, E., Cifuentes, A., 2012. Foodomics: MS-based strategies in modern food science and nutrition. Mass Spectrometry Reviews 31, 49–69. Copyright 2012 Wiley.

the "horse meat scandal." This problem has shown that robust and validated analytical methods to verify the authenticity of meat-based foods are urgently needed (Claydon et al., 2015). To this end, several authors have focused on the development of sensitive methods for detection of horse in different meat products. For instance, Claydon et al. (2015) developed a shotgun proteomics method using nanoflow-LC-HRMS (high-resolution mass spectrometry) to analyze whole protein extracts from various meat preparations. First, proteins from two commercially available beef-containing products (baby food and corned beef) were analyzed to identify proteins that resist industrial processing. Species-specific peptides from these proteins were consequently used for analysis of LC-MS/MS data from various samples to prove the concept of species identification in mixtures of meats. Second, the amino acid sequences of the most confidently identified proteins from horse, beef, and pork preparations were aligned across a range of species (horse, cow, pig, sheep, goat, chicken, turkey, rabbit, and donkey) and peptides unique to each species were selected to create a database of potential marker peptides for the various species. Mixtures of meats containing decreasing amounts of horse meat were then investigated using shotgun proteomics analysis in combination with this bespoke database to determine the sensitivity of the method. Using this method, processed and raw horse meats were detected at levels as low as 0.5% (w/w) (Claydon et al., 2015).

Assessment of meat authenticity by means of targeted peptide biomarkers and HRMS was described by Orduna et al. (2015). Meat-specific authenticity was performed using a well-defined proteogenomic annotation, surrogate tryptic peptides, and analysis using HRMS. Selected mammalian meat samples (beef, horse, pork, and lamb) were homogenized and proteins extracted and digested with trypsin followed by LC separation and HRMS detection in full-scan mode; MS/MS spectra were collected for selected proteotypic peptides, that is, peptides found in only a single known protein and that therefore serve to identify that protein. Fig. 7.4 shows extracted ion chromatograms of y_{14} and y_{13} product ions for mammalian meat samples demonstrating very high specificity to each of the targeted species. Using this targeted method allowed for comprehensive meat speciation down to 1% (w/w) of the undesired product (Orduna et al., 2015).

Identification of porcine-specific peptide markers from thermally processed meat that could differentiate pork from beef, chevon, and chicken meat was reported by Sarah et al. (2016). Markers of tryptic protein digests of chilled, boiled, and autoclaved pork were identified using LC-QTOFMS. Seven porcine-specific peptides were consistently detected and used for a targeted LC-MRM-MS/MS method to verify the method. Out of the seven listed peptides, however, only four peptides were consistently detected with a clean and specific signal. The remaining three peptides produced chromatograms with a considerably high amount of noise, interfering peaks, and nonspecific signals. These four peptides were recommended as the most reliable "thermostable" markers for pork detection in meat products (Sarah et al., 2016).

In another study, von Bargen et al. (2013) used a shotgun proteomics approach to detect trace contaminations of horse meat and pork and demonstrate the specificity of the identified biomarker peptides against chicken, lamb, and beef. For the most sensitive peptides, an LC-MRM-MS/MS method was developed that allowed detection of

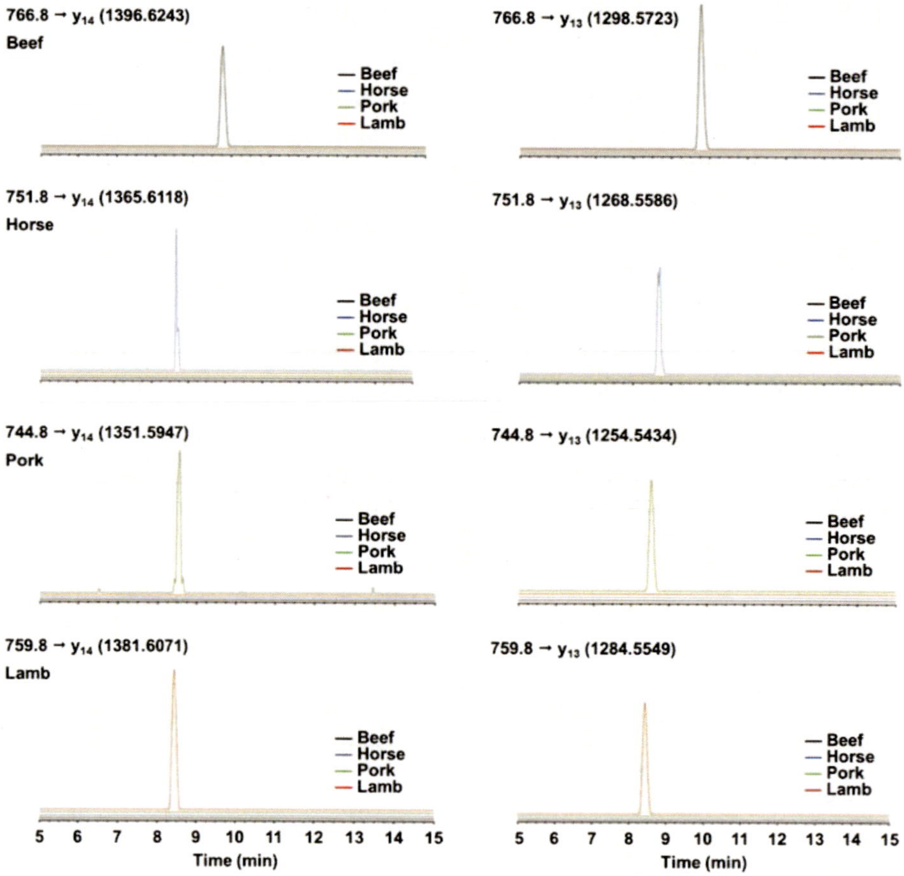

Figure 7.4 Overlay of extracted ion chromatograms of y_{14} and y_{13} product ions of selected mammalian meat samples. After sample homogenization, proteins were extracted and digested with trypsin followed by analysis using LC-HRMS with the acquisition of MS/MS spectra for selected proteotypic peptides.

Reproduced from Orduna, A.R., Husby, E., Yang, C.T., Ghosh, D., Beaudry, F., 2015. Assessment of meat authenticity using bioinformatics, targeted peptide biomarkers and high-resolution mass spectrometry. Food Additives and Contaminants Part A-Chemistry Analysis Control Exposure & Risk Assessment 32, 1709–1717. Copyright 2015 Taylor & Francis.

0.55% (w/w) horse or pork in a beef matrix. To enhance sensitivity, MRM^3 was used, permitting detection down to 0.13% (w/w) pork contamination in beef (von Bargen et al., 2013). In the follow-up study, streamlining of extraction and sample preparation allowed the authors to drastically decrease extraction time to 2 min. Other advantages of this method are that (1) no special proteomics infrastructure, such as two-dimensional polyacrylamide gel electrophoresis or OFFGEL fractionation, is necessary for prefractionation of samples and (2) that separation and detection are performed on conventional RPLC-C18 columns and QqQ instrumentation. This protocol can therefore be easily implemented in most laboratories (von Bargen et al., 2014).

Species-specific peptides for the authentication of processed meat products from beef, pork, horse, chicken, and turkey were reported by Montowska et al. (2015) who applied ambient MS with liquid extraction surface analysis (LESA). A set of 25 species and protein-specific heat stable peptide markers derived from myofibrillar and sarcoplasmic proteins was identified. The LESA-MS technique required minimal sample preparation without fractionation and enabled the unambiguous and simultaneous identification of skeletal muscle proteins and peptides as well as other components of animal origin, including milk proteins such as casein alpha-S1, in whole meat product digests (Montowska et al., 2015).

7.3.1.2 Fish, Shellfish, and Seafood

Species-specific peptides can also be used as proteomics markers for fish, shellfish, and seafood authentication in addition to identification of species of origin in processed products. This is particularly important when the head has been removed and/or the muscle tissues have been processed (Zhou et al., 2012). For instance, Mazzeo et al. (2008) applied MALDI-TOFMS with a simple sample preparation protocol [extraction of the fish sample with water containing 0.1% (v/v) trifluoroacetic acid] for fish authentication. For 25 different fish species, highly specific proteins with molecular weights of ~11 kDa have been selected as specific biomarkers for unambiguous discrimination (Mazzeo et al., 2008). Ortea et al. (2009a,b) presented a proteomic approach for identification of commercially relevant shrimp species using 2-DE and MALDI-TOFMS (Ortea et al., 2009a,b). Differentiation of the species studied was reported to be feasible. Also four samples of commercial origin obtained in local markets were analyzed to validate the methodology (Ortea et al., 2009a).

7.3.1.3 Milk and Cheese

Substitution of milk by lower-cost milk and the undeclared use of milk from different species for the production of traditional cheeses are frequent practices in the dairy industry. To detect such fraudulent practices, proteomics is an important tool because whey proteins can be used as biomarkers. Chen et al. (2004) described a simple procedure for quantification of cow's milk present as an adulterant in goat's milk using LC-MS. The milk sample is mixed with aqueous acetic acid and dichloromethane followed by centrifugation and LC-MS analysis of the upper whey protein fraction after its previous dilution with water. The presence of cow's milk was determined using β-lactoglobulin whey protein as the molecular marker and this method was able to detect the addition of cow's milk to goat's milk at levels as low as 5% (v/v) (Chen et al., 2004).

Use of whey proteins, α-lactalbumin and β-lactoglobulin, as molecular markers to detect the presence of cow's milk in either raw ewe or water buffalo milk samples employed in industrial processes and the addition of powdered milk to samples of fresh raw milk was reported by Cozzolino et al. (2001). Samples were diluted at a ratio of 1:100 (v/v) with 0.1% (v/v) trifluoroacetic acid to decrease the sensitivity of casein, followed by mixing the aliquot with sinapinic acid solution and analysis using

MALDI-TOFMS. The protocol was able to detect the addition of cow's milk to water buffalo milk and ewe's milk at levels as low as 5% (w/w) and 10% (w/w), respectively (Fig. 7.5), and identify added powdered milk (Cozzolino et al., 2001).

She-donkey's milk and goat's milk are commonly used in newborn and infant feeding because they are less allergenic than other milk types. Therefore it is important to avoid adulteration and contamination by other milk allergens. Di Girolamo et al. (2014) focused on she-donkey's and goat's milk adulterations. Raw milk samples

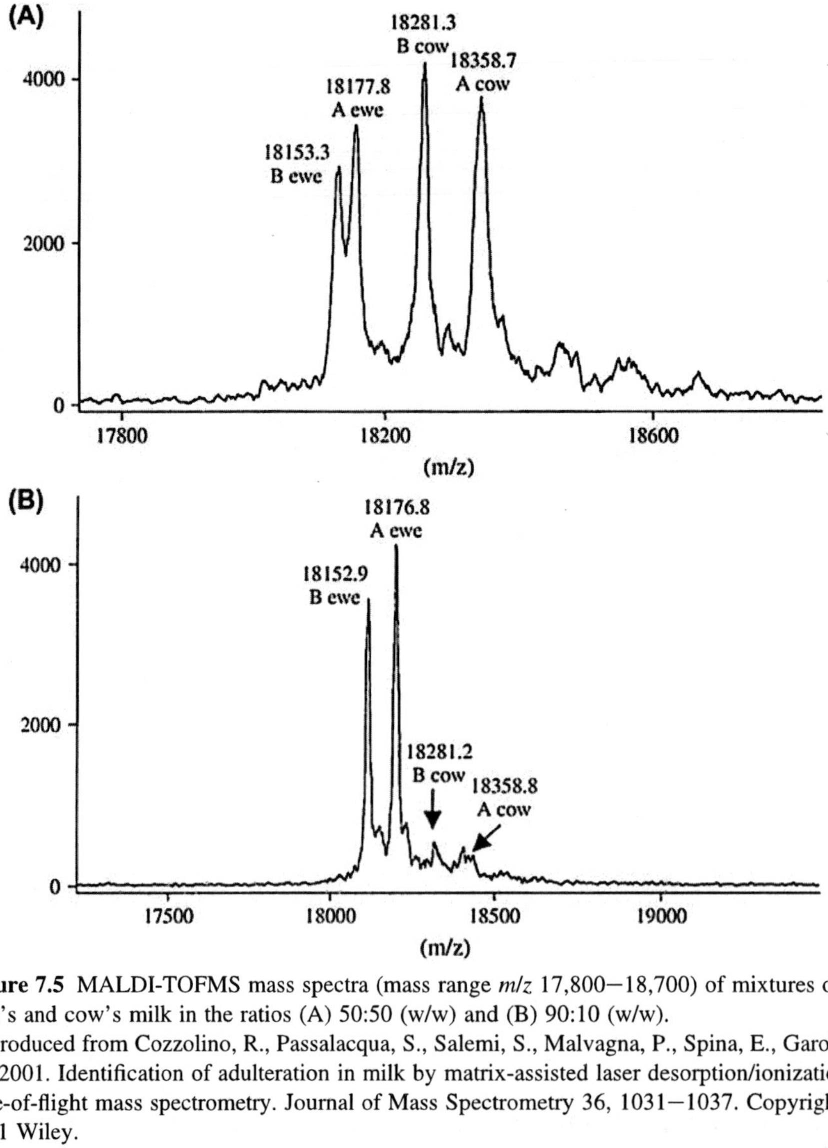

Figure 7.5 MALDI-TOFMS mass spectra (mass range *m/z* 17,800−18,700) of mixtures of ewe's and cow's milk in the ratios (A) 50:50 (w/w) and (B) 90:10 (w/w).
Reproduced from Cozzolino, R., Passalacqua, S., Salemi, S., Malvagna, P., Spina, E., Garozzo, D., 2001. Identification of adulteration in milk by matrix-assisted laser desorption/ionization time-of-flight mass spectrometry. Journal of Mass Spectrometry 36, 1031−1037. Copyright 2001 Wiley.

were defatted by centrifugation and analyzed by MALDI-TOFMS, a workflow that allowed the identification of she-donkey's milk and goat's milk adulteration at levels of 0.5% (v/v) (Di Girolamo et al., 2014).

In the dairy field, a common fraud found is that of cheeses produced by adding milk from animals other than those declared. This might be because of economic, technical, or availability reasons and may have legal, commercial, or medical implications. Guarino et al. (2010) developed a method for detection of undeclared sheep's milk in goat cheeses and cow's milk in sheep cheeses. In a simple procedure, caseins are extracted from cheeses, solubilized, digested with plasmin, and subsequently analyzed by LC-MS/MS. This method permitted detection of 2% (v/w) of sheep's milk in cheeses based on the sheep-specific peptide (Guarino et al., 2010).

In another study, Russo et al. (2012) developed an LC-MS/MS method for detection of buffalo mozzarella adulteration by cow's milk. Mozzarella exudates were diluted in bicarbonate buffer in deionized water followed by trypsin hydrolysis. Raw buffalo and cow's milk were prepared in the same way. After dilution and centrifugation, the samples were analyzed using LC-MS/MS by monitoring specific transitions of the phosphorylated bovine β-casein f33-48 peptide, identified as a novel species-specific marker. Using this method of detection, adulteration levels as low as 0.001% (v/v) bovine milk with respect to buffalo were feasible. The developed method was used for the analysis of seven water buffalo mozzarella samples declared as "Mozzarella di Bufala Campana DOP" (protected designation of origin, PDO) and therefore supposed to be exclusively produced with buffalo milk. As a negative control, two mozzarella samples produced with cow's milk were also analyzed. In addition, samples of bovine and buffalo milk were included in the analysis to ascertain the applicability of the method to raw starting materials. The buffalo marker was not detected in either bovine mozzarella samples or milk. Interestingly, the bovine marker was detected in five out of the seven DOP samples analyzed, with percentages in the range 0.4–4.6% (v/v exudate), indicating the addition of or contamination by cow's milk in the production process of these cheeses (Russo et al., 2012).

In addition to detection of undeclared use of milk from different species, the addition of powdered derivatives represents another process of adulteration. Because high temperatures (180–200°C) are used for milk powder production, the occurrence of some protein modifications (eg, glycation, lactosylation, oxidation, deamidation, or dehydration) can be expected. Indeed, Calvano et al. (2013) used MALDI-TOFMS to analyze tryptic digests resulting from samples of raw liquid (without heat treatment), commercial liquid, and powdered cow's milk. Whey and casein fractions of milk samples were digested in solution followed by MALDI-MS analysis with α-cyano-4-chlorocinnamic acid as a matrix, which enhances the detection of more acid (lactosylated) peptides. Liquid milk samples were adulterated with powdered milk at different percentages and diagnostic peptides were detected down to an adulteration level of 1% (w/v) (Calvano et al., 2013).

Detection of adulterations involving addition of plant material to skimmed milk powder (SMP) was reported by Cordewener et al. (2009). Tryptic digests of SMP and SMP adulterated with soy protein isolate (5%, w/w) or pea protein isolate (5%, w/w) were analyzed using LC-HRMS. The comparative LC-MS approach enabled unequivocal discrimination of those SMP samples containing soy and pea protein from nonadulterated SMP. Numerous peptides originating from the major seed proteins of soy (glycinin, β-conglycin) and pea (legumin, vicilin) were identified in this approach (Cordewener et al., 2009).

7.3.1.4 Other Matrices

Durum wheat (*Triticum turgidum* ssp. *durum* L.) suited for pasta manufacturing processes is commonly adulterated with cheaper common wheat (*Triticum aestivum* L.), the price of which is about 25% lower. Russo et al. (2014) developed an LC-MS/MS method for the selective and sensitive detection and quantification of durum wheat adulteration. The targeted analysis was performed by monitoring specific transitions of a species-specific marker derived from a tryptic peptide of puroindoline a (Pin-a), a cysteine-rich protein present only in common wheat. In addition, two transitions of a reference peptide belonging to purothionin A-1, present in both species, were also monitored. Using this method, detection as low as 0.01% (w/w) of common wheat in durum wheat was feasible. The identified Pin-a marker was also found to be highly diagnostic for the quantification of common wheat in raw materials (kernels) and processed products (pasta) (Russo et al., 2014).

Gelatine is a component of a wide range of foods and accurate labeling is important because different sources (bovine, porcine, chicken) are used for its production. Grundy et al. (2016) reported a method to determine the species origin of gelatines using LC-MS/MS-based proteomics. Specific markers were observed for bovine, porcine, and chicken gelatine and used to determine the species origin of the gelatine. Interestingly, some of the commercial gelatines were found to contain undeclared species (eg, bovine and porcine mix declared on the product label as bovine) (Grundy et al., 2016).

Proteomics has also been applied to alcoholic beverages such as wine (Cereda et al., 2010), beer (Colgrave et al., 2013), and aperitif (Fasoli et al., 2012) but mainly for their characterization or detection of selected proteins (eg, the addition of casein during white wine production).

7.3.2 Metabolomics and Lipidomics

Metabolomics and lipidomics analysis consists of several steps including sample preparation, metabolite extraction, derivatization, metabolite separation, ionization, detection, and data treatment (Fig. 7.6). However, factors such as sample type, an isolated fraction of metabolites, and instrumental platform used in the analysis predetermine the final metabolomics/lipidomics workflow (Cevallos-Cevallos et al., 2009).

For food authenticity and fraud detection, metabolomics and lipidomics are usually used for matrices such as alcohol beverages (beer, wine, spirits), honey, olive oil, milk and cheese products, meat, spices, and juices. Food authenticity studies that we have reviewed have focused on the application potential of a particular instrumental technique or demonstrated proof-of-concept. Compared to proteomics/peptidomics, a few metabolomics or lipidomics studies have also focused on the analysis of large

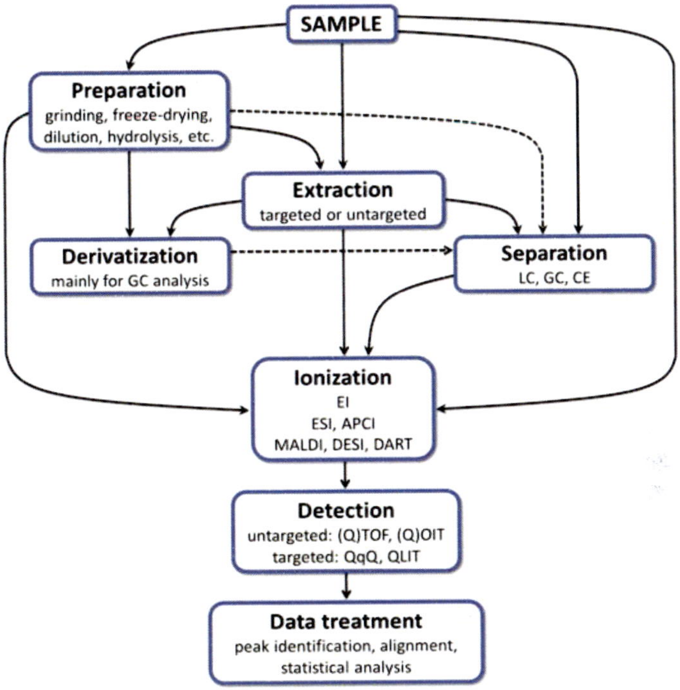

Figure 7.6 Schematic representation of the process of metabolomic and lipidomic analysis. Modified and redrawn from Cevallos-Cevallos, J.M., Reyes-De-Corcuera, J.I., Etxeberria, E., Danyluk, M.D., Rodrick, G.E., 2009. Metabolomic analysis in food science: a review. Trends in Food Science & Technology 20, 557–566. Copyright 2009 Elsevier.

numbers of samples (>100) to obtain robust statistical models. These studies are highlighted in the next sections along with studies in which high selectivity of detection of food adulteration was reported.

7.3.2.1 Alcoholic Beverages

Beer, wine, and spirits represent alcoholic beverages consisting of hundreds of low-molecular-weight volatiles and polar metabolites that can be used for authenticity.

SPME-GC-MS profiling of beer volatiles of 265 specialty beer samples collected over a 1-year period, thus covering possible seasonal variability of the products, was used by Cajka et al. (2010b). Statistical models were tested with the aim of distinguishing: (1) beers labeled as Rochefort 8; (2) a group consisting of Rochefort 6, 8, 10 beers; and (3) Trappist beers. The best prediction ability (100%) was obtained for the model that distinguished a group of Rochefort 6, 8, 10 beers from the rest of the beers (Cajka et al., 2010b). The same set of beers was also examined using DART-TOFMS operated in positive and negative ion mode (Cajka et al., 2011). Again, the best prediction ability (98%) was obtained for the model that differentiated the group of Rochefort 6, 8, 10 beers from the rest of the beers. Both SPME-GC-MS and DART-MS were suggested for monitoring batch-to-batch fluctuation of characteristic component profiles to assess the constancy of the beer production process. The sample throughput time of SPME-GC-MS was 30 min including SPME incubation/extraction and GC-MS analysis of beer volatiles. Concurrently, less than 1 min was needed for DART-TOFMS analysis of a single sample in one ion polarity (Cajka et al., 2010b, 2011). Fig. 7.7 shows a comparison of DART-TOFMS profiles of Rochefort 8 (Trappist) and Primator 24 (non-Trappist) beer samples acquired in positive and negative ionization mode demonstrating differences between acquired profiles of polar metabolites.

Mattarucchi et al. (2010) used LC-MS fingerprinting on 232 beers to distinguish three classes of beers: (1) Rochefort 8; (2) Rochefort 6 and Rochefort 10; and (3) non-Rochefort. The Rochefort beers were clearly distinguished from non-Rochefort beers (100% prediction ability) while only 3.5% of beers were wrongly classified when Rochefort 8 samples were compared to other types of beer from the same Trappist brewery (Rochefort 6 and Rochefort 10). No single variable was able to distinguish Rochefort 8 from the other types of Rochefort beers (Rochefort 6 and Rochefort 10). Therefore the group of Rochefort beers can be well defined by a few variables, while the different types of Rochefort beers (eg, Rochefort 8 vs Rochefort 10) can be discriminated only on the basis of a particular pattern of many variables (ie, the whole fingerprint) (Mattarucchi et al., 2010).

LC-MS and DART-MS techniques for untargeted metabolic fingerprinting and polyphenol profiling of 343 red and white wine samples have been reported (Rubert et al., 2014). Samples were analyzed either without any pretreatment or after liquid–liquid extraction using ethyl acetate to isolate phenolic compounds. Best results were achieved for LC-MS fingerprinting, which permitted discrimination of (1) Sauvignon Blanc, Riesling, and Silvaner (100% correct classification); (2) Riesling, Chardonnay

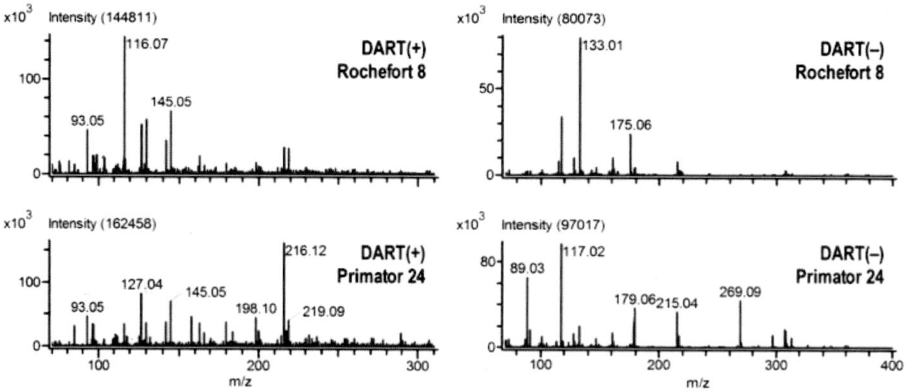

Figure 7.7 Comparison of DART-MS profiles of Rochefort 8 (Trappist) and Primator 24 (non-Trappist) beer samples.
Reproduced from Cajka, T., Riddellova, K., Tomaniova, M., Hajslova, J., 2011. Ambient mass spectrometry employing a DART ion source for metabolomic fingerprinting/profiling: a powerful tool for beer origin recognition. Metabolomics 7, 500–508. Copyright 2011 Springer.

Blanc, and Silvaner (99% correct classification); (3) Pinot Noir, Tempranillo, and Merlot (96% correct classification); and (4) Pinot Noir, Tempranillo, and Shiraz (95% correct classification). Comparison of LC-MS and DART-MS for both untargeted fingerprinting and polyphenol profiling was provided for Merlot and Tempranillo. In general, polyphenol profiling was slightly less efficient for sample discrimination than untargeted fingerprinting. Further, DART-MS showed less discrimination power than LC-MS but the analysis time was significantly reduced (Rubert et al., 2014).

An SPME-GC-MS-based method was also used for the analysis of volatile and semivolatile components of ice wines that originated from Canada and the Czech Republic. Using Kohonen self-organizing maps, a clear discrimination of the 137 samples according to their Canadian and Czech origins was obtained from a 300-cell trained map, without any outlying sample or analysis constituent (Giraudel et al., 2007).

A large set of wines ($n = 334$) originating from South Africa and characterized according to grape variety (Sauvignon Blanc, Chardonnay, Pinotage, Shiraz, Cabernet Sauvignon, Merlot) was analyzed using stir bar sorptive extraction-GC-MS. Using LDA, a correct prediction ability of 100% was obtained for the model distinguishing white and red wines. The same prediction ability was reached for the model distinguishing Sauvignon Blanc and Chardonnay. A correct classification of 97% was obtained for the model distinguishing Pinotage and the rest of the red wines; 3-methylbutyl acetate and ethyl octanoate were seen as influential in this differentiation (Weldegergis et al., 2011).

Ziółkowska focused on determination of the origin of 138 raw spirits obtained from rye, corn, and potato using SPME-GC-MS. The main groups of volatiles detected were fatty acid ethyl esters. Using LDA, a correct prediction ability of 97.4% was obtained for classification of raw spirits according to their origin. Compounds with the best discriminating power were identified to be ethyl dodecanoate, ethyl tetradecanoate, ethyl hexadecanoate, and 3-methylbutan-1-ol (Ziolkowska and Jelen, 2012).

7.3.2.2 Honey

Botanical and/or geographical origin predetermines the price of honey. Unifloral honeys are the most expensive and a higher price is also commanded by honey produced in a specific geographical location.

Ampuero et al. (2004) used (1) static HS-MS, (2) HS-SPME-MS, and (3) inside-needle dynamic extraction (INDEX)-MS for differentiation of 100 unifloral honeys. Generated fingerprints were submitted to discriminating factor analysis and correct classification rates of 92%, 98%, and 98% for static HS-MS, HS-SPME-MS, and INDEX-MS, respectively, were achieved for the model that distinguished acacia, chestnut, fir, and rape honeys. The most discriminating variables (*m/z* fragments) were *m/z* 44, 47, 54, 58, 94 for static HS-MS, *m/z* 59, 76, 94, 104, 144, 145, 157 for HS-SPME-MS, and *m/z* 48, 57, 58, 64, 74, 94, 104 for INDEX-MS (Ampuero et al., 2004).

SPME-GC×GC-TOFMS profiling was used to obtain volatile profiles of 374 honey samples collected over two production seasons in Corsica and other European countries with the aim of distinguishing honeys labeled as "Corsica" (PDO) from all the other honeys. Using ANNs, the prediction ability of the models for the first and second harvest was 93% and 92%, respectively. When the model created for the first harvest (2006) was used to predict samples from the second harvest (2007) the correct prediction ability using this external (validation) set was somewhat lower (81%). This can be explained by a large variation in the profiles of honey volatiles between these two years, possibly caused by different weather conditions. A low correct prediction ability (82%) was also achieved when the model from the second harvest (2007) was applied to predict samples from the first harvest (2006). Therefore the data of this 2-year sampling were merged and subsets used for training and testing thus contained representative samples from both harvests. Using this approach, a correct classification accuracy of 95% was obtained (Cajka et al., 2009). The same honey sample datasets were also statistically evaluated by Stanimirova et al. (2010). Using merged datasets from two harvests, a correct prediction ability of 85%, 87%, 64%, and 92% was obtained for LDA, PLS-DA, SIMCA, and SVM chemometric approaches, respectively (Stanimirova et al., 2010).

7.3.2.3 Olive Oil and Other Vegetable Oils

Studies dealing with edible oil authenticity are usually focused on the investigation of botanical or geographical origin. In both cases, the selection of compounds with discriminating power is quite challenging because the composition of edible oils is the result of complex interaction between botanical variety, environmental conditions, fruit ripening, and oil extraction technology (Montealegre et al., 2010).

Zunin et al. (2005) used HS-GC-MS to detect volatile terpenoid hydrocarbons in 105 olive oil samples to trace their geographical origin (West Liguria, Puglia, Greece, Spain, Tunisia). The analysis of volatile terpenoid hydrocarbons appears to be a straightforward and powerful tool for tracing the geographical origin of extra virgin olive oils from West Liguria. Three individual terpenoid hydrocarbons (α-copaene, α-muurolene, α-farnesene) permitted the distinction of West Liguria oils by a simple decision tree approach. Multivariate analysis of the eight detected terpenoids (α-pinene, limonene, (*Z*)-β-ocimene, (3*E*)-4,8-dimethylnona-1,3,7-triene, α-copaene, eremophyllene, α-muurolene, α-farnesene) facilitated the construction of class models with high correct predictive ability (>95%) (Zunin et al., 2005).

SPME-GC-MS was used to obtain volatile profiles of 914 olive oil samples collected over three production seasons in northwestern Italy (Liguria and other regions) and the rest of Italy, Spain, France, Greece, Cyprus, and Turkey with the aim of distinguishing the olive oils labeled as "Ligurian" (PDO) from all the others ("non-Ligurian"). Initial principal component analysis showed relatively large interannual variability in sample composition from particular regions, although some overlap of data from the three harvests (3 years) was observed (Fig. 7.8). Because the model developed for a single year dataset was not fully applicable for other sampling years, a model that consisted of the 3-year sampling data was used. A correct prediction ability of 81% and 62% was obtained for ANN and LDA, respectively, using this approach (Cajka et al., 2010a).

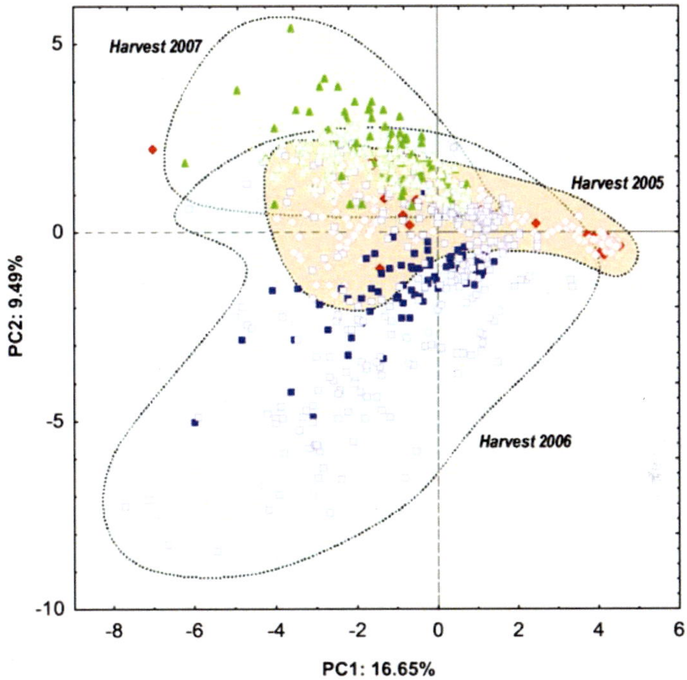

Figure 7.8 Principal component analysis clustering of olive oil samples: harvest 2005 (◆ Liguria, ◇ non-Liguria); harvest 2006 (■ Liguria, □ non-Liguria); harvest 2007 (▲ Liguria, △ non-Liguria).

Reproduced from Cajka, T., Riddellova, K., Klimankova, E., Cerna, M., Pudil, F., Hajslova, J., 2010a. Traceability of olive oil based on volatiles pattern and multivariate analysis. Food Chemistry 121, 282–289. Copyright 2010 Elsevier.

Use of DART-TOFMS to detect triacylglycerols and phenolic compounds to assess the authenticity of extra virgin olive oil was reported by Vaclavik et al. (2009). For triacylglycerols, samples were 50 times diluted with toluene, while a methanol–water mixture (80:20, v/v) was used to extract phenolic compounds followed by DART analysis (<1 min). In addition to the differentiation of various olive oil grades (extra virgin olive oil, olive oil, olive pomace oil), detection of adulteration by hazelnut oil at levels as low as 6% (v/v) was feasible based on the polar analyte fraction (Vaclavik et al., 2009). The pattern of triacylglycerols was seen to be less successful to detect adulteration of extra virgin olive oil with hazelnut oil.

A similar observation was reported by Calvano et al. (2012) who used MALDI-TOFMS for detection of extra virgin olive oil adulteration with hazelnut oil. There is a high degree of similarity between the two oils as regards triacylglycerol composition but phospholipids are usually present at significantly different concentrations for extra virgin olive oil and hazelnut oil. Employing the combination of tributylamine and α-cyano-4-hydroxycinnamic acid as an extraction solvent enriched phospholipids from extra virgin olive oil and hazelnut oil samples. Extracts were analyzed using MALDI-TOFMS using the same ionic liquid (tributylamine and α-cyano-4-hydroxycinnamic) as a MALDI matrix. The analysis of extra virgin olive oil samples progressively adulterated with variable quantities of hazelnut oil permitted detection down to 1% (v/v) contamination level (Calvano et al., 2012).

Zhang et al. (2014) conducted GC-MS analysis on 298 edible oils (soybean, peanut, sunflower, rapeseed, sesame) to obtain fatty acid profiles. In total, 28 fatty acids were identified and used to classify edible oils using principal component analysis, hierarchical cluster analysis, and random forest algorithms. Results showed that fatty acid profiles were able to differentiate these edible vegetable oil groups. In the next step, 300 blended oils were prepared by mixing five oils in random proportions. Furthermore, 60 adulterated mixtures were prepared for each kind of edible vegetable oil by blending with the rest of the vegetable oils at a ratio of 1:9 (w/w) providing in total 300 adulterated mixtures to test whether fatty acid profiles could serve to facilitate detection. Simulated data tests indicated that fatty acid profiles could be used to detect adulteration by 10% (w/w) or a little more than 10% (w/w) of other oils in the case of peanut, sunflower, rapeseed, and sesame oil (Zhang et al., 2014).

7.3.2.4 Milk and Cheese

In a comprehensive study, Hrbek et al. (2014) employed DART-orbital ion trap MS for (1) discrimination between milk samples from different species (cow, $n = 150$; goat, $n = 18$; sheep, $n = 18$), (2) classification of cow's milk produced in organic ($n = 68$) and conventional ($n = 82$) farming, and (3) detection of vegetable oil added to soft cheese. Milk samples were collected over a 4-year period. The nonpolar fraction of milk containing mainly triacylglycerols was isolated using toluene followed by centrifugation and instrumental analysis. To construct an LDA model, milk samples were divided into three groups: cow's milk ($n = 150$), goat's/sheep's milk ($n = 36$), and mixtures with adulteration levels of 50% and 10% (v/v) ($n = 24$). Only a low correct prediction ability (77.6%) was obtained using this set of samples. After removing the mixtures prepared at an adulteration level of 10% (v/v) from the dataset, all samples were classified correctly (prediction ability 100%). Thus, using DART-MS profiling of triacylglycerols, the LDA method enabled reliable detection of goat's/sheep's milk adulteration by cow's milk at a level of 50% (v/v). In the case of discrimination of organic and conventional cow's milk, LDA allowed for classification of samples with low correct prediction ability (66.5%). For detection of vegetable oil (rapeseed, sunflower, and soybean) in the soft cheese samples, adulteration by vegetable oil at a level as low as 1% (w/w) was feasible based on the pattern of triacylglycerols. As an example, Fig. 7.9 shows DART-MS spectra of the extracts of soft cheese adulterated with different vegetable oils (Hrbek et al., 2014).

Detection of bovine milk powder adulteration with vegetable oils or fats using MALDI-MS was conducted by Garcia et al. (2012). After extraction with hexane, extracts were spotted on the MALDI plate, allowed to dry at room temperature, and then MALDI analysis was performed with 2,5-dihydroxybenzoic acid being used as the matrix solution. Both nonadulterated milk powders and powders adulterated by potential adulterants [soybean oil, palm oil, hydrogenated soybean oil, and animal fat (cow

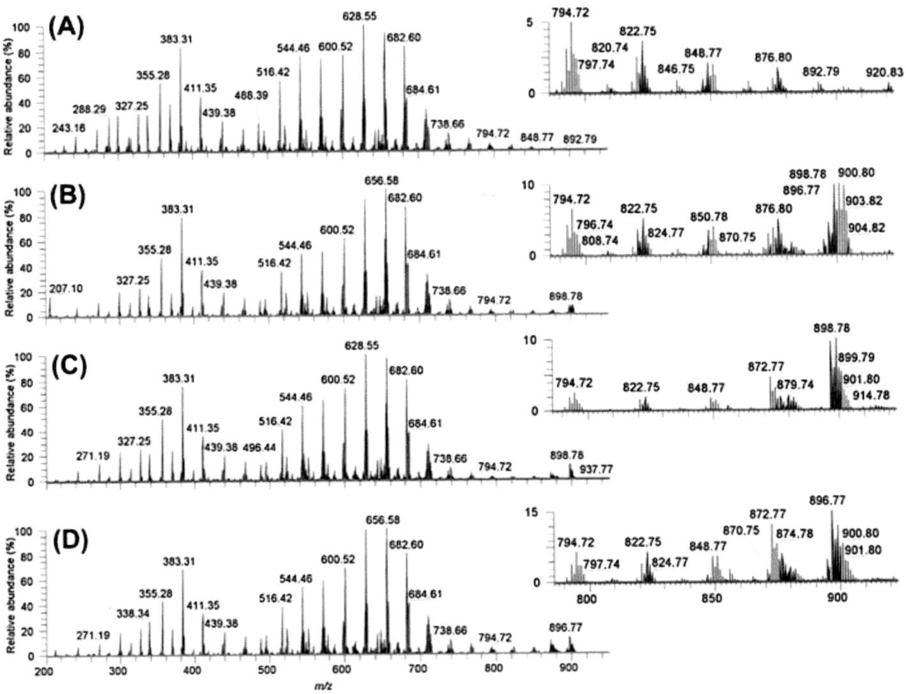

Figure 7.9 DART(+)-MS spectra of soft cheese extracts. (A) No vegetable oil added (reference), (B) addition of rapeseed oil (10%, w/w), (C) addition of sunflower oil (10%, w/w), and (D) addition of soybean oil (10%, w/w).
Reproduced from Hrbek, V., Vaclavik, L., Elich, O., Hajslova, J., 2014. Authentication of milk and milk-based foods by direct analysis in real time ionization-high resolution mass spectrometry (DART-HRMS) technique: a critical assessment. Food Control 36, 138–145. Copyright 2014 Elsevier.

tallow and pork lard)] were examined first. Compared to nonadulterated milk powders, adulterated samples received from the state authority showed a different pattern of triacylglycerols similar to hydrogenated soybean oil (Garcia et al., 2012).

Pisano et al. (2016) applied a GC-MS-based metabolomics approach to characterize polar metabolites of Italian mozzarella cheese produced with buffalo and cow's milk. OPLS-DA was used to identify metabolites that discriminate (1) mozzarella cheese produced with buffalo milk and whey starter cultures ($n = 20$), (2) mozzarella cheese produced with pasteurized cow's milk and commercial starter cultures ($n = 14$), and (3) mozzarella cheese produced with pasteurized cow's milk and citric acid ($n = 4$). Results indicated that metabolite pools reflect the different production protocols and microbial complexity of these dairy products. Among them, orotic acid was discriminating for cow's mozzarella cheeses, while threonine, lactic acid dimer, and serine were discriminating for buffalo mozzarella cheeses (Pisano et al., 2016).

An SPME-MS method was used for determination of the authenticity of PDO cheese (Oscypek) by Majcher et al. (2015). In total, 37 authentic Oscypek cheeses produced from ewe's milk from shepherd huts according to traditional technology, 36 Oscypek-like cheeses produced from cow's milk according to traditional technology, 18 Oscypek-like cheeses produced from ewe's milk in a small dairy factory according to an industrial method, and 22 Oscypek-like cheeses produced from cow's milk in a dairy factory according to an industrial method were analyzed. Collected data were treated using PCA, LDA, SIMCA, and SVM. All applied models showed good efficiency in the separation of original Oscypek (100% correct classification) from other Oscypek-like cheeses. Lower classification ability (58−97%) was observed between the groups of Oscypek-like cheeses indicating similarities in their SPME-MS profiles (Majcher et al., 2015).

7.3.2.5 Other Matrices

An LC-MS-based metabolomics approach for classification of fruit juice and adulteration detection was used by Vaclavik et al. (2012). For analysis, orange ($n = 19$), apple ($n = 16$), and grapefruit ($n = 16$) juices were used, among them samples representing both freshly pressed juices ($n = 8$) and juices prepared from concentrate ($n = 43$). In addition, to simulate adulteration, admixtures of expensive and cheap fruit juices were prepared. The LDA classification model was able to detect 15% (v/v) addition of apple or grapefruit juice to orange juice (Vaclavik et al., 2012).

Guijarro-Diez et al. (2015) focused on authenticity markers of saffron using LC-MS-based metabolomic fingerprinting; authentic saffron samples ($n = 10$) were compared to saffron samples suspected of being adulterated ($n = 10$). Extraction using an ethanol−borate buffer mixture at pH 9.0 (50:50, v/v) followed by RPLC-MS analysis obtained the highest number of significant components, which differed between authentic and adulterated saffron. OPLS-DA allowed discrimination between authentic and suspected saffron samples and also between different geographical origins. Six characteristic compounds of saffron (kaempferol 3-*O*-glucoside, kaempferol 3-*O*-sophoroside, kaempferol 3,7-*O*-diglucoside, kaempferol 3,7,4′-*O*-triglucoside, kaempferol 3-*O*-sophoroside-7-*O*-glucoside, and geranyl-*O*-glucoside) were proposed as novel markers for saffron authenticity (Guijarro-Diez et al., 2015).

SPME-GC-TOFMS was used to determine 29 volatiles for differentiation of Arabica coffee samples ($n = 26$) of different origins. Principal component analysis revealed clustering of samples based on geographical origin (coffees from South and Central America, Africa, and Asia) and compositional changes that coffee undergoes because of the limited shelf-life stability over extensive storage conditions (Risticevic et al., 2008).

DART-TOFMS was also used in a chicken meat metabolomics study aimed at the retrospective control of feed fraud. Samples ($n = 100$) representing meat from chickens fed by feed with and without the addition of banned chicken bone meal (5−8%, w/w) were extracted using a procedure enabling simultaneous isolation of polar and nonpolar metabolites. Differentiation of chicken muscle according to diet (feed with and without the addition of chicken bone meal) was feasible. Experiments conducted after 6 months with additional samples ($n = 16$) confirmed the applicability of this approach. Although correct classification was obtained for both polar and nonpolar extract fingerprints, the analysis of nonpolar extracts showed that the pattern of triacylglycerols was more prone to seasonal variability and/or type of raw materials used during feed preparation, which obscures the bone meal impact to some extent (Cajka et al., 2013).

7.4 Future Trends

Advances in MS-based omics sciences have led to the introduction of high-throughput analytical platforms permitting complex analysis of foods. Both metabolomics/lipidomics and proteomics/peptidomics have been shown to be promising tools for food authenticity and detection of adulteration. Future directions in MS-based food omics can be expected in the following areas:

1. emphasis on rapid and easy sample preparation methods;
2. increasing sample throughput in the case of LC-MS by using microfluidic devices;
3. use of advanced full spectra collection MS systems with increased mass resolving power, enabling polarity switching or collection of both MS^1 and MS/MS without significant loss of signal intensity;
4. improving tools for data mining and data interpretation/visualization;
5. increasing the number of metabolites in publicly accessible MS/MS libraries to improve metabolite identification;
6. increasing the number of samples used for particular studies, covering also seasonal variability, to improve the statistical models and avoid overoptimistic sample classification;
7. attempting to achieve a level of stability enabling interlaboratory comparison in ring trials;
8. focusing on validation of potential biomarkers from the untargeted analysis;
9. merging of targeted (contaminant analysis) and untargeted analysis (food authenticity and detection of unexpected compounds);
10. focusing on methods that can be performed with conventional MS instrumentation so that the protocol can be easily implemented in routine or commercial laboratories.

Acknowledgments

This work was supported by the US National Institutes of Health (NIH) grant U24 DK097154.

References

Ampuero, S., Bogdanov, S., Bosset, J.O., 2004. Classification of unifloral honeys with an MS-based electronic nose using different sampling modes: SHS, SPME and INDEX. European Food Research and Technology 218, 198–207.

von Bargen, C., Brockmeyer, J., Humpf, H.U., 2014. Meat authentication: a new HPLC-MS/MS based method for the fast and sensitive detection of horse and pork in highly processed food. Journal of Agricultural and Food Chemistry 62, 9428–9435.

von Bargen, C., Dojahn, J., Waidelich, D., Humpf, H.U., Brockmeyer, J., 2013. New sensitive high-performance liquid chromatography tandem mass spectrometry method for the detection of horse and pork in halal beef. Journal of Agricultural and Food Chemistry 61, 11986–11994.

Berrueta, L.A., Alonso-Salces, R.M., Heberger, K., 2007. Supervised pattern recognition in food analysis. Journal of Chromatography A 1158, 196–214.

Bjerrum, J.T., 2015. Metabonomics: analytical techniques and associated chemometrics at a glance. Methods in Molecular Biology 1277, 1–14. New York: Springer.

Cajka, T., 2013. Gas chromatography–time-of-flight mass spectrometry in food and environmental analysis. In: Ferrer, I., Thurman, E. (Eds.), Comprehensive Analytical Chemistry: Advanced Techniques in Gas Chromatography–Mass Spectrometry (GC–MS–MS and GC–TOF–MS) for Environmental Chemistry. Amsterdam: Elsevier.

Cajka, T., Danhelova, H., Zachariasova, M., Riddellova, K., Hajslova, J., 2013. Application of direct analysis in real time ionization-mass spectrometry (DART-MS) in chicken meat metabolomics aiming at the retrospective control of feed fraud. Metabolomics 9, 545–557.

Cajka, T., Fiehn, O., 2014. Comprehensive analysis of lipids in biological systems by liquid chromatography-mass spectrometry. TrAC-Trends in Analytical Chemistry 61, 192–206.

Cajka, T., Fiehn, O., 2016. Toward merging untargeted and targeted methods in mass spectrometry-based metabolomics and lipidomics. Analytical Chemistry 88, 524–545.

Cajka, T., Hajslova, J., Pudil, F., Riddellova, K., 2009. Traceability of honey origin based on volatiles pattern processing by artificial neural networks. Journal of Chromatography A 1216, 1458–1462.

Cajka, T., Riddellova, K., Klimankova, E., Cerna, M., Pudil, F., Hajslova, J., 2010a. Traceability of olive oil based on volatiles pattern and multivariate analysis. Food Chemistry 121, 282–289.

Cajka, T., Riddellova, K., Tomaniova, M., Hajslova, J., 2010b. Recognition of beer brand based on multivariate analysis of volatile fingerprint. Journal of Chromatography A 1217, 4195–4203.

Cajka, T., Riddellova, K., Tomaniova, M., Hajslova, J., 2011. Ambient mass spectrometry employing a DART ion source for metabolomic fingerprinting/profiling: a powerful tool for beer origin recognition. Metabolomics 7, 500–508.

Calvano, C.D., De Ceglie, C., D'accolti, L., Zambonin, C.G., 2012. MALDI-TOF mass spectrometry detection of extra-virgin olive oil adulteration with hazelnut oil by analysis of phospholipids using an ionic liquid as matrix and extraction solvent. Food Chemistry 134, 1192–1198.

Calvano, C.D., Monopoli, A., Loizzo, P., Faccia, M., Zambonin, C., 2013. Proteomic approach based on MALDI-TOF MS to detect powdered milk in fresh cow's milk. Journal of Agricultural and Food Chemistry 61, 1609–1617.

Carcea, M., Brereton, P., Hsu, R., Kelly, S., Marmiroli, N., Melini, F., Soukoulis, C., Ding, W.P., 2009. Food authenticity assessment: ensuring compliance with food legislation and traceability requirements. Quality Assurance and Safety of Crops & Foods 1, 93–100.

Cereda, A., Kravchuk, A.V., D'amato, A., Bachi, A., Righetti, P.G., 2010. Proteomics of wine additives: mining for the invisible via combinatorial peptide ligand libraries. Journal of Proteomics 73, 1732–1739.

Cevallos-Cevallos, J.M., Reyes-De-Corcuera, J.I., Etxeberria, E., Danyluk, M.D., Rodrick, G.E., 2009. Metabolomic analysis in food science: a review. Trends in Food Science & Technology 20, 557–566.

Chen, R.K., Chang, L.W., Chung, Y.Y., Lee, M.H., Ling, Y.C., 2004. Quantification of cow milk adulteration in goat milk using high-performance liquid chromatography with electrospray ionization mass spectrometry. Rapid Communications in Mass Spectrometry 18, 1167–1171.

Claydon, A.J., Grundy, H.H., Charlton, A.J., Romero, M.R., 2015. Identification of novel peptides for horse meat speciation in highly processed foodstuffs. Food Additives and Contaminants Part A-Chemistry Analysis Control Exposure & Risk Assessment 32, 1718–1729.

Cody, R.B., Laramee, J.A., Durst, H.D., 2005. Versatile new ion source for the analysis of materials in open air under ambient conditions. Analytical Chemistry 77, 2297–2302.

Colgrave, M.L., Goswami, H., Howitt, C.A., Tanner, G.J., 2013. Proteomics as a tool to understand the complexity of beer. Food Research International 54, 1001–1012.

Cordewener, J.H.G., Luykx, D.M.A.M., Frankhuizen, R., Bremer, M.G.E.G., Hooijerink, H., America, A.H.P., 2009. Untargeted LC-Q-TOF mass spectrometry method for the detection of adulterations in skimmed-milk powder. Journal of Separation Science 32, 1216–1223.

Cozzolino, R., Passalacqua, S., Salemi, S., Malvagna, P., Spina, E., Garozzo, D., 2001. Identification of adulteration in milk by matrix-assisted laser desorption/ionization time-of-flight mass spectrometry. Journal of Mass Spectrometry 36, 1031–1037.

Cunsolo, V., Muccilli, V., Saletti, R., Foti, S., 2014. Mass spectrometry in food proteomics: a tutorial. Journal of Mass Spectrometry 49, 768–784.

Dettmer, K., Aronov, P.A., Hammock, B.D., 2007. Mass spectrometry-based metabolomics. Mass Spectrometry Reviews 26, 51–78.

Draper, J., Lloyd, A.J., Goodacre, R., Beckmann, M., 2013. Flow infusion electrospray ionisation mass spectrometry for high throughput, non-targeted metabolite fingerprinting: a review. Metabolomics 9, S4–S29.

Di Girolamo, F., Masotti, A., Salvatori, G., Scapaticci, M., Muraca, M., Putignani, L., 2014. A sensitive and effective proteomic approach to identify she-donkey's and goat's milk adulterations by MALDI-TOF MS fingerprinting. International Journal of Molecular Sciences 15, 13697–13719.

De Livera, A.M., Sysi-Aho, M., Jacob, L., Gagnon-Bartsch, J.A., Castillo, S., Simpson, J.A., Speed, T.P., 2015. Statistical methods for handling unwanted variation in metabolomics data. Analytical Chemistry 87, 3606–3615.

Fasoli, E., D'amato, A., Citterio, A., Righetti, P.G., 2012. Anyone for an aperitif? Yes, but only a Braulio DOC with its certified proteome. Journal of Proteomics 75, 3374–3379.

Fekete, S., Schappler, J., Veuthey, J.L., Guillarme, D., 2014. Current and future trends in UHPLC. TrAC-Trends in Analytical Chemistry 63, 2–13.

Garcia, J.S., Sanvido, G.B., Saraiva, S.A., Zacca, J.J., Cosso, R.G., Eberlin, M.N., 2012. Bovine milk powder adulteration with vegetable oils or fats revealed by MALDI-QTOF MS. Food Chemistry 131, 722–726.

Gika, H.G., Theodoridis, G.A., Plumb, R.S., Wilson, I.D., 2014. Current practice of liquid chromatography-mass spectrometry in metabolomics and metabonomics. Journal of Pharmaceutical and Biomedical Analysis 87, 12–25.

Giraudel, J.L., Setkova, L., Pawliszyn, J., Montury, M., 2007. Rapid headspace solid-phase microextraction-gas chromatographic-time-of-flight mass spectrometric method for qualitative profiling of ice wine volatile fraction – III. Relative characterization of Canadian and Czech ice wines using self-organizing maps. Journal of Chromatography A 1147, 241–253.

Gonzalez-Arjona, D., Lopez-Perez, G., Gonzalez, A.G., 1999. Performing procrustes discriminant analysis with HOLMES. Talanta 49, 189–197.

Grundy, H.H., Reece, P., Buckley, M., Solazzo, C.M., Dowle, A.A., Ashford, D., Charlton, A.J., Wadsley, M.K., Collins, M.J., 2016. A mass spectrometry method for the determination of the species of origin of gelatine in foods and pharmaceutical products. Food Chemistry 190, 276–284.

Guarino, C., Fuselli, F., La Mantia, A., Longo, L., Faberi, A., Marianella, R.M., 2010. Peptidomic approach, based on liquid chromatography/electrospray ionization tandem mass spectrometry, for detecting sheep's milk in goat's and cow's cheeses. Rapid Communications in Mass Spectrometry 24, 705–713.

Guijarro-Diez, M., Nozal, L., Marina, M.L., Crego, A.L., 2015. Metabolomic fingerprinting of saffron by LC/MS: novel authenticity markers. Analytical and Bioanalytical Chemistry 407, 7197–7213.

Guillarme, D., Ruta, J., Rudaz, S., Veuthey, J.L., 2010. New trends in fast and high-resolution liquid chromatography: a critical comparison of existing approaches. Analytical and Bioanalytical Chemistry 397, 1069–1082.

Han, X.L., Yang, K., Gross, R.W., 2012. Multi-dimensional mass spectrometry-based shotgun lipidomics and novel strategies for lipidomic analyses. Mass Spectrometry Reviews 31, 134–178.

Herrero, M., Simo, C., Garcia-Canas, V., Ibanez, E., Cifuentes, A., 2012. Food omics: MS-based strategies in modern food science and nutrition. Mass Spectrometry Reviews 31, 49–69.

Hirayama, A., Wakayama, M., Soga, T., 2014. Metabolome analysis based on capillary electrophoresis-mass spectrometry. TrAC-Trends in Analytical Chemistry 61, 215–222.

Holcapek, M., Jirasko, R., Lisa, M., 2012. Recent developments in liquid chromatography-mass spectrometry and related techniques. Journal of Chromatography A 1259, 3–15.

Hrbek, V., Vaclavik, L., Elich, O., Hajslova, J., 2014. Authentication of milk and milk-based foods by direct analysis in real time ionization-high resolution mass spectrometry (DART-HRMS) technique: a critical assessment. Food Control 36, 138–145.

Ibanez, C., Garcia-Canas, V., Valdes, A., Simo, C., 2013. Novel MS-based approaches and applications in food metabolomics. TrAC-Trends in Analytical Chemistry 52, 100–111.

Li, D.X., Gan, L., Bronja, A., Schmitz, O.J., 2015. Gas chromatography coupled to atmospheric pressure ionization mass spectrometry (GC-API-MS): review. Analytica Chimica Acta 891, 43–61.

Majcher, M.A., Kaczmarek, A., Klensporf-Pawlik, D., Pikul, J., Jelen, H.H., 2015. SPME-MS-based electronic nose as a tool for determination of authenticity of PDO cheese, Oscypek. Food Analytical Methods 8, 2211–2217.

Mattarucchi, E., Stocchero, M., Moreno-Rojas, J.M., Giordano, G., Reniero, F., Guillou, C., 2010. Authentication of Trappist beers by LC-MS fingerprints and multivariate data analysis. Journal of Agricultural and Food Chemistry 58, 12089–12095.

Mazzeo, M.F., De Giulio, B., Guerriero, G., Ciarcia, G., Malorni, A., Russo, G.L., Siciliano, R.A., 2008. Fish authentication by MALDI-TOF mass spectrometry. Journal of Agricultural and Food Chemistry 56, 11071–11076.

Montealegre, C., Alrgre, M.L.M., Garcia-Ruiz, C., 2010. Traceability markers to the botanical origin in olive oils. Journal of Agricultural and Food Chemistry 58, 28–38.

Montowska, M., Alexander, M.R., Tucker, G.A., Barrett, D.A., 2015. Authentication of processed meat products by peptidomic analysis using rapid ambient mass spectrometry. Food Chemistry 187, 297–304.

Orduna, A.R., Husby, E., Yang, C.T., Ghosh, D., Beaudry, F., 2015. Assessment of meat authenticity using bioinformatics, targeted peptide biomarkers and high-resolution mass spectrometry. Food Additives and Contaminants Part A-Chemistry Analysis Control Exposure & Risk Assessment 32, 1709–1717.

Ortea, I., Canas, B., Calo-Mata, P., Barros-Velazquez, J., Gallardo, J.M., 2009a. Arginine kinase peptide mass fingerprinting as a proteomic approach for species identification and taxonomic analysis of commercially relevant shrimp species. Journal of Agricultural and Food Chemistry 57, 5665–5672.

Ortea, I., Canas, B., Gallardo, J.M., 2009b. Mass spectrometry characterization of species-specific peptides from arginine kinase for the identification of commercially relevant shrimp species. Journal of Proteome Research 8, 5356–5362.

Parker, C.E., Warren, M.R., Mocanu, V., 2009. Mass spectrometry for proteomics. In: Alzate, O. (Ed.), Neuroproteomics. CRC Press, Boca Raton, FL.

Pisano, M.B., Scano, P., Murgia, A., Cosentino, S., Caboni, P., 2016. Metabolomics and microbiological profile of Italian mozzarella cheese produced with buffalo and cow milk. Food Chemistry 192, 618–624.

Pischetsrieder, M., Baeuerlein, R., 2009. Proteome research in food science. Chemical Society Reviews 38, 2600–2608.

Ramautar, R., Heemskerk, A.A.M., Hensbergen, P.J., Deelder, A.M., Busnel, J.M., Mayboroda, O.A., 2012. CE-MS for proteomics: advances in interface development and application. Journal of Proteomics 75, 3814–3828.

Rebane, R., Leito, I., Yurchenko, S., Herodes, K., 2010. A review of analytical techniques for determination of Sudan I-IV dyes in food matrixes. Journal of Chromatography A 1217, 2747–2757.

Riedl, J., Esslinger, S., Fauhl-Hassek, C., 2015. Review of validation and reporting of non-targeted fingerprinting approaches for food authentication. Analytica Chimica Acta 885, 17–32.

Risticevic, S., Carasek, E., Pawliszyn, J., 2008. Headspace solid-phase microextraction-gas chromatographic-time-of-flight mass spectrometric methodology for geographical origin verification of coffee. Analytica Chimica Acta 617, 72–84.

Rovina, K., Siddiquee, S., 2015. A review of recent advances in melamine detection techniques. Journal of Food Composition and Analysis 43, 25–38.

Rubert, J., Lacina, O., Fauhl-Hassek, C., Hajslova, J., 2014. Metabolic fingerprinting based on high-resolution tandem mass spectrometry: a reliable tool for wine authentication? Analytical and Bioanalytical Chemistry 406, 6791–6803.

Russo, R., Cusano, E., Perissi, A., Ferron, F., Severino, V., Parente, A., Chambery, A., 2014. Ultra-high performance liquid chromatography tandem mass spectrometry for the detection of durum wheat contamination or adulteration. Journal of Mass Spectrometry 49, 1239–1246.

Russo, R., Severino, V., Mendez, A., Lliberia, J., Parente, A., Chambery, A., 2012. Detection of buffalo mozzarella adulteration by an ultra-high performance liquid chromatography tandem mass spectrometry methodology. Journal of Mass Spectrometry 47, 1407–1414.

Sarah, S.A., Faradalila, W.N., Salwani, M.S., Amin, I., Karsani, S.A., Sazili, A.Q., 2016. LC–QTOF-MS identification of porcine-specific peptide in heat treated pork identifies candidate markers for meat species determination. Food Chemistry 199, 157–164.

Stanimirova, I., Ustun, B., Cajka, T., Riddelova, K., Hajslova, J., Buydens, L.M.C., Walczak, B., 2010. Tracing the geographical origin of honeys based on volatile compounds profiles assessment using pattern recognition techniques. Food Chemistry 118, 171–176.

Takats, Z., Wiseman, J.M., Gologan, B., Cooks, R.G., 2004. Mass spectrometry sampling under ambient conditions with desorption electrospray ionization. Science 306, 471–473.

Vaclavik, L., Cajka, T., Hrbek, V., Hajslova, J., 2009. Ambient mass spectrometry employing direct analysis in real time (DART) ion source for olive oil quality and authenticity assessment. Analytica Chimica Acta 645, 56–63.

Vaclavik, L., Cajka, T., Zhou, W.L., Wang, P.G., 2014a. Survey of Mass Spectrometry-Based High-Throughput Methods in Food Analysis. In: High-Throughput Analysis for Food Safety, vol. 179, pp. 15–72.

Vaclavik, L., Krynitsky, A.J., Rader, J.I., 2014b. Mass spectrometric analysis of pharmaceutical adulterants in products labeled as botanical dietary supplements or herbal remedies: a review. Analytical and Bioanalytical Chemistry 406, 6767–6790.

Vaclavik, L., Rosmus, J., Popping, B., Hajslova, J., 2010. Rapid determination of melamine and cyanuric acid in milk powder using direct analysis in real time-time-of-flight mass spectrometry. Journal of Chromatography A 1217, 4204–4211.

Vaclavik, L., Schreiber, A., Lacina, O., Cajka, T., Hajslova, J., 2012. Liquid chromatography-mass spectrometry-based metabolomics for authenticity assessment of fruit juices. Metabolomics 8, 793–803.

Vera, L., Acena, L., Guasch, J., Boque, R., Mestres, M., Busto, O., 2011. Characterization and classification of the aroma of beer samples by means of an MS e-nose and chemometric tools. Analytical and Bioanalytical Chemistry 399, 2073–2081.

Wachsmuth, C.J., Hahn, T.A., Oefner, P.J., Dettmer, K., 2015. Enhanced metabolite profiling using a redesigned atmospheric pressure chemical ionization source for gas chromatography coupled to high-resolution time-of-flight mass spectrometry. Analytical and Bioanalytical Chemistry 407, 6669–6680.

Weldegergis, B.T., De Villiers, A., Crouch, A.M., 2011. Chemometric investigation of the volatile content of young South African wines. Food Chemistry 128, 1100–1109.

Wishart, D.S., 2008. Metabolomics: applications to food science and nutrition research. Trends in Food Science & Technology 19, 482–493.

Wolfender, J.L., Marti, G., Thomas, A., Bertrand, S., 2015. Current approaches and challenges for the metabolite profiling of complex natural extracts. Journal of Chromatography A 1382, 136–164.

Zhang, L.X., Li, P.W., Sun, X.M., Wang, X.F., Xu, B.C., Wang, X.P., Ma, F., Zhang, Q., Ding, X.X., 2014. Classification and adulteration detection of vegetable oils based on fatty acid profiles. Journal of Agricultural and Food Chemistry 62, 8745–8751.

Zhou, X.X., Ding, Y.T., Wang, Y.B., 2012. Proteomics: present and future in fish, shellfish and seafood. Reviews in Aquaculture 4, 11–20.

Ziolkowska, A., Jelen, H.H., 2012. Differentiation of raw spirits of rye, corn and potato using chromatographic profiles of volatile compounds. Journal of the Science of Food and Agriculture 92, 2630–2637.

Zunin, P., Boggia, R., Salvadeo, P., Evangelisti, F., 2005. Geographical traceability of West Liguria extravirgin olive oils by the analysis of volatile terpenoid hydrocarbons. Journal of Chromatography A 1089, 243–249.

Advances in Electronic Noses and Tongues for Food Authenticity Testing

8

M. Śliwińska, P. Wiśniewska, T. Dymerski, W. Wardencki, J. Namieśnik
Gdansk University of Technology, Gdańsk, Poland

Chapter Outline

8.1 Introduction

Currently there is an increased consumer awareness about the quality and authenticity of food (Broski, 2010; Śliwińska et al., 2014). One of the important factors in the selection of food products by consumers is the name, origin, and information about the ingredients used in the manufacture of the product. All this information provides evidence about the quality and safety of products (Cajka and Hajslova, 2011; Hrbek et al., 2014). However, with the increase in sales of regional products, the market has seen the increased sale of products at competitive prices but that are not always produced according to traditional recipes. The use of cheap ingredients or mismatched proportions of ingredients, false information about the source of components (geographical origin, botanical, or animal) may lead to incorrect labeling of food

(Hrbek et al., 2014; Oliveri et al., 2010). Incorrect or incomplete information on food products may negatively affect the health of consumers, and, to prevent this there are regulations concerning the protection of consumer health (EU Regulation 178/2002) (Cajka and Hajslova, 2011; European Commission, 2002; Food Standard Agency, 2015). In addition, the European Union supports the promotion of regional products that are reported to be characterized by unique sensory properties (Śliwińska et al., 2015). Therefore, a set of guidelines for the protection of botanical and geographical origin of food products have been introduced. In addition, such products can be labeled with protected designation of origin, protected geographical indication, and traditional specialty guaranteed statements (Majcher et al., 2015; European Commission, 2006). Examples of such products include Spanish Lechazo de Castilla y León, Polish Oscypek cheese, Italian Pasta di Gragnano, and French cider (EU Agricultural Product Quality Policy).

Tests to confirm the authenticity of food are carried out by a variety of analytical techniques: sensory analysis, chromatographic (gas and liquid chromatography coupled with different detectors, such as: mass spectrometer, time-of-flight mass spectrometer, olfactometric detector, flame ionization detector), spectroscopic (infrared spectroscopy, Raman spectroscopy, nuclear magnetic resonance, ultraviolet—visible, fluorescence spectrophotometry or mass spectrometry), and spectrometric (Lees, 2003). The advantages of these techniques are, inter alia, precision, selectivity, and the ability to identify the groups of compounds contained in the sample (Wardencki et al., 2009). In most cases the main disadvantages are the high cost of analysis, and long analysis times of chemical or data analysis (Lees, 2003; Śliwińska et al., 2014). Since the 1980s, however, there has been steady progress in the development of electronic sensors, which require less time to perform single analysis. So far, these devices have been used for general food analysis but also for testing of the quality and authenticity of products (Śliwińska et al., 2014).

The aim of this chapter is to present the principles of electronic noses and tongues as a potential future tool for testing of the authenticity of food. Additionally the advantages and disadvantages of using these sensors will be discussed along with their application to food authenticity testing of the following groups of food products: dairy and meat products, fruits and vegetables, oils and vinegars, teas and coffees, nonalcoholic and alcoholic beverages, and others.

8.2 Electronic Nose

An electronic nose is an analytical device that mimics the principles of the operation of human olfaction (Fig. 8.1). It is mainly used for fast detection, identification, and differentiation of gaseous mixtures. It is capable of analyzing the headspace of food samples in different physical states: gas, liquid, or solid. Volatile components in samples investigated are detected by sensors that mimic olfactory cells present in the nose; each device uses a set of specific sensors that generates a characteristic odor profile called a fingerprint. Odor profiles are created in response to

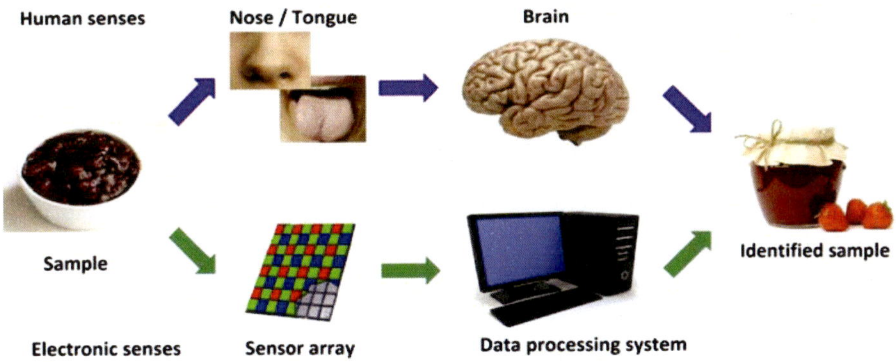

Figure 8.1 Comparison of the principles of operation of the senses of taste and smell with electronic tongue and electronic nose on a strawberry jam sample.

the interaction of the sensors with volatile compounds—headspace of sample. An odor profile thus created is sent to the data recognition system that simulates brain functions. Chemometric methods are used for data analysis; comparison of a collected odor profile with odor profile standards allows for the identification of components in a mixture (Śliwińska et al., 2014; Dymerski et al., 2011).

8.2.1 Types of Electronic Noses

Sensor arrays most commonly used in electronic noses are conductometric and piezoelectric sensors.

The principle of operation of a conductometric sensor is based on changes (resulting from interactions with volatile compounds) in conductivity. Despite the fact that various materials are used, the construction and distribution of specific elements in conductometric sensors are very similar (Śliwińska et al., 2014). Fig. 8.2 shows a simple schematic design of a conductometric sensor, of which

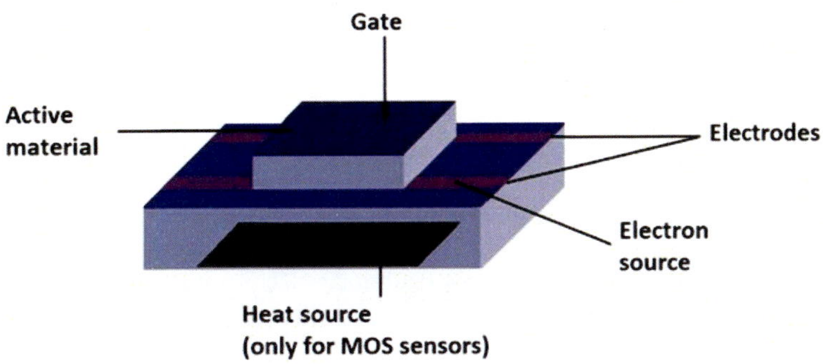

Figure 8.2 Schematic design of a conductometric sensor.

there are three main types: conductive polymer (CP) sensors, metal oxide semiconductors (MOS), and metal oxide semiconductor field-effect transistors (MOSFET).

The main advantages of CP sensors are their fast response and low price; susceptibility to humidity is their main disadvantage (Ciosek and Wróblewski, 2007). Such sensors have been used in an electronic nose in food analysis to identify stages of wine fermentation (Pinheiro et al., 2002), detection of spoiled beef (Panigrahi et al., 2006), and in authenticity studies of identification of beer brands (Pearce et al., 1993) or discrimination of soy sauces (Oshita et al., 2006).

Among the different types of available sensors, the most common and widely used are MOS sensors as they are inexpensive, easy to use, and very sensitive (Dymerski et al., 2011; Du et al., 2002). Their main disadvantage is poor long-term reliability, which therefore necessitates systematic recalibrations and high working temperatures (Oh et al., 2008; Ghasemi-Varnamkhasti and Aghbashlo, 2014). These sensors have been used in many food authenticity tests including discrimination of geographical origin of sweet cherries (Longobardi et al., 2015), classification by geographical origin and grade level of green tea (Huo et al., 2014), and discrimination and classification of virgin and nonvirgin olive oil and seed oil (Martın et al., 2001). Commercial electronic noses are mostly equipped with MOS sensors, for example, different types of FOX and PEN electronic noses.

MOSFET sensors are small and inexpensive; however, their main disadvantage is low sensitivity to ammonia and carbon dioxide together with drifting baselines (Sujatha et al., 2012; Śliwińska et al., 2014). These sensors have been employed in electronic noses that were used in authenticity studies involving discrimination of geographical varieties of extra-virgin olive oil (Cosio et al., 2006). The NST commercial electronic noses employ MOSFET-type sensors.

Main advantages of piezoelectric sensors are their low unit cost, simplicity of fabrication, small size, high sensitivity, and their linearity and rapid response-recovery feature (Sharma et al., 2015). The quartz crystal microbalance (QCM) is principally based on the piezoelectric effect. These sensors were used in electronic noses for authenticity studies to discriminate between products made from Iberian and other kinds of pig (Gonzalez-Martin et al., 2000) and to discriminate between cheese varieties (Pais et al., 2012).

Nowadays more authenticity studies of food are conducted with the use of electronic noses based on fast gas chromatography. It simulates the work of nose by using systems consisting of hundreds of orthogonal sensors that allow for precise separation of volatile compounds in the investigated sample (Śliwińska et al., 2014). This type of equipment uses FID and MS detectors. Results obtained with chromatographic analyses are then used as an input data for statistical analysis.

Short analysis times, precision, and ability to analyze many different volatile compounds are the main advantages of this equipment. The main disadvantages are high cost, large size that considerably reduces portability, constant need for cleaning of chromatographic columns, and low durability. This type of electronic nose was used in studies of discrimination between spirits of different botanical origins (Wiśniewska et al., 2015) and authenticity assessment of *nalewka* liqueurs (Śliwińska et al., 2016).

8.3 Electronic Tongue

An electronic tongue is an analytical device that mimics the principles of the operation of human taste (Fig. 8.1). It is used for recognition, classification, and quantification of components of liquid samples. Information about samples is obtained by sensors that mimic the membrane of gustatory cells present in the taste buds of the tongue (Medina-Plaza et al., 2014; Ghasemi-Varnamkhasti et al., 2011; Polshin et al., 2010). In this device, a set of specific sensors is used that generate a characteristic digital chemical fingerprint (Wei and Wang, 2014). A profile thus created serves as input data for the data recognition system, which simulates brain functions, based on pattern recognition and/or other multivariate data analysis procedures (Śliwińska et al., 2014; Medina-Plaza et al., 2014).

8.3.1 Types of Electronic Tongues

Three most popular types of e-tongues consist of following types of sensors: voltammetric, potentiometric, and impedimetric.

Analysis with an electronic tongue using voltammetric sensors is based on reading the current between two electrodes (working and reference) in an electrochemical cell (Medina-Plaza et al., 2014). Electrodes prepared from metals (Alcañiz et al., 2012; Banerjee(Roy) et al., 2012), carbon paste (Apetrei et al., 2007, 2011; Medina-Plaza et al., 2014), and conducting polymers (Pigani et al., 2000; Parra et al., 2006) are currently used. The advantages of voltammetric sensors include versatility, simplicity, and robustness (Winquist et al., 2002) together with the possibility to combine different analytical principles such as cyclic, stripping, or pulsed voltammetry. On the other hand, these types of sensors exhibit a lack of selectivity (Winquist et al., 2002; Śliwińska et al., 2014). These sensors were used in many food authenticity tests including discrimination of wines based on geographical origin (Parra et al., 2004), discrimination based on grape variety and geographical origin (Rodríguez-Méndez et al., 2008), discrimination and classification of oils (extra virgin olive, sunflower, corn, and soybean oils) (Apetrei and Apetrei, 2014).

The operation of potentiometric sensors is based on the voltage measurement at null current. The main advantages of this kind of sensor are low cost, ease of commercial production, and the availability of a large number of different membranes with different selectivity properties such as glass membranes or lipid layers (Winquist et al., 2002; Śliwińska et al., 2014). This technique unfortunately has a major disadvantage as it is limited to measure charged species only (Winquist et al., 2002). Potentiometric sensors were used in electronic tongues for authenticity studies such as determination of ethanol content in alcohols from different sources (Lvova et al., 2006), discrimination of beer types and beer bitterness (Rudnitskaya et al., 2009), and authentication of fresh cherry tomato juices adulterated with different levels of overripe tomato juices (Hong and Wang, 2014). The most popular commercial electronic tongues that use potentiometric measurement (Astree) are made by ALPHA M.O.S. company.

Measurement of impedance by means of impedance spectroscopy at constant frequency or a set frequency spectrum is the principle of operation of impedimetric sensors (Śliwińska et al., 2014; Escuder-Gilabert and Peris, 2010). These are occasionally used in electronic tongues. Unfortunately there is little information about the application of this equipment in food authenticity tests, although one report has described their use to discriminate between brands of red wines in an electronic tongue (Riul et al., 2004).

There are more and more reports describing research into food quality and authenticity measurement using electronic tongues containing arrays of biosensors. This type of device is called a bioelectronic tongue and it employs enzymes that are selective for specific compounds (Fernandes et al., 2011; Medina-Plaza et al., 2014, 2015). Biosensor data are then input to chemometric tools for data processing (Fig. 8.3). Most often bioelectronic tongues are used to study alcoholic beverages (Ghasemi-Varnamkhast et al., 2012; Zeravik et al., 2009) and fruits (Medina-Plaza et al., 2014, 2015). Biosensor arrays display high selectivity due to enzyme—substrate interactions, and their efficiency can be improved by facilitate the transfer of electrons from the enzyme to the electrode (Apetrei et al., 2010; Śliwińska et al., 2014).

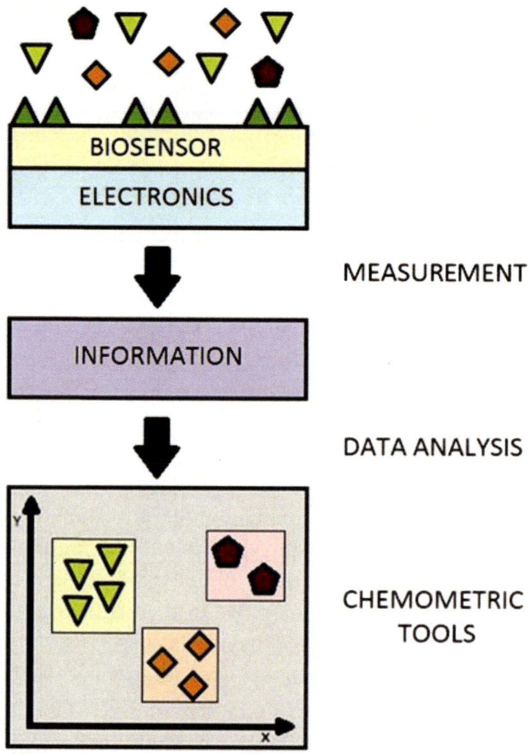

Figure 8.3 Simplified schematic of the principles of operation of biotongues.

8.4 Application of Electronic Nose and Tongue in Food Authenticity Studies

Electronic noise and tongue devices have broad application in food research food process monitoring, evaluation of food freshness, testing the shelf life of food, stability testing of food, and authentication of food. There are still many reports appearing that describe the modification of sensor arrays to increase their areas of application. Examples of the application of electronic nose and electronic tongue in food authenticity tests of many types of foods and food products are presented in Table 8.1.

8.4.1 Dairy Products

Dairy products represent one of the most frequently studied food groups. This group is very diverse and consists of many types of products such as milk, yogurt, and cheese. Dairy products are examined in terms of monitoring of food processing, evaluation of food freshness, and authentication of products (Śliwińska et al., 2014).

An electronic nose has been used for the classification of milk (Brudzewski et al., 2004) and Emmental cheese (Pillonel et al., 2003). An electronic nose based on tin oxide gas sensors was used for the discrimination of milk with different types and contents of fat. For analysis of different types of milk, four types of milk (3.2% v/v), two UHT, and two pasteurized (180 samples of each type of milk), in addition to a pure water reference and a milk reference baseline, were used. Principal component analysis (PCA) was used for data visualization and preliminary analysis. When using a water reference, milks were not distinguished, but when milk was used as a reference, three groups of milk could be distinguished. For analysis of milks with different fat contents, four types of milk were used containing 0% v/v, 0.5% v/v, 2% v/v, and 3.2% v/v. There were, however, difficulties in distinguishing milk with 2% v/v and 3.2% v/v content of fat (Brudzewski et al., 2004). The electronic nose in combination with chemometric analysis proved to be effective for distinguishing milk of different types, ie, pasteurized or UHT treated. The method needs improvement due to the reported difficulty in distinguishing milk of different fat contents and it is possible that the use of a different statistical analysis method would allow for differentiation of all tested samples.

Twenty samples of Emmental cheese made in France, Finland, Switzerland, Austria, and Germany were analyzed by electronic nose (Smart Nose) and GC–MS to identify cheeses on the basis of their geographical origin. For data analysis, PCA was used. Two analyses were performed using the electronic nose: discrimination of Emmental Switzerland from the other samples grouped as one region and discrimination of three Emmental cheeses originating from three regions, ie, Finland, Brittany (France), and Vorarlberg (Austria). In the first case, correct classification was achieved for 90% of the Swiss samples and 91% of the non-Swiss material. In the second case, 100% correct classification was achieved (Pillonel et al., 2003). Although chemometric analysis combined with GC–MS produced a 100% correct classification for both these cases, the Smart Nose turned out to be an interesting alternative for the classification of Emmental cheese in terms of their geographical origin. Advantages

Table 8.1 Examples of the Application of an Electronic Nose and Electronic Tongue in Food Authenticity Tests

Type of Food	Type of Samples	Object of Investigation	Artificial Senses	Type of Artificial Senses	References
Dairy product	Milk	Discrimination by heat treatment	E-nose	Tin oxide-based gas sensors	Brudzewski et al. (2004)
	Emmental cheese	Discrimination of geographic origin	E-nose	Smart Nose	Pillonel et al. (2003)
	Yogurt	Discrimination of yogurt types	E-tongue	Voltammetric electronic tongue based on various potential waveforms	Wei et al. (2013)
Fish and meat products	Anchovies	Analysis of freshness	E-nose	Six tin-oxide gas sensor	Amari et al. (2014)
	Spoiled beef	Identification of spoiled beef	E-nose	Cyranose-320™ based on conducting polymer	Panigrahi et al. (2006)
	Sea bream	Analysis of freshness	E-tongue	16 Potentiometric electrodes	Gil et al. (2008)
Fruit and vegetables	Apricot	Discrimination of different varieties	E-tongue	α-Astree I	Kantor et al. (2008)
	Mango fruit	Differentiation of mango fruits according to cultivar, size, and maturity at harvest	E-nose	FOX 4000: 18MOS	Lebrun et al. (2008)
	Sweet cherries	Discrimination of geographical origin	E-nose	PEN3 10 MOS	Longobardi et al. (2015)
	Tomato	Differentiation between different cultivars	E-tongue	18 Potentiometric sensors, α-Astree	Beullens et al. (2008)

Oils and vinegar	Oils	Discrimination and classification of oils	E-nose	6 MOS	Martın et al. (2001)
	Moroccan virgin olive oils	Differentiation of olives oils according to geographical origin	E-nose	5 MOS	Haddi et al. (2013)
			E-tongue	3 Voltammetric sensors	
	Extra virgin olive oil	Discrimination of different varieties of olives and geographical origin	E-tongue	Print-screen potentiometric devices,	Dias et al. (2014)
Teas and coffees	Green tea	Discrimination of green tea quality	E-nose	8 MOS	Chen et al. (2008)
	Green and black teas	Discrimination between green and black teas	E-tongue	Voltammetric sensors based on MOS sensors	Liu et al. (2014)
	Coffee	Discrimination between coffees of different origins and different varieties	E-tongue	Sensors based on artificial lipid membranes,	Buratti et al. (2014)
			E-nose	PEN2 (10 MOS)	
Nonalcoholic beverages	Cherry tomato juice	Authentication of fresh cherry tomato juices adulterated with different levels of overripe tomato juices	E-nose	PEN2 e-nose (10MOS)	Hong and Wang (2014)
			E-tongue	α-Astree (7 liquid cross-sensitive electrodes)	
	Fruit juices	Differentiation of juices according to botanical origin	E-nose	5 MOS	Haddi et al. (2014)
			E-tongue	6 Potentiometric chemical sensors	
	Citrus juice	Differentiation between juice according to fruit	E-nose	FOX 3000, 12 MOS	Reinhard et al. (2008)
Alcoholic beverages	Spanish wine	Differentiation and classification of red wines	E-nose	16 MOS	García et al. (2006)
	Spanish wine	Discrimination by aging process	E-nose	16 MOS	Lozano et al. (2008)

Continued

Table 8.1 **Examples of the Application of an Electronic Nose and Electronic Tongue in Food Authenticity Tests—cont'd**

Type of Food	Type of Samples	Object of Investigation	Artificial Senses	Type of Artificial Senses	References
	Chinese spirits	Classification according to flavor type	E-nose	PEN3	Liu et al. (2012)
	Wines, beers, whisky	Determination of alcoholic content in beverages made from different source materials	E-tongue	8 Potentiometric solvent polymeric membrane sensors	Lvova et al. (2006)
	Chinese rice wine	Differentiation according to vintage year	E-tongue	α-Astree	Yu et al. (2015)
	Spirits	Differentiation between spirits according to botanical origin	E-nose	Heracles II	Wiśniewska et al. (2015)
Others	Portuguese honey	Discrimination of honey according to predominant pollen	E-tongue	20 All-solid-state potentiometric sensors	Dias et al. (2008)
	Honey	Differentiation by botanical origin	E-nose	Fox 4000 (3 metal oxide sensors chambers equipped with 18 sensors)	Huang et al. (2015)
	Cocoa beans	Discrimination by geographical origin	E-tongue	α-Astree (7 potentiometric chemical sensors)	Teye et al. (2014)
	Spanish honey	Discrimination of honey according to botanical origin	E-tongue	Seven metallic electrodes were used as potentiometric sensors	Escriche et al. (2012)

included a shorter analysis time and easier handling of an electronic nose. After refining the method to achieve a higher correct classification rate, the electronic nose may possibly be used for this type of research instead of GC−MS.

Electronic tongues were used for the discrimination of yogurt types (Wei et al., 2013). Six categories of yogurts of different flavors and produced by four companies were analyzed by a voltammetric electronic tongue (VE-tongue) combined with chemometric methods such as PCA and discriminant function analysis (DFA). Three applied potential waveforms (multifrequency hackle pulse voltammetry, MHPV; multifrequency rectangle pulse voltammetry, MRPV; and multifrequency staircase pulse voltammetry, MSPV) were used for analysis with best results being obtained by VE-tongue based on MSPV. All samples were classified correctly using PCA and DFA, but six categories of yogurts of different flavors clustered separately by PCA (Fig. 8.4). Worst results were obtained by a VE-tongue based on MHPV; none of the samples could be separated by PCA or classified by DFA (Wei et al., 2013).

8.4.2 Fish and Meat Products

Fish and meat products are mainly analyzed by electronic noses, with analysis of these product types via an electronic tongue is less frequent because of more complex preparation required. Electronic nose has been used to analyze the freshness of anchovies (Amari et al., 2014) and to identify spoiled beef (Panigrahi et al., 2006). In the first case, an electronic nose based on six inexpensive commercial tin dioxide gas sensors combined with chemometric methods such as PCA, linear discriminant analysis (LDA), and support vector machine (SVM) were used. Fresh anchovies were kept in a refrigerator at a constant temperature of $4 \pm 1°C$ and they were analyzed after 1, 3, 5, 7, 9, 11, 13, and 15 days of storage. Results obtained by chemometric methods have allowed the samples to be grouped into three states of freshness: fresh (from day 1 to day 3), medium (from day 5 to day 7), and aged (from day 9 to day 15). LDA allowed for discrimination of three states of freshness of anchovies. In the case of SVM, three samples were misclassified (Amari et al., 2014). Those studies illustrate the potential of this approach to determine the freshness of anchovies, but further studies using other chemometric methods are required before commercial use of the method for freshness determination of this food.

An electronic nose (Cyranose-320™) based on a conducting polymer, coupled with artificial neural network (ANN) and PCA was used for the identification of spoiled beef. Meat samples were stored at two storage temperatures, ie, 10°C to expedite the spoilage of meat and 4°C to represent typical storage temperature of meat in retail stores. PCA did not reveal differential clustering of spoiled and unspoiled meat while ANN allowed discrimination of spoiled and unspoiled meat with 97% correct classification for a storage temperature of 10°C and 83% for 4°C stored samples (Panigrahi et al., 2006).

Fillets of cultured sea bream (*Sparus auratus*) were analyzed in term of their freshness over 14 days using an electronic tongue based on 16 potentiometric electrodes.

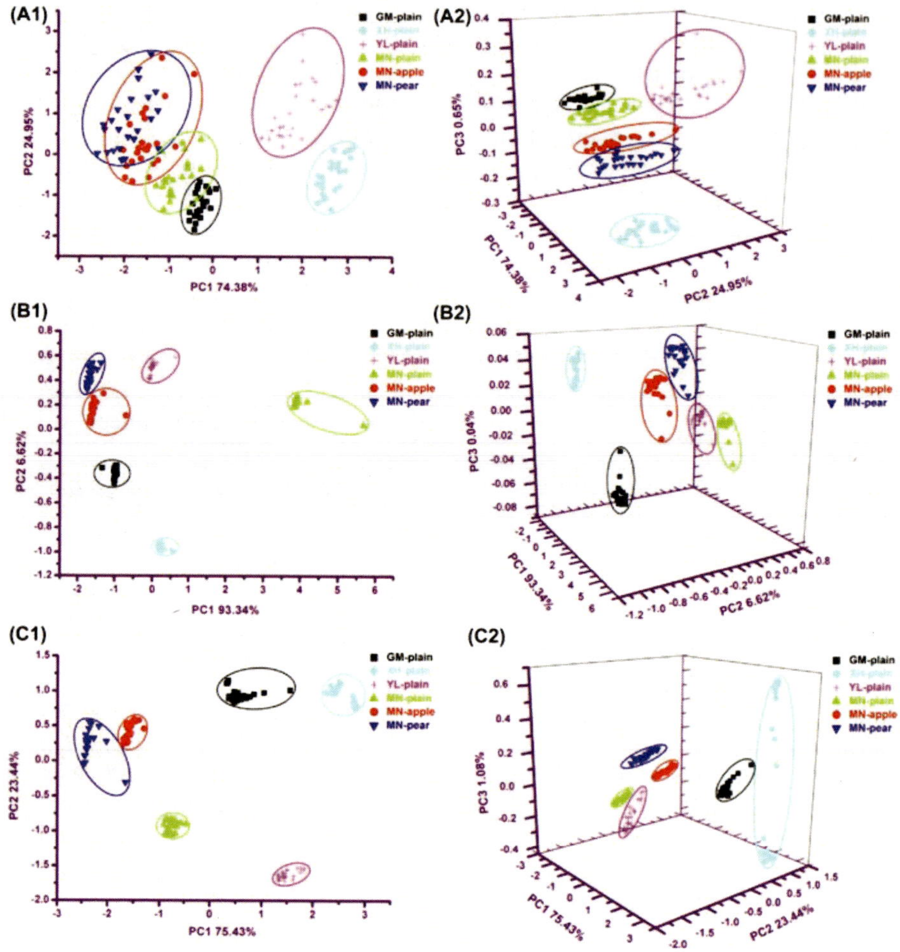

Figure 8.4 PCA score plots for data obtained from set yogurts by the VE-tongue based on MHPV, MRPV, and MSPV. MHPV: (A1) two-dimensional plot (A2) three-dimensional plot; MRPV: (B1) two-dimensional plot and (B2) three-dimensional plot; MSPV: (C1) two-dimensional and (C2) three-dimensional plot MHPV.
Reprinted from Wei, Z., Wang, J., Jin, W., 2013. Evaluation of varieties of set yogurts and their physical properties using a voltammetric electronic tongue based on various potential waveforms. Sensors and Actuators B: Chemical 177, 684–694. Copyright (2013) with permission from Elsevier.

Fuzzy ARTMAP electronic tongue, PCA and multilayer perceptron (MLP) type of ANN were used for data analysis. The fuzzy ARTMAP method allowed classification of fillets with respect to time of storage. A combination of electronic tongue and chemometric data analysis methods can be used to complement sensory analysis and replace other high-cost and time-consuming methodologies (Gil et al., 2008) in similar applications.

8.4.3 *Fruits and Vegetables*

Fruits and vegetables, just as fish and meat products, are mainly investigated by the electronic nose rather than the electronic tongue. An electronic nose was used, for example, for characterization of the geographical origin of Italian sweet cherries (Longobardi et al., 2015) and for the discrimination of mango fruit on the basis of maturity (Lebrun et al., 2008), while an electronic tongue was used for sensing the taste changes of apricots during storage (Kantor et al., 2008) and the analysis of tomato taste (Beullens et al., 2008).

Sweet cherries from two Italian regions were analyzed using an electronic nose (PEN3 based on 10 MOS) and isotope ratio mass spectrometry (IRMS) to distinguish them based on their geographic origin. PCA and LDA were used for data analysis. PCA did not show any clustering of samples based on region of origin, and the best correct classification figures obtained for electronic nose results after LDA ranged from 85.9% to 89.7% using internal validation. These results were worse than those produced using IRMS (Longobardi et al., 2015). However, the electronic nose combined with LDA may be considered as a good instrument for this type of analysis as, compared to IRMS, it is cheaper and the time of analysis is shorter. It is possible that, through the use of more selective sensors, an electronic nose would be able to obtain better results.

An electronic nose (FOX 4000 based on 18 MOS) and GC–MS were used for the discrimination of two types of mangoes based on their maturity; DFA was used for data analysis. Two different analyses were conducted. The first focused on separation of ripe from green Cogshall fruit from different harvest maturities, and the second on separation of different size classes for both green and ripe fruit in the case of Kent and Keitt mangoes. Electronic nose was able to distinguish between green and ripe Cogshall mangoes from each of different harvest maturities and to separate Keitt mango samples immediately after harvest and after 1 week of ripening. Electronic nose was also able to discriminate intact Kent mangoes harvested at different sizes, representing different maturities. In comparison with GC–MS, results obtained from electronic nose for the discrimination of intact ripe Kent and Keitt mangoes were better because groups were located further form each other (Fig. 8.5) (Lebrun et al., 2008).

Two electronic tongues, the first developed at the Saint Petersburg State University, Russia comprised of 18 potentiometric sensors and the second an ASTREE electronic tongue developed by Alpha M.O.S. (Toulouse, France) that consists of 7 commercially available sensors, were used for the analysis of tomato taste. Six tomato cultivars were selected based on their difference in taste. PCA, canonical discriminant analysis (CDA), and partial least squares (PLS) methods were used for data analysis. Electronic tongues were used for two types of analysis. Firstly, both electronic tongues classified tomato on the basis of cultivar. Secondly, an analysis was designed to try to predict tomato taste by relating electronic tongue data with sensory panel evaluations. PLS models were built using the sensory panel evaluations of sweetness, sourness, saltiness, and umami as references. Both electronic tongues were able to quantify tomato's most important taste compounds and to classify tomato cultivars based on their sugar, acid, and mineral contents. In the

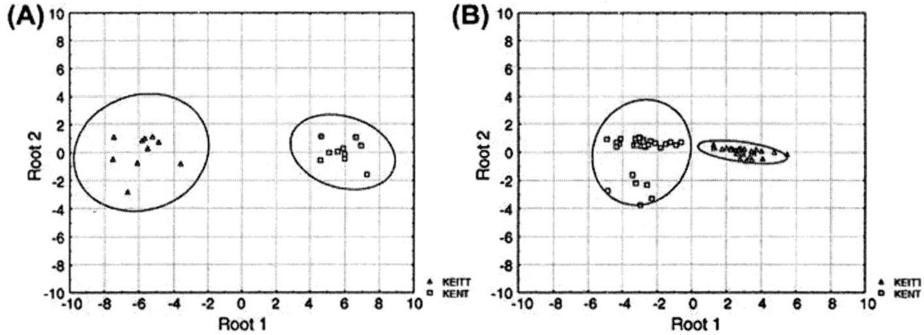

Figure 8.5 Separation of intact ripe Kent and Keitt mangoes by (A) enose and (B) GC. Reprinted from Lebrun, M., Plotto, A., Goodner, K., Ducamp, M.N., Baldwin, E., 2008. Discrimination of mango fruit maturity by volatiles using the electronic nose and gas chromatography. Postharvest Biology and Technology 48(1), 122–131. Copyright (2008) with permission from Elsevier.

case of sample preparation, the electronic tongue developed at the Saint Petersburg State University, Russia was better because of the short sample preparation time and relatively small amount of sample required (Beullens et al., 2008).

An α-Astree I potentiometric electronic tongue combined with analysis of variance (ANOVA), CDA, and PLS analysis was used to distinguish between different apricot varieties and to detect taste changes resulting from 1-methylcyclopropene and controlled atmosphere storage. Six groups (three control and three treated samples) were correctly classified at a level of 71.9% after 4 days, 83.9% after 2 weeks, and 92.9% after 4 weeks of storage. Comparison of electronic nose and sensory analyses revealed that the instrumental measurement was more sensitive to differences between apricots under 1-methylcyclopropene and controlled atmosphere storage than the sensory analysis (Kantor et al., 2008).

8.4.4 Oils and Vinegar

Among this group of products, luxury and traditional products such as olive oils are most frequently analyzed because of the possibility of adulteration of expensive products with cheaper alternatives. Olive oils are very often analyzed by both electronic nose and electronic tongue. An electronic nose based on six metal oxide semiconductor sensors was used for the classification of vegetable oils such as virgin olive oil, nonvirgin olive oil, and seed oil. K-nearest neighbors (KNN), LDA, quadratic discriminant analysis (QDA), soft independent modeling of class analogy (SIMCA), and ANN were used for data analysis. In the case of KNN, percentages of correct classification are not high, ie, for classification virgin, nonvirgin olive oil and seed oil it was less than 80%. Results obtained by LDA were definitely better because the correct classification ranged between 97% and 100%, while with QDA, correct classification rates of between 89% and 94% were achieved. SIMCA gave results higher than 80%, but lower than results obtained with LDA and QDA. ANN analysis gave slightly higher results than LDA. Interestingly, the authors of the articles performed the comparison process in two steps (olive oil/seed oil and virgin olive oil/nonvirgin olive oil) rather than in a one-step process (seed oil/virgin olive oil/nonvirgin olive oil) (Martín et al., 2001).

Five virgin olive oils from different geographical areas of Morocco were classified according to their origin by electronic nose based on a five metal oxide sensors and voltammetric electronic tongue. Data analysis was made using PCA, cluster analysis (CA) and SVM coupled with ANOVA variable selection. Unfortunately, separate use of the electronic nose and electronic tongue did not produce results of the desired accuracy, but fusion of data from these two instruments and a combination of chemometric methods allowed for complete distinction of Moroccan virgin olive oils based on their geographical origin (Haddi et al., 2013).

An electronic tongue comprised of 18 potentiometric sensors was used to classify oils obtained from single olive cultivars (Portuguese cvs. Cobrançosa, Madural, and Verdeal Transmontana; Spanish cvs. Arbequina, Hojiblanca, Picual). Linear discriminant analysis using simulated annealing (LDA-SA) variable selection algorithm, multivariate analysis of variance (MANOVA), and ANOVA were used for data analysis. LDA-SA allowed, in a first analysis, the discrimination of three cultivars of Portuguese olive oils and, in a second analysis, the discrimination of three cultivars of Spanish olive oils. Discrimination between Portuguese and Spanish monovarietal olive oils was a more difficult task. The LDA-SA model did not allow the distinction of Portuguese varieties from Spanish varieties. The authors of the article reported a classification of analysis performance for each Spanish monovarietal virgin olive oils vs the three Portuguese monovarietal virgin olive oils. This solution allowed distinction of Hojiblanca and Picual varieties from Portuguese varieties, but in the case of discrimination of Arbequina cultivar from Portuguese cultivars there was only 61% of correct classification of samples (Dias et al., 2014).

8.4.5 Teas and Coffees

Teas and coffees are mainly analyzed to distinguish between specific types, quality levels, and brands because of the great diversity and presence of varieties. Teas have been analyzed by electronic nose (Chen et al., 2008) and electronic tongue (Liu et al., 2014) to detect varieties and grade levels. Four green tea grade levels were identified by an electronic nose based on seven MOS combined with PCA, KNN, and ANN data analysis methods. PCA analysis did not reveal any cluster separation in the case of green tea grade level. Five principal components were used to create KNN and ANN models, and the percentage of correct identification of grade levels was 97.5% and 100% for KNN and back propagation artificial neural network (BP-ANN), respectively (Chen et al., 2008).

Voltammetric electronic tongue was used for the classification of green and black teas. PCA and SVM were used for data analysis. Four different metallic oxide-modified electrodes were studied: SnO_2, TiO_2, Bi_2O_3, and ZnO. The best PCA results were obtained with a Bi_2O_3-modified nickel foam electrode that performed as the working electrode. For SVM analysis, the input data were PCs that explained 98%

of the total information. Again, Bi_2O_3-modified electrode showed the best classification results (Liu et al., 2014). None of the electrodes allowed for 100% discrimination of black tea from green tea although the discrimination of teas with 98% efficiency for SVM analysis is a good result.

Both electronic nose and electronic tongue were used to characterize aroma and taste profiles of coffees (Arabica, Robusta, and washed Arabica). The electronic nose analyses were performed on 25 samples belonging to the Arabica variety, 25 belonging to the washed Arabica variety, and 25 belonging to the Robusta variety of ground, roasted coffee samples. Electronic tongue analyses were performed on coffee beverages made from the same samples. Electronic nose PEN2 based on 10 metal oxide semiconductor sensors, and electronic tongue based on sensors with a surface combined with artificial lipid membranes, were used. PCA and LDA were used for data analysis. Electronic tongue combined with PCA allowed for the visual separation of Arabica and Robusta varieties in PC score plots but discrimination of the two different Arabica coffees was impossible. LDA was used to classify coffee samples into three classes: washed Arabica, natural Arabica, and Robusta. For electronic nose, the average value of correctly classified samples was 81.8%, while for electronic tongue the corresponding average value was 78.8%. In both cases, Robusta coffees were better classified (100% correctly classified samples) than washed (less than 82% correctly classified samples) and natural Arabica samples (less than 77% correctly classified samples) (Buratti et al., 2014). In this case, the best classification of coffee samples was obtained using the near infrared spectroscopy. The application of electronic senses could assume the role of investigating techniques to present aroma and taste of coffee samples (Buratti et al., 2014).

8.4.6 Nonalcoholic Beverages

The analysis of alcohol-free beverages is a very common application of electronic sensors. A MOS-based electronic nose and SPME-GC-MS were used in the analysis of commercial and self-prepared citrus juices on the basis of fruit type, cultivar, and treatment. LDA was used for data analysis. The first analysis was to distinguish fresh and commercial orange and grapefruit juices while a second step concerned the discrimination of freshly prepared citrus juices, ie, lemon, lime, grapefruit, mandarin, and orange juices. A third analysis was about categorization of orange juices according to their appearance while the last was the discrimination of orange juices according to their processing (fresh, concentrate, not concentrate). In all cases, better results were obtained with SPME-GC-MS analysis. The groups were smaller and distances between the groups were larger than in the case of results obtained with the electronic nose (Reinhard et al., 2008).

Fruit juices made from mango, pear, apple, orange, pineapple, and a multivitamins juice (orange, pear, peach, grapes, apricot) were analyzed by electronic nose and electronic tongue combined with PCA, CA, and Fuzzy ARTMAP to confirm their origins. The electronic nose used in this research was based on five metal oxide sensors while the electronic tongue was based on six potentiometric chemical sensors. PCA analysis performed on 11 fruit juices with data gathered using the electronic nose only allowed visual separation of one orange and two mango juices from the others. Analysis of juices with electronic tongue gave better results, allowing the discrimination of two orange, one pineapple, and one apple juice. After low-level data fusion, which is a simple concatenation of data from different instruments, in this case electronic nose and electronic tongue results, it was possible to distinguish between all juices apart from one orange and one apple juice, the results of which overlapped (Haddi et al., 2014).

An electronic nose (PEN2) based on 10 MOS sensors and an α-Astree electronic tongue based on seven liquid cross-sensitive electrodes or sensors were used for the authentication of fresh cherry tomato juices adulterated with different levels of overripe tomato juices: 0−30% (w/w). PCA, CDA, and SVM were used for data analysis. Better results from electronic nose were obtained with CDA method than with PCA method. In the case of the electronic tongue, single analysis without data fusion allowed for the discrimination of two groups; the other two groups were close to each other on the CDA plot, which caused problems with discrimination. The best results were obtained with low-level data fusion of results from electronic tongue and electronic nose. In each case, all groups were completely discriminated (Hong and Wang, 2014).

8.4.7 Alcoholic Beverages

Alcoholic beverages, especially wines, are among the products that have been most frequently analyzed by means of electronic senses. An electronic nose based on 16 metal oxide semiconductor sensors has been used to classify 4 types of red wines made from the same grape variety and various aging processes. Two different extraction sample methods (static and dynamic headspace) were studied while PCA and probabilistic neural network (PNN) were used for data analysis. Dynamic headspace allowed for a better discrimination of different wines (about 95% correct classification) than the static headspace (about 80% correct classification) (García et al., 2006). The same type of electronic nose was used for the discrimination of wines based on wine aging. Two sets of samples were used, ie, wines from the same cellar aging in wood barrels from American and French wood that were analyzed before aging, after 3, 6, and 12 months of aging in oak barrels and wines from different cellars after 6 months of aging. Following PCA analysis, most wines aged for different times were clearly separated on score plots. The exceptions were wine samples before aging and wine samples after 6 months of aging in American barrels, which were not discriminated (Lozano et al., 2008).

Characterization of Chinese rice wines based on their taste attributes and vintage years was conducted with the α-Astree electronic tongue, HPLC, and by sensory evaluation. LDA was used for data analysis. Electronic tongue discriminated between Chinese wines from different vintage years (2003, 2005, 2008, and 2010), with the smallest distances on the relevant LDA plot being observed between samples of vintages 2008 and 2010; in fact, all the samples were distinguished from each other (Fig. 8.6) (Yu et al., 2015).

Electronic tongue was also used for the discrimination between and determination of alcoholic strength in several commercial alcoholic beverages types: wine, beer,

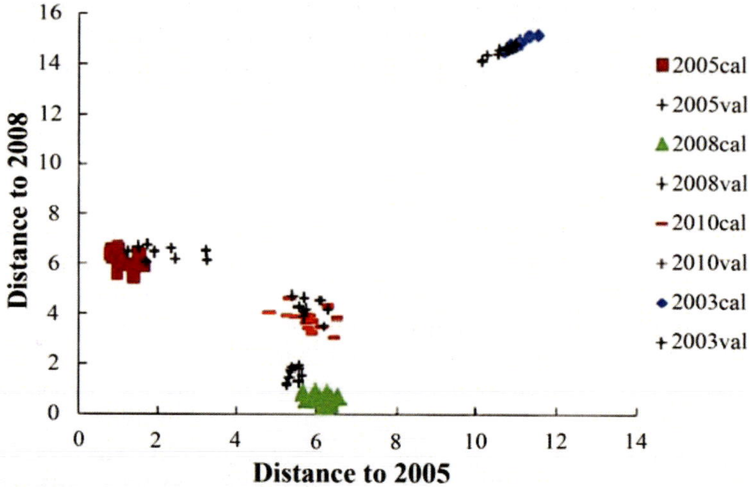

Figure 8.6 LDA discrimination plot for Chinese rice wine samples sourced from the 2003, 2005, 2008, and 2010 vintage years based on the e-tongue response data.
Reprinted from Yu, H., Zhao, J., Li, F., Tian, H., Ma, X., 2015. Characterization of Chinese rice wine taste attributes using liquid chromatographic analysis, sensory evaluation, and an electronic tongue. Journal of Chromatography B 997, 129–135. Copyright (2015) with permission from Elsevier.

grappa, and whiskey. Electronic tongue used in this research was based on potentiometric polymeric membrane electrodes, while PCA was used for the discrimination of samples on the basis of botanical origin. Samples made from barley were successfully distinguished from samples made from grape. Models to predict the alcoholic strength of chosen alcoholic beverages were evaluated and most exhibited a good correlation with actual alcohol content (correlation coefficient $R = 0.952$) except samples of "Ceres" beer and Ballantine's whiskey (Lvova et al., 2006).

Electronic nose was also used for the discrimination of raw spirits based on their botanical origin (Wiśniewska et al., 2015) and discrimination of Chinese spirits as per their flavor types (Liu et al., 2012). Electronic nose based on the technology of ultra-fast gas chromatography was used for the discrimination of raw spirits made from rye, maize, triticale, and wheat according to their botanical origins. Four chemometric methods—PCA, DFA, SIMCA, and statistical quality control (SQC)—were used for data analysis. PCA and SQC did not allow for the discrimination of all samples. Both DFA and SIMCA analyses allowed for the differentiation between agricultural distillates (Wiśniewska et al., 2015).

Electronic nose (PEN 3) was used for the discrimination of 20 Chinese spirits according to eight types of flavor (Jiang, Strong, Mild, Feng, Zhima, Nong jiang, Fougere, Laobaigan). PCA, CA, LDA, SVM, and ANN were used for data analysis. None of the chosen chemometric methods allowed discrimination of samples of five flavor types from each other although the best method was SVM, with the classification accuracy of the test data set of 83.3%. Most erroneous classifications of three prediction models (SVM, ANN, LDA) occurred in analysis of Jiang and Mild flavors (Liu et al., 2012). Chemometric methods used during the study were very diverse, which indicates a thorough examination of chemometric data analysis.

8.4.8 Others

Besides the aforementioned applications, the electronic tongue was used for the discrimination of honeys on the basis of their botanical origin (Dias et al., 2008; Escriche et al., 2012). Fifty-two commercial Portuguese honeys from different regions were analyzed by a potentiometric electronic tongue to identify the predominant pollen. PCA, LDA, and ANOVA were used for data analysis but none were able to distinguish honeys according to their botanical origin (Dias et al., 2008). In this case, the electronic tongue has not proved to be a good replacement for traditional techniques for determining the botanical origin of honeys. A potentiometric electronic tongue was also compared with traditional methodologies for the discrimination of honey according to the botanical origin (Escriche et al., 2012). Four Spanish honeys (citrus, rosemary, polyfloral, and honeydew) were used in this research. PCA, PLS, and ANN were used for data analysis. The best method was ANN, which allowed identification of citrus, rosemary, and honeydew honey with 95.83% accuracy and polyfloral honey with 100% accuracy. In comparison with traditional methodologies, electronic tongue proved to be a good and relatively cheap replacement for the discrimination of honey on the basis of its botanical origin (Escriche et al., 2012).

Honeys were also analyzed by the Fox 4000 electronic nose based on 18 MOS sensors. Honeys used in this research were from 2 geographical and 14 botanical origins. PCA, DFA, and least squares support vector machines (LS-SVM) were used for data analysis with LS-SVM producing the best results for the discrimination of both geographical and botanical origins. Electronic nose combined with this nonlinear chemometric method therefore enabled the discrimination of honeys on the basis of their botanical and geographical origins (Huang et al., 2015). The selection of only those data analysis methods that had a significant impact on differentiation of samples turned out to be a good idea.

Electronic tongue (α-Astree) was also used for the identification of cocoa beans as per their geographical origin. Cocoa beans used in a study originated in seven different areas of Ghana. PCA, FDA, KNN, and SVM were used for data analysis. The best results were obtained with SVM analysis that discriminated cocoa beans with a 100% correct identification rate. The worst results were obtained using PCA, but this is an unsupervised method, not typically used for the discrimination of samples (Teye et al., 2014).

8.5 Conclusions

Consumers are increasingly aware of authentication issues with certain food groups and they are willing to pay for more expensive products when the origin and ingredients are properly determined. Due to these facts, there is an increasing demand among companies and institutes for devices allowing rapid analysis of food products. A number of techniques and methods are used for authenticity assessment. One of these is sensory analysis, which is carried out by groups of panelists. The main disadvantage of this method is the fact that it is not always reflecting the true state of the studied product and in some cases can be subjective. The alternative chromatographic techniques coupled with olfactometric detection require long analysis times, and very often the results obtained are unreliable. The main problem with sophisticated analytical techniques is the high price of equipment and high-maintenance costs. In industry, one of the important factors influencing the choice of analytical method is the price for a single analysis. In spite of the many disadvantages of electronic sensors, such as complicated calibration, poor selectivity of sensors, and complicated data analysis, these devices are increasingly used for food analysis and in other branches of daily life such as with perfume, the pharmaceutical industry, and forensic operations. In addition, there is a trend to combine data from the electronic nose and tongue for authenticity assessments that facilitate the evaluation of taste and smell at the same time. This approach is closest in approach to the sensory analysis provided by panelists. Such systems are more reliable for food authenticity assessment. Year after year, new types of electronic sensors are appearing employing new types of sensors and biosensors. In order to enhance the areas of research, instrument manufacturers constantly improve sensor and biosensor materials and performance.

References

Alcañiz, M., Vivancos, J.L., Masot, R., Ibañez, J., Raga, M., Soto, J., Martínez-Máñez, R., 2012. Design of an electronic system and its application to electronic tongues using variable amplitude pulse voltammetry and impedance spectroscopy. Journal of Food Engineering 111, 122–128.

Amari, A., El Bari, N., Bouchikhi, B., 2014. Electronic nose for anchovy freshness monitoring based on sensor array and pattern recognition methods: principal components analysis, linear discriminant analysis and support vector machine. International Journal of Computing 6 (3), 61–67.

Apetrei, C., Apetrei, I.M., De Saja, J.A., Rodriguez-Mendez, M.L., 2011. Carbon paste electrodes made from different carbonaceous materials: application in the study of antioxidants. Sensors 11, 1328–1344.

Apetrei, C., Apetrei, I.M., Nevares, I., del Alamo, M., Parra, V., Rodriguez-Mendez, M.L., de Saja, J.A., 2007. Using an e-tongue based on voltammetric electrodes to discriminate among red wines aged in oak barrels or aged using alternative methods: correlation between electrochemical signals and analytical parameters. Electrochimica Acta 52 (7), 2588–2594.

Apetrei, C., Apetrei, I.M., Villanueva, S., de Saja, J.A., Gutierrez-Rosales, F., Rodriguez-Mendez, M.L., 2010. Combination of an e-nose, an e-tongue and an e-eye for the characterisation of olive oils with different degree of bitterness. Analytica Chimica Acta 663 (2), 91–97.

Apetrei, I.M., Apetrei, C., 2014. Detection of virgin olive oil adulteration using a voltammetric e-tongue. Computers and Electronics in Agriculture 108, 148–154.

Banerjee(Roy), R., Tudu, B., Shaw, L., Jana, A., Bhattacharyya, N., Bandyopadhyay, R., 2012. Instrumental testing of tea by combining the responses of electronic nose and tongue. J. Food Eng 110, 356–363.

Beullens, K., Mészáros, P., Vermeir, S., Kirsanov, D., Legin, A., Buysens, S., Cap, N., Nicolaï, B.M., Lammertyn, J., 2008. Analysis of tomato taste using two types of electronic tongues. Sensors and Actuators B: Chemical 131 (1), 10–17.

Broski, G., 2010. Addressing food authenticity challenges. In: Food Quality & Safety. http://www.foodqualityandsafety.com/article/addressing-food-authenticity-challenges/.

Brudzewski, K., Osowski, S., Markiewicz, T., 2004. Classification of milk by means of an electronic nose and SVM neural network. Sensors and Actuators B: Chemical 98 (2), 291–298.

Buratti, S., Sinelli, N., Bertone, E., Venturello, A., Casiraghi, E., Geobaldo, F., 2014. Discrimination between washed *Arabica*, natural *Arabica* and *Robusta* coffees by using near infrared spectroscopy, electronic nose and electronic tongue analysis. Journal of the Science of Food and Agriculture 95 (11), 2192–2200.

Cajka, T., Hajslova, J., 2011. Volatile compounds in food authenticity and traceability testing. In: Jeleń, H.H. (Ed.), Food Flavors: Chemical, Sensory and Technological Properties (Boca Raton, FL, United States).

Chen, Q., Zhao, J., Vittayapadung, S., 2008. Identification of the green tea grade level using electronic tongue and pattern recognition. Food Research International 41 (5), 500–504.

Ciosek, P., Wróblewski, W., 2007. Sensor arrays for liquid sensing – electronic tongue systems. Analyst 132, 963–978.

Cosio, M.S., Ballabio, D., Benedetti, S., Gigliotti, C., 2006. Geographical origin and authentication of extra virgin olive oils by an electronic nose in combination with artificial neural networks. Analytica Chimica Acta 567, 202–210.

Dias, L.A., Peres, A.M., Vilas-Boas, M., Rocha, M.A., Estevinho, L., Machado, A.A., 2008. An electronic tongue for honey classification. Microchimica Acta 163 (1–2), 97–102.

Dias, L.G., Fernandes, A., Veloso, A.C., Machado, A.A., Pereira, J.A., Peres, A.M., 2014. Single-cultivar extra virgin olive oil classification using a potentiometric electronic tongue. Food Chemistry 160, 321–329.

Du, W.X., Lin, C.M., Huang, T., Kim, J., Marshall, M., Wei, C.I., 2002. Potential application of the electronic nose for quality assessment of salmon fillets under various storage conditions. Journal of Food Science 67 (1), 307–313.

Dymerski, T.M., Chmiel, T.M., Wardencki, W., 2011. Invited review article: an odor-sensing system – powerful technique for foodstuff studies. Review of Scientific Instruments 82 (11), 111101–111132.

Escriche, I., Kadar, M., Domenech, E., Gil-Sánchez, L., 2012. A potentiometric electronic tongue for the discrimination of honey according to the botanical origin. Comparison with traditional methodologies: physicochemical parameters and volatile profile. Journal of Food Engineering 109 (3), 449–456.

Escuder-Gilabert, L., Peris, M., 2010. Review: highlights in recent applications of electronic tongues in food analysis. Analytica Chimica Acta 665 (1), 15–25.

EU Agricultural Product Quality Policy, http://ec.europa.eu/agriculture/quality/index_en.htm.

European Commission, 2002. Council Regulation (EC) No. 178/2002. http://eur-lex.europa.eu/homepage.html.

European Commission, 2006. Council Regulation (EC) No. 510/2006. http://eur-lex.europa.eu/homepage.html.

Fernandes, E.G.R., Brazaca, L.C., Rodríguez-Mendez, M.L., de Saja, J.A., Zucolotto, V., 2011. Immobilization of lutetium bisphthalocyanine in nanostructured biomimetic sensors using the LbL technique for phenol detection. Biosensors and Bioelectronics 26, 4715–4719.

Food Standard Agency, 2015. http://www.food.gov.uk/.

García, M., Aleixandre, M., Gutiérrez, J., Horrillo, M.C., 2006. Electronic nose for wine discrimination. Sensors and Actuators B: Chemical 113 (2), 911–916.

Ghasemi-Varnamkhasti, M., Aghbashlo, M., 2014. Electronic nose and electronic mucosa as innovative instruments for real-time monitoring of food dryers. Trends in Food Science & Technology 38, 158–166.

Ghasemi-Varnamkhasti, M., Rodríguez-Méndez, M.L., Mohtasebi, S.S., Apetrei, C., Lozano, J., Ahmadi, H., Razavi, S.H., de Saja, J.A., 2012. Monitoring the aging of beers using a bioelectronic tongue. Food Control 25 (1), 216–224.

Ghasemi-Varnamkhasti, M., Mohtasebi, S.S., Rodríguez-Méndez, M.L., Siadat, M., Ahmadia, H., Razavid, S.H., 2011. Electronic and bioelectronic tongues, two promising analytical tools for the quality evaluation of non alcoholic beer. Trends in Food Science & Technology 22 (5), 245–248.

Gil, L., Barat, J.M., Escriche, I., Garcia-Breijo, E., Martínez-Máñez, R., Soto, J., 2008. An electronic tongue for fish freshness analysis using a thick-film array of electrodes. Microchimica Acta 163 (1–2), 121–129.

Gonzalez-Martin, I., Perez-Pavon, J.L., Gonzalez-Perez, C., Hernandez-Mendez, J., Alvarez-Garcia, N., 2000. Differentiation of products derived from Iberian breed swine by electronic olfactometry (electronic nose). Analytica Chimica Acta 424 (2), 279–287.

Ha, D., Sun, Q., Su, K., Wan, H., Li, H., Xu, N., Sun, F., Zhuang, L., Hu, N., Wang, P., 2015. Recent achievements in electronic tongue and bioelectronic tongue as taste sensors. Sensors and Actuators B: Chemical 207, 1136–1146.

Haddi, Z., Alami, H., El Bari, N., Tounsi, M., Barhoumi, H., Maaref, A., Jaffrezic-Renault, N., Bouchikhi, B., 2013. Electronic nose and tongue combination for improved classification of Moroccan virgin olive oil profiles. Food Research International 54 (2), 1488–1498.

Haddi, Z., Mabrouk, S., Bougrini, M., Tahri, K., Sghaier, K., Barhoumi, H., El Bari, N., Maaref, A., Jaffrezic-Renault, N., Bouchikhi, B., 2014. E-Nose and e-Tongue combination for improved recognition of fruit juice samples. Food Chemistry 150, 246–253.

Hong, X., Wang, J., 2014. Detection of adulteration in cherry tomato juices based on electronic nose and tongue: comparison of different data fusion approaches. Journal of Food Engineering 126, 89–97.

Hrbek, V., Vaclavik, L., Elich, O., Hajslova, J., 2014. Authentication of milk and milk-based foods by direct analysis in real time ionization-high resolution mass spectrometry (DART-HRMS) technique: a critical assessment. Food Control 36 (1), 138–145.

Huang, L., Liu, H., Zhang, B., Wu, D., 2015. Application of electronic nose with multivariate analysis and sensor selection for botanical origin identification and quality determination of honey. Food and Bioprocess Technology 9 (2), 359–370.

Huo, D., Wu, Y., Yang, M., Fa, H., Luo, X., Hou, C., 2014. Discrimination of Chinese green tea according to varieties and grade levels using artificial nose and tongue based on colorimetric sensor arrays. Food Chemistry 145, 639–645.

Kantor, D.B., Hitka, G., Fekete, A., Balla, C., 2008. Electronic tongue for sensing taste changes with apricots during storage. Sensors and Actuators B: Chemical 131 (1), 43–47.

Lebrun, M., Plotto, A., Goodner, K., Ducamp, M.N., Baldwin, E., 2008. Discrimination of mango fruit maturity by volatiles using the electronic nose and gas chromatography. Postharvest Biology and Technology 48 (1), 122–131.

Lees, M., 2003. Food Authenticity and Traceability. Woodhead Publishing Limited, Abington Hall, CB.

Liu, M., Han, X., Tu, K., Pan, L., Tud, J., Tang, L., Liu, P., Zhan, G., Zhong, Q., Xiong, Z., 2012. Application of electronic nose in Chinese spirits quality control and flavour assessment. Food Control 26, 564–570.

Liu, N., Liang, Y., Bin, J., Zhang, Z., Huang, J., Shu, R., Yang, K., 2014. Classification of green and black teas by PCA and SVM analysis of cyclic voltammetric signals from metallic oxide-modified electrode. Food Analytical Methods 7, 472–480.

Longobardi, F., Casiello, G., Ventrella, A., Mazzilli, V., Nardelli, A., Sacco, D., Catucci, L., Agostiano, A., 2015. Electronic nose and isotope ratio mass spectrometry in combination with chemometrics for the characterization of the geographical origin of Italian sweet cherries. Food Chemistry 170, 90–96.

Lozano, J., Arroyo, T., Santos, J.P., Cabellos, J.M., Horrillo, M.C., 2008. Electronic nose for wine ageing detection. Sensors and Actuators B: Chemical 113 (1), 180–186.

Lvova, L., Paolesse, R., Di Natale, C., D'Amico, A., 2006. Detection of alcohols in beverages: an application of porphyrin-based electronic tongue. Sensors and Actuators B: Chemical 118 (1), 439–447.

Majcher, M.A., Kaczmarek, A., Klensporf-Pawlik, D., Pikul, J., Jeleń, H.H., 2015. SPME-MS-based electronic nose as a tool for determination of authenticity of PDO cheese, Oscypek. Food Analytical Methods 8 (9), 2211–2217.

Martín, Y.G., Oliveros, M.C.C., Pavón, J.L.P., Pinto, C.G., Cordero, B.M., 2001. Electronic nose based on metal oxide semiconductor sensors and pattern recognition techniques: characterisation of vegetable oils. Analytica Chimica Acta 449 (1), 69–80.

Medina-Plaza, C., García-Hernández, C., de Saja, J.A., Fernández-Escudero, J.A., Barajas, E., Medrano, G., García-Cabezón, C., Martin-Pedrosa, F., Rodriguez-Mendeza, M.L., 2015. The advantages of disposable screen-printed biosensors in a bioelectronic tongue for the analysis of grapes. LWT – Food Science and Technology 62 (2), 940–947.

Medina-Plaza, C., Revilla, G., Muñoz, R., Fernández-Escudero, J.A., Barajas, E., Medrano, G., de Saja, J.A., Rodriguez-Mendez, M.L., 2014. Electronic tongue formed by sensors and biosensors containing phthalocyanines as electron mediators. Application to the analysis of red grapes. Journal of Porphyrins and Phthalocyanines 18, 76–86.

Oh, S.Y., Shin, H.D., Kim, S.J., Hong, J., 2008. Rapid determination of floral aroma compounds of lilac blossom by fast gas chromatography combined with surface acoustic wave sensor. Journal of Chromatography A 1183 (1–2), 170–178.

Oliveri, P., Di Egidio, V., Woodcock, T., Downey, G., 2010. Application of class-modelling techniques to near infrared data for food authentication purposes. Food Chemistry 125 (4), 1450–1456.

Oshita, S., Arase, H., Seo, Y., Kawagoe, Y., Haruta, K., Amitani, H., Kawana, S., Makino, Y., 2006. Odor recognition of soy sauce by semiconducting polymer sensors. Transactions of the ASABE 49 (6), 1839–1844.

Pais, V.F., Oliveira, J.A.B.P., Gomes, M.T.S.R., 2012. An electronic nose based on coated piezoelectric quartz crystals to certify ewes' cheese and to discriminate between cheese varieties. Sensors 12 (2), 1422–1436.

Panigrahi, S., Balasubramanian, S., Gu, H., Logue, C., Marchello, M., 2006. Neural-network-integrated electronic nose system for identification of spoiled beef. LWT-Food Science and Technology 39 (2), 135–145.

Parra, V., Arrieta, Á.A., Fernández-Escudero, J.A., Rodríguez-Méndez, M.L., De Saja, J.A., 2006. Electronic tongue based on chemically modified electrodes and voltammetry for the detection of adulterations in wines. Sensors and Actuators B: Chemical 118 (1–2), 448–453.

Parra, V., Hernando, T., Rodríguez-Méndez, M.L., de Saja, J.A., 2004. Electrochemical sensor array made from bisphthalocyanine modified carbon paste electrodes for discrimination of red wines. Electrochimica Acta 49 (28), 5177–5185.

Pearce, T.C., Gardner, J.W., Friel, S., Bartlett, P.N., Blair, N., 1993. Electronic nose for monitoring the flavor of beers. Analyst 118, 371–377.

Pigani, L., Focab, G., Ulrici, A., Ionescu, K., Martina, V., Terzi, F., Vignali, M., Zanardi, C., Seeber, R., 2000. Classification of red wines by chemometric analysis of voltammetric signals from PEDOT-modified electrodes. Analytica Chimica Acta 643, 67–73.

Pillonel, L., Ampuero, S., Tabacchi, R., Bosset, J., 2003. Analytical methods for the determination of the geographic origin of Emmental cheese: volatile compounds by GC/MS-FID and electronic nose. European Food Research and Technology 216 (2), 179–183.

Pinheiro, C., Rodrigues, C.M., Schäfer, T., Crespo, J.G., 2002. Monitoring the aroma production during wine-must fermentation with an electronic nose. Biotechnology and Bioengineering 77 (6), 632–640.

Polshin, E., Rudnitskaya, A., Kirsanov, D., Legin, A., Saison, D., Delvaux, F., Delvaux, F.R., Nicolaï, B.M., Lammertyn, J., 2010. Electronic tongue as a screening tool for rapid analysis of beer. Talanta 81 (1–2), 88–94.

Reinhard, H., Sager, F., Zoller, O., 2008. Citrus juice classification by SPME-GC-MS and electronic nose measurements. LWT-Food Science and Technology 41 (10), 1906–1912.

Riul, A., de Sousa, H.C., Malmegrim, R.R., dos Santos, D.S., Carvalho, A.C.P.L.F., Fonseca, F.J., Oliveira, O.N., Mattoso, L.H.C., 2004. Wine classification by taste sensors made from ultra-thin films and using neural networks. Sensors and Actuators B: Chemical 98 (1), 77–82.

Rodríguez-Méndez, M.L., Parra, V., Apetrei, C., Villanueva, S., Gay, M., Prieto, N., Martínez, J., de Saja, J.A., 2008. Electronic tongue based on voltammetric electrodes modified with materials showing complementary electroactive properties. Applications. Microchimica Acta 163, 23–31.

Rudnitskaya, A., Polshin, E., Kirsanov, D., Lammertyn, J., Nicolai, B., Saison, D., Delvaux, F.R., Delvaux, F., Legin, A., 2009. Instrumental measurement of beer taste attributes using an electronic tongue. Analytica Chimica Acta 646 (1–2), 111–118.

Sharma, P., Ghosh, A., Tudu, B., Sabhapondit, S., Baruah, B.D., Tamuly, P., Bhattacharyya, N., Bandyopadhyaya, R., 2015. Monitoring the fermentation process of black tea using QCM sensor based electronic nose. Sensors and Actuators B 219, 146–157.

Śliwińska, M., Wiśniewska, P., Dymerski, T., Wardencki, W., Namieśnik, J., 2015. The flavour of fruit spirits and fruit liqueurs: a review. Flavour and Fragrance Journal 30 (3), 197–207.

Śliwińska, M., Wiśniewska, P., Dymerski, T., Namieśnik, J., Wardencki, W., 2014. Food analysis using artificial senses. Journal Agricultural and Food Chemistry 62 (7), 1423–1448.

Śliwińska, M., Wiśniewska, P., Dymerski, T., Wardencki, W., Namieśnik, J., 2016. Application of Electronic Nose Based on Fast GC for Authenticity Assessment of Polish Homemade Liqueurs Called *Nalewka*. Food Analytical Methods. http://dx.doi.org/10.1007/s12161-016-0448-z.

Sujatha, G., Dhivya, N., Ayyadurai, K., Thyagarajan, D., 2012. Advances in electronic-nose technologies. International Journal of Engineering Research and Applications 2 (4), 2248–9622.

Teye, E., Huang, X., Han, F., Botchway, F., 2014. Discrimination of cocoa beans according to geographical origin by electronic tongue and multivariate algorithms. Food Analytical Methods 7 (2), 360–365.

Wardencki, W., Biernacka, P., Chmiel, T., Dymerski, T., 2009. Instrumental techniques used for assessment of food quality. Proceedings of ECOpole 3 (2), 273–279.

Wei, Z., Wang, J., 2014. Tracing floral and geographical origins of honeys by potentiometric and voltammetric electronic tongue. Computers and Electronics in Agriculture 108, 112–122.

Wei, Z., Wang, J., Jin, W., 2013. Evaluation of varieties of set yogurts and their physical properties using a voltammetric electronic tongue based on various potential waveforms. Sensors and Actuators B: Chemical 177, 684–694.

Winquist, F., Krantz-Rülcker, C., Lundström, I., 2002. Electronic tongues and combinations of artificial senses. Sensors Update 11 (1), 279–306.

Wiśniewska, P., Śliwińska, M., Dymerski, T., Wardencki, W., Namieśnik, J., 2015. Differentiation between spirits according to their botanical origin. Food Analytical Methods. http://dx.doi.org/10.1007/s12161-015-0280-x.

Yu, H., Zhao, J., Li, F., Tian, H., Ma, X., 2015. Characterization of Chinese rice wine taste attributes using liquid chromatographic analysis, sensory evaluation, and an electronic tongue. Journal of Chromatography B 997, 129–135.

Zeravik, J., Hlavacek, A., Lacina, K., Skládal, P., 2009. State of the art in the field of electronic and bioelectronic tongues – towards the analysis of wines. Electroanalysis 21 (23), 2509–2520.

Advances in Isotopic Analysis for Food Authenticity Testing

9

K.H. Laursen [1], *L. Bontempo* [2], *F. Camin* [2], *A. Roßmann* [3]
[1]University of Copenhagen, Copenhagen, Denmark; [2]Research and Innovation Centre, Trentino, Italy; [3]Isolab GmbH Laboratory for Stable Isotopes, Schweitenkirchen, Germany

Chapter Outline

9.1 Introduction

Adulteration of food and beverages is an increasing global problem and new fraud cases are frequently reported. This is, for example, evident from the large number of fraud cases revealed in the yearly Europol/Interpol operations (see, eg, Operation Opson IV—2014/2015). Fraud and adulteration can be related to the geographical or vintage origin (wine), the agricultural production method (eg, "conventional" or "organic," "free-range" or "barn-raised"), the processing method, or cases in which products have been diluted (watered) or in which chemical food components have been substituted by cheaper imitations (eg, undeclared sugar or acid addition).

Consequently, consumers are becoming increasingly aware of food quality and safety and demand documentation of the authenticity of food products. The request for analytical methods that can correctly verify the authenticity of food products is therefore greater than ever. Stable isotope ratio analysis (SIRA) represents one of the most well-established and acknowledged methods for authenticity testing; the major advantage of this methodology is its ability to differentiate substances that are chemically identical. Today, SIRA is, for example, routinely used for verifying the authenticity of wine, fruit juices, olive oil, honey, etc (Drivelos and Georgiou, 2012; Roßmann, 2013; Camin et al., 2015b). In this section, we will give a short theoretical background to stable isotope analysis including the major fractionation processes that make isotopic signatures suitable for authenticity testing.

9.1.1 Stable Isotopes

The first analytical instrument for isotope analysis was developed more than 100 years ago (Sulzman, 2007). At a much later stage (approximately in 1975), SIRA was utilized for food authentication for the first time to reveal adulteration of products like honey, maple syrup, and fruit juices (Rossmann, 2001). In the 1970s, SIRA was very time consuming because of tedious procedures for sample preparation and analysis. Today, new analytical developments, such as elemental analyzer-continuous flow-isotope-ratio mass spectrometry (EA-CF-IRMS), allow simultaneous SIRA of several elements on a fully automated routine basis. The majority of SIRA-based food authentications are focused on the low mass elements hydrogen (H), carbon (C), nitrogen (N), oxygen (O), and sulfur (S) and, in some cases, elements from the high mass range such as strontium (Sr) (Table 9.1). For these elements, two or more stable isotopes exist and these differ regarding their number of neutrons and can thereby be measured individually by advanced analytical techniques (Section 9.2.2). The lighter isotopes of each element are often found to be the most abundant in nature. Nitrogen, for example, has two stable isotopes, ^{14}N and ^{15}N whereof ^{14}N constitutes the majority of the earth's atmosphere. The elements H, C, N, O, and S dominate biological material and can be converted into gases for analysis (H_2, CO_2, N_2, CO, and SO_2, respectively). Furthermore, the percentage increase in mass caused by the addition of a single neutron is great in the case of these elements, which make them highly suitable for SIRA. The relative mass difference between ^2H and ^1H is, for example, 100%, while it is 8.3%, 7.1%, 12.5%, and 6.3% for $^{13}C/^{12}C$, $^{15}N/^{14}N$, $^{18}O/^{16}O$, and $^{34}S/^{32}S$, respectively. However, the stable isotopes of heavier elements such as $^{87}Sr/^{86}Sr$ with a lower mass difference (1.2%) have also been the focus of many studies and have, for example, been used for authenticating plants according to their geographical origin (Asfaha et al., 2011; Zampella et al., 2011; Trincherini et al., 2014).

Stable isotope compositions are normally reported as delta values (δ) according to Eq. (9.1):

$$X = \left(\frac{R_s - R_{std}}{R_{std}}\right) \tag{9.1}$$

Table 9.1 Selected Elements, Their Stable Isotopes, Relative Abundances, Corresponding Delta Notation, and Selected Fractionation Processes Relevant for Authenticity Testing (Kelly et al., 2005; Sulzman, 2007; Berglund and Wieser, 2011; Brand et al., 2014)

Element	Isotopes	Natural Abundance	Delta Notation	Fractionation Processes	Information
Hydrogen	^{1}H	99.98	$\delta^{2}H$	Evaporation, condensation, precipitation, transpiration	Geography, water usage, fertilization rate
	^{2}H	0.02			
Carbon	^{12}C	98.9	$\delta^{13}C$	CO_2 assimilation, stomatal conductance	Water use efficiency, fertilization rate
	^{13}C	1.1			
Nitrogen	^{14}N	99.6	$\delta^{15}N$	N transformation processes, atmospheric loss	Fertilizer type and rate
	^{15}N	0.4			
Oxygen	^{16}O	99.76	$\delta^{18}O$[a]	Evaporation, condensation, precipitation, transpiration	Geography, water usage, fertilization rate
	^{17}O	0.04			
	^{18}O	0.2			
Sulfur	^{32}S	95.0	$\delta^{34}S$[a]	S transformation processes, sea spray	Geography, fertilizer type
	^{33}S	0.75			
	^{34}S	4.2			
	^{36}S	0.015			
Strontium	^{84}Sr	0.6	$\delta^{87}Sr$[a]	Radiogenic decay of ^{87}Rb	Geography, geology
	^{86}Sr	9.9			
	^{87}Sr	7.0			
	^{88}Sr	82.6			

[a]The $R(^{18}O/^{16}O)$, $R(^{34}S/^{32}S)$, and $R(^{87}Sr/^{86}Sr)$ ratios are the most common targets for stable isotope determinations of O, S, and Sr, respectively.

and are subsequently presented in units of parts per mil (‰). R_s and R_{std} are the molar ratios of the heavy isotope relative to the light isotope in the sample and a standard, respectively. X can, for example, be $\delta^{2}H$, $\delta^{13}C$, $\delta^{15}N$, $\delta^{18}O$, $\delta^{34}S$, or $\delta^{87}Sr$ and R values are the corresponding isotope ratios: $^{2}H/^{1}H$, $^{13}C/^{12}C$, $^{15}N/^{14}N$, $^{18}O/^{16}O$, $^{34}S/^{32}S$, or $^{87}Sr/^{86}Sr$, respectively. δ(‰) values are normally reported relative to the internationally agreed standards (R_{std}): Vienna-Standard Mean Ocean Water (V-SMOW) for δ^2H and $\delta^{18}O$, Vienna-Pee Dee Belemnite (V-PDB) for $\delta^{13}C$, air for $\delta^{15}N$, Vienna-Canyon Diablo Troilite for $\delta^{34}S$, and strontium carbonate (National Institute of Standards and Technology Standard Reference Material 987) for $\delta^{87}Sr$ (Brand et al., 2014). A positive δ(‰) value indicates that the sample has relatively more of the heavy isotope than does the standard while a negative δ(‰) value indicates that the sample has relatively less of the heavy isotope compared to the standard (Sulzman, 2007; Carter and Barwick, 2011). The biological, biochemical, and climatic causes of these delta value differences are addressed in the following section.

9.1.2 Isotope Fractionation Processes

The use of stable isotope analysis for food authentication is based on the fact that several processes and reactions (biological, biochemical, physical, chemical, etc.) cause isotope fractionation and consequently generate unique isotopic signatures. Stable isotopes of an element have slightly different chemical and physical properties because of their differences in atomic mass. As a consequence, the strength of chemical bonds involving these different isotopes is usually different. A molecule that contains the heavy mass isotope (eg, ^{13}C) is usually more stable than a molecule that contains the light mass isotope (^{12}C) (Kendall and Caldwell, 1998; Sulzman, 2007). In nature, isotopic fractionations are primarily caused by two mechanisms denoted equilibrium (also called thermodynamic or exchange) or kinetic fractionation. In equilibrium fractionation reactions, the distribution of isotopes differs between chemical substances (reactant vs product) or phases (eg, vapor vs liquid) when a reaction is in equilibrium. It is thus assumed that reactants and products are in contact in a closed system, in which reactions are reversible. In equilibrium exchange reactions, the heavier isotope tends to accumulate where bonds are strongest, that is, in the most dense phase, in the phase with the highest oxidation state, or in the compound having the largest molecular mass (Kendall and Caldwell, 1998; Sulzman, 2007). An example of fractionation during phase changes is the condensation of water vapor in rain clouds, which become enriched in the heavier isotopes ^2H and ^{18}O in the water phase, while the light isotopes ^1H and ^{16}O remain in the vapor phase (Kendall and Caldwell, 1998). These fractionation processes can be of great importance for geographical authentications of food commodities based on water isotopes.

The second mechanism—kinetic fractionation—occurs in irreversible or unidirectional reactions. An example is evaporation of water from an open system or loss of N as ammonia (NH_3) to the atmosphere when applying organic fertilizers rich in ammonium (NH_4^+) to agricultural crops. Bond strength and isotope velocity are important in kinetic fractionation reactions, which means that lighter isotopes accumulate in products and residual reactants become enriched in the heavy isotope. Kinetic fractionations are normally associated with processes such as evaporation, diffusion, dissociation reactions, and enzymatic effects and are often much larger than those caused by equilibrium fractionation (Sulzman, 2007). Thus isotopic signatures caused by kinetic fractionations can be important for authentication of food products according to their agricultural production system (eg, organically grown plant products—Section 9.3.2). An overview of selected elements, their stable isotopes, and relative abundances and the corresponding delta notation is shown in Table 9.1. In addition, a selection of the major fractionation processes and the available associated information of relevance to food authenticity testing is presented. As a very general rule, hydrogen and oxygen isotopic data in food products are linked to the hydrogen and oxygen isotope data of water from the specific geographical origin. Carbon is linked to the climatic conditions and the water use efficiency of crops (including C3- or C4-plant species) while nitrogen isotopes are more related to agricultural practices. Sulfur isotopes are affected by geology, volcanic activity, the distance from the sea, and certain anthropogenic effects. Strontium is affected by other fractionation processes than the bioelements and is more related to geology. In addition, SIRA of several other elements has also proven suitable for authentication such as boron (B), magnesium (Mg), and lead (Pb); these have been described elsewhere (Serra et al., 2005; Drivelos and Georgiou, 2012; Laursen et al., 2013).

The fractionation processes described often cause unique isotopic signatures of plant-based food products. These signatures are often sufficiently strong to verify the authenticity of a product as described in detail in Section 9.3. In addition, isotopic signatures have been investigated for assessing the dietary history in animal ecology and thereby for authenticating animal products such as meat, eggs, and dairy products (Capuano et al., 2013; Inácio and Chalk, 2015). In the following section the principles behind stable isotope analysis and recent technological developments will be addressed.

9.2 Measurements, Instrumentation, and Applications

Analytical instrumentation for SIRA has improved during the past decade and today a number of analytical techniques can deliver sufficient mass resolution and precision. Instruments are becoming increasingly user-friendly and novel software developments are automating previously time-consuming and challenging tasks such as instrument tuning and data analysis. EA-CF-IRMS is often the preferred instrument choice for food authentications as it allows efficient sample conversion from organic to gas form and a precision that is often comparable to dual inlet systems. Novel EA-CF-IRMS instruments increasingly allow simultaneous SIRA of several elements (eg, CNS, HCNS, or HO) because of new sample inlet design, improved gas species separation techniques, larger linear dynamic ranges, etc. In addition, the possibility for hyphenating IRMS with different analytical techniques is increasing, which directs SIRA from traditional bulk tissue analysis toward analysis of specific food compounds. Liquid chromatography (LC)-MS-IRMS is, for example, used for C isotope analysis for honey authenticity testing and several applications of gas chromatography-combustion (GC)-C-IRMS such as determination of synthetic or natural food ingredients are appearing (van Leeuwen et al., 2014). In addition, other analytical techniques for stable isotope analysis such as nuclear magnetic resonance (NMR), inductively coupled plasma (ICP)-based mass spectrometry, thermal ionization mass spectrometry (TIMS), etc. and the increasing use of multivariate statistics for data analysis will also be described in the following sections.

9.2.1 Measurement Principles

Despite its many years of use for food authentication, the overall principle of SIRA is more or less the same. For IRMS-based analysis the following steps must be conducted: (1) sample preparation (including preparation of calibration samples), (2) instrument tuning, (3) analyte conversion (often from organic to gas form), (4) analyte analysis, (5) data analysis, and (6) interpretation of analytical results (Fig. 9.1).

In the sample preparation phase, the most common procedure for solid samples is drying and homogenization prior to sample weighing. Sometimes removal of lipids is included (depending on sample type), as, for example, carbohydrates, proteins, and lipids from the same source possess systematically different hydrogen and carbon isotope ratios. As the instrument must be tuned for the highest sensitivity, stability, and linearity, the sample weight is, in principle, of minor importance as long as it produces signals comparable to reference gases and calibration standards. However, for the best analytical results it is recommended that sample weights are comparable and that duplicate (or even triplicate in the case of S) analysis of each sample is conducted. If possible, it is recommended that calibration standards are of the same type as the test samples (matrix matched) (further details in Section 9.2.3). The sample sequence should include blank samples and several calibration standards (in-house reference materials) covering a wide delta range at the beginning and the end of each sequence. In addition, the same sample should be repeated across the sequence to enable drift correction. It is also recommended that reference gas peaks for each sample are included to correct for instrument stability (Carter and Barwick, 2011). As previously mentioned, SIRA of several elements can be conducted simultaneously, but if sample concentrations of each element differ too much, several weight amounts of each sample must be included. This can be the case for simultaneous CNS analysis of plant tissue as the ratio of, for example, C and S can be ~400. Post-analysis, data quality is evaluated using blanks, calibration standards, and drift controls. Subsequently, the delta values obtained are compared to data available in the literature or reference sample databases and interpretations are made (further detailed later). Several deviations of the described measurement procedure exist. An example is H and O isotope analysis of liquids where an H_2 or CO_2 equilibration procedure,

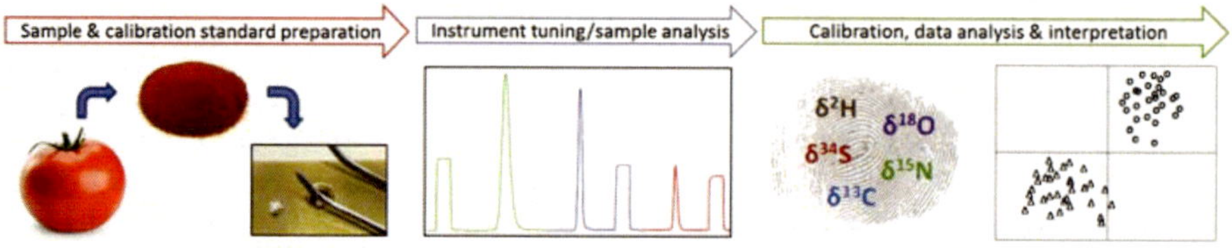

Figure 9.1 Exemplified work flow of traditional stable isotope ratio analysis (SIRA).

respectively, is often utilized (eg, for wine authenticity testing) (Christoph et al., 2015). For a description of LC-IRMS and GC-C-IRMS analysis we refer the reader to review articles by Godin and McCullagh (2011) and van Leeuwen et al. (2014).

9.2.2 Instrumentation

As analytical food authenticity testing is conducted at the natural abundance isotope level (nonenriched samples), specific requirements regarding sample resolution and precision must be accommodated. In this section, the main analytical techniques for the low mass range elements (H, C, N, O, and S) will first be discussed. Subsequently, techniques for SIRA of high mass elements such as Sr will be discussed and finally recent developments regarding compound-specific isotope analysis will be presented. Stable isotope analysis of H, C, N, O, and S is normally conducted by EA-CF-IRMS (Table 9.2). Continuous flow (CF) refers to the fact that sample gases are carried into the source of the mass spectrometer by a continuous helium carrier gas flow. Prior to ionization, mass separation, and ion detection, simple gases of H, C, N, O, or S are produced (H_2, CO_2, N_2, CO, and SO_2, respectively). Conversion to gases is most often conducted by Dumas combustion at 1050−1150° (for CNS) or pyrolysis at 1350−1450° (for HO). The use of a dedicated magnetic sector field for separation and discrete Faraday cups for simultaneous quantification of several ion beams allows

Table 9.2 Selected Analytical Methods for Stable Isotope Analysis and the Parameters Traditionally Measured in Authenticity Studies Using These Techniques (Godin and McCullagh, 2011; Drivelos and Georgiou, 2012; Vanhaecke and Degryse, 2012; Laursen et al., 2014; Van Leeuwen et al., 2014)

Analytical Technique	Abbreviation	Elements Often Measured
Elemental analyzer-continuous flow-isotope ratio mass spectrometry	EA-CF-IRMS[a]	H, C, N, O, S
Gas chromatography-combustion-IRMS	GC-C-IRMS	H, C, N, O
Liquid chromatography-IRMS	LC-IRMS	C
Inductively coupled plasma-mass spectrometry	ICP-MS	B, Sr, Pb
Multicollector-ICP-MS	MC-ICP-MS	B, Mg, Sr, Os, Pb
Thermal ionization mass spectrometry	TIMS	B, Sr, Pb
High-resolution-nuclear magnetic resonance	HR-NMR	H, C
Site-specific isotopic fractionation-nuclear magnetic resonance	SNIF-NMR	H, C

[a]Often referred to as EA-IRMS or simply IRMS.

isotope ratio precisions in the range of 0.01−0.2‰. IRMS is thus highly suitable for natural abundance stable isotope analysis (Table 9.2). However, for elements that cannot be converted to gases (eg, B, Sr) other analytical techniques must be used.

Inductively coupled plasma-mass spectrometry (ICP-MS) also allows stable isotope analysis although superior isotope precisions are obtained by high-resolution instruments [eg, multicollector (MC)-ICP-MS]. The use of several ion collectors, each dedicated to specific isotopes, makes IRMS and MC-ICP-MS superior to quadrupole ICP-MS. However, because of high backgrounds and the specific sample preparations used for ICP-based instruments, SIRA of H, N, and O is not possible. Instead, ICP-based instruments are used for elements such as B, Mg, and high mass range elements such as Sr and Pb. However, MC-ICP-MS analysis often relies on careful sample preparation prior to analysis involving chromatographic steps to remove elements that might otherwise cause spectral interferences (Bolou-Bi et al., 2009; Yang, 2009; Asfaha et al., 2011). Significantly higher operational costs are therefore associated with MC-ICP-MS analyses compared to IRMS. For Sr isotope analysis, the most widely used analytical techniques are TIMS and MC-ICP-MS. Because Sr is isobarically interfered with Kr and Rb, TIMS is especially suitable for ^{87}Rb and ^{87}Sr as both elements can be separated from the filament by stepwise heating. Further details regarding stable isotope analysis of elements in the high mass range can be found elsewhere (Vanhaecke and Degryse, 2012). High-resolution NMR and site-specific natural isotope fractionation (SNIF)-NMR have also proven valuable for authenticity testing of food products (for H and C isotope analysis in different sites of a given molecule). In the following section specific challenges associated with some of the most popular approaches for measuring stable isotope ratios will be discussed.

9.2.3 Bulk Tissue Analysis and Applications

The most common analytical technique for SIRA-based authenticity testing is EA-CF-IRMS. Stable isotope analysis can be applied to bulk samples, consisting of a group of compounds (bulk stable isotope analysis, BSIA) or on specific individual compounds (compound-specific isotope analysis, CSIA, see Section 9.2.4). Of these two, BSIA is the most straightforward because, normally, it does not require complicated sample preparation prior to analysis. Most often freeze-drying of the bulk sample or defatting and freeze-drying is required prior to homogenization and analysis. SIRA is ideally conducted using reference materials that have chemical and physical properties, including isotopic composition, similar to that of the measured samples. Furthermore, samples and standards should be processed in the same manner during preparation and analysis (identical treatment principle) (Brand et al., 2014). The sample preparation process can vary between samples and standards and could be a significant source of isotopic fractionation and/or contamination. Another challenge is that well-calibrated isotopic reference materials for all types of sample compounds and matrices are not available. In practice, primary and secondary isotopic reference materials are therefore used. Primary reference materials define the zero or anchor point of a scale and have assigned stable isotope values that are internationally recognized with no associated uncertainty. Secondary isotopic reference materials have values normally determined within intercollaborative studies involving several laboratories but their certified values cannot be permanently fixed as they could be updated according to improved methods and instrumentation. Normally, in routine laboratories, working standards, possibly of the same matrix as the samples, are used. These are calibrated against primary or secondary reference materials and are used in each sample sequence. For the normalization of data and to assure linearity, two reference materials or calibrated working standards with isotope values covering the variability range of the samples should ideally be used for each element, as suggested by the International Union of Pure and Applied Chemistry (Brand et al., 2014). In particular, for δ^2H and $\delta^{18}O$, data should be normalized against the V-SMOW–SLAP (Standard Light Antarctic Precipitation, International Atomic Energy Agency, IAEA) scale, and, for $\delta^{13}C$, to the V-PDB-LSVEC (lithium carbonate) scale.

Currently, several isotope reference materials are available for each of the elements H, C, N, O, and S [for a list of stable isotope reference material suppliers, we refer the reader to Brand et al. (2014)]. However, at the moment there are no suitable reference materials applicable for multi-isotopic analysis. This could significantly improve the time and costs associated with such analyses. In the case of δ^2H analysis by IRMS, the H atoms in exchangeable positions (ie, when bound to O as in protein-rich material) have to be taken into account, as they could exchange with atmospheric water vapor, leading to potentially erroneous results if not considered. A number of methods have been developed to overcome this problem: the comparative equilibration technique (Wassenaar and Hobson, 2003), standard ambient temperature equilibration (Qi and Coplen, 2011), and steam equilibration (Meier-Augenstein et al., 2013) but the debate on this issue is still ongoing (Coplen and Qi, 2013). Furthermore, for δ^2H analysis of nonwater samples, only a few reference materials exist at the moment (NBS 22—mineral oil ($\delta^2H = -119.6‰$), NBS 30—biotite ($-65.7‰$), IAEA CH7—polyethylene foil ($-100.3‰$)) and only a few organic reference materials with exchangeable H atoms are available and recognized for the determination of δ^2H (U.S. Geological Survey, USGS 42—Tibetan human hair ($-78.5‰$), USGS 43—Indian human hair ($-50.3‰$), CBS—Caribou Hoof Standard ($-197.0‰$) and KHS—Kudu Horn Standard ($-54.1‰$)). Further developments regarding stable isotope reference materials are thus required.

When isotope ratio analysis is being used for authentication or traceability purposes, comparison with a reference dataset is required. Crucial aspects of the database are that the samples collected have to be surely authentic, available in a statistically sufficient number, and representative of the "situation" to be considered (eg, geographical area or agricultural practice). Some examples of databanks currently used are the official EU wine databank, databanks created within the framework of specific projects (eg, the EU projects PURE JUICE and TRACE) or on a requirement to detect specific fraud cases (eg, butter circular trade or caviar), as well as databanks built by private associations or consortia [eg, the European Fruit Juice Association (AIJN) for fruit juices or Grana Padano Protected Designation of Origin (PDO) cheese]. However, for most food commodities, databanks are not available and this should represent a future point of action as is, for example, the case for the current FoodIntegrity project (www.foodintegrity.eu).

A number of isotopic methods have been officially recognized since 1987 for the detection of food frauds in several commodities (some of them are listed in Table 9.3). Specifically, $(D/H)_I$ determination in ethanol obtained by the fermentation of wine, must, and fruit juice (OIV-MA-AS311-05, AOAC 995.17) has been officially recognized for the determination of fraudulent chaptalization using beet-derived sugar. Determination of $\delta^{13}C$ in ethanol from the fermentation of wine, must, and fruit juice (OIV-MA-AS312-07, AOAC 2004.01) has been shown to be suitable for verifying the addition of sugar derived from C4 plants. Similarly, AOAC method 998.12 allows comparison of $\delta^{13}C$ determined in honey and in proteins extracted from honey and is used as an internal standard to highlight the addition of exogenous sugars from C4 plants. Determination of $\delta^{18}O$ of vegetal water of wine, must, and fruit juices (OIV-MA-AS2-12, ENV 12141) has been officially recognized for the detection of the illegal watering down of these products. Regarding vinegar, methods based on SNIF-NMR and IRMS have been officially accepted for determining the botanical origin of acetic acid and for revealing addition of synthetic acetic acid (OIV-OENO-527-2015, OIV-OENO-510-2013). In addition, $\delta^{18}O$ of water is acknowledged as a method for determining if vinegar has been produced from fresh grapes or from dried grapes with subsequent water addition (OIV-OENO-511-2013). Finally, the isotopic signature of Grana Padano cheese has been officially recognized in its PDO production protocol and has been used for the detection of mislabeled products (EU Reg. 584/2011).

9.2.4 Compound-Specific Stable Isotope Analysis and Applications

One of the very recent trends in SIRA-based food authenticity testing is compound-specific isotope analysis (CSIA). It has been observed in several studies that, compared to bulk samples, additional isotopic information can be obtained by focusing on isotopic signatures of specific food compounds. CSIA can be based on both off-line and online compound isolation prior to isotope analysis. A well-known and long-used application is the carbon isotopic composition of bulk honey versus honey protein (AOAC 998.12). Another example is the carbon isotopic composition of sugars, pulp, and acids derived from fruit juices (method of internal standardization). Compound-specific analysis of oxygen, relying on off-line isolation of the compounds of interest prior to introduction into the IRMS, has also recently shown promise for food authentication. It has been demonstrated that $\delta^{18}O$ analysis of plant-derived nitrate can generate information suitable for authenticating organic plant products (Laursen et al., 2013; Mihailova et al., 2014). In these studies, it was demonstrated that CSIA of nitrate eliminated limitations of bulk tissue $\delta^{15}N$ analyses when attempting to discriminate conventional plant products, fertilized with synthetic fertilizers, from organic plant products, fertilized with legume-based green manures (further details in Section 9.3.2). Methods have also been developed for online compound separation and isotope analysis for organic authentication. GC-C-IRMS was, for example, recently used for C and N isotope analysis of amino acids and proved superior to bulk tissue analysis for authenticity testing of organic wheat (Paolini et al., 2015). GC-C-IRMS analysis of C isotopes has also been used for detecting non-natural

Table 9.3 Selected Acknowledged Methods for Authenticity Testing of Certain Food Matrices

Method	Matrix	Parameters Measured	Analytical Method	Databank	References
OIV-MA-AS311-05	Wine, must	$(D/H)_I$ and $(D/H)_{II}$ of ethanol	^{2}H-SNIF-NMR	EU wine databank	EU Reg. 555/2008
OIV-MA-AS312-07	Wine, must	$^{13}C/^{12}C$ of ethanol	IRMS	EU wine databank	EU Reg. 555/2008
OIV-MA-AS2-12	Wine, must	$^{18}O/^{16}O$ of water	IRMS	EU wine databank	EU Reg. 555/2008
CEN-ENV 12140	Fruit juice	$^{13}C/^{12}C$ of sugar	IRMS	AIJN, literature	Kornexl et al. (1996), Martin et al. (1996), Rossmann et al. (1997), Simpkins et al. (2000), Rummel et al. (2010), Bontempo et al. (2014a)
CEN-ENV 13070	Fruit juice	$^{13}C/^{12}C$ of pulp	IRMS	AIJN, literature	
CEN-ENV 12141	Fruit juice	$^{18}O/^{16}O$ of water	IRMS	AIJN, literature	
AOAC 995.17	Fruit juice	$(D/H)_I$ and $(D/H)_{II}$ of ethanol	^{2}H-SNIF-NMR	AIJN, literature	
AOAC 2004.01	Fruit juice, maple syrup	$^{13}C/^{12}C$ of ethanol	IRMS	AIJN, literature	
CEN, EN 16466-1:2012; OIV-OENO-527-2015	Vinegar	$(D/H)CH_3$ of acetic acid	^{2}H-SNIF-NMR	EU wine databank	EU Reg. 555/2008
CEN, EN 16466-2:2012; OIV-OENO-510-2013	Vinegar	$^{13}C/^{12}C$ of acetic acid	IRMS	EU wine databank	EU Reg. 555/2008
CEN, EN 16466-3:2012; OIV-OENO-511-2013	Vinegar	$^{18}O/^{16}O$ of water	IRMS	EU wine databank	EU Reg. 555/2008
Camin et al. (2015a)	Cheese	$^{13}C/^{12}C$, $^2H/^1H$, $^{15}N/^{14}N$, $^{34}S/^{32}S$ of defatted cheese	IRMS	PDO Grana Padano and Parmigiano Reggiano databank	EU Reg. 584/2011
AOAC 998.12	Honey	$^{13}C/^{12}C$ in honey and extracted proteins	IRMS	Literature	White et al. (1998)

$(D/H)_I$ and $(D/H)_{II}$ refers to the isotopic composition at specific sites of a given molecule.
AIJN, European Fruit Juice Association; *AOAC*, Association of Official Analytical Chemists; *CEN*, European Committee for Standardization; *OIV*, International Organisation of Vine and Wine.

strawberry aromas in food (Schipilliti et al., 2011) and for authenticating lemon essential oils (Schipilliti et al., 2012). This work was further developed in a recent study that focused on GC-C-IRMS analysis of citrus essential oils. It was demonstrated that the nature of orange flavor in food products, liqueurs, beverages, etc. can be evaluated using $\delta^{13}C$ values of volatiles (Schipilliti et al., 2015). One study on extra virgin olive oils (EVOOs) demonstrated that $\delta^{13}C$ values of fatty acids in combination with $\delta^{13}C$ of bulk oils are reliable and powerful markers of the geographical origin of olive oils (Faberi et al., 2014). Combined with multivariate statistics, the $\delta^{13}C$ values of bulk oil and individual fatty acids provided a superior discrimination between samples of different geographical origins compared to the fatty acid composition. Because of the often superior discriminative power of CSIA compared to BSIA, further method developments are expected in the future along with fundamental studies aimed at unraveling the key processes controlling the isotopic composition of specific chemical compounds in food products.

9.2.5 *Multivariate Statistics—Chemometrics*

It is increasingly acknowledged that single isotope parameters can rarely supply reliable information for food authentication alone. Instead, several stable isotope parameters and the combination with data from other analytical techniques require multivariate methods of data evaluation. Today, multivariate statistics (chemometrics) is often applied to data as a standard procedure for extraction of latent information and to provide a fast data overview prior to univariate statistical analysis or multivariate classification analysis (Berrueta et al., 2007; Oulhote et al., 2011). This approach has been used efficiently in numerous food authenticity studies and, for example, for investigating the geographical or agricultural origin of samples. Chemometric methods can be roughly divided into two categories: (1) unsupervised and (2) supervised methods. The unsupervised methods include principal component analysis and cluster analysis. These methods are primarily descriptive of the underlying data structure, while supervised methods such as linear discriminant analysis, canonical discriminant analysis, soft independent modeling of class analogy, and partial least squares discriminant analysis can be used to sort samples into predefined classes and subsequently to enable classification of unknown samples. Supervised methods thus rely on prior assumptions regarding sample groupings (Berrueta et al., 2007). It is common to both unsupervised and supervised methods that the multivariate models must be carefully validated to avoid overfitting and overoptimistic classification results (Kjeldahl and Bro, 2010). This represents one of the pitfalls in authenticity studies. Even though numerous examples of applications of chemometrics are described in the scientific literature for food authentications, there is still no harmonization and agreement for assessing and validating results of such multivariate analyses. Nevertheless, multivariate data evaluation is currently considered a valuable and powerful screening tool. Furthermore, the importance of combining an isotopic signature with other variables (eg, minerals or metabolite profiles) should not be overlooked, as they often provide invaluable additional information assisting with interpretation of the data.

In addition to chemometrics, geospatial modeling is increasingly being used to authenticate the geographical origin of food products (Van Der Veer, 2013).

The term "isoscapes" refers specifically to geospatial prediction models based on stable isotopes. These are geographical models based on stable isotope ratios that can be used to describe patterns expected for certain regions (West et al., 2010). They are based on databases but also on geological and climatic information. At least for elements such as hydrogen and oxygen in water, they must be updated yearly to take into account variation caused by climatic differences and climate change, even if attempts have been described for prediction of these stable isotope data from temperature, air humidity, and amount of precipitation. Recent examples of the use of isoscapes for food authentication are especially linked to water isotopes in wine (Hermann and Voerkelius, 2008; Camin et al., 2015b), coffee (Carter et al., 2015b), milk (Ehtesham et al., 2013), and strontium isotopes in water and beef (Kelly, 2007; Voerkelius et al., 2010). Application of isoscapes, even on a larger scale, has been described for human hair with regard to sulfur isotopes in the United States (Valenzuela et al., 2011) and nitrogen and carbon isotopes worldwide (Hulsemann et al., 2015). Despite these initial and promising studies, one should keep in mind that for a reliable assignment of geographical origin, which should, for example, be used in court cases too, a database of authentic samples is still required and isoscapes may only indicate if there is a chance that the isotopic ratios of certain elements can differentiate products from different origins.

9.3 Case Studies

SIRA is now routinely used in several laboratories for food authenticity testing. Numerous commercial laboratories perform authenticity testing of a wide array of food commodities and suspected fraud cases. However, interpretation of the generated data is still challenging as databases of authentic samples are lacking or are restricted as proprietary know-how of individual laboratories. Consequently, private companies and public bodies (eg, public food control institutes) are building their own databases and large EU projects such as the FoodIntegrity project (www.foodintegrity.eu) aim to assemble and make such data publically available. In the following section, we will present examples of cases in which stable isotope analysis has been used for verifying the authenticity of food. We will focus on geographical origin (Table 9.4), agricultural production form (Table 9.5), and a few other cases (for selected food commodities) (Table 9.6). The lists will be representative of the current trends and possibilities using stable isotopes but will not be exhaustive. The combination with other analytical methods such as multielemental analysis or metabolomic profiling is also outside the scope of this chapter and has been reviewed elsewhere (Drivelos and Georgiou, 2012; Capuano et al., 2013; Laursen et al., 2014).

9.3.1 Stable Isotope Analysis for Verifying Geographical Origin

Stable isotope analysis, especially if applied as multielement stable isotope analysis, has been used for several years to detect the geographical origin of raw materials and premium products by linking the stable isotope pattern of products with those

Table 9.4 Selected Food Commodities for Which Geographical Origin Has Been Authenticated Using SIRA

Food Commodity	Analytical Technique	Parameters Measured	References
Extra virgin olive oil	IRMS, GC-C-IRMS	H, C, O	Camin et al. (2010a,b), Faberi et al. (2014)
PDO cheese	IRMS	H, C, N, S	Bontempo et al. (2012), Camin et al. (2012)
Meat	IRMS	H, C, N, S	Schmidt et al. (2005), Camin et al. (2007), Heaton et al. (2008), Perini et al. (2009), Bong et al. (2010), Osorio et al. (2011)
Honey	IRMS	H, C, N, S	Kropf et al. (2010a,b), Schellenberg et al. (2010)
Fruits and vegetables	IRMS	H, C, N, O, S	Meylahn et al. (2006), Longobardi et al. (2015), Mimmo et al. (2015)
Tomatoes	TIMS	Sr	Trincherini et al. (2014)
Seafood	IRMS	H, C, N, O	Carter et al. (2015a), Ortea and Gallardo (2015)

Table 9.5 Selected Food Commodities for Which the Agricultural Origin Has Been Authenticated Using SIRA

Food Commodity	Analytical Technique	Parameters Measured	References
Cereals	IRMS, MC-ICP-MS	H, C, N, O, S, Mg	Laursen et al. (2013)
Wheat	GC-C-IRMS (CSIA)	C, N (amino acids)	Paolini et al. (2015)
Fruits	IRMS	H, C, N, O, S,	Camin et al. (2011), Bat et al. (2012)
Vegetables	IRMS	N	Sturm et al. (2011), Flores et al. (2013)
Vegetables	IRMS (CSIA)	N, O (nitrate)	Laursen et al. (2013), Mihailova et al. (2014)
Eggs	IRMS	C, N	Rogers et al. (2015)
Milk	IRMS	C, N	Molkentin and Giesemann (2010), Chung et al. (2014)
Meat (cattle)	IRMS	C, N, S	Bahar et al. (2008)
Fish	IRMS	C, N	Molkentin et al. (2015)

Table 9.6 Selected Recent Adulteration Case Studies Other Than Geographical or Agricultural Origin Determination

Food Commodity	Authenticity Case	Analytical Technique	Parameters Measured	References
Fruit juice	Sugar addition	IRMS	C	Tosun (2014)
Vinegar	Sugar/water addition, synthetic acetic acid	IRMS/SNIF-NMR	H, C, O	Thomas and Jamin (2009), Camin et al. (2013)
Tomato passata	Water addition	IRMS	O	Bontempo et al. (2014b)
Caffeine	Synthetic caffeine addition	GC-C-IRMS	C	Zhang et al. (2012)
Cider	CO_2 addition	GC-C-IRMS	C	Gaillard et al. (2013)
Vanillin	Synthetic vanillin addition	GC-C-IRMS	C	Greule et al. (2010)
Essential oils	Synthetic or natural adulterants	GC-C-IRMS	C	Schipilliti et al. (2010, 2011, 2012, 2015)

of the natural environments from which they are derived or purport to be derived (Rossmann, 2001; Kelly et al., 2002, 2005). Claims of geographical origin of particular food premium products have "legal" basis within the Regulations on Protected Designations of Origin (PDO), Protected Geographical Indication (PGI), and Traditional Speciality Guaranteed (TSG) stated by EC Regulation 2081/92/EEC and subsequent amendments (510/2006/EC and 1151/2012/EC). These EU Regulations provide a set of common rules across countries to register and protect geographical names used to identify food products and traditional production processes. Furthermore, mandatory rules on origin labeling currently exist in Europe for several sectors, such as honey (EU Reg. 1308/2013), fruits and vegetables (EC Reg. 1234/2007), fish (EU Reg. 1379/2013), beef and beef products (EC Reg. 1760/2000), olive oil (EU Reg. 29/2012), wine (EC Reg. 1234/2007), eggs (EC Reg. 589/2008), and meat of swine, sheep, goat, and poultry (EU Reg. 1337/2013). In parallel with the legislation on the geographical origin of food products, the number of studies on this topic applying stable isotope ratio analysis has also grown (Table 9.4). An example involves PDO cheeses that can cost more than twice the generic imitation cheeses and can be distinguished from the cheaper products on the basis of the isotopic fingerprint (Bontempo et al., 2012; Camin et al., 2012). Furthermore, in the specific case of Grana Padano, the isotopic method has been officially recognized for the authentication of the product (EU Reg. 584/2011). Extra virgin olive oil (EVOO) is another "premium" product that by law has the geographical origin compulsorily declared on the product label. Studies carried out on it showed that the combination of $\delta^{13}C$ with $\delta^{18}O$ and $\delta^{2}H$ in bulk oil (Camin et al., 2010a,b) or with $\delta^{13}C$ of EVOO fatty acids (Faberi et al., 2014) were effective, even if not always completely, in differentiating the geographical origin of European and Italian EVOOs. Some recent applications on the determination of the geographical origin of vegetables and fruits included the combination of $\delta^{13}C$ and $\delta^{15}N$ of fruits and subcomponents (peel, seeds, pulp) that allowed differentiation of the geographical origin of apples produced in two regions of Northern Italy (Mimmo et al., 2015) as well as of $\delta^{2}H$, $\delta^{13}C$, $\delta^{15}N$, $\delta^{18}O$, and $\delta^{34}S$ to distinguish Canadian and Italian lentils (Longobardi et al., 2015). Using the $\delta^{2}H$ and $\delta^{18}O$ of asparagus juice and protein combined with $\delta^{13}C$ of proteins and cellulose of asparagus, a differentiation between asparagus from the German region Beelitz and from Poland was possible (Meylahn et al., 2006). The isotope ratio of $\delta^{87}Sr$ was successfully applied to differentiate Italian and Chinese tomatoes (Trincherini et al., 2014). Regarding honey, Schellenberg et al. (2010) determined the stable isotope ratios of H, C, N, and S in honey proteins and found that the last two parameters provided the maximum discrimination in determining the origin of honey from 20 European regions. Kropf et al. (2010a,b) differentiated honeys from Slovenian macroregions using C and N isotope ratios.

With regard to meat, $\delta^{13}C$ and $\delta^{15}N$ of fat and protein in lambs were able to discriminate lamb from Italy, France, Spain, the United Kingdom, Greece, and Iceland reared with the same feeding regime (Piasentier et al., 2003). Beef samples were differentiated "globally" (Argentina vs. Germany) using $\delta^{2}H$ and $\delta^{18}O$ of meat water (Boner and Forstel, 2004), and "locally" (various German farms) using $\delta^{13}C$, $\delta^{15}N$, and $\delta^{34}S$ of defatted meat. Significant differences were found between $\delta^{2}H$, $\delta^{13}C$, $\delta^{15}N$, $\delta^{18}O$, and $\delta^{34}S$ of defatted meat of lamb samples from different European regions (Camin et al., 2007; Perini et al., 2009), and between beef from several European and non-European countries (Osorio et al., 2011). $\delta^{2}H$ and $\delta^{18}O$ of beef lipid were found to be well correlated with the latitude of the production region (Heaton et al., 2008). Bong et al. (2010) determined $\delta^{13}C$, $\delta^{15}N$, and $\delta^{18}O$ in defatted beef meat and did generally achieve successful discrimination between samples of different global origins circulating on the Korean markets. Finally, poultry from different countries was distinguished on the basis of $\delta^{18}O$ of water extracted from meat (Franke et al., 2008). Two of the more recent applications of SIRA for geographical authentication have focused on seafood (Carter et al., 2015a; Ortea and Gallardo, 2015). Ortea and Gallardo (2015) obtained discrimination between wild and farmed shrimps, different species, and different geographical origins, using $\delta^{13}C$ and $\delta^{15}N$ with or without inclusion of the elemental composition. Carter et al. (2015a) determined $\delta^{2}H$, $\delta^{13}C$, $\delta^{15}N$, and $\delta^{18}O$ in the shells, chitin, and meat of Australian prawns and Asian prawns imported into Australia and found strong differences between geographical origins for all the measured parameters.

9.3.2 *Stable Isotope Analysis for Verifying Agricultural Origin*

In this section we will primarily focus on the use of stable isotope analysis for authenticity testing of organic products. The organic sector has steadily increased during recent decades and now holds significant market shares of numerous food products in several European countries (Lernoud and Willer, 2015). Organic products are often sold at premium prices compared to their conventional counterparts and are thus at risk of fraudulent activities and adulteration. However, no analytical methods are officially recognized as being able to verify if all regulations of organic production have been followed. Organic products within the European Union are produced according to the European Community Council Regulation EC No. 834/2007 and Commission Regulation EC No. 889/2008 (www.ec.europa.eu). Similar regulations are found in other countries, such as the National Organic Program in the United States (www.ams.usda.gov). According to these regulations and programs, synthetic fertilizers and pesticides are prohibited in organic plant production. Instead, such production is based on the use of organic fertilizers including composts, animal manures, and green manures (often legumes). Consequently, the regulations of organic plant products do potentially represent significant differences in fertilizer type and amount compared to conventional agriculture. On this basis, numerous studies have investigated the possibility of using stable isotope analysis for authentication of organic plant products (Table 9.5).

The majority of studies based on SIRA for organic authentication of plant products have focused on nitrogen and it has generally been concluded that $\delta^{15}N$ is the best marker for revealing the fertilization history of a plant (Camin et al., 2011; Sturm et al., 2011; Bat et al., 2012; Flores et al., 2013). Laursen et al. (2013) did, for example, use $\delta^{15}N$ for discriminating organic and conventional wheat, barley, and potatoes that had been fertilized with either animal manure or synthetic fertilizers, respectively. Synthetic fertilizers often have $\delta^{15}N$ values close to 0.0‰ because of the atmospheric origin of N in such fertilizers. In comparison, $\delta^{15}N$ values of organic manures are often higher because of significant isotopic fractionation occurring during storage, application, and biological N transformation processes. A strong isotopic discrimination against ^{15}N does, for example, occur because of ammonia volatilization, denitrification, and nitrification prior to plant uptake (Choi et al., 2003). On this basis, $\delta^{15}N$ has been utilized for discriminating organic and conventional plant products in numerous studies. However, as demonstrated by Laursen et al. (2013), $\delta^{15}N$ values are biased by fertilization of organic plants with legume-based green manures. The ability of legumes to fix nitrogen from the atmosphere results in $\delta^{15}N$ values similar to those obtained from plants grown with synthetic fertilizers and thus disqualifies $\delta^{15}N$ as a reliable marker for organic authentication in some cases. Consequently, a few studies have investigated the possibility of using CSIA of nitrate ($\delta^{15}N$, $\delta^{18}O$) (Laursen et al., 2013; Mihailova et al., 2014) and amino acids ($\delta^{13}C$, $\delta^{15}N$) (Paolini et al., 2015) to eliminate the bias caused by specific growth systems. In addition, it is increasingly acknowledged that multiisotopic analysis (H, C, N, O, S) is required to reliably authenticate the agricultural origin of plants.

Authenticity testing of organic animal products using SIRA has also been tested in several studies. Despite promising results being obtained for some animal products, it has been concluded that SIRA-based authenticity testing is more complicated than for organic plant products. For ruminants, $\delta^{13}C$ seems to be a promising marker to discriminate organic and conventional animal products because of the frequent use of maize (C4 plant) in conventional feed. This often results in lower $\delta^{13}C$ values in organic cattle and dairy products. This trend has, for example, been observed for organic and conventional milk (Molkentin and Giesemann, 2010). $\delta^{15}N$ signatures of sheep and cattle have been related to diet signatures with some variability between farms and years although the reasons for $\delta^{15}N$ differences found between organic and conventional milk are still unclear. Promising $\delta^{15}N$ results have been obtained for organic versus conventional eggs with a clear correlation between $\delta^{15}N$ of egg whites and the feeding regimen (Rogers et al., 2015). The stable isotope parameters $\delta^{2}H$, $\delta^{18}O$, and $\delta^{34}S$ have not proven valuable for authenticity testing of animal products. For further information regarding the use of SIRA for authenticity testing of animal products we refer the reader to reviews by Capuano et al. (2013) and Inácio and Chalk (2015). It should be emphasized that, at the present time, no accepted analytical method for authentication of organic animal products exists and further developments regarding new stable isotope markers, CSIA, combinations with other analytical techniques, and database developments are thus required in the future.

9.3.3 Stable Isotope Analysis for Other Food Authenticity Cases

While authenticity testing of the geographical or agricultural origin of food products using stable isotopes is fairly new, several other authenticity cases exist (Table 9.6). Some of the very first fraud cases in the 1970s, in which stable isotope analysis was used, focused on revealing adulteration of honey, fruit juice, or maple syrup with cheaper extenders, such as sugar syrup made from maize or cane carbohydrates, industrially produced acids, or simply water (Rossmann, 2001). Today, stable isotope analysis is still utilized for these fraud cases while several others have arisen. New examples are related to processing, substitution, quality, etc. One of the more extensively investigated matrices in recent years has been vinegar. Thomas and Jamin (2009) coordinated an interlaboratory study and recommended the determination of $^{2}H/^{1}H$ ratio analysis of the methyl site of acetic acid by SNIF-NMR coupled with that of the $^{13}C/^{12}C$ ratio by IRMS to collect complementary information on the botanical origin of acetic acid and to detect adulterations of vinegar using synthetic acetic acid. Furthermore, in the case of wine vinegar, they proposed the determination of $^{18}O/^{16}O$ in water to differentiate wine vinegar from vinegars made from dried grapes. Subsequently, these aspects have been developed in more detail and Camin et al. (2013) proposed two threshold limits for $\delta^{18}O_{water}$ ($-2‰$ and $-5‰$), defined for raw and diluted vinegars produced from fresh grapes, to detect if a vinegar was obtained by fermenting dried grapes and with subsequent rehydration by tap water, a practice not allowed by European Regulations. In addition, $\delta^{18}O$ determined in ethanol has enabled detection of the watering of wine and in some cases of the origin of the ethanol (eg, from grapes, other fruits, or by synthesis) (Camin et al., 2013).

Similar to vinegar, $\delta^{18}O$ determination of vegetal water resulted in a highly effective discrimination of genuine tomato passata from watered-down paste, also in the case of passata previously concentrated up to 11.9°Brix (Bontempo et al., 2014b). In particular, two lower threshold values were proposed: −1.4‰ for "raw" passata and −2.9‰ for passata previously concentrated up to 11.9°Brix. $\delta^{13}C$ was confirmed to be effective in determining the addition of high-fructose corn syrup and glucose syrup from corn starch in mulberry juices (Tosun, 2014). $\delta^{13}C$ also enabled discrimination between natural and synthetic caffeine (Zhang et al., 2012). In particular, two distinguishable groups of caffeine $\delta^{13}C$ values were determined: natural caffeine presented a range of values between −25 and −32‰ whereas lower values were found for synthetic caffeine (−33 and −38‰). Similarly, $\delta^{2}H$ and $\delta^{13}C$ of vanillin, in combination with $\delta^{2}H$ and $\delta^{13}C$ of vanillin methoxyl groups, proved to be reliable parameters for determining vanillin samples from different origins including natural and synthetic samples (Greule et al., 2010). $\delta^{13}C$ of carbon dioxide determined in French ciders effectively determined if the CO_2 was natural or obtained by carbonation with technical CO_2 (Gaillard et al., 2013), a practice not allowed for organic PDO ciders. One last example of recent SIRA applications is the determination of $\delta^{13}C$ of volatile compounds in essential oils such as lemon, bergamot, mandarin, and sweet orange frequently used in the food industry; this approach has been effective in detecting the sophistication of these high-value products with synthetic or natural adulterants (Schipilliti et al., 2010, 2011, 2012, 2015).

9.4 Conclusion and Future Trends

Stable isotope ratio analysis has played a major role in food authenticity testing worldwide. Its applicability to a wide range of food products and the continuous method developments, instrument improvements, and increasing number of fraud cases indicate that its role will become even greater in the future. It is expected that progress in instrument developments will result in more rapid and precise simultaneous multielement stable isotope determinations. New method developments regarding compound-specific isotope ratio analyses are also likely to generate even more specific information that ultimately will lead to more reliable food authentications and improved protection of consumers, honest producers, food processors, retailers, etc. However, as new types of adulterations will inevitably appear, the need for complementation by other analytical techniques may arise. It is therefore expected that future food authentications will be increasingly based on multivariate datasets generated by several analytical techniques (SIRA, NMR, metabolomics, elemental fingerprinting, etc.). The use of chemometrics is therefore expected to increase in the future. Methods based on untargeted screening can help to select suspicious samples that justify application of multielement stable isotope analysis and other highly sophisticated and expensive analytical methods. Finally, development of reference sample databases is currently making food authentication more reliable and comparable. However, further efforts to establish, maintain, and share databases must be undertaken in both the stable isotope community and food sector.

Sources of Further Information

1. Drivelos, S.A., Georgiou, C.A., 2012. Multi-element and multi-isotope-ratio analysis to determine the geographical origin of foods in the European Union. TrAC—Trends in Analytical Chemistry 40, 38–51.
2. Laursen, K.H., et al., 2014. Authentication of organically grown plants—advantages and limitations of atomic spectroscopy for multi-element and stable isotope analysis. TrAC—Trends in Analytical Chemistry 59, 73–82.
3. Roßmann, A., 2013. 3—New approaches for verifying the geographical origin of foods. *New Analytical Approaches for Verifying the Origin of Food*. P. Brereton, Woodhead Publishing: 41–59.
4. Van Leeuwen et al., 2014. Gas chromatography-combustion-isotope ratio mass spectrometry for traceability and authenticity in foods and beverages. Comprehensive Reviews in Food Science and Food Safety 13, 814–837.

Abbreviations

BSIA	Bulk stable isotope analysis
CSIA	Compound-specific isotope analysis
EA-CF-IRMS	Elemental analyzer-continuous flow-isotope ratio mass spectrometry
GC-C-IRMS	Gas chromatography-combustion-IRMS
HR-NMR	High-resolution-nuclear magnetic resonance
LC-IRMS	Liquid chromatography-IRMS
MC-ICP-MS	Multicollector-inductively coupled plasma-mass spectrometry
SIRA	Stable isotope ratio analysis
SNIF-NMR	Site-specific natural isotope fractionation-nuclear magnetic resonance
TIMS	Thermal ionization mass spectrometry

Acknowledgments

The authors acknowledge the financial support provided by the European Union Seventh Framework Programme (FP7/2007–2013) under the grant agreement number 613688 (FoodIntegrity) and the Danish Council for Independent Research—Technology and Production Sciences via the COM-ISO project (DFF-1337-00055).

References

Asfaha, D.G., Quetel, C.R., Thomas, F., Horacek, M., Wimmer, B., Heiss, G., Dekant, C., Deters-Itzelsberger, P., Hoelzl, S., Rummel, S., Brach-Papa, C., Van Bocxstaele, M., Jamin, E., Baxter, M., Heinrich, K., Kelly, S., Bertoldi, D., Bontempo, L., Camin, F., Larcher, R., Perini, M., Rossmann, A., Schellenberg, A., Schlicht, C., Froeschl, H., Hoogewerff, J., Ueckermann, H., 2011. Combining isotopic signatures of n((87)Sr)/n((86) Sr) and light stable elements (C, N, O, S) with multi-elemental profiling for the authentication of provenance of European cereal samples. Journal of Cereal Science 53, 170–177.

Bahar, B., Schmidt, O., Moloney, A.P., Scrimgeour, C.M., Begley, I.S., Monahan, F.J., 2008. Seasonal variation in the C, N and S stable isotope composition of retail organic and conventional Irish beef. Food Chemistry 106, 1299–1305.

Bat, K.B., Vidrih, R., Necemer, M., Vodopivec, B.M., Mulic, I., Kump, P., Ogrinc, N., 2012. Characterization of Slovenian apples with respect to their botanical and geographical origin and agricultural production practice. Food Technology and Biotechnology 50, 107–116.

Berglund, M., Wieser, M.E., 2011. Isotopic compositions of the elements 2009 (IUPAC technical report). Pure and Applied Chemistry 83, 397–410.

Berrueta, L.A., Alonso-Salces, R.M., Héberger, K., 2007. Supervised pattern recognition in food analysis. Journal of Chromatography A 1158, 196–214.

Bolou-Bi, E.B., Vigier, N., Brenot, A., Poszwa, A., 2009. Magnesium isotope compositions of natural reference materials. Geostandards and Geoanalytical Research 33, 95–109.

Boner, M., Forstel, H., 2004. Stable isotope variation as a tool to trace the authenticity of beef. Analytical and Bioanalytical Chemistry 378, 301–310.

Bong, Y.-S., Shin, W.-J., Lee, A.R., Kim, Y.-S., Kim, K., Lee, K.-S., 2010. Tracing the geographical origin of beefs being circulated in Korean markets based on stable isotopes. Rapid Communications in Mass Spectrometry 24, 155–159.

Bontempo, L., Lombardi, G., Paoletti, R., Ziller, L., Camin, F., 2012. H, C, N and O stable isotope characteristics of alpine forage, milk and cheese. International Dairy Journal 23, 99–104.

Bontempo, L., Caruso, R., Fiorillo, M., Gambino, G.L., Perini, M., Simoni, M., Traulo, P., Wehrens, R., Gagliano, G., Camin, F., 2014a. Stable isotope ratios of H, C, N and O in Italian citrus juices. Journal of Mass Spectrometry 49, 785–791.

Bontempo, L., Ceppa, F.A., Perini, M., Tonon, A., Gagliano, G., Marianella, R.M., Marega, M., Trifiro, A., Camin, F., 2014b. Use of delta O-18 authenticity thresholds to differentiate tomato passata from diluted tomato paste. Food Control 35, 413–418.

Brand, W.A., Coplen, T.B., Vogl, J., Rosner, M., Prohaska, T., 2014. Assessment of international reference materials for isotope-ratio analysis (IUPAC Technical Report). Pure and Applied Chemistry 86, 425–467.

Camin, F., Bontempo, L., Heinrich, K., Horacek, M., Kelly, S.D., Schlicht, C., Thomas, F., Monahan, F.J., Hoogewerff, J., Rossmann, A., 2007. Multi-element (H, C,N,S) stable isotope characteristics of lamb meat from different European regions. Analytical and Bioanalytical Chemistry 389, 309–320.

Camin, F., Larcher, R., Nicolini, G., Bontempo, L., Bertoldi, D., Perini, M., Schlicht, C., Schellenberg, A., Thomas, F., Heinrich, K., Voerkelius, S., Horacek, M., Ueckermann, H., Froeschl, H., Wimmer, B., Heiss, G., Baxter, M., Rossmann, A., Hoogewerff, J., 2010a. Isotopic and elemental data for tracing the origin of European olive oils. Journal of Agricultural and Food Chemistry 58, 570–577.

Camin, F., Larcher, R., Perini, M., Bontempo, L., Bertoldi, D., Gagliano, G., Nicolini, G., Versini, G., 2010b. Characterisation of authentic Italian extra-virgin olive oils by stable isotope ratios of C, O and H and mineral composition. Food Chemistry 118, 901–909.

Camin, F., Perini, M., Bontempo, L., Fabroni, S., Faedi, W., Magnani, S., Baruzzi, G., Bonoli, M., Tabilio, M.R., Musmeci, S., Rossmann, A., Kelly, S.D., Rapisarda, P., 2011. Potential isotopic and chemical markers for characterising organic fruits. Food Chemistry 125, 1072–1082.

Camin, F., Wehrens, R., Bertoldi, D., Bontempo, L., Ziller, L., Perini, M., Nicolini, G., Nocetti, M., Larcher, R., 2012. H, C, N and S stable isotopes and mineral profiles to objectively guarantee the authenticity of grated hard cheeses. Analytica Chimica Acta 711, 54–59.

Camin, F., Bontempo, L., Perini, M., Tonon, A., Breas, O., Guillou, C., Moreno-Rojas, J.M., Gagliano, G., 2013. Control of wine vinegar authenticity through delta O-18 analysis. Food Control 29, 107–111.

Camin, F., Bertoldi, D., Santato, A., Bontempo, L., Perini, M., Ziller, L., Stroppa, A., Larcher, R., 2015a. Validation of methods for H, C, N and S stable isotopes and elemental analysis of cheese: results of an international collaborative study. Rapid Communications in Mass Spectrometry 29, 415–423.

Camin, F., Dordevic, N., Wehrens, R., Neteler, M., Delucchi, L., Postma, G., Buydens, L., 2015b. Climatic and geographical dependence of the H, C and O stable isotope ratios of Italian wine. Analytica Chimica Acta 853, 384–390.

Capuano, E., Boerrigter-Eenling, R., Van Der Veer, G., Van Ruth, S.M., 2013. Analytical authentication of organic products: an overview of markers. Journal of the Science of Food and Agriculture 93, 12–28.

Carter, J., Barwick, V. (Eds.), 2011. Good Practice Guide for Isotope Ratio Mass Spectrometry. Forensic Isotope Ratio Mass Spectrometry (FIRMS) Network.

Carter, J.F., Tinggi, U., Yang, X., Fry, B., 2015a. Stable isotope and trace metal compositions of Australian prawns as a guide to authenticity and wholesomeness. Food Chemistry 170, 241–248.

Carter, J.F., Yates, H.S.A., Tinggi, U., 2015b. Isotopic and elemental composition of roasted coffee as a guide to authenticity and origin. Journal of Agricultural and Food Chemistry 63, 5771–5779.

Choi, W.-J., Ro, H.-M., Lee, S.M., 2003. Natural ^{15}N abundances of inorganic nitrogen in soil treated with fertilizer and compost under changing soil moisture regimes. Soil Biology & Biochemistry 35, 1289–1298.

Christoph, N., Hermann, A., Wachter, H., 2015. 25 years authentication of wine with stable isotope analysis in the European Union – review and outlook. In: Jeanmarie, A. (Ed.), 38th World Congress of Vine and Wine.

Chung, I.M., Park, I., Yoon, J.Y., Yang, Y.S., Kim, S.H., 2014. Determination of organic milk authenticity using carbon and nitrogen natural isotopes. Food Chemistry 160, 214–218.

Coplen, T.B., Qi, H.P., 2013. Recognizing the potential pitfalls of hydrogen isotopic analysis of keratins with steam equilibration to infer origins of wildlife, food, and people. Rapid Communications in Mass Spectrometry 27, 2569.

Drivelos, S.A., Georgiou, C.A., 2012. Multi-element and multi-isotope-ratio analysis to determine the geographical origin of foods in the European Union. TrAC-Trends in Analytical Chemistry 40, 38–51.

Ehtesham, E., Baisden, W.T., Keller, E.D., Hayman, A.R., Van Hale, R., Frew, R.D., 2013. Correlation between precipitation and geographical location of the delta H-2 values of the fatty acids in milk and bulk milk powder. Geochimica Et Cosmochimica Acta 111, 105–116.

Faberi, A., Marianella, R.M., Fuselli, F., La Mantia, A., Ciardiello, F., Montesano, C., Mascini, M., Sergi, M., compagnone, D., 2014. Fatty acid composition and delta C-13 of bulk and individual fatty acids as marker for authenticating Italian PDO/PGI extra virgin olive oils by means of isotopic ratio mass spectrometry. Journal of Mass Spectrometry 49, 840–849.

Flores, P., Lopez, A., Fenoll, J., Hellin, P., Kelly, S., 2013. Classification of organic and conventional sweet peppers and lettuce using a combination of isotopic and bio-markers with multivariate analysis. Journal of Food Composition and Analysis 31, 217–225.

Franke, B.M., Hadorn, R., Bosset, J.O., Gremaud, G., Kreuzer, M., 2008. Is authentication of the geographic origin of poultry meat and dried beef improved by combining multiple trace element and oxygen isotope analysis? Meat Science 80, 944–947.

Gaillard, L., Guyon, F., Salagoity, M.H., Medina, B., 2013. Authenticity of carbon dioxide bubbles in French ciders through multiflow-isotope ratio mass spectrometry measurements. Food Chemistry 141, 2103–2107.

Godin, J.P., Mccullagh, J.S.O., 2011. Review: current applications and challenges for liquid chromatography coupled to isotope ratio mass spectrometry (LC/IRMS). Rapid Communications in Mass Spectrometry 25, 3019–3028.

Greule, M., Tumino, L.D., Kronewald, T., Hener, U., Schleucher, J., Mosandl, A., Keppler, F., 2010. Improved rapid authentication of vanillin using delta C-13 and delta H-2 values. European Food Research and Technology 231, 933–941.

Heaton, K., Kelly, S.D., Hoogewerff, J., Woolfe, M., 2008. Verifying the geographical origin of beef: the application of multi-element isotope and trace element analysis. Food Chemistry 107, 506–515.

Hermann, A., Voerkelius, S., 2008. Meteorological impact on oxygen isotope ratios of German wines. American Journal of Enology and Viticulture 59, 194–199.

Hulsemann, F., Lehn, C., Schneider, S., Jackson, G., Hill, S., Rossmann, A., Scheid, N., Dunn, P.J.H., Flenker, U., Schanzer, W., 2015. Global spatial distributions of nitrogen and carbon stable isotope ratios of modern human hair. Rapid Communications in Mass Spectrometry 29, 2111–2121.

Inácio, C.T., Chalk, P.M., 2015. Principles and limitations of stable isotopes in differentiating organic and conventional foodstuffs: 2. Animal products. Critical Reviews in Food Science and Nutrition.

Kelly, S., Baxter, M., Chapman, S., Rhodes, C., Dennis, J., Brereton, P., 2002. The application of isotopic and elemental analysis to determine the geographical origin of premium long grain rice. European Food Research and Technology 214, 72–78.

Kelly, S., Heaton, K., Hoogewerff, J., 2005. Tracing the geographical origin of food: the application of multi-element and multi-isotope analysis. Trends in Food Science & Technology 16, 555–567.

Kelly, S., 2007. The British Beef Origin Project (BBOP). Food & Environment research Agency.

Kendall, C., Caldwell, E.A., 1998. Fundamentals of isotope geochemistry. In: Kendall, C., Mcdonnell, J.J. (Eds.), Isotope Tracers in Catchment Hydrology. Elsevier, Amsterdam.

Kjeldahl, K., Bro, R., 2010. Some common misunderstandings in chemometrics. Journal of Chemometrics 24, 558–564.

Kornexl, B.E., Rossmann, A., Schmidt, H.L., 1996. Improving fruit juice origin assignment by combined carbon and nitrogen isotope ratio determination in pulps. Zeitschrift Fur Lebensmittel-untersuchung Und-forschung 202, 55–59.

Kropf, U., Golob, T., Necemer, M., Kump, P., Korosec, M., Bertoncelj, J., Ogrinc, N., 2010a. Carbon and nitrogen natural stable isotopes in Slovene honey: adulteration and botanical and geographical aspects. Journal of Agricultural and Food Chemistry 58, 12794–12803.

Kropf, U., Korosec, M., Bertoncelj, J., Ogrinc, N., Necemer, M., Kump, P., Golob, T., 2010b. Determination of the geographical origin of Slovenian black locust, lime and chestnut honey. Food Chemistry 121, 839–846.

Laursen, K.H., Mihailova, A., Kelly, S.D., Epov, V.N., Berail, S., Schjoerring, J.K., Donard, O.F.X., Larsen, E.H., Pedentchouk, N., Marca-Bell, A.D., Halekoh, U., Olesen, J.E., Husted, S., 2013. Is it really organic? – Multi-isotopic analysis as a tool to discriminate between organic and conventional plants. Food Chemistry 141, 2812–2820.

Laursen, K.H., Schjoerring, J.K., Kelly, S.D., Husted, S., 2014. Authentication of organically grown plants – advantages and limitations of atomic spectroscopy for multi-element and stable isotope analysis. TrAC-Trends in Analytical Chemistry 59, 73–82.

Lernoud, J., Willer, H., 2015. Organic agriculture worldwide: current statistics. In: Willer, H., Lernoud, J. (Eds.), The World of Organic Agriculture. Statistics and Emerging Trends 2015. FiBL-IFOAM Report. Research Institute of Organic Agriculture (FiBL), Frick, and IFOAM - Organics International, Bonn.

Longobardi, F., Casiello, G., Cortese, M., Perini, M., Camin, F., Catucci, L., Agostiano, A., 2015. Discrimination of geographical origin of lentils (Lens culinaris Medik.) using isotope ratio mass spectrometry combined with chemometrics. Food Chemistry 188, 343–349.

Martin, G.G., Hanote, V., Lees, M., Martin, Y.L., 1996. Interpretation of combined H-2 SNIF/NMR and C-13 SIRA/MS analyses of fruit juices to detect added sugar. Journal of AOAC International 79, 62–72.

Meier-Augenstein, W., Hobson, K.A., Wassenaar, L.I., 2013. Critique: measuring hydrogen stable isotope abundance of proteins to infer origins of wildlife, food and people. Bioanalysis 5, 751–767.

Meylahn, K., Rucker, A., Wolf, E., 2006. Provenience analysis of asparagus using isotope relation mass spectrometry. Deutsche Lebensmittel-rundschau 102, 523–526.

Mihailova, A., Pedentchouk, N., Kelly, S.D., 2014. Stable isotope analysis of plant-derived nitrate – novel method for discrimination between organically and conventionally grown vegetables. Food Chemistry 154, 238–245.

Mimmo, T., Camin, F., Bontempo, L., Capici, C., Tagliavini, M., Cesco, S., Scampicchio, M., 2015. Traceability of different apple varieties by multivariate analysis of isotope ratio mass spectrometry data. Rapid Communications in Mass Spectrometry 29, 1984–1990.

Molkentin, J., Giesemann, A., 2010. Follow-up of stable isotope analysis of organic versus conventional milk. Analytical and Bioanalytical Chemistry 398, 1493–1500.

Molkentin, J., Lehmann, I., Ostermeyer, U., Rehbein, H., 2015. Traceability of organic fish – authenticating the production origin of salmonids by chemical and isotopic analyses. Food Control 53, 55–66.

Ortea, I., Gallardo, J.M., 2015. Investigation of production method, geographical origin and species authentication in commercially relevant shrimps using stable isotope ratio and/or multi-element analyses combined with chemometrics: an exploratory analysis. Food Chemistry 170, 145–153.

Osorio, M.T., Moloney, A.P., Schmidt, O., Monahan, F.J., 2011. Multielement isotope analysis of bovine muscle for determination of international geographical origin of meat. Journal of Agricultural and Food Chemistry 59, 3285–3294.

Oulhote, Y., Le Bot, B., Deguen, S., Glorennec, P., 2011. Using and interpreting isotope data for source identification. TrAC-Trends in Analytical Chemistry 30, 302–312.

Paolini, M., Ziller, L., Laursen, K.H., Husted, S., Camin, F., 2015. Compound-specific delta N-15 and delta C-13 analyses of amino acids for potential discrimination between organically and conventionally grown wheat. Journal of Agricultural and Food Chemistry 63, 5841–5850.

Perini, M., Camin, F., Bontempo, L., Rossmann, A., Piasentier, E., 2009. Multielement (H, C, N, O, S) stable isotope characteristics of lamb meat from different Italian regions. Rapid Communications in Mass Spectrometry 23, 2573–2585.

Piasentier, E., Valusso, R., Camin, F., Versini, G., 2003. Stable isotope ratio analysis for authentication of lamb meat. Meat Science 64, 239–247.

Qi, H.P., Coplen, T.B., 2011. Investigation of preparation techniques for delta H-2 analysis of keratin materials and a proposed analytical protocol. Rapid Communications in Mass Spectrometry 25, 2209–2222.

Rogers, K.M., Van Ruth, S., Alewijn, M., Philips, A., Rogers, P., 2015. Verification of egg farming systems from The Netherlands and New Zealand using stable isotopes. Journal of Agricultural and Food Chemistry 63, 8372–8380.

Rossmann, A., Koziet, J., Martin, G.J., Dennis, M.J., 1997. Determination of the carbon-13 content of sugars and pulp from fruit juices by isotope-ratio mass spectrometry (internal reference method) — a European interlaboratory comparison. Analytica Chimica Acta 340, 21—29.

Rossmann, A., 2001. Determination of stable isotope ratios in food analysis. Food Reviews International 17, 347—381.

Roßmann, A., 2013. 3-New approaches for verifying the geographical origin of foods. In: Brereton, P. (Ed.), New Analytical Approaches for Verifying the Origin of Food. Woodhead Publishing.

Rummel, S., Hoelzl, S., Horn, P., Rossmann, A., Schlicht, C., 2010. The combination of stable isotope abundance ratios of H, C, N and S with Sr-87/Sr-86 for geographical origin assignment of orange juices. Food Chemistry 118, 890—900.

Schellenberg, A., Chmielus, S., Schlicht, C., Camin, F., Perini, M., Bontempo, L., Heinrich, K., Kelly, S.D., Rossmann, A., Thomas, F., Jamin, E., Horacek, M., 2010. Multielement stable isotope ratios (H, C, N, S) of honey from different European regions. Food Chemistry 121, 770—777.

Schipilliti, L., Tranchida, P.Q., Sciarrone, D., Russo, M., Dugo, P., Dugo, G., Mondello, L., 2010. Genuineness assessment of mandarin essential oils employing gas chromatography-combustion-isotope ratio MS (GC-C-IRMS). Journal of Separation Science 33, 617—625.

Schipilliti, L., Dugo, P., Bonaccorsi, I., Mondello, L., 2011. Headspace-solid phase micro-extraction coupled to gas chromatography-combustion-isotope ratio mass spectrometer and to enantioselective gas chromatography for strawberry flavoured food quality control. Journal of Chromatography A 1218, 7481—7486.

Schipilliti, L., Dugo, P., Bonaccorsi, I., Mondello, L., 2012. Authenticity control on lemon essential oils employing gas chromatography-combustion-isotope ratio mass spectrometry (GC-C-IRMS). Food Chemistry 131, 1523—1530.

Schipilliti, L., Bonaccorsi, I., Cotroneo, A., Dugo, P., Mondello, L., 2015. Carbon isotope ratios of selected volatiles in Citrus sinensis and in orange-flavoured food. Journal of the Science of Food and Agriculture 95, 2944—2950.

Schmidt, O., Quilter, J.M., Bahar, B., Moloney, A.P., Scrimgeour, C.M., Begley, I.S., Monahan, F.J., 2005. Inferring the origin and dietary history of beef from C, N and S stable isotope ratio analysis. Food Chemistry 91, 545—549.

Serra, F., Guillou, C.G., Reniero, F., Ballarin, L., Cantagallo, M.I., Wieser, M., Iyer, S.S., Heberger, K., Vanhaecke, F., 2005. Determination of the geographical origin of green coffee by principal component analysis of carbon, nitrogen and boron stable isotope ratios. Rapid Communications in Mass Spectrometry 19, 2111—2115.

Simpkins, W.A., Patel, G., Harrison, M., Goldberg, D., 2000. Stable carbon isotope ratio analysis of Australian orange juices. Food Chemistry 70, 385—390.

Sturm, M., Kacjan-Marsic, N., Lojen, S., 2011. Can $d^{15}N$ in lettuce tissues reveal the use of synthetic nitrogen fertiliser in organic production? Journal of the Science of Food and Agriculture 91, 262—267.

Sulzman, E.W., 2007. Stable isotope chemistry and measurement: a primer. In: Michener, R., Lajtha, K. (Eds.), Stable Isotopes in Ecology and Environmental Science, second ed. Blackwell Publishing, Oxford.

Thomas, F., Jamin, E., 2009. H-2 NMR and C-13-IRMS analyses of acetic acid from vinegar, O-18-IRMS analysis of water in vinegar: international collaborative study report. Analytica Chimica Acta 649, 98—105.

Tosun, M., 2014. Detection of adulteration in mulberry pekmez samples added various sugar syrups with C-13/C-12 isotope ratio analysis method. Food Chemistry 165, 555—559.

Trincherini, P.R., Baffi, C., Barbero, P., Pizzoglio, E., Spalla, S., 2014. Precise determination of strontium isotope ratios by TIMS to authenticate tomato geographical origin. Food Chemistry 145, 349–355.

Valenzuela, L.O., Chesson, L.A., O'grady, S.P., Cerling, T.E., Ehleringer, J.R., 2011. Spatial distributions of carbon, nitrogen and sulfur isotope ratios in human hair across the central United States. Rapid Communications in Mass Spectrometry 25, 861–868.

Van Der Veer, G., 2013. Development and application of geospatial models for verifying the geographical origin of food. In: Brereton, P. (Ed.), New Analytical Approaches for Verifying the Origin of Food. Woodhead Publ Ltd, Abington Hall Abington, Cambridge Cb1 6ah, Cambs, UK.

Van Leeuwen, K.A., Prenzler, P.D., Ryan, D., Camin, F., 2014. Gas chromatography-combustion-isotope ratio mass spectrometry for traceability and authenticity in foods and beverages. Comprehensive Reviews in Food Science and Food Safety 13, 814–837.

Vanhaecke, F., Degryse, P. (Eds.), 2012. Isotopic Analysis. Fundamentals and Applications Using ICP-MS. Wiley-VCH Verlag & Co, Weinheim, Germany.

Voerkelius, S., Lorenz, G.D., Rummel, S., Quetel, C.R., Heiss, G., Baxter, M., Brach-Papa, C., Deters-Itzelsberger, P., Hoelzl, S., Hoogewerff, J., Ponzevera, E., Van Bocxstaele, M., Ueckermann, H., 2010. Strontium isotopic signatures of natural mineral waters, the reference to a simple geological map and its potential for authentication of food. Food Chemistry 118, 933–940.

Wassenaar, L.I., Hobson, K.A., 2003. Comparative equilibration and online technique for determination of non-exchangeable hydrogen of keratins for use in animal migration studies. Isotopes in Environmental and Health Studies 39, 211–217.

West, J.B., Bowen, G.J., Dawson, T.E., Tu, K.P. (Eds.), 2010. Isoscapes – Understanding Movement, Pattern, and Process on Earth Through Isotope Mapping, Dordrecht. Springer, Heidelberg, London, New York.

White, J.W., Winters, K., Martin, P., Rossmann, A., 1998. Stable carbon isotope ratio analysis of honey: validation of internal standard procedure for worldwide application. Journal of AOAC International 81, 610–619.

Yang, L., 2009. Accurate and precise determination of isotopic ratios by MC-ICP-MS: a review. Mass Spectrometry Reviews 28, 990–1011.

Zampella, M., Quetel, C.R., Paredes, E., Asfaha, D.G., Vingiani, S., Adamo, P., 2011. Soil properties, strontium isotopic signatures and multi-element profiles to authenticate the origin of vegetables from small-scale regions: illustration with early potatoes from southern Italy. Rapid Communications in Mass Spectrometry 25, 2721–2731.

Zhang, L., Kujawinski, D.M., Federherr, E., Schmidt, T.C., Jochmann, M.A., 2012. Caffeine in your drink: natural or synthetic? Analytical Chemistry 84, 2805–2810.

Advances in Chromatographic Techniques for Food Authenticity Testing

10

C. Fanali, L. Dugo, L. Mondello
Università Campus Bio-Medico of Rome, Rome, Italy

Chapter Outline

10.1 Introduction

Chromatography is a technique of great importance in the field of separation science which was pioneered in the early 20th century when Ramsey realized separation of mixtures of gases and vapors of adsorbent materials such as coal and Tswett (1906) separated some plant pigments by liquid chromatography.

Chromatography is a common name for techniques based on the adsorption and/ or partition of molecules to be separated between a mobile and a stationary phase. Separation is the result of selective distribution of molecules between the two phases. Stationary phases are generally solids (inorganic or organic) while mobile phases are liquids or gases. Chromatographic techniques are classified according to the character of both the stationary and the mobile phases, the form of the stationary phase, and the forces driving separation. Methods most frequently used in food analysis are gas chromatography (GC) and high-performance liquid chromatography (HPLC). The most commonly used detectors for chromatographic techniques involve UV–visible (UV–vis), fluorescence, electrochemical, flame ionization detector (FID), electron capture detector (ECD), mass spectrometer (MS), etc. The principal disadvantage of chromatographic techniques is their inherently complex operation, which requires special training to ensure that the technique is performed correctly (Ornelas-Soto et al., 2011).

The objectives of this chapter are the compilation and concise survey of the most important results in the field of the application of various GC and HPLC methodologies for the assessment of food authenticity and traceability, the brief elucidation of the theoretical principles, and the critical discussion of the practical results. Basic knowledge of the principles of GC and HPLC is included (Forgács and Cserháti, 2003).

10.2 Process of Using Chromatographic Techniques in the Analysis of Food

Chromatographic techniques are one of the more active areas in food analysis. Because of their high separation capacity, chromatographic procedures have found increasing employment in food science for the qualitative and quantitative analysis of a large number of molecules such as normal constituents of foods, additives, pollutants, etc.

Separations based on liquid chromatography are the most numerous as can be deduced from the many works published on the use of different formats of LC to detect nonvolatile food compounds such as proteins, amino acids, phenolic compounds, carbohydrates, additives, triglycerides, phospholipids, chiral compounds and pigments (Ibañez and Señoráns, 2005). On the other hand, GC still has an important role in food analysis for the determination of naturally volatile or semivolatile compounds like fatty acids, alcohols, sterols, etc.

10.2.1 Chromatographic Separation Principles and Technologies

Elution chromatography is a technique in which the mobile phase is passed continuously through the entire length of the chromatographic bed (column) while the sample is introduced into the system in defined amounts. It is introduced onto the column as a narrow zone through an injection system. Afterward the zone is transported through the column by the mobile phase moving at a previously selected velocity. The chromatographic process is described by either equilibrium or kinetic theories. Analytes are in continuous equilibrium between mobile and stationary phase and, after a certain time, they separate from each other and leave the column outlet as separate narrow bands. The result appears as a chromatogram showing the time or mobile phase volume vs detector signal typically displayed graphically on x- and y-axes, respectively. Analytes appear as peaks that ideally have a Gaussian distribution of compound concentrations in the mobile phase.

The tendency of a given component to interact with the stationary phase is described in chemical terms through an equilibrium constant known as a distribution constant, or even partition coefficient (K_c), which is the ratio of the concentration of the solute molecules in the stationary phase (c_S) to that in the mobile phase (c_M):

$$K_c = \frac{c_S}{c_M} \tag{10.1}$$

Hence, the greater the value of K_c is for a sample component, the higher is its solubility, and therefore the longer its retention time in the stationary phase.

The time that any solute spends in the mobile phase, which is the unretained peak time (t_M) summed with the so-called adjusted retention time ($t_{R'}$) that corresponds to the time the solute spends distributed in the stationary phase, is equivalent to the retention time (t_R):

$$t_R = t_M + t_{R'} \tag{10.2}$$

Solute retention can also be expressed in terms of a retention factor (k), also called a capacity factor, that indicates the time spent by the solute in contact with the stationary phase compared with the time spent in contact with the mobile phase, according to the following equation:

$$k = \frac{t_{R'}}{t_M} \tag{10.3}$$

Among other parameters to be considered in a chromatographic process, the separation factor (α) is also very important. The separation factor for two components is calculated as follows:

$$\alpha = \frac{k_B}{k_A} = \frac{t_{B'}}{t_{A'}} \tag{10.4}$$

where k_B and k_A are the relative retention factor of two studied analytes (the earlier eluting compound A and the later eluting B).

It is worth highlighting that the separation factor is a useful measure of relative peak position in the chromatogram; however, since it does not contain any information about peak widths, it is not adequate on its own to describe peak separations.

The chromatographic process can be described using the theory of distillation. A chromatographic system can be imagined as being similar to a distillation column, which is composed of a series of thin layers called theoretical plates. The balance of distribution of the solute between stationary and mobile phase is achieved in each of these plates of the column. The terms theoretical plates (N) and plate height (height equivalent to theoretical plate, HETP) are commonly used in chromatography to describe the performance of chromatographic systems.

The number of theoretical plates is calculated by the following equation:

$$N = 16\left(\frac{t_R}{w_b}\right)^2 \text{ or } 5.545\left(\frac{t_R}{w_h}\right)^2 \tag{10.5}$$

where w_b is the width at the base of peak and w_h the width at half height.

Resolution (R_S) is a quantitative measure of the degree of separation between two chromatographic peaks, A and B; it is defined as the ratio between the difference of retention times and the average of the peak width at the baseline:

$$R_s = 2\frac{\Delta t}{w_A + w_B} \tag{10.6}$$

where w_A and w_B are the widths at the base of peak A and B, respectively. The degree of separation between two chromatographic peaks improves with an increase of R_S.

If we consider two chromatographic peaks A and B which have the same base width ($w_A = w_B = w$), the following alternative expression for the resolution can be considered:

$$R_s = \frac{\sqrt{N}}{4}\left(\frac{\alpha - 1}{\alpha}\right)\left(\frac{1 + k_m}{k_m}\right) \tag{10.7}$$

where $k_m = 1/2 \times (k_B + k_A)$.

As can be observed from this equation, resolution is influenced by two main parameters, namely efficiency N and selectivity (a function of α and k). Selectivity more strongly affects R_s (Fanali et al., 2013b).

10.2.2 Gas Chromatography

Gas chromatography is a technique suitable for the analysis of volatile and semivolatile substances. It facilitates vaporization of the sample and its subsequent transport in the mobile phase (carrier gas) through a column containing the stationary phase. A subclassification of the technique is based on the physical condition of the stationary phase: if the stationary phase is a solid, the technique is called gas–solid chromatography (GSC); if it is a liquid, it is called gas–liquid chromatography (GLC). GLC is by far the most widely used and facilitates separation of sample components from each other on the basis of their different vapor pressures and relative affinity for the particular stationary phase. Sample component partition into the stationary liquid phase is based on their solubility at the given operating temperature. Compounds with lower vapor pressure (higher volatility) are partitioned to a greater extent in a mobile phase and eluted earlier than compounds with higher vapor pressure (lower volatility) or that strongly interact with the stationary phase (Cordero et al., 2012).

Important characteristics of molecules that may be analyzed using this method are vapor pressure at temperatures below 350–400°C and thermostability without decomposition during vaporization. Components of a gas chromatographic system are: a carrier gas system, injector, gas chromatographic column, detector, and data processing unit (Forgács and Cserháti, 2003). Common carrier gases are hydrogen, helium, and nitrogen, gases that behave almost ideally at low pressures and temperatures typically used in GC systems. Choice of the carrier gas is important because it affects the sensitivity of the detection and the separation characteristics of the system. Injectors deliver the sample to the head of the GC column and can be classified into two major groups: vaporization and on-column injectors. The sample to be analyzed is introduced by a syringe into the thermostated injection chamber at high temperature (100–300°C), which enables rapid vaporization of the sample that is then mixed with the carrier gas and transported onto the column. On-column injectors allow the injection of a liquid sample directly into the column without a separate vaporization step. Molecules of the injected sample are then separated in the column.

There are two main types of GC columns used for the analysis: packed and capillary columns (ie, the open-tubular column (OTC)). Packed columns are made of stainless steel or glass and contain small particles of an inert and porous support covered by a thin layer of stationary phase. The most common solid supports are diatomaceous earths, fluorocarbons, graphitized carbon black and glass beads. These columns are usually 0.5–3 m long with an internal diameter greater than 2 mm packed with adsorbent or liquid-coated support particles of 100–250 μm diameter (Forgács and Cserháti, 2003).

Capillary column are columns in which the stationary phase is coated as a thin film on the inner wall of the capillary. The internal walls of a wall-coated open-tubular (WCOT) column are coated with an absorbing, liquid polymer film. The internal walls of a porous-layer open-tubular (PLOT) column are covered with a solid porous layer having large adsorbing surface (Dorman and Dawes, 2012). In food analysis, the commonly adopted analytical columns consist of fused silica tubing with an inner diameter ranging from 0.1 to 0.53 mm. The amount of stationary phase in a capillary column is denoted by its film thickness, which is typically 0.1–5 μm (Cordero et al., 2012). Open tubular columns provide much lower flow resistance and consequently can be used in longer lengths to obtain very high plate numbers as compared to packed columns. Columns have to be thermostated at constant temperature (isothermal separation mode) or by varying the temperature during analysis time (temperature gradient mode) for compound separation.

Separated compounds exit from the column and transfer to the detectors. A number of detectors have been developed for GC that can be classified as universal or selective. Among the universal detectors, those most commonly used in food analysis are FID and MS. FID is a mass-sensitive and destructive detector and its response is stable and linear with solute concentrations up to seven orders of magnitude. MS detectors operate on the principle of ionization of a compound followed by the physical separation of charged ions and their detection. Typically, ion sources coupled to GC equipment are electron impact (EI) or chemical ionization (CI). Low- and high-resolution mass analyzers are employed such as single (Q) or triple quadrupole (QqQ) and time-of-flight (ToF). Among selective detectors, electron capture detectors

(ECDs) are nondestructive, highly sensitive to all electron-reacting compounds containing halogen, nitro, or carbonyl group (ie, pesticides) (Klee, 2012).

GC has been employed for several food composition applications and is an important tool for the analysis of fatty acids, sterols, alcohols, aroma compounds, and off-flavors. Other polar compounds may also be analyzed by GC after prior chemical derivation such as amino acids, hydroxy (poly)carboxylic acids, fatty acids, phenolic compounds, sugars, vitamins, etc (Lehotay, 2002).

10.2.3 High-performance Liquid Chromatography

In high-performance or high-pressure liquid chromatography, the mobile phase is a liquid that is pumped through the column. A HPLC instrument comprises solvent reservoirs, a solvent delivery system (pumps), an injector system, a column, a detector and a data-acquisition system. Column characteristics are very important for compound separation. HPLC columns are classified based on their dimensions; analytical columns have an internal diameter (I.D.) ranging from 4.6 to 1 mm while their length fluctuates from 30 to 300 mm. The trend is to reduce the size of the columns by employing capillary columns with an I.D. ranging from 500 to 10 μm, which are referred to as capillary or nano-LC. Columns are packed with particles of different diameter made of silica and modified-silica, polymeric, or carbon adsorbents, and adsorbents based on metal oxides (titanium, zirconium, and aluminium) that are used as stationary phases. Columns using smaller particle sizes exhibit a great increase in efficiency. However, the smaller the particle diameter, the greater is the resistance of the column to the flow of the mobile phase. Particle sizes range between 3 and 10 μm; columns with a particle size lower than 2 μm require special instrumentation, which are referred to as ultra-high-pressure liquid chromatography (UHPLC) instruments. An alternative to reducing particle size in order to improve separation efficiencies and speed is the use of superficially porous particles, also termed core-shell or fused-core particles. These particles are composed of a 1.7-μm solid core enrobed in a 0.5-μm porous silica layer (dp = 2.7 μm or lower) to reduce mass transfer and increase peak efficiency. Advantages of this technology include (1) the ability to reach high peak efficiency and (2) a requirement for only short analysis times without using very-high-pressure LC instrumentation necessary for sub-2-μm column particles. Nowadays, more than 90% of applications employ particle packed columns with 4.6 and 4.0 mm internal diameter, 150 and 250 mm length, and 3−5 μm particle size (Unger et al., 2013).

Samples are injected through an injection valve fitted with a sample loop of a few μL volume. The choice of stationary and mobile phases is a key parameter that influences retention and selectivity (Yashin and Yashin, 2012).

Many of the separation modes used today in HPLC were described prior to 1960. Reversed (RP) and normal (NP) phase are the main retention mechanisms widely used in current chromatographic separations. In normal phase liquid chromatography (NP-HPLC), a polar-bonded stationary phase is employed such as diol, amino, and cyano phases. Polar and moderately polar compounds are well separated by NP-HPLC techniques. In reversed-phase liquid chromatography (RP-HPLC), the stationary phase is hydrophobic and the mobile phase is highly polar. A great number of reversed-phase columns are available; among them C_8 and C_{18} silica-bonded stationary phases are the most used. Mobile phases consist of a mixture of water plus an organic solvent such as methanol, acetonitrile, or tetrahydrofuran. A wide range of compounds can be separated by RP-HPLC. Other LC methods include ion-exchange chromatography (IEC) used for the separation of a mixture of ions (anions or cations), size-exclusion chromatography employed for the separation of macromolecules based on their molecular weights, and chiral chromatography that is applied to the analysis of isomer mixtures such as enantiomers by use of a chiral stationary phase (Nollet, 2003). In the 1970s, hydrophilic-interaction chromatography (HILIC) was developed and later improved for separating polar compounds (Buszewski and Noga, 2012).

Several detectors have been used in HPLC, most commonly optical, luminescent, electrochemical, and mass spectrometric systems (Zhang et al., 2008). The most widely used is the UV—vis absorbance detector. Other photometric detectors include photodiode array (PDA), and fluorescence detectors. A refractive index (RI) detector is popular for size-exclusion chromatography while evaporative light-scattering (ELSD) and charged-aerosol (CAD) detectors now represent a better choice as a universal detector than their RI counterpart (Snyder and Dolan, 2013).

Mass spectrometry applied to food analysis has evolved in recent years; it has mainly been used for identification and quantification of food compounds. Atmospheric pressure chemical ionization (APCI) and electrospray ion source (ESI) have been employed as interfaces between LC systems and the mass analyzer (Nollet, 2003).

Mass analyzers are characterized by high resolution, which makes separation of two ions possible. Those most commonly used in LC are the single quadrupole, triple quadrupole, and ion-trap (IT) systems. Recently, high-resolution MS instrumentation allowing exact mass determination, such as ToF or orbitrap or hybrid instruments like Q-TOF, IT-TOF, have been commercialized and applied to food analysis (Fanali et al., 2013b).

On analysis of food components by HPLC, there are hundreds of books and reviews that are published with applications to different compound classes like vitamins, carbohydrates, proteins, amino acids, lipids like triglycerides, and minor bioactive substances like phenolic compounds and pigments.

10.2.4 Recent Developments in Chromatography

Monodimensional (one column) chromatography has been employed in food analysis to a great extent in the past. Recently, the necessity to enhance the separation power of chromatographic systems has resulted in the development of multidimensional chromatography. This allows the combination of two or more independent or nearly independent separation processes, significantly increasing the separation power and peak capacity of the corresponding one-dimensional techniques. Different chromatographic couplings have been realized and applied to food analysis, among them multidimensional gas chromatography (MDGC), multidimensional liquid chromatography (MDLC), and multidimensional LC-GC. MDGC consists of an arrangement of two or more columns in which eluent fractions from the first column are injected in the second one. Heart cut valves or the more sophisticated modulators are employed to transfer one or a few eluting fractions (typical in MDGC) or the whole eluted fraction (comprehensive GC × GC) from the first to the second dimension, respectively (Marriott et al., 2012). MDLC techniques can be classified into three different groups based on the fraction transfer method from the first to the second dimension: off-line MDLC, online MDLC, and comprehensive LC (LC × LC). In off-line MDLC, fractions from the first dimension are collected, concentrated, and reinjected in the second dimension. In online MDLC, special systems are used to automatically transfer selected fractions from the first to the second dimension; in comprehensive LC, all of the compounds separated in the first dimension are transferred in the second dimension by employing specific interfaces able to collect the entire first fraction and reinject it (Herrero et al., 2009). LC-GC couplings have been developed in both online and off-line modes. Advantages of such a coupling are the high sample capacity, the wide range of separation mechanisms of the LC, and the high efficiency of the GC. Disadvantages arise from the requirement for relatively complex instrumentation due to the use of different interfaces used to couple LC and GC equipment (Purcaro et al., 2012).

Food analysis applications of multidimensional chromatography have been reviewed in some recently published papers (Dugo et al., 2008; Herrero et al., 2009; Tranchida et al., 2004).

The main disadvantage of these approaches is the long total analysis time, and these methods are therefore only recommended for highly detailed characterization of complex samples and not for routine quality control, which is typically of lower complexity.

Although conventional analytical techniques remain the choice for determining a wide number of compounds of interest in food chemistry, recently miniaturization has been studied and also proposed for this purpose. In these techniques, analyte separations take place in capillary columns of narrow I.D. containing only a few mg of a selected stationary phase (SP) (packed columns); alternatively, the SP can be directly polymerized into the capillary (monolithic) or bonded on the column wall (Fanali et al., 2013a). In all cases, compounds are eluted by a selected mobile phase (MP) at reduced flow rate (μL/min or nL/min). Highest and lowest flow rates are applied in capillary liquid chromatography (CLC) and nano-liquid chromatography (nano-LC), respectively. Although unified nomenclature has not yet been agreed upon, these two microfluidic techniques can also be classified considering the I.D. of the capillary used, eg, nano-LC I.D. <100 μm while CLC I.D. is in the range 100–320 μm (Fanali et al., 2011a).

Considering the column dimensions and the flow rates used with these techniques, extra-column band broadening effects must be minimized in order to avoid negative influences on the separation efficiency. Therefore, special attention must be placed on the selection of some important parameters such as injected sample volume, detection, and tube connections. Usually only 7–60 nL and 1–4 μL of sample are injected in nLC or CLC applications, respectively, while on-column detection is performed when a UV–vis detector is employed. MS detectors were also successfully used in order to obtain higher sensitivity and in addition to enable compound characterization. It is noteworthy that hyphenation of CLC/n-LC with MS can be easily done employing nano-spray interfaces because a relatively low flow of MP is involved. Finally, tube connection is done using capillaries, and the capillary column is often directly connected to the injection valve (Fanali et al., 2013a). Among other features of CLC/nano-LC that must be considered are that because of the low flow rate, high mass sensitivity can be obtained due to the lower peak dilution but low sample volumes are necessary. Finally, reduced costs are expected due to the low volumes of organic solvent used and reduced waste.

CLC or nano-LC techniques have been successfully applied to food analysis for the determination of several compounds, eg, phenolic compounds (Fanali et al., 2011b; Si-Ahmed et al., 2010), amino acids (D'Orazio et al., 2008; Dominguez-Vega et al., 2011), peptides and proteins (Rizzello et al., 2009; De Angelis et al., 2006; Kwon, 2004), allergens (Monaci et al., 2010; Weber et al., 2006), amines and polyamines (Hernandez-Borges et al., 2007; Rosales-Conrado et al., 2008), phytosterols and vitamins (Rocco and Fanali, 2009; Calvano et al., 2010; Cerretani et al., 2010), toxins (Aqai et al., 2011; Timperio et al., 2006), and organic compounds (Fanali et al., 2005).

The determination of the herein-mentioned compounds could be very important to investigations into food quality, adulteration, and authenticity testing.

10.3 Adulterations Which can be Detected by Using Chromatographic Techniques

Sometimes, reading the list of ingredients or the nutrition facts label on a foodstuff may not tell the real story. Moore et al. (2012) reported the definition of food adulteration, or food fraud, as "a collective term that encompasses the deliberate substitution, addition, tampering, or misrepresentation of food, food ingredients, or food packaging, or false or misleading statements made about a product for economic gain." Often, adulteration is motivated by economic reasons, eg, maximizing profit by adding a cheaper ingredient. Addressing a more specific type of fraud, the United States Pharmacopeial (USP) Expert Panel on Food Ingredient Intentional Adulterants defined the intentional or economically motivated adulteration of food ingredients as "the fraudulent addition of non-authentic substances or removal or replacement of authentic substances without the purchaser's knowledge for economic gain of the seller" (Moore et al., 2012).

Chromatographic-based methods are able to detect different kinds of food adulteration that can be classified as resulting from ingredient replacement and addition. Based on the type of fraud, they can be listed as follows:

- Complete or partial substitution of a food ingredient or one authentic food by a similar but cheaper one. Examples include substituting bonito for tuna, sea trout for salmon, or addition of seed oils to extra virgin olive oil.
- Adding food with a cheaper base material. Examples include adding water, sugar, acids, and coloring to fruit juices and addition of melamine to milk to artificially increase apparent protein content.
- False declaration of geographic, species, botanical, or varietal origin. Examples include substitution of less-expensive cow's milk for sheep or goat's milk; substitution of common

wheat for durum wheat; substitution of Greek or Turkish olive oil for Italian olive oil; and substitution of synthetically produced vanillin for botanically derived natural vanillin.

- False declaration of raw material origin or production process used to manufacture a food.
- Nondeclaration or false declaration of processes. Examples include fraudulent labeling of a synthetically derived flavor chemical as being naturally derived; food falsely labeled as organically produced; poor quality, filtered honey or a honey substitute product labeled as honey.
- Addition of a nonauthentic substance to mask an inferior quality ingredient for color and/or taste enhancement. An example is the addition of a color additive (such as Sudan Red dyes) to enhance the color of poor quality paprika.

Table 10.1 reports some examples of chromatographic methods applied to food authenticity and fraud analysis reported in recently published papers.

The most important examples of chromatographic analysis of this kind of adulteration will be reported in the following sections.

10.4 Foodstuffs Suitable for Testing Using Chromatographic Techniques

Separation techniques are one of the more active areas in food analysis. Applications based on liquid chromatography are the most numerous as can be deduced from the many papers published on the use of different HPLC formats. GC also has an important role in food analysis but is limited to volatile or semivolatile compounds. Almost all foods can be tested using these techniques, which are able to perform qualitative and quantitative analysis of different classes of food constituents.

Moore et al. (2012) recently reviewed and analyzed data on food adulteration collected from publicly available articles. Results summarized comprise a database that was published in the US Pharmacopeial Convention's Food Chemicals Codex (8th edition) (United States Pharmacopeia, 2012). They reported the top 25 foods with the greatest number of reports; among them, seven foods represented more than 50% of the scholarly records: olive oil, milk, honey, saffron, orange juice, coffee, and apple juice. HPLC and GC were among the most common analytical detection procedures (Moore et al., 2012).

10.5 Case Studies

10.5.1 Case Study on Edible Vegetable Oils

Oils and fats constitute one of the major classes of food products, with edible vegetable oils having largely supplanted animal fats in processed food formulations. For this reason, their authenticity has become an important issue (Aparicio and Aparicio-Ruiz, 2000). Among those previously mentioned, olive oil is the most studied. A wide variety of methods has been developed to confirm the authenticity or detect the adulteration of olive

Table 10.1 **Type of Food Fraud and Chromatographic Detection Methods**

Fraud Type	Specific Topic	Example	Compound Studied	Instrumental Chromatographic Technique	References
Ingredient substitution	Substituting one milk type for another one	Mixing cow's milk with buffalo milk before production of buffalo mozzarella cheese	β-Lactoglobulin proteins	RP-HPLC/UV	Enne et al. (2005)
			β-Lactoglobulin proteins	HPLC-ESI-MS	Czerwenka et al. (2010)
			β-Casein tryptic peptides	UHPLC-ESI-Q/TOF-MS/MS	Russo et al. (2012)
		Addition of milk of different species	Casein proteins	HPLC-PDA	Bramanti et al. (2003)
			Casein proteins	HPLC-UV	Veoloso et al. (2002)
			β-Lactoglobulin proteins	HPLC-UV	Ferreira and Caçote (2003)
			β-Lactoglobulin proteins	RP-HPLC-ESI-MS	Chen et al. (2004)
		Addition of vegetable or animal fat to milk fat	FAs	GC-FID	Ulberth (2003)
			Sterols	online GC-HPLC	Kamm et al. (2002)
	Partial substitution of high-price oils with lower-price oils	Adulteration of virgin olive oil with other seed oils (eg, maize, cottonseed, hazelnut, rapeseed, and sunflower)	TAGs	GC	Andrikopoulos et al. (2001)

Continued

Table 10.1 **Type of Food Fraud and Chromatographic Detection Methods—cont'd**

Fraud Type	Specific Topic	Example	Compound Studied	Instrumental Chromatographic Technique	References
			TAGs	HPLC-APCI-MS-MS	Fasciotti and Annibal (2010)
			Sterols fraction	online coupled LC−GC−FID	Grob et al. (1994)
			Sterol fraction	GC × GC-FID/MS	Purcaro et al. (2015)
		Adulteration of argan oil by lower-price vegetable oils like olive oil, soybean oil, or sunflower oil	TAGs profile	HPLC−ELSD	Salghi et al. (2014)
		Adulteration of virgin olive oil with lower-grade oil (eg, refined olive oil, deodorized virgin olive oils, olive pomace oil)			
		Adulteration of seed oils	FAs	GC-MS and multivariate statistical analysis	Zhang et al. (2014)
		Adulteration of sesame oils with perilla oil	TAGs profile	RP-HPLC-RID	Lee et al. (2001)
	Partial substitution of expensive fruit juices with cheaper ones	Adulteration of orange juice	Phenolic compounds	HPLC−DAD-ESI−MS/MS and HPLC−DAD	Abad-Garcia et al. (2014)

		Addition of grape juice to expensive juices	Organic acids	HPLC-MS/MS	Ehling and Cole (2011)
False declaration of geographic, species, botanical, or varietal origin		Authentication of honey's floral origin	Phenolic compounds	HPLC-DADUV	Cavazza et al. (2013)
			Phenolic acids and abscissic acid	HPLC-DAD-UV	Yao et al. (2004)
		Authentication of honey geographical origin	Volatile compounds	GC–MS	Allissandrakis et al. (2007)
Addition of non-authentic food compounds		Adulteration of milk with small nitrogen-containing compounds	Melamine and nitrogen compounds	HPLC-ESI-MS with a HILIC column	Abernethy and Higgs (2013)
		Addition of syrups to honey	Fructose and glucose and oligosaccharides	GC-FID and HPAEC-PAD	Cotte et al. (2003)
			Maltooligosaccharides	HPAEC-PAD	Morales et al. (2008)
			Marker syrup compound	HPLC-RID	Wang et al. (2015)
			Maltooligosaccharides	UHPLC-ELSD	Zhou et al. (2014)
		Addition of aromas to commercial fruit juices	Volatile chiral compounds	GC–MS	Ruiz Del Castillo et al. (2003)

oils. Fat and oil authentication by means of the analysis of different component lipid classes by both HPLC and GC analysis can facilitate detection of their adulteration.

Profiles of different classes of lipids are characteristic of individual plant species and, to a lesser extent, of edible vegetable oils origin; these include triacylglycerols, fatty acids, sterols, and other minor compounds (Tsimidou and Boskou, 2003).

"Fatty acidomics", the entire fatty acid family of an edible fat, is a key marker of and quality parameter for these food matrices. They are usually analyzed by GC–MS after derivatization to fatty acid methyl esters (FAMEs) and identified by comparison of their mass spectra and retention indices of standards and/or using mass spectra libraries (Zhang et al., 2014). The percentage values for each fatty acid are compared with those recognized by national and international organizations, and increases or decreases in the levels of certain fatty acids may indicate adulteration. Fatty acid patterns could be useful, even if not highly distinctive, for authenticity purposes especially for the analysis of pure oils.

For example, detection of high percentages of palmitic acid indicate the presence of palm oil, while the presence of erucic acid in trace amounts can be used to identify the presence of rapeseed oil. In the case of blends involving oils of different botanical origin, the FA composition is so complex, in part also to chromatographic peak merging, that it cannot be used for authentication. It has been recognized that fatty acid profile is only a part of the oil composition; additional analysis of other macro- and microcomponents of oils is sometimes necessary (Osorio et al., 2014).

Triglyceride (TAG) profiles follow a specific pattern for different oils. Such a profile is considered to be a good fingerprint for the purpose of detecting adulteration due to fatty acids being distributed on glycerol molecules according to a certain position-specific pattern. TAG analysis can be performed by HPLC or high temperature GC (Ruiz-Samblás et al., 2012), with the former being the most common technique (Aparicio and Aparicio-Ruiz, 2000). A great number of HPLC methods employing different stationary and mobile phases, columns, and detectors have been developed and applied to TAG analysis. RP-HPLC separation has been largely used for TAG analysis in which components are separated according to the combined effect of the chain lengths of the FA moieties contained in a given TAG species plus their degree of unsaturation (Buchgraber et al., 2004). The parameter used to classify them is the "equivalent carbon number" (ECN) defined as $ECN = CN - 2DB$, where CN is the number of carbons in the FAs chains and DB is the total number of double bonds present in the FAs. RP-HPLC combined with RID is also used in the official method adopted by IUPAC (1987) (Method 2.323, 1987) and A.O.C.S. (1997). Detectors such as ELSD and CAD have been employed and demonstrated to be universal detectors that are very useful for TAG analysis. MS detectors provide elucidation of the regio-isomer composition of TAGs in fats and oils together with FA composition (Bosque-Sendra et al., 2012). APCI-MS in combination with HPLC has proven to be a very valuable technique for analysis of different lipids from a variety of sources. Nonaqueous reversed-phase (NARP) HPLC with APCI-MS detection has been recently applied to characterization and quantification of TAGs in different plant oils. In this technique, TAGs are separated according to ECN, and separation of almost all TAGs within one ECN group or of TAGs with different DB positions is possible. The method was applied to the analysis of 26 plant oils important in food, nutrition, and cosmetic industries. Chromatograms were used as plant oil fingerprints for qualitative analysis, while quantitative analysis was assessed by relative concentrations for all TAGs and FAs in individual samples. The method provided high separation selectivity with a high number of positively identified TAGs. A fingerprint of the different oils was obtained from chromatographic profiles together to precise quantitative analysis including low abundant TAGs (Lisa and Holcapek, 2008). An off-line 2D combination of NARP and silver-ion HPLC coupled with APCI-MS in the analysis of complex TAG samples containing FAs with different acyl chain lengths, different numbers, positions, and geometry of DBs, and different regioisomer positions of FAs on the glycerol skeleton is a very recent and powerful combination of methods. A high number of TAGs can be separated and identified. This method is useful for very complex samples like blackcurrant oil as example of a highly complex plant oil containing both α- and γ-Ln and beef tallow as representative of animal fats containing also *trans*-FAs. However it requires long analysis time, therefore it is not recommended for routine quality control analysis of oils and fats of low complexity (Holcapek et al., 2009).

TAG analysis can be used for adulteration detection by two different approaches: determination of specific markers (specific TAGs or TAG ratio), or application of chemometric analysis of TAG fingerprints. As an example of the first approach, Park et al. (2010) used specific TAG targets to detect sesame oil adulteration with soybean oil. L/S, O/Ln, and L/Ln ratio from fatty acids analysis or LLL/OOO ratio from TAGs analysis could be useful indicators. Moreover, LLLn peak and percentage of linolenic acid, which mainly come from soybean oil, are valuable markers. The authors concluded that TAG analysis by HPLC-ELSD together with fatty acids determination by GC-FID can be a useful tool to detect the mixture of sesame oil with other edible oils containing high linolenic acid.

As an example of the second approach, the TAG profiles of various oils, obtained through HPLC-CAD analysis, were investigated using multivariate analysis. Different categories of olive oils (extra virgin, virgin, refined, and pomace) and various vegetable oils (sunflower, rapeseed, corn, soybean, canola, seed, and grape-seed) were analyzed at different mixed percentages. Detection of olive oil adulteration by different seed oils (errors not exceeding 10% reported) was possible (De la Mata-Espinosa et al., 2011). A wider summary of authenticity studies using TAG composition is given in a recent review (Bosque-Sendra et al., 2012).

TAG profile analysis has been also used to detect different kinds of edible vegetable oil substitutions such as olive oil adulteration by different vegetable oils (Andrikopoulos et al., 2001) or by soybean oil (Fasciotti and Annibal, 2010); argan oil adulteration with common vegetable oils (Salghi et al., 2014); and sesame oil adulteration with perilla oil (Lee et al., 2001).

Analysis of minor compounds, constituents of the unsaponifiable fraction such as tocopherols and phytosterols, has been shown to aid authenticity confirmation in vegetable oils. Identification and determination of phytosterols, which comprise a major portion of the unsaponifiable matter, are mainly used to reveal the presence of vegetable fats in animal fats or admixtures of vegetable fats. Qualitative and quantitative differences between phytosterol fractions are well established for a great variety of vegetable fats. Their presence and concentration may vary depending on the type of plant, its geographic origin and harvesting period, etc. GC coupled to different detectors is the prevalent chromatographic technique employed for their analysis (Aparicio and Aparicio-Ruiz, 2000). Other chromatographic approaches include online coupled LC-GC-FID analysis (Grob et al., 1994), and recently a nano-LC application has also been proposed (Rocco and Fanali, 2009). The official GC sterol analysis of olive oil is used as an indicator for the detection of seed oils. Some sterols are characteristic of seed oils. The profile of sterols is often decisive in clarifying the adulteration of vegetable oils with other cheaper oils; several examples are reviewed by Aparicio and Aparicio-Ruiz (2000). Moreover, sterol analysis can be useful to detect adulteration of virgin oil (olive oil) with refined oils (Osorio et al., 2014) or other plant oils (Al-Ismail et al., 2010). The detection of the adulteration of refined olive oil with refined hazelnut oil was performed by quantification of free and esterified phytosterols (Bowadt and Aparicio, 2003). Recently, Baocheng et al. (2014) developed classification and adulteration identification methods for different vegetable oils on the basis of free sterols analysis by GC × GC coupled to TOF-MS. A comprehensive GC × GC method, employing a simultaneous dual detection (FID and MS) to generate a chemical fingerprint of minor compounds in edible oil, was developed and optimized. In particular, the profiles of extra virgin olive oil samples were compared to a hazelnut oil sample, highlighting that the latter was characterized by a large number of compounds completely absent in the extra virgin olive oil samples, making this approach suitable for adulteration detection (Purcaro et al., 2015).

Rocco and Fanali (2009) optimized and validated a nano-LC method for the analysis of brassicasterol, stigmasterol, campesterol, cholesterol, and sitosterol in extra virgin olive oil (EVOO). The analysis was done in about 20 min employing a capillary column packed with a C18-RP (sub-2 -μm particles) stationary phase for 15 cm, using methanol as a mobile phase. Quantitative analysis was carried out with a UV detector while molecular weight determination was done using a mass spectrometer. Analysis of EVOOs of different origin revealed the presence of β-sitosterol, which indicated the absence of adulteration. The detection of brassicasterol would indicate the presence of rapeseed oil, while high concentrations of cholesterol may indicate the addition of animal fat. In the EVOOs analyzed, these two markers were present at very low concentration. Fig. 10.1 shows a nano-LC separation with online ESI-MS detection of phytosterols.

Few authentication studies are based on tocopherol determination (Aparicio and Aparicio-Ruiz, 2000). Tocopherols and tocotrienols are most frequently analyzed by HPLC coupled with fluorescence detection. Several parameters affect the concentration of these compounds in vegetable oils, and, for this reason, in authentication or adulteration studies they are considered as analytes that can provide information complementary to other compounds (Osorio et al., 2014). However, recently Chen et al. (2011) proposed a method for measuring tocopherols (α-, (β + γ)-, and δ-tocopherols) in vegetable oils by RP-HPLC with fluorescence detection. The ratio of α- and

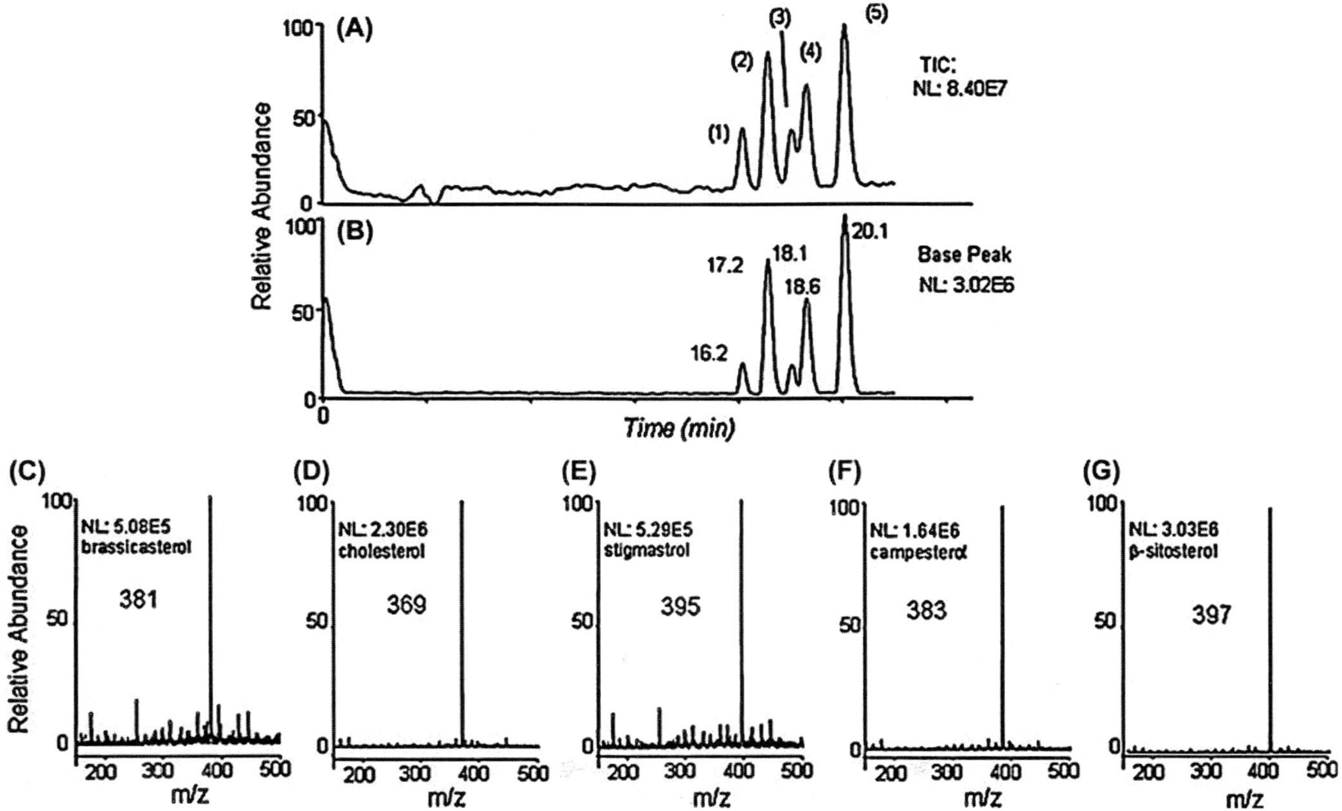

Figure 10.1 Nano-LC separation with online ESI-MS detection of (1) brassicasterol, (2) cholesterol, (3) stigmasterol, (4) campesterol, and (5) β-sitosterol. (A) Total ion chromatogram (TIC), (B) base peak chromatogram, and (C–G) full-scan mass spectra of the studied phytosterols. Reproduced from Rocco, A., Fanali, S., 2009. Analysis of phytosterols in extra-virgin olive oil by nanoliquid chromatography. Journal of Chromatography A 1216, 7173–7717 with permission of Elsevier.

($\beta + \gamma$)-tocopherols (named α/β tocopherol ratio) of different vegetable oils was systematically measured and proposed as a marker of authenticity.

10.5.2 Case Study on Milk and Dairy Products

As is the case with vegetable oils, the qualitative and quantitative determination of lipids of dairy products may detect foreign fat in milk fat. Among milk fat products, butter is the most important because of its widespread use. For this reason, its quality is very important; it has always been subjected to adulteration by addition of cheaper vegetable or animal fats. Detection of foreign fat in milk fat can be performed by studying FAs, TAGs, and minor lipid compounds of the unsaponifiable fraction (De La Fuente and Juárez, 2005). Addition of vegetable oils to milk fat can be detected by quantifying single FAs or the concentration ratio of two or more FAs following GC analysis. FA ratios have also been used in past years to discriminate between milk fat of different species (eg, bovine, ovine, and caprine; Ulberth, 2003). Limitations of FA analysis are due to the difficulty of detecting low incorporation concentrations of vegetable oils in milk fat or to the natural variability of milk FA composition. TAG analysis using GC analysis of classes of compounds with identical numbers of acyl-C atoms has been proposed and applied (De La Fuente and Juárez, 2005). Analysis of minor compounds can be very useful for authentication purposes. Analysis of free sterols or trimethylsilyl derivatives by silica column GC was performed and permitted detection of adulteration of milk fat by vegetable oils (Alonso et al., 1997). Determination by HPLC has been also reported; an online GC-HPLC method has been applied to the detection of vegetable oils in milk fat using β-sitosterol as a marker compound (Kamm et al., 2002).

A comprehensive GC × GC method, with dual MS/FID detection, for the qualitative and quantitative analysis of the unsaponifiable fraction of milk lipids (cow butter, buffalo, ewe, and goat milks) was developed and optimized. GC-high-resolution ToF MS analysis was employed to confirm identification of detected compounds. A large number of compounds were separated and identified demonstrating the usefulness of such a method for dairy product authenticity studies (Tranchida et al., 2013). Fig. 10.2 shows a GC × GC–FID chromatogram of the unsaponifiable fraction of buffalo milk.

Detection of adulteration by the substitution of one milk type for another has been achieved principally by protein analysis (Borkovà and Snášelová, 2005). HPLC analysis has been employed to determine individual milk proteins due to the fact that different chromatographic profiles are obtained for milk from different species. This analysis has been employed to verify milk and cheese authenticity, especially for protected denomination of origin (PDO) cheeses. In comparison with bovine dairy products, those from goats, ewes, and buffalos are more expensive, and authentication also in this case is an economic matter. Ion exchange, reversed phase and hydrophobic interactive chromatography columns have been used to separate both casein and whey protein fractions of milk. Milk casein proteins were analyzed in milk from different animal species by hydrophobic interaction HPLC coupled to a PDA detector (Bramanti et al., 2003) and RP-HPLC coupled to a UV detector (Veoloso et al., 2002).

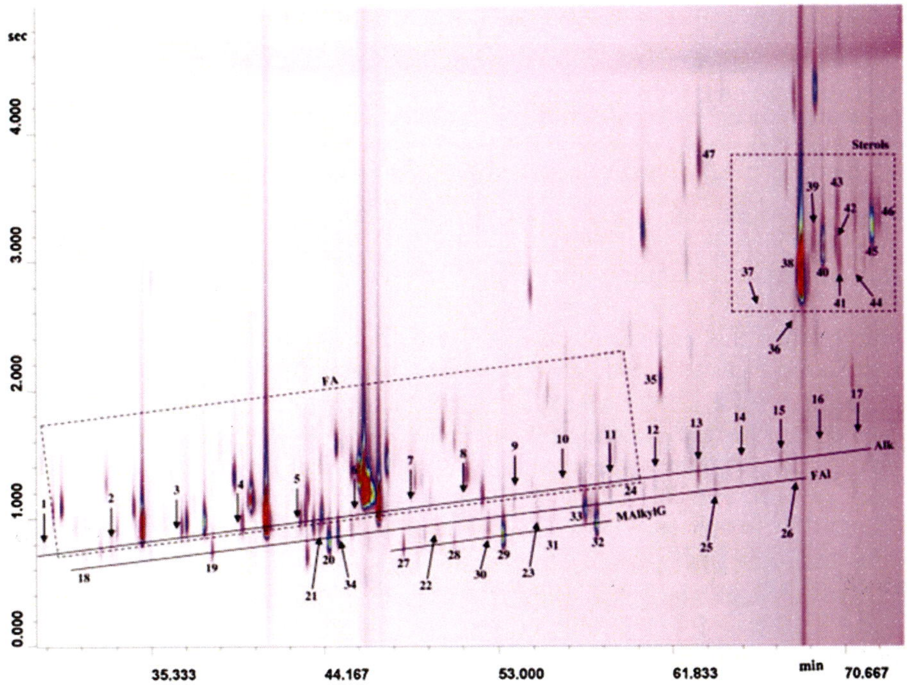

Figure 10.2 GC × GC-FID chromatogram relative to the analysis of the unsaponifiable fraction of buffalo milk.
Reproduced from Tranchida, P.Q., Salivo, S., Bonaccorsi, I., Rotondo, A., Dugoa, P., Mondello, L., 2013. Analysis of the unsaponifiable fraction of lipids belonging to various milk-types by using comprehensive two-dimensional gas chromatography with dual mass spectrometry/flame ionization detection and with the support of high resolution time-of-flight mass spectrometry for structural elucidation. Journal of Chromatography A 1313, 194–201 with permission of Elsevier.

Bramanti et al. (2003) demonstrated that hydrophobic interaction HPLC was a good tool for separation and quantitation of caseins in milk samples. The validated method, fast, versatile, and specific, was applied to their analysis in raw milk, from cow, goat, ewe, and buffalo, their mixtures and cheeses. Results showed different elution profiles of casein's fraction of the different analyzed milk types. The authors proposed the ratio of the area of selected peaks of casein (α_{s1}/κ, α_{s2}/β, β/κ, and α_{s2}/α_{s1}) for prediction of composition of milk mixtures suggesting the employment of the method to detection of goat's or ewe's milk adulteration with cow's milk.

A HPLC-UV method was also proposed as suitable for routine separation and quantification of k-, α-, and β-caseins in raw and processed milks. Good accuracy, precision, and rapidity were achieved. The method was applied to the analysis of bovine, ovine, and caprine milks although it was only possible to detect and quantify additions of 5% or more of bovine to caprine milk. With respect to detection of milk adulterations, gel electrophoresis was more sensitive (Veoloso et al., 2002).

Analysis of whey proteins was performed by RP-HPLC coupled to a UV detector (Ferreira and Caçote, 2003; Enne et al., 2005). Ferreira and Caçote (2003) developed a qualitative and quantitative method for the analysis of β-lactoglobulins by RP-HPLC in bovine, ovine, and caprine milk mixtures and fresh and ripened cheeses. Different chromatographic patterns were obtained for the three milk types. The method proved to be very sensitive and accurate for detecting milk type in fresh and ripened cheeses made from binary mixtures of bovine, ovine, or caprine raw milks. It allowed quantification of milk species within the concentration range of 5−95%. Commercial PDO cheeses were analyzed for their authenticity evaluation. Enne et al. (2005) developed an RP-HPLC-UV method for the measurement of quantity ratios within β-lactoglobulin protein family on raw milk, cheese matrix, and cheese governing liquid to detect adulteration of water buffalo mozzarella by bovine milk's addition. The developed method allowed to detect the addition of cow's milk down to 0.5%. An important successful point was the use of proper calibration curves to eliminate matrix-dependent biases. The possibility to perform analysis on governing liquid samples, bypassing whey proteins' extraction from cheese matrix, lowered analysis time.

HPLC-MS methods for β-lactoglobulin analysis of milk and cheese have been also published (Chen et al., 2004; Czerwenka et al., 2007, 2010). Chen et al. (2004) developed a simple method based on solvent extraction followed by RP-HPLC-ESI-MS analysis of intact β-lactoglobulin to detect adulteration of goat's with cow's milk. The method allowed to detect cow's milk addition as low as 5% (v/v).

Czerwenka et al. (2010) employed HPLC-ESI-MS for the first time for the detection of the adulteration of water buffalo milk and mozzarella by cow's milk. The method allowed fast analysis with the advantage of a fully qualitative identification of variants of intact β-lactoglobulin. However, the authors evidenced critical points regarding quantitative analysis because the concentration of the marker compounds can vary between and within the milks mixed together for adulteration. Commercial buffalo mozzarella samples from Austria were analyzed showing some products adulterated with high levels of cow's milk.

Recently, a UHPLC-ESI-Q/TOF tandem mass spectrometry (MS/MS) method for peptide analysis in order to detect buffalo mozzarella adulteration has been reported. The quantitative analysis was performed by multiple reaction monitoring (MRM) scan function of specific transitions of phosphorylated β-casein tryptic peptide. The selectivity and sensitivity of MRM scan offer powerful capabilities in detecting adulteration of dairy products (Russo et al., 2012).

A method to aid in the detection of adulteration of fresh milk with a range of different small, nitrogen-containing compounds including melamine has been recently developed; this procedure employs HPLC with a HILIC column coupled to ESI-MS. The developed method was rapid and proposed as alternative to infrared instruments to reduce the numbers of samples identified as outliers (Abernethy and Higgs, 2013).

10.5.3 Case Study on Honey

Honey adulteration is a complex problem, which currently has a significant economic impact as well as nutritional and organoleptic consequences. Several types of economically motivated adulteration have been identified in the honey industry; chromatographic methods have been reported to have a role in addition of less expensive syrups and false declaration of botanical and geographical origins of honey. Several authors have proposed studying carbohydrates, the main constituents of honey, by chromatographic techniques. Some of this work has aimed to confirm honey authenticity in terms of its botanical or geographical origin (Ouchemoukh et al., 2010) while some others are related to honey adulteration by addition of different syrups (Cordella et al., 2005; Morales et al., 2008; Wang et al., 2015; Zhou et al., 2014; Cotte et al., 2003; Ruiz-Matute et al., 2010). The common inexpensive sweeteners added as adulterants to honey include corn syrup (CS), high-fructose corn syrup (HFCS), invert syrup (IS), or high-fructose inulin syrup (HFIS). A fingerprint profile of honey oligosaccharides has been obtained through different methods: a high-performance anion-exchange chromatography pulsed amperometric detection (HPAEC-PAD) system (Morales et al., 2008), HPLC equipped with a common RID detector (Wang et al., 2015), and simultaneously GC-FID and HPAEC-PAD analysis (Cotte et al., 2003). Morales et al. (2008) applied a simple HPAEC-PAD method for quantitative analysis of maltooligosaccharides to detect honey adulterations with CS and HFCS. The method was based on activated charcoal sample treatment to fractionate honey carbohydrates followed by their analysis. Different honey and CS and HFCS samples were analyzed and oligosaccharides quantified. Adulterated samples were prepared by adding 5%, 10%, and 20% of syrup to a honey sample. The method demonstrated to be a useful tool to detect adulterations of honey with industrial syrups. Cotte et al. (2003) employed HPAEC-PAD to assay fructose and glucose and GC-FID for the determination of the entire profile of di- and trisaccharides. The results of the two techniques were combined with a statistical processing. This approach was tested to demonstrate the addition of syrup to acacia, chestnut, and lavender honeys. A database of oligosaccharides using authentic honey samples was created. A great number (141) of commercial monofloral French honeys were analyzed. The limits of detection were very good, between 5% and 10% for tested monofloral honeys.

In a different way, Wang et al. (2015) proposed a simple, low-cost, environmental, and precise method for the detection of honey adulteration with starch syrup employing HPLC-RID instrument. Any sample preparation was adopted. Twelve pure honey samples from different nectar sources and geographical origins in China and different adulterated honey with HSF samples were analyzed. The analysis was based on detection of an indicator peak of starch syrup on chromatograms able to determine a detectable syrup content near to 2.5% (w/w). Recently, Zhou et al. (2014) reported a UPLC separation together with ELSD detection method to effectively identify honey adulterated with maltooligosaccharides. This method allowed the separation of six different maltooligosaccharides from honey samples using a simple liquid—liquid extraction procedure followed by fast analysis (less than 6 min). The method was applied to 290 honey samples collected from apiaries, supermarkets, and traditional agri-product markets. The UPLC-ELSD method provided a superior sensitivity to maltooligosaccharides analysis in honey with respect to the traditional HPLC-RID method.

Analysis of phenolic compounds in honey samples has been proposed for the evaluation of authenticity of unifloral honeys and for their classification. Cavazza et al. (2013) reported a chromatographic fingerprint analysis of phenolic compounds in monofloral honeys of different botanical origin employing HPLC-DAD/UV equipment after solid phase extraction. Chemometric data analysis was applied in order to select a limited number of phenolic compounds able to differentiate honeys according to their botanical origin. A method based on solid phase extraction (SPE) and isocratic liquid chromatographic separation using a central composite design was developed for the analysis of flavonoid markers quercetin, hesperetin, and chrysin found in north Iranian citrus honey samples. This method was fully validated and applied to analysis of different samples (Hadjmohammadi et al., 2009). Analysis of phenolic acids and abscissic acid of monofloral eucalyptus honeys from Australia was assessed for their potential use as floral markers and to detect the occurrence of species-specific markers. HPLC separation of phenolic acids employing an RP-C18 column coupled to a PDA detector was developed. Profiles of phenolic acids and abscissic acid appeared to be promising for objective confirmation of the authenticity of the floral origin of Australian honeys (Yao et al., 2004).

Also, free amino acid profile analysis was proposed for the determination of botanical or geographical origin of honey. Cometto et al. (2003) proposed an RP-HPLC-UV quantitative analysis of amino acids in 56 honey samples from three different Argentine regions, each with characteristic apiarian flora. Statistical analysis of data showed evidence of clusters related to apiarian flora around apiaries. Rebane and Herodes (2008) developed a HPLC-UV method with precolumn derivatization by diethyl ethoxymethylenemalonate for the analysis of free amino acids in 61 unifloral and polyfloral honey samples from Estonia. Statistical analysis revealed that some amino acids were more powerful indicators of honey botanical origin than others. Results obtained showed the utility of such an approach for assessing the botanical origin of Estonian honeys.

Use of the volatiles composition of thyme honeys was proposed as a means of establishing a discriminant model for their geographical origin. Twenty-eight samples were analyzed by means of solid-phase microextraction coupled to a GC-MS instrument. A discriminant analysis was assessed in order to classify samples. Results of statistical analysis showed good discrimination among samples being promising to establish a discrimination model for honeys with these geographical regions origins (Allissandrakis et al., 2007).

10.5.4 Case Study on Fruit Juices

Fruit juices, in particular orange and apple juice, are among the top seven foods reported between 1980 and 2010 as the most common targets of adulteration (Moore et al., 2012). In addition, false use of geographical indications by unauthorized parties is detrimental to consumers and legitimate producers. For fruit juice, the main authenticity issues involve (1) simple dilution with water; (2) addition of sugars different from those contained in the actual fruit; (3) addition of pulp wash and peel-derived by-products; (4) blending of expensive fruit juices with juices extracted from lower-value fruits; and (5) false labeling of products in terms of their cultivar or geographical origin (Vaclavik et al., 2011).

These procedures may be applied alone or in combination in order to make the detection of adulteration more difficult. The complexity in detection and prevention of fruit juice adulteration arises from several parameters that affect fruit composition such as cultivar, geographical origin, stage of maturity, environmental growth conditions, storage and fruit picking conditions, as well as the juice extraction system (Fugel et al., 2005). Until now, a number of methods have been developed to tackle various aspects of fruit juice authenticity. The most established approaches are based on analysis of carbohydrates, phenolic compounds, carotenoids, amino acids, or other organic acids using different chromatographic methods.

Phenolic compounds are very promising markers for the determination of food authenticity due to their taxonomic specificity. Their analysis by chromatographic techniques has been applied especially to orange juice adulteration. Sweet orange (*Citrus sinensis*) juices, the consumption of which has significantly increased in recent years, may be adulterated with tangerine (*Citrus reticulate*), lemon (*Citrus limon*) and/or grapefruit (*Citrus paradisi*). Abad-Garcia et al. (2014) developed an HPLC-DAD/ESI-MS/MS and HPLC-DAD for characterization and quantification respectively of phenolic compounds in citrus juices. These phenolic compound profiles, being representative of the Spanish citrus fruit juice production, were studied with the aim of differentiating citrus juices according to the species used for their elaboration: sweet orange, tangerine, lemon, or grapefruit. Statistical and chemometric methods were applied to identify possible markers and develop classification models. Classification models correctly identified all sweet orange and tangerine juices. The presented model seems to be promising for detecting sweet orange juice adulterations with tangerine juice although it required an external validation.

A method for authenticity control of apple and pear juices was developed by Schieber et al. (2001) involving HPLC and HPLC-ESI-MS. It was applied to the characterization and quantification of phenolic constituents in apple juice, apple pomace, and extracts of pear fruits. Furthermore, blends of apple juice with pear juice and vice versa were analyzed. The resulting method was suitable for authenticity control of apple and pear juice by determining characteristic quercetin and isorhamnetin glycosides, and dihydrochalcones, respectively. However, only a small number of samples were analyzed.

An LC-ESI-MS/MS method was developed for the analysis and authentication of fruit-based products and fruit-based pharmaceutical preparations. The proposed method was then applied to the analysis of polyphenols in 23 grape-based and cranberry-based natural products and pharmaceutical preparations. Concentration data were analyzed by multivariate statistical analysis. Results from this statistical analysis revealed that concentration data for such phenolic compounds allowed the samples analyzed to be clustered according to their source fruit. The method showed a good performance with low limits of detection and with very good precisions and accuracies. The polyphenols concentration determined using this approach could be used as discriminating elements for samples classification (Puigventós et al., 2015).

Stander et al. (2013) developed a non-targeted method to detect adulteration of fruit juices by the addition of sugar or other less-expensive fruit juices as well as preservatives, artificial sweeteners, and colors. They employed hydrophilic-interaction liquid chromatography—mass spectrometry (HILIC-MS) using electrospray ionization in the negative mode and UV detection. This study focused on the main types of fruit juices consumed on the South African market and included apple, orange, grape, and blends of these juices with other fruits like mango, pear, and guava. The developed nontargeted method allowed the detection of polyphenolic marker compounds such as hesperidin and naringin as well as sugars and artificial sweeteners in 14 -min analysis time. Different fruit juices were differentiated by the content of marker compounds such as sorbitol, certain phenolic molecules and their saccharide profile. Statistical data analysis identified possible juice adulteration and a need to submit samples to further investigations.

Organic acids are another class of compounds that play an important role in the authenticity testing of fruit juices. As an example, tartaric acid is usually considered an indicator of the addition of grape juice to a more expensive juice. Similarly, excess malic and/or quinic acid can be used as an indicator of apple juice addition to a more expensive juice. A method based on stable isotope dilution HPLC-MS/MS was developed for citric, malic, quinic, and tartaric acid analysis in fruit juices and applied to six types of juice. Marker organic acids like tartaric acid are usually considered an indicator of grape juice addition to a more expensive juice. Similarly, organic acids ratios are indicators of juice additions to expensive ones. The proposed method enabled their determination for fruit juices discrimination. Moreover, results confirmed the presence of low levels of tartaric acid and quinic acid in pomegranate juice, with important implications for authenticity studies (Ehling and Cole, 2011).

Amino acid profiles of commercially available fruit juices were also studied for the purpose of evaluating their authenticity. Amino acids were derivatized with OPA/MPA and analyzed by HPLC coupled to a fluorescence detector (Asadpoor et al., 2014). Gomez-Ariza et al. (2005) developed an LC-ESI-MS/MS method based on the use of a normal-phase chromatographic column for the identification and quantification of 20 amino acids. The method was applied to different kinds of orange juice: commercial orange juice from both frozen concentrates and freshly squeezed oranges and fresh, hand-squeezed sweet orange juice. An evaluation of differences in composition between the juices and the potential adulteration assessment has been performed. The comparison of amino acids profile of commercial orange juice with fresh hand-squeezed ones enabled confirmation of their authenticity.

Orange juice contains L-amino acids and therefore the presence of their D-isomers may indicate adulteration, microbiological contamination, uncontrolled fermentation processes, etc. Therefore, the analysis of amino acid enantiomers could be used to assess not only their quality but also adulterations. A nano-LC method for the analysis of these compounds in orange juices has been proposed in which compounds were derivatized with fluorescein isothiocyanate (FITC), separated in a laboratory-made capillary column (75 μm I.D.), packed with vancomycin-modified silica-diol particles, and detected with a mass spectrometer. Samples were preconcentrated in a C18 cartridge. Neither of the two samples tested (commercial and fresh juice) contained the D-amino acids (D'Orazio et al., 2008).

Analysis of volatile chiral compounds was also proposed to differentiate natural compounds from those of synthetic origin in fruit juice. Ruiz Del Castillo et al. (2003) developed a method to determine the origin of aromas as well as to detect their addition to commercial fruit beverages on the basis of the enantiomeric composition of certain chiral terpenes. Aroma compounds were extracted by SPME and separated by GC employing a chiral column coupled to an FID detector. Determination of the enantiomeric distribution of chiral terpenes, mainly limonene, linalool, and R terpineol, was shown to be useful for detection of the addition of aromas to fruit beverages. These authors demonstrated that alteration of the defined percentage of their enantiomeric distribution may be attributable to the addition of aromas (Ruiz Del Castillo et al., 2003).

Analysis of the enantiomeric distribution of chiral compounds in fruit juices was also performed by developing a method based on the use of online coupling RP-HPLC-GC-MS to evaluate juice authenticity. The aim of this work was to propose and evaluate a different experimental setup for the RPLC-GC system. The proposed method allowed efficient chromatographic separation and high sensitivity for chiral compounds analysis. It was tested on a small number of real samples (two commercial beverages containing a variety of fruit juices) as an example of application (Caja et al., 2004).

10.6 Future Trends

One of the most important emerging trends is the miniaturization of analytical systems. For this reason, micro- and nano-columns have been developed for HPLC analysis as described through the chapter. However, so far, few applications on food analysis and specifically on food authentication have been developed using such miniaturized equipment. In the context of miniaturization, microfluidic analytical systems have also shown interesting applications. Such miniaturized systems, called micrototal analysis systems (μTAS), also include nano-LC instrumentation. These instruments offer smaller footprints, lower energy demands, ultra-fast analysis, and high throughput than any other equipment. Most importantly, they open the door to portable instrumentation, alleviating critical sampling and sample-integrity challenges. Miniaturized systems and their applications in food analysis are expected to grow.

With regard to multidimensional chromatography methods, few applications have so far been published on food analysis. Limitations are due to instrumental costs, and the necessity for highly trained personnel and dedicated laboratories. Mature techniques, such as GC × GC and LC × LC, will continue to be developed and refined. Two-dimensional combinations, such as LC × GC, LC × CE, and CE × CE, have already been explored, and the proof of concept for three-dimensional approaches (GC × GC × GC, LC × LC × LC) has been demonstrated.

Sources of Further Information

USP Food Fraud Database: https://www.foodfraud.org/node.

References

Abad-García, B., Garmón-Lobato, S., Sánchez-Ilárduya, M.B., Berrueta, L.A., Gallo, B., Vicente, F., Alonso-Salces, R.M., 2014. Polyphenolic contents in citrus fruit juices: authenticity assessment. European Food Research and Technology 238, 803–818.

Abernethy, G., Higgs, K., 2013. Rapid detection of economic adulterants in fresh milk by liquid chromatography–tandem mass spectrometry. Journal of Chromatography A 1288, 10–20.

Al-Ismail, K.M., Alsaed, A.K., Ahmad, R., 2010. Detection of olive oil adulteration with some plant oils by GLC analysis of sterols using polar column. Food Chemistry 121, 1255–1259.

Allissandrakis, E., Tarantilis, P.A., Harizanis, P.C., Pollisiou, M., 2007. Comparison of the volatile composition in thyme honeys from several origins in Greece. Journal of Agricultural and Food Chemistry 55, 8152–8157.

Alonso, L., Fontecha, J., Lozada, L., Juárez, M., 1997. Determination of mixtures in vegetable oils and milk fat by analysis of sterol fraction by gas chromatography. Journal of the American Oil Chemists' Society 74, 131–135.

Andrikopoulos, K.N., Giannakis, G.I., Tzamtis, V., 2001. Analysis of olive oil and seed oil triglycerides by capillary gas chromatography as a tool for the detection of the adulteration of olive oil. Journal of Chromatographic Science 39, 137–145.

Aparicio, R., Aparicio-Ruız, R., 2000. Authentication of vegetable oils by chromatographic techniques. Journal of Chromatography A 881, 93–104.

Aqai, P., Peters, J., Gerssen, A., Haasnoot, W., Nielen, M.W.F., 2011. Immunomagnetic microbeads for screening with flow cytometry and identification with nanoliquid chromatography mass spectrometry of ochratoxins in wheat and cereal. Analytical and Bioanalytical Chemistry 400, 3085–3096.

Asadpoor, M., Ansarin, M., Nemati, M., 2014. Amino acid profile as a feasible tool for determination of the authenticity of fruit juices. Advanced Pharmaceutical Bulletin 4, 359–362.

Baocheng, X., Zhang, L.X., Wang, H., Luo, D., Li, P., 2014. Characterization and authentication of four important edible oils using free phytosterol profiles established by GC-GC-TOF/MS. Analytical Methods 6, 6860–6870.

Borková, M., Snášelová, J., 2005. Possibilities of different animal milk detection in milk and dairy products – a review. Czech Journal of Food Sciences 23, 41–50.

Bowadt, S., Aparicio, R., 2003. The detection of the adulteration of olive oil with hazelnut oil: a challenge for the chemists. Inform 14, 342–344.

Bosque-Sendra, J.M., Cuadros-Rodríguez, L., Ruiz-Samblás, C., Paulina de la Mata, A., 2012. Combining chromatography and chemometrics for the characterization and authentication of fats and oils from triacylglycerol compositional data-Review. Analytica Chimica Acta 724, 1–11.

Bramanti, E., Sortino, C., Onor, M., Beni, F., Raspi, G., 2003. Separation and determination of denatured α_{s1}-, α_{s2}-, β- and k-caseins by hydrophobic interaction chromatography in cows', ewes' and goats' milk, milk mixtures and cheeses. Journal of Chromatography A 994, 59–74.

Buszewski, B., Noga, S., 2012. Hydrophilic interaction liquid chromatography (HILIC)-a powerful separation technique. Analytical and Bioanalytical Chemistry 402, 231–247.

Buchgraber, M., Ulberth, F., Emons, H., Anklam, E., 2004. Triacylglycerol profiling by using chromatographic techniques. European Journal of Lipid Science and Technology 106, 621–648.

Caja, M.M., Blanch, G.P., Herraiz, M., Ruiz del Castillo, M.L., 2004. On-line reversed–phase liquid chromatography-gas chromatography coupled to mass spectrometry for enantiomeric analysis of chiral compounds in fruit beverages. Journal of Chromatography A 1054, 81–85.

Calvano, C.D., Aresta, A., Zambonin, C.G., 2010. Detection of hazelnut oil in extra virgin olive oil by analysis of polar components by micro-solid phase extraction based on hydrophilic liquid chromatography and MALDI-TOF mass spectrometry. Journal of Mass Spectrometry 45, 981–988.

Cavazza, A., Corradini, C., Musci, M., Salvadeo, P., 2013. High-performance liquid chromatographic phenolic compound fingerprint for authenticity assessment of honey. Journal of the Science of Food and Agriculture 93, 1169–1175.

Cerretani, L., Lerma-Garcia, M.J., Herrero-Martinez, J.M., Gallina-Toschi, T., Simo-Alfonso, E.F., 2010. Determination of tocopherols and tocotrienols in vegetable oils by nanoliquid chromatography with ultraviolet-visible detection using a silica monolithic column. Journal of Agricultural and Food Chemistry 58, 757–761.

Chen, H., Angiuli, M., Ferrari, C., Tombari, E., Salvetti, G., Bramanti, E., 2011. Tocopherol speciation as first screening for the assessment of extra virgin olive oil quality by reversed-phase high-performance liquid chromatography/fluorescence detector. Food Chemistry 125, 1423–1429.

Chen, R.-K., Chang, L.-W., Chung, Y.-Y., Lee, M.-H., Ling, Y.-C., 2004. Quantification of cow milk adulteration in goat milk using high-performance liquid chromatography with electrospray ionization mass spectrometry. Rapid Communications in Mass Spectrometry 18, 1167–1171.

Cometto, P., Faye, M.P.F., Naranjo, R.D., Rubio, M.A., Aldao, M.A.J., 2003. Comparison of free amino acids profile in honey from three Argentinian regions. Journal of Agricultural and Food Chemistry 51, 5079–5087.

Cordella, C., Militā, J.S.L.T., Clement, M.-C., Drajnudel, P., Cabrol-Bass, D., 2005. Detection and quantification of honey adulteration via direct incorporation of sugar syrups or bee-feeding: preliminary study using high-performance anion exchange chromatography with pulsed amperometric detection (HPAEC-PAD) and chemometrics. Analytica Chimica Acta 531, 239–248.

Cordero, C., Liberto, E., Sgorbini, B., Rubiolo, P., Bicchi, C., 2012. Gas chromatography. In: Picò, Y. (Ed.), Chemical Analysis of Food: Techniques and Applications. Academic Press, San Diego, CA, pp. 311–374.

Cotte, J.F., Casabianca, H., Chardon, S., Lheritier, J., Grenier-Loustalot, M.F., 2003. Application of carbohydrate analysis to verify honey authenticity. Journal of Chromatography A 1021, 145–155.

Czerwenka, C., Maier, I., Potocnik, N., Pittner, F., Lindner, W., 2007. Absolute quantitation of beta-lactoglobulin by protein liquid chromatography mass spectrometry and its application to different milk products. Analytical Chemistry 79, 5165–5172.

Czerwenka, C., Muller, L., Lindner, W., 2010. Detection of the adulteration of water buffalo milk and mozzarella with cow's milk by liquid chromatography–mass spectrometry analysis of b-lactoglobulin variants. Food Chemistry 122, 901–908.

De Angelis, M., Rizzello, C.G., Fasano, A., Clemente, M.G., De Simone, C., Silano, M., De Vincenzi, M., Losito, I., Gobbetti, M., 2006. VSL#3 probiotic preparation has the capacity to hydrolyze gliadin polypeptides responsible for Celiac Sprue. Biochimica et Biophysica Acta 1762, 80–93.

De La Fuente, M.A., Juárez, M., 2005. Authenticity assessment of dairy products. Critical Reviews in Food Science and Nutrition 45, 563–585.

De la Mata-Espinosa, P., Bosque-Sendra, J.M., Bro, R., Cuadros-Rodríguez, L., 2011. Olive oil quantification of edible vegetable oil blends using triacylglycerols chromatographic fingerprints and chemometric tools. Talanta 85, 177−182.

D'Orazio, G., Cifuentes, A., Fanali, S., 2008. Chiral nano-liquid chromatography-mass spectrometry applied to amino acids analysis for orange juice profiling. Food Chemistry 108, 1114−1121.

Dominguez-Vega, E., Crego, A.L., Lomsadze, K., Chankvetadze, B., Marina, M.L., 2011. Enantiomeric separation of FMOC-amino acids by nano-LC and CEC using a new chiral stationary phase, cellulose tris(3-chloro-4-methylphenylcarbamate). Electrophoresis 32, 2700−2707.

Dorman, F.L., Dawes, P., 2012. Column technology: open tubular columns. In: Poole, C.F. (Ed.), Gas Chromatography. Elsevier, New York.

Dugo, P., Kumm, T., Cacciola, F., Dugo, G., Mondello, L., 2008. Multidimensional liquid chromatographic separations applied to the analysis of food samples. Journal of Liquid Chromatography & Related Technologies 31, 1758−1807.

Ehling, S., Cole, S., 2011. Analysis of organic acids in fruit juices by liquid chromatography-mass spectrometry: an enhanced tool for authenticity testing. Journal of Agricultural and Food Chemistry 59, 2229−2234.

Enne, G., Elez, D., Fondrini, F., Bonizzi, I., Feligini, M., Aleandri, R., 2005. High-performance liquid chromatography of governing liquid to detect illegal bovine milk's addition in water buffalo Mozzarella: comparison with results from raw milk and cheese matrix. Journal of Chromatography A 1094, 169−174.

Fanali, S., Aturki, Z., D'Orazio, G., Raggi, M.A., Quaglia, M.G., Sabbioni, C., Rocco, A., 2005. Use of nano-liquid chromatography for the analysis of glycyrrhizin and glycyrrhetic acid in licorice roots and candies. Journal of Separation Science 28, 982−986.

Fanali, C., Asensio-Ramos, M., Hernandez-Borges, J., Rocco, A., Fanali, S., 2011a. Nano-liquid chromatographic separations. In: Byrdwell, W.C., Holcapek, M. (Eds.), Extreme Chromatography. AOCS Press, Urbana, IL, USA, pp. 301−380.

Fanali, C., Dugo, L., D'Orazio, G., Lirangi, M., Dachá, M., Dugo, P., Mondello, L., 2011b. Analysis of anthocyanins in commercial fruit juices by using nano-liquid chromatography-electrospray-mass spectrometry and high-performance liquid chromatography with UV-vis detector. Journal of Separation Science 34, 150−159.

Fanali, C., Dugo, L., Dugo, P., Mondello, L., 2013a. Capillary-liquid chromatography (CLC) and nano-LC in food analysis. Trends in Analytical Chemistry 52, 226−238.

Fanali, C., Dugo, P., Mondello, L., D'Orazio, G., Fanali, S., 2013b. Recent developments in high-performance liquid chromatography. In: Nollet, L.M.L., Toldrà, F. (Eds.), Food Analysis by HPLC, third ed. CRC Press, USA, pp. 1−31.

Fasciotti, M., Annibal, D.P.N., 2010. Optimization and application of methods of triacylglycerol evaluation for characterization of olive oil adulteration by soybean oil with HPLC-APCI-MS-MS. Talanta 81, 1116−1125.

Ferreira, I.M.P.L.V.O., Caçote, H., 2003. Detection and quantification of bovine, ovine and caprine milk percentages in protected denomination of origin cheeses by reversed-phase high-performance liquid chromatography of beta-lactoglobulins. Journal of Chromatography A 1015, 111−118.

Forgács, E., Cserháti, T., 2003. Gas chromatography. In: Lees, M. (Ed.), Food Authenticity and Traceability. CRC Press, Boca Raton, FL, pp. 197−217.

Fügel, R., Carle, R., Schieber, A., 2005. Quality and authenticity control of fruit purées, fruit preparations and jams-a review. Trends in Food Science & Technology 16, 433−441.

Gómez-Ariza, J.L., Villegas-Portero, M.J., Bernal-Daza, V., 2005. Characterization and analysis of amino acids in orange juice by HPLC—MS/MS for authenticity assessment. Analytica Chimica Acta 540, 221—230.

Grob, K., Giuffre, A.M., Leuzzi, U., Mincione, B., 1994. Fat Science Technology. 96, 286.

Hadjmohammadi, M.R., Nazari, S., Kamel, K., 2009. Determination of flavanoid markers in honey with SPE and LC using experimental design. Chromatographia 69, 1291—1297.

Hernandez-Borges, J., D'Orazio, G., Aturki, Z., Fanali, S., 2007. Nano-liquid chromatography analysis of dansylated biogenic amines in wines. Journal of Chromatography A 1147, 192—199.

Herrero, M., Ibánez, E., Cifuentes, A., Bernal, J., 2009. Multidimensional chromatography in food analysis. Journal of Chromatography A 1216, 7110—7129.

Holcapek, M., Velinská, H., Lisa, M., Cesla, P., 2009. Orthogonality of silver-ion and non-aqueous reversed-phase HPLC/MS in the analysis of complex natural mixtures of triacylglycerols. Journal of Separation Science 32, 3672—3680.

Ibañez, E., Señoráns, F.J., 2005. Liquid chromatography: food applications. In: Worsfold, P., Townshend, A., Poole, C. (Eds.), Encyclopedia of Analytical Science, second ed.

Kamm, W., Dionisi, F., Hischenhuber, C., Schmarr, H.-G., Engel, K.-H., 2002. Rapid detection of vegetable oils in milk fat by on-line LC-GC analysis of β-sitosterol as marker. European Journal of Lipid Science and Technology 104, 756—761.

Klee, M.S., 2012. Detectors. In: Poole, C.F. (Ed.), Gas Chromatography. Elsevier, New York.

Kwon, S.W., 2004. Profiling of soluble proteins in wine by nano-high-performance liquid chromatography/tandem mass spectrometry. Journal of Agricultural and Food Chemistry 52, 7258—7263.

Lee, D.-S., Lee, E.-S., Kim, H.-J., Kim, S.-O., Kim, K., 2001. Reversed phase liquid chromatographic determination of triacylglycerol composition in sesame oils and the chemometric detection of adulteration. Analytica Chimica Acta 429, 321—330.

Lehotay, S.J., 2002. Application of gas chromatography in food analysis. Trends in Analytical Chemistry 21, 686—697.

Lisa, M., Holcapek, M., 2008. TGs profiling in plant oils important in food industry, dietetics and cosmetics using HPLC/APCI—MS. Journal of Chromatography A 1198, 115—130.

Marriott, P.J., Chin, S.-T., Maikhunthod, B., Schmarr, H.-G., Bieri, S., 2012. Multidimensional gas chromatography. Trends in Analytical Chemistry 34, 1—20.

Method 2.323. In: Paquot, C., Hautfenne, A. (Eds.), 1987. Standard Methods for the Analysis of Oils and Derivatives, seventh ed. Blackwell Publishing, Oxford.

Monaci, L., Losito, I., Palmisano, F., Visconti, A., 2010. Identification of allergenic milk proteins markers in fined white wines by capillary liquid chromatography electrospray ionization-tandem mass spectrometry. Journal of Chromatography A 1217, 4300—4305.

Moore, J.C., Spink, J., Lipp, M., 2012. Development and application of a database of food ingredient fraud and economically motivated adulteration from 1980 to 2010. Journal of Food Science 77, R118—R126.

Morales, V., Corzo, N., Sanz, M.L., 2008. HPAEC-PAD oligosaccharide analysis to detect adulterations of honey with sugar syrups. Food Chemistry 107, 922—928.

Nollet, L.M.L., 2003. High-pressure liquid chromatography (HPLC). In: Lees, M. (Ed.), Food Authentication, Food Authenticity and Traceability. CRC Press, Boca Raton, FL, pp. 218—238.

Ornelas-Soto, N., Barbosa-Garcia, O., Lopez-de-Alba, P.L., 2011. In: Shoyama, Y. (Ed.), Procedures of Food Quality Control: Analysis Methods, Sampling and Sample Pretreatment, Quality Control of Herbal Medicines and Related Areas. InTech, ISBN 978-953-307-682-9.

Osorio, M.T., Haughey, S.A., Elliott, C.T., Koidis, A., 2014. Evaluation of methodologies to determine vegetable oil species present in oil mixtures: proposition of an approach to meet the EU legislation demands for correct vegetable oils labeling. Food Research International 60, 66–67.

Ouchemoukh, S., Schweitzer, P., Bey, M.B., Djoudad-Kadji, H., Louaileche, H., 2010. HPLC sugar profiles of Algerian honeys. Food Chemistry 121, 561–568.

Park, Y.W., Chang, P.-S., Lee, J.H., 2010. Application of triacylglycerol and fatty acid analyses to discriminate blended sesame oil with soybean oil. Food Chemistry 123, 377–383.

Puigventós, L., Navarro, M., Alechaga, É., Núñez, O., Saurina, J., Hernández-Cassou, S., Puignou, L., 2015. Determination of polyphenolic profiles by liquid chromatography-electrospray-tandem mass spectrometry for the authentication of fruit extracts. Analytical and Bioanalytical Chemistry 407, 597–608.

Purcaro, G., Moret, S., Conte, L., 2012. Hyphenated liquid chromatography–gas chromatography technique: recent evolution and applications. Journal of Chromatography A 1255, 100–111.

Purcaro, G., Barp, L., Beccarissa, M., Conte, L.S., 2015. Fingerprinting of vegetable oil minor components by multidimensional comprehensive gas chromatography with dual detection. Analytical and Bioanalytical Chemistry 407, 309–319.

Rebane, R., Herodes, K., 2008. Evaluation of the botanical origin of Estonian unifloral and polyfloral honeys by amino acid content. Journal of Agricultural and Food Chemistry 56, 10716–10720.

Rizzello, C.G., Coda, R., De Angelis, M., Di Cagno, R., Carnevali, P., Gobbetti, M., 2009. Long-term fungal inhibitory activity of water-soluble extract from *Amaranthus* spp. seeds during storage of gluten-free and wheat flour breads. International Journal of Food Microbiology 131, 189–196.

Rocco, A., Fanali, S., 2009. Analysis of phytosterols in extra-virgin olive oil by nanoliquid chromatography. Journal of Chromatography A 1216, 7173–7178.

Rosales-Conrado, N., Leon-Gonzales, M.E., Perez-Arribas, L.V., Polo-Diez, L.M., 2008. Determination of heterocyclic aromatic amines by capillary high performance liquid chromatography with diode array detection in ready-to-eat cooked ham treated with electron-beam irradiation. Analytical and Bioanalytical Chemistry 391, 1433–1442.

Ruiz del Castillo, M.L., Caja, M.M., Herraiz, M., 2003. Use of the enantiomeric composition for the assessment of the authenticity of fruit beverages. Journal of Agricultural and Food Chemistry 51, 1284–1288.

Ruiz-Matute, A.I., Rodríguez-Sánchez, S., Sanz, M.L., Martínez-Castro, I., 2010. Detection of adulterations of honey with high fructose syrups from inulin by GC analysis. Journal of Food Composition and Analysis 23, 273–276.

Ruiz-Samblás, C., Marini, F., Cuadros-Rodríguez, L., González-Casado, A., 2012. Quantification of blending of olive oils and edible vegetable oils by triacylglycerol fingerprint gas chromatography and chemometric tools. Journal of Chromatography B 910, 71–77.

Russo, R., Severino, V., Mendez, A., Lliberia, J., Parente, A., Chambery, A., 2012. Detection of buffalo mozzarella adulteration by an ultra-high performance liquid chromatography tandem mass spectrometry methodology. Journal of Mass Spectrometry 47, 1407–1414.

Salghi, R., Armbruster, W., Schwack, W., 2014. Detection of argan oil adulteration with vegetable oils by high-performance liquid chromatography–evaporative light scattering detection. Food Chemistry 153, 387–392.

Schieber, A., Keller, P., Carle, R., 2001. Determination of phenolic acids and flavonoids of apple and pear by high-performance liquid chromatography. Journal of Chromatography A 910, 265–273.

Si-Ahmed, K., Tazerouti, F., Badjah-Hadj-Ahmed, A.Y., Aturki, Z., D'Orazio, G., Rocco, A., Fanali, S., 2010. Analysis of hesperetin enantiomers in human urine after ingestion of blood orange juice by using nano-liquid chromatography. Journal of Pharmaceutical and Biomedical 51, 225–229.

Snyder, L.R., Dolan, J.W., 2013. Milestones in the development of liquid chromatography. In: Liquid Chromatography Fundamentals and Instrumentation. Elsevier, Waltham, MA, USA.

Stander, M.A., Kühn, W., Hiten, N.F., 2013. Survey of South African fruit juices using a fast screening HILIC-MS method. Food Additives & Contaminants: Part A 30, 1473–1484.

Timperio, A.M., Magro, P., Chilosi, G., Zolla, L., 2006. Assay of ochratoxin A in grape by high-pressure liquid chromatography coupled on line with an ESI–mass spectrometry. Journal of Chromatography B 832, 127–133.

Tranchida, P.Q., Dugo, P., Dugo, G., Mondello, L., 2004. Comprehensive two-dimensional chromatography in food analysis. Journal of Chromatography A 1054, 3–16.

Tranchida, P.Q., Salivo, S., Bonaccorsi, I., Rotondo, A., Dugoa, P., Mondello, L., 2013. Analysis of the unsaponifiable fraction of lipids belonging to various milk-types by using comprehensive two-dimensional gas chromatography with dual mass spectrometry/flame ionization detection and with the support of high resolution time-of-flight mass spectrometry for structural elucidation. Journal of Chromatography A 1313, 194–201.

Tsimidou, M., Boskou, D., 2003. Adulteration of foods: detection. In: Trugo, L., Finglas, P.M. (Eds.), Encyclopedia of Food Sciences and Nutrition, second ed. Acadamic Press, pp. 47–55.

Tswett, M., 1906. Physikalisch-Chemische Studien über das Chlorophyll. Die Adsorption (Physical-chemical studies chlorophyll. Adsorption). Berichte der Deutschen botanischen Gesellschaft 24, 316–326.

Ulberth, F., 2003. Milk and dairy products. In: Lees, M. (Ed.), Food Authenticity and Traceability. CRC Press, Boca Raton, FL.

Unger, K.K., Lamotte, S., Machtejevas, E., 2013. Milestones in the development of liquid chromatography. In: Liquid Chromatography Fundamentals and Instrumentation. Elsevier, Waltham, MA, USA.

United States Pharmacopeia, 2012. Food Chemicals Codex, eighth ed. The United States Pharmacopeial Convention, Rockville, Md.

Vaclavik, L., Schreiber, A., Lacina, O., Cajka, T., Hajslova, J., 2011. Liquid chromatography–mass spectrometry-based metabolomics for authenticity assessment of fruit juices. Metabolomics 8, 793–803.

Veloso, A.C.A., Teixeira, N., Ferreira, I.M.P.L.V.O., 2002. Separation and quantification of the major casein fractions by reverse-phase high-performance liquid chromatography and urea–polyacrylamide gel electrophoresis detection of milk adulterations. Journal of Chromatography A 967, 209–218.

Wang, S., Guo, Q., Wang, L., Lin, L., Shi, H., Cao, H., Cao, B., 2015. Detection of honey adulteration with starch syrup by high performance liquid chromatography. Food Chemistry 172, 669–674.

Weber, D., Raymond, P., Ben-Rejeb, S., Lau, B., 2006. Development of a liquid chromatography-tandem mass spectrometry method using capillary liquid chromatography and nanoelectrospray ionization-quadrupole time-of-flight hybrid mass spectrometer for the detection of milk allergens. Journal of Agricultural and Food Chemistry 54, 1604–1610.

Yashin, Y.I., Yashin, A.Y., 2012. Liquid chromatography. In: Picò, Y. (Ed.), Chemical Analysis of Food: Techniques and Applications. Academic Press, San Diego, CA, pp. 311–374.

Yao, L., Jiang, Y., Singanusong, R., Datta, N., Raymont, K., 2004. Phenolic acids and abscisic acid in Australian Eucalyptus honeys and their potential for floral authentication. Food Chemistry 86, 169–177.

Zhang, B., Li, X., Yan, B., 2008. Advances in HPLC detection—towards universal detection. Analytical and Bioanalytical Chemistry 390, 299–301.

Zhang, L., Li, P., Sun, X., Wang, X., Xu, B., Wang, X., Ma, F., Zhang, Q., Ding, X., 2014. Classification and adulteration detection of vegetable oils based on fatty acid profiles. Journal of Agricultural and Food Chemistry 62, 8745–8751.

Zhou, J., Qi, Y., Ritho, J., Duan, L., Wu, L., Dia, Q., Li, Y., Zhao, J., 2014. Analysis of maltooligosaccharides in honey samples by ultra-performance liquid chromatography coupled with evaporative light scattering detection. Food Research International 56, 260–265.

Advances in Polymerase Chain Reaction Technologies for Food Authenticity Testing

11

E. Maestri, N. Marmiroli
University of Parma, Parma, Italy

Chapter Outline

11.1 Introduction

The horse meat scandal of 2013 has to be considered a turning point for DNA analysis in food authenticity. The discovery of horse meat as a fraudulent addition to beef meat preparations across Europe, such as burgers and lasagne, brought to the attention of consumers, law enforcers, and regulators the need for reliable, rapid, and effective tools for detection of such cases of adulteration (http://ec.europa.eu/food/safety/official_controls/food_fraud/horse_meat/index_en.htm). It was evident that the only way to detect the presence of horse meat was through analysis of DNA extracted from food, but the methods to be applied could be a matter for discussion (Busby and Burns, 2014); they can in fact be based on detection of nuclear or mitochondrial loci, in a qualitative or quantitative approach, with multitarget or simple approaches. The effectiveness and sensitivity of the methods determine the limit of detection (LOD), the threshold that defines the limits for applicability of the technique; below this limit, adulteration is not detectable.

An extensive collection of material from the literature before 2010 (Moore et al., 2012) identified the main categories of fraud and adulteration in food. The possible types of frauds have been categorized into three groups: the "replacement" of an ingredient with a different substance or ingredient that is less expensive; and the "addition" of non-authorized, non-authentic substances; the "removal" of a component that is authentic. By definition, the fraud is economically motivated (Manning and Soon, 2014), so the examples reported by Moore et al. refer to cases in which the manipulation of the food product lowered the costs with respect to the authentic product. In some instances, the authenticity of a food product, and the fraudulent substitution of ingredients, can affect the health of consumers. One such example is the use of fish species that contain specific lipid compounds with known laxative properties, like escolar, *Lepidocybium flavobrunneum* (Dalama et al., 2015).

According to Moore et al. (2012), the food categories in which ingredients are more often subjected to fraud include oils, milk, fruit juices, and spices. The most recent report of the newly instituted Food Fraud Network (European Commission, 2015) identified in the European Union (EU) 60 cases of cross-border fraudulent events in 2014; meat and fish were the categories most affected in this survey. Apparently there is a discrepancy between the focus of research efforts and the types of frauds in the food business.

The EU has invested millions of euro for research on food safety, quality, traceability, and recently "integrity" of the food supply chains; the "What's for Lunch?" conference in 2011 summarized the main results (http://ec.europa.eu/research/agriculture/wfl/index_en.html). The research project FoodIntegrity (www.foodintegrity.eu) is currently coordinating efforts for organizing and harmonizing the knowledge gathered in the past years, building knowledge bases and guidelines for analysts, researchers, and stakeholders. Among the many different analytical techniques, amplification of DNA through the polymerase chain reaction (PCR; Mullis et al., 1986) has a central role as a tool for analysis in food authenticity issues. Table 11.1 reports some examples of issues connected to frauds in food production-which can be addressed with analytical approaches based on PCR amplification; some of these will be mentioned or discussed in this chapter. The examples are classified into two groups according to the type of analytical approach that is required: (1) the verification of presence/absence of specific ingredients; (2) the identification of the ingredients (species determination). Both types of analyses are needed to detect instances of replacement, addition or substitution. The results of a literature search

Table 11.1 Examples Illustrating Food Authenticity Issues That Can Be Addressed With Polymerase Chain Reaction–Based Analyses

Food Category or Product	Verification of Presence of Declared Ingredient or Absence of Specified Ingredients	Species Identification
Meats	• Beef instead of buffalo • Pork in halal or kosher foods • Presence of ostrich meat • Beef of Korean breed • Meat from male animals (beef) • Ingredients specific for traditional products • Soybean in meat preparations	• Game meat, game birds • Multiple species in complex foods • Diversity of fermentation organisms
Seafood	• Scombroid mislabeling • Presence of Salmonidae, adulteration with trout • Perch instead of grouper • Substitution of anglerfish (*Lophius* spp.) • Ingredients from shark • Presence of true sardines • Presence of flying fish	• Identification of threatened species • Tuna species identification • Identification of scallops • Identification of jellyfish • Labeling of shrimps • Ingredients in sushi or sashimi
Dairy products and milk	• Buffalo or yak milk • Cow milk in hypoallergenic products • Breed in traditional products	• Identification of microbial strains in cheese production • Fingerprinting of microbiota for geographical origin
Cereals	• Ingredients from no gluten cereals • Adulteration of spelt with wheat • Varietal identification in protected designations of origin	• Identification of cereals in flour • Identification of fragrant rice
Oils	• Varietal identification in protected designations of origin	• Identification of adulterants from different species
Coffee, tea, chocolate, wine, fruit juices	• Identification of variety or cultivar (eg, Arabica and Robusta coffee) • Presence of a variety from a specific area (Ecuadorian cocoa) • Dilution of orange juice with mandarin juice	• Identification of yeast strains in wine • Identification of allergenic ingredients (eg, nuts)
Mushrooms	• Presence of *Boletus edulis*	
Marzipan	• Use of apricot or peach kernel instead of almond	

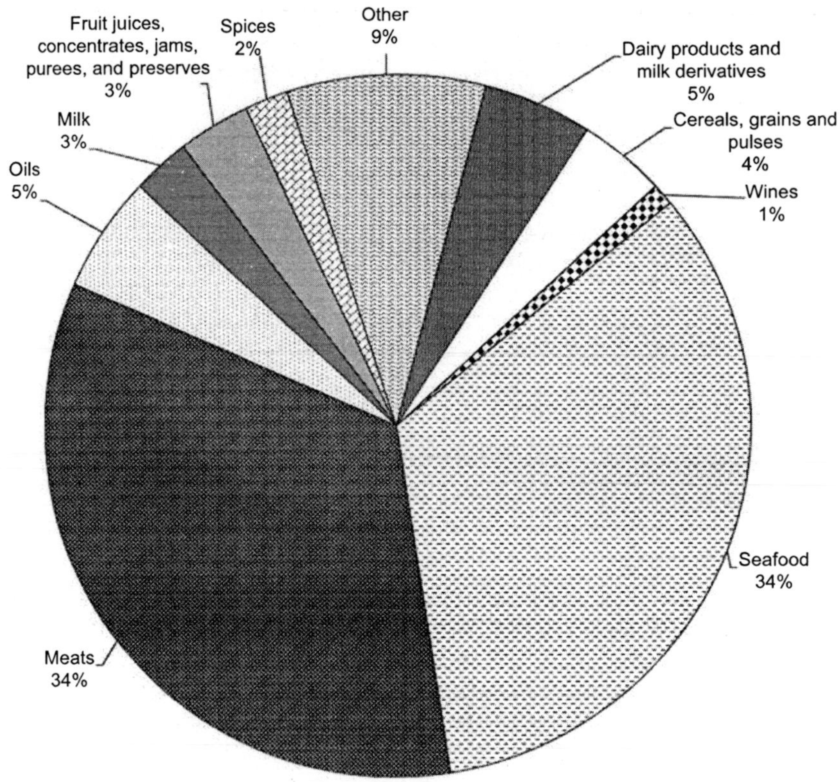

Figure 11.1 Percent distribution of scholarly record citations based on food ingredient category (as of April 2015). Categories are according to Moore et al. (2012).

(Web of Science, performed in April 2015, 1993–2015) covering 300 papers on the use of PCR in food analysis show that authenticity of seafood and meat are the main targets (Fig. 11.1). This is in agreement with the current occurrence of frauds in the food sector (European Commission, 2015).

The chapter will address the critical steps and requirements in PCR analysis of food products, reporting on the recent literature for consolidated approaches and innovative solutions.

11.2 Process of Using PCR Technologies in the Analysis of Food

11.2.1 Procedures for DNA Extraction and Purification

The extraction of DNA from cellular structures is a critical step in the utilization of PCR for food authenticity procedures. The experiments reported in the literature are performed either with commercial kits or with in-house methods, showing differences in efficacy, cost, and ease of execution (Pirondini et al., 2010; Turci et al., 2010; Pafundo et al., 2011; Ramos-Gómez et al., 2014). Examples of commercial kits often utilized for food products are: Wizard Genomic DNA (Promega), DNeasy Blood and Tissue kit (Qiagen), DNeasy Plant Kit (Qiagen), QIAamp DNA Stool kit (Qiagen), NucleoSpin Food (Macherey—Nagel), and NucleoSpin Plant (Macherey—Nagel).

The in-house protocols are usually based on the use of detergents (Demeke and Jenkins, 2010), such as hexadecyltrimethylammonium bromide (CTAB), polyvinylpyrrolidone (PVP), sodium dodecyl sulphate (SDS), Tween-20, guanidine hydrochloride, and guanidine isothiocyanate.

It is a fact that the tissues and organs of animals or plants affect the efficiency of DNA extraction differently. The modular approach introduced by Holst-Jensen and Berdal (2004) for detection of genetically modified organisms brings a separate validation for each step of the procedure. For each different matrix, the procedure of DNA extraction must be validated, evaluating the effectiveness in purifying DNA of acceptable quality and quantity. The choice of DNA extraction method might be based on previous experience, literature data, and the preparation of suitable control samples. A discriminating factor is also the requirements for a skilled labor force and expensive resources, when the aim of the analysis is the application in the food industry.

In recent years, the development of extraction-less or direct PCR methods, without prior DNA purification (Mercier et al., 1990; Kitpipit et al., 2014), has been proposed to achieve time and cost savings, but also to increase recovery of DNA molecules and assay sensitivity. Extraction-less methods are frequently used in medicine and diagnostics, but their application to food matrices still requires development. An advantage of these protocols is that dilution of the sample allows the dilution of inhibitors (see Section 11.4.2). Commercial kits can be exploited in this procedure, such as Phire Direct PCR kits (Life Technologies).

11.2.2 Concerns About DNA Copy Number and Representation of Genomic Information

The degree of ploidy could be a relevant issue when analyzing complex food products and identifying materials from different species or different tissues. Several examples of polyploid cells can be found in animals (liver, muscle) and plants (endosperm, pericarp). Polyploidy usually refers to the nuclear genome, but it must be considered that the number of genome copies from mitochondria and chloroplasts is also variable. Floren et al. (2015) recently estimated the proportion of mitochondrial vs nuclear gene markers in different tissues from bovines; muscle and liver cells contained over 1000 copies of mitochondrial targets per each copy of nuclear target, whereas fat and tendons contained about 200. It is therefore evident that reliable quantification of food components must consider the degree of ploidy and the number of copies of the target genes.

It has been reported that the determination of DNA content in food products requires a case-by-case approach to account for effects due to the matrix. A solution proposed by Drummond et al. (2013) requires the generation of standard curves in the analyzed matrix, for instance milk—this should account for differences in amplificability of DNA from the species of interest.

11.2.3 Nuclear vs Organellar Genomes as Targets for Analysis

The application of PCR approaches in the analyses for food authenticity relies essentially on the concept of "DNA barcoding," that is, the amplification of short gene sequences exhibiting high-interspecific variability (between species) and low-intraspecific variability (within species; Hebert et al., 2003). Modifications of this basic approach concern the choice of targets and the methodology for discriminating between variants. According to the principles of DNA barcoding (www.barcodeoflife.org), the standard target for animal species is the 5′ region of the mitochondrial gene for cytochrome c oxidase subunit 1 (*COI* or *COX1*); for plant species, two chloroplast genes are chosen: ribulose-bisphosphate carboxylase oxygenase (*rbcL*) and maturase K (*matK*). The Barcode of Life Data Systems server (www.boldsystems.org) provides a service for identification of species from sequences of these target genes, although the number of plant species is limited.

The chloroplast genome (cpDNA) can be exploited for definite identification of food from plants also in complex mixtures, since the gene order is conserved and the number of copies per cell is high. By appropriately choosing the target fragment for analysis, amplification of cpDNA can provide identification of the plant species, exploiting sequence variations in coding sequences or introns (see Table 11.2). Additional targets have been suggested to improve the approach when amplification of *rbcL* and *matK* fails, such as the intergenic region *trnH*(GUG)-*psbA*, between the genes for tRNA-histidine and the photosystem II protein D1 (Pang et al., 2012). A common marker is also a fragment including the intraspacer region *trnL*(UAA)-*trnF*(GAA), or the intron of *trnL*, in which specific polymorphisms can be recognized and exploited (James and Schmidt, 2004).

Markers from the mitochondrial DNA (mtDNA) are usually preferred in analysis of food of animal origin (Table 11.2 and Fig. 11.2). The small dimension of mtDNA and the presence of multiple copies in each cell increase the chances of finding the targets when analyzing processed products. From the genetic point of view, the availability of sequence data, together with the extent of inter- and intraspecies variability, has led to identification of suitable markers: cytochrome b (*CYTB*), *COX1*, NADH dehydrogenase subunit 5 (*ND5*) and subunit 2 (*ND2*), ATPase subunit 6 and 8, D-loop, and 16S rRNA. In several applications, and for the Barcode of Life, the *COX1* gene has been chosen as target due to its low intraspecific variability (eg, Dalama et al., 2015; for fish identification). The consensus primers for the *COX1* gene may fail to amplify DNA in some species (eg, in Scombridae, Abdullah and Rehbein, 2014), and so alternative target genes are studied (see, eg, Marín et al., 2015).

However, when a quantification of the contribution for each species is required, mtDNA cannot be the marker of choice, since the number of mitochondrial genomes in cells is variable (see Section 11.2.2). For this purpose, a nuclear DNA marker is required, present in single copy and assessed with quantitative real-time PCR (qPCR), using external standards for precise quantification (see Section 11.2.4).

Table 11.2 Examples of Genes and Markers Applied to Analysis of Main Food Products for Identification of Species or Varieties

Main Food Category or Product	Genome Localization of the Marker	Marker Gene or Locus (Gene Symbol)[a]
Meats	Mitochondrial	Cytochrome b (*CYTB*)
		ATP synthase F0 subunit 6 (*ATP6*)
		ATP synthase F0 subunit 8 (*ATP8*)
		Cytochrome c oxidase subunit I (*COX1*)
		Cytochrome c oxidase subunit II (*COX2*)
		12S rRNA
		16S rRNA
		D-loop
	Nuclear	Coagulation factor II (*F2*)
		Myostatin (*MSTN*)
		18S rRNA (*RN18S1*)[b]
Seafood	Mitochondrial	Cytochrome b (*CYTB*)
		tRNA-Glu, tRNA-Thr
		Cytochrome c oxidase subunit I (*COX1*)
		16S rRNA gene, 5′ end
	Nuclear	Rhodopsin (*RH1*)
		28S rRNA[b]
Dairy products and milk	Mitochondrial	D-loop
		Cytochrome b (*CYTB*)
		12S rRNA
Cereals	Chloroplast	*trnL*(UAA) intron
	Nuclear	Barley: γ-hordein
		Rice: phospholipase D (*PLD*), betaine aldehyde dehydrogenase (*BAD2*)
		Wheat: Acetyl-CoA carboxylase (*Acc-1*)
		Wheat D genome: γ-gliadin
		ITS1 region in rRNA gene
Coffee, tea, chocolate, wine, fruit juices	Chloroplast	*trnL*(UAA) intron
		trnL(UAA)-*trnF*(GAA) intraspacer region
		trnH(GUG)-*psbA* intergenic region

Continued

Table 11.2 Continued

Main Food Category or Product	Genome Localization of the Marker	Marker Gene or Locus (Gene Symbol)[a]
Oils	Chloroplast	*trnL*(UAA) intron
		Ribulose 1,5-bisphosphate carboxylase large subunit (*rbcL*)
	Nuclear	Plasma intrinsic protein (*pip1*)
		Fatty acid desaturase 2 (*fad2*)
		Oleosin
		Cycloartenol synthase 2 (*OEX*)
		Lupeol synthase (*lup*)
Microbiota of food products	Bacterial genome	16-23S ribosomal intergenic transcribed spacer phenylalanyl-tRNA synthase (*pheS*)

[a]Gene symbols as reported in NCBI (www.ncbi.nlm.nih.gov).
[b]Genes utilized as positive control of amplification.

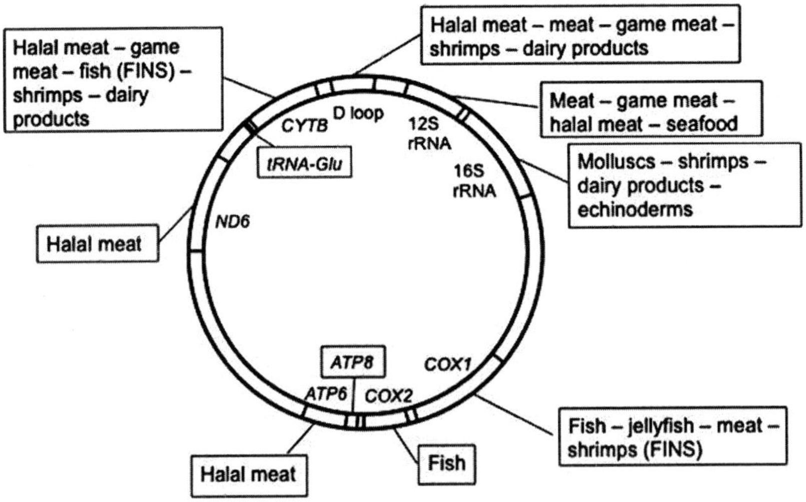

Figure 11.2 Schematic representation of a mitochondrial genome from animal organisms, with indication of the genes mainly used for species identification. For each gene, indication of recent applications to food analysis is provided in external boxes.

One such gene is the myostatin gene, which is present in all mammals and also in bird species.

When using nuclear genes for identification, one objective could be the maximization of differences between breeds or species. In this case, after choosing a gene present in single copy in all species of interest, highly variable regions of the gene should be targeted, such as introns or regulatory regions. Table 11.2 lists some of the genes commonly utilized for different food products. An alternative is to use highly polymorphic molecular markers (Martins-Lopes et al., 2013), such as microsatellites (simple sequence repeat regions) or single nucleotide polymorphisms (SNPs). Based on the polymorphic information content (PIC), a panel of markers is usually required to achieve certain identification of the cultivars present in the sample (Consolandi et al., 2007; Vietina et al., 2011; Bazakos et al., 2012; Savo Sardaro et al., 2013). SNPs can be also used as markers for the mtDNA, to trace maternal lineages in animals. In the mtDNA of pigs, 63 polymorphic positions can discriminate between Asian and European descent for the recognition of rustic breeds of European origin (van Asch et al., 2011).

For the purpose of recognizing ingredients with allergenic potential, a specific marker gene is required for each species of concern (eg, in Pafundo et al., 2009, 2011) together with a common reference gene.

A control gene for verification of amplificability of DNA is sometimes utilized. Suitable marker genes are the 18S rRNA gene (Amaral et al., 2015) and the 28S rRNA gene (Armani et al., 2014).

The existence of intraspecies variation in the sequences chosen as targets can become a problem when looking for adulteration, by hindering the annealing of primers in PCR reactions, or increasing the complexity of the fingerprinting results. Optimization of each panel of primers is a prerequisite for the design of an effective test, as demonstrated in Castigliego et al. (2015).

11.2.4 End Point vs Real-Time PCR

End point PCR can provide sufficient data when the assay is developed for qualitative purposes, for instance, determining the presence or absence of a specific target. It can be effective when combined (hyphenated) with innovative methods for visualization of amplicons without gel electrophoresis (see Section 11.5.1).

Real-time PCR is currently widely used in place of end point PCR. Several books and reviews have described the principles and technical modifications of qPCR and the applications to quantification of template DNA (eg, see Marmiroli and Maestri, 2007; Navarro et al., 2015). The main approaches for quantitative detection of amplicons rely either on dyes that intercalate in double-stranded DNA, like SybrGreen I, or on specific oligonucleotide probes labeled with fluorescent dyes. An extensive description of the different chemistries is out of the purpose of this chapter. Often, tests for food authenticity are developed with intercalating dyes, since they are less expensive than tests based on specific probes, both for reagents and for equipment.

In developing a method based on qPCR for food analysis, critical parameters should be subjected to optimization to achieve sensitivity and specificity: concentration of primers and probes, annealing temperature, and quantity of the template DNA. A requirement for PCR efficiency ranging between 90% and 110% is often mandatory, which corresponds to the slope in reference curves between −3.1 and −3.6 (Codex Alimentarius Commission, 2010).

The LOD for qPCR applications can be as low as 3 pg of template DNA and is estimated considering the lowest concentration of template DNA that corresponds to successful amplification with 95% confidence. The LOD value is critical in determining the applicability of a technique or method, and affects the regulator's choice about the threshold above which the substitution can be considered "intentional adulteration." Busby and Burns (2014) performed a comparison of LOD values obtained with different PCR approaches in mixtures of horse and beef meat. They highlighted an important problem that is observable when comparing results from the literature: there is extreme heterogeneity of measurement units in LOD values, as weight percentage, or number of genome copies, or picograms of DNA. In the process of quantification, it should be necessary to convert the results expressed as copy number or concentration into a measure that provides information about the adulteration or mixture, such as percentage based on weight or volume. A description of such a procedure is provided by Druml et al. (2015) for mixtures of game meat and identification of deer species.

Repeatability, robustness, and reproducibility are other parameters for defining the reliability of the method, and they can be estimated by assessing the standard deviation of repeated measures in different conditions: thermal cycler models, DNA extraction procedure, operator, volumes of reaction, and reagent concentrations.

End point PCR is often followed by sequencing for confirmation of the target amplicon. Real-time PCR can be combined with the melting curve analysis (MCA), where the kinetics of denaturation of the amplicons can provide information about the sequence, in appropriate conditions. The test must ensure that the target amplicons are well discriminated by their melting temperatures (eg, in Castigliego et al., 2015).

Optimization of PCR reactions, in any case, requires trials and comparisons in a number of different conditions for primer sequences and concentrations, DNA concentration, reagents concentrations, Taq polymerase, temperature conditions, and equipment (Codex Alimentarius Commission, 2010).

11.2.5 Multiplex Analyses and Multitarget Analyses

Analyses for food authenticity rarely require amplification of a single target. More often the identification of ingredients requires multiple comparisons. The development of assays with simultaneous amplification of different target genes is therefore an active field of research (Ali et al., 2014).

11.2.5.1 Multiplex PCR

Multiplexing endpoint PCR protocols requires an accurate optimization phase, necessary to avoid nonspecific amplification due to the presence of multiple primer pairs in the reaction mixture. The main decisions for optimization concern the concentrations of DNA template, primers, $MgCl_2$, deoxynucleotides, Taq polymerase, and the temperature regime. A recent example of optimization with complete description of the procedure can be found in Armani et al. (2014) for a PCR reaction including six primer pairs.

11.2.5.2 Dual-Probe Assay

Dual-probe assay is a qualitative assay designed to detect the presence of two species or entities in mixtures. The target gene is amplified from conserved primers, whereas two TaqMan probes, labeled with different fluorophores, are designed to target a specific polymorphism present in the amplified fragments, discriminating between two species or breeds (eg, orange and mandarin, Pardo, 2015). The fluorescence for both dyes measured at end point identifies the composition of the sample through an appropriate software for genotyping. If the target gene is in the nuclear genome, it can be adapted for quantitative purposes.

11.2.5.3 Triplex qPCR

This is a quantitative assay designed to compare the amount of the target gene against two calibrator genes specific for the species of interest; the three amplicons are detected with TaqMan probes labeled with different dyes. In the approach described by Iwobi et al. (2015) the target gene is myostatin, compared with two probes targeting coding sequences of genes specific for beef and pork, respectively, cyclic-GMP-phosphodiesterase and β-actin. Two reference curves are constructed by considering the genome equivalents of the two species. The authors suggest that this approach overcomes the problems in DNA quantification in complex mixtures where different tissues are combined together.

11.3 Application of PCR Technologies to Detect Adulteration

The main issue in food authenticity is "origin" at large, which can be geographical origin or the source of raw matter, ie, the organisms used for production. PCR approaches are targeted to biological components of food, derived from the organisms that contributed to production or processing, and therefore they are ideally suited both for verification of claims and for fingerprinting of unknown components (Table 11.1). On the other hand, identification of the country or location of origin has been addressed through other systems, targeting other components of food products besides DNA, eg, proportions of stable isotopes (Chapter 12 this volume). A possible contribution of PCR to determination of geographical origin has made use of bacterial diversity as a marker of territorial specificity. For example, Połka et al. (2015) have fingerprinted the bacterial flora involved in fermentation of typical salami combining PCR, denaturing gradient gel electrophoresis (PCR-DGGE), and sequencing of 16S rRNA genes. The bacterial communities can be indicative of a specific region but they can also indicate compliance with the technical specification of certified products: protected designation of origin (PDO), protected geographical indication (PGI) in Europe. The bacterial biodiversity in milk samples can be related to the production site or farm, as in Feligini et al. (2015). The identity and proportion of bacteria is of high relevance also in the case of fermented dairy products, cheese, yogurt, and such. Bottari et al. (2013) developed a multiplex assay in qPCR followed by MCA, for fingerprinting the starters in the production of PDO cheese Parmigiano Reggiano. PCR-DGGE of 16S and 26S rRNA genes have also been used to describe the microbial communities responsible for fermentation of cocoa, as biological markers associated to the quality of the food product (Hamdouche et al., 2015).

Based on this approach, the fingerprinting of microbial communities in food has been proposed as a way of tracing the farming type, organic or conventional; Bigot et al. (2015) applied PCR-DGGE as a "biological signature" for yeasts and bacteria associated to nectarines and peaches, discriminating the fruits according to their origin.

11.4 Case Studies

The application of PCR-based methods to authenticity analyses is affected by the complexity of the food product in terms of ingredients, and by the amount of processing required for its production. Acid pH, high temperature, and mechanical treatments can lead to chemical and physical modifications of DNA molecules (Peano et al., 2004). These factors will affect the length of the DNA molecules recovered and the presence of inhibitors to the PCR reactions. Therefore, the choice of the most appropriate method for sample treatment must be performed on a case-by-case basis (Scarano and Rao, 2014).

The method of choice for DNA extraction and purification should provide sufficient amounts of DNA, of sufficient quality to allow amplification, eliminating potential inhibitors that might be present in the food product (Pirondini et al., 2010; Turci et al., 2010).

Several substances present in food can behave as inhibitors of polymerase reactions: polysaccharides, polyphenols, tannins, fatty acids, lipids, and minerals can be present in food products, particularly in those of plant origin (Demeke and Jenkins, 2010). A recent review (Schrader et al., 2012) illustrates the mechanisms of inhibition of PCR reactions and possible procedures for elimination of inhibitors; dilution is often the method of choice in food analysis, and new approaches take this into consideration (see Section 11.5).

The length of the amplicons is a critical issue in planning a PCR method for food authenticity and choosing target genes. It has been well demonstrated that transformation and processing in food production affects the integrity of macromolecular components, altering proteins and DNA as well (Gryson, 2010). In samples containing highly degraded DNA, amplicons should be designed to be about 100 bp in length. It has been reported, in fact, that thermal treatments at 65°C and 126°C led to fragmentation of meat DNA into 100 bp pieces (Lopez-Andreo et al., 2012), whereas in maize only fragments of 133 bp could be reproducibly amplified in processed products (tacos, crackers; Peano et al., 2004).

11.4.1 Seafood

There is currently a paradox in seafood and fish markets worldwide. The health benefits of fish in comparison to other source of proteins, mainly meat, has led to an increased demand, which has resulted in increased pressure on fish populations and unsustainability of fisheries in general (Ye et al., 2013). The impact of illegal, unregulated, unreported (IUU) fishery is increasing steadily, and seafood authenticity has become a widespread problem; substitution of premium fish species with cheaper or more common species is the most common type of fraud (European Commission, 2015; Table 11.1). Identification of species based on visual inspection cannot be achieved when the material is sold in fillets and prepared food. Considering that the substitution often involves closely related species, the requirements for species-specific markers for DNA barcoding are stringent (Rasmussen and Morrissey, 2008).

Additionally, regulations in different countries require that labeling of fish products includes the scientific name of the species, creating a requirement for unequivocal identification in processed products: in the EU, Regulation (EC) No. 2065/2001 (Commission Regulation, 2001). Mislabeling of fish products could represent a risk for health as well, since cheaper sources of fish usually come from areas with higher water pollution, like the Mekong River.

For fish species identification, the Fish Barcode of Life (FISH-BOL, www.fishbol.org) represents a specific resource, currently numbering over 10,000 species (as of May 2015). Identification of fish species has been achieved with amplification of short fragments of the mitochondrial genome (Table 11.2). The *COX1* gene sequence (Fig. 11.2) was shown to be appropriate for DNA barcoding since unique sequences characterize different species of the genuses *Lates*, *Pangasius*, *Pangasianodon*, *Tilapia*, and *Oreochromis* (Galal-Khallaf et al., 2014).

A recent example where several fish species were compared concerned the presence of anglerfish (*Lophius* spp.) and substitution with other cheaper species (Castigliego et al., 2015). In this case multiplex qPCR followed by MCA was chosen as a suitable test and the target for amplification was the mitochondrial gene *CYTB*.

The same approaches are valid also for other kinds of seafood, like jellyfish, which might be present in Asian food products. Starting from the sequences of the DNA barcoding effort, a multiplex PCR for five targets was recently developed (Armani et al., 2014), using the *COX1* gene as target. The primer pairs were developed to amplify five sequences of different lengths from Asian and Mediterranean species. To achieve this, the reverse primers were positioned in polymorphic regions, whereas the forward primer with degenerated sequence was common to all species, yielding fragments of 50–200 bp.

Scallops are common food material, also affected by mislabeling and fraud; due to the failure in DNA amplification of the *COX1* gene, the 16S rRNA gene has been proposed as target for species identification, exploiting the variability in the 5′ end (Marín et al., 2015). Also in Scombridae the *COX1* gene barcoding fails to identify correctly the species of *Thunnus*, and additional polymorphisms in the nuclear gene for rhodopsin have been suggested for a correct identification (Abdullah and Rehbein, 2014).

Due to the specificities of authenticity issues in fish species, deriving from identification of related species in highly processed products, the forensically informative nucleotide sequencing (FINS) technique has been shown to be successful. In this approach, the target gene is amplified with universal primers and the amplicons are then sequenced on both strands. The sequences obtained from samples are aligned and subjected to phylogenetic analysis including as reference other sequences obtained from databases. If the phylogenetic tree supports the clustering of the species of interest and their discrimination from other species, the technique is validated for use in solving authenticity issues. A recent example is described by Espiñeira and Vieites (2015) for identification of mullet species, using as target the mitochondrial *CYTB* gene (Fig. 11.2).

Application of FINS requires, however, the existence of discriminating SNPs, sequencing facilities and a high level of knowledge on genomic sequences of the relevant species, as has been illustrated for Gadoides (Lago et al., 2013). A limit of the FINS approach is also the high level of homology between closely related species, which could make discrimination impossible as in the case of *CYTB* fragments sequenced from *Gadus ogac* and *Gadus microcephalus* (Lago et al., 2013).

11.4.2 Meat

Labeling of meat products in the EU requires the indication of the species of origin and the relative quantity in a mixture of species. For this reason, the analytical method of choice must enable the recognition of species-specific markers, proteins, or DNA fragments, but with a quantitative result (see Kumar et al., 2015 for a review).

Identification of animal species in meat is performed through DNA barcoding with mtDNA markers, as described in Section 11.2.3 (Table 11.2 and Fig. 11.2). In contrast with identification of seafood products, the FINS approach has been rarely applied.

A common authenticity issue concerns the composition of traditional foods, where specific types of meat must be utilized. One such example is the Alheira sausage of Portugal, requiring expensive ingredients based on game meat, which could be substituted with cheaper meat from pork or beef (Amaral et al., 2015). In these cases, species-specific target genes are required for identifying ingredients and adulterants; if quantification is not required, mitochondrial markers are the appropriate choice (Table 11.2).

One authenticity issue of high relevance for meat products concerns the labeling of food according to the halal or kosher attributes (Table 11.1); the presence of pork meat or ingredients is a common problem in both instances, but also other types of meat should be absent (eg, dog, cat, monkey). For this kind of analysis, species-specific markers are chosen in the mtDNA (Table 11.2 and Fig. 11.2), which can be analyzed in simplex or multiplex assays from complex processed food (eg, Ali et al., 2015). A hexaplex reaction for detection of pork and horse meat was developed by Kitpipit et al. (2014) starting directly from samples without any DNA extraction, based on amplification of mtDNA markers: *CYTB*, *COX1*, 12S rRNA. The assay is amenable to application in processed foods containing degraded DNA.

In other instances, it is necessary to identify the breed of the animal, for instance, when it is more expensive (eg, Angus beef) or for reasons of compliance with the technical specification of a PDO or PGI product. In this case, DNA barcoding is not applicable, whereas highly polymorphic genetic markers are required, as microsatellites and SNPs (as in Negrini et al., 2010).

A very peculiar authenticity issue is the recognition of beef meat coming from male animals, since this kind of meat is more expensive than other beef meat types. In this case, all the markers based on organelle genomes fail. Only nuclear genes located on the Y chromosome can be considered for this purpose; the assay is tiered, because at first a PCR reaction based on *CYTB* is required to confirm the presence of beef meat, and a second PCR reaction will detect two loci of the Y chromosome (Herrero et al., 2013).

11.4.3 Dairy Products

Dairy products are characterized by high lipid content and harsh processing procedures, all of which may hinder the recovery of DNA for successful amplification (Pirondini et al., 2010). One of the main authenticity issues is the addition of bovine milk to milk from other species, due to higher availability and economic gain. This fraudulent behavior can affect human health in the case of hypoallergenic milk deriving from goat or donkey. Detection of cow DNA can be easily performed with analyses based on mitochondrial genes (*CYTB*, 12S rRNA; Fig. 11.2) or nuclear genes (casein isoforms). Agrimonti et al. (2015) developed a quadruplex PCR system for identification of species origin in milk and cheese: cow, sheep, goat, and buffalo were recognized through amplification of short fragments of *CYTB* and 12S rRNA genes, ranging from 50 to 100 bp. Amplification of DNA from cheese was less efficient, as compared to milk.

Dairy products, as meat products, can have issues linked to the technical specifications of PDO and PGI products, requiring identification of breeds rather than of species. Discrimination of bacterial species in the natural whey starter can also be critical for authenticity of PDO cheeses, as is the case of Parmigiano Reggiano and Grana Padano (Bottari et al., 2013). Fingerprinting techniques like PCR-DGGE can be relevant in these cases to ensure authenticity of fermented products.

Traceability of microbiota components through DNA barcoding has been applied to connect the product to the production site, considering that milk and dairy products usually contain a microbiota that is essential in the production process and contributes to the main qualities of the product. DNA extracted from raw milk samples can be analyzed with fingerprinting techniques based on amplification of the 16S-23S intergenic transcribed spacers and identification of length polymorphisms. The bacterial communities of milk samples can be correlated to the farm of origin (Feligini et al., 2015).

11.4.4 Cereals

Authenticity issues for cereal-based food have been recently reviewed (Gullì et al., 2013). The main problems are connected to species identification for quality of bread and pasta (Table 11.1), but the discrimination of Triticeae species can be particularly difficult due to the high levels of gene homology. Identification of cereal species is also essential for verification of gluten-free products developed to assist patients affected by celiac disease; species to be avoided include wheat, rye, barley, and oat, whereas rice and maize are safe. Discrimination of these species in commercial food products has been performed through qPCR based on the ITS1 region of the nuclear ribosomal DNA gene—23% of food products declaring no traces of cereals contained detectable contents according to qPCR (Pegels et al., 2015).

A specific case concerns protected denominations, like PDO bread—the technical specification requires that flour comes from specific cultivars. Identification of cultivars can be performed with highly polymorphic markers, usually microsatellite loci (Pasqualone et al., 2010). The presence of three genomes, A, B, and D, gives rise to homeologous genes containing specific polymorphisms; one example is the SNP in the γ-gliadin of the D genome, which discriminates bread wheat varieties from spelt varieties (Mayer et al., 2012).

In the case of rice and derived products, there are premium varieties like Basmati or Thai Jasmine, which can be identified with molecular markers (Bucher et al., 2014) or targeted analyses; amplification focuses on a target gene involved in the production of fragrant metabolites, characteristic feature of those varieties, encoding for betaine aldehyde dehydrogenase (*BAD2*; Ganopoulos et al., 2011). A deletion of 8 bp is characteristic of the fragrant rice.

11.4.5 Olive Oil

The EU recently invested millions in efforts to protect the market of olive oil from fraud, and it has been assessed that this product has high levels of counterfeiting (Moore et al., 2012). The existence of certified olive oils, labeled as PDO or PGI, requires specific methods to detect the presence of unwanted material, or cheap oil, oil from different botanical sources (Agrimonti et al., 2011). The main problem for authenticity analysis in olive oil relies in the difficulty of extracting acceptable amounts of DNA from the lipid matrix. A series of methods, based on commercial kits and in-house-developed protocols, have been tried and evaluated (Agrimonti et al., 2011; Ramos-Gómez et al., 2014). The difficulty in extracting DNA from olive oil, and the presence of PCR inhibitors, decrease the efficiency of PCR amplification, and thereby the recognition of allelic differences required for identification of cultivars. The choice of short amplicons, shorter than 100 bp, is crucial to the reliability of PCR reactions (Vietina et al., 2011).

Detection of alien species in olive oil can be performed by amplifying a common target gene (Table 11.2), like chloroplast *rbcL*, and detecting sequence differences with high resolution melting analysis (Ganopoulos et al., 2013; Vietina et al., 2013).

Concerning the identification of varieties or cultivars, the most common approaches involve polymorphic nuclear genome markers such as microsatellites or SNPs (reviewed in Agrimonti et al., 2011). The applicability of informative markers such as SNPs is increased by developing a rapid assay based on recognition of the polymorphic base pair, as in PCR-restriction fragment length polymorphism (RFLP) or cleaved amplified polymorphic sequence (CAPS) (Uncu et al., 2015) or developing a high-throughput platform for simultaneous recognition of many amplicons

(Consolandi et al., 2007). The most recent development in this trend is the assay proposed by Kalogianni et al. (2015) with detection of SNPs by primer extension reaction followed by hybridization on microspheres and analysis with a flow cytometer. The advantage of this system is in the possibility of high-throughput analysis to multiplex genotyping of 50 SNPs.

A problem often reported for olive oil analysis concerns the genetic constituents in the drupe; the pulp cells contain the same genetic information as the mother plant, whereas the embryo cells in the seed contain genetic material from the pollinator plant, which could belong to a different variety. Even though the contribution of the embryo to the oil production is limited, the presence of additional alleles in oil, with respect to the mother plant, has been reported (Raieta et al., 2015).

11.4.6 Other Examples

Identification of plant species or cultivars could be highly relevant in processed products such as sauces, fruit juices, and complex food products. Often the identification of plant species such as maize, soybean, and rapeseed can be instrumental as preliminary to traceability of genetically modified organisms (GMOs; Marmiroli et al., 2008).

Tomato is consumed worldwide, as fresh product or in processed products and as ingredients. In Italy some varieties have been labeled with PDO or PGI, and identification of cultivars can also be relevant for industrial processing. Discrimination among cultivars of the same species in plants requires the use of polymorphic markers, obtained through amplification of short fragments of DNA to increase the likelihood of successful amplification in products subjected to harsh mechanical, chemical, or thermal treatments; microsatellite loci of the nuclear genome are ideal for this purpose, due to the high-polymorphism-information content, and to stability along the food chain (Savo Sardaro et al., 2013).

A commodity with issues in food authenticity is coffee, where discrimination of varieties Arabica and Robusta can be relevant for pricing and consumer trust. Spaniolas et al. (2014) have addressed this need by analyzing SNPs differences in the plastid genome. The SNaPshot technique, based on primer extension from the polymorphic site, can analyze just one SNP at a time, whereas pyrosequencing of amplicons can detect all polymorphisms at the same time. The performance of pyrosequencing was better in terms of precision and sensitivity, but its application can be limited by available resources for sequencing.

11.5 Future Trends

11.5.1 Hyphenating PCR With Other Techniques

"Hyphenated" approaches combine PCR with other analytical tools or detection systems to improve applicability, sensitivity, or efficacy.

Combination of PCR with immunological detection in the format of enzyme-linked immunosorbent assay is called PCR-ELISA (Musiani et al., 2007); after a PCR reaction performed with digoxigenin-labeled primers, the amplicons are recognized by hybridization to probes and detected by antibodies linked to horseradish peroxidase. The enzyme activity is then detected with colorimetric, fluorescent, or chemiluminescent substrates. The advantages of this approach are the reproducibility, low cost, and ease, with possibilities for automation (eg, see Santaclara et al., 2015). Modifications of this technique have been proposed to increase its applicability outside of the analytical laboratories, for instance, by developing isothermal methods that do not require the use of thermal cyclers (Santiago-Felipe et al., 2014).

Endpoint PCR can be combined with digestion with restriction enzymes in PCR-RFLP to identify allelic variants and SNPs. Bazakos et al. (2012) have applied this approach to olive oil authenticity, to discriminate among 10 Greek varieties with five SNPs in two nuclear genes. The presence of SNPs gives a different outcome in the digestion, and capillary electrophoresis can be used to fractionate an amplicon and its fragments.

PCR combined with capillary electrophoresis after denaturation of the amplicons allows the analysis of single-strand conformation polymorphism. A target sequence amplified in DNA from different species using consensus primers will show different conformations and therefore different peaks in the electropherograms. To discriminate between olive and alien species in oil extracts, Zhang et al. (2012) have chosen two amplicons from the chloroplast *rbcL* gene.

Isothermal amplification can be performed without the need for cycling between different temperatures for denaturation, annealing, and extension; denaturation of dsDNA is obtained through the use of helicase or recombinase enzymes. A method that can be used in food analysis is the loop-mediated isothermal amplification (Tomita et al., 2008); the mechanism involves four primers annealing on six regions of the target DNA and specific DNA polymerase enzymes that can perform displacement of DNA strands. This technique can amplify DNA without changes in temperature and without a denaturation step. Additionally, amplicon formation can be detected in different simple ways, amenable to implementation outside of laboratories; Vaagt et al. (2013) report about the detection of amplicons using lateral flow dipsticks, requiring the use of one primer labeled with biotin and a hybridization probe labeled with fluorescein isothiocyanate, recognized by specific antibodies. Alternatively, detection can be performed by visual inspection (Focke et al., 2013).

Recent developments in analytical techniques could simplify the analysis of amplicons from food products. A modification of the dipstick detection makes use of hybridization to probes conjugated to gold nanoparticles for visualization of the amplified products (Trantakis et al., 2012). An innovative application of surface-enhanced Raman spectroscopy has allowed the detection of SNPs in long amplicons by exploiting melting of the target DNA hybridized to immobilized probes (Papadopoulou et al., 2015). Even though the authors show an application to genomic DNA of pathogen bacteria, the approach could be feasible for any situation in which a SNP can discriminate between two targets. Other recognition systems based on electrical and electrochemical procedures have been recently described (Goda et al., 2015) in the context of point-of-care testing; this testifies to a trend toward the development of methods for DNA amplification that could be applied outside of a laboratory, for instance, near line or at line in the food supply chain.

In a different approach, Ponzoni et al. (2013) have proposed the adaptation to food analysis of the xMAP assay, used in biomedicine and diagnostics, to detect amplicons of the polymorphic plant β-tubulin intron; up to five different plant species could be identified in complex food products, exploiting the hybridization of the amplicons to specific capture probes immobilized on magnetic beads. This application is an example of the development of innovative analytical techniques in food analysis starting from techniques applied in other diagnostic or forensic fields.

11.5.2 Digital PCR and Lab-on-Chip Approach

Digital PCR (dPCR) is a newly developed technique that increases the sensitivity of PCR in samples containing low amounts of DNA, a situation that often occurs in food analysis. The concept of dPCR is to perform the amplification in several cells or tubes (up to thousands or millions), with statistical analysis of the percentage of success with endpoint PCR; this can be related to the quantity of template in the original sample (Baker, 2012). The performance of dPCR allows the detection of DNA in very diluted samples, decreasing the impact of PCR inhibitors; a value of the limit of quantification 10 times lower than qPCR has been reported for meat mixtures (Floren et al., 2015). Whereas the higher sensitivity of dPCR is appropriate in medicine and diagnostics for detection of small differences among samples, in food analysis its main advantage would be the possibility for analyzing diluted samples containing inhibitors. A further modification, droplet dPCR (ddPCR) is more suitable for relative quantification, as has been demonstrated in the case of GMO detection (Morisset et al., 2013). However, the dynamic range of dPCR is lower than in qPCR, which makes it suitable for highly diluted samples.

A further development of PCR relies on microfluidic devices, which can allow the applicability on-site for food analyses. The "lab-on-a-chip" approach should provide high throughput in conditions of low availability of samples, decreasing the time required for amplification. The recent development of systems requiring no external pumps for movement of the fluids should provide additional flexibility and portability of these devices (Tachibana et al., 2015). Most recent approaches that could be transferred to food analysis are based on discs (lab-on-disc) to exploit centrifugal forces, and these could include the whole analytical platform from DNA extraction to PCR amplification and amplicon analysis, as exemplified in Roy et al. (2015).

Sources of Further Information and Conclusions

Information about the use of PCR for food analysis is largely available in many specialized scientific journals and books (see references list). Additionally, Websites of potential interest (active as of May 2015) are:

1. www.ec.europa.eu/jrc/en/research-topic/food-authenticity-and-quality—Website of the Joint Research Centre of the European Commission. It provides links to related topics and publications.

2. www.codexalimentarius.org—Website of Codex Alimentarius, the reference hub for all official information on protocols and standards in food analysis.
3. www.foodintegrity.eu—Website of the project of the European Commission Seventh Framework Programme FoodIntegrity. It will contain databases and guidelines on analytical techniques when they are developed during the project activity.
4. www.moniqa.org—Website of the MoniQA Association for facilitation of research, funded after the end of the MoniQA Network of Excellence (EU funded in Sixth Framework Programme).
5. www.foodfraud.msu.edu—Website of the Food Fraud Initiative, providing e-learning courses.
6. www.foodfraud.org—A database on fraud events, hosted by the United States. Pharmacopeial Convention (Moore et al., 2012).
7. www.foodqualitynews.com—An example of a newsletter providing news and information about frauds and technological developments.
8. www.ec.europa.eu/food/safety/official_controls/food_fraud/index_en.htm —Website hosting information on the Food Fraud Network of the European Commission and EU policies.

The information available, and the recent examples reported in the present chapter, highlight the strong need for harmonization and integration. Even if each food matrix can be seen as a specific new challenge, requiring ad hoc approaches and development or optimization of techniques for DNA analysis, harmonized protocols are essential. The plethora of protocols, methods for data analysis, measurement units, and performance parameters can hinder the progress in research and in implementation of tools essential for fighting food fraud, and for protecting consumers (Manning and Soon, 2014). The relevance of research efforts funded by governmental institutions, joining together scientists and operators from different countries, is also essential, because food fraud and crimes are transboundary in nature.

Acknowledgments

All authors acknowledge funding by the University of Parma, local funds. Author Elena Maestri acknowledges the contribution of the project FOODINTEGRITY, which has received funding from the EU's Seventh Framework Programme for research, technological development, and demonstration under grant agreement No. 613688.

References

Abdullah, A., Rehbein, H., 2014. Authentication of raw and processed tuna from Indonesian markets using DNA barcoding, nuclear gene and character-based approach. European Food Research and Technology 239, 695–706.

Agrimonti, C., Pirondini, A., Marmiroli, M., Marmiroli, N., 2015. A quadruplex PCR (qxPCR) assay for adulteration in dairy products. Food Chemistry 187, 58–64.

Agrimonti, C., Vietina, M., Marmiroli, N., 2011. The use of food genomics to ensure the traceability of olive oil. Trends in Food Science & Technology 22, 237–244.

Ali, M.E., Razzak, M.A., Hamid, S.B.A., 2014. Multiplex PCR in species authentication: probability and prospects - a review. Food Analytical Methods 7, 1933–1949.

Ali, M.E., Razzak, M.A., Hamid, S.B.A., Rahman, M.M., Amin, M.A., Rashid, N.R.R., Asing, 2015. Multiplex PCR assay for the detection of five meat species forbidden in Islamic foods. Food Chemistry 177, 214–224.

Amaral, J.S., Santos, C.G., Melo, V.S., Costa, J., Oliveira, M.B.P.P., Mafra, I., 2015. Identification of duck, partridge, pheasant, quail, chicken and turkey meats by species-specific PCR assays to assess the authenticity of traditional game meat Alheira sausages. Food Control 47, 190–195.

Armani, A., Giusti, A., Castigliego, L., Rossi, A., Tinacci, L., Gianfaldoni, D., Guidi, A., 2014. Pentaplex PCR as screening assay for jellyfish species identification in food products. Journal of Agricultural and Food Chemistry 62, 12134–12143.

Baker, M., 2012. Digital PCR hits its stride. Nature Methods 9, 541–544.

Bazakos, C., Dulger, A.O., Uncu, A.T., Spaniolas, S., Spano, T., Kalaitzis, P., 2012. A SNP-based PCR-RFLP capillary electrophoresis analysis for the identification of the varietal origin of olive oils. Food Chemistry 134, 2411–2418.

Bigot, C., Meile, J.-C., Kapitan, A., Montet, D., 2015. Discriminating organic and conventional foods by analysis of their microbial ecology: an application to fruits. Food Control 48, 123–129.

Bottari, B., Agrimonti, C., Gatti, M., Neviani, E., Marmiroli, N., 2013. Development of a multiplex real time PCR to detect thermophilic lactic acid bacteria in natural whey starters. International Journal of Food Microbiology 160, 290–297.

Bucher, T.B., Fridez, F., Köppel, R., 2014. Duplex real-time PCR for the determination of non-Basmati rice in Basmati rice (*Oryza sativa*). European Food Research and Technology 238, 417–423.

Busby, E., Burns, M., 2014. Method verification of the LOD associated with PCR approaches for the detection of horse meat. Journal of the Association of Public Analysts 42, 001–017.

Castigliego, L., Armani, A., Tinacci, L., Gianfaldoni, D., Guidi, A., 2015. Two alternative multiplex PCRs for the identification of the seven species of anglerfish (*Lophius* spp.) using an end-point or a melting curve analysis real-time protocol. Food Chemistry 166, 1–9.

Codex Alimentarius Commission, 2010. Guidelines on Performance Criteria and Validation of Methods for Detection, Identification and Quantification of Specific DNA Sequences and Specific Proteins in Foods, CAC/GL 74–2010.

Commission Regulation (EC) No. 2065/2001 of 22 October 2001 Laying Down Detailed Rules for the Application of Council Regulation (EC) No. 104/2000 as Regards Informing Consumers about Fishery and Aquaculture Products. OJ L, 278, October 23, 2001, pp. 6–8.

Consolandi, C., Palmieri, L., Doveri, S., Maestri, E., Marmiroli, N., Reale, S., Lee, D., Baldoni, L., Tosti, N., Severgnini, M., De Bellis, G., Castiglioni, B., 2007. Olive variety identification by ligation detection in a universal array format. Journal of Biotechnology 129, 565–574.

Dalama, J., Vieites, J.M., Espineira, M., 2015. Detection of the causal agents of Keriorrhea (*Lepidocybium flavobrunneum* and *Ruvettus pretiosus*) by means of real time PCR. Food Chemistry 174, 326–329.

Demeke, T., Jenkins, G.R., 2010. Influence of DNA extraction methods, PCR inhibitors and quantification methods on real-time PCR assay of biotechnology-derived traits. Analytical and Bioanalytical Chemistry 396, 1977–1990.

Druml, B., Grandits, S., Mayer, W., Hochegger, R., Cichna-Markl, M., 2015. Authenticity control of game meat products – a single method to detect and quantify adulteration of fallow deer (*Dama dama*), red deer (*Cervus elaphus*) and sika deer (*Cervus nippon*) by real-time PCR. Food Chemistry 170, 508–517.

Drummond, M.G., Brasil, B.S.A.F., Dalsecco, L.S., Brasil, R.S.A.F., Teixeira, L.V., Oliveira, D.A.A., 2013. A versatile real-time PCR method to quantify bovine contamination in buffalo products. Food Control 29, 131–137.

Espiñeira, M., Vieites, J.M., 2015. Genetic system for traceability of goatfishes by FINS methodology and authentication of mullets (*Mullus barbatus* and *Mullus surmuletus*) by RT-PCR. European Food Research and Technology 240, 423–429.

European Commission, 2015. Food Fraud Network Activity Report 2014. Available from: http://ec.europa.eu/food/safety/official_controls/food_fraud/index_en.htm.

Feligini, M., Panelli, S., Sacchi, R., Ghitti, M., Capelli, E., 2015. Tracing the origin of raw milk from farm by using Automated Ribosomal Intergenic Spacer Analysis (ARISA) fingerprinting of microbiota. Food Control 50, 51–56.

Floren, C., Wiedemann, I., Brenig, B., Schütz, E., Beck, J., 2015. Species identification and quantification in meat and meat products using droplet digital PCR (ddPCR). Food Chemistry 173, 1054–1058.

Focke, F., Haase, I., Fischer, M., 2013. Loop-mediated isothermal amplification (LAMP): methods for plant species identification in food. Journal of Agricultural and Food Chemistry 61, 2943–2949.

Galal-Khallaf, A., Ardura, A., Mohammed-Geba, K., Borrell, Y.J., Garcia-Vazquez, E., 2014. DNA barcoding reveals a high level of mislabeling in Egyptian fish fillets. Food Control 46, 441–445.

Ganopoulos, I., Argiriou, A., Tsaftaris, A., 2011. Adulteration in Basmati rice detected quantitatively by combined use of microsatellite and fragrance typing with High Resolution Melting (HRM) analysis. Food Chemistry 129, 652–659.

Ganopoulos, I., Bazakos, C., Madesis, P., Kalaitzis, P., Tsaftaris, A., 2013. Barcode DNA high-resolution melting (Bar-HMR) analysis as a novel close-tubed and accurate tool for olive oil forensic use. Journal of the Science of Food and Agriculture 93, 2281–2286.

Goda, T., Tabata, M., Miyahara, Y., 2015. Electrical and electrochemical monitoring of nucleic acid amplification. Frontiers in Bioengineering and Biotechnology 3 article 29.

Gryson, N., 2010. Effect of food processing on plant DNA degradation and PCR-based GMO analysis: a review. Analytical and Bioanalytical Chemistry 396, 2003–2022.

Gullì, M., Visioli, G., Marmiroli, M., Malcevschi, A., Maestri, E., 2013. Authenticity of cereals and cereal-based products: protecting tradition in bread- and pasta-making with modern analytical techniques. In: Sforza, S. (Ed.), Food Authentication Using Bioorganic Molecules. DesTech Publications, Inc., Lancaster, PA, pp. 129–150.

Hamdouche, Y., Guehi, T., Durand, N., Kedjebo, K.B.D., Montet, D., Melie, J.C., 2015. Dynamics of microbial ecology during cocoa fermentation and drying: towards the identification of molecular markers. Food Control 48, 117–122.

Hebert, P.D.N., Cywinska, A., Ball, S.L., deWaard, J.R., 2003. Biological identifications through DNA barcodes. Proceedings of the Royal Society of London 270, 313–321.

Herrero, B., Royo, L.J., Lago, F.C., Vieites, J.M., Espiñeira, M., 2013. Authentication of male beef by multiplex fast real-time PCR. Food Additives & Contaminants 30, 218–225.

Holst-Jensen, A., Berdal, K.G., 2004. The modular analytical procedure and validation approach and the units of measurement for genetically modified materials in foods and feeds. Journal of AOAC International 87, 927–936.

Iwobi, A., Sebah, D., Kraemer, I., Losher, C., Fischer, G., Busch, U., Huber, I., 2015. A multiplex real-time PCR method for the quantification of beef and pork fractions in minced meat. Food Chemistry 169, 305–313.

James, D., Schmidt, A., 2004. Use of an intron region of a chloroplast tRNA gene (*trn*L) as a target for PCR identification of specific food crops including sources of potential allergens. Food Research International 37, 395–402.

Kalogianni, D.P., Bazakos, C., Boutsika, L.M., Targem, M.B., Christopoulos, T.K., Kalaitzis, P., Ioannou, P.C., 2015. Olive oil fingerprinting by multiplex SNP genotyping on fluorescent microspheres. Journal of Agricultural and Food Chemistry 63, 3121–3128.

Kitpipit, T., Sittichan, K., Thanakiatkrai, P., 2014. Direct-multiplex PCR assay for meat species identification in food products. Food Chemistry 163, 77–82.

Kumar, A., Kumar, R.R., Sharma, B.D., Gokulkrishnan, P., Mendiratta, S.K., Sharma, D., 2015. Identification of species origin of meat and meat products on the DNA basis: a review. Critical Reviews in Food Science and Nutrition 55, 1340–1351.

Lago, F.C., Vieites, J.M., Espiñeira, M., 2013. Authentication of gadoids from highly processed products susceptible to include species mixtures by means of DNA sequencing methods. European Food Research and Technology 236, 171–180.

Lopez-Andreo, M., Aldeguer, M., Guillen, I., Gabaldon, J.A., Puyet, A., 2012. Detection and quantification of meat species by qPCR in heat-processed food containing highly fragmented DNA. Food Chemistry 134, 518–523.

Manning, L., Soon, J.M., 2014. Developing systems to control food adulteration. Food Policy 49, 23–32.

Marín, A., Fujimoto, T., Arai, K., 2015. The variable 5' end of the 16S rRNA gene as a novel barcoding tool for scallops (Bivalvia, Pectinidae). Fisheries Science 81, 73–81.

Marmiroli, N., Maestri, E., 2007. Polymerase chain reaction (PCR). In: Picò, Y. (Ed.), Food Toxicant Analysis - Techniques, Strategies and Developments. Elsevier, Amsterdam, the Netherlands, pp. 147–187.

Marmiroli, N., Maestri, E., Gullì, M., Malcevschi, A., Peano, C., Bordoni, R., De Bellis, G., 2008. Methods for detection of GMOs in food and feed. Analytical and Bioanalytical Chemistry 392, 369–384.

Martins-Lopes, P., Gomes, S., Pereira, L., Guedes-Pinto, H., 2013. Molecular markers for food traceability. Food Technology and Biotechnology 51, 198–207.

Mayer, F., Haase, I., Graubner, A., Heising, F., Paschke-Kratzin, A., Fischer, M., 2012. Use of polymorphisms in the γ-gliadin gene of spelt and wheat as a tool for authenticity control. Journal of Agricultural and Food Chemistry 60, 1350–1357.

Mercier, B., Gaucher, C., Feugeas, O., Mazurier, C., 1990. Direct PCR from whole blood, without DNA extraction. Nucleic Acids Research 18, 5908.

Moore, J.C., Spink, J., Lipp, M., 2012. Development and application of a database of food ingredient fraud and economically motivated adulteration from 1980 to 2010. Journal of Food Science 77, R118–R126.

Morisset, D., Štebih, D., Milavec, M., Gruden, K., Žel, J., 2013. Quantitative analysis of food and feed samples with droplet digital PCR. PLoS One 8 (5), e62583.

Mullis, K., Faloona, F., Scharf, S., 1986. Specific enzymatic amplification of DNA in vitro: the polymerase chain reaction. Cold Spring Harbor Symposium Quantitative Biology 51, 263–273.

Musiani, M., Vanturoli, S., Gallinella, G., Zerbini, M., 2007. Qualitative PCR-ELISA protocol for the detection and typing of viral genomes. Nature Protocols 2, 2502–2510.

Navarro, E., Serrano-Heras, G., Castaño, M.J., Solera, J., 2015. Real-time PCR detection chemistry. Clinica Chimica Acta 439, 231–250.

Negrini, R., Nicoloso, L., Crepaldi, P., Milanesi, E., Marino, R., Perini, D., Pariset, L., Dunner, S., Leveziel, H., Williams, J.L., Ajmone Marsan, P., 2010. Traceability of four

European protected geographic indication (PGI) beef products using single nucleotide polymorphism (SNP) and Bayesian statistics. Meat Science 80, 1212–1217.

Pafundo, S., Gullì, M., Marmiroli, N., 2009. SYBR® GreenER™ real-time PCR to detect almond in traces in processed food. Food Chemistry 116, 811–815.

Pafundo, S., Gullì, M., Marmiroli, N., 2011. Comparison of DNA extraction methods and development of duplex PCR and Real-Time PCR to detect tomato, carrot, and celery in food. Journal of Agricultural and Food Chemistry 59, 10414–10424.

Pang, X., Liu, C., Shi, L., Liu, R., Liang, D., Li, H., Cherny, S.S., Chen, S., 2012. Utility of the *trnH–psbA* intergenic spacer region and its combinations as plant DNA barcodes: a meta-analysis. PLoS One 7 (11), e48833.

Papadopoulou, E., Goodchild, S.A., Cleary, D.W., Weller, S.A., Gale, N., Stubberfield, M.R., Brown, T., Bartlett, P.N., 2015. Using surface-enhanced Raman spectroscopy and electrochemically driven melting to discriminate *Yersinia pestis* from *Y. pseudotubercolosis* based on single nucleotide polymorphisms within unpurified polymerase chain reaction amplicons. Analytical Chemistry 87, 1605–1612.

Pardo, M.A., 2015. Evaluation of a dual-probe real time PCR system for detection of mandarin in commercial orange juice. Food Chemistry 172, 377–384.

Pasqualone, A., Alba, V., Mangini, G., Blanco, A., Montemurro, C., 2010. Durum wheat cultivar traceability in PDO Altamura bread by analysis of DNA microsatellites. European Food Research and Technology 230, 723–729.

Peano, C., Samson, M.C., Palmieri, L., Gullì, M., Marmiroli, N., 2004. Qualitative and quantitative evaluation of the genomic DNA extracted from GMO and non-GMO foodstuffs with four different extraction methods. Journal of Agricultural and Food Chemistry 52, 6962–6968.

Pegels, N., Gonzalez, I., Garcia, T., Martin, R., 2015. Authenticity testing of wheat, barley, rye and oats in food and feed market samples by real-time PCR assays. LWT – Food Science and Technology 60, 867–875.

Pirondini, A., Bonas, U., Maestri, E., Visioli, G., Marmiroli, M., Marmiroli, N., 2010. Yield and amplificability of different DNA extraction procedures for traceability in the dairy food chain. Food Control 21, 663–668.

Połka, J., Rebecchi, A., Pisacane, V., Morelli, L., Puglisi, E., 2015. Bacterial diversity in typical Italian salami at different ripening stages as revealed by high-throughput sequencing of 16S rRNA amplicons. Food Microbiology 46, 342–356.

Ponzoni, E., Breviario, D., Mautino, A., Gianì, S., Morello, L., 2013. A multiplex, bead-based array for profiling plant-derived components in complex food matrixes. Analytical and Bioanalytical Chemistry 405, 9849–9858.

Raieta, K., Muccillo, L., Colantuoni, V., 2015. A novel reliable method of DNA extraction from olive oil suitable for molecular traceability. Food Chemistry 172, 596–602.

Ramos-Gómez, S., Busto, M.D., Perez-Mateos, M., Ortega, N., 2014. Development of a method to recovery and amplification DNA by real-time PCR from commercial vegetable oils. Food Chemistry 158, 374–383.

Rasmussen, R.S., Morrissey, M.T., 2008. DNA-based methods for the identification of commercial fish and seafood species. Comprehensive Reviews in Food Science and Food Safety 7, 280–295.

Roy, E., Stewart, G., Mounier, M., Malic, L., Peytavi, R., Clime, L., Madou, M., Bossinot, M., Bergeron, M.G., Veres, T., 2015. From cellular lysis to microarray detection, an integrated thermoplastic elastomer (TPE) point of care Lab on a Disc. Lab on a Chip 15, 406–416.

Santaclara, F.J., Velasco, A., Perez-Martin, R.I., Quinteiro, J., Rey-Mendez, M., Pardo, M.A., Jimenez, E., Sotelo, C.G., 2015. Development of a multiplex PCR–ELISA method for the genetic authentication of *Thunnus* species and *Katsuwonus pelamis* in food products. Food Chemistry 180, 9–16.

Santiago-Felipe, S., Tortajada-Genaro, L.A., Puchades, R., Maquieira, A., 2014. Recombinase polymerase and enzyme-linked immunosorbent assay as a DNA amplification-detection strategy for food analysis. Analytica Chimica Acta 811, 81–87.

Savo Sardaro, M.L., Marmiroli, M., Maestri, E., Marmiroli, N., 2013. Genetic characterization of Italian tomato varieties and their traceability in tomato food products. Food Science & Nutrition 1, 54–62. http://dx.doi.org/10.1002/fsn3.8.

Scarano, D., Rao, R., 2014. DNA markers for food products authentication. Diversity 6, 579–596.

Schrader, C., Schielke, A., Ellerbroek, L., Johne, R., 2012. PCR inhibitors - occurrence, properties and removal. Journal of Applied Microbiology 113, 1014–1026.

Spaniolas, S., Bazakos, C., Tucker, G.A., Bennett, M.J., 2014. Comparison of SNP-based detection assays for food analysis: coffee authentication. Journal of AOAC International 97, 1114–1120.

Tachibana, H., Saito, M., Tsuji, K., Yamanaka, K., Hoa, L.Q., Tamiya, E., 2015. Self-propelled continuous-flow PCR in capillary-driven microfluidic device: microfluidic behavior and DNA amplification. Sensors and Actuators B: Chemical 206, 303–310.

Tomita, N., Mori, Y., Kanda, H., Notomi, T., 2008. Loop-mediated isothermal amplification (LAMP) of gene sequences and simple visual detection of products. Nature Protocols 3, 877–882.

Trantakis, I.A., Spaniolas, S., Kalaitzis, P., Ioannou, P.C., Tucker, G.A., Christopoulos, T.K., 2012. Dipstick test for DNA-based food authentication. Application to coffee authenticity assessment. Journal of Agricultural and Food Chemistry 60, 713–717.

Turci, M., Savo Sardaro, M.L., Visioli, G., Maestri, E., Marmiroli, M., Marmiroli, N., 2010. Evaluation of DNA extraction procedures for traceability of various tomato products. Food Control 21, 143–149.

Uncu, A.T., Frary, A., Doganlar, S., 2015. Cultivar origin and admixture detection in Turkish olive oils by SNP-based CAPS assays. Journal of Agricultural and Food Chemistry 63, 2284–2295.

Vaagt, F., Haase, I., Fischer, M., 2013. Loop-mediated isothermal amplification (LAMP)-based method for rapid mushroom species identification. Journal of Agricultural and Food Chemistry 61, 1833–1840.

van Asch, B., Silva Santos, L., Carneiro, J., Pereira, F., Amorim, A., 2011. Identification of mtDNA lineages of *Sus scrofa* by multiplex single base extension for the authentication of processed food products. Journal of Agricultural and Food Chemistry 59, 6920–6926.

Vietina, M., Agrimonti, C., Marmiroli, M., Bonas, U., Marmiroli, N., 2011. Applicability of SSR markers to the traceability of monovarietal olive oils. Journal of the Science of Food and Agriculture 91, 1381–1391.

Vietina, M., Agrimonti, C., Marmiroli, N., 2013. Detection of plant oil DNA using high resolution melting (HRM) post PCR analysis: a tool for disclosure of olive oil adulteration. Food Chemistry 141, 3820–3826.

Ye, Y., Cochrane, K., Bianchi, G., Willmann, R., Majkowski, J., Tandstad, M., Carocci, P., 2013. Rebuilding global fisheries: the World Summit goal, costs and benefits. Fish and Fisheries 14, 174–185.

Zhang, H., Wu, Y., Li, Y., Wang, B., Han, J., Ju, X., Chen, Y., 2012. PCR-CE-SSCP used to authenticate edible oils. Food Control 27, 322–329.

Advances in Differential Scanning Calorimetry for Food Authenticity Testing

12

T. Nur Azira [1], *I. Amin* [2]
[1]International Islamic University Malaysia, Kuala Lumpur, Malaysia; [2]Universiti Putra Malaysia, Serdang, Selangor, Malaysia

Chapter Outline

12.1 Introduction

Differential scanning calorimetry (DSC) is a thermoanalytical technique that measures the difference between the amount of heat required to increase the temperature of a sample and suitable reference material as a function of temperature. This differential heat flow is then recorded as a peak. The enthalpy change is directly proportional to the area under the peak, and this indicates whether the thermal event is exothermic (energy producing) or endothermic (energy consuming). DSC has played an important role in the analysis of the thermal behavior of fats, oils, carbohydrates, and proteins, particularly in the field of food science and technology. Moreover, DSC is a rapid and simple technique as, in most cases, no specific sample preparation is needed. It is also well known as an environmentally friendly technique as it does not require any chemical or solvent utilization.

DSC was first developed in the early 1960s by Watson and O'Neill (1962) and introduced commercially at the Pittsburgh Conference on Analytical Chemistry and Applied Spectroscopy in 1963. During the 1970s, its potential for use in food research become obvious as reviewed by Biliaderis (1983). Examples of these applications have involved the thermal effect of food ingredients or components in a food system, evaluation of starch gelatinization and protein degradation, innovation of technological treatments in order to improve food characteristics or shelf life, and detection of adulteration. It records thermal processes such as melting, heat capacity, crystallization, glass transition temperature, and enthalpy of foods and their components. Such measurements can provide both qualitative and quantitative data on physical and chemical changes that involve exothermic (eg, freezing, crystallization, and oxidation) and endothermic (eg, melting, denaturation, gelatinization, and evaporation) processes or changes in heat capacity.

In the case of food component interactions, thermal events deduced from DSC may be elimination or appearance of a new exothermic or endothermic peak. Additionally, any changes of peak onset, peak shape, peak maximum, or peak offset temperature and relative height might be considered. Lai and Lo (2008) reviewed eight factors that may influence the results of DSC namely scanning rate, furnace atmosphere, calibration of the instrument, sample mass, particle size and packing, diluent, sample vessel, and purge gas. In order to ensure good-quality results, all these factors should be carefully considered. Depending on operating principle, there are two types of DSC systems: (1) power-compensated DSC, in which the sample and reference are heated in two separate furnace blocks; and (2) heat flux DSC, in which the sample and reference are heated in the same furnace block furnace block. Although the instrumentation is fundamentally different, both provide the same information. There are published reviews (Farkas and Mohacsi-Farkas, 1996; Clas et al., 1999; Chauhan and Mittu, 2012) on the fundamental concepts, instrumentation, and general applications of DSC. Although numerous reports have been published on the applications of DSC in food analysis, limited information on food authentication testing using DSC is available. Therefore the aim of this chapter is to report various DSC applications in foods, with an emphasis on authenticity testing. The potential use of this technique in tackling some issues akin to adulteration, contamination, cultivar, and geographical origin are comprehensively reviewed. In addition, several examples of current trends, limitations, and prospects of this technique are also highlighted.

12.2 Uses of Differential Scanning Calorimetry in the Analysis of Foods

Currently, DSC is used in a large number and variety of applications. It is suitable for analysis of food systems as they are often exposed to cooling or heating during processing; indeed, data obtained can be directly used to examine the thermal transition of a food system. In addition, the availability of a wide range of DSC sample pans enables researchers to study material either in solid or liquid forms (Elmer, 2013; Clas et al., 1999). Several applications of DSC in different type of foods testing are shown in Table 12.1.

Despite its wide application in food testing, the use of statistical tools such as chemometrics in processing DSC data is rare. Commonly, chemometric tools are applied to indicate or classify the differences and similarities of different food components and their chemical composition. The first paper based on the combination of DSC with chemometrics was published by Bergner and Albano (1993). They performed partial least

Table 12.1 Application of Differential Scanning Calorimetry in Food Testing (2010–2016)

Application	Food	References
Authenticity	Honey, butter, olive oil, coconut oil	Nikolova et al. (2012), Nurrulhidayah et al. (2015), Chatziantoniou et al. (2014), Mansor et al. (2012), and Tomaszewska-Gras (2016)
Gelatinization properties	Gluten-free flour doughs, rice, potato, tapioca, and jackfruit starches	Bosmans et al. (2016), Zhang et al. (2016), Moreira et al. (2015), Li et al. (2013), and Eguchi et al. (2014)
Protein degradation	Fish fillet	Matos et al. (2011)
Shelf life	Tilapia fish burger, fillet	Bainy et al. (2015) and Korzeniowska et al. (2013)
Oxidative stability	Rose hip oil, vegetable oil, seed oil, flaxseed oil, chia oil	Grajzer et al. (2015), Pardauil et al. (2011), Qi et al. (2016), Naik et al. (2014), and Zanqui et al. (2015a,b)
Characterization of fat	Blends of mango seed fat and palm oil	Jahurul et al. (2014)
Effect of processing	Dried button mushroom	Dinani et al. (2015)
Food packaging		Arrieta et al. (2013), Blanco and Siracusa (2013), and Abdorreza et al. (2011)

squares (PLS) regression using DSC data in order to predict 15 chemical and physical components in peat. Several examples of DSC applications adopted for the detection of adulterants and quality control by using a particular chemometric strategy have been reported as follows.

Jensen and Jorgensen (2003) used DSC to measure thermal denaturation in fillets during storage of cod muscle. Thermal denaturation profiles of samples were then subjected to PLS in order to identify effects of various storage treatments. Bertram et al. (2006) have applied PLS to DSC and nuclear magnetic resonance (NMR) data to study the relationship between thermal denaturation of proteins/protein structures and heat-induced changes in water mobility during heating of pork. Cerretani et al. (2011) developed a novel strategy based on PLS coupled with unfolded DSC data for the determination of fatty acid composition in olive oil. Results obtained were statistically similar to those produced by conventional official procedures and even more rapid. In addition, the same authors adopted the same strategy by coupling principal component analysis (PCA) with DSC profiles to measure the degree of thermal stress of extra virgin olive oil (Maggio et al., 2012). They also demonstrated a combined high-pressure liquid chromatography (HPLC)-DSC-PLS procedure to examine the influence of triacylglycerol (TAG) composition on the cooling curve shape of extra virgin olive oil from different Mediterranean areas. Results from 69 samples showed that cooling transitions were markedly influenced by triolein (OOO), dioleoyl-linoleoyl-glycerol (OLO), and dioleoyl-palmitoyl-glycerol + stearoyl-oleoyl-linoleoyl-glycerol (OOP + SLO), which are the most typical TAGs in extra virgin olive oil (Maggio et al., 2014). A study by Chiavaro et al. (2013) demonstrated that the application of PCA to thermal properties was useful in evaluating lipid degradation in virgin olive oil, while Caponio et al. (2013) used PCA to discriminate between samples of olive oil at different refining stages and/or oxidation level correlating to thermal and chemical properties.

Recently, DSC combined with chemometric data analysis has been used in some food authentication studies. Working on detection of lard adulteration, Dahimi et al. (2014) have used this approach in differentiating lard from beef and chicken fats and their mixtures using PCA. In this study, the extracted chicken fat (CF), lard (LD), beef fat (BF), and a series of 14 samples consisting of 0.5−10% w/w of LD were adulterated with CF and BF separately and analyzed using DSC. As shown in Fig. 12.1, PCA successfully differentiated BT and CF from LD less than 1% based on heating profiles, although it should be pointed out that PCA is not a modeling method but merely revels structure in a data collection and cannot be used in a predictive sense.

In another study, Mansor et al. (2012) applied stepwise multiple linear regression analysis (SMLR) for quantitatively estimating the percentage of LD adulteration in virgin coconut oil (VCO) (1−30% v/v of LD in VCO). Temperature peaks such as onset, endset, melting, and cooling range were assembled as independent predictors in SMLR analysis. Even though fatty acid (FA) and TAG analysis by gas chromatography−flame ionization detector (GC−FID) and HPLC, respectively, were able to detect LD adulteration in VCO, they did not provide a qualitative analysis and are restricted by the need for chemicals and highly trained staff to run the systems. A similar approach has been adopted by Tomaszewska-Gras (2016) and Nurulhidayah et al. (2015) to detect palm oil and lard, respectively, in butter as well as palm kernel and soybean oil detection in VCO by Marina et al. (2009b). Bayes-Garcia et al. (2016) revealed that the thermal profiles of two Iberian hams, namely *Cebo* (sample c1) and *Bellota* (sample b1), were almost identical (Fig. 12.2). However, following data processing using PLS discriminant analysis (PLS-DA), both heating and cooling thermograms successfully discriminated between the ham categories (Fig. 12.3).

Furthermore, there are also several studies that manipulated the chemometric approach with DSC in determining the varietal and geographical origin of foods such as olive oil (Chatziantoniou et al., 2014; Chiavaro et al., 2011) and almond (Sanahuja et al., 2011). Based on previous studies described, a strategy based on coupling DSC to chemometric data analysis could be an appropriate tool to aid understanding of food properties. Some examples are summarized in Table 12.2.

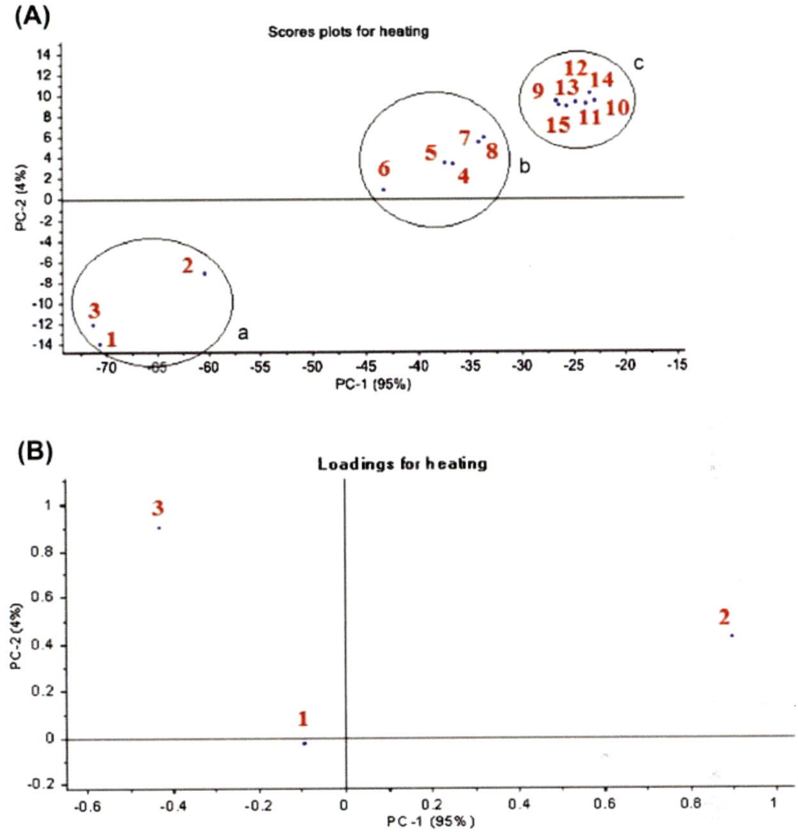

Figure 12.1 PCA score plot (A) and loading plot (B) of heating thermograms of pure and adulterated samples. (1) BT; (2) LD; (3) CF; (4) BT + 0.5% LD; (5) BT + 1% LD; (6) BT + 2% LD; (7) BT + 3% LD; (8) BT + 4% LD; (9) BT + 5% LD; (10) CF + 0.5% LD; (11) CF + 1% LD; (12) CF + 2% LD; (13) CF + 3% LD; (14) CF + 4% LD; and (15) CF + 5% LD in score plot. a: (1, 2 and 3) referred to pure BT, pure LD and pure CF respectively; b: (4, 5, 6, 7 and 8) referred to BT + LD; and c: (9, 10, 11, 12, 13, 14 and 15) referred to CF + LD. (1) Onset temperature; (2) enthalpy; and (3) end set temperature in loading plot (Dahimi et al., 2014).

12.3 Uses of Differential Scanning Calorimetry in Food Authenticity Testing

Authenticity testing is one of the main areas utilizing DSC. Most applications are focused on oil and fat-containing samples. DSC is a well-known method that has been applied for oil characterization (Tan and Che Man, 2000, 2002; Che Man and Tan, 2002; Tan et al., 2002; Barba et al., 2013). Generally, researchers studied the effects of cooling and heating rates on the crystallization and melting properties, generally as a quality control tool. Apart from this, there are numerous studies published

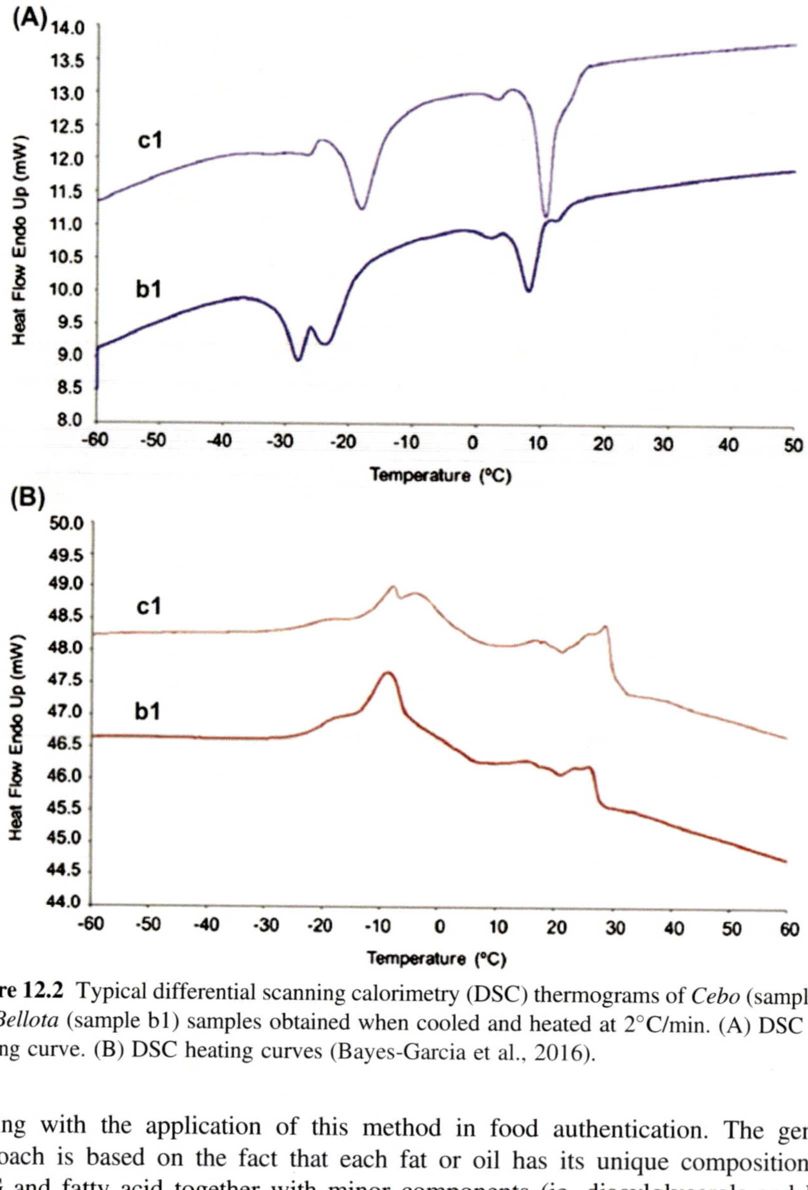

Figure 12.2 Typical differential scanning calorimetry (DSC) thermograms of *Cebo* (sample c1) and *Bellota* (sample b1) samples obtained when cooled and heated at 2°C/min. (A) DSC cooling curve. (B) DSC heating curves (Bayes-Garcia et al., 2016).

dealing with the application of this method in food authentication. The general approach is based on the fact that each fat or oil has its unique compositions of TAG and fatty acid together with minor components (ie, diacylglycerols and lipid oxidation products), which enable identification by their unique crystallization or melting curve properties. This information can be utilized for assessing, for example, cultivar, geographic origin, commercial categories, and adulteration.

In the context of oil authenticity, most of the published work deals with olive oil. Olive oil is a traditional Mediterranean food product that is obtained solely from the fruit of the olive tree (*Olea europaea* L.). It is produced by physical operations such as milling, pressing, centrifugation, and filtration and is reported to have a

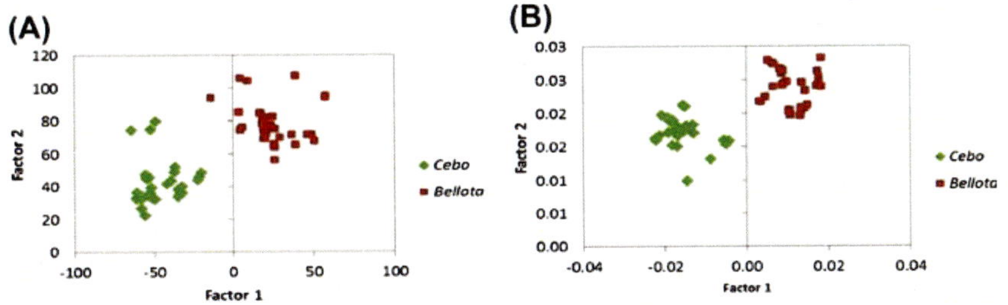

Figure 12.3 PLS discriminant analysis (PLS-DA) score plot: first two factors of the PLS-DA models based on (A) the cooling thermograms (from 25 to −45°C; data correspond to first derivative and scaling of variables to unit variance, three measurements per sample); (B) heating thermograms (from −30 to 40°C; data correspond to first derivative and scaling of variables to unit variance, three measurements per sample; Bayes-Garcia et al., 2016).

high-nutritional value (Garcia-Gonzalez and Aparicio, 2010; Bendini et al., 2007). Due to its high-economic value, it has always been exposed to potential adulteration. In a review published by Aparicio et al. (2013), several official methods and promising alternatives have been reported to deal with authenticity of olive oil; these include spectroscopic, isotopic, and chromatographic techniques, and most of the official methods are based on chromatographic methods. The instruments are quite expensive, the analysis is time consuming, requires skilled and experienced operators, therefore justifying development of other more rapid and simple methods such as DSC.

Research groups have applied DSC to many problems involving olive oil including discriminating commercial categories (Chiavaro et al., 2008a), differentiation of different cultivars and geographical origin (Kotti et al., 2009; Chiavaro et al., 2010, 2011), and detection of olive oil adulteration with cheaper oils (Chiavaro et al., 2008b, 2009). The relationship between thermal properties and chemical components was evaluated. Chiavaro et al. (2010) determined the statistical correlations between cooling transition, oxidative stability index (OSI values), and chemical components (TAG, FA, DAG, and FFA) of monovarietal extra virgin olive oils from different Italian regions. DSC cooling curves were used as they are well-known outputs able to be simply understood as well as avoid problems related to fat polymorphism, which is a common phenomenon observed during the melting process of fats. In another study, Chiavaro et al. (2011) suggested that a combination of DSC (cooling curves), GC, and isotope analysis with LDA was efficient in the confirmation of extra virgin olive oil cultivars and geographical origin. Chiavaro et al. (2008a) differentiated five distinct commercial categories of extra virgin olive oil, olive oil, refined olive oil, olive-pomace oil, and refined olive-pomace oil based on cooling and heating profiles. However, differentiation on basis of heating profile was found to be troublesome as the thermograms were more complex.

Kotti et al. (2009) discriminated extra virgin olive oils on the basis of cultivar–environment interaction in the case of Tunisian samples from two different cultivars (Chetoui and Chemlali) and different geographical production origins by means of cooling and heating profiles as well as chemical composition. Cooling and heating

Table 12.2 Differential Scanning Calorimetry Studies Combined With Chemometrics in Foods

Food Product	Multivariate Analysis	Aim of the Study	References
Olive oil	Linear discriminant analysis (LDA)	Determination of the varietal and geographical origin	Chatziantoniou et al. (2014) and Chiavaro et al. (2011)
	Partial least squares (PLS) regression	Evaluation of triacylglycerol composition on cooking profiles	Maggio et al. (2014)
		Evaluation of fatty acid composition	Cerretani et al. (2011)
	Principal component analysis (PCA)	Evaluation of lipid degradation	Chiavaro et al. (2013)
		Evaluation of oxidative levels	Caponio et al. (2013)
		Evaluation of thermo-oxidation	Maggio et al. (2012)
Virgin coconut oil	Stepwise multiple linear regression (SMLR)	Detection of lard adulteration	Mansor et al. (2012)
		Detection of palm kernel and soybean oil adulteration	Marina et al. (2009b)
Palm oil	LDA	Identification of palm, palm kernel, and coconut oil	Dyszel and Baish (1992)
Canola oil	SMLR	Detection of lard stearin	Marikkar and Rana (2014)
Butter	Multiple linear regression (MLR)	Determination of palm oil adulterant	Tomaszewska-Gras (2016)
	SMLR	Detection of lard adulteration	Nurrulhidayah et al. (2015)
Chicken and beef fats	PCA	Detection of lard adulteration	Dahimi et al. (2014)
Cod muscle	PLS	Identification of possible effects of various storage treatments	Jensen and Jorgensen (2003)

Table 12.2 Differential Scanning Calorimetry Studies Combined With Chemometrics in Foods—cont'd

Food Product	Multivariate Analysis	Aim of the Study	References
Pork	PCA and PLS discriminant analysis	Discrimination between Iberian dry-cured ham categories	Bayes-Garcia et al. (2016)
		Investigation of protein denaturation	Bertram et al. (2006)
Almond	LDA	Discrimination among different cultivars	Sanahuja et al. (2011)

thermograms of all samples are shown in Fig. 12.4. Two very clear events were exhibited in cooling profiles and the same events were also observed in previous study of different categories (Chiavaro et al., 2008a) and cultivars (Chiavaro et al., 2007) of olive oils. Heating profiles displayed more complex thermograms than cooling because of the presence of multiple events. They appeared more distinctive than cooling as differences were noticeable not only among oil samples of the same cultivar from different geographical origins but also between samples of Chetoui and Chemlali cultivars.

Furthermore, Laddomada et al. (2013) promoted the application of a modulated adiabatic scanning calorimeter in temperature-scanning mode with a tailor-made time-temperature protocol for analysis at various points along the olive oil supply chain. Compared with conventional DSC, this equipment was simpler, compact, and portable. Additionally, the time-temperature protocol was successful in origin differentiation of extra virgin olive oils. Additionally, a potential use of fast DSC was evaluated in order to replace traditional DSC for adulteration detection. The results obtained are comparable yet not always distinguishable (van Wetten et al., 2014).

With regard to adulteration with other vegetable oils, Chiavaro et al. (2008b) suggested that DSC may be useful in detecting extra virgin oil adulteration with hazelnut oil. Due to their similar chemical compositions (ie, TAG, FA, and total sterols), hazelnut oil is often used as an adulterant in extra virgin olive oil. This admixture is difficult to detect, especially when the concentration of hazelnut oil is below 20%. From results obtained, these authors concluded that DSC is able to detect at least 5% of refined hazelnut oil in extra virgin olive oil on the basis of alterations of both heating and cooling thermogram profiles of pure extra virgin olive oil. Cooling thermograms (ie, enthalpy and T_{on} of transition) are affected by hazelnut oil adulteration at a concentration as low as 5%. Nevertheless, they are not able to discriminate the exact percentage of hazelnut oil adulterated as thermal properties did not exhibit significant difference in the range of 5–20% and 30–40%, respectively (Fig. 12.5). In addition, heating thermograms may offer a qualitative method for assessing the adulteration by evaluating the line shape of the thermograms (Fig. 12.6). Bodurov et al. (2013) and

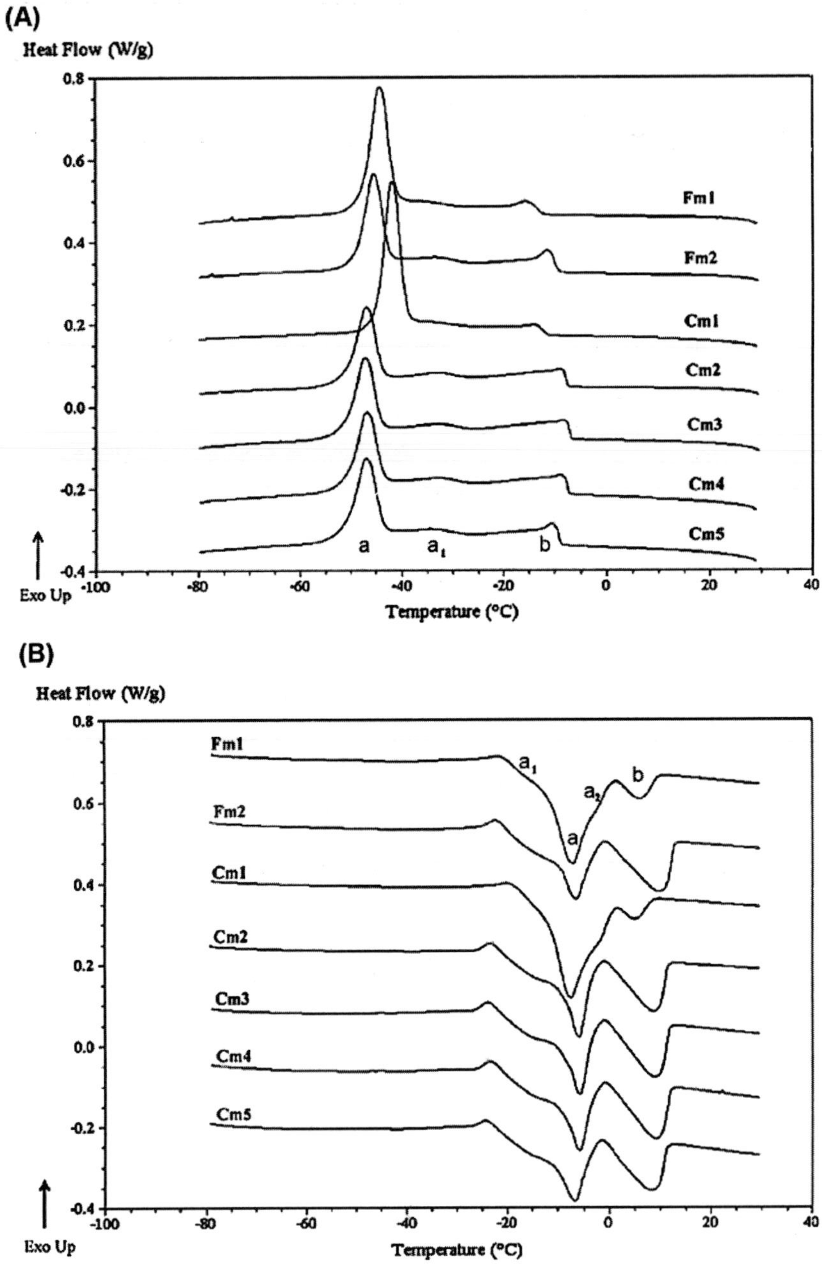

Figure 12.4 Cooling and heating thermograms of different cultivars of Tunisian olive oils. (A) Major and minor exothermic events are indicated with a, a_1, and b, respectively; (B) Major and minor endothermic events are indicated with a, a_1, a_2, and b, respectively. Fm1: Chetoui from Tunis; Fm2: Chemlali from Sfax; Cm1: Chetoui from El Kef; Cm2: Chemlali from Sfax; Cm3: Chemlali from Messadine; Cm4: Chemlali from Moknine; and Cm5: Menzel hayet (Kotti et al., 2009).

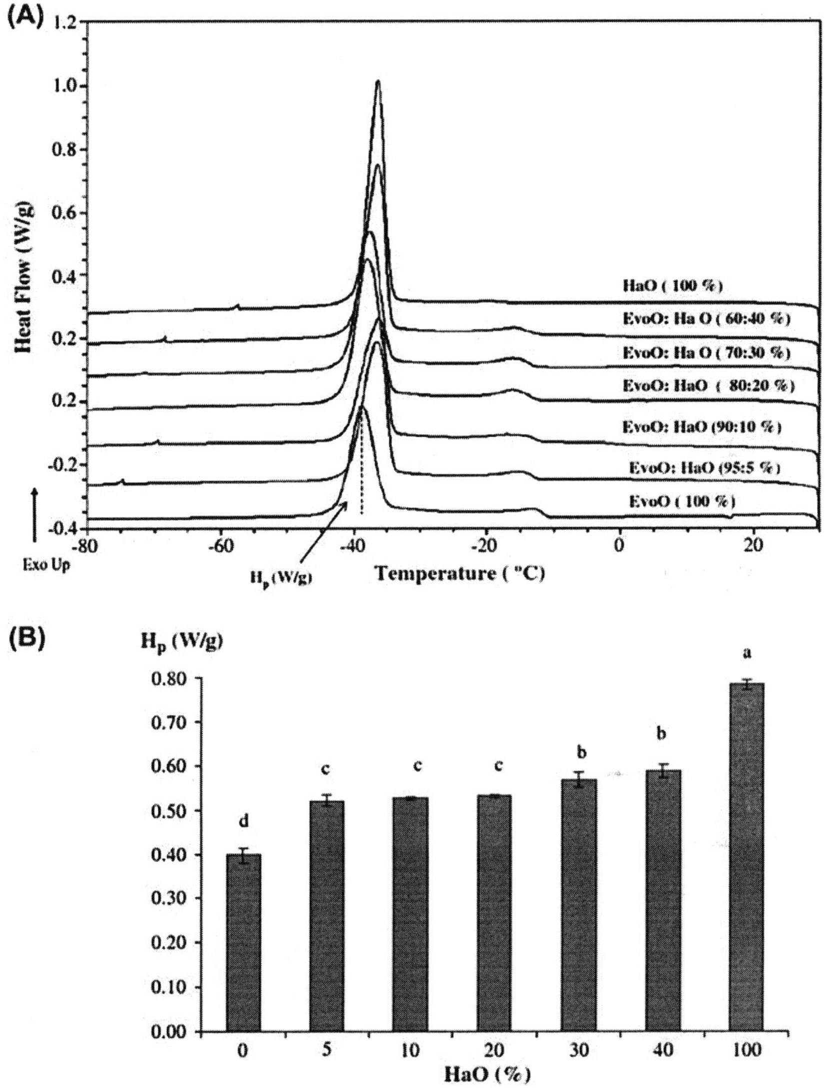

Figure 12.5 (A) Representative differential scanning calorimetry cooling thermograms of extra virgin olive oil (EvoO) and hazelnut olive oil (HaO) and their admixtures. (B) Peak height (W/g) of the major exothermic event (*dotted line A*) of cooling thermograms at different HaO percentage added. *Error bars* represent ±1SD ($n = 3$). Bars with the same letters are not significantly different ($p < .05$) (Chiavaro et al., 2008b).

Jafari et al. (2009) have also applied DSC to detect the presence of soybean, sunflower, or canola oils in olive oil.

Coconut (*Cocos nucifera*) is a fruit that is abundant in tropical and subtropical countries such as the Philippines, Malaysia, Indonesia, and India. Virgin coconut oil (VCO) is obtained from the fresh and mature kernel of the coconut without going

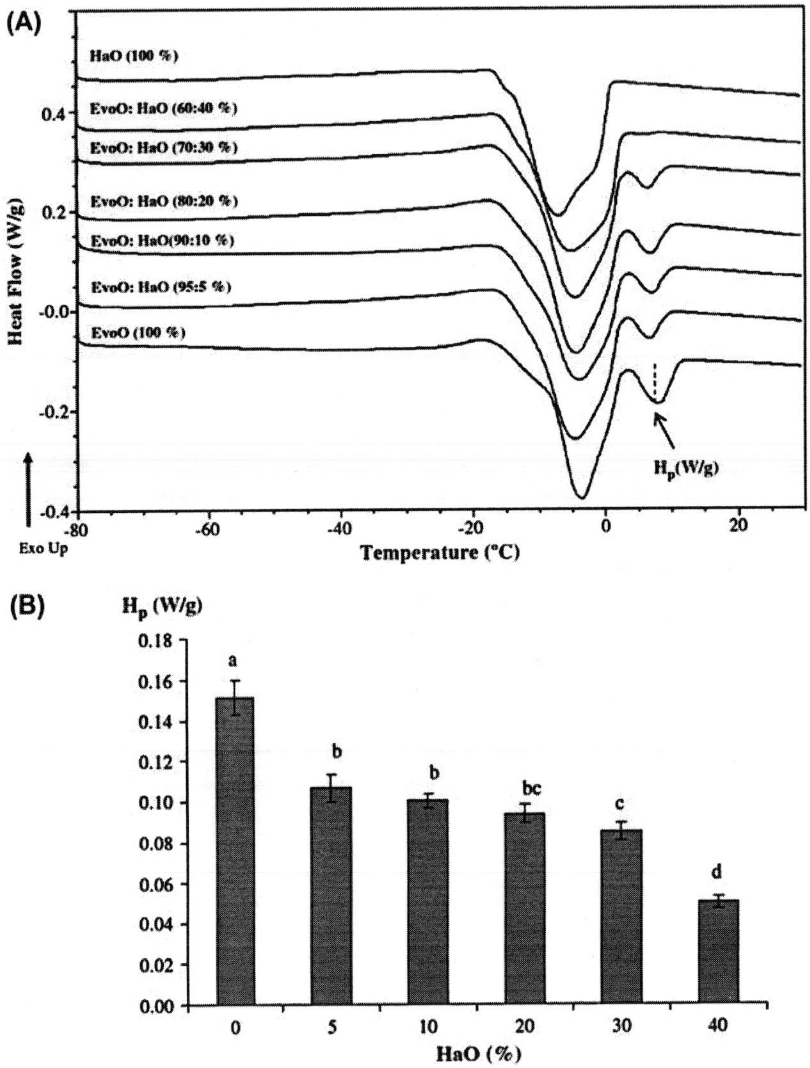

Figure 12.6 (A) Representative differential scanning calorimetry heating thermograms of extra virgin olive oil (EvoO) and hazelnut olive oil (HaO) and their admixtures. (B) Peak height (W/g) of the major exothermic event (*dotted line A*) of cooling thermograms at different HaO percentage added. *Error bars* represent ±1SD ($n = 3$). Bars with the same letters are not significantly different ($p < .05$) (Chiavaro et al., 2008b).

through any chemical refining, bleaching, and deodorizing (RBD) process (Marina et al., 2009a). It is gaining popularity as a cooking oil and a functional food supplement. Although the physical properties of VCO and lard are almost similar, they contain different amounts of saturated and unsaturated TAG and FA. Mansor et al. (2012) used both cooling and melting profiles in determining lard adulteration in

VCO. The appearance of multiple endothermic and exothermic peaks was explained by the arrangements and saturation levels of TAG; the less saturated the TAG, the lower the melting point and vice versa. Therefore, as lard has more unsaturated FA and TAG than VCO, lard heating thermograms exhibit two major endothermic peaks with lower melting points at −3.93 and 18.83°C (Fig. 12.7).

As shown in Fig. 12.8, the heating thermograms of adulterated VCO exhibited one major endothermic peak (peak A) together with a smaller shoulder peak embedded in the major peak. DSC was reported as being able to qualitatively detect lard adulteration when VCO is successively adulterated with lard from 1% to 30%, on the basis of the endothermic max T peak A, which increased in magnitude as lard percentage increased.

The existence of the two major exothermic peaks in VCO can be related to crystallization of the TAG (Fig. 12.9). Similar patterns were obtained in the cooling thermograms as related to crystallization. The curves exhibited slight changes, the size of peak

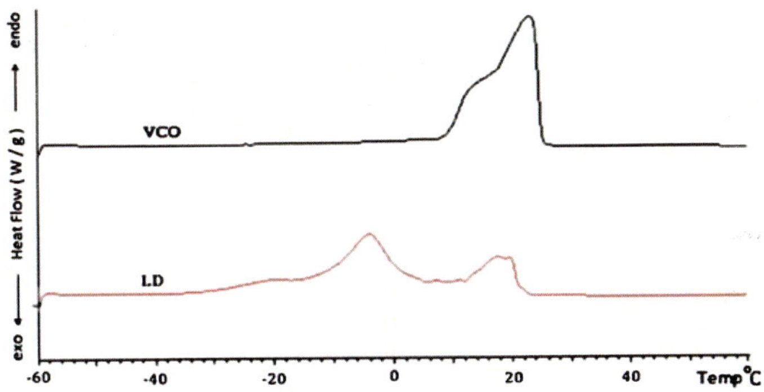

Figure 12.7 Differential scanning calorimetry heating thermograms of pure virgin coconut oil (VCO) and pure lard (LD) (Mansor et al., 2012).

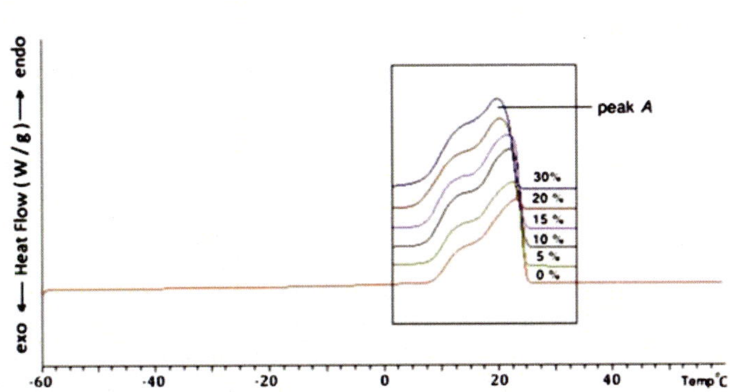

Figure 12.8 Differential scanning calorimetry heating thermograms of virgin coconut oil (VCO) adulterated with lard (LD) (v/v) (Mansor et al., 2012).

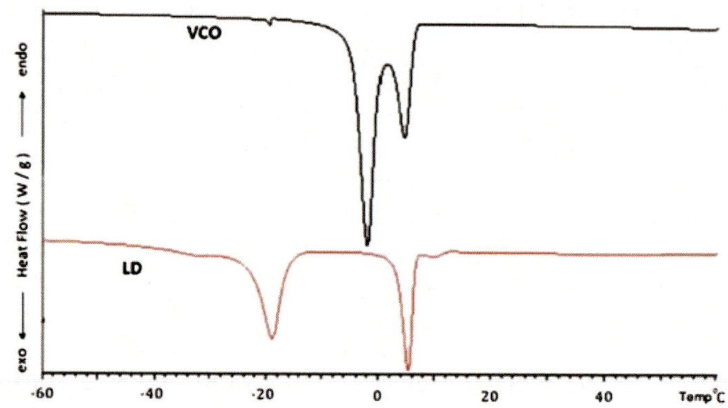

Figure 12.9 Differential scanning calorimetry cooling thermograms of pure virgin coconut oil (VCO) and pure lard (LD) (Mansor et al., 2012).

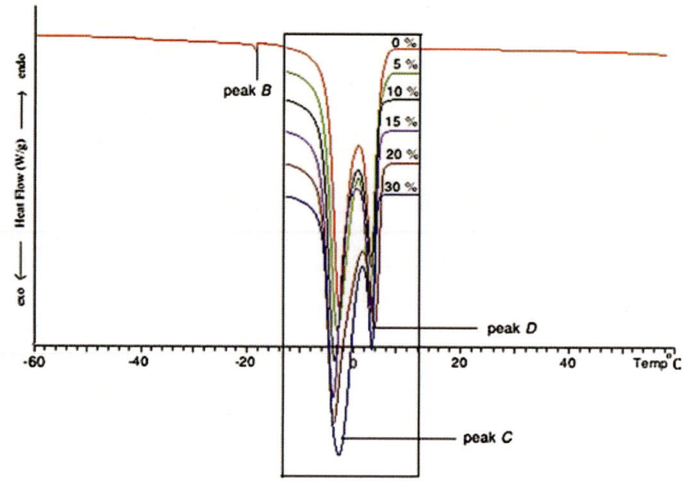

Figure 12.10 Differential scanning calorimetry cooling thermograms of virgin coconut oil (VCO) adulterated with lard (LD) (v/v) (Mansor et al., 2012).

C increased and there was reduction in the height of peak D and a smoothing effect on shoulder peak A when the percentage of LD adulteration increased (Fig. 12.10).

In another study, Marikkar and Rana (2014) aimed to detect and quantify lard stearin in canola oil. Pure canola oil samples were spiked with lard stearin ranging from 5% to 15% (w/w) and the cooling and heating profiles obtained were analyzed. According to the results, the authors concluded that the canola oil cooling curve at −19.5°C was strongly influenced by lard stearin and displayed significant variations when adulteration levels reached 5% (w/w). Applications of DSC in oil authentication are summarized in Table 12.3. In addition, the application of DSC in fats, nuts, honey, etc. are summarized in Tables 12.4−12.7, respectively.

Table 12.3 Differential Scanning Calorimetry Studies of Vegetable Oil Authenticity

Product	Issue	Sub-issue	Aim of the Study	References
Olive oil	Adulteration	Addition of other vegetable oil	Detection of sunflower oil in olive oil	van Wetten et al. (2014)
	Cultivar and geographical origin	Varietal olive oil and inexact label	Determination of the varietal and geographical origin of Greek extra virgin olive oils	Chatziantoniou et al. (2014)
	Adulteration	Addition of other vegetable oil	Detection of sunflower, soybean, and canola oils in olive oil	Bodurov et al. (2013) and Jafari et al. (2009)
	Geographical origin	Inexact label	Characterization of extra virgin olive oils of different provenance	Laddomada et al. (2013)
	Adulteration	Addition of other vegetable oil	Detection of high oleic sunflower oil in extra virgin olive oil	Chiavaro et al. (2009)
	Adulteration	Addition of other vegetable oil	Detection of refined hazelnut oil in extra virgin olive oil	Chiavaro et al. (2008b)
	Commercial categories	Inexact label	Discrimination among olive oils of different commercial categories (extra virgin olive oil, olive oil, refined olive oil, olive-pomace oil, and refined olive-pomace oil)	Chiavaro et al. (2008a)
	Cultivar and geographical origin	Traceability	Discrimination among olive oils of different cultivar and geographical origin	Chiavaro et al. (2011)
	Cultivar and geographical origin	Traceability	Differentiation of olive oils of different cultivars and/or geographical provenance	Kotti et al. (2009)
	Geographical origin	Traceability	Discrimination among olive oils of different geographical origin	Chiavaro et al. (2010)

Continued

Table 12.3 Differential Scanning Calorimetry Studies of Vegetable Oil Authenticity—cont'd

Product	Issue	Sub-issue	Aim of the Study	References
	Geographical origin/ adulteration	Traceability	Screening quality and origin of olive oil	Angiuli et al. (2006) and Ferrari et al. (2007)
	Adulteration	Addition of other vegetable oil	Detection of sunflower and corn oils in extra virgin oil	Torrecilla et al. (2011)
Palm oil	Adulteration	Addition of animal fat	Determination of genuine lard, chicken fat, and beef tallow in palm olein	Marikkar et al. (2003a)
	Adulteration	Addition of animal fat	Detection of lipase-catalyzed interesterified lard in refined-bleached deodorized (RBD) palm oil	Marikkar et al. (2002a)
	Adulteration	Addition of animal fat	Detection of lard and randomized lard in RBD palm oil	Marikkar et al. (2001)
	Commercial categories	Inexact label	Identification of palm, palm kernel, and coconut oils	Dyszel and Baish (1992)
Coconut oil	Adulteration	Addition of animal fat	Detection of lard in virgin coconut oil	Mansor et al. (2012)
	Adulteration	Addition of other vegetable oil	Detection of palm kernel oil and soybean oil in virgin coconut oil	Marina et al. (2009b)
Canola oil	Adulteration	Addition of animal fat	Detection of lard stearin in canola oil	Marikkar and Rana (2014)
	Adulteration	Addition of animal fat	Detection of genuine lard, beef tallow, and chicken fat in canola oil	Marikkar et al. (2002b)
Sesame oil	Adulteration	Addition of other vegetable oil	Detection of corn oil and sunflower oil in sesame oil	Fahimdanesh et al. (2014)
Sunflower oil	Adulteration	Contamination of animal fat	Detection of lard and beef tallow in sunflower oil	Marikkar et al. (2012)

Table 12.4 Differential Scanning Calorimetry Studies of Fat Authenticity

Product	Issue	Sub-issue	Aim of the Study	References
Confectionery fats (cocoa butter equivalents)	Adulteration	Addition of other natural edible fats	Classification of types of confectionery fat	Cebula and Smith (1992)
Butter	Adulteration	Addition of vegetable fat	Detection of palm oil in butter	Tomaszewska-Gras (2016)
	Adulteration	Addition of other animal fat	Detection of lard in butter	Nurrulhidayah et al. (2015)
	Adulteration		Detection of butter adulteration with water	Tomaszewska-Gras (2012)
	Adulteration	Addition of other animal and vegetable fats	Detection of beef body fat and margarine in butter	Aktas and Kaya (2001)
	Adulteration	Addition of other animal fat	Detection of chicken fat in butter	Coni et al. (1994)
	Adulteration	Addition of other animal fat	Detection of pig and buffalo body fats in cow and buffalo butter	Lambelet and Ganguli (1983)
	Adulteration	Addition of other animal fat	Detection of goat body fat in butter	Lambelet et al. (1980)
Beef tallow and chicken fat	Adulteration	Cross-contamination of other animal fat	Detection of lard in mixture systems containing beef tallow and chicken fat separately	Dahimi et al. (2014)

Table 12.5 **Differential Scanning Calorimetry Studies of Nut Authenticity**

Product	Issue	Sub-issue	Aim of the Study	References
Almond (Spanish Guara and Marcona and American Butte)	Cultivar	Varietal almonds	Discrimination among different almond cultivars	Sanahuja et al. (2011)
Macadamia	Geographical origin	Inexact label	Identification of macadamia nuts grown in South Africa	Dyszel (1990)
Pistachio nut	Geographical origin	Inexact label	Determination of country of origin	Dyszel and Pettit (1990)
Peanut	Geographical origin	Inexact label	Determination of country of origin	Dyszel (1993)

Table 12.6 **Differential Scanning Calorimetry Studies of Honey Authenticity**

Product	Issue	Sub-issue	Aim of the Study	References
Lime bee honey	Adulteration	Addition of glucose	Detection of glucose in honey	Nikolova et al. (2012)
	Adulteration	Addition of syrup	Detection of syrup in honey	Cordella et al. (2003)
Lavandula, Robinia, and Fir honeys	Adulteration	Addition of industrial sugar syrup	Detection of industrial sugar syrup in honey	Cordella et al. (2002)

Table 12.7 Differential Scanning Calorimetry Studies of Others

Product	Issue	Sub-issue	Aim of the Study	References
Shark	Adulteration	Inexact label	Differentiation between smoked and unsmoked of shark muscle	Schubring (2007)
Fried tempeh, chicken, and beef products	Adulteration	Religious issue	Detection of lard in fried products	Marikkar et al. (2003b)
Edible waxes	Adulteration	Health issue	Differentiation between edible waxes and wax esters that are used to coat apples	Ritter et al. (2001)
Meat	Commercial categories	Inexact label	Discrimination between Iberian dry-cured ham categories	Bayes-Garcia et al. (2016)

12.4 Conclusions and Future Perspectives

Authenticity determination by DSC displays undisputable advantages, such as ease of measurement, speed, and environmental friendliness. However, its application as a sole technique is often not definitive as some thermal transitions are very weak or complex, making evaluation troublesome. Currently, a growing interest has been shown in combining DSC results with chemometric tools. By considering all the data obtained, chemometrics makes better results possible. Several authenticity aspects analyzed with DSC included discrimination of cultivars, geographical origin, and commercial categories as well as detection of adulteration. Based on the literature, the most common samples that have been analyzed using DSC are oils and fats. This increasing interest in DSC suggests that its application in authentication is reliable and suitable for screening purposes to reduce the time and cost prior to verification with other highly sophisticated confirmatory methods.

Sources of Further Information

1. Haines, P.J., Wilburn, F.W., 1995. Differential thermal analysis and differential scanning calorimetry. In: Haines, P.J. (Ed.), Thermal Methods of Analysis Principles, Applications and Problems. Chapman and Hall.
2. Haines, P.J., Reading, M., Wilburn, F.W., 1998. Differential thermal analysis and differential scanning calorimetry. In: Brown, M.E. (Ed.), Handbook of Thermal Analysis and Calorimetry. In: Principles and Practice, vol. I. Elsevier Science B.V.

3. Laye, P.G., 2002. Principles of thermal analysis and calorimetry. In: Haines, P.J. (Ed.), Principles of Thermal Analysis and Calorimetry. Royal Society of Chemistry, Cambridge.
4. Brown, M.E., 1998. Handbook of Thermal Analysis and Calorimetry. In: Principles and Practice, vol. 1. Elsevier.
5. Burlett, J.D., 2008. Quality control. In: Brown, M.E., Gallagher, P.K. (Eds.), Handbook of Thermal Analysis and Calorimetry. In: Recent Advances, Techniques and Applications, vol. 5. Elsevier B.V.
6. Kaletunc, G., 2009. Calorimetry in Food Processing: Analysis and Design of Food Systems. Wiley-Blackwell.

References

Abdorreza, M.N., Cheng, L.H., Karim, A.A., 2011. Effects of plasticizers on thermal properties and heat sealability of sago starch films. Food Hydrocolloids 25, 56–60.

Aktas, N., Kaya, M., 2001. Detection of beef body fat and margarine in butterfat by differential scanning calorimetry. Journal of Thermal Analysis and Calorimetry 66, 795–801.

Angiuli, M., Ferrari, C., Lepori, L., Matteoli, E., Salvetti, G., Tombari, E., Banti, A., Minnaja, N., 2006. On testing quality and traceability of virgin olive oil by calorimetry. Journal of Thermal Analysis and Calorimetry 84, 105–112.

Aparicio, R., Morales, M.T., Aparicio-Ruiz, R., Tena, N., Garcia-Gonzalez, D.L., 2013. Authenticity of olive oil: mapping and comparing official methods and promising alternatives. Food Research International 54, 2025–2038.

Arrieta, M., Lopez, J., Ferrandiz, S., Peltzer, M.A., 2013. Characterization of PLA-limonene blends for food packaging applications. Polymer Testing 32, 760–768.

Bainy, E.M., Corazza, M.L., Lenzi, M.K., 2015. Measurement of freezing point of tilapia fish burger differential scanning calorimetry (DSC) cooling curve method. Journal of Food Engineering 161, 82–86.

Barba, L., Arrighetti, G., Calligaris, S., 2013. Crystallization and melting properties of extra virgin olive oil studied by synchrotron XRD and DSC. European Journal of Lipid Science and Technology 115, 322–329.

Bayes-Garcia, L., Tres, A., Vichi, S., Calvet, T., Cuevas-Diarte, M.A., Codony, R., Boatella, J., Caixact, J., Ueno, S., Guardiola, F., 2016. Authentication of Iberian dry-cured ham: new approaches by polymorphic fingerprint and ultrahigh resolution mass spectrometry. Food Control 60, 370–377.

Bendini, A., Cerretani, L., Carrasco-Pancorbo, A., Gomez-Caravaca, A.M., Segura-Carretero, A., Fernandez-Gutierrez, A., Lercker, G., 2007. Phenolic molecules in virgin olive oils: a survey of their sensory properties, health effects, antioxidant activity and analytical methods. An overview of the last decade. Molecules 12, 1679–1719.

Bergner, K., Albano, C., 1993. Thermal analysis of peat. Analytical Chemistry 65, 204–208.

Bertram, H.C., Wu, Z., van den Berg, F., Anderson, H.J., 2006. NMR relaxometry and differential scanning calorimetry during meat cooking. Meat Science 74, 684–689.

Biliaderis, C.G., 1983. Differential scanning calorimetry in food research – a review. Food Chemistry 10, 239–265.

Blanco, I., Siracusa, V., 2013. Kinetic study of the thermal and thermos-oxidative degradations of polylactide-modified films for food packaging. Journal of Thermal Analysis and Calorimetry 112, 1171–1177.

Bodurov, I., Vlaeva, I., Marudova, M., Yovcheva, T., Nikolova, K., Eftimov, T., Plachkova, V., 2013. Detection of adulteration in olive oils using optical and thermal methods. Bulgarian Chemical Communications 45, 81–85.

Bosmans, G.M., Pareyt, B., Delcour, J.A., 2016. Non-additive response of blends of rice and potato starch during heating at intermediate water contents: a differential scanning calorimetry and proton nuclear magnetic resonance study. Food Chemistry 192, 568–595.

Caponio, F., Chiavaro, E., Paradiso, V.M., Paciulli, M., Summo, C., Cerratani, L., Gomes, T., 2013. Chemical and thermal evaluation of olive oil refining at different oxidative levels. European Journal of Lipid Science and Technology 115, 1146–1154.

Cebula, D.J., Smith, K.W., 1992. Differential scanning calorimetry of confectionery fats: part II – effects of blends and minor components. Journal of the American Oil Chemists' Society 69, 992–998.

Cerretani, L., Maggio, R.M., Barnaba, C., Toschi, T.G., Chiavaro, E., 2011. Application of partial least square regression to differential scanning calorimetry data for fatty acid quantitation in olive oil. Food Chemistry 127, 1899–1904.

Chatziantoniou, S.E., Triantafillou, D.J., Karayannakidis, P.D., Diamantopoulos, E., 2014. Traceability monitoring of Greek extra virgin olive oil by different scanning calorimetry. Thermochimica Acta 576, 9–17.

Chauhan, A., Mittu, B., 2012. Modern approach to research by DSC and its advancements. Pharmaceutica Analytica Acta Journal 3, 8.

Che Man, Y.B., Tan, C.P., 2002. Comparative differential scanning calorimetric analysis of vegetable oils: II. Effects of cooling rate variation. Phytochemical Analysis 13, 142–151.

Chiavaro, E., Cerretani, L., Matteo, A.D., Barnabe, C., Bendini, A., Iacumin, P., 2011. Application of a multidisciplinary approach for the evaluation of traceability of extra virgin olive oil. European Journal of Lipid Science and Technology 113, 1509–1519.

Chiavaro, E., Cerretani, L., Paradiso, V.M., Summo, C., Paciulli, M., Toschi, T.G., Caponio, F., 2013. Thermal and chemical evaluation of naturally auto-oxidised virgin olive oils: a correlation study. Journal of the Science of Food and Agriculture 93, 2909–2916.

Chiavaro, E., Rodriguez-Estrada, M.T., Barnaba, C., Vittadini, E., Cerretani, L., Bendini, A., 2008a. Differential scanning calorimetry: a potential tool for discrimination of olive commercial categories. Analytical Chimica Acta 625, 215–226.

Chiavaro, E., Vittadini, E., Rodriguez-Estrada, M.T., Cerretani, L., Bendini, A., 2008b. Differential scanning calorimeter application to the detection of refined hazelnut oil in extra virgin olive oil. Food Chemistry 110, 248–256.

Chiavaro, E., Rodriguez-Estrada, M.T., Bendini, A., Cerretani, L., 2010. Correlation between thermal properties and chemical composition of Italian virgin olive oils. European Journal of Lipid Science and Technology 112, 580–592.

Chiavaro, E., Vittadini, E., Rodriguez-Estrada, M.T., Cerretani, L., Capelli, L., Bendini, A., 2009. Differential scanning calorimetry detection of high oleic sunflower oil as adulterant in extra-virgin olive oil. Journal of Food Lipids 16, 227–244.

Chiavaro, E., Vittadini, E., Rodriguez-Estrada, M.T., Cerretani, L., Bonoli, M., Bendini, A., Lercker, G., 2007. Monovarietal extra virgin olive oils: correlation between thermal properties and chemical composition. Journal of Agricultural and Food Chemistry 55, 10779–10786.

Clas, S.D., Dalton, C.R., Hancock, B.C., 1999. Differential scanning calorimetry: applications in drug development. Pharmaceutical Science & Technology Today 2, 311–320.

Coni, E., di Pasquale, M., Coppolelli, P., Bocca, A., 1994. Detection of animal fats in butter by differential scanning calorimetry: a pilot study. Journal of the American Oil Chemists' Society 71, 807–810.

Cordella, C., Antinelli, J.F., Aurieres, C., Faucon, J.P., Cabrol-Bass, D., Sbirrazzuoli, N., 2002. Use of differential scanning calorimetry (DSC) as a new technique for detection of adulteration in honeys. 1. Study of adulteration effect on honey thermal behavior. Journal of Agricultural and Food Chemistry 50, 203–208.

Cordella, C., Faucon, J.P., Cabrol-Bass, D., Sbirrazzuoli, N., 2003. Application of DSC as a tool for honey floral species characterization and adulteration detection. Journal of Thermal Analysis and Calorimetry 71, 279–290.

Dahimi, O., Rahim, A.A., Abdulkarim, S.M., Hassan, M.S., Hashari, S.B.T., Siti Mashitoh, A., Saadi, S., 2014. Multivariable statistical analysis treatment of DSC thermal properties for animal fat adulteration. Food Chemistry 158, 132–138.

Dinani, S.T., Hamdami, N., Shahedi, M., Havet, M., Queveau, D., 2015. Influence of the electrohydrodynamic process on the properties of dried button mushroom slices: a differential scanning calorimetry (DSC) study. Food and Bioproducts Processing 95, 83–95.

Dyszel, S.M., 1990. Characterization of macadamia nuts by differential scanning calorimetry for country of origin. Thermochimica Acta 166, 291–300.

Dyszel, S.M., 1993. Characterization of peanuts by DSC for country of origin. Thermochemica Acta 226, 265–274.

Dyszel, S.M., Baish, S.K., 1992. Characterization of tropical oils by DSC. Thermochimica Acta 212, 39–49.

Dyszel, S.M., Pettit, B.C., 1990. Determination of the country of origin of pistachio nuts by DSC and HPLC. Journal of the American Oil Chemists' Society 67, 947–951.

Eguchi, S., Kitamoto, N., Nishinari, K., Yoshimura, M., 2014. Effects of esterified tapioca starch on the physical and thermal properties of Japanese white salted noodles prepared partly by residual heat. Food Hydrocolloids 35, 198–208.

Elmer, P., 2013. Guide to Selection of DSC Sample Pans. Technical Note, Waltham, MA, USA.

Fahimdanesh, M., Bahrami, M.E., Zargani, M., 2014. 66 Check fraud sesame (*Sesamus Indicum*) oil using different scanning calorimetry (DSC) analysis. International Journal of Plant, Animal and Environmental Sciences 4, 554–560.

Farkas, J., Mohacsi-Farkas, C., 1996. Application of differential scanning calorimetry in food research and food quality assurance. Journal of Thermal Analysis 47, 1787–1803.

Ferrari, C., Angiuli, M., Tombari, E., Righetti, M.C., Matteoli, E., Salvetti, G., 2007. Promoting calorimetry for olive oil authentication. Thermochimica Acta 459, 58–63.

Garcia-Gonzalez, D.L., Aparicio, R., 2010. Research in olive oil: challenges for the near future. Journal of Agricultural and Food Chemistry 58, 12569–12577.

Grajzer, M., Prescha, A., Korzonek, K., Wojakowska, A., Dziadas, M., Kulma, A., Grajeta, H., 2015. Characteristics of rose hip (*Rose canina* L.) cold-pressed oil and its oxidative stability studied by the differential scanning calorimetry method. Food Chemistry 188, 456–466.

Jafari, M., Kadivar, M., Keramat, J., 2009. Detection of adulteration in Iranian olive oils using instrumental (GC, NMR, DSC) methods. Journal of the American Oil Chemists' Society 86, 103–110.

Jahurul, M.H.A., Zaidul, I.S.M., Norulaini, N.A.N., Sahena, F., Abedin, M.Z., Ghafoor, K., Mohd Omar, A.K., 2014. Characterization of crystallization and melting profiles of blends of mango seed fat and palm oil mid-fraction as cocoa butter replacers using differential scanning calorimetry and pulse nuclear magnetic resonance. Food Research International 55, 103–109.

Jensen, K.N., Jorgensen, B.M., 2003. Effect of storage conditions on differential scanning calorimetry profiles from thawed cod muscle. Lebensmittel-Wissenschaft und-Technologie 36, 807–812.

Korzeniowska, M., Cheung, I.W.Y., Li-Chan, E.C.Y., 2013. Effects of fish protein hydrolysate and freeze-thaw treatment on physicochemical and gel properties of natural actomyosin from Pacific cod. Food Chemistry 138, 1967–1975.

Kotti, F., Chiavaro, E., Cerretani, L., Barnaba, C., Gargouri, M., Bendini, A., 2009. Chemical and thermal characterization of Tunsian extra virgin olive oil from Chetoui and Chemlali cultivars and different geographical origin. European Food Research and Technology 228, 735–742.

Laddomada, B., Colella, G., Tufariello, M., Durante, M., Angiuli, M., Salvetti, G., Mita, G., 2013. Application of a simplified calorimetric assay for the evaluation of extra virgin olive oil quality. Food Research International 54, 2062–2068.

Lai, O.M., Lo, S.K., 2008. Thermal technique: differential scanning calorimetry (DSC). In: Sun, D.W. (Ed.), Modern Techniques for Food Authentication. Elsevier Inc., Amsterdam, the Netherlands.

Lambelet, P., Ganguli, N.C., 1983. Detection of pig and buffalo body fat in cow and buffalo ghees by differential scanning calorimetry. Journal of the American Oil Chemists' Society 5, 1005–1008.

Lambelet, P., Singhal, O.P., Ganguli, N.C., 1980. Detection of goat body fat in Ghee by differential thermal analysis. Journal of the American Oil Chemists' Society 57, 364–366.

Li, Q., Xie, Q., Yu, S., Gao, Q., 2013. New approach to study starch gelatinization applying a combination of hot-stage light microscopy and differential scanning calorimetry. Journal of Agricultural and Food Chemistry 61, 1212–1218.

Maggio, R.M., Barnaba, C., Cerretani, L., Paciulli, M., Chiavaro, E., 2014. Study of the influence of triacylglycerol composition on DSC cooling curves of extra virgin olive oil by chemometric data processing. Journal of Thermal Analysis and Calorimetry 115, 2037–2044.

Maggio, R.M., Cerretani, L., Barnaba, C., Chiavaro, E., 2012. Application of differential scanning calorimetry-chemometric coupled procedure to the evaluation of thermos-oxidation on extra virgin olive oil. Food Biophysics 7, 114–123.

Mansor, T.S.T., Che Man, Y.B., Shuhaimi, M., 2012. Employment of differential scanning calorimetry in detecting lard adulteration in virgin coconut oil. Journal of the American Chemical Society 89, 485–496.

Marikkar, J.M.N., Rana, S., 2014. Use of differential scanning calorimetry to detect canola oil (*Brassica napus* L.) adulterated with lard stearin. Journal of Oleo Science 63, 867–873.

Marikkar, J.M.N., Dzulkifly, M.H., Nor Nadiha, M.Z., Che Man, Y.B., 2012. Detection of animal fat contaminations in sunflower oil by differential scanning calorimetry. International Journal of Food Properties 15, 683–690.

Marikkar, J.M.N., Ghazali, H.M., Che Man, Y.B., Lai, O.M., 2003a. Differential scanning calorimetric analysis for determination of some animal fats as adulterants in palm olein. Journal of Food Lipids 10, 63–79.

Marikkar, J.M.N., Ghazali, H.M., Long, K., Lai, O.M., 2003b. Lard uptake and its detection in selected food products deep-fried in lard. Food Research International 36, 1047–1060.

Marikkar, J.M.N., Lai, O.M., Ghazali, H.M., Che Man, Y.B., 2001. Detection of lard and randomized lard as adulterants in refined-bleached-deodorized palm oil by differential scanning calorimetry. Journal of the American Oil Chemists' Society 78, 1113–1119.

Marikkar, J.M.N., Lai, O.M., Ghazali, H.M., Che Man, Y.B., 2002a. Compositional and thermal analysis of RBD palm oil adulterated with lipase-catalyzed interesterified lard. Food Chemistry 76, 246–258.

Marikkar, J.M.N., Ghazali, H.M., Che Man, Y.B., Lai, O.M., 2002b. The use of cooling and heating thermograms for monitoring of tallow, lard and chicken fat adulterations in canola oil. Food Research International 35, 1007–1014.

Marina, A.M., Che Man, Y.B., Amin, I., 2009a. Virgin coconut oil: emerging functional food oil. Trends in Food Science and Technology 20, 481–487.

Marina, A.M., Che Man, Y.B., Nazimah, S.A.H., Amin, I., 2009b. Monitoring the adulteration of virgin coconut oil by selected vegetable oils using differential scanning calorimetry. Journal of Food Lipids 16, 50–61.

Matos, E., Silva, T.S., Tiago, T., Aureliano, M., Dinis, M.T., Dias, J., 2011. Effect of harvesting stress and storage conditions on protein degradation in fillets of farmed gilthead seabream (*Sparus aurata*): a differential scanning calorimetry study. Food Chemistry 126, 270–276.

Moreira, R., Chenlo, F., Arufe, F.C., 2015. Starch transitions of different gluten free flour doughs determined by dynamic thermal mechanical analysis and differential scanning calorimetry. Carbohydrate Polymers 127, 160–167.

Naik, A., Meda, V., Lele, S.S., 2014. Application of EPR spectroscopy and DSC for oxidative stability studies of *Nigella sativa* and *Lepidium sativum* seed oil. Journal of the American Oil Chemists' Society 91, 935–941.

Nikolova, K., Panchev, I., Sainov, S., Gentscheva, G., Ivanova, E., 2012. Selected physical properties of lime bee honey in order to discriminate between pure honey and honey adulterated with glucose. International Journal of Food Properties 15, 1358–1368.

Nurrulhidayah, A.F., Arieff, S.R., Rohman, A., Amin, I., Shuhaimi, M., Khatib, A., 2015. Detection of butter adulteration with lard using differential scanning calorimetry. International Food Research Journal 22, 832–839.

Pardauil, J.J.R., Sauza, L.K.C., Molfetta, F.A., Zamian, J.R., Filho, G.N.R., da Costa, C.E.F., 2011. Determination of the oxidative stability by DSC of vegetable oils from the Amazonian area. Bioresource Technology 102, 5873–5877.

Qi, B., Zhang, Q., Sui, X., Wang, Z., Li, Y., Jiang, L., 2016. Differential scanning calorimetry study: assessing the influence of composition of vegetable oils on oxidation. Food Chemistry 194, 601–607.

Ritter, B., Schulte, J., Schulte, E., Thier, H.P., 2001. Detection of coating waxes on apples by differential scanning calorimetry. European Food Research and Technology 212, 603–607.

Sanahuja, A.B., Teruel, N.G., Carratala, M.L.M., Selva, M.C.G., 2011. Characterization of almond cultivars by the use of thermal analysis techniques. Application to cultivar authenticity. Journal of the American Oil Chemists' Society 88, 1687–1693.

Schubring, R., 2007. DSC measurements on sharks. Thermochimica Acta 458, 124–131.

Tan, C.P., Che Man, Y.B., 2000. Differential scanning calorimetric analysis of edible oils: comparison of thermal properties and chemical composition. Journal of the American Oil Chemists' Society 77, 143–155.

Tan, C.P., Che Man, Y.B., 2002. Comparative differential scanning calorimetric analysis of vegetable oils: I. Effects of heating rate variation. Phytochemical Analysis 13, 129–141.

Tan, C.P., Che Man, Y.B., Selamat, J., Yusoff, M.S.A., 2002. Comparative studies of oxidative stability of edible oils by differential scanning calorimetry and oxidative stability index methods. Food Chemistry 76, 385–389.

Tomaszewska-Gras, J., 2012. Detection of butter adulteration with water using differential scanning calorimetry. Journal of Thermal Analysis and Calorimetry 108, 433–438.

Tomaszewska-Gras, J., 2016. Rapid quantitative determination of butter adulteration with palm oil using the DSC technique. Food Control 60, 629–635.

Torrecilla, J.S., Garcia, J., Garcia, S., Rodriguez, F., 2011. Quantification of adulterant agents in extra virgin oil by models based on its thermophysical properties. Journal of Food Engineering 103, 211–218.

van Wetten, I.A., van Herwaarden, A.W., Splinter, R., van Ruth, S.M., 2014. Oil analysis by fast DSC. Procedia Engineering 87, 280–283.

Watson, E., O'Neill, M., 1962. Differential Microcalorimeter. US3263484A.

Zanqui, A.B., de Morais, D.R., de Silva, C.M., Santos, J.M., Gomes, S.T.M., Visentainer, J.V., Eberlin, M.N., Cardozo-Filho, L., Matsushita, M., 2015a. Subcritical extraction of flaxseed oil with n-propane: composition and purity. Food Chemistry 188, 452–458.

Zanqui, A.B., de Morais, D.R., de Silva, C.M., Santos, J.M., Chiavelli, L.U.R., Bittencourt, P.R.S., Eberlin, M.N., Visentainer, J.V., Cardozo-Filho, L., Matsushita, M., 2015b. Subcritical extraction of *Salvia hispanica* L. oil with *N*-propane: composition, purity and oxidation stability as compared to the oils obtained by conventional solvent extraction methods. Journal of the Brazilian Chemical Society 26, 282–289.

Zhang, Y., Zhu, K., He, S., Tan, L., Kong, X., 2016. Characterizations of high purity starches isolated from five different jackfruit cultivars. Food Hydrocolloids 52, 785–794.

Part Two

Advances in Authenticity Testing

Advances in Authenticity Testing of Geographical Origin of Food Products

13

A.M. Pustjens, M. Muilwijk, Y. Weesepoel, S.M. van Ruth
Wageningen University and Research Centre, Wageningen, The Netherlands

Chapter Outline

13.1 Introduction

Authentication of food and feed is a topic of ongoing interest. On the one hand, consumers demand safe, honest, and properly labeled food. On the other hand, producers need to ensure that their raw materials are safe and their products have an added value to distinguish them from competitors' products. One of the authenticity topics of interest is the geographical origin of food products, which arises for economic, safety, and sustainability reasons. Therefore, European legislation has been enacted to protect consumers from false and misleading information and producers from dishonest competition (Xiaobing and Kireeva, 2011). Specifications for geographical indications of food products are laid down in Regulation (EC) No. 510/2006. Registration of geographical names is divided into three classes: protected designation of origin (PDO), protected geographical indication (PGI), and traditional specialties guaranteed (TSG). Furthermore, in European legislation, additional attention is paid to correct labeling of the geographical origin of some specific food products, eg, Regulation (EU) No. 1379/2013 concerning the origin of fish and aquaculture products.

In this chapter an update is presented on the advances in authenticity testing of geographical origin of food products from late 2008 until early 2015. Developments that took place before 2008 were previously reported by Luykx et al. (2008). The updated analysis methods for determining the geographical origin comprise isotopic analysis (Section 13.2), elemental analysis (Section 13.3), compositional analysis (Section 13.4), nondestructive analysis (Section 13.5), and a varied collection of other techniques (Section 13.6). Within these sections, individual techniques are discussed and illustrated using several food product cases as examples.

13.2 Techniques for Analyzing Isotopes

All food products have their own isotopic composition. The stable isotope ratios of food products are determined by the metabolic turnover of the plant or animal species that makes them up. Biological material, like food, is made of many elements, among others carbon, hydrogen, nitrogen, oxygen, sulfur, and strontium. Their isotopic ratios can be used as an indication of the geographical origin of a product, although usually a combination of isotope ratios is needed to determine the geographical origin depending on the type of food product (Vinci et al., 2013). In general, isotopic analyses to confirm the provenance of food products are performed on bulk, ie, the whole sample. However, in some cases, only a certain fraction or even an individual component of the food product is of interest, eg, proteins or lipids. This fraction can therefore be extracted from the whole food in a separate preliminary step. It is also possible to couple the isotope ratio mass spectrometer to gas or liquid chromatography equipment for the isotopic analysis of individual compounds. This approach is used, for example, to distinguish natural and synthetic hormones, although reports of its application for the determination of geographical origin of food are rare. GC-IRMS may, for example, be used to discriminate geographical origin of fermentation of raw materials based on the hydrogen isotope ratios of acetic acid present in vinegar (Hattori et al., 2010).

Hydrogen and oxygen isotopes in water are partly dependent on climatic conditions. Plants take up water with a certain isotopic composition from the soil. Within the leaves, evapotranspiration takes place, causing an enrichment of the heavier isotope of hydrogen and oxygen in the water present in the leaf. The $^{18}O/^{16}O$ ratio of biomass arises from the cell water and the organically bound oxygen. However, in food analysis it is often only the water fraction of a liquid food product that is analyzed, thereby excluding the contribution of organically bound oxygen from any subsequent data interpretation. Analysis of oxygen isotope ratios is very valuable for the determination of the geographical origin of wines and fruit juices (Krivachy et al., 2015). Carbon isotope ratios ($^{13}C/^{12}C$) allow discrimination between plants using different photosynthetic pathways, namely C3 and C4 plants, and thereby enable discrimination of an animal's diet. In animal products, feeding regime history can also be determined when analyzing the $^{13}C/^{12}C$ ratio of nails and hooves (Vinci et al., 2013).

The nitrogen isotope ratio ($^{15}N/^{14}N$) is determined by the trophic level of plant or animal species and agricultural practices (whether or not nitrogen-containing synthetic fertilizer has been applied to the land); it is also able to distinguish between marine and terrestrial plants. In animal products, this ratio is mainly determined by the animal's diet (Vinci et al., 2013). In nature, sulfur exists in four stable isotopes, of which ^{34}S and ^{32}S are the most common. The sulfur isotope ratio ($^{34}S/^{32}S$) in plant species is determined by the soil composition of the area in which the plant is growing, atmospheric SO_2, and the use of sulfur-containing synthetic fertilizer. This makes the analysis of sulfur isotope ratios especially valuable for the determination of the geographical origin of plants. To enable analysis of animal products, specific organs or tissues should be selected on the basis of the abundance of certain sulfur-containing proteins and proteoglycans (Krivachy et al., 2015). Strontium is naturally present in rocks and soil and can be taken up by plants during germination. The isotopic composition of strontium ($^{87}Sr/^{86}Sr$) is linked to the nature, age, and origin of the material and can thus help in the verification of the geographical origin of food products (Medini et al., 2015).

Usually, a combination of isotope ratios is analyzed; this strategy has been successfully used in the determination of the geographical origin of milk, cheese, butter, animal products, vegetables, natural flavors, honey, wines, and fruit (juices) (Luykx and van Ruth, 2008). Since then, isotope ratio mass spectrometry (IRMS), nuclear magnetic resonance (NMR), and thermal ionization mass spectrometry (TIMS) are used regularly in the verification of the geographical origin of food products, as discussed in the following sections.

13.2.1 Isotope Ratio Mass Spectrometry

The most common apparatus used to determine stable isotope ratios is IRMS. Two types of IRMS apparatus exist, namely a continuous-flow IRMS (CF-IRMS) and a dual-input IRMS (DI-IRMS). For DI-IRMS, gasses are prepared off-line while for CF-IRMS these are prepared online. CF-IRMS can be coupled to another interface, eg, an elemental analyzer (EA-IRMS), gas chromatography (GC-IRMS), or liquid chromatography (LC-IRMS).

Using EA-IRMS to analyze the $^{13}C/^{12}C$ ratio of different cereals has revealed significant differences ($p < .05$) for different geographical origins (Wu et al., 2015). These authors have analyzed rice, soybean, millet, wheat, and corn from the United States, Canada, Australia, and three provinces in China. Also, dried distillers grains with solubles (a by-product from bioethanol production that is used in animal feed) originating from the United States, Canada, European Union (EU), and China can be distinguished using EA-IRMS analysis of $^{2}H/^{1}H$, $^{13}C/^{12}C$, $^{15}N/^{14}N$, and $^{18}O/^{16}O$. Using a cross-validated canonical discriminant analysis (CDA) model, the origin could be predicted with a sensitivity of 80−100% and a specificity of 92−100% (Nietner et al., 2014). The $^{34}S/^{32}S$ isotope ratio alone did not allow discrimination of samples from the selected countries. A combination of $^{13}C/^{12}C$ and $^{15}N/^{14}N$ enabled classification of the geographical origin of different types of fish and crustaceans, namely croaker (Chaguri et al., 2015), shrimps (Ortea and Gallardo, 2015), mackerel, yellow croaker, and pollock (Kim et al., 2015).

To differentiate extra virgin olive oil from eight Mediterranean countries, n-alkanes were extracted and analyzed by GC-IRMS for their $^{13}C/^{12}C$ and $^{2}H/^{1}H$ ratios. The n-C29 alkane showed the highest discriminating power and enabled correct classification of 93.4% of the olive oil from northern and southern Mediterranean countries using a cross-validated CDA model (Mihailova et al., 2015). Verification of the geographical origin of wine has already been successfully demonstrated; however, it was disputed whether this would still be possible when wines from different vintage years were analyzed. Raco et al. (2015) showed that analysis of $^{2}H/^{1}H$ and $^{18}O/^{16}O$ using CF-IRMS can indeed verify wine geographical origin independent of vintage year. Using $^{13}C/^{12}C$ this was not possible.

13.2.2 Thermal Ionization Mass Spectrometry

TIMS is a technique in which a sample is heated, thereby ionizing elements present in a food product. The ionized elements are then passed through a magnetic field to detect the mass-to-charge ratio of the different ions, thereby enabling separation of different isotopes. This technique is mainly used for analyzing isotopes with relatively low ionization energy, such as strontium. Based on strontium isotope ratio analysis by TIMS, tomato and tomato products from China and Italy were found to be significantly different ($p < .01$; Trincherini et al., 2014). However, differentiation of Lambrusco wines from different locations in the Modena district in Italy was not possible using strontium isotope ratios (Durante et al., 2015). In addition, $^{87}Sr/^{86}Sr$ ratios have been determined by TIMS to determine the geographical origin of olive oils after extraction of strontium using a novel extraction protocol specific for a lipid matrix (Medini et al., 2015).

13.2.3 Nuclear Magnetic Resonance

In addition to IRMS, NMR is also used in the analysis of stable isotopes, especially ^{1}H and ^{13}C. Site-specific natural isotope fractionation NMR (SNIF-NMR) is often used in food analysis. The principle behind NMR is the fact that many nuclei have an associated spin and all nuclei are electrically charged. In the presence of an applied external magnetic field, an energy transfer occurs that can be measured at different wavelengths. NMR is used to analyze the purity or the molecular structure of a sample. A combination of ^{1}H NMR and an externally validated linear discriminant analysis (LDA) model has been able to correctly classify 94.6% of Italian sweet cherries originating from three areas within Italy (Longobardi et al., 2013). Additionally, the geographical origin of cocoa beans from Ecuador, Grenada, and African regions could be correctly classified using the application of ^{1}H NMR combined with a cross-validated stepwise discriminant analysis model (Caligiani et al., 2014).

The potential of ^{1}H SNIF-NMR in the differentiation of wines from locations within Romania was evaluated. The calculation of the D/H ratio of both methyl and methylene groups of ethanol in these wines considerably improved the ability to differentiate (Bejjani et al., 2014). When the ^{1}H NMR analysis was combined with inductively coupled plasma atomic emission spectroscopy or mass spectrometry (ICP-AES/ICP-MS) multielement analysis, the geographical origin of two types of medicinal herbs from three locations in Korea and three others in China could be determined. Using a cross-validated partial least squares discriminant analysis (PLS-DA), 83–97% of the analyzed medicinal herbs could be correctly classified (Kwon et al., 2014).

To verify the geographical origin of fermented honey, EA-IRMS analysis of $^{13}C/^{12}C$ alone was not sufficient; however, when these data were combined with SNIF-NMR analysis of the D/H ratio related to the photosynthetic sugar metabolism of plants, samples from eight different locations within Romania could be distinguished (Dinca et al., 2014).

13.3 Techniques for Analyzing Elements

The concentration of organic compounds present is not only related to the geographical origin but also very much dependent on, eg, seasonal changes and climate conditions in the year of cultivation. Therefore, it can be very useful to look at inorganic compounds present in food. For example, the content of certain elements is highly correlated with the growing conditions in a particular environment (Drivelos et al., 2014). This information is applicable both to plant and animal products, in which the elemental composition of the feed will determine the mineral composition in certain animal tissues.

Inductively coupled plasma analysis can be linked to a mass spectrometer (ICP-MS), an atomic emission spectrometer (ICP-AES), or optical emission spectroscopic equipment (ICP-OES). With all three types of equipment, a relatively quick screening of elements can be performed. With ICP-AES, up to 60 different elements can be quantified while ICP-MS can yield information on over 70 elements.

Until 2008, ICP-AES analysis was successfully used to determine the geographical origin of honey and wines. Furthermore, ICP-MS analysis was successfully applied for the determination of geographical origin of vegetables, tea, and wines (Luykx and van Ruth, 2008). Since then, the geographical origin of olive oil has been determined using ICP-MS analysis of the elements tungsten (W), iron (Fe), magnesium (Mg), manganese (Mn), calcium (Ca), barium (Ba), lithium (Li), and bismuth (Bi). Using a combination of these elements, 93% of the olive oils from orchards located in four different municipalities in southern Spain could be correctly classified (Beltrán et al., 2015). The geographical origin of saffron was confirmed by analyzing boron (B), sodium (Na), strontium (Sr), and rubidium (Rb) by ICP-MS also. In this way saffron from three regions in Italy could be distinguished (D'Archivio et al., 2014). Using ICP-AES analysis of eight different elements, cumin from four countries could be distinguished: China, India, Syria, and Turkey. The elements involved were Ca, Mg, K, Fe, Na, Mn, Sr, and Zn (Hondrogiannis et al., 2012).

Data produced separately by ICP-AES and ICP-MS can also be combined, for example, when verifying the geographical origin of vinegar. Scandium (Sc), chromium (Cr), cobalt (Co), nickel (Ni), arsenic (As), yttrium (Y), molybdenum (Mo), cadmium (Cd), cesium (Cs), Ba, lanthanum (La), cerium (Ce), and lead (Pb) were analyzed by ICP-MS while data on the content of Al, Fe, Mn, Zn, Ca, K, Mg, and Na were measured by ICP-AES. In this way vinegar from five regions in China could be distinguished (Zheng et al., 2014). Apart from applications to food products of plant origin, the geographical origin of shrimps has been investigated by a combination of ICP-OES, to analyze P and S, and ICP-MS, to analyze As, Cd, and Pb. Using these elements, wild shrimp from six areas in the world could be distinguished (Ortea and Gallardo, 2015).

Another way to determine elemental composition is X-ray fluorescence. This has been used, for example, to distinguish soybeans that were grown in Japan from imported soybeans from other locations in the world (Otaka et al., 2014). In addition, X-ray fluorescence and ICP-MS data have been combined to determine the geographical origin of vanilla from Madagascar, Uganda, India, Indonesia, and Papua New Guinea (Hondrogiannis et al., 2013).

13.4 Separation Techniques for Compositional Analysis

Food products originating from different geographical locations often have differences in phytochemical, protein, fat, carbohydrate, and volatile content. Due to growing conditions at the designated region, subtle differences may be present within the complex mixture of a particular group of compounds that might have structural similarities. In order to exploit these differences, one possible strategy is to separate the compound class of interest into its individual components. Subsequently, chromatogram shapes or peak areas of individual compounds can be analyzed by multivariate data analysis in order to expose principal component vectors for geographical origin. The "classical" techniques to achieve such a separation are ((ultra-)high performance) liquid chromatography ((U)HP)LC, gas chromatography (GC), and capillary electrophoresis (CE). Depending on the compound class(es) of interest, availability of equipment, sample pretreatment, and detection techniques (DAD, MS, ELSD, etc.), one of these three techniques will be most appropriate for the provenance problem being studied. In Table 13.1 an overview of the latest reports concerning LC, GC, and CE techniques for confirming the geographical origin of foods is presented. It is apparent that there is no single best solution for each individual food product; this is due to the availability of a large variety of analytical techniques and progress in technique development. For example, confirming the provenance of oils and fats can be performed by either LC, GC, or CE by analyzing polyphenols, triacylglycerides, and (semi-)volatiles, respectively. Similar options exist in the case of honey and propolis (Table 13.1). It is interesting to see that the main categories of compounds investigated are phytonutrients,

Table 13.1 Condensed Overview of the Latest Peer-reviewed Work on LC, GC, and CE Separation Techniques Applied to Geographical Provenance Confirmation in Food

Food class	Food subclass	Geographical regions	Separation and detection technique	Chemical markers of interest	Statistical or MVA method	Min-max % success	Reference
Chocolate	Cocoa and chocolate	Ecuador, Ghana	GC–MS	Fatty acids	3-factor ANOVA, Tukey's test	N.R.	Torres-Moreno et al. (2015)
Coffee	Arabica coffee	Brazil, Colombia, Costa Rica, Guatemala, Ethiopia, Indonesia	HS-SPME-GC-TOF-MS	(Semi-)volatiles	PCA	N.R.	Risticevic et al. (2008)
Fruits	Goji berry	Mongolia, China, Tibet	LC-qTOF-MS	Flavonol glycosides, coumaric acid	PCA, PLS-DA	N.R.	Bondia-Pons et al. (2014)
Herbs and spices	Saffron	Greece, Iran, Italy, Spain	GC–MS and FID	Isophorones, C_{13}-norisoprenoids	ANOVA, discriminant analysis	94–96	Anastasaki et al. (2009)
	Red Ginseng	Korea, China	LC-MS/MS	Ginsenosides	Discriminant function analysis	N.R.	Moon et al. (2014)
	Ginger	China, India, Malaysia, Thailand, Vietnam	LC-DAD	Gingerols and 6 related compounds	HCA, PCA, LDA	N.R.	Yudthavorasit et al. (2014)

Continued

Table 13.1 Condensed Overview of the Latest Peer-reviewed Work on LC, GC, and CE Separation Techniques Applied to Geographical Provenance Confirmation in Food—cont'd

Food class	Food subclass	Geographical regions	Separation and detection technique	Chemical markers of interest	Statistical or MVA method	Min-max % success	Reference
Honey and propolis	Honey	Corsica, France (non-Corsican), Italy, Austria, Germany	HS-SPME-GCxGC-TOF-MS	(Semi-)volatiles	LDA, PLS-DA, SIMCA, SVM	45–87	Stanimirova et al. (2010)
		8 regions in Santa Catarina (Brazil)	CE-DAD	Cations	PCA	N.R.	Rizelio et al. (2012)
	Propolis	10 provinces in China	LC-DAD	Flavonoids	Similarity analysis	N.R.	Zhou et al. (2008)
		4 regions in China	DHS-GC-MS	Volatile acids, esters, alcohols, terpenes, other aromatics	PCA	N.R.	Cheng et al. (2013)
Oils and fats	Extra virgin olive oil	PDO Chianti Classico (Italy), PDO Sierra de Segura (Spain)	CE-DAD	Polyphenols	Tukey's test, PCA	N.R.	Carrasco-Pancorbo et al. (2009)

		Croatia, Italy, Spain	CE-DAD	Polyphenols	LDA	N.R.	Lerma-García et al. (2009)
	Virgin Oueslati olive oil	7 regions in Tunisia	HS-SPME-GC-MS and FID	(Semi-)volatiles	PCA, HCA	N.R.	Youssef et al. (2011)
	Extra virgin Chemlali olive oil	13 regions in Tunisia	LC-ESI-TOF-MS	Phenolics	CDA	Max 100	Taamalli et al. (2012)
	Palm oil	South East Asia, Africa, South America	LC-DAD HTGC-MS	Triacylglycerols	PLS-DA	83–100 71–100	Ruiz-Samblás et al. (2013)
Sweeteners	*Stevia rebaudiana*	Brazil, Paraguay, Italy	LC-ESI-MS/MS	Steviol glycosides	Two-way ANOVA PCA	N.R.	Montoro et al. (2013)
Vegetables	Olive	Several regions in Spain, 'other countries'	CE-DAD	Proteins	Discriminant analysis	Max 79	Montealegre et al. (2012)
	Olive leaves (*Olea europaea*)	3 cities in Italy	LC-ESI-MS/MS	Phenolics	LDA, SIMCA, KNN	93–100	Di Donna et al. (2010)
	Potato	3 regions in Italy	HS-SPME-GC-MS	(Semi-)volatiles	Discriminant analysis	Max 100	Longobardi et al. (2011)
	Fresh tomato, tomato paste	4 regions in Italy	HS-SPME-GC-MS	(Semi-)volatiles	PCA SIMCA LDA	94–96 (fresh) 97–100 (paste)	Feudo et al. (2011)

Continued

Table 13.1 Condensed Overview of the Latest Peer-reviewed Work on LC, GC, and CE Separation Techniques Applied to Geographical Provenance Confirmation in Food—cont'd

Food class	Food subclass	Geographical regions	Separation and detection technique	Chemical markers of interest	Statistical or MVA method	Min-max % success	Reference
Wheat	Distillers dried grains and solubles	Europe, China, USA	GC-FID	Fatty acids	PCA, PLS-DA	100–100	Alba Tres et al. (2014)
Wine	Sauvignon blanc wine	New Zealand, France, Austria	HS-SPME-GC-MS/MS	Key volatile compounds	ANOVA	N.R.	Green et al. (2011)
	Argentinian red wine	3 regions in Argentina	LC-MS	Anthocyanins	PLS-DA UPLS-DA	100–100	Pisano et al. (2015)

N.R., Not reported.

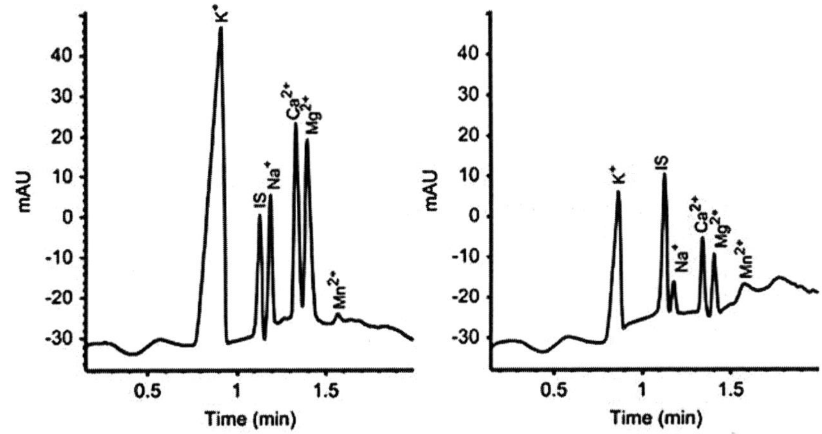

Figure 13.1 Electropherogram of cations present in two Brazilian (Santa Catarina) honey samples analyzed by capillary electrophoresis. Left: "Florianopolis" region, right: "São Miguel do Oeste" region.
Adapted from Rizelio, V.M., Gonzaga, L.V., Borges, G.D.C., Maltez, H.F., Costa, A.C.O., Fett, R., 2012. Fast determination of cations in honey by capillary electrophoresis: a possible method for geographic origin discrimination. Talanta 99, 450–456.

using LC, and (semi-)volatiles and fatty acids using GC. Recent developments around the technique of CE are opening up new opportunities such as, for example, in provenance confirmation of honey by cation analysis (Fig. 13.1) and of olives on the basis of protein analysis. Although trends in separation techniques emerge from time to time, for example, supercritical fluid chromatography, researchers tend to stay with the classical approach as, to the best of our knowledge, no reports describing the use of supercritical fluid separation in geographical provenance problems are available.

13.5 (Semi-)Nondestructive Techniques

Often sample preparation represents a costly and time-consuming process before the actual analysis starts. Therefore, more and more attention is being paid to so-called nondestructive techniques. Although the definition of *(semi-)nondestructive* can be debated, this term is to be understood to mean that virtually no sample preparation is required nor is the sample destroyed by extraction, drying, etc. In this section, three groups of such analytical techniques are discussed.

13.5.1 Proton Transfer Reaction Mass Spectrometry

Proton transfer reaction mass spectrometry (PTR-MS) assesses the volatile organic compounds (VOCs) present in the headspace of a closed sample container under controlled temperature and gas flows. Headspace VOCs are chemically ionized by reaction with hydroxonium ions (H_3O^+), a step that is regarded as a "soft-ionization" practice. The H_3O^+ ions are produced from pure water vapor in an external glow discharge ion source. After acceleration in an electrical field, which can also lead to dissociation of the VOC ions by gas collision, a quantitative ion chromatogram is obtained that serves as the fingerprint of the sample (Luykx and van Ruth, 2008). PTR-MS devices can be equipped with different types of mass analyzers. An ion trap mass analyzer is suitable for simultaneous investigation of VOCs from a complex gas mixture while, very recently, a time-of-flight (TOF) detector has been introduced to the market; this has the advantage that the mass detector resolution is higher than for the ion traps making possible, for example, the analysis of isobaric compounds (Zardin et al., 2014). Quadrupole mass analyzers are also available, but in the specific case of PTR-MS, this technique suffers from disadvantages compared to ion trap and TOF mass analyzers. In separate developments, NO^+, O_2^+, Kr^+, and Xe^+ ions are being introduced for the detection of compounds such as ethylene and acetylene, which cannot be ionized by H_3O^+ (Cappellin et al., 2013).

PTR-MS, as a relatively new technique, has already proven itself to be very effective in correctly identifying the region of origin of several high-value products like olive oil, truffles, Grana Padano cheese, etc. (Luykx and van Ruth, 2008). New developments in the usage of PTR-MS for the geographical origin classification of different European olive oils showed correct prediction percentages as high as 86% using PLS-DA classification (Araghipour et al., 2008). In the field of crude palm oils, PTR-MS in combination with PLS-DA was successfully used for the separation of South East Asian from non-South East Asian samples. Furthermore, a similar model with high success rates was produced to discriminate African from South American crude palm oil (Tres et al., 2013). For dairy products, PTR-MS was also applied to geographical provenance problems. Maçatelli et al. (2009) analyzed 83 commercial European butters by PTR-MS to predict country of origin; an average success rate of 88% was reported. For artisanal farmers' cumin cheese from Leiden (the Netherlands) with EU PDO, PTR-MS was employed to develop authentication models in order to discriminate these from commercial Dutch cumin cheese brands (Galle et al., 2011). Dry cured hams produced in specific PDOs from Iberia (Spain) and three Italian regions could be discriminated from each other by PTR-MS followed by data preprocessing and visualization by principal component analysis (PCA) (del Pulgar et al., 2011). Also for mono-origin (Brazil, Ethiopia, and Guatemala) coffees (*Coffea arabica*), significant differences were found in volatile profiles by PTR-MS and PCA (Yener et al., 2014). For alcoholic beverages like wines, the high concentration of ethanol in the headspace leads to depletion of H_3O^+ ions and therefore less ionization of other VOCs. Although, for example, dilution of the wine sample could effectively tackle this problem, a rapid chromatographic step (FastGC) prior to PTR-MS was recently used to eliminate it (Fig. 13.2). In combination with PCA visualization, PTR-MS was used successfully in discriminating the region of origin of several red wines (Romano et al., 2014). A more exotic example of recent developments is the analysis of sea urchin volatiles from different geographic regions in New Zealand (Phillips et al., 2010). Finally, although not a food product, the geographical provenance of the flower bulb lily of the valley (*Convallaria majalis*) could be discriminated

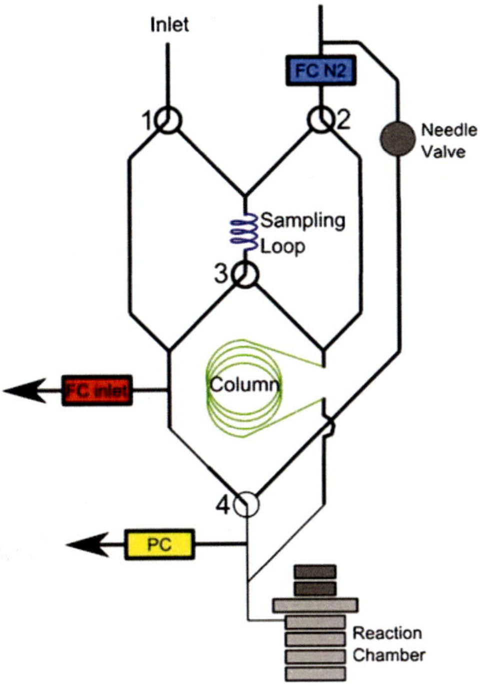

Figure 13.2 Schematic drawing of a PTR-ToF-MS inlet system with a FastGC setup, in order to tackle analysis problems with foods containing a high level of alcohol such as wines.
Adapted from Romano, A., Fischer, L., Herbig, J., Campbell-Sills, H., Coulon, J., Lucas, P., Cappellin, L., Biasioli, F., 2014. Wine analysis by FastGC proton-transfer reaction-time-of-flight-mass spectrometry. International Journal of Mass Spectrometry 369 (0), 81−86.

with PTR-MS (van Ruth and de Visser, 2015). This may pave the way for future determination of the provenance other edible *Allium* species such as garlic.

To conclude this section, VOCs present in the headspace of food products are of course not only affected by their geographical origin. Several other factors should be taken into account as they can strongly influence the outcome of a geographical provenance test. For example, in the case of fruits and vegetables, the maturity of a product strongly influences the VOC composition, as was recently investigated for olive fruits (Masi et al., 2014) and apple ripening (Soukoulis et al., 2013). VOCs found upon different postharvest processing of grape must were different for differing processing temperatures (Cappellin et al., 2013). Finally, in the case of meat, the rearing system to which an animal was exposed influences the headspace VOCs. Pigs with different diets, which were used to produce Iberian dry-cured ham, showed clearly different VOCs (Sánchez del Pulgar et al., 2013).

13.5.2 Sensor Technology: Electronic Nose and Electronic Tongue

The term *sensor technology* is often used to refer to the electronic nose technology, which employs the VOCs contained in a sample as the basis of analysis. However, the electronic tongue, which can be used in liquids, can be seen as a technique based on a similar concept. Both techniques use an array of semi-selective sensors (eg, metal oxide semiconductors or polymers) to generate analytical data that, combined with chemometrics, may determine, for example, the geographical origin of a product.

In the case of the electronic nose or e-nose, no prior separation of the VOCs is required and the individual sensor responses are interpreted by chemometrics. One type of sensor array reacts upon absorption of a volatile compound and causes a change in physical properties of the sensor. This can be, for example, changes in electrical conductivity (eg, moisture content), changes in reflectance and surface energy (oxidative reactions), etc. More recently, electronic noses based on mass spectrometry have become popular. VOCs contained in a sample are ionized and led into a mass spectrometer, which produces a global mass spectrum serving as a fingerprint (Berna et al., 2009; Luykx and van Ruth, 2008). The use of the e-nose for geographical provenance confirmation has increased over the last five years. Raw propolis from four different geographical regions in China could be discriminated by this method (Cheng et al., 2013). For different Polish honey types, separation was also possible, although no different geographical regions were defined (Dymerski et al., 2014). For wines, the e-nose with mass spectrometry–based detection seems to be ideal, as interfering ethanol fragment ions can be filtered out. For sensors based on metal oxide, the ethanol has to be removed. In the case of Sauvignon Blanc wines, the e-nose in combination with LDA could divide wines from three countries and six regions into three classes (Berna et al., 2009). For Tempranillo wines, e-nose with mass spectrometry detection was used to discriminate between Australian and Spanish products with a correct classification rate of up to 86% (Cynkar et al., 2010). For discrimination of olive oil from different PDOs from the Liguria region of Italy, the e-nose was employed as part of a three-way combinatorial approach that also involved UV–Vis and near infrared spectroscopy to build a class model for this specific olive oil (Casale et al., 2010). For Italian sweet cherries from the Apulia and Emilia Romagna regions, the e-nose in combination with LDA analysis was successfully used for confirming regional provenance; additional IRMS analysis and the combination of data improved the results (Longobardi et al., 2015). For liquorice roots (*Glycyrrhiza glabra* L.), the e-nose can be used to confirm geographical origin as an alternative to destructive GC–MS techniques. By odorprinting, liquorice roots from China, Iran, different Italian regions, and Turkey could be discriminated by multivariate statistics (Russo et al., 2014). Finally, Korean and Chinese red ginseng variants could be discriminated by a mass spectrometer–based e-nose (Moon et al., 2014).

The application of the electronic tongue or e-tongue, multivariate statistics, and geographical provenance has also increased in recent years. As for the e-nose, there is an array of different sensors available that can be applied in a (crude) liquid. These mostly potentiometric and voltammetric sensors respond or react to one or more chemical substances in the sample liquid (Tahara and Toko, 2013). In addition to these, there are numerous other types of sensors being developed for a wide array of applications (Ha et al., 2015). The e-tongue finds its geographical provenance application especially in the field of tea. Green and black teas originating from different regions in China could be distinguished by this approach (He et al., 2009). Furthermore, the provenance of Chinese green tea with PDO from three Longjing subareas could be determined accurately (Xu et al., 2013). The e-tongue has also shown very good results in the case of origin confirmation of mineral, spring, and tap waters from different origins (Sipos et al., 2012), and a similar conclusion can be drawn for white wines (Gutierrez et al., 2011). When looking to more apolar liquids such as oils, the e-tongue can be also applied after addition of supporting electrolytes to provide conductivity information (Oliveri et al., 2009). In the case of honey, recent advances in potentiometric and electronic e-tongue have been made to classify its geographical origin (Wei and Wang, 2014; Wei et al., 2009). Finally, e-tongue methods have also been developed for confirming the provenance of cocoa beans, although this method is destructive. Ground cocoa beans were dissolved in water, filtered, and subsequently measured by e-tongue. In this case, a support vector machine algorithm was sufficient for accurate classification (Teye et al., 2014).

13.5.3 Spectroscopic Techniques

Mid-infrared (MIR), near infrared (NIR), and Raman vibrational spectroscopy are generally fast analytical techniques (seconds), have low running costs, require little sample preparation, and are in most cases nondestructive. Miniaturization of the these types of spectrometers makes this technique especially suitable for operation in the field (Downey, 2013). Though it goes beyond the scope of this chapter to fully explain the principles of each type of spectroscopy technique, in general, MIR and NIR operate in the 2500–25,000 nm (4000–400 cm^{-1}) and 780–2500 nm (12,820–4000 cm^{-1}), respectively, reflecting the fact that IR spectra mostly reflect molecular vibrations involving changes in dipole moment. Raman equipment is often high-intensity and laser operated, and the vibrational information is retrieved from light that is scattered from the sample. Raman is especially sensitive to alterations in polarizability. For more in-depth reading, see Downey (2013).

Virtually any type of food, fresh or processed, can be analyzed by spectroscopic techniques, in either a nondestructive or destructive way. For geographical provenance of food this is no different, though the success rates for classification very much depend on the selection of the sample set, type of spectroscopic technique used, type of data pretreatment applied, and type of chemometric algorithm used. In Table 13.2, a condensed overview is presented with recent examples of peer-reviewed work using spectroscopy and multivariate analysis for the determination of geographical origin of food. From Table 13.2 it also becomes clear that the definition of "geographical regions" is very much dependent on the product that needs to be distinguished from similar products produced in other regions. For products with a PDO status like Swiss cheeses and extra virgin olive oils, selection of several regions in addition to the PDO production site is often observed. Recently, a paper was published on determining geographical origin of Alpine agricultural products like apples, meats, and cheeses using nondestructive NIR spectroscopy (Huck-Pezzei et al., 2014). In Fig. 13.3, apples from the Alpine region were separated by PCA on the basis of NIR spectra collected by surface scanning with a customized sample rotation tool. The NIR spectra were subsequently averaged prior to PCA. For more mainstream products, a worldwide sample selection is often employed. Multivariate data analysis methods for the interrogation of the spectroscopic data are numerous and can be specially

Table 13.2 Condensed Overview of the Latest Peer-reviewed Work on Spectroscopic Analysis and Geographical Provenance Confirmation of Food

Food class	Food subclass	Geographical regions	Spectroscopic technique(s)	MVA method	Min-max % success	References
Dairy	Butter	3 Moroccan regions	FT-MIR	PCA and PLS-DA	98–100	Bassbasi et al. (2014)
	Cheese (Gruyère PDO and L'Etivaz PDO)	Several production altitudes in Switzerland	ATR-MIR	PCA and FDA	90–91	Karoui et al. (2007)
Fish	Tilapia	4 Chinese regions	NIR	SIMCA	75–80	Liu et al. (2015)
Fruit	Persimmon	7 Spanish regions	NIR	LS-SVM	Max 98	Khanmohammadi et al. (2014)
Herbs and spices	Saffron	Iran, Greece, Spain	NIR	PLS-DA	88–100	Zalacain et al. (2005)
Honey	Unifloral honeys	Switzerland, Germany, France	ATR-FT-MIR	LDA	76–100	Ruoff et al. (2006)
	Filtered and unfiltered honeys	Ireland, Argentina, Czech, Hungary, Mexico	NIR	SIMCA PLSR	100 (unfiltered) 96–100 (filtered)	Woodcock et al. (2007)
	Unprocessed mixed floral types	Galicia (Spain) and commercial samples	NIR	SIMCA	93–100	Herrero Latorre et al. (2013)
	Unifloral and mixed floral types	Italy, "east Europe," Spain	microRaman	PCA	N.R.	Corvucci et al. (2015)

Olive oil	Extra virgin olive oil	Italy (PDO-Liguria), France, Spain, Greece, Cyprus, Turkey	ATR-FT-IR	PLS-DA FDA	70–80	Hennessy et al. (2009)
		Italy (PDO-Liguria), Italy, Spain	NIR (UV–Vis, e-nose)	UNEQ-QDA SIMCA	100	Casale et al. (2010)
		Italy (PDO-Sabina), Italy, "Mediterranean countries"	MIR NIR	PLS-DA SIMCA	Up to 100	Bevilacqua et al. (2012)
	N.R.	Spain, Turkey, Italy	Vis-NIR	DOSC-GA-PLSR	Up to 97	Lin et al. (2012)
Rice	Indica and Japonica rice	Different Chinese regions	Raman	SIMCA PLS-DA KNN SVM	90–100	Feng et al. (2013)
Tea	Yerba mate (*Ilex paraguayensis* St. Hil.)	Brazil, Argentina, Brazil–Uruguay blend	NIR	PLS-DA LDA	100	Cozzolino et al. (2010)
	White tea	China (Anji and non-Anji produce)	NIR	OCPLS SIMCA	Up to 93	Xu et al. (2012)
	Green and black tea	Argentina, Brazil, Sri Lanka	NIR	SIMCA PLS-DA SPA-LDA	88–100	Diniz et al. (2014)
	Black tea	3 Chinese provinces, India, Kenya, Sri Lanka, Burma	FT-NIR	PLS	Max 94	Ren et al. (2013)

Continued

Table 13.2 Condensed Overview of the Latest Peer-reviewed Work on Spectroscopic Analysis and Geographical Provenance Confirmation of Food—cont'd

Food class	Food subclass	Geographical regions	Spectroscopic technique(s)	MVA method	Min-max % success	References
Vegetables	West Lake Lotus root powder	Different Chinese regions	NIR	PLSCM SVDD	85–92	Xu et al. (2012)
	Lentil seeds	Greece and "other countries"	DR-FTIR	Discriminant analysis	N.R.	Kouvoutsakis et al. (2014)
Wheat	Multiple varieties	Different Chinese regions	NIR	PLS-DA LDA	Up to 100	Zhao et al. (2013)
		Different Chinese regions	NIR	PLS-DA	73–95	Zhao et al. (2014)
	Distillers dried grains and solubles	Canada, China, EU, India, United States	FT-IR	LDA SIMCA	Max 94 (China – USA)	Nietner et al. (2013)
		Canada, United States, Europe China	ATR-FT-MIR	PLS-DA	Multiple comparisons made between regions	Vermeulen et al. (2015)
		China, United States, Europe	NIR	PLS-DA OPLS-DA	N.R.	Zhou et al. (2014)

N.R., Not reported.

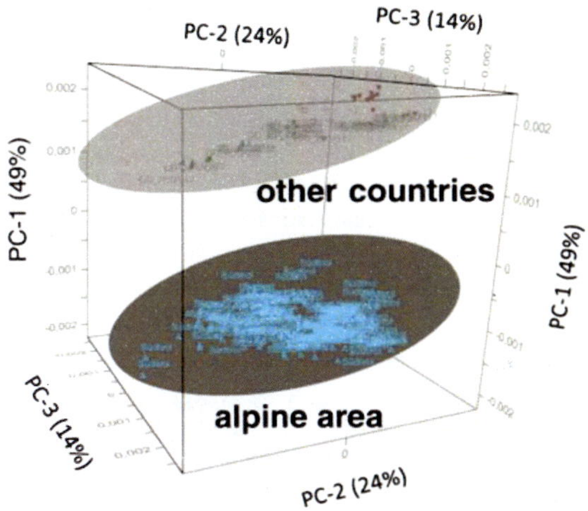

Figure 13.3 Principal component analysis score plot revealing a separation of Alpine area apples (160 Golden Delicious apples South Tyrol, Südtirol) and apples grown in 20 different countries (235 Golden Delicious apples) by nondestructive NIR spectroscopy.
Adapted from Huck-Pezzei, V.A., Seitz, I., Karer, R., Schmutzler, M., De Benedictis, L., Wild, B., Huck, C.W., 2014. Alps food authentication, typicality and intrinsic quality by near infrared spectroscopy. Food Research International 62, 984–990.

customized to cope with specific equipment or samples. Furthermore, when a combination of different techniques is used, data may be fused prior to chemometric processing as was done, for example, by Casale et al. (2010). Further reading on chemometrics in the context of food origin confirmation or discrimination can be found in Vandeginste and Brereton (2013).

13.6 Other Techniques

13.6.1 DNA Technology

The polymerase chain reaction (PCR) to analyze the genetic origin of food products is widely used; in the literature, it is also claimed that it can be used to determine geographical origin. Prior to 2008, PCR has been successfully used to determine the geographical origin of buffalo mozzarella, whey cultures, grapes, and olive oils (Luykx and van Ruth, 2008). Differentiation is possible due to the presence of different microorganisms in the food product. Since 2008, a link has been shown between the geographical origin and microbial flora for fish (Takashima et al., 2014), Minas cheese (Arcuri et al., 2013), fruits (El Sheikha et al., 2011), and marine salts (Dufossé et al., 2013). Attempts have also been made to determine the geographical origin of meat, although these are still at a very early stage and more research is required (Montowska and Pospiech, 2012).

13.6.2 Sensory Analysis

In sensory analysis or sensory evaluation, trained judges or sensory panels are used as the instruments with which to detect deviations from a quality standard. The responses of the panel are recorded, and by means of statistical analysis it is determined whether a product meets specific standards. This tool has already been effectively applied in geographical provenance work for many decades (Luykx and van Ruth, 2008). As performed traditionally, wine is one of the products in which sensory panel analysis accounts for the majority of reported applications. Sensory tests for special properties of olive oil, like the geographical origin, were even included in regulations. Recently, a new study on geographical provenance of Sauvignon Blanc wines using sensory evaluation was performed. Professional wine tasters were able to correctly determine the origin of New Zealand, French, and Austrian wines (Green et al., 2011) while a similar procedure was followed for PDO artichokes (Di Salvo et al., 2014). Finally, for propolis provenance confirmation, combined GC-MS-olfactometry methods were used to determine characteristic regional volatile profiles by trained panel sniffing (Cheng et al., 2013).

13.7 Conclusions

In this chapter, an update on the advances in authenticity testing of geographical origin of food products from late 2008 until early 2015 has been presented. The analytical methods that have been shown to be most successful in provenance testing of food products are isotopic analysis, analysis of multiple elements, compositional analysis, volatile compound profiling, sensor technology, spectroscopic methods, DNA technology, and sensory analysis. Products tested in recent years are oils, dairy products, honey, wines, vegetables, fruits, coffee, tea, herbs, and spices. Some products of animal origin have also been tested such as shrimps and meat cuts. Determining the geographical origin of food products will continue to be a very important scientific topic. Analytical methods that will be of particular interest are methods that can be used to analyze every batch of raw material that enters a food processing factory, therefore, the methods have to be quick and reliable. Methods are preferably nondestructive, especially for expensive food products like herbs and spices. Finally, provenance confirmation of more complex products, such as ready-to-eat meals, will be the topic of investigation in the near future as convenience products remain popular among consumers.

List of Abbreviations of Analytical Equipment

ATR	Attenuated total reflectance
CE	Capillary electrophoresis
CF-IRMS	Continuous flow IRMS
DI-IRMS	Dual input IRMS

DF-FTIR	Diffuse reflectance Fourier transform infrared spectroscopy
DHS-GC-MS	Dynamic headspace GC–MS
EA-IRMS	Elemental analyzer IRMS
ESI	Electrospray ionization
FID	Flame ionization detection
GC	Gas chromatography
GC-IRMS	Gas chromatography IRMS
GCxGC	Two-dimensional gas chromatography
HS-SPME-...	Head-space solid phase micro-extraction-...
HTGC-MS	High temperature GC–MS
ICP	Inductively coupled plasma
ICP-AES	ICP atomic emission spectroscopy
ICP-MS	ICP mass spectrometry
ICP-OES	ICP optical emission spectroscopy
IRMS	Isotope ratio mass spectrometry
LC or CE-DAD	LC or CE - Diode array detector
LC	Liquid chromatography
LC-CAD	LC - Charged aerosol detector
MS/MS	Tandem mass spectrometry
MS	Mass spectrometry
NMR	Nuclear magnetic resonance
qTOF	Quadrupole time of flight
SNIF-NMR	Site-specific natural isotope fractionation NMR
TIMS	Thermal ionization mass spectrometry
TOF	Time of flight
(U)HPLC	(Ultra-)High-performance liquid chromatography

List of Abbreviations of (Multivariate) Statistical Analysis

ANOVA	Analysis of variance
CDA	Canonical discriminant analysis
DOSC-GA-PLSR	Direct orthogonal signal correction - genetic algorithms - PLSR
FDA	Factorial discriminant analysis
HCA	Hierarchical cluster analysis
KNN	K-nearest neighbors
LDA	Linear discriminant analysis
OCPLS	One-class partial least squares
OPLS-DA	Orthogonal partial least squares discriminant analysis
PCA	Principal component analysis
PLSCM	Linear partial least squares class model
PLS-DA	Partial least squares discriminant analysis
PLSR	Partial least squares regression
SIMCA	Soft independent modeling of class analogy
SPA-LDA	Successive projections algorithm associated with linear discriminant analysis
SVDD	Non-linear support vector data description
SVM	Support vector machine

UNEQ-QDA Unequal-quadratic discriminant analysis
UPLS-DA Unfolded PLS-DA

References

Anastasaki, E., Kanakis, C., Pappas, C., Maggi, L., del Campo, C.P., Carmona, M., Alonso, G.L., Polissiou, M.G., 2009. Geographical differentiation of saffron by GC–MS/FID and chemometrics. European Food Research and Technology 229 (6), 899–905.

Araghipour, N., Colineau, J., Koot, A., Akkermans, W., Rojas, J.M.M., Beauchamp, J., Wisthaler, A., Märk, T.D., Downey, G., Guillou, C., Mannina, L., van Ruth, S., 2008. Geographical origin classification of olive oils by PTR-MS. Food Chemistry 108 (1), 374–383.

Arcuri, E.F., El Sheikha, A.F., Rychlik, T., Piro-Métayer, I., Montet, D., 2013. Determination of cheese origin by using 16S rDNA fingerprinting of bacteria communities by PCR–DGGE: preliminary application to traditional Minas cheese. Food Control 30 (1), 1–6.

Bassbasi, M., De Luca, M., Ioele, G., Oussama, A., Ragno, G., 2014. Prediction of the geographical origin of butters by partial least square discriminant analysis (PLS-DA) applied to infrared spectroscopy (FTIR) data. Journal of Food Composition and Analysis 33 (2), 210–215.

Bejjani, J., Balaban, M., Rizk, T., 2014. A sharper characterization of the geographical origin of Lebanese wines by a new interpretation of the hydrogen isotope ratios of ethanol. Food Chemistry 165 (0), 134–139.

Beltrán, M., Sánchez-Astudillo, M., Aparicio, R., García-González, D.L., 2015. Geographical traceability of virgin olive oils from south-western Spain by their multi-elemental composition. Food Chemistry 169 (0), 350–357.

Berna, A.Z., Trowell, S., Clifford, D., Cynkar, W., Cozzolino, D., 2009. Geographical origin of Sauvignon Blanc wines predicted by mass spectrometry and metal oxide based electronic nose. Analytica Chimica Acta 648 (2), 146–152.

Bevilacqua, M., Bucci, R., Magrì, A.D., Magrì, A.L., Marini, F., 2012. Tracing the origin of extra virgin olive oils by infrared spectroscopy and chemometrics: a case study. Analytica Chimica Acta 717 (0), 39–51.

Bondia-Pons, I., Savolainen, O., Törrönen, R., Martinez, J.A., Poutanen, K., Hanhineva, K., 2014. Metabolic profiling of Goji berry extracts for discrimination of geographical origin by non-targeted liquid chromatography coupled to quadrupole time-of-flight mass spectrometry. Food Research International 63 (Part B), 132–138.

Caligiani, A., Palla, L., Acquotti, D., Marseglia, A., Palla, G., 2014. Application of 1H NMR for the characterisation of cocoa beans of different geographical origins and fermentation levels. Food Chemistry 157 (0), 94–99.

Cappellin, L., Loreto, F., Aprea, E., Romano, A., del Pulgar, J., Gasperi, F., Biasioli, F., 2013. PTR-MS in Italy: a multipurpose sensor with applications in environmental, agri-food and health science. Sensors 13 (9), 11923–11955.

Carrasco-Pancorbo, A., Gomez-Caravaca, A.M., Segura-Carretero, A., Cerretani, L., Bendini, A., Fernandez-Gutierrez, A., 2009. Use of capillary electrophoresis with UV detection to compare the phenolic profiles of extra-virgin olive oils belonging to Spanish and Italian PDOs and their relation to sensorial properties. Journal of the Science of Food and Agriculture 89 (12), 2144–2155.

Casale, M., Casolino, C., Oliveri, P., Forina, M., 2010. The potential of coupling information using three analytical techniques for identifying the geographical origin of Liguria extra virgin olive oil. Food Chemistry 118 (1), 163–170.

Chaguri, M.P., Maulvault, A.L., Nunes, M.L., Santiago, D.A., Denadai, J.C., Fogaça, F.H., Sant'Ana, L.S., Ducatti, C., Bandarra, N., Carvalho, M.L., Marques, A., 2015. Different tools to trace geographic origin and seasonality of croaker (*Micropogonias furnieri*). LWT – Food Science and Technology 61 (1), 194–200.

Cheng, H., Qin, Z.H., Guo, X.F., Hu, X.S., Wu, J.H., 2013. Geographical origin identification of propolis using GC–MS and electronic nose combined with principal component analysis. Food Research International 51 (2), 813–822.

Corvucci, F., Nobili, L., Melucci, D., Grillenzoni, F.-V., 2015. The discrimination of honey origin using melissopalynology and Raman spectroscopy techniques coupled with multivariate analysis. Food Chemistry 169 (0), 297–304.

Cozzolino, D., Restaino, E., Fassio, A., 2010. Discrimination of yerba mate (*Ilex paraguayensis* St. Hil.) samples according to their geographical origin by means of near infrared spectroscopy and multivariate analysis. Sensing and Instrumentation for Food Quality and Safety 4 (2), 67–72.

Cynkar, W., Dambergs, R., Smith, P., Cozzolino, D., 2010. Classification of Tempranillo wines according to geographic origin: combination of mass spectrometry based electronic nose and chemometrics. Analytica Chimica Acta 660 (1–2), 227–231.

D'Archivio, A.A., Giannitto, A., Incani, A., Nisi, S., 2014. Analysis of the mineral composition of Italian saffron by ICP-MS and classification of geographical origin. Food Chemistry 157 (0), 485–489.

Di Donna, L., Mazzotti, F., Naccarato, A., Salerno, R., Tagarelli, A., Taverna, D., Sindona, G., 2010. Secondary metabolites of *Olea europaea* leaves as markers for the discrimination of cultivars and cultivation zones by multivariate analysis. Food Chemistry 121 (2), 492–496.

Di Salvo, R., Fadda, C., Sanguinetti, A.M., Naes, T., Del Caro, A., 2014. Effect of harvest time and geographical area on sensory and instrumental texture profile of a PDO artichoke. International Journal of Food Science and Technology 49 (4), 1231–1237.

Dinca, O.-R., Ionete, R., Popescu, R., Costinel, D., Radu, G.-L., 2014. Geographical and botanical origin discrimination of Romanian honey using complex stable isotope data and chemometrics. Food Analytical Methods 1–12.

Diniz, P., Gomes, A., Pistonesi, M., Band, B., de Araújo, M., 2014. Simultaneous classification of teas according to their varieties and geographical origins by using NIR spectroscopy and SPA-LDA. Food Analytical Methods 7 (8), 1712–1718.

Downey, G., 2013. 6-Vibrational spectroscopy in studies of food origin. In: Brereton, P. (Ed.), New Analytical Approaches for Verifying the Origin of Food. Woodhead Publishing, pp. 94–116.

Drivelos, S.A., Higgins, K., Kalivas, J.H., Haroutounian, S.A., Georgiou, C.A., 2014. Data fusion for food authentication. Combining rare earth elements and trace metals to discriminate "*Fava santorinis*" from other yellow split peas using chemometric tools. Food Chemistry 165 (0), 316–322.

Dufossé, L., Donadio, C., Valla, A., Meile, J.-C., Montet, D., 2013. Determination of speciality food salt origin by using 16S rDNA fingerprinting of bacterial communities by PCR–DGGE: an application on marine salts produced in solar salterns from the French Atlantic Ocean. Food Control 32 (2), 644–649.

Durante, C., Baschieri, C., Bertacchini, L., Bertelli, D., Cocchi, M., Marchetti, A., Manzini, D., Papotti, G., Sighinolfi, S., 2015. An analytical approach to Sr isotope ratio determination in Lambrusco wines for geographical traceability purposes. Food Chemistry 173 (0), 557–563.

Dymerski, T., Gebicki, J., Wardencki, W., Namieśnik, J., 2014. Application of an electronic nose instrument to fast classification of polish honey types. Sensors 14 (6), 10709–10724.

El Sheikha, A.F., Métayer, I., Montet, D., 2011. A biological bar code for determining the geographical origin of fruit by using 28S rDNA fingerprinting of fungal communities by PCR-DGGE: an application to *Physalis* fruits from Egypt. Food Biotechnology 25 (2), 115–129.

Feng, X., Zhang, Q., Cong, P., Zhu, Z., 2013. Preliminary study on classification of rice and detection of paraffin in the adulterated samples by Raman spectroscopy combined with multivariate analysis. Talanta 115 (0), 548–555.

Feudo, G.L., Macchione, B., Naccarato, A., Sindona, G., Tagarelli, A., 2011. The volatile fraction profiling of fresh tomatoes and triple concentrate tomato pastes as parameter for the determination of geographical origin. Food Research International 44 (3), 781–788.

Galle, S.A., Koot, A., Soukoulis, C., Cappellin, L., Biasioli, F., Alewijn, M., van Ruth, S.M., 2011. Typicality and geographical origin markers of protected origin cheese from The Netherlands revealed by PTR-MS. Journal of Agricultural and Food Chemistry 59 (6), 2554–2563.

Green, J.A., Parr, W.V., Breitmeyer, J., Valentin, D., Sherlock, R., 2011. Sensory and chemical characterisation of Sauvignon blanc wine: influence of source of origin. Food Research International 44 (9), 2788–2797.

Gutierrez, M., Llobera, A., Ipatov, A., Vila-Planas, J., Minguez, S., Demming, S., Buettgenbach, S., Capdevila, F., Domingo, C., Jimenez-Jorquera, C., 2011. Application of an E-tongue to the analysis of monovarietal and blends of white wines. Sensors 11 (5), 4840–4857.

Ha, D., Sun, Q.Y., Su, K.Q., Wan, H., Li, H.B., Xu, N., Sun, F., Zhuang, L.J., Hu, N., Wang, P., 2015. Recent achievements in electronic tongue and bioelectronic tongue as taste sensors. Sensors and Actuators B-Chemical 207, 1136–1146.

Hattori, R., Yamada, K., Shibata, H., Hirano, S., Tajima, O., Yoshida, N., 2010. Measurement of the isotope ratio of acetic acid in vinegar by HS-SPME-GC-TC/C-IRMS. Journal of Agricultural and Food Chemistry 58 (12), 7115–7118.

He, W., Hu, X., Zhao, L., Liao, X., Zhang, Y., Zhang, M., Wu, J., 2009. Evaluation of Chinese tea by the electronic tongue: correlation with sensory properties and classification according to geographical origin and grade level. Food Research International 42 (10), 1462–1467.

Hennessy, S., Downey, G., O'Donnell, C.P., 2009. Confirmation of food origin claims by Fourier transform infrared spectroscopy and chemometrics: extra virgin olive oil from Liguria. Journal of Agricultural and Food Chemistry 57 (5), 1735–1741.

Herrero Latorre, C., Peña Crecente, R.M., García Martín, S., Barciela García, J., 2013. A fast chemometric procedure based on NIR data for authentication of honey with protected geographical indication. Food Chemistry 141 (4), 3559–3565.

Hondrogiannis, E., Peterson, K., Zapf, C.M., Roy, W., Blackney, B., Dailey, K., 2012. The use of wavelength dispersive X-ray fluorescence and discriminant analysis in the identification of the elemental composition of cumin samples and the determination of the country of origin. Food Chemistry 135 (4), 2825–2831.

Hondrogiannis, E., Rotta, K., Zapf, C.M., 2013. The use of wavelength dispersive x-ray fluorescence in the identification of the elemental composition of vanilla samples and the determination of the geographic origin by discriminant function analysis. Journal of Food Science 78 (3), C395–C401.

Huck-Pezzei, V.A., Seitz, I., Karer, R., Schmutzler, M., De Benedictis, L., Wild, B., Huck, C.W., 2014. Alps food authentication, typicality and intrinsic quality by near infrared spectroscopy. Food Research International 62, 984–990.

Karoui, R., Mazerolles, G., Bosset, J.-O., de Baerdemaeker, J., Dufour, E., 2007. Utilisation of mid-infrared spectroscopy for determination of the geographic origin of Gruyère PDO and L'Etivaz PDO Swiss cheeses. Food Chemistry 105 (2), 847–854.

Khanmohammadi, M., Karami, F., Mir-Marqués, A., Bagheri Garmarudi, A., Garrigues, S., de la Guardia, M., 2014. Classification of persimmon fruit origin by near infrared spectrometry and least squares-support vector machines. Journal of Food Engineering 142 (0), 17–22.

Kim, H., Suresh Kumar, K., Shin, K.-H., 2015. Applicability of stable C and N isotope analysis in inferring the geographical origin and authentication of commercial fish (Mackerel, Yellow Croaker and Pollock). Food Chemistry 172 (0), 523–527.

Kouvoutsakis, G., Mitsi, C., Tarantilis, P.A., Polissiou, M.G., Pappas, C.S., 2014. Geographical differentiation of dried lentil seed (*Lens culinaris*) samples using diffuse reflectance Fourier transform infrared spectroscopy (DRIFTS) and discriminant analysis. Food Chemistry 145 (0), 1011–1014.

Krivachy, N., Rossmann, A., Schmidt, H.-L., 2015. Potentials and caveats with oxygen and sulfur stable isotope analyses in authenticity and origin checks of food and food commodities. Food Control 48 (0), 143–150.

Kwon, Y.-K., Bong, Y.-S., Lee, K.-S., Hwang, G.-S., 2014. An integrated analysis for determining the geographical origin of medicinal herbs using ICP-AES/ICP-MS and 1H NMR analysis. Food Chemistry 161 (0), 168–175.

Lerma-García, M.J., Lantano, C., Chiavaro, E., Cerretani, L., Herrero-Martínez, J.M., Simó-Alfonso, E.F., 2009. Classification of extra virgin olive oils according to their geographical origin using phenolic compound profiles obtained by capillary electrochromatography. Food Research International 42 (10), 1446–1452.

Lin, P., Chen, Y., He, Y., 2012. Identification of geographical origin of olive oil using visible and near-infrared spectroscopy technique combined with chemometrics. Food and Bioprocess Technology 5 (1), 235–242.

Liu, Y., Ma, D.-H., Wang, X.-C., Liu, L.-P., Fan, Y.-X., Cao, J.-X., 2015. Prediction of chemical composition and geographical origin traceability of Chinese export tilapia fillets products by near infrared reflectance spectroscopy. LWT – Food Science and Technology 60 (2 Part 2), 1214–1218.

Longobardi, F., Casiello, G., Sacco, D., Tedone, L., Sacco, A., 2011. Characterisation of the geographical origin of Italian potatoes, based on stable isotope and volatile compound analyses. Food Chemistry 124 (4), 1708–1713.

Longobardi, F., Casiello, G., Ventrella, A., Mazzilli, V., Nardelli, A., Sacco, D., Catucci, L., Agostiano, A., 2015. Electronic nose and isotope ratio mass spectrometry in combination with chemometrics for the characterization of the geographical origin of Italian sweet cherries. Food Chemistry 170 (0), 90–96.

Longobardi, F., Ventrella, A., Bianco, A., Catucci, L., Cafagna, I., Gallo, V., Mastrorilli, P., Agostiano, A., 2013. Non-targeted 1H NMR fingerprinting and multivariate statistical analyses for the characterisation of the geographical origin of Italian sweet cherries. Food Chemistry 141 (3), 3028–3033.

Luykx, D.M.A.M., van Ruth, S.M., 2008. An overview of analytical methods for determining the geographical origin of food products. Food Chemistry 107 (2), 897–911.

Maçatelli, M., Akkermans, W., Koot, A., Buchgraber, M., Paterson, A., van Ruth, S., 2009. Verification of the geographical origin of European butters using PTR-MS. Journal of Food Composition and Analysis 22 (2), 169–175.

Masi, E., Romani, A., Pandolfi, C., Heimler, D., Mancuso, S., 2014. PTR-TOF-MS analysis of volatile compounds in olive fruits. Journal of the Science of Food and Agriculture 1428–1434.

Medini, S., Janin, M., Verdoux, P., Techer, I., 2015. Methodological development for 87Sr/86Sr measurement in olive oil and preliminary discussion of its use for geographical traceability of PDO Nîmes (France). Food Chemistry 171 (0), 78–83.

Mihailova, A., Abbado, D., Kelly, S.D., Pedentchouk, N., 2015. The impact of environmental factors on molecular and stable isotope compositions of n-alkanes in Mediterranean extra virgin olive oils. Food Chemistry 173 (0), 114–121.

Montealegre, C., Garcia, M.C., del Rio, C., Marina, M.L., Garcia-Ruiz, C., 2012. Separation of olive proteins by capillary gel electrophoresis. Talanta 97, 420–424.

Montoro, P., Molfetta, I., Maldini, M., Ceccarini, L., Piacente, S., Pizza, C., Macchia, M., 2013. Determination of six steviol glycosides of *Stevia rebaudiana* (Bertoni) from different geographical origin by LC–ESI–MS/MS. Food Chemistry 141 (2), 745–753.

Montowska, M., Pospiech, E., 2012. Is authentication of regional and traditional food made of meat possible? Critical Reviews in Food Science and Nutrition 52 (6), 475–487.

Moon, J., Han, H., Park, S., Dong, H., Han, K.-Y., Kim, H., Bang, K.-H., Choi, J., Noh, B., 2014. Discrimination of the origin of commercial red ginseng concentrates using LC-MS/MS and electronic nose analysis based on a mass spectrometer. Food Science and Biotechnology 23 (5), 1433–1440.

Nietner, T., Haughey, S.A., Ogle, N., Fauhl-Hassek, C., Elliott, C.T., 2014. Determination of geographical origin of distillers dried grains and solubles using isotope ratio mass spectrometry. Food Research International 60 (0), 146–153.

Nietner, T., Pfister, M., Glomb, M.A., Fauhl-Hassek, C., 2013. Authentication of the botanical and geographical origin of distillers dried grains and solubles (DDGS) by FT-IR spectroscopy. Journal of Agricultural and Food Chemistry 61 (30), 7225–7233.

Oliveri, P., Baldo, M.A., Daniele, S., Forina, M., 2009. Development of a voltammetric electronic tongue for discrimination of edible oils. Analytical and Bioanalytical Chemistry 395 (4), 1135–1143.

Ortea, I., Gallardo, J.M., 2015. Investigation of production method, geographical origin and species authentication in commercially relevant shrimps using stable isotope ratio and/or multi-element analyses combined with chemometrics: an exploratory analysis. Food Chemistry 170 (0), 145–153.

Otaka, A., Hokura, A., Nakai, I., 2014. Determination of trace elements in soybean by x-ray fluorescence analysis and its application to identification of their production areas. Food Chemistry 147 (0), 318–326.

Phillips, K., Niimi, J., Hamid, N., Silcock, P., Delahunty, C., Barker, M., Sewell, M., Bremer, P., 2010. Sensory and volatile analysis of sea urchin roe from different geographical regions in New Zealand. LWT – Food Science and Technology 43 (2), 202–213.

Pisano, P.L., Silva, M.F., Olivieri, A.C., 2015. Anthocyanins as markers for the classification of Argentinean wines according to botanical and geographical origin. Chemometric modeling of liquid chromatography–mass spectrometry data. Food Chemistry 175 (0), 174–180.

del Pulgar, J.S., Soukoulis, C., Biasioli, F., Cappellin, L., García, C., Gasperi, F., Granitto, P., Märk, T.D., Piasentier, E., Schuhfried, E., 2011. Rapid characterization of dry cured ham produced following different PDOs by proton transfer reaction time of flight mass spectrometry (PTR-ToF-MS). Talanta 85 (1), 386–393.

Raco, B., Dotsika, E., Poutoukis, D., Battaglini, R., Chantzi, P., 2015. O–H–C isotope ratio determination in wine in order to be used as a fingerprint of its regional origin. Food Chemistry 168 (0), 588–594.

Ren, G.X., Wang, S.P., Ning, J.M., Xu, R.R., Wang, Y.X., Xing, Z.Q., Wan, X.C., Zhang, Z.Z., 2013. Quantitative analysis and geographical traceability of black tea using Fourier transform near-infrared spectroscopy (FT-NIRS). Food Research International 53 (2), 822–826.

Risticevic, S., Carasek, E., Pawliszyn, J., 2008. Headspace solid-phase microextraction–gas chromatographic–time-of-flight mass spectrometric methodology for geographical origin verification of coffee. Analytica Chimica Acta 617 (1–2), 72–84.

Rizelio, V.M., Gonzaga, L.V., Borges, G.D.C., Maltez, H.F., Costa, A.C.O., Fett, R., 2012. Fast determination of cations in honey by capillary electrophoresis: a possible method for geographic origin discrimination. Talanta 99, 450–456.

Romano, A., Fischer, L., Herbig, J., Campbell-Sills, H., Coulon, J., Lucas, P., Cappellin, L., Biasioli, F., 2014. Wine analysis by FastGC proton-transfer reaction-time-of-flight-mass spectrometry. International Journal of Mass Spectrometry 369 (0), 81–86.

Ruiz-Samblás, C., Arrebola-Pascual, C., Tres, A., van Ruth, S., Cuadros-Rodríguez, L., 2013. Authentication of geographical origin of palm oil by chromatographic fingerprinting of triacylglycerols and partial least square-discriminant analysis. Talanta 116 (0), 788–793.

Ruoff, K., Luginbühl, W., Künzli, R., Iglesias, M.T., Bogdanov, S., Bosset, J.O., von der Ohe, K., von der Ohe, W., Amadò, R., 2006. Authentication of the botanical and geographical origin of honey by mid-infrared spectroscopy. Journal of Agricultural and Food Chemistry 54 (18), 6873–6880.

Russo, M., Serra, D., Suraci, F., Di Sanzo, R., Fuda, S., Postorino, S., 2014. The potential of e-nose aroma profiling for identifying the geographical origin of licorice (*Glycyrrhiza glabra* L.) roots. Food Chemistry 165 (0), 467–474.

van Ruth, S., de Visser, R., 2015. Provenancing flower bulbs by analytical fingerprinting: *Convallaria majalis*. Agriculture 5 (1), 17–29.

Sánchez del Pulgar, J., Soukoulis, C., Carrapiso, A.I., Cappellin, L., Granitto, P., Aprea, E., Romano, A., Gasperi, F., Biasioli, F., 2013. Effect of the pig rearing system on the final volatile profile of Iberian dry-cured ham as detected by PTR-ToF-MS. Meat Science 93 (3), 420–428.

Sipos, L., Kovacs, Z., Sagi-Kiss, V., Csiki, T., Kokai, Z., Fekete, A., Heberger, K., 2012. Discrimination of mineral waters by electronic tongue, sensory evaluation and chemical analysis. Food Chemistry 135 (4), 2947–2953.

Soukoulis, C., Cappellin, L., Aprea, E., Costa, F., Viola, R., Märk, T., Gasperi, F., Biasioli, F., 2013. PTR-ToF-MS, a novel, rapid, high sensitivity and non-invasive tool to monitor volatile compound release during fruit post-harvest storage: the case study of apple ripening. Food and Bioprocess Technology 6 (10), 2831–2843.

Stanimirova, I., Üstün, B., Cajka, T., Riddelova, K., Hajslova, J., Buydens, L.M.C., Walczak, B., 2010. Tracing the geographical origin of honeys based on volatile compounds profiles assessment using pattern recognition techniques. Food Chemistry 118 (1), 171–176.

Taamalli, A., Arráez Román, D., Zarrouk, M., Segura-Carretero, A., Fernández-Gutiérrez, A., 2012. Classification of 'Chemlali' accessions according to the geographical area using chemometric methods of phenolic profiles analysed by HPLC–ESI-TOF–MS. Food Chemistry 132 (1), 561–566.

Tahara, Y., Toko, K., 2013. Electronic tongues – a review. IEEE Sensors Journal 13 (8), 3001–3011.

Takashima, Y., Iguchi, J., Namikoshi, A., Yamashita, Y., Yamashita, M., 2014. DNA analysis for identification of species and geographical origins of fishery products. Bunseki Kagaku 63 (10), 797–807.

Teye, E., Huang, X., Han, F., Botchway, F., 2014. Discrimination of cocoa beans according to geographical origin by electronic tongue and multivariate algorithms. Food Analytical Methods 7 (2), 360–365.

Torres-Moreno, M., Torrescasana, E., Salas-Salvadó, J., Blanch, C., 2015. Nutritional composition and fatty acids profile in cocoa beans and chocolates with different geographical origin and processing conditions. Food Chemistry 166 (0), 125–132.

Tres, A., Heenan, S.P., van Ruth, S., 2014. Authentication of dried distilled grain with solubles (DDGS) by fatty acid and volatile profiling. LWT – Food Science and Technology 59 (1), 215–221.

Tres, A., Ruiz-Samblas, C., van der Veer, G., van Ruth, S.M., 2013. Geographical provenance of palm oil by fatty acid and volatile compound fingerprinting techniques. Food Chemistry 137 (1–4), 142–150.

Trincherini, P.R., Baffi, C., Barbero, P., Pizzoglio, E., Spalla, S., 2014. Precise determination of strontium isotope ratios by TIMS to authenticate tomato geographical origin. Food Chemistry 145 (0), 349–355.

Vandeginste, B., Brereton, P., 2013. 7-Chemometrics in studies of food origin. In: New Analytical Approaches for Verifying the Origin of Food. Woodhead Publishing, pp. 117–145.

Vermeulen, P., Fernández Pierna, J.A., Abbas, O., Dardenne, P., Baeten, V., 2015. Origin identification of dried distillers grains with solubles using attenuated total reflection Fourier transform mid-infrared spectroscopy after in situ oil extraction. Food Chemistry. http://dx.doi.org/10.1016/j.foodchem.2014.09.103.

Vinci, G., Preti, R., Tieri, A., Vieri, S., 2013. Authenticity and quality of animal origin food investigated by stable-isotope ratio analysis. Journal of the Science of Food and Agriculture 93 (3), 439–448.

Wei, Z., Wang, J., 2014. Tracing floral and geographical origins of honeys by potentiometric and voltammetric electronic tongue. Computers and Electronics in Agriculture 108, 112–122.

Wei, Z., Wang, J., Liao, W., 2009. Technique potential for classification of honey by electronic tongue. Journal of Food Engineering 94 (3–4), 260–266.

Woodcock, T., Downey, G., Kelly, J.D., O'Donnell, C., 2007. Geographical classification of honey samples by near-infrared spectroscopy: a feasibility study. Journal of Agricultural and Food Chemistry 55 (22), 9128–9134.

Wu, Y., Luo, D., Dong, H., Wan, J., Luo, H., Xian, Y., Guo, X., Qin, F., Han, W., Wang, L., Wang, B., 2015. Geographical origin of cereal grains based on element analyser-stable isotope ratio mass spectrometry (EA-SIRMS). Food Chemistry 174 (0), 553–557.

Xiaobing, Y., Kireeva, I., 2011. QandA Manual: China Legislation on Geographical Indications. EU-China Project for the Protection of Intellectual Property Rights (IPR-2). www.ipr2.com. last visited 23rd May, 2015.

Xu, L., Shi, P.-T., Ye, Z.-H., Yan, S.-M., Cai, C.-B., Zhong, W., Yu, X.-P., 2012a. Rapid geographical origin analysis of pure West Lake lotus root powder (WL-LRP) by near-infrared spectroscopy combined with multivariate class modeling techniques. Food Research International 49 (2), 771–777.

Xu, L., Yan, S.-M., Ye, Z.-H., Fu, X.-S., Yu, X.-P., 2013. Combining electronic tongue array and chemometrics for discriminating the specific geographical origins of green tea. Journal of Analytical Methods in Chemistry 2013, 350801.

Xu, L., Ye, Z.-H., Yan, S.-M., Shi, P.-T., Cui, H.-F., Fu, X.-S., Yu, X.-P., 2012b. Combining local wavelength information and ensemble learning to enhance the specificity of class modeling techniques: identification of food geographical origins and adulteration. Analytica Chimica Acta 754 (0), 31–38.

Yener, S., Romano, A., Cappellin, L., Märk, T.D., Sánchez del Pulgar, J., Gasperi, F., Navarini, L., Biasioli, F., 2014. PTR-ToF-MS characterisation of roasted coffees (*C. arabica*) from different geographic origins. Journal of Mass Spectrometry 49 (9), 929–935.

Youssef, O., Guido, F., Manel, I., Youssef, N.B., Luigi, C.P., Mohamed, H., Daoud, D., Mokhtar, Z., 2011. Volatile compounds and compositional quality of virgin olive oil from Oueslati variety: influence of geographical origin. Food Chemistry 124 (4), 1770–1776.

Yudthavorasit, S., Wongravee, K., Leepipatpiboon, N., 2014. Characteristic fingerprint based on gingerol derivative analysis for discrimination of ginger (*Zingiber officinale*) according to geographical origin using HPLC-DAD combined with chemometrics. Food Chemistry 158 (0), 101–111.

Zalacain, A., Ordoudi, S.A., Díaz-Plaza, E.M., Carmona, M., Blázquez, I., Tsimidou, M.Z., Alonso, G.L., 2005. Near-infrared spectroscopy in saffron quality control: determination of chemical composition and geographical origin. Journal of Agricultural and Food Chemistry 53 (24), 9337–9341.

Zardin, E., Tyapkova, O., Buettner, A., Beauchamp, J., 2014. Performance assessment of proton-transfer-reaction time-of-flight mass spectrometry (PTR-TOF-MS) for analysis of isobaric compounds in food-flavour applications. LWT – Food Science and Technology 56 (1), 153–160.

Zhao, H., Guo, B., Wei, Y., Zhang, B., 2013. Near infrared reflectance spectroscopy for determination of the geographical origin of wheat. Food Chemistry 138 (2–3), 1902–1907.

Zhao, H., Guo, B., Wei, Y., Zhang, B., 2014. Effects of grown origin, genotype, harvest year, and their interactions of wheat kernels on near infrared spectral fingerprints for geographical traceability. Food Chemistry 152 (0), 316–322.

Zheng, Y., Ruan, G., Li, B., Xiong, C., Chen, S., Luo, M., Li, Y., Du, F., 2014. Multi-composition analysis and pattern recognition of Chinese geographical indication product: vinegar. European Food Research and Technology 238 (2), 337–344.

Zhou, J., Li, Y., Zhao, J., Xue, X., Wu, L., Chen, F., 2008. Geographical traceability of propolis by high-performance liquid-chromatography fingerprints. Food Chemistry 108 (2), 749–759.

Zhou, X., Yang, Z., Haughey, S.A., Galvin-King, P., Han, L., Elliott, C.T., 2014. Classification the geographical origin of corn distillers dried grains with solubles by near infrared reflectance spectroscopy combined with chemometrics: a feasibility study. Food Chemistry. http://dx.doi.org/10.1016/j.foodchem.2014.09.104.

Advances in Authenticity Testing for Meat Speciation

14

J. Amaral, L. Meira, M.B.P.P. Oliveira, I. Mafra
University of Porto, Porto, Portugal

Chapter Outline

14.1 Introduction

Nowadays, and particularly after the horse meat scandal in Europe, consumers are increasingly aware of the problem of food adulteration and consequently demand clear and reliable information about the composition of foods they are buying and eating. Meat, a highly appreciated premium source of protein, is among the foods most prone to suffer adulteration for economic gain. According to EU legislation laying down the general principles and requirements of food law (European Commission, 2002) and EU labeling regulations (European Commission, 2001), meat products should be accurately labeled regarding their species content, with food adulteration and misleading information being considered illegal. However, because of its high demand and value, frauds in the meat industry and retail markets have become a widespread problem, especially in ground and comminuted meat products. Adulteration in the meat sector encompasses many issues, including the substitution of high-quality muscle proteins by other, lower-value meat species or by vegetable proteins, the addition of undeclared ingredients such as constituents of animal origin (eg, blood plasma, offal), the addition of nonmeat components such as water and additives, mislabeling regarding the quantity of meat ingredients, the geographical origin of meats and/or the animal feeding regime, and undeclared processing methods in meat products, such as irradiation and thawed meat (Ballin, 2010; Montowska and Pospiech, 2011a). All these practices are of concern, either for economic reasons, as they lead to unfair competition among producers and deceive consumers, or for health reasons since traceability is compromised. Additionally, they restrict consumers' freedom of choice, in particular for those who choose to follow strict diets for religious motives since the consumption of certain species is not allowed in some religions. For example, pork and its derivatives (among other species) are strictly forbidden to Muslims and Jews who can only consume halal or kosher meat, respectively. For those consumers, the presence of certain animal species, which are undeclared on the product label, is perhaps of most concern.

Adulteration of meat and meat products because of species substitution is also of major importance in the case of traditional products and/or game meat (Montowska and Pospiech, 2012a; Costa et al., 2016a) since both types of products are frequently more expensive and perceived by consumers as being of superior quality. In the case of game meat, its consumption has been increasing in recent years, mainly because of its particular taste and flavor but also because it may be considered a healthier and less-fat meat, obtained from animals free of hormones and drugs such as antibiotics. However, game meat supply depends on animal availability and can sometimes be restricted to hunting seasons. This, together with its generally higher price, makes game meat and products thereof very prone to adulteration by fraudulent substitution of meat species (Amaral et al., 2014, 2015). Traditional foods, frequently considered as delicacies, are another type of product that is highly susceptible to meat species substitution. Among the regional and traditional products in the European Union labeled with the logos of protected designation of origin (PDO), protected geographical indication (PGI), or traditional specialty guaranteed (TSG), there are currently 146 registered products in the category of "Fresh meat and offal" and 155 in "Meat products (cooked, salted, smoked, etc.)." From those, several are produced from specific breeds as described in the specifications accompanying the application for registration. For example, the Portuguese meat products "Morcela de Estremoz e Borba" (PGI) and "Presunto de Barrancos" (PDO) are produced from pork meat exclusively from the Alentejana breed (*Sus ibericus*), and the lamb meat "Cordeiro Mirandês" refers exclusively to the Churra Galega Mirandesa breed. Many other examples, similar to these, from other countries could be mentioned. Since products holding PDO, PGI, or TSG logos generally command higher prices than other comparable meat products, they are susceptible targets for economic fraud through undeclared substitution of the specified meat by other meat from a similar breed.

Considering the relevance of species substitution in the subject of meat adulteration, this chapter intends to provide an updated overview, attempting to have a global world coverage on the most recent research studies regarding the development of methodologies for meat and meat product authenticity testing with respect to speciation and the applicability to the identification of meat species in commercial products.

14.2 Protein-Based Methods

In each species, the genes (genome) predetermine the amino acid composition of the expressed proteins, their quantity, and rate of synthesis (Montowska and Pospiech, 2011a). Since the proteome of an organism is the result of the expression of its genome, the analysis of proteins has been frequently suggested for species identification purposes. As a result, different protein-based methodologies, including electrophoretic, chromatographic, and immunochemical techniques, have been proposed for meat and meat product authentication studies. However, when evaluating the suitability of these methods, it should be taken into account that protein composition can vary, not only among species, but also with many other factors, including tissue type, animal's age and sex, meat processing treatments, and storage period. Therefore the application of protein-based methods generally gives better results when applied to species identification in raw than in processed meat products. In this case the difficulties to overcome are related to the complexity and variability of foods, as well as the type of processing that can frequently induce protein denaturation or degradation.

14.2.1 Electrophoretic Techniques

Electrophoresis is a powerful technique based on the use of an electric field for the separation of proteins into distinctive patterns. It includes different electrokinetic separation techniques according to the principle used for protein separation, such as differences in electrophoretic mobility, isoelectric point, molecular size, or a combination of these. Electrophoresis can be conducted either on gel, such as the case of polyacrylamide gel electrophoresis (PAGE) and its modification using sodium dodecyl sulfate as a denaturing agent (SDS-PAGE), isoelectric focusing (IEF), and, more recently, two-dimensional electrophoresis (2-DE), or in small narrow capillaries, such as the case of capillary zone electrophoresis and capillary isoelectric focusing among others. Apart from being routinely used as a tool in different DNA-based methods and being very useful in proteomic studies performed by mass spectrometry (MS), electrophoretic methods per se have also been applied for meat species identification. There are only a few reports on meat authentication by protein gel electrophoresis, despite being considered a well-known and frequently used technique for species identification in raw fish and control of marine products (Montowska and Pospiech, 2007, 2012a; Etienne et al., 2000). The first studies used SDS-PAGE and IEF on polyacrylamide gel to identify meat cuts of different species (cow, sheep, lamb, goat, red deer, and rabbit) and obtained somewhat ambiguous results (Hofmann, 1985 referred in Montowska and Pospiech, 2007). Since several factors, other than the animal species, can affect the results achieved by SDS-PAGE, this technique frequently presents some constraints when applied for species authentication purposes, in particular regarding meat mixtures and processed meat products, because of its lack of reproducibility and low discriminating power. IEF has also been used for species identification in raw meat (Kaiser et al., 1980; Slattery and Sinclair, 1983; Kim and Shelef, 1986; Skarpeid et al., 1998). Compared to SDS-PAGE, IEF generally presents better band resolution, but gives more complicated and less consistent patterns, which also advises against its use for the authentication of processed meat products. Better results can be achieved by means of 2-DE coupled to image analysis software since it allows the separation of thousands of proteins in one gel and analysis of changes in protein expression levels, such as isoforms and posttranslational modifications (Montowska and Pospiech, 2012b). Species-specific differences in the molecular weight and isoelectric point of skeletal muscle myosin light chain (MLC) isoforms of six species, namely, cow, pork, chicken, turkey, duck, and goose, were revealed by 2-DE (Montowska and Pospiech, 2011b). The authors concluded that each species showed a characteristic pattern on 2-DE gels that can be used for species identification in raw meat mixtures since even a 2% difference in the sequences of MLC resulted in different electrophoretic mobilities. Later, the same methodology was applied to investigate if the interspecies differences noticed in the expression of MLC isoforms in raw meat were also observed in minced meat and meat products (frankfurters and sausages) produced from the same six species (Montowska et al., 2012b). The results showed that the MLC suffered only a relatively small degradation after processing, enabling species identification in all samples when the combination of all the three MLC isoforms was taken into account, and as long as the content of meat of one species in the mixture was not lower than 10%. Thus, the authors concluded that MLC isoforms have the potential to be used as markers for the authentication of meat products made from the analyzed species.

As an alternative to gel electrophoresis, capillary electrophoresis (CE) has also been applied to meat species authentication studies since it offers high resolving power and sensitivity in protein analysis. A CE-SDS methodology, developed by Cota-Rivas and Vallejo-Cordoba (1997) for the analysis of sarcoplasmic proteins, revealed the existence of qualitative and quantitative differences in raw beef, pork, and turkey meat. Linear discriminant analysis (LDA) was later used by the same authors for the interpretation of the quantitative data obtained by CE-SDS (Vallejo-Cordoba and Cota-Rivas, 1998). The correct classification given by LDA on water-soluble protein data was 100% for all meat species except pork (94%). The same group also proposed the use of CE for the discrimination of bovine and ostrich meats (Vallejo-Cordoba et al., 2010). Although the applicability of CE methodology for meat species differentiation was suggested, in both studies the authors only tested a limited number of meat samples ($n = 42$ in total for beef, pork, and turkey samples and $n = 20$ for beef and ostrich), thus further work should be performed using samples from different animals and tissues to confirm these results. Since only fresh meat was used in both studies, the proposed CE methodologies seem to be applicable only for the authentication of raw meat. Moreover, they do not seem adequate for species identification or quantification in meat mixtures since species discrimination was mainly based on quantitative profiles of proteins that are common to different species.

14.2.2 Immunochemical Techniques

Immunochemical assays are based on the specific reaction between antibodies and antigens and are frequently used for meat species authentication. The enzyme-linked immunosorbent assay (ELISA) is the most widely used immunochemical technique. ELISA presents several advantages, such as its simplicity and easy implementation because it does not require expensive equipment or specialized technicians, it has high specificity, high sensitivity, and high throughput, and is thus very suitable for routine application in quality control laboratories (Asensio et al., 2008). On the other hand, the performance of the assay depends on the availability and specificity of the chosen antibody to detect a particular species. Both polyclonal and monoclonal antibodies have been used in ELISA for food authentication. The former offers the advantage of recognizing different epitopes of the antigens, being more tolerant to small changes in the nature of the antigen, but more prone to cross-reactivity with other species, in particular with those that are closely related. This explains the differences between different commercial kits available for the detection of poultry meat, instead of specifically identifying the presence of chicken or turkey. Another limitation of ELISA regards the identification of species in processed meat products since proteins can suffer denaturation that leads to specific epitope alterations (Hird et al., 2005) and consequent decreased sensitivity or even false negatives. Moreover, potential target proteins for ELISA are often irreversibly aggregated, insoluble, and difficult to extract in highly processed products (Taylor et al., 2009; Kotoura et al., 2012). To overcome this drawback, the use of antibodies raised against heat-resistant muscle proteins, such as skeletal muscle protein troponin I, has been proposed in different reports (Chen et al., 1998; Chen and Hsieh, 2000; Djurdjevic et al., 2005; Liu et al., 2006; Zvereva et al., 2015). Currently, polyclonal antibodies raised against heat-resistant species-specific muscle-related glycoproteins are included in several commercial kits, which are being used by regulatory agencies to detect meat species adulteration and to enforce national and transnational laws and regulations (Asensio et al., 2008). These kits are, in general, marketed to meet or exceed the United States Department of Agriculture Food Safety and Inspection Service protocol standards for the Cooked Meat Species ELISA. Nonetheless, commercial kits should be used only for qualitative purposes because limits of detection in processed foods can vary with fat content, degree of thermal processing, tissue, and maturation of meat. Giovannacci et al. (2004) applied different commercial ELISA kits for the identification of beef, sheep, pork, and poultry in 40 commercial canned products and found that half of those were in good agreement with the label, while the others failed because of the presence of undeclared species. Similarly, López et al. (2011) applied different commercial ELISA kits for meat species identification in several cooked meat products, including sausages and hams, either produced in pilot plants or acquired in supermarkets. The methodology allowed identification of all animal species described on the labels. The same samples were also evaluated by SDS-PAGE, which failed to detect some of the species in some of the samples, possibly because they were only present in low amounts.

A later study by Kotoura et al. (2012) proposed the use of different monoclonal antibodies, raised to detect SDS-denatured proteins, to accurately determine the beef content in model processed foods and some commercial foods. The proposed method comprised a sandwich ELISA using two types of monoclonal antibodies, one raised against denatured beef myoglobin and another against a unique amino acid sequence of beef myoglobin. This system allowed the determination of beef content in chicken or pork meats, irrespective of the processing conditions; no cross-reactivity with other food proteins, such as pork, chicken, egg, milk, wheat, buckwheat, peanut, shrimp, and crab was detected, though some cross-reactivity occurred with lamb.

14.2.3 Chromatographic and Mass Spectrometry Techniques

As alternative protein-based methods, several studies suggest the use of chromatographic techniques, mainly high-performance liquid chromatography (HPLC) coupled with different detectors and liquid chromatography (LC) hyphenated with different MS detectors. Giaretta et al. (2013) proposed an anionic exchange ultra-performance liquid chromatography (UPLC) coupled with diode-array detection for the separation of myoglobin from raw meat samples of beef, chicken, horse, ostrich, pork, and water buffalo. Previous to the UPLC analysis, samples were treated with sodium nitrite to transform oxymyoglobin and deoxymyoglobin to the more stable metmyoglobin and desalified on a PD-10 column. This methodology allowed the detection of 5% (w/w) of pork in raw beef burgers. Although exhibiting low sensitivity and possibly being only suited for the analysis of raw meat, the authors pointed out the simplicity of the method and the use of equipment that is commonly present in quality control laboratories as advantages. HPLC coupled to electrochemical analysis was proposed by Hung et al. (2011) to directly detect peptides and amino acids that exhibit little or no chromogenic behavior. The authors used a novel copper nanoparticle-plated screen-printed electrode, which allowed the selective detection of amino acids and small peptides in protein-rich matrices, while being insensitive to large proteins. This methodology allowed the differentiation of ostrich from pork, beef, and chicken meat based on the chromatographic profiles that presented characteristic peaks of lysine, glutamine, carnosine, and anserine. However, this work only described its application to differentiate raw meats, each containing single species and without mentioning the number of samples used for each species and other variability factors (eg, with different age, sex, breeds) within each species.

More recently, modern proteomics has taken advantage of equipment advances, namely, the development of soft ionization techniques, such as matrix-assisted laser desorption ionization (MALDI) and electrospray ionization (ESI) that allow the accurate analysis of peptides by MS methods and, consequently, their use as reliable biomarkers for meat authentication purposes (Sentandreu and Sentandreu, 2014). Although other protein-based methods present drawbacks regarding the analysis of processed meat products, the use of specific peptide markers is related to the primary structure of proteins, which is known to be relatively resistant to processing (Buckley et al., 2013; Sentandreu and Sentandreu, 2011). Authentication methods based on peptide identification by MS can also allow differentiation between tissues of the same species when targeting tissue-specific peptide sequences (Sentandreu and Sentandreu, 2014). Moreover, since high mass accuracy and high sensitivity can be achieved with modern mass spectrometers, this approach generally allows the detection of low amounts of undeclared species in meat products (Sentandreu and Sentandreu, 2014). Nevertheless, the high cost of equipment, the need for specialized technicians, and the duration of the analysis, very important in the case of perishable foods, are seen as disadvantages.

The use of MS for peptide identification is frequently coupled to a previous separation step by LC. Sentandreu et al. (2010) proposed a methodology for the detection of chicken meat in mixed meats that comprised the extraction of myofibrillar proteins, the enrichment of target proteins by OFFGEL isoelectric focusing, in-solution trypsin digestion of MLC3, and the analysis of the generated peptides by LC-MS/MS. Based on the results obtained by SDS-PAGE and MALDI-TOF MS analysis, MLC3 was selected because of its heat stability. An enrichment step by OFFGEL fractionation was included to lower the detection limit of the method. Selection of heat-stable peptides from chicken MLC3 and the use of stable isotope-labeled peptides allowed the quantitative detection of 0.5% (w/w) of chicken in mixtures with pork meat. The authors considered that, once optimized, the whole protocol has the potential to be carried out within 3–4 days, which is still a very long period when compared to the most commonly used DNA-based methods.

The use of LC-MS/MS with a multiple reaction monitoring (MRM) method for the identification of specific peptides was also proposed for the identification of horse and pork in halal beef (von Bargen et al., 2013) and in highly processed foods (von Bargen et al., 2014). The method allowed detection of 0.55% (w/w) of horse or pork in beef, or down to 0.13% pork in beef when MRM^3 and a micro-LC system were applied (von Bargen et al., 2013). Since the selected marker peptides were proven to be sufficiently stable to heat processing, the same methodology was further used for the identification of pork and horse meat in highly processed foods (von Bargen et al., 2014). In this study, the authors also developed a rapid 2-min extraction protocol that allowed an efficient protein extraction from many types of sample, including highly processed foods. The method was able to detect pork and horse meat down to 0.24% (w/w) in a beef meat matrix and was further applied to commercial products, including salami, sausages, meatballs, canned meat, and Frikandeln. All samples were found to be in agreement with the labeled information, with the exception of one declaring only beef in which horse-specific peptides were detected and further confirmed by droplet digital PCR. The authors suggested that the proposed methodology could be easily applicable in routine control laboratories since it is fast and does not require any sample pretreatment or concentration by SDS-PAGE or OFFGEL fractionation.

The use of ambient MS techniques, namely, liquid extraction surface analysis mass spectrometry (LESA-MS) using tandem electrospray MS, without needing previous chromatographic separation, was proposed as fast approaches for the discrimination of five meat species, namely, pork, beef, horse, chicken, and turkey (Montowska et al., 2014a,b; Fig. 14.1). LESA-MS/MS allowed the identification of species in mixtures of cooked meat, namely, the detection of 10% (w/w) of cooked pork, horse, or turkey meats in a beef matrix and 5% (w/w) of chicken in beef. The method involved a washing step to remove salts and fats that interfere with efficient ionization, followed by digestion and direct ionization of dried in-solution tryptic digests from a polymer surface by LESA-MS, which was significantly faster than other proteomic approaches. According to the authors, the time of analysis could be shortened to approximately 1 h by applying microwaves or ultrasonication during the digestion process. On the other

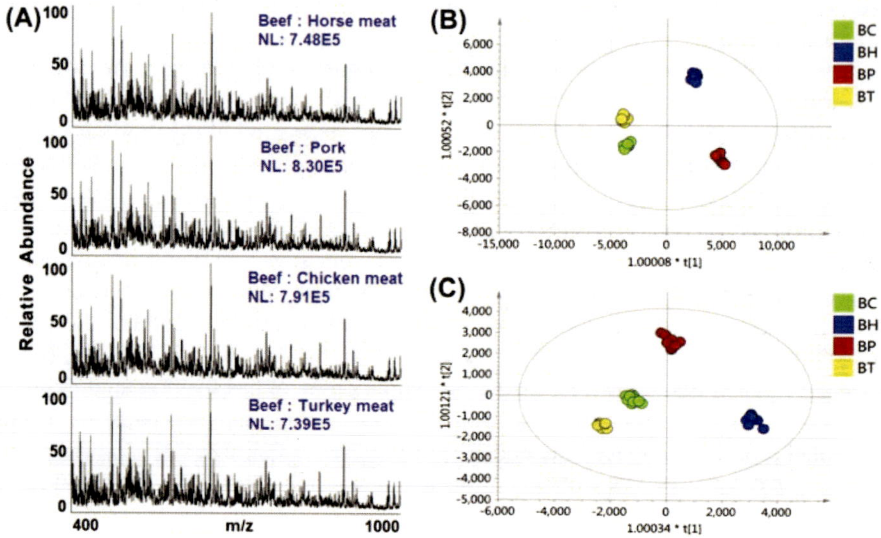

Figure 14.1 Distinguishing meat species in cooked beef. (A) Liquid extraction surface analysis mass spectrometry (LESA-MS) average mass spectra of tryptic digests of cooked meat mixtures of beef spiked with 1% (w/w) of horse, pork, chicken, and turkey meat. Orthogonal partial least squares discriminant analysis (OPLS-DA) score plots of datasets collected from beef spiked with 10% (B) and 1% (C) of the second meat species, *m/z* 400–1000, $n = 50$. *BC*, Beef/chicken meat; *BH*, beef/horse meat; *BP*, beef/pork; *BT*, beef/turkey meat. Reprinted with permission from Montowska, M., Alexander, M.R., Tucker, G.A., Barrett, D.A., 2014b. Rapid detection of peptide markers for authentication purposes in raw and cooked meat using ambient liquid extraction surface analysis mass spectrometry. Analytical Chemistry (86), 10257–10265. Copyright © 2014 American Chemical Society.

hand, the sensitivity of this methodology was much lower when compared to LC-MS/MS (Table 14.1). Applicability of the LESA-MS/MS method was later assessed by the same group to identify different peptide markers in several types of processed meat products, including commercial samples and in-house prepared reference sausages. Results showed that three samples were mislabeled, one pork sausage declaring veal that presented only peptide markers for pork species and two cocktail sausage samples that declared turkey that was not detected. Nevertheless, the authors stated that, considering the low sensitivity of the LESA-MS/MS method, the possibility that the meat content was below the limit of detection could not be excluded. Additionally, a sample of horse sausage was also positive for pork meat.

14.3 DNA-Based Methods

Analytical techniques relying on DNA-based methods have rapidly evolved during recent years as alternatives to overcome the limitations of protein analysis. Compared to protein-based methods, they present several advantages, specifically the ubiquity of

Table 14.1 Summarized Information About Protein-Based Methods Applied to Meat Species Detection

Method	Target Species	Target Molecule	Type of Product	Sensitivity	References
2-DE	Cattle, pork, chicken, turkey, duck, and goose	Myosin light chain isoforms	Raw meat	–	Montowska and Pospiech (2011b)
2-DE	Cattle, pork, chicken, turkey, duck, and goose	Myosin light chain isoforms	Minced meat mixtures, processed meat products (frankfurters and sausages)	Not determined, but content of meat of one species in the mixture should be <10% (w/w)	Montowska and Pospiech (2012b)
CE	Cattle and ostrich	Water-soluble protein and salt soluble protein fractions	Raw meat	–	Vallejo-Cordoba et al. (2010)
ELISA with monoclonal antibodies	Chicken and turkey	Thermostable soluble muscle proteins in chicken (35, 30, 25, and 23.5 kDa) and turkey (29.5, 26, 24.5, and 22 kDa)	Cooked (100°C, 15 min) mammalian meat (pork, cattle, lamb, horse, deer)	1% (chicken in cooked beef or chicken in cooked pork)	Djurdjevic et al. (2005)
Sandwich ELISA with monoclonal antibodies	Pork	Skeletal muscle troponin I	Raw and heat-processed meat mixtures	0.05% (w/w) (raw, cooked, or autoclaved pork in chicken), 0.05% (w/w) (raw pork in beef), and 0.1% (w/w) (cooked or autoclaved pork in beef mixtures)	Liu et al. (2006)
ELISA with monoclonal antibodies	Cattle	SDS-denatured beef myoglobin and peptide with an amino acid sequence unique to beef myoglobin	Raw and cooked meat	9.5 ng/mL (detection); 12.8 ng/mL (quantification)	Kotoura et al. (2012)
Sandwich ELISA	Mammalian (cattle, pork, lamb, and horse)	Skeletal muscle protein troponin I	Raw meat and meat products	4.8 ng/mL (detection); 8.7–52 ng/mL (quantification range)	Zvereva et al. (2015)

Continued

Table 14.1 Summarized Information About Protein-Based Methods Applied to Meat Species Detection—cont'd

Method	Target Species	Target Molecule	Type of Product	Sensitivity	References
OFFGEL isoelectric focusing fractionation and LC-ESI-MS/MS	Chicken	Two peptides (DQGTFEDFVEGLR and ALGQNPTNAEINK) from myosin light chain 3	Raw and cooked meat	0.5% (w/w) (chicken in pork meat; quantification using stable isotope-labeled peptides as internal standard)	Sentandreu et al. (2010)
LC-MS/MS and micro LC-MS/MS using MRM and MRM^3	Horse and pork	Peptides YDIINLR from troponin T, TLAFLFAER from myosin-4, and EFEIGNLQSK from myosin-2	Raw meat	0.55% (w/w) (horse or pork in beef), 0.13% (w/w) (pork in beef using micro-LC and MRM^3)	Von Bargen et al. (2013)
HPLC-MS/MS using MRM and MRM^3	Horse and pork	Peptides YDIINLR from troponin T, TLAFLFAER from myosin-4, SALAHAVQSSR from myosin-1 and -4, EFEIGNLQSK from myosin-2, and LVNDLTGQR from myosin-1	Processed food matrices	0.24% (w/w) (horse or pork in beef)	Von Bargen et al. (2014)
LESA-MS/MS	Horse, pork, chicken, and turkey	Several heat-stable peptides from MLC1/3f, MLC2f, troponin C, myoglobin, myosin-1, or myosin-4	Cooked meat	10% (w/w) (cooked pork, horse, or turkey meat), 5% (w/w) (chicken meat in beef)	Montowska et al. (2014b)
LESA-MS/MS	Horse, pork, chicken, turkey, and cattle	25 species-specific heat-stable peptides	Processed meat products	–	Montowska et al. (2015)

2-DE, Two-dimensional electrophoresis; *CE*, capillary electrophoresis; *ELISA*, enzyme-linked immunosorbent assay; *HPLC-MS/MS*, high-performance liquid chromatography tandem mass spectrometry; *LC-MS/MS*, liquid chromatography tandem mass spectrometry; *LC-ESI-MS/MS*, liquid chromatography electrospray ionization tandem mass spectrometry; *LESA-MS/MS*, liquid extraction surface analysis tandem mass spectrometry; *MLC*, myosin light chain; *MRM*, multiple reaction monitoring; *SDS*, sodium dodecyl sulfate.

nucleic acids in every type of cell and their greater stability than proteins. Most DNA-based methods rely on the polymerase chain reaction (PCR) technique for its specificity, sensitivity, simplicity, and rapidity, allowing the identification of species of origin even in complex and processed foods. Specificity of PCR assays is related to the target sequences based on the appropriate primer choice. For accurate species identification, the primers should be designed or selected after adequate in silico and in vitro analysis to confirm their specificity. Both nuclear and mitochondrial genes can be targeted as species-specific DNA markers. Mitochondrial DNA (mtDNA) is several-fold more abundant than nuclear, increasing the sensitivity of PCR assays because of the high number of mtDNA copies per cell. Besides, mtDNA evolves much faster than nuclear DNA, containing more sequence diversity that enables the identification of phylogenetically related taxa (Fajardo et al., 2010; Girish et al., 2005).

PCR amplification is based on hybridization of specific primers that flank a target DNA sequence followed by in vitro synthesis to form millions of copies. DNA amplification followed by agarose gel electrophoresis to verify fragment size is the simplest PCR approach to detect the presence of a certain meat species (Fajardo et al., 2010). Depending on the genetic marker or the aim of the analysis, additional methods can complement the analysis of PCR products, such as sequencing and restriction fragment length polymorphism (RFLP). The vast majority of PCR methods is based on species-specific primers by means of end-point PCR, multiplex PCR, and real-time PCR (Ballin et al., 2009; Fajardo et al., 2010). The use of short arbitrary primers to generate fingerprint patterns of random amplified polymorphic DNA (RAPD) has been applied to species identification of meats, taking advantage of the fact that prior knowledge of the target sequence is not required (Arslan et al., 2005; Calvo et al., 2001; Rastogi et al., 2007). However, difficulties in obtaining reproducible patterns and the inappropriateness of analyzing admixed meat species make the applicability of RAPD of limited scope in the case of processed foods (Fajardo et al., 2010). Other fingerprint DNA-based methods, such as single sequence repeats (SSRs) or microsatellites, single nucleotide polymorphisms (SNPs), and PCR with single-strand conformation polymorphisms (SSCPs) have also been used for meat species differentiation. Analysis of SSR markers facilitated the discrimination of pork from wild boar, both of which belong to the same species (*Sus scrofa*) and therefore are very difficult to differentiate (Conyers et al., 2012). SNP represents a promising molecular method for meat species traceability, as described by Yang et al. (2014). PCR-SSCP with capillary electrophoresis targeting the mitochondrial 12S rRNA gene was successfully developed and applied to differentiate eight avian species based on their distinct patterns (Tisza et al., 2016).

14.3.1 PCR-RFLP

PCR followed by RFLP analysis relies on specific restriction sites recognized by the restriction enzymes, allowing species identification based on the different patterns obtained (Ballin et al., 2009). This technique has been largely applied to meat and meat product speciation and has the ability to differentiate closely related species (Fajardo et al., 2010). The advantages of PCR-RFLP are related to its simplicity, low cost, and suitability for routine analysis (Pfeiffer et al., 2004). On the contrary, the possible existence of intraspecific mutations at restriction sites (Pereira et al., 2008), the presence of mixed species, and processing are likely to constrain the application of PCR-RFLP in meat product authentication (Fajardo et al., 2010).

Table 14.2 summarizes the most relevant information from reported PCR-RFLP methods, from which it can be inferred that mtDNA markers are mostly targeted to differentiate domestic and game meat species. Most PCR-RFLP methods use gel

Table 14.2 Summarized Information About Methods of PCR-RFLP Applied to Meat Species Detection

Target Species	Application	Target Gene	Sensitivity	References
Pork, cattle, wild boar, buffalo, sheep, goat, horse, chicken, turkey, red deer, roe deer, moose, antelope, chamois, mouflon, and kangaroo	Sausages, marinated and heat-treated meats	Cytochrome b	<1% (w/w) (pork)	Meyer et al. (1995)
Red deer and sika deer	Raw and heat-treated meats	Cytochrome b	–	Matsunaga et al. (1998)
Buffalo, cattle, sheep, goat, hare, red deer, fallow deer, moose, antelope, gazelle, wildebeest, chamois, Pyrenean ibex, and kangaroo	Frozen meat and lyophilized protein extracts	Cytochrome b	–	Wolf et al. (1999)
Pork	Meat, mortadella, pork sausage, and dry-cured ham	D-loop	5% (w/w) (pork)	Montiel-Sosa et al. (2000)
Ostrich	Raw and heat-treated meats	Cytochrome b	–	Abdulmawjood and Buelte (2002)
Cattle, goat, sheep, pork, quail, wild boar, chicken, turkey, red deer, and roe deer	Chicken nuggets, hamburgers, croquettes, sausages, ham, tortellini, moussaka, pâté, ravioli, and cannelloni	Cytochrome b	–	Pascoal et al. (2004)

Table 14.2 Summarized Information About Methods of PCR-RFLP Applied to Meat Species Detection—cont'd

Target Species	Application	Target Gene	Sensitivity	References
Cattle, sheep, goat, red deer, and roe deer	Blood and tissue	D-loop	–	Pfeiffer et al. (2004)
Cattle, buffalo, sheep, and goat	Raw and heat-treated meats, and fried meat products	12S rRNA	–	Girish et al. (2005)
Pork	Raw meats and fats (halal)	Cytochrome b	–	Aida et al. (2005)
Cattle, sheep, goat, red deer, fallow deer, and roe deer	Raw and heat-treated meats	12S rRNA	–	Fajardo et al. (2006)
Cattle, sheep, goat, pork, horse, poultry, and deer	Raw meats	Cytochrome b	1% (w/w) (beef and horse)	Maede (2006)
Chicken, duck, turkey, guinea fowl, and quail	Raw meats, heat-treated meats, and fried croquettes	12S rRNA	–	Girish et al. (2007)
Chamois, Pyrenean ibex, mouflon, cattle, sheep, and goat	Raw and heat-treated meats	12S rRNA, D-loop	–	Fajardo et al. (2007a)
Pork and wild boar	Raw meats	MC1R	–	Fajardo et al. (2008)
Quail, pheasant, red-legged partridge, guinea fowl, capercaillie, Eurasian woodcock, woodpigeon, and song thrush	Raw meats	12S rRNA	–	Rojas et al. (2008)
Red deer, fallow deer, roe deer, chamois, mouflon, Pyrenean ibex, goat, cattle, sheep, and swine	Raw meats	12S rRNA	–	Fajardo et al. (2009a,b)
Quail, pheasant, red-legged partridge, chukar partridge, guinea fowl, capercaillie,	Raw meats	D-loop	–	Rojas et al. (2009a)

Continued

Table 14.2 Summarized Information About Methods of PCR-RFLP Applied to Meat Species Detection—cont'd

Target Species	Application	Target Gene	Sensitivity	References
Eurasian woodcock, and woodpigeon				
Cattle, pork, buffalo, quail, chicken, goat, and rabbit	Raw meats	Cytochrome b	–	Murugaiah et al. (2009)
Chicken, turkey, duck, goose, pheasant, partridge, woodcock, ostrich, quail, and song thrush	Raw and heat-treated meats	12S rRNA, Cytochrome b	–	Stamoulis et al. (2010)
Cattle, chicken, turkey, sheep, pork, buffalo, camel, and donkey	Raw meats and blood	Cytochrome c oxidase subunit 1	–	Haider et al. (2012)
Pork	Meatballs, streaky beacon, frankfurters, and burgers	Cytochrome b	0.01% (w/w) (pork) 0.0001 ng (pork DNA)	Ali et al. (2012a)
Cattle, buffalo, goat, sheep, and pork	Raw meats	Cytochrome b	–	Kumar et al. (2014)
Cattle, sheep, pork, chicken, donkey, and horse	Raw meats, sausages, frankfurters, hamburgers, and hams	Cytochrome b	–	Doosti et al. (2014)
Cat	Raw, heat-treated meats and meatballs	18S rRNA	0.01% (w/w)	Ali et al. (2015a)
Dog	Burger formulations and commercial burgers	Cytochrome b	0.01% (w/w) 0.0001 ng (dog DNA)	Rahman et al. (2015)

MC1R, Melanocortin receptor 1 gene; *PCR-RFLP*, polymerase chain reaction restriction fragment length polymorphism.

electrophoresis as a simple and economic strategy to analyze fragment patterns. More recently, chip-based capillary electrophoresis has emerged as an alternative to conventional electrophoresis for RFLP analysis for meat authentication, producing higher resolution band patterns, shorter analysis times, higher versatility, reproducibility, and suitability for automation (Ali et al., 2012a, 2015a; Fajardo et al., 2009a; Rahman et al., 2015).

14.3.2 Species-Specific PCR

Species-specific PCR has been increasingly used because of its simplicity, high specificity, and high sensitivity; it is suitable for meat authentication studies even in complex and processed foods. It relies on accurate marker selection (Genbank, http://www.ncbi.nlm.nih.gov/) and design of specific primers that, after adequate method optimization, are able to produce one single PCR product from the target species. Species-specific PCR is mainly based on conventional PCR analyzed after 30–40 amplification cycles by agarose gel electrophoresis, known as qualitative or end-point PCR. Since amplification products are analyzed by the latter phases of amplification (plateau phase), the results are considered as qualitative, being quantitative or semiquantitative only in certain cases after cycle number optimization and normalization (Soares et al., 2010). Table 14.3 summarizes the wide number of species-specific PCR methods applied to meat species detection, which target mostly mtDNA markers as verified also in PCR-RFLP methods. A great advantage of species-specific PCR methods is the ability to provide results on relative and absolute sensitivity, contrary to most PCR-RFLP methods and other fingerprint techniques.

By the use of two or more specific primer pairs in the same PCR amplification and after adequate method optimization, we can easily advance to multitarget PCR. Multiplex end-point assays are very similar to single target PCR methods, with the great advantage of allowing simultaneous multitarget detection and becoming therefore cost-effective and high-throughput methods. Ali et al. (2014b) reported a comprehensive review on the multiplex PCR methods applied to species authentication, relating the important steps for method development. Table 14.3 also summarizes the reported multiplex PCR methods for meat species identification in foods.

14.3.3 PCR-Sequencing

Sequencing of PCR fragments allows collection of the full nucleotide information, which is then compared with a comprehensive reference database to achieve species identification. Ideally, the target DNA region must consist of a variable sequence that should be sufficiently informative for species differentiation. Additionally, the sequence should be flanked by highly conserved regions that are ideal for the design of universal PCR primers that amplify in a large number of species (Pereira et al., 2008). As for other PCR-based methods, mtDNA, such as cytochrome b, 12S, and 16S rRNA genes, have been widely used for species discrimination by PCR-sequencing (Fajardo et al., 2010; Pereira et al., 2008). Regions with considerably high mutation ratios, such as most animal mtDNA sequences, are recommended to achieve discrimination of closely related species (Pereira et al., 2008). Currently, the mitochondrial gene coding for cytochrome c oxidase subunit I (COI) is considered a reliable DNA barcode for the discrimination of animal species.

PCR-sequencing targeting cytochrome b was used to detect goose species (*Anser anser*) in Italian "Mortara" salami (Colombo et al., 2002) and chamois (*Rupicapra rupicapra*) meat (Colombo et al., 2004). Horreo et al. (2013) designed universal primers based on the nucleotide sequences of the 16S rRNA gene of 40 animal species

Table 14.3 **Summarized Information About Methods of Species-Specific PCR Applied to Meat Species Detection**

Technique	Target species	Application	Target Gene	Sensitivity	References
Species-specific PCR	Pork	Raw meats, heat-treated meats and sausages	Porcine growth hormone	0.1% (w/w)	Meyer et al. (1994)
	Goat, chicken, cattle, sheep, pig, and horse	Raw and heat-treated meats	Cytochrome b	–	Matsunaga et al. (1999)
	Cattle, pork, chicken, and ruminants	Ground meats and sausages	Short interspersed elements	0.5 pg (cattle DNA), 0.05 pg (pork DNA), 5 pg (chicken DNA) 0.005% (w/w) (cattle), 0.0005% (w/w) (pork), 0.05% (chicken) (w/w)	Walker et al. (2003)
	Chicken, pork, goose, and mule duck	Binary liver/foie gras mixtures	α-Actin	0.1% (w/w)	Rodríguez et al. (2003a)
	Chicken, pork, goose, turkey, and mule duck	Raw meats, livers, and binary liver/foie gras mixtures	12S rRNA	1% (w/w)	Rodríguez et al. (2003b)
	Pork, cattle, sheep, and goat	Raw and heat-treated meat mixtures	12S rRNA	1% (w/w)	Rodríguez et al. (2004)
	Cattle	Raw meats, heat-treated meats, beef in wheat flour, tortellini, sausages, and ravioli	Cytochrome b	0.025% (w/w)	Pascoal et al. (2005)
	Cattle, sheep, goat, and deer	Raw meats, heat-treated meats, and meat meals	12S rRNA–$tRNA^{val}$–16S rRNA	0.05% (w/w)	Ha et al. (2006)
	Horse, dog, cat, bovine, sheep, porcine, and goat	Binary raw meat mixtures	Cytochrome b	0.1% (w/w)	Ilhak and Arslan (2007)

	Horse, donkey, and pork	Binary raw meat mixtures	ATPase 8/ATPase 6, ND2 and ND5 (dehydrogenase subunits 2 and 5)	0.1% (w/w) 0.01 ng DNA	Kesmen et al. (2007)
	Cattle, sheep, and goat	Raw and heat-treated meats	12S rRNA	0.1% (w/w)	Martín et al. (2007a)
	Muscovy duck, mallard duck, mule duck, and common teal	Raw meats, binary raw meat mixtures, and heat-treated meats	12S rRNA	0.1% (w/w) (Muscovy duck and mule duck in raw and heat-treated meats)	Martín et al. (2007b)
	Red deer, fallow deer, and roe deer	Raw and heat-treated meats, hams, sausages, and cooked meats	12S rRNA	–	Fajardo et al. (2007b)
	Chamois, Pyrenean ibex, and mouflon	Raw meats, binary raw meat mixtures, and heat-treated meats	D-loop	0.1% (w/w)	Fajardo et al. (2007c)
	Rabbit	Binary raw and heat-treated mixtures of rabbit meat in oats	12S rRNA	0.1% (w/w) (raw and heat-treated)	Martín et al. (2009)
	Quail, pheasant, partridge, and guinea fowl	Binary raw meat mixtures, pâtés, braised meats, pickled meats, and minced meats	12S rRNA	0.1% (w/w) (raw and heat-treated)	Rojas et al. (2009b)
	Turkey, chicken, duck, and guinea fowl	Liquid and powder eggs	Cytochrome b	0.1% (w/w)	Nau et al. (2009)
	Chicken, duck, pigeon, and pork	Raw and heat-treated meats, blood	Cytochrome b, D-loop	–	Haunshi et al. (2009)

Continued

Table 14.3 **Summarized Information About Methods of Species-Specific PCR Applied to Meat Species Detection—cont'd**

Technique	Target species	Application	Target Gene	Sensitivity	References
	Chicken	Raw and heat-treated meats, binary meat mixtures (patty, kebab, and block)	D-loop	1% (w/w)	Mane et al. (2009)
	Quail, pheasant, partridge and guinea fowl, pigeon, Eurasian woodcock, and song thrush	Binary raw meat mixtures	D-loop	0.1% (w/w) (raw and heat-treated)	Rojas et al. (2010)
	Chicken, turkey, and pork	Raw meats, binary raw meat mixtures, and heat-treated meats	Cytochrome b	0.1% (w/w) (poultry)	Hernández-Chávez et al. (2011)
	Cattle	Raw and heat-treated meats, binary meat mixtures (patty, kebab, and block)	D-loop	<1% (w/w)	Mane et al. (2012a)
	Buffalo	Raw and heat-treated meats, binary meat mixtures (patty, kebab, and block)	D-loop	1% (w/w)	Mane et al. (2012b)
	Hare	Binary raw meat mixtures	Cytochrome b	0.01% (w/w)	Santos et al. (2012)
	Chicken	Raw meats, blood, and binary raw and heat-treated meat mixtures	5-Aminolevulinate synthase	0.1% (w/w) 10 pg (chicken DNA)	Karabasanavar et al. (2013)
	Pork	Raw meats, blood, and binary meats mixtures	D-loop	0.1% (w/w) 10 pg (pork DNA)	Karabasanavar et al. (2014)

	Dog	Raw and heat-treated meats, spiked frankfurters	Cytochrome b	0.1% (w/w) 0.02 ng (dog DNA)	Ali et al. (2014a)
	Cattle, pork, sheep, and chicken	Binary meat mixtures, animal meals, pork lard, blood, whey, casein, and hemoglobin	12S rRNA, Cytochrome c oxidase subunit I, 16S rRNA	0.09% (w/w) (cattle, pork, and sheep), 0.08% (w/w) (chicken)	Natonek-Wiśniewska et al. (2013)
	Cattle, hare, rabbit, red deer, and pork	Binary meat mixtures, game meat Alheiras	Cytochrome b, 12S rRNA	0.01% (w/w) (rabbit, cattle, and hare), 0.1% (w/w) (red deer and pork)	Amaral et al. (2014)
	Duck, partridge, pheasant, quail, chicken, and turkey	Binary meat mixtures, game meat Alheiras	Cytochrome b, 12S rRNA	0.01% (w/w)	Amaral et al. (2015)
	Cattle, sheep, chicken, and donkey	Raw meats, ground meats, and binary meat mixtures	D-loop, Cytochrome c oxidase subunit II, 12S rRNA, ND2	0.1% (w/w) (chicken and donkey)	Mousavi et al. (2015)
Multiplex PCR	Goat, chicken, cattle, sheep, pig, and horse	Raw and heat-treated meats	Cytochrome b	0.25 ng DNA	Matsunaga et al. (1999)
	Ruminant, poultry, fish, and pork	Raw and heat-treated meats, feedstuff, and baby food	12S rRNA, tRNA-Val, and 16S rRNA	0.002% (w/w) (ruminants)	Dalmasso et al. (2004)
	Ruminant, poultry, and pork	Raw meats, ground meats, and sausages	16S rRNA, 12S rRNA, 12S rRNA–tRNA-Val	–	Ghovvati et al. (2009)

Continued

Table 14.3 Summarized Information About Methods of Species-Specific PCR Applied to Meat Species Detection—cont'd

Technique	Target species	Application	Target Gene	Sensitivity	References
	Pork and chicken	Binary raw meat mixtures	Cytochrome b, 12S rRNA	0.1% (w/w) (pork detection) 1% (w/w) (pork quantification)	Soares et al. (2010)
	Cattle, sheep, pork, and poultry	Blood and different tissues	tRNA-Val–16S rRNA, tRNA-Lys-ATPase 8, 12S rRNA–tRNA-Val, and 12S rRNA	1 ng (pork and sheep DNA), 5 ng (poultry DNA), 0.5 ng (cattle DNA)	Zha et al. (2010)
	Sika deer, wapiti, red deer, and reindeer	Blood	D-loop, 16S rRNA	0.05 ng (sika deer and wapiti DNA), 0.1 ng (red deer DNA), 0.5 ng (red deer DNA), 0.02 ng (reindeer DNA)	Zha et al. (2011)
	Chicken, beef, pork, and mutton	Half-cooked and cooked meats, processed foods	Cytochrome b	1 ng DNA	Zhang (2013)
	Soybean, poultry, horse, and pork	Reference sausages	Lectin, 12S rRNA, Cytochrome b, ATPase 6	0.01% (w/w)	Safdar et al. (2014)
	Cattle, chicken, goat, camel, and donkey	Raw meats and sausages	Cytochrome b, 12S rRNA, ND2	–	Nejad et al. (2014)

	Chicken, duck, and goose	Raw and heat-treated meats, meat mixtures, sausage, kebab, dry meat, jerky, and shredded beef	12S rRNA, Cytochrome b, D-loop	1% (w/w) 0.05 ng DNA	Hou et al. (2015)
	Donkey, mule, and horse	Raw and heat-treated meats	ATPase 8/6, ND2	1% (w/w)	Chen et al. (2015)
	Cattle, sheep, goat, and fish	Raw meats, raw and heat-treated meat mixtures in soybean meal	ATPase 8, tGlu/cytb, 12S rRNA	0.1% (w/w)	Safdar and Junejo (2015)
	Horse, soybean, sheep, poultry, pork, and cow	Raw meats, meat mixtures, sausages, meatballs, and cikofte	Cytochrome b, lectin, 12S rRNA, ATPase 6/8	0.01% (w/w)	Safdar and Junejo (2016)
Multiplex PCR with CGE	Badger, cat, cow, dog, donkey, fox, goat, guinea pig, harvest mouse, hedgehog, horse, house mouse, human, pig, rabbit, rat, red deer, and sheep	Tissue, hair, or buccal cells	Cytochrome b	40,000 copies (~1.36 pg)	Tobe and Linacre (2008)
	Cat, dog, pork, monkey, and rat	Raw meats, binary raw and heat-treated meatballs	ND5, ATPase 6, Cytochrome b	1% (w/w) 0.01–0.02 ng DNA	Ali et al. (2015b)

CGE, Capillary gel electrophoresis; *PCR*, polymerase chain reaction.

that belonged to seven different taxonomic classes (Actinopterygii, Gasteropoda, Cephalaspidomorphi, Amphibia, Chondrichthyes, Aves, and Mammalia), obtaining PCR amplicons ranging from 80 to 125 bp. Sequencing analyses confirmed the differences among species and, although very short, they were considered very informative and enabled clustering of samples into their respective taxonomic group.

The mitochondrial 12S rRNA gene was first targeted by Girish et al. (2004) for the differentiation of cattle (*Bos indicus*), buffalo (*Bubalus bubalis*), sheep (*Ovis aries*), goat (*Capra hircus*), and mithun (*Bos frontalis*). The method was successfully applied to authenticate processed meat products (patties, steam cooked blocks, croquettes, and autoclaved blocks). Later on, the same authors used the same target gene and sequencing as a tool for further development of PCR-RFLP methods for meat species differentiation (Girish et al., 2005, 2007). In fact, sequencing of PCR products has been frequently used as an intermediate step during the development of several methods of PCR-RFLP (Fajardo et al., 2006; Rojas et al., 2009a), species-specific PCR (Haunshi et al., 2009; Santos et al., 2012), and real-time PCR (Laube et al., 2007; Santos et al., 2012; Kane and Hellberg, 2016).

The major limitation of PCR-sequencing is its unsuitability for identification of species in meat mixtures, producing ambiguous sequence results (Girish et al., 2004). The use of large sequence fragments is not recommended in the case of species identification in processed food products that contain low amounts of and degraded DNA (Pereira et al., 2008).

14.3.4 DNA Barcoding

DNA barcoding relies on sequence variation within a short and standardized region of the genome, designated as a "barcode," to provide accurate species identification. This approach is based on the analysis of the variability within a standard DNA barcode region, which is useful to establish taxonomic relationships. It involves the PCR amplification and sequencing of fragments of 400—800 bp by the use of consensus primers (Hebert et al., 2003). The Barcode of Life Data Systems (BOLD) is designed to support the generation and application of DNA barcode data, providing a data retrieval interface that enables searching public records by the use of multiple search criteria. An ideal DNA barcode should clearly enable a greater interspecies than intraspecies variability, allowing fast, reliable, automatable, and cost-effective species identification (Hebert et al., 2003). The COI barcoding region has been preferred among the mitochondrial protein-coding genes as the core molecular diagnostic system for animal species identification (Hebert et al., 2003; Luo et al., 2011).

The introduction of DNA barcoding represents a promising approach for food authentication, being broadly applied in fish species. DNA barcoding has been successful when applied to seafood because the number of species is high in comparison to other animal sources, such as cattle, sheep, goat, and horse, enhancing the effectiveness of the approach. Moreover, the classical identification methods are not useful in many cases, such as processed foods, and in the case of seafood, more than in other groups, it is possible to go further than the level of species identification (Galimberti et al., 2013).

Although few applications have been published, DNA barcoding has emerged in recent years as a tool for the authentication of meats and meat products, including game. Quinto et al. (2016) performed a survey on game meat products sold in the United States in which the COI gene was successfully used as DNA barcoding to detect mislabeling. The same research group used the same DNA barcode approach to verify the labeling of ground meat products sold in the United States (Kane and Hellberg, 2016). In both studies, BOLD was used to identify sequences at the species level. In South Africa a DNA barcoding approach was effectively used to confirm that the reliability of commercial labeling of game meat is very poor (D'Amato et al., 2013) and for species identification in forensic wildlife cases (Dalton and Kotze, 2011). In spite of the advantages of DNA barcoding, currently it is not able to identify multiple species in meat mixtures, requiring the use of other methods, such as real-time PCR or next-generation sequencing (Hellberg and Morrissey, 2011; Kane and Hellberg, 2016). Another limitation is related to the use of relatively large fragment sizes ($\sim$650 bp), which can disable the barcode amplification when analyzing highly processed foods containing degraded DNA (Fajardo et al., 2010).

14.3.5 Real-Time PCR

Real-time PCR is the method of choice in many laboratories for diagnostic tests and food analysis. It merges PCR chemistry with the use of fluorescent reporter molecules to monitor the PCR products along amplification cycles. The combination of high sensitivity and specificity, with reproducibility, low level of cross-contamination, and reduced time of analysis are advantages that make real-time PCR an attractive alternative to conventional PCR (Navarro et al., 2015). Probably the most important benefit of real-time PCR is its capacity to quantify the starting amount of a specific DNA target, which arises from its ability to measure the target product at early stages of amplification (exponential). To monitor the progress of amplification, different real-time PCR chemistries are available and classified into two main groups: double-stranded DNA intercalating molecules or binding dyes, such as SYBR green I and EvaGreen; and fluorophore-labeled oligonucleotides, such as the hydrolysis TaqMan probes (Navarro et al., 2015). The use of DNA binding dyes is the simplest and most economical approach because it does not need the use of any fluorophore-labeled oligonucleotides. However, it leads to specific and also to non-specific amplification products, requiring a melting curve analysis to verify specificity.

The most commonly used real-time PCR universal dye in several research areas, including meat species identification, is the SYBR green I (Ballin et al., 2009; Navarro et al., 2015). More recently, the use of third-generation dyes, such as EvaGreen, offers enhanced fluorescence since it can be used at higher concentrations than SYBR green I, generating greater signals, increased sensitivity, and excellent stability without causing PCR inhibition (Wang et al., 2006). The application of real-time PCR with EvaGreen fluorescent dye has been reported in the identification of Cervidae (Chen et al., 2009) and hare meat species (Santos et al., 2012). The use of EvaGreen, as a saturation dye, offers also the advantage of performing high-resolution melting (HRM) analysis, when using high-resolution instrumentation. HRM analysis involves a more precise temperature control when performing melting curve analysis and an enhanced data acquisition system as compared to current equipment. HRM analysis has already demonstrated its potential in food analysis, particularly in differentiating closely related species and plant cultivars (Druml and Cichna, 2014). In pork meat traceability, HRM analysis targeting SNP detection was successfully applied as a genotyping method (Yang et al., 2014). The report showed that results of HRM genotyping were accurate and, in general, consistent with PCR-RFLP and real-time PCR with TaqMan probes data, but at a much lower cost.

The real-time PCR approach with hydrolysis TaqMan probes has been widely applied to several areas of research (Navarro et al., 2015), as the most common being in food authentication, genetically modified organism quantification, and allergen detection (Ali et al., 2014b; Ballin et al., 2009; Costa et al., 2016b; Mafra et al., 2008). Hydrolysis probes are designed to bind to a specific region of the target DNA, with mechanism of action that relies on the 5—3′ exonuclease activity of Taq polymerase, which degrades the bound probe during amplification. TaqMan probes contain a donor fluorescent moiety at the 5′-end and an acceptor fluorescent moiety at the 3′-end that quenches the fluorescence emitted from the donor molecule because of their close proximity. Advantages of using TaqMan probes are related to their relatively simple design and multiplexing capacity, without requiring melting curve analysis (Navarro et al., 2015). Table 14.4 summarizes the reported real-time PCR methods for meat species identification in foods, in which can be seen the extensive use of TaqMan probes, targeting mostly mtDNA.

14.5.6 Next-Generation Sequencing

In recent years, enormous progress has been made in DNA sequencing technologies. Next-generation sequencing (NGS) technologies have revolutionized the analysis of DNA, in terms of speed, read length, and throughput, along with a sharp reduction in cost per-base. Compared to first-generation sequencing methods, such as Sanger sequencing, the new methods share three major improvements: (1) they rely on the preparation of NGS libraries in a cell-free system, without requiring bacterial cloning of DNA fragments; (2) they produce thousands to several millions of sequencing reactions in parallel, instead of hundreds; and (3) the sequencing output is directly detected without the need for postreaction analysis, such electrophoresis, and the nucleotide base query is performed cyclically and in parallel (van Dijk et al., 2014; Fig. 14.2). NGS is becoming a standard approach in a large number of studies in all species and in many different fields, including resequencing or de novo sequencing of large and small genomes, metagenomics, and transcriptomics among many other research and applied areas (Bertolini et al., 2015; Buermans and den Dunnen, 2014; van Dijk et al., 2014). The huge number of reads generated by NGS has enabled the sequencing of entire genomes with exceptional speed. This has become possible in part because of significant advances in data handling by bioinformatic tools.

Despite the high potential of NGS for species identification, only a few studies have been reported regarding meat species differentiation. Tillmar et al. (2013) described a DNA-typing method for the determination of mammal species using targeted,

Table 14.4 **Summarized Information About Methods of Real-Time PCR Applied to Meat Species Detection**

Technique	Target Species	Application	Target Gene	Sensitivity	References
Real-time PCR with TaqMan probes	Cattle, pork, lamb, chicken, and turkey	Binary raw meat mixtures	Cytochrome b	0.5% (w/w)	Dooley et al. (2004)
	Horse and donkey	Model raw meat mixtures and commercial products (horse sausage, horse steak, horse burger, horse ham, and horse salami)	Cytochrome b	1 pg (donkey DNA) or 25 pg (horse DNA)	Chisholm et al. (2005)
	Duck (mallard and Muscovy duck)	Roasted duck, smoked duck, duck pâté, game casserole, and feed samples	Cytochrome b	Estimated as 0.0001% (w/w)	Hird et al. (2005)
	Pork	Binary mixtures of raw and sterilized pork in beef muscles	12S rRNA	0.01 ng (pork DNA), 0.5% (w/w) (pork in beef mixtures)	Rodríguez et al. (2005)
	Cattle, pork, lamb, goat, chicken, turkey, and duck	Home canned food, normal cans, cans for use under tropical conditions, and ultra-high heat-treated cans with an amount of at least 0.1% of the respective species	Cyclic guanosine monophosphate phosphodiesterase, ryanodine receptor, and interleukin-2 precursor	10 genome copies	Laube et al. (2007)
	Cattle	Raw meats, processed meat products, milk, and cheese	Cytochrome b	35 pg (cattle DNA)	Zhang et al. (2007)
	Cattle, pork, horse, mutton, chicken, and turkey	Processed meat products	Satellite IV DNA for cattle and cytochrome b for the other species	0.05% (w/w) (pork, lard, horse, mutton, chicken, and turkey), 0.1% (cattle)	Jonker et al. (2008)

Continued

Table 14.4 Summarized Information About Methods of Real-Time PCR Applied to Meat Species Detection—cont'd

Technique	Target Species	Application	Target Gene	Sensitivity	References
	Chamois and Pyrenean ibex	Raw and heat-treated binary mixtures	12S rRNA and D-loop	–	Fajardo et al. (2009a,b)
	Donkey, pork, and horse	Raw and cocked patty samples prepared with binary meat mixtures in beef	Mitochondrial ND2, ND5, and ATPase 6/8	0.0001% (w/w) 0.0001 ng DNA	Kesmen et al. (2009)
	Pork	Model meatballs spiked with pork meat, commercial meatballs of pork, beef, chicken, mutton, and chevon/goat	Cytochrome b	0.01% (w/w)	Ali et al. (2012b)
	Pork	Model chicken nuggets spiked with pork meat, commercial nuggets of pork, beef, chicken, mutton, and chevon	Cytochrome b	0.01% (w/w)	Ali et al. (2012c)
	Rabbit and hare	Binary mixtures of processed muscles [rabbit, hare, and rabbit plus hare (1:1, w/w)] in oat matrix; commercial dog and cat foods labeled as containing rabbit	12S rRNA	0.1% (w/w) (processed muscles), 0.01 ng/μL (each target DNA)	Pegels et al. (2013)
	Fallow deer, red deer, and sika deer	Meat products labeled as containing deer or game, model game sausage	Epidermal growth factor pseudogene	0.5% (w/w) (fallow deer and red deer), 0.1% (w/w) (sika deer)	Druml et al. (2015a)
	Roe deer	Raw binary meat mixtures with pork, game model sausage	Lactoferrin	0.03% (w/w)	Druml et al. (2015c)
	Cat and dog	Samples of pet food, farm animal products, and raw materials	Cytochrome oxidase subunit I	2 pg (cat DNA), 0.2 pg (dog DNA)	Espiñeira and Vieites (2015)
	Horse	Heat-processed binary mixtures of horse in bovine meat, meat-based products, and pet foods	12S rRNA	1 pg horse DNA	Pegels et al. (2015)

	Horse	Raw binary mixtures of horse meat in beef	Equine growth hormone receptor	≤0.1% (w/w)	Nixon et al. (2015)
	Camel	Braised camel meat and charqui	Cytochrome b	0.01% (w/w) 5 fg/μL camel DNA	Wu et al. (2015)
	Dog	Model chicken nuggets with known amounts of dog meat, halal commercial chicken nuggets	Cytochrome b	0.01% (w/w)	Rahman et al. (2016)
Multiplex real-time PCR with TaqMan probes	Chicken, duck, and pork	Ternary mixtures of pork, duck, and goose blood	Beta-actin, transforming growth factor, T-cell growth factor	1% (w/w) (three target species in ternary mixtures), 0.15 ng for all species	Cheng et al. (2014)
	Roe deer and deer (the sum of fallow deer, red deer, and sika deer)	Raw binary meat mixtures with pork, several meat species mixtures, model game sausage	Lactoferrin, exon 21 of epidermal growth factor pseudogene	–	Druml et al. (2015b)
	Cattle and pork	Raw binary meat mixtures, minced meat products, and meat products	Cyclic-guanosine monophosphate -phosphodiesterase, β-actin	20 genome equivalents	Iwobi et al. (2015)
	Murine (lab rat, lab mouse, and wild mouse)	Binary meat mixture of murine meat in mutton, meat products spiked with murine meat	Cytochrome b	0.1% (w/w), 1 pg of DNA per reaction	Fang and Zhang (2016)
	Duck, goose, chicken, turkey, and pork	Model liver pâté (containing goose, duck, and chicken liver and turkey and pork meat), liver–meat products	Cytochrome b, D-loop	2% (w/w) (turkey), 1% (w/w) (duck, goose, and chicken), 1% (w/w) (pork)	Köppel et al. (2013)

Continued

Table 14.4 Summarized Information About Methods of Real-Time PCR Applied to Meat Species Detection—cont'd

Technique	Target Species	Application	Target Gene	Sensitivity	References
Real-time PCR with TaqMan minor groove binding probes	Cattle and pork	Raw and cooked/sterilized meatballs prepared with binary mixtures of beef and pork	t-Glu-cytb	1% (w/w) (raw and cooked/ sterilized beef), 1% (w/w) (raw pork), 5% (w/w) (cooked/sterilized pork)	López-Andreo et al. (2012)
Real-time PCR with molecular beacon probe	Pork	Raw meat mixtures	Cytochrome b	0.1% (w/w) (pork in pork—beef mixtures), 0.0001 ng pork DNA	Yusop et al. (2012)
Real-time PCR with TaqMan probes and real-time with SYBR green I dye	Capercaillie	Raw and sterilized binary mixtures of capercaillie in chicken meat	12S rRNA	0.1% (w/w)	Rojas et al. (2011)
	Cattle and buffalo	Milk- and meat-derived food products	Cytochrome b, 16S rRNA	—	Drummond et al. (2013)
Real-time PCR with SYBR green I dye	Pork	Different mixtures of pork, cattle, camel, horse, and chicken raw meats, halal-labeled beef, and chicken products	Mitochondrial DNA	0.1 ng (pork DNA)	Farrokhi and Joozani (2011)
	Pork	Raw binary mixtures in poultry meat, frankfurters, barbecue sausages, hamburgers, and nuggets	Cytochrome b	0.1% (w/w) 5 pg (pork DNA)	Soares et al. (2013)
Real-time PCR with EvaGreen dye	Hare	Binary raw meat mixtures	Cytochrome b	1 pg (hare DNA)	Santos et al. (2012)
Multiplex real-time PCR with EvaGreen dye	Cattle and soybean	Model sausages and commercial sausages	ATPase 8, lectin	0.003% (w/w) (beef), 0.001% (w/w) (soybean)	Safdar and Abasıyanık (2013)

PCR, Polymerase chain reaction.

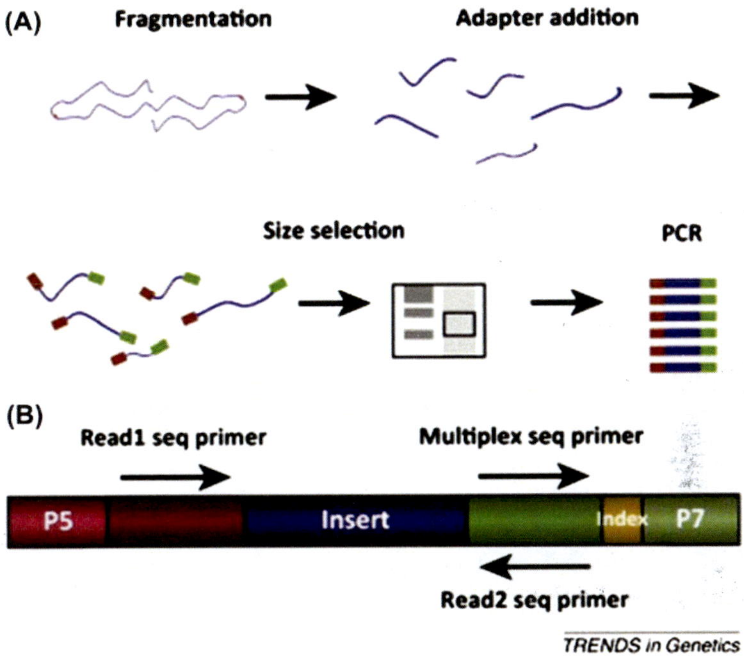

Figure 14.2 (A) Simplified representation of a typical next-generation sequencing (NGS) library preparation workflow. (B) Architecture of a standard Illumina NGS library. Adapters are indicated in two-tone red and green, the insert is in blue. An index or barcode is indicated in yellow. Sequencing primers are indicated by arrows. Shown is an Illumina library in which "P5" and "P7" are the sequences used for flow cell attachment and amplification. In other technologies the names of these terminal sequences are different, but the principle is the same. Reprinted with permission from van Dijk, E.L., Auger, H., Jaszczyszyn, Y., Thermes, C., 2014. Ten years of next-generation sequencing technology. Trends in Genetics (30), 418–426. Copyright © 2014 Elsevier.

massively parallel sequencing of a short mtDNA sequence by means of NGS. The method was designed through phylogenetic analyses of DNA reference sequences of more than 300 mammal species, using binary DNA mixtures. Results obtained were promising since they allowed discrimination of over 99.9% of mammal species, with the ability to detect minor components at concentrations as low as 1% (w/w) in mixed samples (Tillmar et al., 2013). A major advantage of NGS cited by the authors was the use of short PCR amplicons, which facilitates the analysis of degraded and poor-quality DNA. The use of universal PCR primers, without requiring prior species or sequence information and the possibility of detecting minute amounts of DNA, is an additional advantage of NGS, particularly in the case of forensic and food analysis.

The report of Ripp et al. (2014) showed that NGS of total DNA derived from foodstuff material can readily identify and quantify species components with high accuracy by a single experimental assay. Sequence data simulation and real-case Illumina sequencing of DNA from reference sausages composed of mammalian (pig, cow, horse, sheep) and avian (chicken, turkey) species were able to correctly quantify material at the 1% (w/w) level via a read counting approach. The same authors performed an additional metagenomic step to facilitate identification of traces from animal, plant, and microbial DNA, including unexpected species, which is prospectively important for the detection of food allergens and pathogens.

In the report by Bertoloni et al. (2015), the potential of the next-generation semiconductor-based sequencing technology (Ion Torrent Personal Genome Machine) was evaluated for the identification of DNA from meat species (pig, horse, cattle, sheep, rabbit, chicken, turkey, pheasant, duck, goose, and pigeon), as well as from human and rat, in DNA mixtures, using different universal primers to target the mitochondrial 12S and 16S rRNA genes. The approach allowed the detection of low levels of pork and horse DNA from reads obtained with different universal primer pairs, which could overcome the potential problems of amplification competition among species.

14.3.7 Biosensors

Recently, DNA biosensors and DNA biochip technology have been suggested as high-throughput alternative genetic approaches. Ali et al. (2011) developed a novel nanobiosensor based on a 3 nm diameter citrate—tannate-coated gold nanoparticle functionalized with a fluorophore-labeled probe consisting of a 27-nucleotide *Alu*I-fragment of pork cytochrome b gene. This biosensor was able to detect 0.5% and 1% (w/w) of pork in, respectively, raw and autoclaved beef binary meat mixtures, in a single step without any separation or washing. Considering that the degree of fluorescence depends on the degree of target binding, the method has the potential for quantitation by the use of a standard curve generated with known concentrations of probes and targets (Ali et al., 2011). The same methodology was further applied for the quantitative estimation of spiked pork in burger formulations (Ali et al., 2012d) and in mixed meatball preparations (Ali et al., 2014c), both with more than 90% accuracy.

DNA biochips rely on the use of microarray analysis and exploit the principle of hybridization of PCR-amplified fragments on specific probes bound onto the arrays. The technique presents, in general, the major advantage of allowing for simultaneous detection of multiple targets, saving time and reducing costs, but it can be limited by the overall proficiency of the PCR amplification (Iwobi et al., 2011). Iwobi et al. (2011) tested and compared two commercially available animal DNA biochip detection systems, the CarnoCheck Test Kit (Greiner Bio-One) and the MEAT^{species} LCD Array (Chipron), which allow the simultaneous identification of 8 and 14 animal species, respectively (Fig. 14.3). Both test systems are based on the PCR amplification of consensus DNA regions and species-specific probes that exploit differences within the mtDNA of the targeted animal species. The two systems showed a good sensitivity, although this was higher for the LCD array since at least 0.1% of all meat species in the analyzed samples were detectable using this biochip. The two systems were applied to the analysis of 70 commercial samples and the results validated against conventional PCR methods, showing a general good performance of both DNA biochips. A possible disadvantage of the method, in particular for the CarnoCheck Test Kit, is

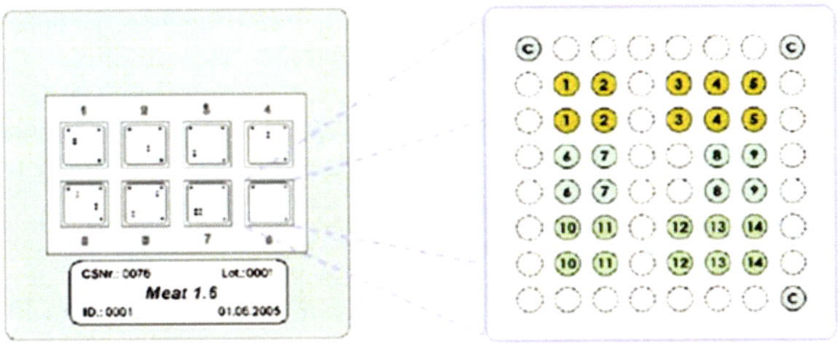

Capture Probes

N°	Probe	Specificity	N°	Probe	Specificity
01	Beef	*Bos taurus*	08	Rabbit	*Oryctolagus cuniculus*
02	Buffalo	*Bubalus bubalis*	09	Hare	*Lepus europaeus*
03	Pork	*Sus scrofa*	10	Chicken	*Gallus gallus*
04	Sheep	*Ovis aries*	11	Turkey	*Meleagris gallopavo*
05	Goat	*Capra hircus*	12	Goose	*Ansa albifrons*
06	Horse	*Equus caballus 1)*	13	Mall. Duck	*Anas platyrhyncos*
07	Donkey	*Equus asinus 1)*	14	Musc. Duck	*Cairina moschata*
			C	Hyb-Contr.	Functional controls (Hybridization + stain)

Figure 14.3 LCD Array Meat 1.6 Test System for meat species identification. The figure shows the spotting pattern of the array while the table lists the capture probes immobilized on each array (Data Sheet MeatSpecies 1.6, V-I-08, Chipron).
Reprinted with permission from Iwobi, A.N., Huber, I., Hauner, G., Miller, A., Busch, U., 2011. Biochip technology for the detection of animal species in meat products. Food Analytical Methods (4), 389–398. Copyright © 2010 Springer Science + Business Media, LLC.

the need for a special scanner and software to analyze results. As a result, a silicon-based optical thin-film biosensor DNA chip was developed for the identification of eight animal species, for which color change results could be interpreted by the naked eye without the need for expensive instruments (Wang et al., 2015).

14.4 Spectroscopic Methods

In recent years, several studies have focused on the possibility of using spectroscopy for meat authentication purposes for several reasons including speed and its nondestructive character, being able to obtain information about the chemical structure of molecules without causing sample alteration. Its simplicity, both in regard to sample preparation and the possibility of being operated by nonexpert technicians, is another advantage. However, an essential point for the successful application of spectroscopy relies on the construction of a suitable spectral database, which should include, ideally, all the possible parameter variations likely to be found in the matrices under evaluation. Based on such databases, useful models can be created, tested, and validated through the use of appropriate multivariate statistical tools. To date, different techniques have been applied to meat authentication studies, including Raman, Fourier-transform infrared (FTIR), near-infrared (NIR), and mid-infrared (MIR) spectroscopy, among others. However, most studies performed so far only comprise the evaluation of raw meats and include, generally, a low number of samples to build up the proposed models. Moreover, several aimed only at differentiating single-species meats, without evaluating the possibility of meat mixtures.

The use of FTIR spectroscopy and partial least square (PLS) calibration was proposed by Rohman et al. (2011) to detect beef meatball adulteration with pork meat. Fat extracted from beef meatball adulterated with 1.0–100.0% (w/w) of pork was analyzed by FTIR spectroscopy in the MIR region (4000–650 cm^{-1}) for quantification purposes. Statistical results, calculated from the prediction samples set as mean difference and standard deviation of difference for determination of accuracy (closeness of agreement between actual data and the predicted data of FTIR results) and precision (measure of the random error in a dataset), indicated that the methodology was appropriate and precise enough to detect adulteration with pork meat. However, the authors stated that beef and pork samples were randomly obtained from five different slaughter houses and that the calibration set comprised pork spiked at concentrations of 1%, 3%, 5%, 10%, and 25% (w/w), but the total number of analyzed samples was not specified. Moreover, instead of using an independent validation dataset, the calibration model was cross-validated using the "leave-one-out" technique by removing one sample spectrum at a time. The same technique was later used by the same research group to detect adulteration of beef meatballs with rat meat (Rahmania et al., 2015). In this work, besides PLS calibration, principal component analysis (PCA) was used, resulting in a clear separation of 100% beef and 100% rat meatballs. For the four commercial samples analyzed in the study, two presented score plots closer to beef meatballs, being classified as beef samples, but PCA analysis failed to classify the other two because they were far away from pure meat samples. Thus, more work is needed to clarify these results, possibly comprising the use of a larger dataset, including also binary meat mixtures.

Raman spectroscopy, combined with chemometrics, has been suggested by Boyacı et al. (2014) for the discrimination of beef and horse meat. Raman spectra were obtained from fat extracted from different parts of horse and beef carcasses and also from laboratory model mixtures containing 25%, 50%, and 75% (w/w) horse meat. A calibration dataset including 14 horse and 25 beef samples was used to create a PCA model based on the preprocessed Raman spectra data. Samples from the validation dataset included four horse and six beef meat samples, which were all correctly identified. The performance of the developed model was then tested using the model meat mixtures adulterated with horse meat, which appeared on the PCA plot separated from the single meat. Even though the authors concluded that the developed Raman method was capable of successfully identifying beef containing 25% of horse meat, they stated that more tests should be performed on a higher number of samples, corroborating the idea that the results from this proof-of-concept study should not be overinterpreted. Raman spectroscopy was also suggested for the classification of frankfurters made of chicken, turkey, and mixed meats (Campos et al., 2014) by the use of training and test sets comprising 38 and 19 samples, respectively. A drawback of this study was the fact that all the samples used to construct the model were commercially acquired, so there was no assurance that they actually contained the meat stated on the labels. Additionally, the proportion of correctly classified samples for the test set was only equal to or higher than 90%, with best results being obtained for the meat mixture frankfurters. A similar approach was performed by Restaino et al. (2011), who aimed at discriminating meat pâtés according to the animal species by means of NIR spectroscopy and chemometrics. Both beef ($n = 5$) and pork pâtés ($n = 7$) were correctly classified using PCA followed by stepwise linear discriminant analysis, while pork and beef mixture pâtés ($n = 18$) only achieved a 72% correct classification. Again, the number of samples used in this study should be considered too low to make any authoritative conclusions. The use of NIR spectroscopy, UV−visible (UV−Vis), and MIR was investigated by Alamprese et al. (2013) for the detection of minced beef adulteration by turkey meat. By comparing the developed PLS regression models in terms of prediction errors, best results tested were obtained with NIR spectra. Nevertheless, considering the root mean square error of prediction values obtained (5.79−9.22), the method was more suited to be used for preliminary sample screening. Mamani-Linares et al. (2012) proposed to use visible and NIR reflectance spectroscopy to discriminate meat and meat juices from beef, llama, and horse. From a total of 79 samples (31 from beef, 21 from llama, and 27 from horse, acquired in different shops to increase sample diversity) most were correctly classified, although a few (six) were classified as uncertain. The authors suggested that broadening the calibration set by including more samples of different years, geographic origin, animal breeds, production systems, and muscles could contribute to develop more robust models.

Recently, the performance of three different methods based on NIR spectroscopy was evaluated for detecting adulteration of pure veal sausages with pork meat or fat, namely, a high-performance Fourier-transform-NIR (FT-NIR) laboratory desktop device, an FT-NIR equipped with a fiber-optic probe suitable for industrial application and a handheld FT-NIR spectrometer for on-site use (Schmutzler et al., 2015). After pretreatment of spectral data, PCA scores were used as input data for support vector machines classification and validation. Both the laboratory setup and the industrial fiber-optic setup were able to detect up to the lowest level of adulteration tested [10% (w/w) pork meat or fat], even when measurements were made through the polymer packaging instead of using a quartz cuvette. Similar results were obtained with the handheld equipment for sausages adulterated with pork meat, though without enabling the detection of pork fat at levels lower than 20% (w/w); measurements through the polymer packaging were possible down to this level.

The use of NIR spectroscopy coupled to image analysis has also been discussed as a fast, low-cost, and proper alternative since hyperspectral imaging integrates both spectroscopic and imaging techniques in one system, providing both spectral and spatial information simultaneously. Kamruzzaman et al. (2013) used NIR hyperspectral imaging for the detection of adulteration in minced lamb meats, as well as to detect the level of horse meat adulteration in minced beef (Kamruzzaman et al., 2015). In each case, the authors selected four important wavelengths that were used to build up a model and an image processing algorithm was developed to apply the model to each pixel in the image. This approach integrates spectroscopy and image analysis, providing both spectral and spatial information simultaneously, thus allowing to detect a particular type of meat and its distribution in the analyzed sample. In both studies, results demonstrated that hyperspectral imaging coupled with multivariate analysis could be successfully applied as a rapid screening technique for meat adulteration detection. Another technique tested for meat authentication is ^{1}H NMR spectroscopy. Jakes et al. (2015) proposed a methodology to distinguish beef from horse meat based on exploiting triglyceride signatures obtained by 60 MHz ^{1}H NMR spectroscopy. The protocol included a simple chloroform extraction and was tested in two different laboratories for horse and beef meat, including freeze-thawed samples. The model developed was then applied to 107 extracts prepared from independent samples resulting in all but one being correctly authenticated. The technique proved to be fast, low cost, and simple to use, being a potential alternative as a high-throughput approach for screening raw meat.

14.5 Final Remarks

Species identification in meats and meat products has been the subject of an increasing number of reports because of its importance in food authentication and to major advances in analytical methods. Both proteins and DNA have been the main target molecules for method development, but the latter have been preferred. Without targeting particular molecules, the spectroscopic methods have also advanced very recently for meat species identification based on Raman, FTIR, NIR, and H^{1} NMR. If, on the one hand, they can offer advantages, such as simple use, speed, low cost, and minimal or no sample extraction/preparation, on the other hand they still lack applicability, mainly to meat mixtures, and mostly rely on chemometrics after constructing suitable spectra databases. Protein-based methods have demonstrated their effectiveness in meat species identification by means of electrophoretic, immunochemical, and chromatographic techniques. Recent advances in MS have prompted the development of proteomic approaches for meat species differentiation based on the high discriminant power of peptide biomarkers, which have enhanced specificity when compared to other protein methods.

DNA-based methods play a crucial role in meat species identification because the advantages of specificity, sensitivity, simplicity, and low cost can be combined with their application to complex and processed food matrices. Species-specific PCR methods targeting mainly mtDNA markers are the most commonly used approaches for meat species detection in a wide range of meat products, covering all the domestic and game meat species used as food. For increased specificity and quantitative purposes, real-time PCR with TaqMan probes have also been extensively applied in meat species identification, being more recently the most reported technique. For high-throughput species identification, DNA chips are emerging as potential tools for multiple-species detection, but still need to improve sensitivity and applicability. Recent technological improvements have revolutionized genomics with the advent of NGS, which has rapidly become a key technology in basic science and only recently applied in meat species identification. The great potential for meat species identification arises from the possibility of identifying more than one species at the same time, including also unexpected or untargeted species, without any previous information about their presence, based on the high-throughput reads and bioinformatics. These advantages are worth exploiting in the near future for forensic food analysis and identifying fraudulent practices in meat and in meat-derived foods.

References

Abdulmawjood, A., Bülte, M., 2002. Identification of ostrich meat by restriction fragment length polymorphism (RFLP) analysis of cytochrome b gene. Journal of Food Science 67, 1688–1691.

Aida, A.A., Che Man, Y.B., Wong, C.M.V.L., Raha, A.R., Son, R., 2005. Analysis of raw meats and fats of pigs using polymerase chain reaction for Halal authentication. Meat Science 69, 47–52.

Alamprese, C., Casale, M., Sinelli, N., Lanteri, S., Casiraghi, E., 2013. Detection of minced beef adulteration with turkey meat by UV-vis, NIR and MIR spectroscopy. LWT-Food Science and Technology 53, 225–232.

Ali, M.E., Al Amin, M., Hamid, S.B.A., Hossain, M.A.M., Mustafa, S., 2015a. Lab-on-a-chip-based PCR-RFLP assay for the confirmed detection of short-length feline DNA in food. Food Additives & Contaminants: Part A 32, 1373–1383.

Ali, M.E., Hashim, U., Dhahi, T.S., Mustafa, S., Man, Y.B.C., Latif, M.A., 2012c. Analysis of pork adulteration in commercial burgers targeting porcine-specific mitochondrial cytochrome B gene by TaqMan probe real-time polymerase chain reaction. Food Analytical Methods 5, 784–794.

Ali, M.E., Hashim, U., Mustafa, S., Che Man, Y., 2012a. Swine-specific PCR-RFLP assay targeting mitochondrial cytochrome b gene for semiquantitative detection of pork in commercial meat products. Food Analytical Methods 5, 613–623.

Ali, M.E., Hashim, U., Mustafa, S., Man, Y.B.C., Adam, T., Humayun, Q., 2014c. Nanobiosensor for the detection and quantification of pork adulteration in meatball formulation. Journal of Experimental Nanoscience 9, 152–160.

Ali, M.E., Hashim, U., Mustafa, S., Man, Y.B.C., Latif, M.A., Islam, K.N., Bakar, M., Rahman, M.M., 2012b. TaqMan real-time polymerase chain reaction for the determination of pork adulteration in meat nuggets. Journal of Food and Nutrition Research 51, 1–12.

Ali, M.E., Hashim, U., Mustafa, S., Man, Y.B.C., Yusop, M.H.M., Kashif, M., Dhahi, T.S., Bari, M.F., Hakim, M.A., Latif, M.A., 2011. Nanobiosensor for detection and quantification of DNA sequences in degraded mixed meats. Journal of Nanomaterials 11. Article ID 781098.

Ali, M.E., Mustafa, S., Hashim, U., Man, Y.B.C., Foo, K.L., 2012d. Nanobioprobe for the determination of pork adulteration in burger formulations. Journal of Nanomaterials 7. Article ID 832387.

Ali, M.E., Rahman, M.M., Hamid, S., Mustafa, S., Bhassu, S., Hashim, U., 2014a. Canine-specific PCR assay targeting cytochrome b gene for the detection of dog meat adulteration in commercial frankfurters. Food Analytical Methods 7, 234–241.

Ali, M.E., Razzak, M.A., Hamid, S., 2014b. Multiplex PCR in species authentication: probability and prospects—a review. Food Analytical Methods 7, 1933–1949.

Ali, M.E., Razzak, M.A., Hamid, S.B.A., Rahman, M.M., Amin, M.A., Rashid, N.R.A., Asing, 2015b. Multiplex PCR assay for the detection of five meat species forbidden in Islamic foods. Food Chemistry 177, 214–224.

Amaral, J.S., Santos, C.G., Melo, V.S., Costa, J., Oliveira, M.B.P.P., Mafra, I., 2015. Identification of duck, partridge, pheasant, quail, chicken and turkey meats by species-specific PCR assays to assess the authenticity of traditional game meat Alheira sausages. Food Control 47, 190–195.

Amaral, J.S., Santos, C.G., Melo, V.S., Oliveira, M.B.P.P., Mafra, I., 2014. Authentication of a traditional game meat sausage (Alheira) by species-specific PCR assays to detect hare, rabbit, red deer, pork and cow meats. Food Research International 60, 140–145.

Arslan, A.L.I., Ilhak, I., Calicioglu, M., Karahan, M., 2005. Identification of meats using random amplified polymorphic DNA (RAPD) technique. Journal of Muscle Foods 16, 37–45.

Asensio, L., Gonzalez, I., Garcia, T., Martin, R., 2008. Determination of food authenticity by enzyme-linked immunosorbent assay (ELISA). Food Control 19, 1–8.

Ballin, N.Z., 2010. Authentication of meat and meat products. Meat Science 86, 577–587.

Ballin, N.Z., Vogensen, F.K., Karlsson, A.H., 2009. Species determination - can we detect and quantify meat adulteration? Meat Science 83, 165–174.

von Bargen, C., Brockmeyer, J., Humpf, H.-U., 2014. Meat authentication: a new HPLC-MS/MS based method for the fast and sensitive detection of horse and pork in highly processed food. Journal of Agricultural and Food Chemistry 62, 9428–9435.

von Bargen, C., Dojahn, J., Waidelich, D., Humpf, H.-U., Brockmeyer, J., 2013. New sensitive high-performance liquid chromatography tandem mass spectrometry method for the detection of horse and pork in Halal beef. Journal of Agricultural and Food Chemistry 61, 11986–11994.

Bertolini, F., Ghionda, M.C., D'Alessandro, E., Geraci, C., Chiofalo, V., Fontanesi, L., 2015. A next generation semiconductor based sequencing approach for the identification of meat species in DNA mixtures. PLoS One 10, e0121701.

Boyaci, I.H., Temiz, H.T., Uysal, R.S., Velioglu, H.M., Yadegari, R.J., Rishkan, M.M., 2014. A novel method for discrimination of beef and horsemeat using Raman spectroscopy. Food Chemistry 148, 37–41.

Buckley, M., Melton, N.D., Montgomery, J., 2013. Proteomics analysis of ancient food vessel stitching reveals >4000-year-old milk protein. Rapid Communications in Mass Spectrometry 27, 531–538.

Buermans, H.P.J., den Dunnen, J.T., 2014. Next generation sequencing technology: advances and applications. Biochimica et Biophysica Acta (BBA) - Molecular Basis of Disease 1842, 1932–1941.

Calvo, J.H., Zaragoza, P., Osta, R., 2001. Random amplified polymorphic DNA fingerprints for identification of species in poultry pâté. Poultry Science 80, 522–524.

Campos, N.D.S., Oliveira, K.S., Almeida, M.R., Stephani, R., de Oliveira, L.F.C., 2014. Classification of frankfurters by FT-Raman spectroscopy and chemometric methods. Molecules 19, 18980–18992.

Chen, A., Wei, C., Chen, G., Zhao, Y., Yang, S., 2015. Duplex PCR approach for the detection and quantification of donkey, horse and mule in raw and heat-processed meat products. International Journal of Food Science & Technology 50, 834–839.

Chen, F.C., Hsieh, Y.H.P., 2000. Detection of pork in heat-processed meat products by monoclonal antibody-based ELISA. Journal of AOAC International 83, 79–85.

Chen, F.C., Hsieh, Y.H.P., Bridgman, R.C., 1998. Monoclonal antibodies to porcine thermal-stable muscle protein for detection of pork in raw and cooked meats. Journal of Food Science 63, 201–205.

Chen, Y., Wu, Y., Wang, J., Xu, B., Zhong, Z., Xia, J., 2009. Identification of cervidae DNA in feedstuff using a real-time polymerase chain reaction method with the new fluorescence intercalating dye EvaGreen. Journal of AOAC International 92, 175–180.

Cheng, X., He, W., Huang, F., Huang, M., Zhou, G., 2014. Multiplex real-time PCR for the identification and quantification of DNA from duck, pig and chicken in Chinese blood curds. Food Research International 60, 30–37.

Chisholm, J., Conyers, C., Booth, C., Lawley, W., Hird, H., 2005. The detection of horse and donkey using real-time PCR. Meat Science 70, 727–732.

Colombo, F., Cardia, A., Renon, P., Cantoni, C., 2004. A note on the identification of *Rupicapra rupicapra* species by polymerase chain reaction product sequencing. Meat Science 66, 753–755.

Colombo, F., Marchisio, E., Pizzini, A., Cantoni, C., 2002. Identification of the goose species (*Anser anser*) in Italian "Mortara" salami by DNA sequencing and a polymerase chain reaction with an original primer pair. Meat Science 61, 291–294.

Conyers, C.M., Allnutt, T.R., Hird, H.J., Kaye, J., Chisholm, J., 2012. Development of a microsatellite-based method for the differentiation of European wild boar (*Sus scrofa scrofa*) from domestic pig breeds (*Sus scrofa domestica*) in food. Journal of Agricultural and Food Chemistry 60, 3341–3347.

Costa, H., Mafra, I., Oliveira, M.B.P.P., Amaral, J.S., 2016a. Game: types and composition. In: Caballero, B., Finglas, P., Toldrá, F. (Eds.), The Encyclopedia of Food and Health, vol. 3. Academic Press, Oxford, pp. 177–183.

Costa, J., Mafra, I., Carrapatoso, I., Oliveira, M.B.P.P., 2016b. Hazelnut allergens: molecular characterisation, detection and clinical relevance. Critical Reviews in Food Science and Nutrition. http://dx.doi.org/10.1080/10408398.2013.826173.

Cota-Rivas, M., Vallejo-Cordoba, B., 1997. Capillary electrophoresis for meat species differentiation. Journal of Capillary Electrophoresis 4, 195–199.

D'Amato, M.E., Alechine, E., Cloete, K.W., Davison, S., Corach, D., 2013. Where is the game? Wild meat products authentication in South Africa: a case study. Investigative Genetics 4, 1–13.

Dalmasso, A., Fontanella, E., Piatti, P., Civera, T., Rosati, S., Bottero, M.T., 2004. A multiplex PCR assay for the identification of animal species in feedstuffs. Molecular and Cellular Probes 18, 81–87.

Dalton, D.L., Kotze, A., 2011. DNA barcoding as a tool for species identification in three forensic wildlife cases in South Africa. Forensic Science International 207, e51–e54.

van Dijk, E.L., Auger, H., Jaszczyszyn, Y., Thermes, C., 2014. Ten years of next-generation sequencing technology. Trends in Genetics 30, 418–426.

Djurdievic, N., Sheu, S.C., Hsieh, Y.H.P., 2005. Quantitative detection of poultry in cooked meat products. Journal of Food Science 70, C586–C593.

Dooley, J.J., Paine, K.E., Garrett, S.D., Brown, H.M., 2004. Detection of meat species using TaqMan real-time PCR assays. Meat Science 68, 431–438.

Doosti, A., Ghasemi Dehkordi, P., Rahimi, E., 2014. Molecular assay to fraud identification of meat products. Journal of Food Science and Technology 51, 148–152.

Druml, B., Cichna-Markl, M., 2014. High resolution melting (HRM) analysis of DNA – its role and potential in food analysis. Food Chemistry 158, 245–254.

Druml, B., Grandits, S., Mayer, W., Hochegger, R., Cichna-Markl, M., 2015a. Authenticity control of game meat products – a single method to detect and quantify adulteration of fallow deer (*Dama dama*), red deer (*Cervus elaphus*) and sika deer (*Cervus nippon*) by real-time PCR. Food Chemistry 170, 508–517.

Druml, B., Hochegger, R., Cichna-Markl, M., 2015b. Duplex real-time PCR assay for the simultaneous determination of the roe deer (*Capreolus capreolus*) and deer (sum of fallow deer, red deer and sika deer) content in game meat products. Food Control 57, 370–376.

Druml, B., Mayer, W., Cichna-Markl, M., Hochegger, R., 2015c. Development and validation of a TaqMan real-time PCR assay for the identification and quantification of roe deer (*Capreolus capreolus*) in food to detect food adulteration. Food Chemistry 178, 319–326.

Drummond, M.G., Brasil, B., Dalsecco, L.S., Brasil, R., Teixeira, L.V., Oliveira, D.A.A., 2013. A versatile real-time PCR method to quantify bovine contamination in buffalo products. Food Control 29, 131–137.

Espiñeira, M., Vieites, J.M., 2015. Detection of dog and cat traces in food, pet food and farm animal feed by real-time PCR. European Food Research and Technology 241, 233–238.

Etienne, M., Jerome, M., Fleurence, J., Rehbein, H., Kundiger, R., Mendes, R., Costa, H., Perez-Martin, R., Pineiro-Gonzalez, C., Craig, A., Mackie, I., Yman, I.M., Ferm, M., Martinez, I., Jessen, F., Smelt, A., Luten, J., 2000. Identification of fish species after cooking by SDS-PAGE and urea IEF: a collaborative study. Journal of Agricultural and Food Chemistry 48, 2653–2658.

European Commission, 2001. Directive 2001/101/EC of 26 November 2001 amending Directive 2000/13/EC of the European Parliament and of the Council on the approximation of 20 March 2000 on the approximation of the laws of the Member States relating to the labelling, presentation and advertising of foodstuffs. Official Journal of the European Communities L310, 19–21.

European Commission, 2002. Regulation (EC) No 178/2002 of the European Parliament and of the Council of 28 January 2002 laying down the general principles and requirements of food law, establishing the European Food Safety Authority and laying down procedures in matters of food safety. Official Journal of the European Communities L 31, 1–24.

Fajardo, V., González, I., Dooley, J., Garret, S., Brown, H.M., García, T., Martín, R., 2009a. Application of polymerase chain reaction–restriction fragment length polymorphism analysis and lab-on-a-chip capillary electrophoresis for the specific identification of game and domestic meats. Journal of the Science of Food and Agriculture 89, 843–847.

Fajardo, V., González, I., López-Calleja, I., Martín, I., Hernández, P.E., Garcia, T., Martín, R., 2006. PCR-RFLP Authentication of meats from red deer (*Cervus elaphus*), fallow deer (*Dama dama*), roe deer (*Capreolus capreolus*), cattle (*Bos taurus*), sheep (*Ovis aries*), and goat (*Capra hircus*). Journal of Agricultural and Food Chemistry 54, 1144–1150.

Fajardo, V., González, I., López-Calleja, I., Martín, I., Rojas, M., Garcia, T., Hernandez, P.E., Martin, R., 2007c. PCR identification of meats from chamois (*Rupicapra rupicapra*), pyrenean ibex (*Capra pyrenaica*), and mouflon (*Ovis ammon*) targeting specific sequences from the mitochondrial D-loop region. Meat Science 76, 644–652.

Fajardo, V., González, I., López-Calleja, I., Martín, I., Rojas, M., Pavón, M.Á., Hernández, P.E., García, T., Martín, R., 2007a. Analysis of mitochondrial DNA for authentication of meats from chamois (*Rupicapra rupicapra*), pyrenean ibex (*Capra pyrenaica*), and mouflon (*Ovis ammon*) by polymerase chain reaction-restriction fragment length polymorphism. Journal of AOAC International 90, 179–186.

Fajardo, V., González, I., López-Calleja, I., Martín, I., Rojas, M., Hernández, P.E., García, T., Martín, R., 2007b. Identification of meats from red deer (*Cervus elaphus*), fallow deer (*Dama dama*), and roe deer (*Capreolus capreolus*) using polymerase chain reaction targeting specific sequences from the mitochondrial 12S rRNA gene. Meat Science 76, 234–240.

Fajardo, V., Gonzalez, I., Martin, I., Rojas, M., Hernandez, P.E., Garcia, T., Martin, R., 2008. Differentiation of European wild boar (*Sus scrofa scrofa*) and domestic swine (*Sus scrofa domestica*) meats by PCR analysis targeting the mitochondrial D-loop and the nuclear melanocortin receptor 1 (MC1R) genes. Meat Science 78, 314–322.
Fajardo, V., Gonzalez, I., Martin, I., Rojas, M., Hernandez, P.E., Garcia, T., Martin, R., 2009b. A LightCycler TaqMan PCR assay for quantitative detection of chamois (*Rupicapra rupicapra*) and pyrenean ibex (*Capra pyrenaica*) in experimental meat mixtures. International Journal of Food Science and Technology 44, 1997–2004.
Fajardo, V., González, I., Rojas, M., García, T., Martín, R., 2010. A review of current PCR-based methodologies for the authentication of meats from game animal species. Trends in Food Science & Technology 21, 408–421.
Fang, X., Zhang, C., 2016. Detection of adulterated murine components in meat products by TaqMan real-time PCR. Food Chemistry 192, 485–490.
Farrokhi, R., Joozani, R.J., 2011. Identification of pork genome in commercial meat extracts for Halal authentication by SYBR green I real-time PCR. International Journal of Food Science and Technology 46, 951–955.
Galimberti, A., De Mattia, F., Losa, A., Bruni, I., Federici, S., Casiraghi, M., Martellos, S., Labra, M., 2013. DNA barcoding as a new tool for food traceability. Food Research International 50, 55–63.
Ghovvati, S., Nassiri, M.R., Mirhoseini, S.Z., Moussavi, A.H., Javadmanesh, A., 2009. Fraud identification in industrial meat products by multiplex PCR assay. Food Control 20, 696–699.
Giaretta, N., Di Giuseppe, A.M.A., Lippert, M., Parente, A., Di Maro, A., 2013. Myoglobin as marker in meat adulteration: a UPLC method for determining the presence of pork meat in raw beef burger. Food Chemistry 141, 1814–1820.
Giovannacci, I., Guizard, C., Carlier, M., Duval, V., Martin, J.L., Demeulemester, C., 2004. Species identification of meat products by ELISA. International Journal of Food Science and Technology 39, 863–867.
Girish, P.S., Anjaneyulu, A.S.R., Viswas, K.N., Anand, M., Rajkumar, N., Shivakumar, B.M., Bhaskar, S., 2004. Sequence analysis of mitochondrial 12S rRNA gene can identify meat species. Meat Science 66, 551–556.
Girish, P.S., Anjaneyulu, A.S.R., Viswas, K.N., Shivakumar, B.M., Anand, M., Patel, M., Sharma, B., 2005. Meat species identification by polymerase chain reaction-restriction fragment length polymorphism (PCR-RFLP) of mitochondrial 12S rRNA gene. Meat Science 70, 107–112.
Girish, P., Anjaneyulu, A., Viswas, K., Santhosh, F., Bhilegaonkar, K., Agarwal, R., Kondaiah, N., Nagappa, K., 2007. Polymerase chain reaction–restriction fragment length polymorphism of mitochondrial 12S rRNA gene: a simple method for identification of poultry meat species. Veterinary Research Communications 31, 447–455.
Ha, J.C., Jung, W.T., Nam, Y.S., Moon, T.W., 2006. PCR identification of ruminant tissue in raw and heat-treated meat meals. Journal of Food Protection 69, 2241–2247.
Haider, N., Nabulsi, I., Al-Safadi, B., 2012. Identification of meat species by PCR-RFLP of the mitochondrial COI gene. Meat Science 90, 490–493.
Haunshi, S., Basumatary, R., Girish, P.S., Doley, S., Bardoloi, R.K., Kumar, A., 2009. Identification of chicken, duck, pigeon and pig meat by species-specific markers of mitochondrial origin. Meat Science 83, 454–459.
Hebert, P.D.N., Cywinska, A., Ball, S.L., de Waard, J.R., 2003. Biological identifications through DNA barcodes. Proceedings of the Royal Society of London. Series B: Biological Sciences 270, 313–321.

Hellberg, R.S.R., Morrissey, M.T., 2011. Advances in DNA-based techniques for the detection of seafood species substitution on the commercial market. Journal of the Association for Laboratory Automation 16, 308–321.

Hernández-Chávez, J.F., González-Córdova, A.F., Rodríguez-Ramírez, R., Vallejo-Cordoba, B., 2011. Development of a polymerase chain reaction and capillary gel electrophoresis method for the detection of chicken or turkey meat in heat-treated pork meat mixtures. Analytica Chimica Acta 708, 149–154.

Hird, H., Chisholm, J., Brown, J., 2005. The detection of commercial duck species in food using a single probe-multiple species-specific primer real-time PCR assay. European Food Research and Technology 221, 559–563.

Hofmann, K., 1985. Principal problems in the identification of meat species of alaughter animals using electrophoretic methods. In: Patterson, R.L.S. (Ed.), Biochemical identification of meat species. Elsevier, London, pp. 9–31.

Horreo, J.L., Ardura, A., Pola, I.G., Martinez, J.L., Garcia-Vazquez, E., 2013. Universal primers for species authentication of animal foodstuff in a single polymerase chain reaction. Journal of the Science of Food and Agriculture 93, 354–361.

Hou, B., Meng, X., Zhang, L., Guo, J., Li, S., Jin, H., 2015. Development of a sensitive and specific multiplex PCR method for the simultaneous detection of chicken, duck and goose DNA in meat products. Meat Science 101, 90–94.

Hung, C.-J., Ho, H.-P., Chang, C.-C., Lee, M.-R., Franje, C.A., Kuo, S.-I., Lee, R.-J., Chou, C.-C., 2011. Electrochemical profiling using copper nanoparticle-plated electrode for identification of ostrich meat and evaluation of meat grades. Food Chemistry 126, 1417–1423.

Ilhak, O.I., Arslan, A., 2007. Identification of meat species by polymerase chain reaction (PCR) technique. Turkish Journal of Veterinary and Animal Sciences 31, 159–163.

Iwobi, A.N., Huber, I., Hauner, G., Miller, A., Busch, U., 2011. Biochip technology for the detection of animal species in meat products. Food Analytical Methods 4, 389–398.

Iwobi, A., Sebah, D., Kraemer, I., Losher, C., Fischer, G., Busch, U., Huber, I., 2015. A multiplex real-time PCR method for the quantification of beef and pork fractions in minced meat. Food Chemistry 169, 305–313.

Jakes, W., Gerdova, A., Defernez, M., Watson, A.D., McCallum, C., Limer, E., Colquhoun, I.J., Williamson, D.C., Kemsley, E.K., 2015. Authentication of beef versus horse meat using 60 MHz ^{1}H NMR spectroscopy. Food Chemistry 175, 1–9.

Jonker, K.M., Tilburg, J., Hagele, G.H., De Boer, E., 2008. Species identification in meat products using real-time PCR. Food Additives and Contaminants 25, 527–533.

Kaiser, K.P., Matheis, G., Kmita-Dürrmann, C., Belitz, H.D., 1980. Qualitative and quantitative analysis of raw binary meat mixtures by means of isoelectric focusing in polyacrylamide gel. Zeitschrift für Lebensmittel-Untersuchung und Forschung 171, 415–419.

Kamruzzaman, M., Makino, Y., Oshita, S., Liu, S., 2015. Assessment of visible near-infrared hyperspectral imaging as a tool for detection of horsemeat adulteration in minced beef. Food and Bioprocess Technology 8, 1054–1062.

Kamruzzaman, M., Sun, D.W., El Masry, G., Allen, P., 2013. Fast detection and visualization of minced lamb meat adulteration using NIR hyperspectral imaging and multivariate image analysis. Talanta 103, 130–136.

Kane, D.E., Hellberg, R.S., 2016. Identification of species in ground meat products sold on the U.S. commercial market using DNA-based methods. Food Control 59, 158–163.

Karabasanavar, N.S., Singh, S.P., Kumar, D., Shebannavar, S.N., 2014. Detection of pork adulteration by highly-specific PCR assay of mitochondrial D-loop. Food Chemistry 145, 530–534.

Karabasanavar, N., Singh, S.P., Kumar, D., Shebannavar, S., 2013. Development and application of highly specific PCR for detection of chicken (*Gallus gallus*) meat adulteration. European Food Research and Technology 236, 129–134.

Kesmen, Z., Gulluce, A., Sahin, F., Yetim, H., 2009. Identification of meat species by TaqMan-based real-time PCR assay. Meat Science 82, 444–449.

Kesmen, Z., Sahin, F., Yetim, H., 2007. PCR assay for the identification of animal species in cooked sausages. Meat Science 77, 649–653.

Kim, H., Shelef, L.A., 1986. Characterization and identification of raw beef, pork, chicken and turkey meats by electrophoretic patterns of their sarcoplasmic proteins. Journal of Food Science 51, 731–735.

Köppel, R., Daniels, M., Felderer, N., Brünen-Nieweler, C., 2013. Multiplex real-time PCR for the detection and quantification of DNA from duck, goose, chicken, turkey and pork. European Food Research and Technology 236, 1093–1098.

Kotoura, S.Y., Murakami-Yamaguchi, K., Kizu, Nakamura, M., Fuchu, H., Miake, K., Sugiyama, M., Narita, H., 2012. Establishment of a sandwich ELISA for the determination of beef content in processed foods by using monoclonal antibodies to myoglobin. Food and Agricultural Immunology 23, 289–301.

Kumar, D., Singh, S.P., Karabasanavar, N., Singh, R., Umapathi, V., 2014. Authentication of beef, carabeef, chevon, mutton and pork by a PCR-RFLP assay of mitochondrial cytb gene. Journal of Food Science and Technology 51, 3458–3463.

Laube, I., Zagon, J., Spiegelberg, A., Butschke, A., Kroh, L.W., Broll, H., 2007. Development and design of a 'ready-to-use' reaction plate for a PCR-based simultaneous detection of animal species used in foods. International Journal of Food Science & Technology 42, 9–17.

Liu, L.H., Chen, F.C., Dorsey, J.L., Hsieh, Y.H.P., 2006. Sensitive monoclonal antibody-based sandwich ELISA for the detection of porcine skeletal muscle in meat and feed products. Journal of Food Science 71, M1–M6.

López, B.L., Binaghi, J.M., Greco, B.C., Mambrín, C.M., Valencia, E.M., 2011. Identificación de especies cárnicas en productos cárnicos cocidos: utilización de SDS-PAGE como método de screening. Revista Chilena de Nutrición 38, 187–196.

López-Andreo, M., Aldeguer, M., Guillén, I., Gabaldón, J.A., Puyet, A., 2012. Detection and quantification of meat species by qPCR in heat-processed food containing highly fragmented DNA. Food Chemistry 134, 518–523.

Luo, A., Zhang, A., Ho, S.Y., Xu, W., Zhang, Y., Shi, W., Cameron, S.L., Zhu, C., 2011. Potential efficacy of mitochondrial genes for animal DNA barcoding: a case study using eutherian mammals. BMC Genomics 12, 1–13.

Maede, D., 2006. A strategy for molecular species detection in meat and meat products by PCR-RFLP and DNA sequencing using mitochondrial and chromosomal genetic sequences. European Food Research and Technology 224, 209–217.

Mafra, I., Ferreira, I.M.P.L.V.O., Oliveira, M.B.P.P., 2008. Food authentication by PCR-based methods. European Food Research and Technology 227, 649–665.

Mamani-Linares, L.W., Gallo, C., Alomar, D., 2012. Identification of cattle, llama and horse meat by near infrared reflectance or transflectance spectroscopy. Meat Science 90, 378–385.

Mane, B.G., Mendiratta, S.K., Tiwari, A.K., 2009. Polymerase chain reaction assay for identification of chicken in meat and meat products. Food Chemistry 116, 806–810.

Mane, B.G., Mendiratta, S.K., Tiwari, A.K., 2012a. Beef specific polymerase chain reaction assay for authentication of meat and meat products. Food Control 28, 246–249.

Mane, B.G., Mendiratta, S.K., Tiwari, A.K., Bhilegaokar, K.N., 2012b. Detection of adulteration of meat and meat products with buffalo meat employing polymerase chain reaction assay. Food Analytical Methods 5, 296–300.

Martín, I., García, T., Fajardo, V., López-Calleja, I., Hernández, P.E., González, I., Martín, R., 2007a. Species-specific PCR for the identification of ruminant species in feedstuffs. Meat Science 75, 120–127.

Martín, I., García, T., Fajardo, V., López-Calleja, I., Rojas, M., Hernández, P.E., González, I., Martín, R., 2007b. Mitochondrial markers for the detection of four duck species and the specific identification of Muscovy duck in meat mixtures using the polymerase chain reaction. Meat Science 76, 721–729.

Martín, I., García, T., Fajardo, V., Rojas, M., Pegels, N., Hernández, P.E., González, I., Martín, R., 2009. Polymerase chain reaction detection of rabbit DNA in food and animal feed. World Rabbit Science 17, 27–34.

Matsunaga, T., Chikuni, K., Tanabe, R., Muroya, S., Nakai, H., Shibata, K., Yamada, J., Shinmura, Y., 1998. Determination of mitochondrial cytochrome b gene sequence for red deer (*Cervus elaphus*) and the differentiation of closely related deer meats. Meat Science 49, 379–385.

Matsunaga, T., Chikuni, K., Tanabe, R., Muroya, S., Shibata, K., Yamada, J., Shinmura, Y., 1999. A quick and simple method for the identification of meat species and meat products by PCR assay. Meat Science 51, 143–148.

Meyer, R., Candrian, U., Lüthy, J., 1994. Detection of pork in heated meat products by the polymerase chain reaction. Journal of AOAC International 77, 617–622.

Meyer, R., Höfelein, C., Lüthy, J., Candrian, U., 1995. Polymerase chain reaction-restriction fragment length polymorphism analysis: a simple method for species identification in food. Journal of AOAC International 78, 1542–1551.

Montiel-Sosa, J.F., Ruiz-Pesini, E., Montoya, J., Roncalés, P., López-Pérez, M.J., Pérez-Martos, A., 2000. Direct and highly species-specific detection of pork meat and fat in meat products by PCR amplification of mitochondrial DNA. Journal of Agricultural and Food Chemistry 48, 2829–2832.

Montowska, M., Pospiech, E., 2007. Species identification of meat by electrophoretic methods. Acta Scientiarum Polonorum Technologia Alimentaria 6, 5–16.

Montowska, M., Pospiech, E., 2011a. Authenticity determination of meat and meat products on the protein and DNA basis. Food Reviews International 27, 84–100.

Montowska, M., Pospiech, E., 2011b. Differences in two-dimensional gel electrophoresis patterns of skeletal muscle myosin light chain isoforms between *Bos taurus*, *Sus scrofa* and selected poultry species. Journal of the Science of Food and Agriculture 91, 2449–2456.

Montowska, M., Pospiech, E., 2012a. Is authentication of regional and traditional food made of meat possible? Critical Reviews in Food Science and Nutrition 52, 475–487.

Montowska, M., Pospiech, E., 2012b. Myosin light chain isoforms retain their species-specific electrophoretic mobility after processing, which enables differentiation between six species: 2DE analysis of minced meat and meat products made from beef, pork and poultry. Proteomics 12, 2879–2889.

Montowska, M., Alexander, M.R., Tucker, G.A., Barrett, D.A., 2014b. Rapid detection of peptide markers for authentication purposes in raw and cooked meat using ambient liquid extraction surface analysis mass spectrometry. Analytical Chemistry 86, 10257–10265.

Montowska, M., Alexander, M.R., Tucker, G.A., Barrett, D.A., 2015. Authentication of processed meat products by peptidomic analysis using rapid ambient mass spectrometry. Food Chemistry 187, 297–304.

Montowska, M., Rao, W., Alexander, M.R., Tucker, G.A., Barrett, D.A., 2014a. Tryptic digestion coupled with ambient desorption electrospray ionization and liquid extraction surface analysis mass spectrometry enabling identification of skeletal muscle proteins in mixtures and distinguishing between beef, pork, horse, chicken, and turkey meat. Analytical Chemistry 6 (86), 4479–4487.

Mousavi, S.M., Jahed Khaniki, G., Eskandari, S., Rabiei, M., Mirab Samiee, S., Mehdizadeh, M., 2015. Applicability of species-specific polymerase chain reaction for fraud identification in raw ground meat commercially sold in Iran. Journal of Food Composition and Analysis 40, 47–51.

Murugaiah, C., Noor, Z.M., Mastakim, M., Bilung, L.M., Selamat, J., Radu, S., 2009. Meat species identification and Halal authentication analysis using mitochondrial DNA. Meat Science 83, 57–61.

Natonek-Wiśniewska, M., Krzyścin, P., Piestrzyńska-Kajtoch, A., 2013. The species identification of bovine, porcine, ovine and chicken components in animal meals, feeds and their ingredients, based on COX I analysis and ribosomal DNA sequences. Food Control 34, 69–78.

Nau, F., Désert, C., Cochet, M.-F., Pasco, M., Jan, S., Baron, F., Lagarrigue, S., Guérin-Dubiard, C., 2009. Detection of turkey, duck, and guinea fowl egg in hen egg products by species-specific PCR. Food Analytical Methods 2, 231–238.

Navarro, E., Serrano-Heras, G., Castaño, M.J., Solera, J., 2015. Real-time PCR detection chemistry. Clinica Chimica Acta 439, 231–250.

Nejad, F.P., Tafvizi, F., Ebrahimi, M.T., Hosseni, S.E., 2014. Optimization of multiplex PCR for the identification of animal species using mitochondrial genes in sausages. European Food Research and Technology 239, 533–541.

Nixon, G.J., Wilkes, T.M., Burns, M.J., 2015. Development of a real-time PCR approach for the relative quantitation of horse DNA. Analytical Methods 7, 8590–8596.

Pascoal, A., Prado, M., Calo, P., Cepeda, A., Barros-Velázquez, J., 2005. Detection of bovine DNA in raw and heat-processed foodstuffs, commercial foods and specific risk materials by a novel specific polymerase chain reaction method. European Food Research and Technology 220, 444–450.

Pascoal, A., Prado, M., Castro, J., Cepeda, A., Barros-Velásquez, J., 2004. Survey of authenticity of meat species in food products subjected to different technological processes, by means of PCR-RFLP analysis. European Food Research and Technology 218, 306–312.

Pegels, N., Garcia, T., Martin, R., Gonzalez, I., 2015. Market analysis of food and feed products for detection of horse DNA by a TaqMan real-time PCR. Food Analytical Methods 8, 489–498.

Pegels, N., Lopez-Calleja, I., Garcia, T., Martin, R., Gonzalez, I., 2013. Detection of rabbit and hare processed material in compound feeds by TaqMan real-time PCR. Food Additives and Contaminants Part A-Chemistry Analysis Control Exposure & Risk Assessment 30, 771–779.

Pereira, F., Carneiro, J., Amorim, A., 2008. Identification of species with DNA-based technology: current progress and challenges. Recent Patents on DNA & Gene Sequences 2, 187–200.

Pfeiffer, I., Burger, J., Brenig, B., 2004. Diagnostic polymorphisms in the mitochondrial cytochrome b gene allow discrimination between cattle, sheep, goat, roe buck and deer by PCR-RFLP. BMC Genetics 5, 30.

Quinto, C.A., Tinoco, R., Hellberg, R.S., 2016. DNA barcoding reveals mislabeling of game meat species on the US commercial market. Food Control 59, 386–392.

Rahman, M.M., Abd Hamid, S.B., Basirun, W.J., Bhassu, S., Rashid, N.R.A., Mustafa, S., Desa, M.N.M., Ali, M.E., 2016. TaqMan probe real-time polymerase chain reaction assay for the quantification of canine DNA in chicken nugget. Food Additives and Contaminants Part A - Chemistry Analysis Control Exposure & Risk Assessment 33, 10–18.

Rahman, M.M., Ali, M.E., Hamid, S., Bhassu, S., Mustafa, S., Al Amin, M., Razzak, M.A., 2015. Lab-on-a-Chip PCR-RFLP Assay for the detection of canine DNA in burger formulations. Food Analytical Methods 8, 1598–1606.

Rahmania, H., Sudjadi, Rohman, A., 2015. The employment of FTIR spectroscopy in combination with chemometrics for analysis of rat meat in meatball formulation. Meat Science 100, 301–305.

Rastogi, G., Dharne, M.S., Walujkar, S., Kumar, A., Patole, M.S., Shouche, Y.S., 2007. Species identification and authentication of tissues of animal origin using mitochondrial and nuclear markers. Meat Science 76, 666–674.

Restaino, E., Fassio, A., Cozzolino, D., 2011. Discrimination of meat patés according to the animal species by means of near infrared spectroscopy and chemometrics. CyTA – Journal of Food 9, 210–213.

Ripp, F., Krombholz, C.F., Liu, Y., Weber, M., Schäfer, A., Schmidt, B., Köppel, R., Hankeln, T., 2014. All-Food-Seq (AFS): a quantifiable screen for species in biological samples by deep DNA sequencing. BMC Genomics 15, 1–11.

Rodríguez, M.A., García, T., González, I., Asensio, L., Hernández, P.E., Martín, R., 2004. PCR identification of beef, sheep, goat, and pork in raw and heat-treated meat mixtures. Journal of Food Protection 67, 172–177.

Rodríguez, M.A., García, T., González, I., Asensio, L., Hernández, P.E., Martín, R., 2003a. Qualitative PCR for the detection of chicken and pork adulteration in goose and mule duck foie gras. Journal of the Science of Food and Agriculture 83, 1176–1181.

Rodríguez, M.A., García, T., González, I., Asensio, L., Mayoral, B., López-Calleja, I., Hernández, P.E., Martín, R., 2003b. Identification of goose, mule duck, chicken, turkey, and swine in foie gras species-specific polymerase chain reaction. Journal of Agricultural and Food Chemistry 51, 1524–1529.

Rodriguez, M.A., Garcia, T., Gonzalez, I., Hernandez, P.E., Martin, R., 2005. TaqMan real-time PCR for the detection and quantitation of pork in meat mixtures. Meat Science 70, 113–120.

Rohman, A., Sismindari, Erwanto, Y., Man, Y.B.C., 2011. Analysis of pork adulteration in beef meatball using Fourier transform infrared (FTIR) spectroscopy. Meat Science 88, 91–95.

Rojas, M., González, I., Fajardo, V., Martín, I., Hernández, P.E., García, T., Martín, R., 2009a. Identification of raw and heat-processed meats from game bird species by polymerase chain reaction-restriction fragment length polymorphism of the mitochondrial D-loop region. Poultry Science 88, 669–679.

Rojas, M., González, I., Fajardo, V., Martín, I., Hernández, P.E., García, T., Martín, R., 2009b. Authentication of meats from quail (*Coturnix coturnix*), pheasant (*Phasianus colchicus*), partridge (*Alectoris* spp.), and guinea fowl (*Numida meleagris*) using polymerase chain reaction targeting specific sequences from the mitochondrial 12S rRNA gene. Food Control 20, 896–902.

Rojas, M., González, I., Fajardo, V., Martín, I., Hernández, P.E., García, T., Martín, R., 2008. Polymerase chain reaction-restriction fragment length polymorphism authentication of raw meats from game birds. Journal of AOAC International 91, 1416–1422.

Rojas, M., González, I., Pavón, M.A., Pegels, N., Hernández, P.E., García, T., Martín, R., 2010. Polymerase chain reaction assay for verifying the labeling of meat and commercial meat products from game birds targeting specific sequences from the mitochondrial D-loop region. Poultry Science 89, 1021–1032.

Rojas, M., González, I., Pavón, M.Á., Pegels, N., Hernández, P.E., García, T., Martín, R., 2011. Development of a real-time PCR assay to control the illegal trade of meat from protected capercaillie species (*Tetrao urogallus*). Forensic Science International 210, 133–138.
Safdar, M., Abasıyanık, M.F., 2013. Development of fast multiplex real-time PCR assays based on EvaGreen fluorescence dye for identification of beef and soybean origins in processed sausages. Food Research International 54, 1652–1656.
Safdar, M., Junejo, Y., 2015. A multiplex-conventional PCR assay for bovine, ovine, caprine and fish species identification in feedstuffs: highly sensitive and specific. Food Control 50, 190–194.
Safdar, M., Junejo, Y., 2016. The development of a hexaplex-conventional PCR for identification of six animal and plant species in foodstuffs. Food Chemistry 192, 745–749.
Safdar, M., Junejo, Y., Arman, K., Abasıyanık, M.F., 2014. A highly sensitive and specific tetraplex PCR assay for soybean, poultry, horse and pork species identification in sausages: development and validation. Meat Science 98, 296–300.
Santos, C.G., Melo, V.S., Amaral, J.S., Estevinho, L., Oliveira, M.B.P.P., Mafra, I., 2012. Identification of hare meat by a species-specific marker of mitochondrial origin. Meat Science 90, 836–841.
Schmutzler, M., Beganovic, A., Boehler, G., Huck, C.W., 2015. Methods for detection of pork adulteration in veal product based on FT-NIR spectroscopy for laboratory, industrial and on-site analysis. Food Control 57, 258–267.
Sentandreu, M.A., Sentandreu, E., 2011. Peptide biomarkers as a way to determine meat authenticity. Meat Science 89, 280–285.
Sentandreu, M.A., Sentandreu, E., 2014. Authenticity of meat products: tools against fraud. Food Research International 60, 19–29.
Sentandreu, M.A., Fraser, P.D., Halket, J., Patel, R., Bramley, P.M., 2010. A proteomic-based approach for detection of chicken in meat mixes. Journal of Proteome Research 9, 3374–3383.
Skarpeid, H.J., Kvaal, K., Hildrum, K.I., 1998. Identification of animal species in ground meat mixtures by multivariate analysis of isoelectric focusing protein profiles. Electrophoresis 19, 3103–3109.
Slattery, W.J., Sinclair, A.J., 1983. Differentiation of meat according to species by the electrophoretic separation of muscle lactate dehydrogenase and esterase isoenzymes and isoelectric focusing of soluble muscle proteins. Australian Veterinary Journal 60, 47–51.
Soares, S., Amaral, J.S., Mafra, I., Oliveira, M.B.P.P., 2010. Quantitative detection of poultry meat adulteration with pork by a duplex PCR assay. Meat Science 85, 531–536.
Soares, S., Amaral, J.S., Oliveira, M.B.P.P., Mafra, I., 2013. A SYBR Green real-time PCR assay to detect and quantify pork meat in processed poultry meat products. Meat Science 94, 115–120.
Stamoulis, P., Stamatis, C., Sarafidou, T., Mamuris, Z., 2010. Development and application of molecular markers for poultry meat identification in food chain. Food Control 21, 1061–1065.
Taylor, S.L., Nordlee, J.A., Niemann, L.M., Lambrecht, D.M., 2009. Allergen immunoassays. Considerations for use of naturally incurred standards. Analytical and Bioanalytical Chemistry 395, 83–92.
Tillmar, A.O., Dell'Amico, B., Welander, J., Holmlund, G., 2013. A universal method for species identification of mammals utilizing next generation sequencing for the analysis of DNA mixtures. PLoS One 8, e83761.
Tisza, Á., Csikós, Á., Simon, Á., Gulyás, G., Jávor, A., Czeglédi, L., 2016. Identification of poultry species using polymerase chain reaction-single strand conformation polymorphism

(PCR-SSCP) and capillary electrophoresis-single strand conformation polymorphism (CE-SSCP) methods. Food Control 59, 430–438.

Tobe, S.S., Linacre, A.M.T., 2008. A multiplex assay to identify 18 European mammal species from mixtures using the mitochondrial cytochrome b gene. Electrophoresis 29, 340–347.

Vallejo-Cordoba, B., Cota-Rivas, M., 1998. Meat species identification by linear discriminant analysis of capillary electrophoresis protein profiles. Journal of Capillary Electrophoresis 5, 171–175.

Vallejo-Cordoba, B., Rodríguez-Ramírez, R., González-Córdova, A.F., 2010. Capillary electrophoresis for bovine and ostrich meat characterisation. Food Chemistry 120, 304–307.

Walker, J.A., Hughes, D.A., Anders, B.A., Shewale, J., Sinha, S.K., Batzer, M.A., 2003. Quantitative intra-short interspersed element PCR species-specific DNA identification. Analytical Biochemistry 316, 259–269.

Wang, W., Chen, K., Xu, C., 2006. DNA quantification using EvaGreen and a real-time PCR instrument. Analytical Biochemistry 356, 303–305.

Wang, W., Zhu, Y., Chen, Y., Xu, X., Zhou, G., 2015. Rapid visual detection of eight meat species using optical thin-film biosensor chips. Journal of AOAC International 98, 410–414.

Wolf, C., Rentsch, J., Hübner, P., 1999. PCR-RFLP Analysis of mitochondrial DNA: a reliable method for species identification. Journal of Agricultural and Food Chemistry 47, 1350–1355.

Wu, Y., Yang, Y., Wang, B., Liu, M., Han, J., Chen, Y., 2015. A real-time PCR method targeting camel ingredient for food authentication. Journal of AOAC International 98, 1640–1644.

Yang, S., Li, C., Wu, Q., Zhu, C., Xu, X., Zhou, G., 2014. High-resolution melting analysis: a promising molecular method for meat traceability. European Food Research and Technology 239, 473–480.

Yusop, M.H.M., Mustafa, S., Man, Y.B.C., Omar, A.R., Mokhtar, N.F.K., 2012. Detection of raw pork targeting porcine-specific mitochondrial cytochrome b gene by molecular beacon probe real-time polymerase chain reaction. Food Analytical Methods 5, 422–429.

Zha, D., Xing, X., Yang, F., 2010. A multiplex PCR assay for fraud identification of deer products. Food Control 21, 1402–1407.

Zha, D.-M., Xing, X.-M., Yang, F.-H., 2011. Rapid identification of deer products by multiplex PCR assay. Food Chemistry 129, 1904–1908.

Zhang, C., 2013. Semi-nested multiplex PCR enhanced method sensitivity of species detection in further-processed meats. Food Control 31, 326–330.

Zhang, C.L., Fowler, M.R., Scott, N.W., Lawson, G., Slater, A., 2007. A TaqMan real-time PCR system for the identification and quantification of bovine DNA in meats, milks and cheeses. Food Control 18, 1149–1158.

Zvereva, E.A., Kovalev, L.I., Ivanov, A.V., Kovaleva, M.A., Zherdev, A.V., Shishkin, S.S., Lisitsyn, A.B., Chernukha, I.M., Dzantiev, B.B., 2015. Enzyme immunoassay and proteomic characterization of troponin I as a marker of mammalian muscle compounds in raw meat and some meat products. Meat Science 105, 46–52.

Advances in Authenticity Testing for Fish Speciation

15

M. Espiñeira, F. Lago
ANFACO-CECOPESCA, Vigo, Spain

Chapter Outline

15.1 Introduction

The demand for transparency in the food chain is growing because consumers demand products that are safe, healthy, and of high and consistent quality. They demand guarantees for important food characteristics, calling for transparency and an effective response if a problem arises (Trienekens et al., 2012). For this reason among others, the concept of traceability has been introduced in the food sector. Traceability, intended to guarantee food quality and sanitary security, is defined in European Regulation 178/2002 as "the ability to trace and follow a food, feed, food-producing animal or substance intended to be, or expected to be incorporated into a food or feed, through all stages of production, processing and distribution" (EC, 2002).

Consequently, development of fast and economical traceability systems is necessary. These systems allow producers ability to control their production process, from acceptance of raw material through processing to release of commercial product, and at the same time guarantee to consumers that the products they have at their disposal on the markets are reliable and of the quality that they expect.

Availability of information to any interested person improves transparency in process management and of the market. All of this benefits the entire production chain, contributes to greater assurance around quality and product certification, and helps prevent consumer fraud.

One of the main supports in guaranteeing traceability of a product through the production and marketing chain is verification of product authenticity. However, to fully understand this concept, the differentiation between different but related terms such as identification, authentication, and species detection is essential. Identification refers to the determination of the fish species present in the sample and answers the question: what species is this? Authentication relates to confirmation that the species present is actually that which is declared on a label answers the question: is this sample the stated species or not? Finally, detection confirms the presence or absence of the fish species of interest and answers the question: is this species present? Verification of the authenticity of fishery products essentially consists of checking the identity of the fish species that are contained in those products.

Fraudulent and deceptive practices involving, for example, the whole or partial substitution of a high-value species with a similar lower-value one is facilitated by great variability in the prices of fish species as well as in the quality of products made from them. Because of this, it is important that both the relevant regulatory authorities and the commercial environment protect consumer interests, ensuring the quality and reliability of products that reach the market. To this end, the European Union (EU) has established Regulation 1379/2013 on the common organization of the markets in fishery and aquaculture products (EU, 2013). This regulation includes standards for the proper labeling of fishery products and mandatory information regarding labeling of fishery products to be marketed in the EU, such as the commercial designation of the species, its scientific name, and the capture or farming zone, among others.

To assess the veracity of fish product labeling, it is necessary to show that the product is marketed under the name of the fish species that it really and also contains the raw material and the ingredient percentages that are declared on the product label. The growth of international trade and the corresponding increase in the number of potentially marketable species, as well as the increase in the number of processing methods, necessitate the development of fast and effective methods to verify species identification in the fishery products.

For years methodologies based on morphological and specific characteristics have been used to identify fish species. In the case of products involving minimal manipulation, such as those that are fresh, chilled, or frozen, species identification based on morphological characters is relatively easy. However, those that have undergone various transformation processes lose these characteristics and their identification by morphological inspection is not possible. This has led to the development of techniques based on intrinsic components of fish tissues, such as proteins and nucleic acids (Lago et al., 2014).

15.2 Methods Used in Fish Speciation

15.2.1 Morphological Methods

Morphological methods for identifying fish species are based on the search for specific external characteristics. Over many years, morphological identification keys for different taxonomic seafood groups have been developed; these keys combine a multitude of features, such as body shape, skin color, size of the specimen, number and position of the fins, size and shape of the flakes, or several measurements on different parts of the body (Fig. 15.1). A sequential combination of these morphological features allows the assignment of a specimen to one species or another on the basis of identification keys.

Reference keys for the identification of fish species are published by the Food and Agriculture Organisation of the United Nations (FAO). These publications include general information about the species, scientific nomenclature, common names, distinguishing features, geographic distribution, commercial importance, and lists of

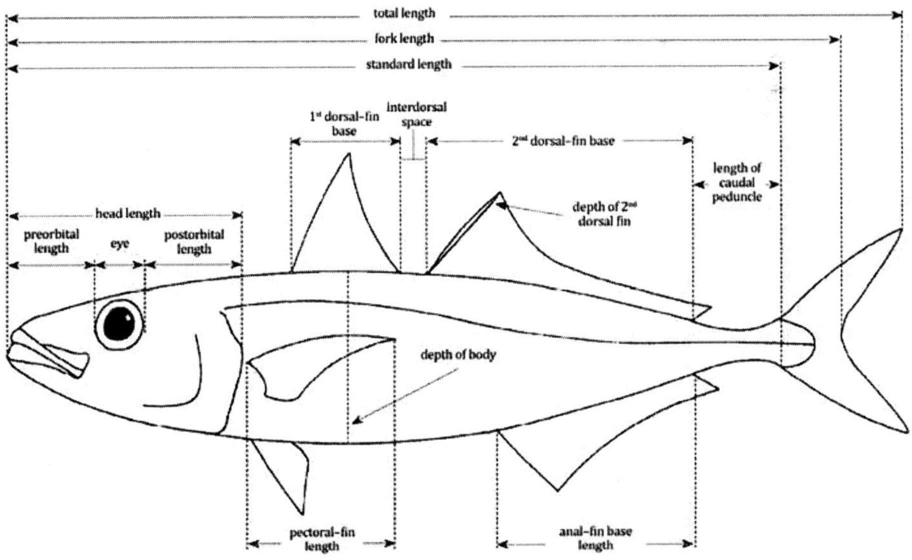

Figure 15.1 Standard measures used in morphological identification of species.
Food and Agriculture Organisation of the United Nations, 1999. The Living Marine Resources of the Western Central Pacific. In: Carpenter, K.E., Niem, V.H., FAO Species Identification Guide for Fishery Purposes vol. 3, pp. 1541, Rome, Italy. http://www.fao.org. Reproduced with permission.

relevant literature. Access to these keys is free through the Website of the FAO: http://www.fao.org/fishery/fishfinder/publications/en.

When a new species of fish is described, new morphological identification keys are identified or maybe existing keys are updated. Generally, keys are focused on a taxonomic group or they are associated with a specific geographical area. A recent example of such work is reported by Lavoué in 2014, who described two new species of African electric fish from the Congo River basin. A key for *Petrocephalus* species from this geographic zone is included in the work (Lavoué and Sullivan, 2014). Another example is the work of Jeong in 2008 who described a new species of skate from China while a key for species of *Dipturus* found in the western North Pacific is also included (Jeong and Nakabo, 2008).

Recent advances in morphological identification are provided by the introduction of new information technologies that represent better dissemination and access to information for all audiences. In this sense, some Websites are focused on providing comprehensive information on the morphology of species of fish, including diagnostic feature cards and visual identification cards (www.fishbase.org; www.pescabase.org; http://www.fao.org). These pages also offer the ability to access morphological identification keys (http://www.fishbase.org/keys/allkeys.php) and even give online access to identification tools (Fig. 15.2).

Advances in software programs have allowed the integration of tools of morphometric measurements and even allowed the coupling of digital gauges to facilitate measurements and their incorporation into the database, after which a possible species

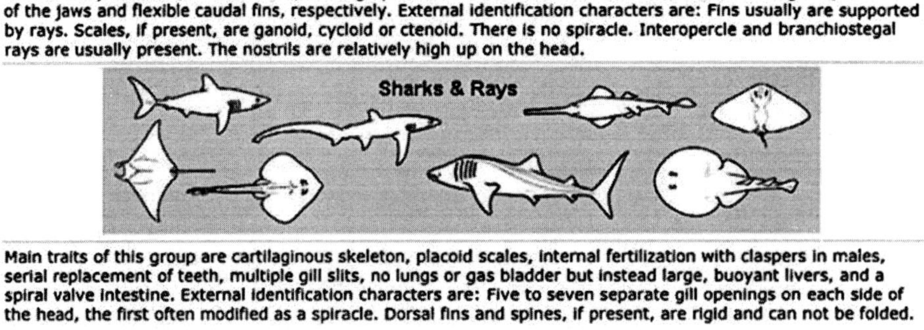

Figure 15.2 Morphological identification tool using physical characteristics.
FishBase, reprinted with permission from FishBase (www.fishbase.org).

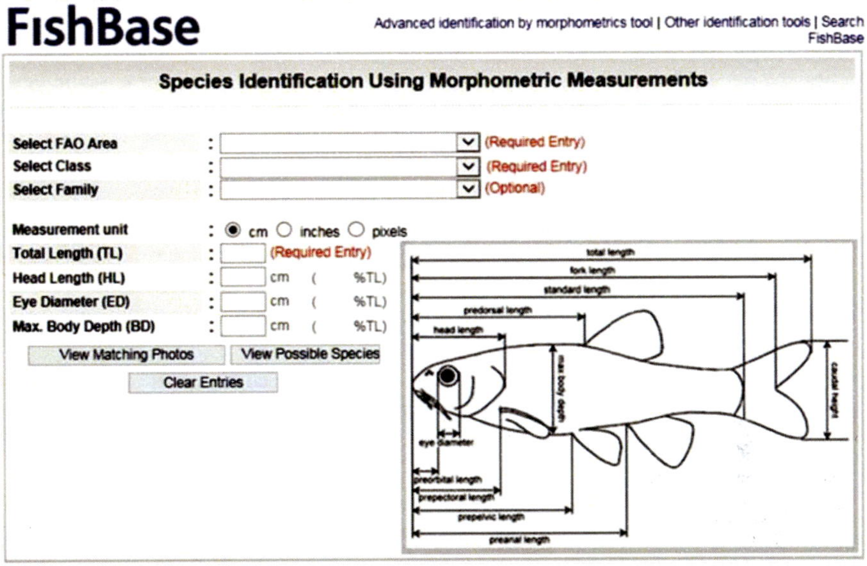

Figure 15.3 Morphological identification tool using morphometric parameters.
Source: FishBase, reprinted with permission from FishBase (www.fishbase.org).

identification is obtained. An example of one species determination tool based on morphometric measurements is found on the Website www.fishbase.org (Fig. 15.3).

Identification of fish species based on morphological characteristics, either through identification using cards with specific descriptions or by morphometric determinations, remains a daily work tool. Companies that produce and market fish products use these tools to ensure that the raw material acquired in the form of whole specimens corresponds to the species demanded. Generally, cards with distinguishing morphological characteristics of the species of interest are used for identification of whole specimens.

All these advances make morphological identification of species one of the most widely used methods of identification for whole specimens of adult fish. However, in early stages of development, morphological identification is very complex because great similarity between some species exists. Therefore, fish in these early developmental stages require appropriate optical systems and specialized personnel for proper identification.

Major drawbacks of morphological fish species identification arise from the high diversity and morphological plasticity of this taxonomic group. Even with whole specimens, there may be a large interspecific variation; additionally, differences between different species can be very small. Identification of a fish specimen based on its physical characteristics is difficult in both such cases (Strauss and Bond, 1990).

Another disadvantage of this fish identification system is the inevitable loss of morphological characteristics during processing treatments (for example, canning or filleting). This makes identification using morphology difficult or even impossible, prompting the development of alternative methods for fish species identification that are independent of morphological features (Teletchea, 2009).

15.2.2 Protein-based Methods

The first protein-based identification methods to be applied to fish species were electrophoresis, isoelectric focusing, and liquid chromatography. All are based on differences in size or charge of the proteins of which fish muscle tissue is comprised; each species exhibits a particular protein profile. Therefore, comparison of protein profiles obtained against a collection of standard species profiles allows identification of the test species (Lundstrom, 1981; Mackie et al., 1999; Osman et al., 1987; Rehbein, 1990).

Subsequently, immunological methods, based on the specificity of the interaction between antibodies and protein antigens in fish species, emerged as an alternative method of protein differentiation applicable to species identification. It is in these particular methodologies that recent advances have been made.

15.2.2.1 Immunological Methods

In the application of immunological methods for fish species identification, antibodies generated against a particular protein or group of proteins of a species are used for its identification. Only in the presence of the target species does antigen–antibody binding take place, a binding that will lead to a detectable signal in the relevant assay.

Recent advances in immunological methods for species identification pursue simplicity and flexibility in the development of assays. Thus, enzyme-linked immunosorbent assay (ELISA) and immunochromatography strip tests are two of the most important to have emerged.

ELISA

One of the most commonly used immunological methods is the ELISA, which consists of the coupling of an enzymatic reaction to the specific binding of antigen and antibody. Thus, the assay combines high specificity, provided by the specific binding of antigen and antibody, with high sensitivity, provided by the enzyme amplification. Enzymatic activity ensures that even a minimal binding of antigen to the appropriate antibody triggers a reaction that generally produces an observable and measurable chromogenic product. Reading of results is performed qualitatively by the observed presence or absence of signal, or quantitatively by use of an optical density reader or a fluorescence detector, depending on the product of the enzymatic reaction. Quantitation is performed from a standard curve obtained from serial dilutions of known concentration of the target analyte (Fig. 15.4) (Gan and Patel, 2013; Lequin, 2005; Thermo-Scientific, 2011).

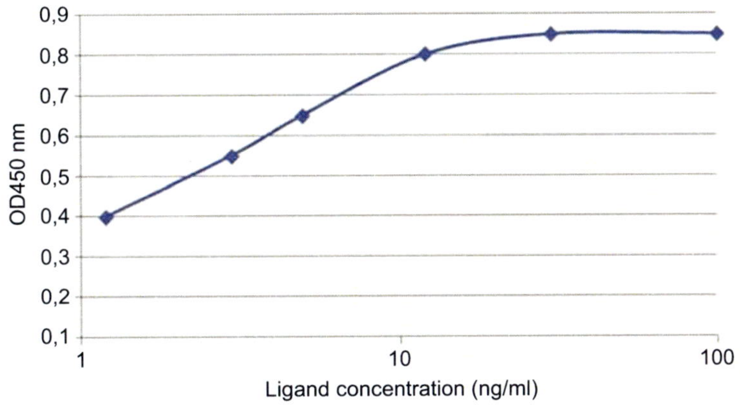

Figure 15.4 Example of a quantification standard curve using the OD450 nm values reported in ng/ml.

Variants of ELISA assays most used in the food sector are the indirect and sandwich methods (Asensio et al., 2008). Indirect ELISA uses a specific primary antibody that binds antigen, and a secondary antibody labeled with the enzyme that binds to the primary antibody. By adding the enzyme substrate, a reaction will take place where the secondary antibody binds and a chromogenic product consequently arises (Fig. 15.5) (Gan and Patel, 2013; Lequin, 2005; Thermo-Scientific, 2011).

Sandwich ELISA uses two specific antibodies: a first capture antibody that is generally immobilized on a surface and binds to the antigen in the first place; and a second detection antibody that binds to a different antigen site. This second antibody may be

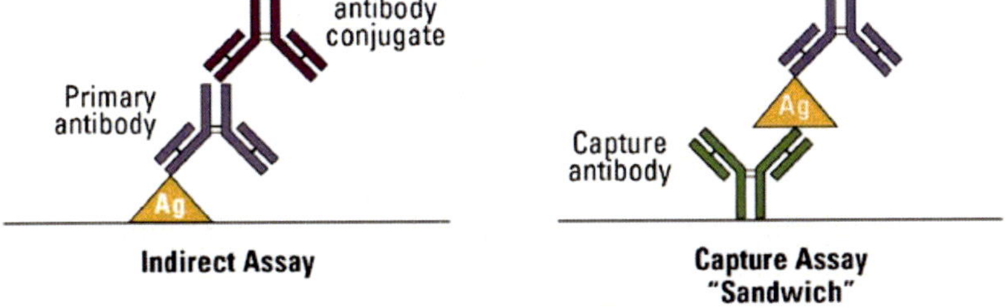

Figure 15.5 Common ELISA formats.
Thermo Fisher Scientific (life technologies), reprinted with permission of Thermo Fisher Scientific, copyright 2015 (https://www.lifetechnologies.com).

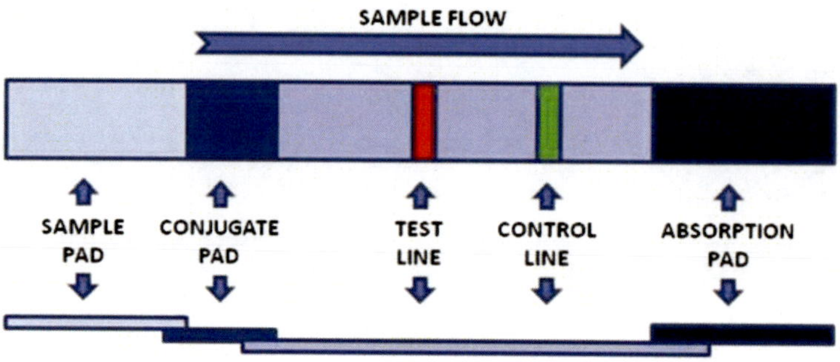

Figure 15.6 Schematic representation of the basic structure of an immunochromatographic strip.

labeled with enzyme but, alternatively, a secondary labeled antibody that binds to the detection antibody could also be used. Thus, the cost of marking specific antibodies used in each test can be avoided. The antibody is specifically captured and detected by two antigens, thus increasing assay specificity (Fig. 15.6) (Gan and Patel, 2013; Lequin, 2005; Thermo-Scientific, 2011).

The main advantages of the ELISA tests are its high specificity and sensitivity. Moreover, ELISA is a rapid procedure that does not require complex equipment, although the analyses need to be performed by experienced personnel as they involve multiple steps. Another advantage is its capacity for quantification by introducing a standard curve developed using known antigen concentrations. Main limitations of the technique are the possibility of cross-reactivity due to nonspecific reactions with antibodies, or interference from sample components, reducing the efficiency of the reaction. Another drawback is the inability to detect analytes at very low concentration, since a low signal may be overlapped and obscured by the baseline signal of the sample and reagent components (Harlow and Lane, 1999).

However, the general specificity, speed, and simplicity of this technique facilitates its application in food control laboratories as a routine tool as a quality control tool for food products (Hsieh et al., 2009). Interest in its application to the identification of fish species has led to the publication of several papers focused on the development and application of this technique. Among the most recent, the work of Carrera et al., in which the authors develop an ELISA test for the identification of *Thunnus alalunga* in fresh and frozen fillets, thus allowing its differentiation from other scombrid species of lesser commercial value, may be mentioned (Carrera et al., 2014). Many other studies have laid the groundwork for development of immunological methods aimed at obtaining specific antibodies for other fish species. Examples include reports of applications to species such as salmon (*Salmo salar*), trout (*Oncorhynchus mykiss*), Pacific herring (*Clupea pallasii*), common carp (*Cyprinus carpio*), rohu (*Labeo rohita*), and Philippine catfish (*Clarias batrachus*) (Carrera et al., 1997; Purcell et al., 2012; Rathore et al., 2008; Sood et al., 2012; Vesely et al., 2006).

Currently, the development of ELISA kits for the identification of species of fish has not yet reached full commercial exploitation. This could be due to the great number of fish species that are marketed, implying a very complex validation of any new methodologies developed, which increases assay cost. Incorporation of new technologies will maximize the commercial development of these kits and their application as a screening tool at wholesale and retail market levels for fisheries products.

Recent advances in this technique are focused on improving the specificity and sensitivity by incorporating new technologies and the development of new detection systems. These involve equipment for coating of assay plates or for automatic washing of assay plates, which simplify and speed up the corresponding steps of the ELISA process. Among the latest developments of this technique is the creation of automated ELISA platforms. These are integrated systems that allow the automatic development of all assay steps, simplifying protocols and reducing analysis times. These automated work platforms integrate a great variety of dispensers and washing systems for microplates with a particular reader or detection system, depending on assay requirements. Some of the more recently developed platforms include new formats of ELISA based on miniaturized systems in plates or microfluidic systems that allow increased sensitivity and reduced interference by sample components. Incorporation of these new technologies and materials allows the development of multiplex assays, thereby increasing the capability of assays so that a multitude of single well analytes can be tested, while also reducing the volume of sample and reagents required to perform the assay. The introduction of ELISA platforms also involves incorporating novel, ultrasensitive detection systems based on different chemicals that allow binding of the particles to immunocomplexes. This results in high sensitivity and stability, eliminating possible interference by reagents and sample components (Comley, 2012). All these additions increase the sensitivity, specificity, simplicity, and speed of the ELISA assays, encouraging its application in many food industry sectors.

Immunochromatographic Test Strips

Immunochromatography systems consist of immunoreagents immobilized on a carrier and fluid flow through that carrier. In the case of a test strip, it is an assembly of several plain, porous carriers impregnated with immunoreagents. On contact with the test strip, a liquid sample flows along the carriers with detectable immune complexes being formed in certain zones of the strip (Dzantiev et al., 2014).

A test strip consists of several zones, typically constituted by segments made of different materials. When a test is run, a sample is added to the proximal end of the strip, the sample pad, at which point it is treated to make it compatible with the rest of the test. This treated sample migrates through this region to the conjugate pad, where a particulate conjugate has been immobilized; this has been conjugated to one of the specific biological components of the assay, either an antigen or antibody depending on the assay format. The sample remobilizes the dried conjugate after which the analyte in the sample interacts with the conjugate as both migrate into the next section of the strip, the reaction matrix. This reaction matrix is a porous membrane, onto which the other specific biological components of the assay have been immobilized. These are typically proteins, either antibody or antigen, which have been laid down in bands in specific areas of the membrane where they serve to capture the analyte and the conjugate as they migrate past the capture line (test line and control line) (O'Farrell, 2009) (Fig. 15.6).

Generally, the control band contains antiimmunoglobulin antibodies that are specific against conjugated particles. Then, it captures the excess conjugate and this acts as a control to indicate that the desired reaction has been carried out correctly. Results are interpreted in terms of the presence or absence of a signal on the control line and in the line of analyte capture. This reading can be detected visually or through specific readers, depending on the marking system used in the reaction.

Principal advantages of the immunochromatographic strips are the speed and the simplicity with which the test, which does not require specialized personnel or complex equipment, is performed. However, its limitations focus on the assay sensitivity, which can be affected by unspecific interactions of the components of the sample with the antibodies of capture lines, resulting in false positives, or by interference in the antigen—antibody binding, leading to false negatives. Another disadvantage of this technique is the inability to analyze more than one species in the same assay because the combination of antibodies of different species may result in unspecific binding reactions, reducing the efficiency of the assay and impeding the interpretation of results.

The development of applications based on this methodology for detection of fish species is growing, although it has not yet achieved a high degree of commercial use. One example of the latest commercial products is the detection test for *Pangasius* genus (*EZ Pangasius, by ELISA Technologies*), the main objective of which is to avoid substitutions by other species when the fish is presented in the form of a fillet without any of the characteristic morphological characteristics.

Advances in this technology are directed to improving aspects such as:

- Development of new material that reduces interactions with the components of the sample, increasing sensitivity and efficiency of the assay.
- Development of a quantitative test, using materials and markers that can be precisely quantified.
- Reduction of the volume of sample required for testing.
- Development of integrated reading systems that allow the capture of data, minimizing mistakes and facilitating the development of quantitative tests.
- Development of multiplex assays that allow simultaneous detection of more than one species (Dzantiev et al., 2014; Sajid et al., 2015).

15.2.3 Gene-based Methods

When morphological characteristics are deleted or modified during the preparation of processed products, identification methods based on these characteristics cannot be applied. Equally, protein-based methods are not suitable for routine sample analysis because proteins lose their biological activity after animal death and their presence and characteristics depend on the cell types included (Asensio, 2007). Moreover, most proteins are thermolabile, so that their structure is denatured when they are subjected to heat treatments such as those undergone by many processed foods, precluding their use as target (Asensio, 2007; Mackie et al., 1999; Rehbein, 1990).

Use of genetic methods for species identification has been extended in recent decades, principally involving DNA-based methods because they have many advantages over protein-based methods. Although DNA is also degraded, eg, during the heat-sterilization step of the canning process, it is still possible to obtain small fragments with sufficient differences in sequence to enable even closely related species to be differentiated and identified (Espiñeira et al., 2010; Lago et al., 201a,b). Another advantage of genetic methods is that DNA can potentially be retrieved from any species in virtually any kind of organic substrate, such as muscle, fin, or blood, because it is present in all cells of an organism (Lockley & Bardsley, 2000; Teletchea, 2009).

Since analytical methods based on DNA have been shown to have several advantages over those based on proteins, numerous genetic methods are currently being investigated for identification of fish species. The most common methods used for it are based on amplification by polymerase chain reaction (PCR); some methods include the use of PCR along with restriction fragment length polymorphism (RFLP), forensically informative nucleotide sequencing (FINS), amplified fragment length polymorphism, or real-time PCR.

15.2.3.1 Real-time PCR

Use of real-time PCR methods for fish identification has increased considerably because this method not only allows identification of species in products containing more than one species but it also enables their quantification. This technique is based on the fact that amplification products are transformed into compounds that fluoresce, and this fluorescence is detected and monitored while the amplification takes place. A previously established linear relationship between the PCR product and fluorescence intensity is used to calculate the amount of target DNA contained in a sample being tested (Lago et al., 2014) (Fig. 15.7).

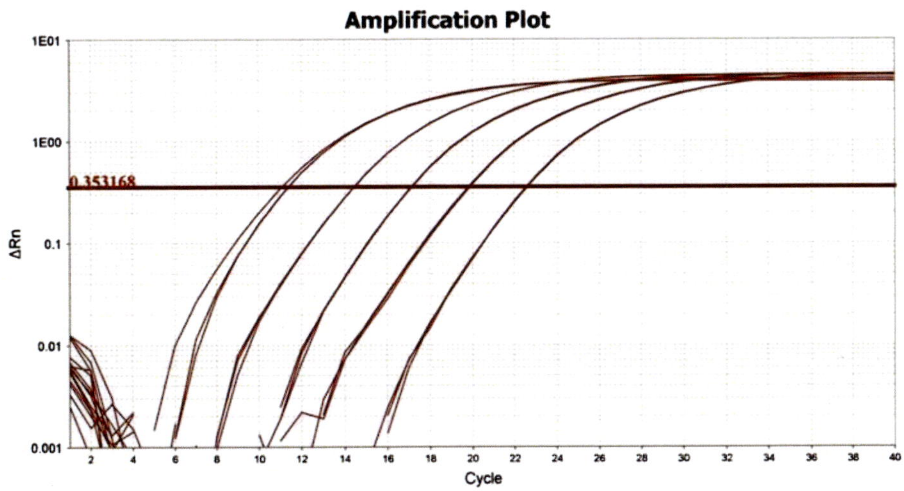

Figure 15.7 Amplification plot obtained by real-time PCR.

The methodology can be more or less specific depending on the chemistry that is used. Two reporter systems are commonly involved, namely, the intercalating SYBR green assay and the TaqMan® probe system. If fluorophores are used as intercalating agents, they will join to the double-stranded DNA sequences indistinctly, both to the target sequence and to primer dimers, generating nonspecific products that would contribute to the fluorescent signal, resulting in an overestimation of the target material. The TaqMan® probe method utilizes a fluorescent-labeled probe that hybridizes to an additional conserved region lying within the target amplicon sequence. This additional specificity afforded by the TaqMan® probe ensures that the fluorescent signal generated during real-time PCR is derived only from amplification of the target sequence (Smith and Osborn, 2009).

Real-time PCR is a technique that addresses the need for both rapid and accurate detection and quantification of small amounts of genetic material. Also, due to its sensitivity, it can be applied to highly processed samples, allowing the amplification of small DNA fragments of less than 200 bp. These features make it a highly effective tool for the detection of fish species in canned and processed products, in which the raw material is subjected to high pressures and temperatures and DNA is partially degraded (Bustin, 2004).

Among other advantages of this technique is the capacity for development of multiplex real-time PCR assays. These include the ability to detect and authenticate various species in the same reaction, implying even greater savings, both economic and in analysis time. However, it is important to emphasize the difficulty of developing multiplex assays, in which the design and setup is more complicated because, while the same conditions should be optimal for detecting each species, this is not always possible.

Despite the advantages of this technique, it is necessary to take into account several different considerations when making a species assignment in a given sample. In species that are closely related phylogenetically, only a few nucleotide differences exist in their DNA sequences and it is then necessary to obtain as much nucleotide information as possible to confidently assign a sample to a given species. Real-time PCR only evaluates the hybridization positions of the probe and primers set, so this must be taken into account in the design of the methodology. In addition, the selected molecular marker should have a high intraspecific conservation to obtain a specific primer/probe set, taking into account all haplotype variation (Lago et al., 2014).

However, the specificity and sensitivity of this technique, combined with its high speed, robustness, reliability, and the possibility of automation, make it acceptable for identification of fish species in fishery products (Asensio, 2007; Lago et al., 2014). Today it is one of the most commonly used techniques for detection and authentication of fish species. A reflection of this may be seen in the development of a multitude of methodologies for a great variety of taxonomic groups of commercial importance: scombrids (Chuang et al., 2012; Dalmasso et al., 2007; Liu et al., 2015; Lopez and Pardo, 2005), salmonids (Herrero et al., 2011c; Hird et al., 2012; Li et al., 2013), sardines (Armani et al., 2012; Herrero et al., 2011b), eels (Espiñeira and Vieites, 2016; Minegishi et al., 2009; Watanabe et al., 2004), anglerfish (Castigliego et al., 2015; Herrero et al., 2011d), flatfish (Herrero et al., 2012), groupers

(Chen et al., 2012; Trotta et al., 2005), gadoids (Fox et al., 2005; Herrero et al., 2010; Hird et al., 2012; Sánchez et al., 2009; Taylor et al., 2002), and swordfish (Herrero et al., 2011a).

Current advances in this technique focus on the application of new technologies that allow greater automation of equipment and in the integration of systems in platforms that expedite both the development of methodologies and the generation of results (Lee et al., 2010). Recent trends are also aimed at the introduction of new chemical and detection systems that reduce analysis time and increase sensitivity of the methodologies (Fang et al., 2012; Lee et al., 2013; Patterson et al., 2013).

Most recent developments involving real-time PCR methods emphasize the integration of microfluidics technologies and techniques involving microelectromechanical systems. This has enabled the introduction of chips as supports to the reactions, reducing the volume of sample and reagents required in addition to the reaction time. One of the great advantages of these new developments centers around its portability, with its small size allowing in situ applications thereby streamlining decision-making after analysis. So far, the results of its application indicate poor limits of detection, low reproducibility, and low yields, but it is a new technology that is still under development and possesses great prospects (Cho et al., 2006; Fang et al., 2009; Lee et al., 2010; Mauk et al., 2015; Oblath et al., 2013; Zhu et al., 2012).

15.2.3.2 PCR-ELISA

This method combines both PCR and ELISA into a single analytical procedure, and its application is very similar to ELISA except that it allows the detection of nucleic acid instead of protein.

PCR-ELISA is an immunological method to quantify the PCR product directly after immobilization of biotinylated DNA on a microplate. The whole method involves three steps: amplification, immobilization, and detection. In the initial step, a gene of interest will be amplified through PCR in the presence of digoxigenin-11-dUTP (DIG-dUTP); DIG-labeled PCR products will then bind to specific oligonucleotide probes, labeled with biotin at their 5′ end. A subsequent step involves immobilizing the gene of interest to the microplate, which is achieved by streptavidin-coated microplates in the presence of biotin on the 5′ end of the formed hybrid. The strong affinity of the avidin-biotin interaction encourages formation of an avidin-biotin complex, thus binding to the microplate only PCR products with the specific gene of interest. All other nonspecific products are washed off. After immobilization, detection of biotinylated DNA is achieved using an anti-DIG-peroxidase conjugate with a substrate to form a chromogenic reaction that is both visible and measured using a spectrophotometer (Fig. 15.8). Another PCR-ELISA detection method involves use of a fluorescein probe; detection is achieved by the use of antifluorescein antibodies conjugated to horseradish peroxidase to detect the hybridized fluorescein-labeled oligonucleotide probe (Gomes et al., 2010; Sue et al., 2014).

This particular technique uses specific probes combined with a colorimetric detection. It provides high sensitivity and specificity, special equipment is not necessary, and it allows screening assays involving large numbers of samples. This means a

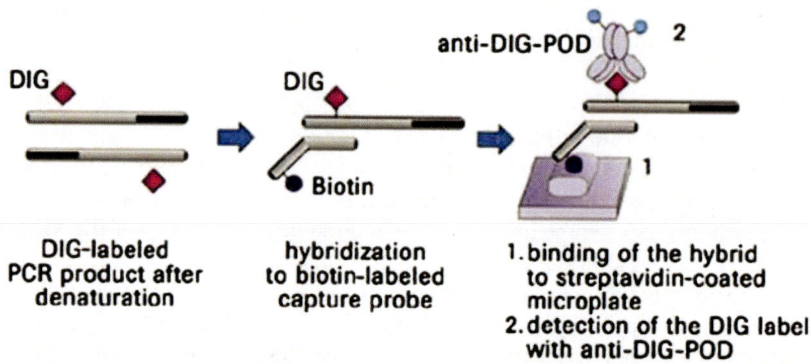

Figure 15.8 Schematic of PCR-ELISA procedure.
Roche Diagnostics, Image is being used with written permission from Roche Molecular Systems, Inc. Further use outside of this publication is prohibited (http://lifescience.roche.com).

reduction in analytical costs. However, its sensitivity has been compared with other molecular techniques, and some studies have concluded that it is lower than results obtained with real-time PCR (Menotti et al., 2010; Seo et al., 2012; Sue et al., 2014).

Among disadvantages associated with this technique are the possibilities of interference by the sample components, leading to false-positive results and reducing the efficiency of the methodology. Furthermore, compounds present in both the sample and the reagents can generate signal. This makes detection of the target analyte difficult when it is present at low concentrations, lead to false negatives and reduces method sensitivity (Menotti et al., 2003; Scotter et al., 2005). Another disadvantage of PCR-ELISA is that its implementation requires equipping for both methodologies, a thermocycler and a plate reader, which increases the cost and makes its application more difficult. Furthermore, this technique requires experienced personnel who are trained to correctly perform the multistep process.

Most applications of this methodology have been focused on the diagnosis and detection of diseases and pathogens that affect humans in medical studies and the food industry (Raji et al., 2011; Tahk et al., 2012; Tahk et al., 2011). Its application for fish species identification is recent, eg, note the work of Santaclara et al., who developed a PCR-ELISA method for authentication of *Thunnus* species, and Taboada et al., who developed PCR-ELISA assays for the identification of Atlantic cod (*Gadus morhua*), Alaska pollock (*Theragra chalcogramma*), and ling (*Molva molva*) (Santaclara et al., 2014; Taboada et al., 2014).

Most recent advances in the PCR-ELISA technique are focused on reduction of test cost and time requirement. Main efforts are focused on the development of multiplex assays, in which several specific sequences may be detected simultaneously and without cross-reactivity. The key challenge for this procedure is to design probes that are highly specific for each of the species of interest without exhibiting any cross-reactions. Another trend of interest is the reduction or elimination of washing steps and incubation times, with the aim of speeding up the assays and reducing reagent costs (Sue et al., 2014).

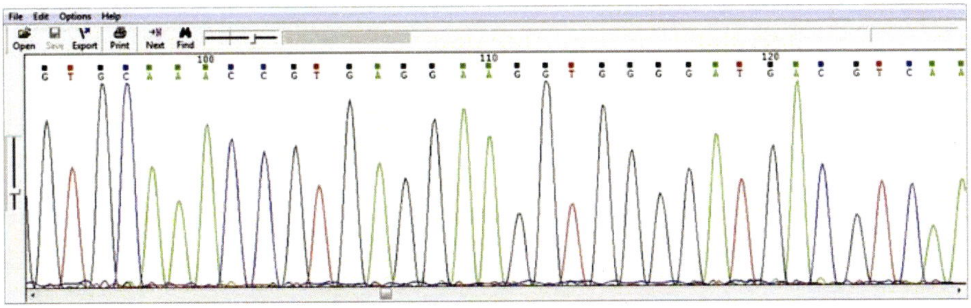

Figure 15.9 Chromatogram of the sequence obtained from an amplified fragment by PCR.

15.2.3.3 PCR and Sequencing

Methods that use PCR sequencing and nucleotide analysis for the identification of species are generally referred to as FINS (Fig. 15.9). The principle behind them involves PCR amplification and sequencing of a specific DNA fragment, followed by analysis of nucleotide variation between the target sequence and reference sequence patterns of known species (Bartlett and Davidson, 1992; Rasmussen and Morrissey, 2011). From the sequences, a distance matrix is constructed; through algorithmic calculations and analysis, a phylogenetic tree is obtained, allowing the assignment of the unknown species to a group according to its genetic distance from such a group.

The greatest advantage of this methodology is that it uses all the nucleotide information of the amplified fragment, which gives it high reliability, specificity, sensitivity, accuracy, and reproducibility. Also, it is not affected by intraspecific variability and allows detection of new species that have not been previously studied (Lago et al., 2014).

Limitations of this methodology include the fact that, in most cases, it does not allow the identification of a mixture of species, although some methodologies that are useful in cases of mixed species have been developed. Lago et al. demonstrated the ability to identify mixtures of species of the *Gadus* genus (*G. morhua* and *Gadus ogac/macrocephalus*) and mixtures of *Sardina pilchardus* and *Sardinella aurita* (Lago et al., 2011a,b, 2013). Other disadvantages are the time required for the assay and the high cost of equipment, reagents, and materials necessary for each analysis. In recent years, costs have been reduced, facilitating greater access to these methodologies by many laboratories.

In recent years, FINS methodology has been widely used for identification of fish species because of its efficiency and reliability. Published reports cover a wide range of taxonomic groups, including many of commercial importance: scombroids (Espiñeira et al., 2009; Infante et al., 2007), anchovies (Jerome et al., 2008; Santaclara et al., 2006), anglerfish (Espiñeira et al., 2008a), salmonids (Espiñeira et al., 2009), sardines (Jerome et al., 2003; Lago et al., 2011a,b), gadoids (Calo-Mata et al., 2003; Lago et al., 2013; Pérez and Presa, 2008), flatfish (Espiñeira et al., 2008b), horse mackerel (Karaiskou et al., 2003, 2007; Lago et al., 2011a,b), and swordfish (Herrero et al., 2011a).

Progress in these methods is focused on reducing the time and cost of sequencing through the integration of new technologies in sequencing systems and analysis programs, resulting in what is known as next-generation sequencing (see Section 15.4.1).

15.3 Case Studies

Several case studies will be detailed to show the application of these genetic techniques in the authentication of fish species.

15.3.1 Real-time PCR

For application of real-time PCR, many reports exist that indicate the effectiveness of this method for detection and authentication of fish species. Among these, the work of Herrero et al., who focused various on this methodology, may be highlighted (Herrero et al., 2011a,b, 2012, 2010). One recent study of Herrero et al. focused on the authentication of European sole (*Solea solea*) and on its differentiation from the most common substitute species. In this study, the authors report the development of a methodology based on a species-specific set of primers and a TaqMan probe that amplifies a 116 bp fragment of the internal transcribed spacer 1 (ITS 1) ribosomal DNA region. Specificity of the methodology was tested extensively with DNA isolates from a wide range of flatfish species and any cross-reaction was observed. Method sensitivity was evaluated using serial dilutions of *S. solea* DNA with DNA of other species of the *Solea* genus; results indicated an efficiency of 100% and a limit of detection of 2.5 ng without any false-positive result. Additionally, the methodology was validated for application to all types of manufactured products to detect the presence of *S. solea*, with successful results. Subsequently, the method was applied to 40 commercial samples to determine whether correct labeling had been employed in the market; the authors reported that 30% of the samples tested were incorrectly labeled. It was demonstrated that the assay is a useful tool for the authentication of *S. solea* in all product types due to its accuracy, sensitivity, specificity, and rapidity; it is also claimed to be useful for monitoring and verifying food labeling regulations (Herrero et al., 2012).

15.3.2 PCR-ELISA

One of the most recent studies in which a PCR-ELISA technique was applied to species authentication is of Santaclara et al., who developed a multiplex PCR-ELISA assay for authentication of *Thunnus* species (Santaclara et al., 2014). In this work, multiple sequential analytical steps allow to determine if a particular sample belongs to the *Thunnus* genus or to another taxonomic group. When this first test is positive (ie, the sample belongs to *Thunnus*), some of the proposed systems allow the assignment of the sample to *Thunnus albacares*, *T. alalunga* or to *Thunnus orientalis* and *Thunnus thynnus*; when it is negative, another system attempts to determine if the sample is *Katsuwonus pelamis*.

The difficulty with the methodology is that it involves several sequential PCR steps and, even in case of fresh and frozen samples, involves steps of visualization and purification in agarose gel. After purification of the amplified fragments by PCR, an ELISA assay is performed for each of them comprising the following steps: (1) hybridization of the DIG-labeled PCR product and the biotinylated probe; (2) binding of the hybridization product to a streptavidin-coated microplate; (3) washing; (4) binding of the antibody anti-DIG to the labeled enzyme; (5) washing; (6) addition of specific substrate to the revealing enzyme; and (7) measurement of absorbance and evaluation of results. Another difficulty associated with this assay is that the realization of the ELISA should be carried out by experienced personnel because variations in washing or incubation times could result in false-positive or false-negative results.

Assay results showed that the technique described by Santaclara et al. is a useful tool to authenticate the species belonging to the *Thunnus* genus and *K. pelamis*. At the same time, it was confirmed that cooking and canning processes do not affect the performance of the method.

15.3.3 PCR and Sequencing

PCR followed by sequencing is one of the most used techniques for identification of fish species. In this field, the Molecular Biology Unit, which has the ENAC accreditation called List of Essays under Accreditation (LEBA) in species identification using this methodology, should be noted. LEBA is an open and growing list that, in addition to fish species, includes other taxonomic groups such as cephalopods, mussels, and meat, and that adds value and international validity to any report issued for identification of these species (Lago et al., 2014).

The Molecular Biology Group of ANFACO-CECOPESCA has several publications that reflect the application of PCR and sequencing to identify fish species (Lago FC., 2012 #37; Lago FC., 2011 #24; Lago FC., 2011 #4; Lago FC., 2011 #6; Herrero B., 2011 #1; Espiñeira M., 2009 #16; Espiñeira M., 2015 #40; Espiñeira M., 2012 #38; Espiñeira M., 2009 #15; Espiñeira M., 2008 #18; Espiñeira M., 2008 #19). Among its most recent publications one paper (Lago et al., 2013) in particular should be noted because of the commercial importance of the target species and their applicability to species mixtures. This methodology allows the correct identification of the main species of gadoid, among which are included more than 15 species of cod and related species, in any form found in the market and regardless of the degree of transformation that they have undergone. In addition, a methodology based on SNP analysis of *Gadus* species that allows detection of mixtures of these species in seafood products has also been designed.

The work is based on amplification of a fragment of mitochondrial cytochrome b (cyt b) marker; subsequent phylogenetic analyses were carried out to authenticate these products and assure their correct labeling. Two fragments of the cyt b gene were amplified, one of 464 bp and another internal fragment to this of 263 bp, to allow the authentication of gadoid species in highly processed products. After sequencing, the phylogenetic analysis of the sequences has established relationships between gadoid species by constructing phylogenetic trees, one for each set of fragments. In both cases, all the sequences belonging to individuals of the same species have grouped in the same cluster and are well differentiated, allowing their identification to species level with high levels of confidence. Also, the authors designed a specific method based on SNP analysis for detection of the mixture of the three *Gadus* species (*G. morhua*, *G. macrocephalus*, and *G. ogac*). These are the species that are most similar, both morphologically and genetically. If the mixture with other species included even some species not listed in this work, the genetic difference would be so obvious that the species mixture would be detected by the appearance of numerous double peaks in the sequence chromatograms. Results obtained for specificity and sensitivity of the methodology show that this technique is highly reliable with a specificity of 100% (Lago et al., 2013).

These results show that the methodology is a very appropriate tool for the authentication of gadoids and detection of species mixtures of the *Gadus* genus in all kind of seafood products; it is applied in the routine work of ANFACO-CECOPESCA Unit of Molecular Biology. Applications of this method are the following: normative control of raw and processed products, particularly for the authenticity of imported species; verification of the traceability of different fishing batches along the commercial chain; correct labeling and protection of the rights of the consumers; fair competition among fishing operators; and control of fisheries (Lago et al., 2013).

15.4 Future Trends

15.4.1 Massive Sequencing

New trends around sequencing point to the next-generation sequencing or massive sequencing. Compared with traditional DNA sequencing based on the dideoxy chain termination technique, next-generation sequencing relies on immobilization of fragmented DNA templates on a solid support system. The spatially separated, immobilized fragments can then be amplified simultaneously by PCR and subjected to massively parallel DNA sequencing. This advance enables rapid sequencing of large stretches of DNA base pairs spanning entire genomes, with the latest instruments capable of producing hundreds of gigabases of data on a single sequencing run (Rasmussen and Morrissey, 2011). The result is a sequencing technology that is simpler, faster, more cost effective, and scalable.

It shows high potential for use in automated, high-throughput identification of seafood species in different product types and for identification of diagnostic nucleotide sites that can be targeted in species-specific PCR assays or for species identification using direct sequencing of diagnostic fragments (Rasmussen and Morrissey, 2011).

Although sequencing platforms that integrate this new technology already exist in the market (*Ion Torrent PGM* from *Life Technologies*, *MiSeq/HiSeq system* from *Ilumina*, or *454 Gs-Junior/GS-FLX* from *Roche*), their implementation is still inaccessible to most laboratories due to their high cost and to the need for highly specialized personnel with specific knowledge of bioinformatics to analyze the information contained in the sequences obtained.

15.4.2 Digital PCR

Digital PCR (dPCR) is a new method for accurate quantification of nucleic acids. It uses a limiting dilution analysis together with Poisson distribution analysis to allow the absolute quantification of the number of copies of target DNA. Digital PCR uses an amplification reaction system similar to a system of standard dPCR. A droplet generator is used to separate each dPCR reaction mixture into 20,000 nL drops with each drop containing zero (negative) and one or more copies of the target DNA (positive). After a conventional PCR procedure, the total number of individual positive or negative droplets is counted and recorded by a drop reader. Finally, the number of precise measurements of genomic targets in copies per microliter on one chip contained in the samples can be calculated directly using the Poisson distribution law. Use of a nanofluidic chip provides a quick and easy mechanism by which to run thousands of parallel PCR reactions (Fig. 15.10).

As a refinement of conventional qPCR, dPCR has the potential to allow a more accurate and sensitive measurement of the number of copies of target DNA, especially for low concentration and composite samples. To date, no direct applications of this technique on the identification of fish species have been published, but its obvious potential is based on the ability to analyze samples containing species mixtures with high sensitivity and in a single trial, performing multiple reactions in parallel.

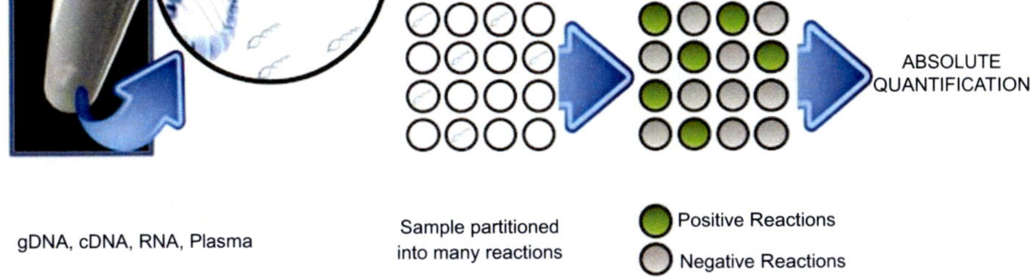

Figure 15.10 Digital polymerase chain reaction (PCR) steps.

Sources of Further Information

Barcode-LIFE

In 2003 researchers at the University of Guelph in Canada published a paper proposing a new system of species identification and discovery using a very short genetic sequence from a standard part of the genome. Their method was similar to the way a supermarket scanner distinguishes products using the black stripes of the Universal Product Code. They called the new molecular identification system "DNA barcoding."

The promise of accurate, rapid, and inexpensive species identification captured the attention of taxonomists, geneticists, and evolutionary biologists around the world. In June of 2007, delegates from 25 countries met to discuss a proposed "United Nations of barcoding," a global collaboration of biodiversity scientists that would create a DNA barcode reference library for all multicellular life.

Efforts began to establish a committee in each country, establishing the administrative structures and finalizing the research plans of the International Barcode of Life (iBOL) project. The formal activation of iBOL was in October 2010 (http://ibol.org/about-us/background/).

This BOL initiative is a global platform, the main aim of which is standardization of protocols for identifying species using PCR and sequencing based on standardized sequences. These are called DNA barcodes and are collected in a public and international database (http://www.barcodeoflife.org). For most species groups, the standard DNA barcode is a 650 bp region of the COI gene, which is relatively highly conserved within species but shows sufficient variation between species to allow for differentiation (Hebert et al., 2003; Ward et al., 2009). An overarching goal of the BOL initiative is the development of a comprehensive reference sequence database containing DNA barcode records for all eukaryotic species. That portion of the project focused on fish is called FISH-BOL (www.fishbol.org) and currently has DNA barcode records for close to 8000 species; numerous studies have been published that show unambiguous species differentiation (Ward et al., 2009).

Latest trends in the use of DNA barcodes include the use of minibarcodes. Minibarcodes are shorter fragments of the full-length DNA barcode and have high potential for use with samples that contain low-quality DNA, such as canned seafood, from which the full-length barcode cannot be recovered. Several minibarcode regions have been identified that allow for differentiation of a range of species, and these regions have been tested in silico to differentiate commercially important salmon and trout species (Galal-Khallaf et al., 2014; Hajibabaei et al., 2006; Meusnier et al., 2008; Rasmussen et al., 2009).

References

Armani, A., Castigliego, L., Tinacci, L., Gianfaldoni, D., Guidi, A., 2012. Multiplex conventional and real-time PCR for fish species identification of Bianchetto (juvenile form of *Sardina pilchardus*), Rossetto (*Aphia minuta*), and Icefish in fresh, marinated and cooked products. Food Chemistry 133 (1), 184–192.

Asensio, L., González, I., García, T., Martín, R., 2008. Determination of food authenticity by enzyme-linked immunosorbent assay (ELISA). Food Control 19 (1), 1–8.

Asensio, L., 2007. PCR-based methods for fish and fishery products authentication. Trends in Food Science & Technology 18 (11), 558–566.

Bartlett, S.E., Davidson, W.S., 1992. Fins (forensically informative nucleotide sequencing): a procedure for identifying the animal origin of biological specimens. Biotechniques 12 (3), 408–411.

Bustin, S.A., 2004. AZ of Quantitative PCR. International University Line La Jolla.

Calo-Mata, P., Sotelo, C.G., Pérez-Martín, R.I., Rehbein, H., Hold, G.L., Russell, V.J., et al., 2003. Identification of gadoid fish species using DNA-based techniques. European Food Research and Technology 217 (3), 259–264.

Carrera, E., García, T., Céspedes, A., González, I., Sanz, B., Hernández, P.E., et al., 1997. Immunostick colorimetric ELISA assay for the identification of smoked salmon, trout and bream. Journal of the Science of Food and Agriculture 74 (4), 547–550.

Carrera, E., Terni, M., Montero, A., Garcí, T., González, I., Martín, R., 2014. ELISA-based detection of mislabeled albacore (*Thunnus alalunga*) fresh and frozen fish fillets. Food and Agricultural Immunology 25 (4), 569–577.

Castigliego, L., Armani, A., Tinacci, L., Gianfaldoni, D., Guidi, A., 2015. Two alternative multiplex PCRs for the identification of the seven species of anglerfish (*Lophius* spp.) using an end-point or a melting curve analysis real-time protocol. Food Chemistry 166, 1–9.

Chen, S., Zhang, J., Chen, W., Zhang, Y., Wang, J., Xu, D., et al., 2012. Quick method for grouper species identification using real-time PCR. Food Control 27 (1), 108–112.

Cho, Y., Kim, J., Lee, Y., Kim, Y., Namkoong, K., Lim, H., et al., 2006. Clinical evaluation of micro-scale chip-based PCR system for rapid detection of hepatitis B virus. Biosensors and Bioelectronics 21 (11), 2161–2169.

Chuang, P., Chen, M., Shiao, J., 2012. Identification of tuna species by a real-time polymerase chain reaction technique. Food Chemistry 133 (3), 1055–1061.

Comley, J., 2012. ELISA Assays – Recent Innovations Take Analyte Detection to New Levels. Fall, 2012. Drug discovery World.

Dalmasso, A., Fontanella, E., Piatti, P., Civera, T., Secchi, C., Bottero, M.T., 2007. Identification of four tuna species by means of real-time PCR and melting curve analysis. Veterinary Research Communications 31, 355–357.

Dzantiev, B.B., Byzova, N.A., Urusov, A.E., Zherdev, A.V., 2014. Immunochromatographic methods in food analysis. TrAC Trends in Analytical Chemistry 55, 81–93.

EC, 2002. Regulation N° 178/2002 of the European Parliament and of the Council of 28 January2002 Laying Down the General Principles and Requirements of Food Law, Establishing the European Food Safety Authority and Laying Down Procedures in Matters of Food Safety.

Espiñeira, M., Vieites, J.M., 2016. Genetic system for an integral traceability of European eel (*Anguilla anguilla*) in aquaculture and seafood products: authentication by fast real time PCR. European Food Research and Technology 242, 25–31.

Espiñeira, M., González-Lavín, N., Vieites, J.M., Santaclara, F.J., 2008a. Authentication of anglerfish species (*Lophius* spp.) by means of polymerase chain reaction-restriction fragment length polymorphism (PCR-RFLP) and forensically informative nucleotide sequencing (fins) methodologies. Journal of Agricultural and Food Chemistry 56 (22), 10594–10599.

Espiñeira, M., González-Lavín, N., Vieites, J.M., Santaclara, F.J., 2008b. Development of a method for the genetic identification of flatfish species on the basis of mitochondrial DNA sequences. Journal of Agricultural and Food Chemistry 56 (19), 8954–8961.

Espiñeira, M., Gonzalez-Lavín, N., Vieites, J.M., Santaclara, F.J., 2009. Development of a method for the identification of scombroid and common substitute species in seafood products by FINS. Food Chemistry 117 (4), 698–704.

Espiñeira, M., Vieites, J.M., Santaclara, F.J., 2009. Development of a genetic method for the identification of salmon, trout, and bream in seafood products by means of PCR-RFLP and FINS methodologies. European Food Research and Technology 229 (5), 785–793.

Espiñeira, M., Vieites, J.M., Santaclara, F.J., 2010. Species authentication of octopus, cuttlefish, bobtail and bottle squids (families Octopodidae, Sepiidae and Sepiolidae) by FINS methodology in seafoods. Food Chemistry 121 (2), 527–532.

EU, 2013. Regulation N° 1379/2013 of the European Parliament and of the Council of 11 December, 2013 on the Common Organisation of the Markets in Fishery and Aquaculture Products, Amending Council Regulations (EC) No 1184/2006 and (EC) No 1224/2009 and Repealing Council Regulation (EC) No 104/2000.

Fang, T.H., Ramalingam, N., Xian-Dui, D., Ngin, T.S., Xianting, Z., Kuan, T.L., et al., 2009. Real-time PCR microfluidic devices with concurrent electrochemical detection. Biosensors and Bioelectronics 24 (7), 2131–2136.

Fang, X., Zhang, H., Zhang, F., Jing, F., Mao, H., Jin, Q., et al., 2012. Real-time monitoring of strand-displacement DNA amplification by a contactless electrochemical microsystem using interdigitated electrodes. Lab on a Chip 12 (17), 3190–3196.

Fox, C.J., Taylor, M.I., Pereyra, R., Villasana, M.I., Rico, C., 2005. TaqMan® DNA technology confirms likely overestimation of cod (*Gadus morhua* L.) egg abundance in the Irish Sea: implications for the assessment of the cod stock and mapping of spawning areas using egg-based methods. Molecular Ecology 14 (3), 879–884.

Galal-Khallaf, A., Ardura, A., Mohammed-Geba, K., Borrell, Y.J., Garcia-Vazquez, E., 2014. DNA barcoding reveals a high level of mislabeling in Egyptian fish fillets. Food Control 46, 441–445.

Gan, S.D., Patel, K.R., 2013. Enzyme immunoassay and enzyme-linked immunosorbent assay. Journal of Investigative Dermatology 133 (9), e12.

Gomes, L.I., dos Santos Marques, L.H., Enk, M.J., de Oliveira, M.C., Coelho, P.M.Z., Rabello, A., 2010. Development and evaluation of a sensitive PCR-ELISA system for detection of schistosoma infection in feces. PLoS Neglected Tropical Diseases 4 (4), e664.

Hajibabaei, M., Smith, M., Janzen, D.H., Rodriguez, J.J., Whitfield, J.B., Hebert, P.N., 2006. A minimalist barcode can identify a specimen whose DNA is degraded. Molecular Ecology Notes 6 (4), 959–964.

Harlow, E., Lane, D., 1999. Using Antibodies: A Laboratory Manual. Cold Spring Harbor Laboratory Press.

Hebert, P.N., Cywinska, A., Ball, S.L., 2003. Biological identifications through DNA barcodes. Proceedings of the Royal Society of London B: Biological Sciences 270 (1512), 313–321.

Herrero, B., Madrinán, M., Vieites, J.M., Espiñeira, M., 2010. Authentication of Atlantic cod (*Gadus morhua*) using real time PCR. Journal of Agricultural and Food Chemistry 58 (8), 4794–4799.

Herrero, B., Lago, F.C., Vieites, J.M., Espiñeira, M., 2011a. Authentication of swordfish (*Xiphias gladius*) by RT- PCR and FINS methodologies. European Food Research and Technology 233 (2), 195–202.

Herrero, B., Lago, F.C., Vieites, J.M., Espiñeira, M., 2011b. Development of a rapid and simple molecular identification methodology for true sardines (*Sardina pilchardus*) and false sardines (*Sardinella aurita*) based on the real-time PCR technique. European Food Research and Technology 233 (5), 851–857.

Herrero, B., Vieites, J.M., Espiñeira, M., 2011c. Authentication of Atlantic salmon (*Salmo salar*) using real-time PCR. Food Chemistry 127 (3), 1268–1272.
Herrero, B., Vieites, J.M., Espiñeira, M., 2011d. Duplex real-time PCR for authentication of anglerfish species. European Food Research and Technology 233 (5), 817–823.
Herrero, B., Lago, F.C., Vieites, J.M., Espiñeira, M., 2012. Real-time PCR method applied to seafood products for authentication of European sole (*Solea solea*) and differentiation of common substitute species. Food Additives & Contaminants: Part A 29 (1), 12–18.
Hird, H.J., Chisholm, J., Kaye, J., Colyer, A., Hold, G., Conyers, C.M., et al., 2012. Development of real-time PCR assays for the detection of Atlantic cod (*Gadus morhua*), Atlantic salmon (*Salmo salar*) and European plaice (*Pleuronectes platessa*) in complex food samples. European Food Research and Technology 234 (1), 127–136.
Hsieh, Y.H.P., Chen, Y.T., Gajewski, K., 2009. Monoclonal antibody-based sandwich ELISA for reliable identification of imported Pangasius catfish. Journal of Food Science 74 (8), C602–C607.
Infante, C., Blanco, E., Zuasti, E., Crespo, A., Manchado, M., 2007. Phylogenetic differentiation between Atlantic *Scomber colias* and Pacific *Scomber japonicus* based on nuclear DNA sequences. Genetica 130 (1), 1–8.
Jeong, C., Nakabo, T., 2008. *Dipturus wuhanlingi*, a new species of skates (*Elasmobranchii*: Rajidae) from China. Ichthyological Research 55 (2), 183–190.
Jerome, M., Lemaire, C., Verrez-Bagnis, V., Etienne, M., 2003. Direct sequencing method for species identification of canned sardine and sardine-type products. Journal of Agricultural and Food Chemistry 51 (25), 7326–7332.
Jerome, M., Martinsohn, J.T., Ortega, D., Carreau, P., Verrez-Bagnis, V., Mouchel, O., 2008. Toward fish and seafood traceability: anchovy species determination in fish products by molecular markers and support through a public domain database. Journal of Agricultural and Food Chemistry 56 (10), 3460–3469.
Karaiskou, N., Apostolidis, A.P., Triantafyllidis, A., Kouvatsi, A., Triantaphyllidis, C., 2003. Genetic identification and phylogeny of three species of the genus *Trachurus* based on mitochondrial DNA analysis. Marine Biotechnology 5 (5), 493–504.
Karaiskou, N., Triantafyllidis, A., Alvarez, P., Lopes, P., Garcia-Vazquez, E., Triantaphyllidis, C., 2007. Horse mackerel egg identification using DNA methodology. Marine Ecology 28 (4), 429–434.
Lago, F.C., Herrero, B., Vieites, J.M., Espineira, M., 2011a. Genetic identification of horse mackerel and related species in seafood products by means of forensically informative nucleotide sequencing methodology. Journal of Agricultural and Food Chemistry 59 (6), 2223–2228.
Lago, F.C., Herrero, B., Vieites, J.M., Espiñeira, M., 2011b. FINS methodology to identification of sardines and related species in canned products and detection of mixture by means of SNP analysis systems. European Food Research and Technology 232 (6), 1077–1086.
Lago, F.C., Vieites, J.M., Espiñeira, M., 2013. Authentication of gadoids from highly processed products susceptible to include species mixtures by means of DNA sequencing methods. European Food Research and Technology 236 (1), 171–180.
Lago, F.C., Alonso, M., Vieites, J.M., Espiñeira, M., 2014. Fish and seafood authenticity—species identification. In: Seafood Processing. John Wiley & Sons, Ltd, pp. 419–452.
Lavoué, S., Sullivan, J.P., 2014. *Petrocephalus boboto* and *Petrocephalus arnegardi*, two new species of African electric fish (Osteoglossomorpha, Mormyridae) from the Congo River basin. ZooKeys 400, 43.
Lee, D., Chen, P.J., Lee, G.B., 2010. The evolution of real-time PCR machines to real-time PCR chips. Biosensors and Bioelectronics 25 (7), 1820–1824.

Lee, D.C., Yip, S.P., Lee, T.M.H., 2013. Simple and sensitive electrochemical DNA detection of primer generation-rolling circle amplification. Electroanalysis 25 (5), 1310–1315.

Lequin, R.M., 2005. Enzyme immunoassay (EIA)/enzyme-linked immunosorbent assay (ELISA). Clinical Chemistry 51 (12), 2415–2418.

Li, X., Li, J., Zhang, S., He, Y., Pan, L., 2013. Novel real-time PCR method based on growth hormone gene for identification of salmonidae ingredient in food. Journal of Agricultural and Food Chemistry 61 (21), 5170–5177.

Liu, S., Xu, K., Wu, Z., Xie, X., Feng, J., 2015. Identification of five highly priced tuna species by quantitative real-time polymerase chain reaction. Mitochondrial DNA (preprint) 1–10.

Lockley, A.K., Bardsley, R.G., 2000. DNA-based methods for food authentication. Trends in Food Science & Technology 11 (2), 67–77.

Lopez, I., Pardo, M.A., 2005. Application of relative quantification TaqMan® real-time polymerase chain reaction technology for the identification and quantification of *Thunnus alalunga* and *Thunnus albacares*. Journal of Agricultural and Food Chemistry 53 (11), 4554–4560.

Lundstrom, R.C., 1981. Rapid fish species identification by agarose gel isoelectric focusing of sarcoplasmic proteins. Journal-Association of Official Analytical Chemists 64 (1), 38–43.

Mackie, I.M., Pryde, S.E., Gonzales-Sotelo, C., Medina, I., Pérez-Martín, R., Quinteiro, J., et al., 1999. Challenges in the identification of species of canned fish. Trends in Food Science & Technology 10 (1), 9–14.

Mauk, M.G., Liu, C., Sadik, M., Bau, H.H., 2015. Microfluidic devices for nucleic acid (NA) isolation, isothermal NA amplification, and real-time detection. Mobile Health Technologies: Methods and Protocols 15–40.

Menotti, J., Vilela, G., Romand, S., Garin, Y.J., Ades, L., Gluckman, E., et al., 2003. Comparison of PCR-enzyme-linked immunosorbent assay and real-time PCR assay for diagnosis of an unusual case of cerebral toxoplasmosis in a stem cell transplant recipient. Journal of Clinical Microbiology 41 (11), 5313–5316.

Menotti, J., Garin, Y.J.F., Thulliez, P., Sérugue, M.C., Stanislawiak, J., Ribaud, P., et al., 2010. Evaluation of a new 5′-nuclease real-time PCR assay targeting the Toxoplasma gondii AF146527 genomic repeat. Clinical Microbiology and Infection 16 (4), 363–368.

Meusnier, I., Singer, G.C., Landry, J., Hickey, D.A., Hebert, P.N., Hajibabaei, M., 2008. A universal DNA mini-barcode for biodiversity analysis. BMC Genomics 9 (1), 214.

Minegishi, Y., Yoshinaga, T., Aoyama, J., Tsukamoto, K., 2009. Species identification of Anguilla japonica by real-time PCR based on a sequence detection system: a practical application to eggs and larvae. ICES Journal of Marine Science: Journal du Conseil 66 (9), 1915–1918.

Oblath, E.A., Henley, W.H., Alarie, J.P., Ramsey, J.M., 2013. A microfluidic chip integrating DNA extraction and real-time PCR for the detection of bacteria in saliva. Lab on a Chip 13 (7), 1325–1332.

O'Farrell, B., 2009. Evolution in lateral flow-based immunoassay systems. In: Lateral Flow Immunoassay. Springer, pp. 1–33.

Osman, M.A., Ashoor, S.H., Marsh, P.C., 1987. Liquid chromatographic identification of common fish species. Journal-association of Official Analytical Chemists 70 (4), 618–625.

Patterson, A.S., Hsieh, K., Soh, H.T., Plaxco, K.W., 2013. Electrochemical real-time nucleic acid amplification: towards point-of-care quantification of pathogens. Trends in Biotechnology 31 (12), 704–712.

Pérez, M., Presa, P., 2008. Validation of a tRNA-Glu-cytochrome b key for the molecular identification of 12 hake species (Merluccius spp.) and Atlantic Cod (*Gadus morhua*) using PCR-RFLPs, FINS, and BLAST. Journal of Agricultural and Food Chemistry 56 (22), 10865–10871.

Purcell, M.K., Bromage, E.S., Silva, J., Hansen, J.D., Badil, S.M., Woodson, J.C., et al., 2012. Production and characterisation of monoclonal antibodies to IgM of Pacific herring (*Clupea pallasii*). Fish & Shellfish Immunology 33 (3), 552–558.

Raji, N., Sadeghizadeh, M., Tafreshi, K.N., Jahanzad, E., 2011. Detection of human Papillomavirus 18 in cervical cancer samples using PCR-ELISA (DIAPOPS). Iranian Journal of Microbiology 3 (4), 177.

Rasmussen, R.S., Morrissey, M.T., 2011. Advances in DNA-based techniques for the detection of seafood species substitution on the commercial market. Journal of the Association for Laboratory Automation 16 (4), 308–321.

Rasmussen, R.S., Morrissey, M.T., Hebert, P.N., 2009. DNA barcoding of commercially important salmon and trout species (Oncorhynchus and Salmo) from North America. Journal of Agricultural and Food Chemistry 57 (18), 8379–8385.

Rathore, G., Kumar, G., Sood, N., Kapoor, D., Lakra, W.S., 2008. Development of monoclonal antibodies to rohu [*Labeo rohita*] immunoglobulins for use in immunoassays. Fish & Shellfish Immunology 25 (6), 761–774.

Rehbein, H., 1990. Electrophoretic techniques for species identification of fishery products. Zeitschrift für Lebensmittel-Untersuchung und Forschung 191 (1), 1–10.

Sajid, M., Kawde, A.N., Daud, M., 2015. Designs, formats and applications of lateral flow assay: a literature review. Journal of Saudi Chemical Society 19 (6), 689–705.

Sánchez, A., Quinteiro, J., Rey-Mendez, M., Perez-Martín, R.I., Sotelo, C.G., 2009. Identification of European hake species (*Merluccius merluccius*) using real-time PCR. Journal of Agricultural and Food Chemistry 57 (9), 3397–3403.

Santaclara, F.J., Cabado, A.G., Vieites, J.M., 2006. Development of a method for genetic identification of four species of anchovies: *E. encrasicolus*, *E. anchoita*, *E. ringens* and *E. japonicus*. European Food Research and Technology 223 (5), 609–614.

Santaclara, F.J., Velasco, A., Pérez-Martín, R.I., Quinteiro, J., Rey-Méndez, M., Pardo, M.A., et al., 2014. Development of a multiplex PCR-ELISA method for the genetic authentication of Thunnus species and *Katsuwonus pelamis* in food products. Food Chemistry 180, 9–16.

Scotter, J.M., Campbell, P., Anderson, T.P., Murdoch, D.R., Chambers, S.T., Nigel, P.W., 2005. Comparison of PCR-ELISA and galactomannan detection for the diagnosis of invasive aspergillosis. Pathology 37 (3), 246–253.

Seo, D.J., Tahk, H., Lee, K.B., Lee, M.H., Son, N.R., Seo, S., et al., 2012. Detecting hepatitis E virus with a reverse transcription polymerase chain reaction enzyme-linked immunosorbent assay. Food and Environmental Virology 4 (1), 14–20.

Smith, C.J., Osborn, A.M., 2009. Advantages and limitations of quantitative PCR (Q-PCR)-based approaches in microbial ecology. FEMS Microbiology Ecology 67 (1), 6–20.

Sood, N., Chaudhary, D.K., Singh, A., Rathore, G., 2012. Monoclonal antibody to serum immunoglobulins of *Clarias batrachus* and its application in immunoassays. Gene 511 (2), 411–419.

Strauss, R.E., Bond, C.E., 1990. Taxonomic Methods: Morphology. Methods for Fish Biology. American Fisheries Society, Bethesda, Maryland, pp. 109–140.

Sue, M.J., Yeap, S.K., Omar, A.R., Tan, S.W., 2014. Application of PCR-ELISA in molecular diagnosis. BioMed Research International 2014, 6.

Taboada, L., Sánchez, A., Velasco, A., Santaclara, F.J., Pérez-Martín, R.I., Sotelo, C.G., 2014. Identification of Atlantic cod (*Gadus morhua*), ling (molva molva), and Alaska pollock (*Gadus chalcogrammus*) by PCR-ELISA using duplex PCR. Journal of Agricultural and Food Chemistry 62 (24), 5699–5706.

Tahk, H., Lee, M.H., Lee, K.B., Cheon, D., Choi, C., 2011. Development of duplex RT-PCR-ELISA for the simultaneous detection of hepatitis A virus and hepatitis E virus. Journal of Virological Methods 175 (1), 137–140.

Tahk, H., Lee, K.B., Lee, M.H., Seo, D.J., Cheon, D., Choi, C., 2012. Development of reverse transcriptase polymerase chain reaction enzyme-linked immunosorbent assay for the detection of hepatitis A virus in vegetables. Food Control 23 (1), 210–214.

Taylor, M.I., Fox, C., Rico, I., Rico, C., 2002. Species-specific TaqMan® probes for simultaneous identification of (*Gadus morhua* L.), haddock (*Melanogrammus aeglefinus* L.) and whiting (*Merlangius merlangus* L.). Molecular Ecology Notes 2 (4), 599–601.

Teletchea, F., 2009. Molecular identification methods of fish species: reassessment and possible applications. Reviews in Fish Biology and Fisheries 19 (3), 265–293.

Thermo-Scientific, 2011. Thermo Scientific Pierce Assay Development Technical Handbook.

Trienekens, J.H., Wognum, P.M., Beulens, J.M., van der Vorst, G.A.J., 2012. Transparency in complex dynamic food supply chains. Advanced Engineering Informatics 26 (1), 55–65.

Trotta, M., Schönhuth, S., Pepe, T., Cortesi, M.L., Puyet, A., Bautista, J.M., 2005. Multiplex PCR method for use in real-time PCR for identification of fish fillets from grouper (*Epinephelus* and *Mycteroperca* species) and common substitute species. Journal of Agricultural and Food Chemistry 53 (6), 2039–2045.

Vesely, T., Reschova, S., Pokorova, D., Hulova, J., Nevorankova, Z., 2006. Production of monoclonal antibodies against immunoglobulin heavy chain in common carp (*Cyprinus carpio* L.). Veterinarni Medicina-Praha 51 (5), 296.

Ward, R.D., Hanner, R., Hebert, P.N., 2009. The campaign to DNA barcode all fishes, FISH-BOL. Journal of Fish Biology 74 (2), 329–356.

Watanabe, S., Minegishi, Y., Yoshinaga, T., Aoyama, J., Tsukamoto, K., 2004. A quick method for species identification of Japanese eel (*Anguilla japonica*) using real-time PCR: an onboard application for use during sampling surveys. Marine Biotechnology 6 (6), 566–574.

Zhu, L., Li, L., An, D., Wang, M., Zhang, L., Wang, Y.K., et al., 2012. An integrated microfluidic real-time PCR system for pathogen detection. In: Paper Presented at the Technical Proceedings of the 2012 NSTI Nanotechnology Conference and Expo. NSTI-Nanotech, California, USA.

Authentication of Cereals and Cereal Products

16

D. Cozzolino
Central Queensland University, Rockhampton, Queensland, Australia

Chapter Outline

16.1 Introduction

Cereal grains are among the most important of the foods we grow; a large proportion of cultivated grains is milled and marketed as flour in order to produce breads, cakes, biscuits, and many other commodities (Xie et al., 2005; Schwartz and Whistler, 2009). Starch is the major component of cereal grains, and changes in its biophysical and biochemical properties, such as amylose and amylopectin content, water uptake, protein quantity and quality, and fatty acids and lipids, will have an effect on its end use properties (eg, baking, malting, brewing, and polymer production) (Xie et al., 2005; Schwartz and Whistler, 2009). Starch stored in the seeds and tubers of various agricultural crops including maize, wheat, rice, barley, among other cereals and cereal products provides the main source of energy in the human diet (Schwartz and Whistler, 2009).

In the developed world, starch is also utilized in the production of food (bread) and beverages (beer, whisky), as well as the manufacturing of adhesives, cosmetics, detergents, paper, and textiles (Schwartz and Whistler, 2009). Starch is also used in the production of biodegradable packing materials and is increasingly seen as an attractive alternative to petroleum-based products (Schwartz and Whistler, 2009). Expansion of dietary and industrial uses of starch is creating an increased industrial demand for it, and with advancements in genetic engineering and modern breeding technologies, it is now possible to modify starch biosynthesis in different plant species, including cereals (Schwartz and Whistler, 2009; Shanon et al., 2009).

Current chemical and physical methods used in research and by the cereal industry to determine composition and monitor quality issues in cereals are slow, destructive, and many are based on empirical relationships. The lack of simple, reliable, and non-destructive methods for the determination of chemical composition in agricultural products has been one of the main obstacles to the development of rapid quality control in both the food industry and commercial trade. Conventional methods of analysis for quality control involve time-consuming, laborious, and costly procedures and chemical reagents (Williams, 2010; Karoui et al., 2010; Weeranantanaphan et al., 2011; Cozzolino, 2009, 2012).

In recent years, the combination of novel instrumentation and chemometric techniques has resulted in the development of rapid methods relating multivariate data, such as near-infrared (NIR) and mid-infrared (MIR) spectra of samples, to the concentration of specific chemical constituents (Karoui et al., 2010; Weeranantanaphan et al., 2011; Cozzolino, 2009, 2012). Infrared radiation is defined as the region of the electromagnetic spectrum between the visible (VIS) and the microwave wavelengths. The nominal range of wavelengths for NIR is between 780 and 2500 nm (12,820 to 4000 cm^{-1}), while for MIR, the spectral range is from 2500 to 25,000 nm (4000 to 400 cm^{-1}) (Subramanian and Rodriguez-Saona, 2009). Solid, liquid, or gaseous samples can absorb some of the incident infrared radiation at specific wavelengths resulting in a "fingerprint" or spectrum (Cozzolino, 2011; Smyth and Cozzolino, 2011, 2013; Subramanian and Rodriguez-Saona, 2009). Spectral "signatures" in the MIR result from absorbances that excite the fundamental stretching, bending, and rotating vibrations of some of the sample molecules, while NIR spectra result from complex overtones and high-frequency combinations at the shorter wavelengths. Although NIR intensities are 10−1000 times lower than those in the MIR range and the absorption peaks concomitantly smaller, highly sensitive spectrometers can nonetheless be built (Cozzolino, 2009, 2011; Subramanian and Rodriguez-Saona, 2009). This allows concentrated bulk or even aqueous materials to be scanned and analyzed quickly and easily. Spectral peaks in the MIR frequencies are often sharper and better resolved than in the NIR, while all the higher overtones (first through sixth) of the O-H, N-H, C-H, and S-H bands from the MIR region are observed in the NIR region, although they are much weaker than the fundamental frequencies in the MIR (Subramanian and Rodriguez-Saona, 2009). In addition to the existence of combination bands (eg, C-O stretch and N-H bend in protein), these overtones give rise to a crowded NIR spectrum with strongly overlapping bands. A major disadvantage of this characteristic overlap and complexity in NIR spectra has been the difficulty of quantification and interpretation of data from NIR spectra. On the other hand, the broad overlapping bands can diminish the need for using a large number of wavelengths in calibration and analysis routines (Cozzolino, 2011; Smyth and Cozzolino, 2011, 2013; Subramanian and Rodriguez-Saona, 2009).

Worldwide interest in food quality and methods of production has increased significantly in recent decades, due in part to changes in eating habits, consumer behavior, and the increased industrialization and globalization of food supply chains. Demand for high levels of quality and safety in agricultural and food crop production requires high standards in quality assurance and process control; satisfying this demand in turn requires appropriate analytical tools for analysis before, during, and after food or food ingredient production (Agelet and Hurburgh, 2010; Karoui et al., 2010; Weeranantanaphan et al., 2011; Cozzolino, 2009, 2011, 2012). Desirable features of such tools include speed, ease of use, minimal or no sample preparation, and the avoidance of sample destruction. These features are characteristic of a range of spectroscopic methods including MIR and NIR spectroscopy (McClure, 2004; Woodcock et al., 2008; Karoui et al., 2010; Weeranantanaphan et al., 2011).

It is well known that the combination of multivariate data analysis (MVA) with instrumental methods such as NIR and MIR spectroscopy can enhance the information extracted from spectra and thereby increase their use for a wide range of applications including composition measurement, traceability, and authenticity (McClure, 2004; Woodcock et al., 2008; Agelet and Hurburgh, 2010; Karoui et al., 2010; Weeranantanaphan et al., 2011; Brereton, 2003, 2007; Cozzolino, 2009). Therefore, the combinations of MVA with analytical instruments has the ability to determine more than one component at a time and can act as a support to establish links to other sample characteristics (McClure, 2004; Woodcock et al., 2008; Karoui et al., 2010; Agelet and Hurburgh, 2010; Weeranantanaphan et al., 2011; Brereton, 2003, 2007; Cozzolino, 2009, 2011, 2012, 2014). The use of MVA on large datasets produced by modern analytical instruments provides the ability to detect patterns in a dataset and to develop mathematical models to predict or monitor composition and other characteristics such as authenticity (McClure, 2004; Agelet and Hurburgh, 2010; Karoui et al., 2010; Weeranantanaphan et al., 2011; Brereton, 2003, 2007; Cozzolino, 2014).

Although both NIR and MIR spectroscopy combined with MVA have been extensively used to measure chemical composition in several cereals and oilseeds (eg, protein, moisture, and oil) (Delwiche, 1995, 1998; Delwiche et al., 1998; Jespersen and Munck, 2009; Himmelsbach, 2010; Agelet et al., 2012), few reports can be found on the use of these methods for varietal discrimination of cereals or authenticity confirmation in cereals and cereal products. In this chapter, an overview of applications of both NIR and MIR spectroscopy combined with multivariate data methods such as principal component analysis (PCA), linear discriminant analysis (LDA), and partial least squares discriminant analysis (PLS-DA) to aid authentication of and traceability systems for cereals are discussed.

16.2 Application of NIR and MIR Spectroscopy to Cereal Grain Authentication

16.2.1 NIR Spectroscopy and Varietal Classification of Wheat, Barley, Rice, and Corn Grains

A number of reports on the use of NIR spectroscopy as an analytical tool for the determination of quality parameters in a wide range of cereals and cereal products can be found in the scientific literature (Miralbes, 2008; Pojic et al., 2008; Pojic and

Martilovic, 2013). In the literature prior to 2001, there were few publications that reported the use of this technique to classify or trace cereals or cereal by-products. Some recent reports state that the ultimate goal of the application of the NIR spectroscopy is not solely to obtain the best estimates of the reference compositional values but a discrimination of the samples on the basis of their functionality or origin (variety, geographical) using their spectral properties (Christy and Kvalheim, 2007; Miralbés, 2008; Pojic et al., 2008; Pojic and Martilovic, 2013). Recent trends on the use and applications of NIR spectroscopy for the testing of seeds for properties such as vigor, disease, and insect pests have been also discussed and reviewed by other authors (Singh et al., 2010; Zhu et al., 2015).

Applications of NIR spectroscopy for classification purposes is based on the assumption that samples with different spectral responses are different in physical and/or chemical properties (Mohan et al., 2005; Christy and Kvalheim, 2007; Miralbés, 2008; Pojic et al., 2008; Pojic and Martilovic, 2013). Such differences in the spectral responses are a consequence of genetics, growing conditions, seasons, disease incidence, etc. (Mohan et al., 2005; Christy and Kvalheim, 2007; Miralbés, 2008; Pojic et al., 2008; Pojic and Martilovic, 2013).

One of the first applications of NIR spectroscopy for classification purposes was reported by Bertrand et al. (1985) for the identification of wheat varieties suitable for bread baking. Delwiche and Norris (1993) reported successful classification of ground samples of hard red winter (HRW) and hard red spring (HRS) wheat varieties. The use of algorithms such as artificial neural networks (ANNs) as tools to classify wheat classes was also reported by several authors (Chen et al., 1995; Song et al., 1995). Delwiche and Massie (1996) reported successful classification of individual kernels into different categories of wheat samples using partial least squares regression (PLS) or multiple linear regression (MLR). Dowell (2000) and Wang et al. (2002) reported the successful application of NIR spectroscopy for classification of vitreous and nonvitreous wheat kernels. The results reported by these authors suggested that the light-scattering effects between kernels was a direct effect of grain hardness, starch and protein content of individual kernels (Dowell, 2000; Wang et al., 1999). The results reported by Dowell (2000) showed that classification of obviously vitreous or non-vitreous kernels by NIR spectroscopy agreed almost perfectly with the reference method. However, with samples that were difficult to classify using the reference method, the NIR method classified only 75% of kernels (Dowell, 2000). According to these authors, the classification rates appear to be affected, at least in part, to scattering effects and to starch and protein differences between vitreous and non-vitreous kernels (Dowell, 2000). Wang and Paliwal (2006) explored the combination of NIR spectroscopy and several pattern recognition (LDA, PCA) and compression techniques (Fourier, discrete wavelet) to discriminate between several Canadian wheat varieties. Cocchi et al. (2005) and Foca et al. (2009) demonstrated the successful application of NIR spectroscopy to the distinction between bread wheats and flours of different baking quality. Another application on the use of NIR spectroscopy for classification purposes was reported by Dowell et al. (2009), which related to the selection and sorting of single wheat kernels (waxy vs nonwaxy) by using an automated single kernel NIR sorting system while Wang et al. (1999) evaluated the use of VIS and NIR to predict the number of dominant alleles in single kernels. Delwiche et al. (1999, 2006, 2011) reported the utilization of NIR spectroscopy for the differentiation of starch waxy genotypes in wheat varieties, obtaining classification accuracies of between 90% and 100%. Two years of breeders' samples (2003 and 2004) corresponding to more than 40 distinctive lines were subdivided about equally into the four genotypes (Delwiche et al., 2006). LDA classification models were developed using four wavelengths and each model consistently demonstrated a high ability (typically >95% of the time) to classify the fully waxy genotype (Delwiche et al., 2006). However, correct classification among the three other genotypes (wild type, wx-A1 null, and wx-B1 null) was generally not possible (Delwiche et al., 2006). A combination of NIR spectroscopy and genetic markers was reported to classify five wheat varieties sourced from Syria (Saleh, 2012), with the author concluding that the combination of NIR with other genetic techniques could be a powerful tool to identify and classify wheat varieties (Saleh, 2012).

Kwon et al. (1998) reported the use of NIR spectroscopy to identify rice varieties, while Delwiche et al. (1995) used NIR and PCA to classify amylose content in different rice varieties. The classification of paddy rice cultivars grown in Central, Eastern, and Southern Taiwan, harvested in three consecutive years (1997, 1998, and 1999), was attempted using discriminant analysis (DA) and a back-propagation neural network (BP-NN) with four wavelength selection methods (Liu et al., 2006). Average classification rates reported by these authors were 98.1% and 92.5%, using DA and BPNN, respectively (Liu et al., 2006).

More recently, Guo et al. (2010) developed a system to discriminate between corn seed varieties using FT-NIR combined with a specific pattern recognition technique—biomimetic pattern recognition. NIR spectroscopy was also reported to discriminate maize hybrid seed samples according to purity from different origins and years (Huang et al., 2014). Spectral acquisition was carried out using FT-NIR combined with different preprocessing methods such as moving window average, first derivative, and vector normalization together with pattern recognition methods including PCA and LDA (Huang et al., 2014). The average correct acceptance of the test and average correct rejection rates reported by the authors were 95% and 85%, respectively (Huang et al., 2014). Five different methods of pattern recognition, namely locally linear embedding (LLE), wavelet transform (WT), PCA, PLS, and support vector machine (SVM), were used to discriminate corn seeds based on their NIR spectra (Liu et al., 2012). Results reported by these authors indicated that, using three different spectral regions, performances of the three methods were as follows: PCA + SVM, LLE + SVM, and PLS + SVM were superior to WT + SVM and SVM methods (Liu et al., 2012). The combination of both NIR spectroscopy and ANN was reported for the classification of corn seeds from four varieties, namely Gaoyou115, Nongda368, Nongda108, and Nongda4967 (Chen et al., 2008). In order to improve the ability of the models to classify samples, the authors reported the use of a novel algorithm—Levenberg—Marquard (LM) (Chen et al., 2008). According to the authors the correct classification rate obtained using the LM algorithm was 95%. The results demonstrated that this identification method was rapid and nondestructive, and could be used for classification (Chen et al., 2008).

In barley, the main application of NIR in relation to classification was related to the discrimination between grains from normal and mutant barley samples (Munck et al., 2001, 2004; Munck and Moller, 2005; Jacobsen et al., 2005). These authors compared different wavelength regions in the NIR range (Munck and Moller, 2005) and reported that the mean spectra from the mutants and normal barleys were different from each other at wavelengths around 2276 nm correlating to starch, at 2294 nm describing amino acids, at 2336 and 2352 nm characteristic of cellulose content, and unsaturated fat at 2347 nm (Munck and Moller, 2005). According to these authors, from this data it was possible to make hypotheses about differences in chemical composition between normal and mutant lines (Munck and Moller, 2005). They concluded that multivariate statistical methods (eg, PCA) are indispensable for the classification of original barley endosperm mutants and their recombinants with standard varieties where different mathematical models should be used for the gamete and zygote levels of biological organization (Munck and Moller, 2005). In addition, classic probability statistics effective on the gene recombination level should be complemented by pattern recognition data analysis (chemometrics) for analyzing gene expression by NIR at the phenotype level (Munck and Moller, 2005).

The use of derivatives of NIR spectra to remove linear trends associated with differing particle size distribution from one sample to the next of the same type of biological material was used to classify barley varieties grown in Australia (Wiley et al., 2009). These authors compared the fourth-derivative spectra of wholemeal flour samples having high-nitrogen content with flour samples from low-nitrogen content allowing the identification of wavelengths in the NIR region at which there were statistically significant differences between the groups (Wiley et al., 2009). In addition, the use of the fourth-derivative spectral comparisons allowed the authors to identify novel biochemical differences between the flour samples analyzed (Wiley et al., 2009). According to these authors, visual assessment of the spectra of all mutants revealed a variable region (1470–1520 nm, corresponding to N-H stretch vibrations) that allowed the identification of extreme samples that differed markedly in hordein content (Wiley et al., 2009).

16.2.2 MIR Spectroscopy and Varietal Classification of Wheat, Barley, Rice, and Corn Grains

Different kinds of cereal flours submitted to various technological treatments were classified on the basis of their MIR spectra using pattern recognition techniques (Cochi et al., 2004). Classification in the wavelet domain was achieved by use of a wavelet packet transform for efficient pattern recognition (WPTER) algorithm, which allowed the most discriminant spectral regions to be identified and used. The use of PCA on the selected features showed an effective clustering of the flours analyzed (Cochi et al., 2004). Classification models were obtained for both training and test samples using improved wheat and wheat for biscuits (Cochi et al., 2004). The classification, sensitivity, and specificity rates reported by the authors were in the ranges of 73–100%, 0–93%, 29–100%, and 48–100% for improved wheat and wheat for biscuits, respectively (Cochi et al., 2004). Furthermore, mixtures of varying composition of the flours studied were distributed in PCA space according to their composition (Cochi et al., 2004). The use of attenuated total reflection Fourier transform infrared (ATR-FTIR) spectroscopy was reported to discriminate flours of several maize landraces from southern Brazil (Kuhnen et al., 2010). PCA applied to the MIR spectral range between 3000 and 600 cm^{-1} (whole spectrum) and 1650−1500 cm^{-1} (fingerprint region of proteins) spectral windows clearly discriminated the *Amarelao* landrace from 25 other maize landraces (Kuhnen et al., 2010). Quantitative and semi-qualitative analysis of proteins extracted from these samples showed a wide compositional and quality range among the fractions, mainly prolamine and glutelin (5.57−30.98 g/kg) contents. These authors concluded that the combination of both ATR-FTIR and PCA could be useful tools for the rapid screening and discrimination of maize with distinct chemical compositions (Kuhnen et al., 2010). Within the last decade, an increasing amount of genetic data has been used to clarify the problems inherent in wheat taxonomy. However, some of these techniques for obtaining and analyzing these types of data are not only cumbersome but also expensive and technically demanding (Demir et al., 2015). MIR spectroscopy was evaluated as a sensitive, rapid, and low-cost phylogenetic analysis tool for wheat seed samples (Demir et al., 2015) by analyzing samples from *Triticum* and *Aegilops* species using ATR-FTIR spectroscopy in combination with hierarchical cluster analysis and PCA (Demir et al., 2015). Results reported indicated that the lignin band (1525−1505 cm^{-1}) discriminated the species at the genus level (Demir et al., 2015). However, the species were clustered according to their genome commonalities when data from the whole spectral range were used (4000−650 cm^{-1}). Successful differentiation of *Triticum* and its closely related genus *Aegilops* clearly demonstrated the power of ATR-FTIR spectroscopy as a suitable tool for phylogenetic research (Demir et al., 2015).

16.2.3 Hyperspectral Imaging Applied to Classify Cereal Grains

Recently the use of NIR hyperspectral spectroscopy was evaluated to classify wheat samples grown in Canada using wavelet texture features (Choudhary et al., 2009). These authors concluded that the wavelet texture analysis of the NIR hyperspectral images of bulk wheat kernels is an effective tool for discrimination of wheat classes (Choudhary et al., 2009). Correct classification rates ranged between 63% and 100% depending on the classification method used by the authors (eg, linear, quadratic, or ANN) (Choudhary et al., 2009). NIR hyperspectral image analysis has been also used to classify individual wheat grains representing different Australian varieties as either sound or discolored by one of the commercially important black point, field fungi, or pink stains (Berman et al., 2007). These authors used a separate training (188 grains) and test set (665 grains) and used penalized discriminant analysis as method of classification in which a simple rule for grain classification was developed (Berman et al., 2007). Overall correct classification accuracies of 95% were reported by the authors using spectral data in the 420−2500 nm wavelength range (training = 97%, validation = 95%) as well as in the attenuated ranges of 420−1000 nm (training = 98%, validation = 95%) and 420−700 nm (training = 95%, validation = 95%) (Berman et al., 2007). These results also indicated that the visible range of the electromagnetic spectrum might be used for classification of wheat samples (Berman et al., 2007). Vitreousness is an important grading factor for durum wheat kernels that is associated with protein content (Gorreta et al., 2006). Hyperspectral reflectance images of wheat kernels at different vitreousness values have been reported using the wavelength range between 650 and 1100 nm (Gorreta et al., 2006). A discrimination method based on latent variables extracted by PLS has enabled satisfactory discrimination results to be obtained, ie, 100% correct separation between vitreous and nonvitreous kernels and a correct classification rate of up to 94% for the discrimination of total and partial starchy kernel classes (Gorreta et al., 2006).

Most authors have suggested that the NIR spectral differences between samples for specific traits was a result of interactions between different chemical (eg, amylose content, lipid—amylose interactions, protein) and physical (eg, scattering) properties of the endosperm. In general, the vast majority of classification models reported have applied PCA or ANN, with ANN models proving to perform better than PCA using a Mahalanobis distance classifier (Mahesh et al., 2008, 2011). Differentiation of wheat classes is one of the important challenges for the Canadian grain industry since, even though some wheat classes may look similar, their chemical composition and consequently the end product quality can vary significantly (Mahesh et al., 2008, 2011). Visual differentiation of wheat classes suffers from disadvantages such as inconsistency, low throughput, and the need for a large labor input. NIR hyperspectral imaging was used to develop classification models to differentiate wheat classes grown in western Canada (Mahesh et al., 2008, 2011). Wheat bulk samples were scanned in the wavelength region between 960 and 1700 nm at 10 nm intervals using an InGaAs NIR camera (Mahesh et al., 2008, 2011). Classification accuracies reported for each of the groups analyzed were 100% in classifying Canada Prairie Spring Red, Canada Western Red Winter, and Canada Western Soft White Spring wheat classes and higher than 94% for the other wheat classes analyzed such as Canada Western Extra Strong, Canada Western Hard White Spring, Canada Western Red Spring, Canada Prairie Spring White, and Canada Western Amber Durum using LDA (Mahesh et al., 2008, 2011). The authors also reported the use of quadratic discriminant analysis with a leave-one-out cross-validation method, producing classification accuracies of higher than 86% for all wheat classes. Overall classification accuracies for models developed using sample set sizes of 60% training—30% testing—10% validation (referred to as 60-30-10) and 70% training—20% testing—10% validation (referred to as 70-20-10) ANN models were above 90% for independent validation sets using three-layer standard and Wardnet back-propagation neural network architectures (Mahesh et al., 2008, 2011). The authors also concluded that one of the major limitations of this technique is the production of a large volume of information that requires appropriate data processing techniques to interpret the results accurately (Mahesh et al., 2008, 2011). The same authors also highlighted the fact that proper calibration methods are needed to remove the inherent and external noise in the system during imaging (Mahesh et al., 2008, 2011; Delwiche et al., 2013).

NIR hyperspectral imaging was reported for the identification of rice seed cultivars applying PLS-DA, soft independent modeling of class analogy (SIMCA), K-nearest neighbor (KNN), SVM, and random forest (RF) techniques (Kong et al., 2013). Spectra of 1039–1612 nm were used in their entirety to build classification models. PLS-DA and KNN models produced over 80% classification accuracy while SIMCA, SVM, and RF models generated 100% classification accuracy in both the calibration and prediction sample sets (Kong et al., 2013). Overall results indicated that hyperspectral imaging could be used for rice seed cultivar identification and that RF is an effective classification technique (Kong et al., 2013).

A system to identify the purity of waxy corn was developed based on the combined spectral, morphological, and textural features extracted from VIS and NIR hyperspectral images (Yang et al., 2015). In order to reduce the dimensions of the spectral dataset, spectral feature vectors were constructed using the successive projections algorithm (Yang et al., 2015). Five morphological features (area, circularity, aspect ratio, roundness, and solidity) and eight texture features (energy, contrast, correlation, entropy, and their standard deviations) were extracted as descriptive appearance characters from every corn kernel (Yang et al., 2015). Both SVM and PLS-DA were used to build classification models for seed variety classification based on different groups of features (Yang et al., 2015). Results reported by these authors demonstrated that, by combining spectral and appearance characteristics, better classification results were obtained (Yang et al., 2015). Recognition accuracy achieved by the SVM model (98.2% and 96.3% for germ side and endosperm side, respectively) were better than those reported using PLS-DA as a classification tool (Yang et al., 2015).

16.2.4 Geographical Origin of Cereals

The feasibility of using NIR spectroscopy combined with chemometrics to discriminate wheat samples from different geographical origins of China has been reported (Zhao et al., 2011, 2013). A total of 240 wheat samples from two growing years from four of the major wheat-producing regions in China was analyzed (Zhao et al., 2011, 2013). Before the classification routines used by the authors, the spectra of both wheat kernel and flour samples were pre-processed (Zhao et al., 2011, 2013). LDA based on PCA scores and PLS-DA techniques were applied to classify samples according to their geographical origin (Zhao et al., 2011, 2013). Classification rates reported by these authors for wheat kernel samples were 82.5–92.5% and 77.5–87.5% using LDA and PLS-DA, respectively (Zhao et al., 2011, 2013). For wheat flour, the classification rates reported were 85.5–87.5% and 72–85% using LDA and PLS-DA, respectively (Zhao et al., 2011, 2013). The authors concluded that NIR spectroscopy combined with chemometrics is a promising method for identifying wheat according to geographical origin; however, according to the authors, the effectiveness of the proposed method should be further validated (Zhao et al., 2011, 2013). In Europe, Miralbés (2008) demonstrated discrimination of wheat varieties that originated from Spain and France, reporting classification rates of 99.5% (calibration) and 94% (validation). Kim et al. (2003) used a modified least squares regression analysis of NIR spectroscopy to verify the authenticity of Korean-grown rice versus imported rice for short and medium-long grains. The results reported by these authors indicated that 100% of the samples were correctly classified (Kim et al., 2003).

According to the authors, although authentication of rice was performed successfully using NIR spectroscopy, further efforts are needed for implementation of this methodology for authentication of rice for industry purposes (Kim et al., 2003).

Instrumental techniques such as NIR spectroscopy are used in industry to monitor product composition and quality (Gonzalez-Martin et al., 2014). As occurs with other food industries, the Chilean flour industry needs simple, rapid techniques to objectively assess the origin of different products, which is often related to their quality (Gonzalez-Martin et al., 2014). NIR spectroscopy has been used in combination with chemometric methods to predict the geographic origin of wheat grain and flour samples produced in different regions of Chile (Gonzalez-Martin et al., 2014). NIR spectral data were analyzed using a supervised pattern recognition method such as PLS-DA and 76% of the wheat grain samples and between 90% and 96% of the flour samples were correctly classified according to their geographic origin (Gonzalez-Martin et al., 2014). Results reported by these authors showed that NIR spectroscopy, together with chemometric methods, can provide a rapid tool for the classification of wheat grain and flour samples according to their geographic origin (Gonzalez-Martin et al., 2014).

Identification of the geographical origin of rice was also attempted by combining pattern recognition techniques with NIR spectroscopy (Xie et al., 2013). Several Xiangshui and non-Xiangshui rice samples grown in different geographical origins were analyzed using agglomerative hierarchical cluster analysis and Fisher's linear discriminant analysis (Xie et al., 2013). Overall, results reported by these authors indicated that Xiangshui rice and non-Xiangshui rice can be correctly classified (100% correct classification) using both classification methods, while correct classification rates for non-Xiangshui rice on the basis of geographic origin were 91.9% by agglomerative hierarchical cluster analysis and 96.7% by Fisher's linear discriminant analysis, respectively (Xie et al., 2013).

16.2.5 Transgenic and Genetically Modified Cereals

Combining these novel phenotyping methods with high-throughput genotyping based on different "omic" technologies and analyzing the data with sophisticated mathematical models promises to provide a major breakthrough in the elucidation of the underlying genetic basis of complex plant traits, such as drought resistance, frost tolerance, or transgenic crops (Rossel et al., 2001; Rui et al., 2005; Alishahi et al., 2010; Cozzolino, 2014). Modern biotechnology, based on recombinant DNA techniques, has made it possible to introduce new traits with great potential for crop improvement (Cozzolino, 2014). However, concerns about unintended effects of gene transformation that possibly threaten the environment or consumer health have persuaded scientists to initiate pre-release tests on genetically modified organisms. Assessment of a "substantial equivalence" concept by comparison of a genetically modified organism to a comparator with a history of safe use could be the first step of a comprehensive risk assessment (Keymanesh et al., 2009; Cozzolino, 2014). One of the main criteria used is the abundance of metabolites or compounds present in the matrix associated with the changes originated from genetic or environmental factors (Keymanesh et al., 2009;

Cozzolino, 2014). Since measurement of all metabolites would be very costly, if indeed it is practically possible, statistical evaluation of processed spectral data recorded on grains could be a time and cost-effective substitution for complex chemical analysis (Keymanesh et al., 2009; Cozzolino, 2014). In recent years, the ability of multivariate statistical techniques combined with molecular spectroscopy (infrared and NMR) were tested as methods to identify transgenic rice (Keymanesh et al., 2009). Results reported by these authors confirmed the capability of multivariate data analysis combined with molecular spectroscopy in applications related with studies of the metabolome (Keymanesh et al., 2009).

Munck et al. (2004) assessed the discriminatory power of NIR spectroscopy combined with PCA to evaluate different lysine mutants in barley. These authors were able to identify different mutants based on the NIR fingerprint of each sample (Munck et al., 2004). It has been shown that it is possible to select improved malting barley genotypes based on NIR spectra that represent a total physicochemical spectral fingerprint of the samples and are interpreted using PCA (Munck et al., 2004, 2001). The use of NIR spectroscopy was also evaluated to discriminate barley flour containing high levels of lysine amino acids (Munck et al., 2004, 2001). It was found that differences between these two barley flours might be observed through interpretation of the PCA scores (Munck et al., 2004, 2001). Thereby, these two variants of barley flour clustered correctly into two groups according to their different NIR spectra. The effect of different environments on transgenic and nontransgenic plant materials measured by NIR spectroscopy was evaluated by the same authors. Several other reports can be found on the use of NIR spectroscopy to discriminate between transgenic and nontransgenic grains (Rossel et al., 2001; Rui et al., 2005; Alishahi et al., 2010). These authors reported that methods such as PCA or discriminant analysis yield good performance in completely separating transgenic from nontransgenic grains. Other reports can be found on the use of NIR spectroscopy to discriminate between transgenic and nontransgenic grains (Hurburgh et al., 2000; Campbell et al., 2000; Ahmed, 2002; Rossel et al., 2001; Rui et al., 2005). These authors also reported that the PCA method completely separated transgenic from nontransgenic grains, concluding that the utilization of NIR spectroscopy as a nondestructive method had a suitable efficiency to detect transgenic grains (Hurburgh et al., 2000; Campbell et al., 2000; Ahmed, 2002; Rossel et al., 2001; Rui et al., 2005; Alishahi et al., 2010). NIR spectroscopy in reflectance mode has been applied to the problem of differentiating four genotypes of durum wheat such as "waxy," Wx A1 null null, wx-B1 null, and wild type (Lavine et al., 2014). Test data consisted of 95 NIR reflectance spectra of wheat samples obtained from a USDA-ARS wheat breeding program (Lavine et al., 2014). The genetic algorithm (GA) pattern recognition method employed both supervised and unsupervised learning to identify wavelet coefficients that optimized clustering of the spectra by genotype in a plot as a function of the main principal components that explain most of the variability of the data (Lavine et al., 2014). According to the authors, by sampling key feature subsets, scoring their PC plots, and tracking those genotypes and samples that were difficult to classify, the pattern recognition GA was able to identify a set of wavelet coefficients, the PC plot of which revealed clustering of wheat samples on the basis of their "waxy" condition (Lavine et al., 2014). An overall correct classification rate of 78% was achieved (Lavine et al., 2014). The combination of NIR and PLS-DA was used to discriminate between transgenic (TCTP and mi166) and wild-type (Zhonghua 11) rice samples (Long et al., 2015). Rice lines transformed with a protein (OsTCTP) and a regulation gene (Osmi166) were also discriminated (Long et al., 2015). The transgenic and wild-type rice were distinguished from each other with a correct classification rate of 100% in the validation test (Long et al., 2015). Transgenic rice TCTP and mi166 were also distinguished from each other in the range with a correct classification rate of 100% (Long et al., 2015). Campbell et al. (2000) combined NIR with PCA analysis to identify and classify the endosperm of maize mutants. These authors have analyzed a total of 1176 grain samples representing 10 different single- and double-mutant genotypic classes of specialty starch corn using NIR transmittance spectroscopy (Campbell et al., 2000). The genotypes used by the authors included amylose-extender, dull, sugary-2, waxy, and the combinations between them (Campbell et al., 2000). Two-class classification models (only two genotypes compared) were developed using PLS while three-way and multiclass models were examined using PCA (Campbell et al., 2000). The effectiveness of the calibrations was evaluated by examining the percentage of unknown grain samples incorrectly classified (Campbell et al., 2000). These authors reported that two-class models performed better than multiclass models. However, they did not show improvement when discriminating between genotypes with overlapping amylose content (Campbell et al., 2000). On the other hand, three-way models including double mutants and their corresponding single-mutant counterparts had misclassification percentages typically higher than 5% using PCA (Campbell et al., 2000). Overall, the best multiclass model using all 10 genotypic classes simultaneously revealed only two classes with misclassification rates higher than 10% (Campbell et al., 2000). This study demonstrated that, depending on the material to be considered, NIR spectroscopy could be useful for segregation of specialty starch hybrid grains from other grain types (Campbell et al., 2000).

16.3 Concluding Remarks

Although both NIR and MIR spectroscopy combined with MVA have been extensively used to measure several biochemical, chemical, and physical compositional parameters in cereals and cereal products (eg, protein, moisture, and oil), few reports can be found on the use of these methods to target varietal discrimination and traceability issues.

It is well recognized by agronomists, breeders, and farmers that adapting and using these technologies is a promising way forward to efficiently and reliably improve important agronomical characteristics of crops, to adapt and develop new varieties, to improve our understanding about crops (eg, physiology, biochemistry, and adaptation), to maintain a sustainable agriculture, as well as to guarantee to consumers the origin of the crops and foods produced.

In recent years infrared and vibrational spectroscopy technologies have been introduced as fingerprinting techniques within the food sector in order to target fraud, traceability, and authentication issues. These techniques are recognized by their main advantages over the traditional chemical and chromatographic methods such as speed, ease of use in routine operations, and minimal or zero sample preparation.

It is clear that the breadth of these types of applications, either in routine use or under development, is showing no sign of diminishing. Overall, the combination of different vibrational spectroscopy techniques (eg, NIR, MIR, Raman) with multivariate methods (eg, PCA, LDA) could be used as tools to fingerprint samples on a large scale (eg, at the farm gate, handling, and storage).

In addition, advances in hardware (eg, optics, instrumentation), such as hyperspectral imaging or handheld instruments, and the developments in chemometrics and data handling (eg, new algorithms), will enhance the applications of vibrational spectroscopy as tools for the traceability and authentication of cereals.

References

Agelet, L.E., Hurburgh, C.R., 2010. A tutorial on near infrared spectroscopy and its calibration. Critical Reviews in Analytical Chemistry 40, 246–260.

Agelet, L.E., Armstrong, P.R., Romagosa Clariana, I., Hurburgh, C.R., 2012. Measurement of single soybean seed attributes by near infrared technologies. A comparative study. Journal of Agriculture Food and Chemistry 60, 8314–8322.

Ahmed, F.E., 2002. Detection of genetically modified organisms in foods. Trends in Biotechnology 20, 215–223.

Alishahi, H., Farahmand, H., Prieto, N., Cozzolino, D., 2010. Identification of transgenic foods using NIR spectroscopy: a review. Spectrochimica Acta Part A: Molecular and Biomolecular Spectroscopy 75, 1–7.

Berman, M., Connor, P.M., Whitbourn, L.B., Coward, D.A., Osborne, B.G., Southan, M.D., 2007. Classification of sound and stained wheat grains using visible and near infrared hyperspectral image analysis. Journal of Near Infrared Spectroscopy 15 (6), 351–358.

Bertrand, D., Robert, P., Loisel, F., 1985. Identification of some wheat varieties by near infrared reflectance spectroscopy. Journal of the Science of Food and Agriculture 36, 1120–1124.

Brereton, R.G., 2003. Chemometrics: Data Analysis for the Laboratory and Chemical Plant. John Wiley & Sons, Ltd, UK.

Brereton, R.G., 2007. Applied Chemometrics for Scientist. John Wiley & Sons, Ltd, UK.

Campbell, M.R., Sykes, J., Glover, D.V., 2000. Classification of single and double-mutant corn endosperm genotypes by near-infrared transmittance spectroscopy. Cereal Chemistry 77, 774–778.

Christy, A.A., Kvalheim, O.M., 2007. Latent-variable analysis of multivariate data in infrared spectrometry. In: Ozaki, et al. (Eds.), Near-infrared Spectroscopy in Food Science and Technology. Wiley, Hoboken, pp. 145–162.

Cocchi, M., Corbellini, M., Foca, G., 2005. Classification of bread wheat flours in different quality categories by a wavelet-based feature selection/classification algorithm on NIR spectra. Analytica Chimica Acta 544, 100–107.

Cocchi, M., Foca, G., Lucisano, M., 2004. Classification of cereal flours by chemometric analysis of MIR spectra. Journal of Agriculture Food and Chemistry 52, 1062–1067.

Chen, Y.R., Delwiche, S.R., Hruschka, W.R., 1995. Classification of hard red wheat by feedforward backpropagation neural networks. Cereal Chemistry 72, 317–319.

Chen, J., Chen, X., Li, W., Wang, J.-H., Han, D.-H., 2008. Study on discrimination of corn seed based on near-infrared spectra and artificial neural network model. Spectroscopy and Spectral Analysis 28, 1806–1809.

Choudhary, R., Mahesh, S., Paliwal, J., Jayas, D.S., 2009. Identification of wheat classes using wavelet features from near infrared hyperspectral images of bulk samples. Biosystems Engineering 102, 115–127.

Cozzolino, D., 2009. Near infrared spectroscopy in natural products analysis. Planta Medica 75, 746–757.

Cozzolino, D., 2011. Infrared methods for high throughput screening of metabolites: food and medical applications. Combinatorial Chemistry & High Throughput Screening 14, 125–131.

Cozzolino, D., 2012. Recent trends on the use of infrared spectroscopy to trace and authenticate natural and agricultural food products. Applied Spectroscopy Reviews 47, 518–530.

Cozzolino, D., 2014. An overview of the use of infrared spectroscopy and chemometrics in authenticity and traceability of cereals. Food Research International 60 (2014), 262–265.

Demir, P., Onde, S., Severcan, F., 2015. Phylogeny of cultivated and wild wheat species using ATR-FTIR spectroscopy. Spectrochimica Acta Part A-Molecular and Biomolecular Spectroscopy 135, 757–763.

Delwiche, S.R., Norris, K.H., 1993. Classification of hard red wheat by near-infrared diffuse reflectance spectroscopy. Cereal Chemistry 70, 29–35.

Delwiche, S.R., 1995. Single wheat kernel analysis by near-infrared transmittance: protein content. Cereal Chemistry 72, 11–16.

Delwiche, S.R., Massie, D.R., 1996. Classification of wheat by visible and near-infrared reflectance spectroscopy. Cereal Chemistry 73, 399–405.

Delwiche, S.R., 1998. Protein content of single kernels of wheat by near infrared reflectance spectroscopy. Journal of Cereal Science 27, 241–254.

Delwiche, R.S., Graybosch, R.A., Peterson, C.J., 1998. Predicting protein composition, biochemical properties, and dough-handling properties of hard red winter wheat by near-infrared reflectance. Cereal Chemistry 75, 412–416.

Delwiche, S.R., Graybosch, R.A., Peterson, C.J., 1999. Identification of wheat lines possessing the 1AL.1RS or 1BL.1RS wheat-rye translocation by near-infrared reflectance spectroscopy. Cereal Chemistry 76, 255–260.

Delwiche, S.R., Graybosch, R.A., Hansen, L.E., Souza, E., Dowell, F.E., 2006. Single kernel near-infrared analysis of tetraploid (Durum) wheat for classification of the waxy condition. Cereal Chemistry 83, 287–292.

Delwiche, S.R., Graybosch, R.A., Amand, P.S., Bai, G., 2011. Starch waxiness in hexaploid wheat (*Triticum aestivum* L.) by NIR reflectance spectroscopy. Journal of Agricultural and Food Chemistry 59, 4002–4008.

Delwiche, S.R., Souza, E.J., Kim, M.S., 2013. Limitations of single kernel near-infrared hyperspectral imaging of soft wheat for milling quality. Biosystems Engineering 115, 260–273.

Dowell, F.E., 2000. Differentiating vitreous and nonvitreous durum wheat kernels by using near-infrared spectroscopy. Cereal Chemistry 77, 155–158.

Dowell, F.E., Maghirang, E.B., Graybosch, R.A., Berzonsky, W.A., Delwiche, S.R., 2009. Selecting and sorting waxy wheat kernels using near-infrared spectroscopy. Cereal Chemistry 86, 251–255.

Foca, G., Cocchi, M., Li Vigni, M., Caramanico, R., Corbellini, M., Ulrici, A., 2009. Different feature selection strategies in the wavelet domain applied to NIR-based quality classification models of bread wheat flours. Chemometrics and Intelligent Laboratory Systems 99, 91–100.

Gonzalez-Martin, I., Moncada, W., Gonzalez-Perez, G., Zapata San Martin, C., Lopez-Gonzalez, N., Lobos Ortega, F., Hernandez-Hierro, I.J.-M., 2014. Chilean flour and wheat grain: tracing their origin using near infrared spectroscopy and chemometrics. Food Chemistry 145, 802–806.

Gorretta, N., Roger, J.M., Aubert, M., Campan, F., Roumet, P., 2006. Determining vitreousness of durum wheat kernels using near infrared hyperspectral imaging. Journal of Near Infrared Spectroscopy 14 (4), 231−239.

Guo, T.-T., Wang, S.-J., Wang, H.-W., Hu, H.-X., An, D., Wu, W.-J., Xia, W., Zhai, Y.-F., 2010. A new discrimination method of maize seed varieties based on near-infrared spectroscopy. Spectroscopy and Spectral Analysis 30, 2372−2376.

Himmelsbasch, D.S., 2010. The analysis of rice by vibrational spectroscopy. In: Li-Chan, E., Griffiths, P.R., Chalmers, J.M. (Eds.), Applications of Vibrational Spectroscopy in Food Science. Wiley and Sons, UK.

Huang, H.-J., Yan, Y.-L., Shen, B.-H., Li, L., An, D., 2014. Near infrared spectroscopy analysis method of maize hybrid seed purity discrimination. Spectroscopy and Spectral Analysis 34 (5), 1253−1258.

Hurburgh, C.R., Rippke, G.R., Heithoff, C., Roussel, S.A., Hardy, C.L., 2000. Detection of genetically modified grains by near-infrared spectroscopy. In: Proceedings PITTCON 2000-Science for the 21st Century, 12−17 March, New Orleans, USA, p. 1431.

Jacobsen, S., Sondergaard, I., Moller, B., Desler, T., Munck, L., 2005. A chemometric evaluation of the underlying physical and chemical patterns that support near infrared spectroscopy of barley seeds as a tool for explorative classification of endosperm, genes and gene combinations. Journal of Cereal Science 42, 281−299.

Jespersen, B.M., Munck, L., 2009. Cereals and cereal products. In: Da Wen Sun Infrared Spectroscopy for Quality Analysis and Control. Elsevier.

Karoui, R., Downey, G., Blecker, C., 2010. Mid-infrared spectroscopy coupled with chemometrics: a tool for the analysis of intact food systems and the exploration of their molecular structure-quality relationships - a review. Chemical Reviews 110, 6144−6168.

Keymanesh, K., Darvishi, M.H., Sardari, S., 2009. Metabolome comparison of transgenic and non-transgenic rice by statistical analysis of FTIR and NMR. Rice Science 16, 119−123.

Kim, S.S., Mee-Ra, R., Kim, M.J., Lee, S.-H., 2003. Authentication of rice using near-infrared reflectance spectroscopy. Cereal Chemistry 80 (3), 346−349.

Kuhnen, S., Ogliari, J., Dias, B., Fernando, P., 2010. ATR-FTIR spectroscopy and chemometric analysis applied to discrimination of landrace maize flours produced in southern Brazil. International Journal of Food Science and Technology 45, 1673−1681.

Kong, W., Zhang, C., Liu, F., Nie, P., He, Y., 2013. Rice seed cultivar identification using near-infrared hyperspectral imaging and multivariate data analysis. Sensors 13 (7), 8916−8927.

Kwon, Y.K., Cho, R.K., Davies, A.M.C., 1998. Identification of rice variety using near infrared spectroscopy. Journal of Near Infrared Spectroscopy vol. 6, A67−A73.

Lavine, B.K., Mirjankar, N., Deiwiche, S., 2014. Classification of the waxy condition of durum wheat by near infrared reflectance spectroscopy using wavelets and a genetic algorithm. Microchemical Journal 117, 178−182.

Liu, C.-C., Shaw, J.-T., Poong, K.-Y., Hong, M.-C., Shen, M.-L., 2006. Wavelength selection for classifying paddy rice by near-infrared spectroscopy. Cereal Chemistry 83, 335−339.

Liu, T.-L., Su, Q.-Y., Sun, Q., Yang, L.-M., 2012. Recognition of corn seeds based on pattern recognition and near infrared spectroscopy technology. Spectroscopy and Spectral Analysis 32 (5), 1209−1212.

Long, Z., Shan-shan, W., Yan-fei, D., Jia-rong, P., Cheng, Z., 2015. Discrimination of transgenic rice based on near infrared reflectance spectroscopy and partial least squares regression discriminant analysis. Rice Science 22 (5), 245−249.

Mahesh, S., Manickavasagan, A., Jayas, D.S., Paliwal, J., White, N.D.G., 2008. Feasibility of near-infrared hyperspectral imaging to differentiate Canadian wheat classes. Biosystems Engineering 101, 50–57.

Mahesh, S., Jayas, D.S., Paliwal, J., White, N.D.G., 2011. Identification of wheat classes at different moisture levels using near-infrared hyperspectral images of bulk samples. Sensing and Instrumentation for Food Quality and Safety 5, 1–9.

McClure, F.W., 2004. 204 years of near infrared technology: 1800–2003. Journal of Near Infrared Spectroscopy 11, 487–498.

Miralbés, C., 2008. Discrimination of European wheat varieties using near infrared reflectance spectroscopy. Food Chemistry 106, 386–389.

Mohan, L.A., Karunakaran, C., Jayas, D.S., White, N.D.G., 2005. Classification of bulk cereals using visible and NIR reflectance characteristics. Canadian Biosystems Engineering 47, 7–14.

Munck, L., Nielsen, J., Møller, B., Jacobsen, S., Søndergaard, I., Engelsen, S.B., Nørgaard, L., Bro, R., 2001. Exploring the phenotypic expression of a regulatory proteome-altering gene by spectroscopy and chemometrics. Analytica Chimica Acta 446, 171–186.

Munck, L., Møller, B., Jacobsen, S., Søndergaard, I., 2004. Near infrared spectra indicate specific mutant endosperm genes and reveal a new mechanism for substituting starch with (1/3, 1/4)-b-glucan in barley. Journal of Cereal Science 40, 213–222.

Munck, L., Moller, B., 2005. Principal component analysis of near infrared spectra as a tool of endosperm mutant characterization and in barley breeding for quality. Czech Journal of Genetics and Plant Breeding 41, 89–95.

Pojić, M., Mastilović, J., Pestorić, M., Radusin, T., 2008. The ensuring of traceability of measurements for cereal quality determination. Food Processing Quality and Safety 35, 11–18.

Pojić, M., Mastilović, J., 2013. Near infrared spectroscopy—advanced analytical tool in wheat breeding, trade, and processing. Food Bioprocess Technology 6, 330–352.

Rossel, S.A., Hardy, C.L., Hurburgh, C.R., Rippke, G.R., 2001. Application of near-infrared diffuse reflectance spectroscopy to the detection and identification of transgenic corn. Applied Spectroscopy 55, 1425–1432.

Rui, Y., Luo, Y., Haung, K., Wang, W., Zhang, L., 2005. Discrimination of transgenic corns using NIR diffuse reflectance spectroscopy and back propagation (BP). Spectroscopy and Spectral Analysis 25, 1581–1592.

Saleh, B., 2012. Biochemical and genetic variation of some Syrian wheat varieties using NIR, RAPD and AFLPs techniques. Journal of Plant Biology Research 1, 1–11.

Shannon, J.C., Garwood, D.L., Charles, D., 2009. Genetics and physiology of starch development. In: Starch: Chemistry and Technology, third ed. Academic Press, Elsevier.

Singh, C.B., Jayas, D.S., Paliwal, J., White, N.D.G., 2010. Identification of insect-damaged wheat kernels using shortwave near-infrared hyperspectral and digital colour imaging. Computers and Electronics in Agriculture 73, 118–125.

Smyth, H.E., Cozzolino, D., 2011. Applications of infrared spectroscopy for quantitative analysis of volatile and secondary metabolites in plant materials. Current Bioactive Compounds 7, 66–74.

Smyth, H.E., Cozzolino, D., 2013. Instrumental methods (spectroscopy, electronic nose and tongue) as tools to predict taste and aroma in beverages: advantages and limitations. Chemical Reviews 113, 1429–1440.

Song, H., Delwiche, S.R., Chen, Y.R., 1995. Neural network classification of wheat using single kernel near-infrared transmittance spectra. Optical Engineering 34, 2927–2934.

Subramanian, A., Rodriguez-Saona, L., 2009. Fourier transform infrared (FTIR) spectroscopy. In: Sun, D.W. (Ed.), Infrared Spectroscopy for Food Quality Analysis and Control. Academic Press, UK, pp. 146–174.

Schwartz, D., Whistler, R.L., 2009. History and future of starch. In: BeMiller, J.N., Whistler, R.L. (Eds.), Starch: Chemistry and Technology, third ed. Academic Press, Elsevier.

Wang, D., Dowell, F.E., Lacey, R.E., 1999. Predicting the number of dominant R alleles in single wheat kernels using visible and near-infrared reflectance spectra. Cereal Chemistry 76, 6–9.

Wang, D., Dowell, F.E., Dempster, R., 2002. Determining vitreous subclasses of hard red spring wheat using visible/near-infrared spectroscopy. Cereal Chemistry 79 (3), 418–422.

Wang, W., Paliwal, J., 2006. Spectral data compression and analyses techniques to discriminate wheat classes. Transactions of the ASABE 49, 1607–1612.

Weeranantanaphan, J., Downey, G., Allen, P., Sun, D.W., 2011. A review of near infrared spectroscopy in muscle food analysis: 2005–2010. Journal of Near Infrared Spectroscopy 19, 61–104.

Wiley, P.R., Tanner, G.J., Chandler, P.M., 2009. Molecular classification of barley (*Hordeum vulgare* L.) mutants using derivative NIR spectroscopy. Journal of Agricultural and Food Chemistry 57, 4042–4050.

Williams, P., 2010. The analysis of wheat by near infrared spectroscopy. In: Li-Chan, E.C.Y., Griffiths, P.R., Chalmers, J.M. (Eds.), Applications of Vibrational Spectroscopy in Food Science. John Wiley and Sons, UK.

Woodcock, T., Downey, G., O'Donnell, C.P., 2008. Better quality food and beverages: the role of near infrared spectroscopy. Journal of Near Infrared Spectroscopy 16, 1–29.

Xie, S., Liu, Q., Cui, S.W., 2005. Starch modification and applications. In: Cui, S. (Ed.), Food Carbohydrates. Taylor and Francis, Boca Raton.

Xie, L.-Y., Shen, S.-G., Liu, Z.-H., Sun, H.-W., 2013. Identification of geographical origins of rice with pattern recognition technique by near infrared spectroscopy. Spectroscopy and Spectral Analysis 33, 102–105.

Yang, X., Hong, H., You, Z., Cheng, F., 2015. Spectral and image integrated analysis of hyperspectral data for waxy corn seed variety classification. Sensors (Switzerland) 15, 15578–15594.

Zhao, H., Guo, B., Wei, Y., Zhang, B., 2013. Near infrared reflectance spectroscopy for determination of the geographical origin of wheat. Food Chemistry 138, 1902–1907.

Zhao, H.Y., Guo, BoL., Wei, YiM., Zhang, B., Sun, S.M., Yan, J.H., Zhang, L., 2011. Identification of geographical origins of wheat with discriminant analysis by near infrared spectroscopy. Scientia Agricultura Sinica 44, 1451–1456.

Zhu, L.-W., Ma Wen-guang, H.J., Zheng, Y.-Y., Tian, Y.-X., Guan, Y.-J., Hu, W.-M., 2015. Advances of NIR spectroscopy technology applied in seed quality detection. Spectroscopy and Spectral Analysis 35, 346–349.

Part Three

Advances in Authenticity Testing for Food Adulteration

Advances in Testing for Adulteration and Authenticity of Dairy Products

17

G.A. Abernethy, J.G. Bendall, S.E. Holroyd
Fonterra Research & Development Centre, Palmerston North, New Zealand

Chapter Outline

17.1 Introduction

Milk and milk products are very rich in nutritional density (Smedman et al., 2010) and, as such, they form a vitally important component of a healthy diet (McDonald, 2008). In 2004 it was conservatively estimated that, if the adult population of the United States were to consume three to four cups of milk per day, the resulting reductions in medical conditions, such as obesity, hypertension, type 2 diabetes, stroke, coronary heart disease, osteoporosis, kidney stones, preeclampsia, and colorectal cancer would result in health care savings in excess of US$200 billion over a five-year period

(McCarron and Heaney, 2004). That study was extended in 2011 to include North and South America, Europe, and Asia/Pacific and the five-year health care savings were estimated to amount to in excess of US$6.9 trillion (McCarron, 2011). As large as they are, those economic benefits do not even begin to include the immeasurable benefits from increased quality of life.

However, these profound benefits are placed at jeopardy if the reputation of milk and milk products as high-quality foods is compromised by unethical behavior arising from, eg, economic motivations. Once farming began on an industrial scale, with centralized distribution supplying milk to large cities, the adulteration of milk (chiefly by adding water) began to occur on a systematic basis, as was realized by the New York Department of Health in 1868 (Weinstein, 1947). Advances in analytical chemistry during the 19th century facilitated both the design of new ways to adulterate food based on knowledge about composition and the means to detect such adulteration, so that, by the early 20th century, adulteration was no longer a common practice in developed countries (Jackson, 2009; Tunick, 2009); however, developing countries still have problems with the prevalence of milk adulteration (Kenny, 2013).

The means to analytically test for the authenticity of dairy products was critically reviewed (de la Fuente and Juárez) in 2005. This chapter describes key developments that have occurred during the last decade for both the adulteration of milk and dairy products and the detection and prevention of adulteration, with additional comments from a commercial and food safety perspective.

17.1.1 Definitions

Codex Alimentarius, the organization whose standards are used by the World Trade Organization as a reference for food control systems, has not set any definition for the word *adulterate*, and various international agencies use the term with different meanings. The definition from the Oxford English Dictionary is used throughout this chapter, that is, to "render (something) poorer in quality by adding another substance."

Because adulterants are deliberately added, they may not necessarily fall within the definition of a contaminant (something that is present inadvertently). The key point is that they are knowingly being added for the purpose of deception.

Codex Alimentarius Standard 193-1995 defines a "contaminant" as being: "Any substance not intentionally added to food, which is present in such food as a result of the production (including operations carried out in crop husbandry, animal husbandry and veterinary medicine), manufacture, processing, preparation, treatment, packing, packaging, transport or holding of such food or as a result of environmental contamination. The term does not include insect fragments, rodent hairs and other extraneous matter."

In the context of food, "authenticity" is the certainty of knowing that a product genuinely is what it claims to be on the label. Codex Alimentarius does not specifically define "authenticity" although its Code of Practice CAC/GL 60-2006 makes it clear that authenticity relates to confidence in the accuracy of the information provided, such as country of origin, organic farming practices, kosher or halal status, etc.

17.2 Types of Dairy Product Adulteration and Nonauthenticity

17.2.1 Adulteration

The driving force for most adulteration is economic gain, whereby there is a profit opportunity from substituting a certain proportion of a high-value product with a lower-value one. Given that risks from prosecution exist at any level of adulteration, together with the outlay of capital required to adulterate at any amount, adulteration at trace levels is generally not worthwhile. At a minimum, economic adulteration requires the substitution of at least 3% (by weight) to provide a reasonable financial return for the adulterators. Less than this and there may not be any net profit from their activities. Adulteration at higher percentages not only means a higher rate of return on the adulterator's investment but also carries a higher risk of detection. A pattern that is often encountered with adulteration is that the deception will start out at a low proportion of substitution and then, as word of the profit opportunity spreads, other adulterators will adulterate at an increasingly higher proportion until greed raises the amount of adulteration to such a level that the deception becomes obvious to the consumer by means of a different appearance, flavor, functionality, or safety of the product. Moore et al. (2012) have noted the creation of a comprehensive database for food ingredient fraud as an effective method of identifying trends in this area.

17.2.2 Adulteration With Water

Dilution with water is the simplest means to adulterate milk. It, along with the adulteration of other foods (Punch, 1855), was a widespread practice during the 19th century in the United Kingdom (Lancet, 1857) as well as in France (Gem, 1857) and the United States (Weinstein, 1947). Although the introduction of testing for solids content helped greatly to prevent the practice of watering-down milk (McConnell, 1908), water addition still occurs even in modern times—albeit a degree of deception is now required to evade detection in countries with mature dairy industries, where testing is routine (Cheese Reporter, 2005). In 2011, a survey of milk in Pakistan found that 88% of all cow's milk was still being adulterated with water, ranging from 10% to 50% by proportion and at an average proportion of 25% (Aziz and Khan, 2013). We would also note that water addition may occur to milk inadvertently during milk collection.

High rates of infant mortality during the 19th century had several interconnected causes: breast-feeding being a strong factor for reducing infant mortality; it was counterbalanced by increased fertility being an important factor that increased infant mortality; and breastfeeding also lowering fertility through lactational amenorrhea, which reinforced the reduction of infant mortality (Woods et al., 1989). Unhygienic cow's milk being fed to infants and causing diarrhea was certainly a large factor in infant mortality, but the widespread watering-down of milk would also have caused infant deaths, both directly for infants who were fed cow's milk and indirectly for infants whose mothers relied on nutritional energy from their own consumption of cow's

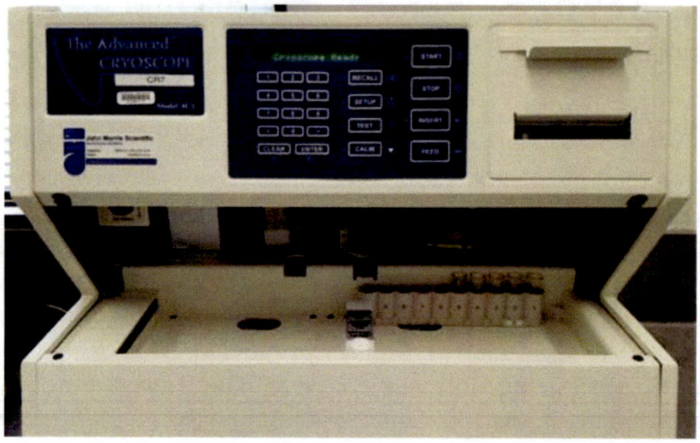

Figure 17.1 Cryoscope apparatus for freezing point measurement of milk.

milk—with the adulterated milk failing to provide sufficient nutritional sustenance to permit the mothers to nurse their infants.

The proportion of any added water in milk can be estimated by routine high-precision measurement of the freezing point of milk (ISO|IDF, 2009). Some variation of milk's freezing point occurs with season and individual cows, but for pooled milk from a farm vat the range in milli °C is usually quite narrow (Fig. 17.1).

17.2.3 Adulteration With Food Materials as Fillers

To evade detection by not having an appropriate solids content, some other cheap filler material must be added to the milk. Even when food materials are used as fillers, the nutritional effects can be severe or fatal, as in the case of infant formula that can be an infant's sole source of nutrition. This proved to be the case in 2004 when infant formula that contained very little protein, because of adulteration with starch or sugar, caused infants in China to suffer from "big head disease," whereby the infants' heads would grow unusually large whereas their torsos remained skeletal (China Daily, 2004). At least 13 infants died and hundreds more required hospitalization during that 2004 event.

Simple alternatives to adulterating milk by watering-down include "recycling" milk that has exceeded its expiry date into ultra-high-temperature-treated milk (Dairy Markets, 2005) or adding reconstituted milk powder into fresh milk (Ohta et al., 2002; Calvano et al., 2013). Because milk is being adulterated with milk ingredients that can have essentially the same chemical components as the milk to which they are being added, this type of adulteration can be difficult to detect. Most importantly, such adulteration will not occur unless there is an economic benefit to the adulterator. That can occur only if the ingredients have spoiled, or have gone beyond their expiry dates, or were otherwise procured at low cost. To help to prevent this last problem, nontoxic tracer compounds, such as vanillin, that can easily be identified by flavor are often added to subsidized dairy products (EU, 2000). Detecting the adulteration of fresh milk with reconstituted milk powder requires either analyzing for furosine content (Ohta et al., 2002) or examining the modified proteins (Calvano et al., 2013).

A progression from adulterating fresh milk with inferior milk is the adulteration of milk with whey. Liquid whey, which is a by-product of cheese making, has lost most of the milk fat and casein (the predominant protein of milk) to the cheese curd. Visually, whey resembles skim milk and is distinctly milky in flavor with a slight cultured aspect. Whey has traditionally been a low-value by-product that was used to feed farm animals, thereby making it an attractive material to use for the economic adulteration of milk. Checks must be put in place to ensure that skim milk powder does not contain rennet or acid whey as a by-product from cheese or casein manufacture (EU, 2009). The detection of added whey in skim milk is usually done by measuring casein macropeptide (Mollé and Léonil, 2005), but other approaches include measuring the content of cysteine (Ballin, 2006), an amino acid that makes up only 0.3% of the composition of casein compared with 3% of the composition of whey (Belitz et al., 2004).

Milk fat commands a price premium over vegetable oils because of its desirable flavor. This creates an incentive to adulterate the milk fat component of butter or ghee with inferior vegetable oils, or even to add vegetable oils to skim milk to pass the adulterated skim milk off as full-fat milk (Ntakatsane et al., 2013). Such adulteration is usually monitored by analysis either of the unique fatty acid profile of the milk fat component of dairy products (ISO|IDF, 2002a) as methyl ester derivatives (ISO|IDF, 2002b) or of the nonderivatized triglycerides (ISO|IDF, 2010a).

The carbohydrate portion of milk powder consists mainly of lactose, which is relatively expensive as a food ingredient. Maltodextrin, which is produced from starch and has generally recognized as safe (GRAS) status, is permitted as a food ingredient and is a much cheaper carbohydrate than lactose. Maltodextrin has been used as an adulterant (Sanvido et al., 2010), in combination with whey and vegetable oils, which provide balance to the protein and fat components of milk powder. The adulteration of milk powder with maltodextrin can be detected using near-infrared spectroscopy (Capuano et al., 2015). As it is a starch product, maltodextrin is permitted for use in infant formula at up to 30% of the carbohydrate portion by Codex Alimentarius Standard 72-1981 and at up to 10% of the carbohydrate portion in Chinese infant formula (China Daily, 2012).

17.2.4 Adulteration With Preservatives

Further bacterial growth in milk that has become spoiled through excessive bacterial numbers can be inhibited by the addition of hydrogen peroxide (Lück, 1956), which acts as a bacteriostatic agent rather than as a bacteriocide at doses below 900 ppm (Demeter et al., 1959). Cases of hydrogen peroxide being added to milk have occurred in northern Italy (Dairy Markets, 2004) and Colombia (Dairy Markets, 2009; Food News, 2009). Small quantities of hydrogen peroxide in milk are not normally a health concern (WHO, 1980) but excessive amounts can cause irritation of the throat and mucous membranes. Codex's Recommended Code of Practice CAC/GL 13-1991 permits the addition of small quantities of both hydrogen peroxide and thiocyanate, to activate the natural lactoperoxidase system in milk, but only in countries that do not have dairy industries with refrigeration infrastructure. Such treated milk is not acceptable for international trade without mutual agreement between the countries concerned, as noted by Codex's CAC/RCP 57-2004.

A consequence of high-bacterial growth in milk is that the lactic acid generated causes a decrease in pH and milk souring. This has been masked by adulterating milk with sodium hydroxide, a practice that has been observed relatively recently (Dairy Markets, 2008). The 2011 survey of milk in Pakistan quoted previously, which found that most milk was adulterated with water, also found that 27% of all surveyed milk was adulterated with carbonate and that 7% was adulterated with hydrogen peroxide (Aziz and Khan, 2013).

17.2.5 Adulteration With Nonfood Materials as Fillers

Milk protein is superior to almost all other food proteins for human nutrition based on its protein digestibility corrected amino acid score (Rutherfurd et al., 2015). As milk protein is more valuable than vegetable protein, milk powder is a potential target for adulteration with cheaper soy or pea protein (ISO|IDF, 2006). Milk powder is also at risk of being adulterated with nonfood-grade proteins, with one recent example of concern being hydrolyzed leather protein (China Daily, 2011). Because leather scraps may contain chromium from the tanning process, hydrolyzed leather protein poses a potential food safety risk if used as an adulterant. Methods for detecting this type of adulteration are mostly based on analysis of the amino acid L-hydroxyproline (Fig. 17.2), which is relatively abundant in collagen, the most abundant protein in skin, tendons, and animal hides (Li and Meng, 2008; Jin et al., 2009; Wang et al., 2009). The natural level of L-hydroxyproline in milk proteins is very low (Li et al., 2011), and analysis for L-hydroxyproline has been used as a means to detect gelatin, which is both a permitted food ingredient in yogurt (Nakano and Ozimek, 2003) and a nonpermitted ingredient of infant formula (Fay et al., 1991).

Milk fat in traditional ghee can be adulterated with mineral oils (unresolved complex mixtures of branched-chain alkyl and aryl hydrocarbons), which are cheaper than vegetable oils; this practice continues to be a problem in parts of India (Parmar et al., 2010). The economic adulteration of fats and oils (including milk fat) with mineral oil can be detected by simple techniques, such as passage through a column of activated alumina (AOCS Official Method Ca 6c-65; AOAC Official Method 966.17) or treating the fat with potassium hydroxide and extracting nonsaponifiable mineral oils (AOAC Official Method 945.102). Milk fat has a natural hydrocarbon component but the amounts are far below the quantities required for economic adulteration, and this component consists mostly of *n*-alkanes from plants rather than the unresolved complex mixtures of branched-chain hydrocarbons that arise from petroleum sources (McCarthy et al., 1964; Povolo et al., 2009).

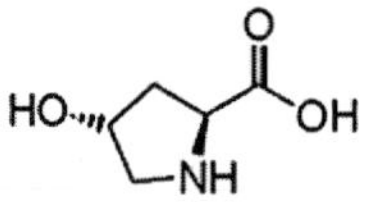

Figure 17.2 Structure of L-hydroxyproline.

17.2.6 Adulteration With Melamine

Adulteration of milk with melamine, which occurred in China during 2008, was one of the largest food contamination incidents of the last decade. The first public report by Western media of a single infant fatality from melamine (Reuters, 2008a) was quickly followed by reports of other deaths as the enormity of the scale of the incident became evident. By the end of November 2008, the Chinese Ministry of Health had confirmed that 294,000 infants had been affected, more than 50,000 infants had been hospitalized, and six infants had died (WHO, 2008). However, as the official number of people affected ceased to be updated beyond October 2008 (New York Times, 2008), the true number of cases could have been higher, especially when considering that a survey of 300,000 infants and young children in Beijing alone found that 25% had been exposed to melamine-contaminated formula (People's Daily Online, 2008).

Melamine did not act as a filler to substitute for any of the vital components of milk. Instead, melamine, which contains 66.7% nitrogen by weight, functioned by elevating the nitrogen content of diluted milk back to the levels of nonadulterated milk. The protein content of foods is not measured directly, but is typically done by measuring nitrogen content using the Kjeldahl or Dumas methods (Wiles et al., 1998; ISO|IDF, 2014) (Fig. 17.3) and then applying a conversion factor. Conversion factors of 6.38 for dairy protein and 5.8 for soy protein are used (IDF, 2006). Nitrogen from melamine

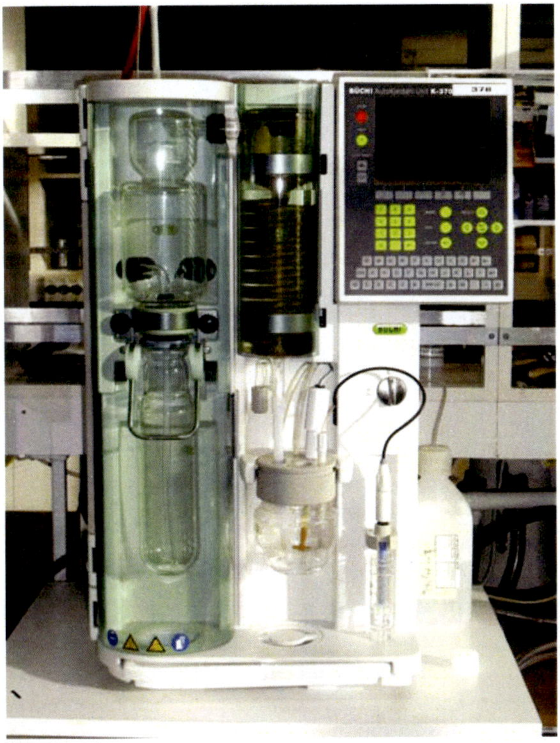

Figure 17.3 Apparatus for Kjeldahl analysis.

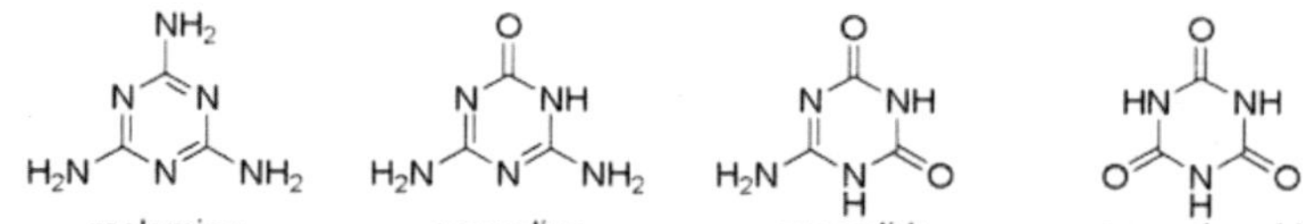

Figure 17.4 Structures of melamine, ammeline, ammelide, and cyanuric acid.

in watered-down milk would falsely indicate to any standard testing that the protein content was correct, and other substances in the melamine concoction (including fats and emulsifiers) would bring the solids content of the adulterated milk back into the range for normal milk (Xin and Stone, 2008).

It would be pointless to add only a small quantity of water, if the watered-down milk remained within the known natural range for milk, and then to mask that illegal practice with a small quantity of melamine, because no economic gain would result and yet the risks from discovery and subsequent law enforcement consequences would still exist. Milk protein content naturally ranges from 2.97% to 3.49% (w/w), depending upon the season and the stage of lactation (Auldist et al., 1998). Therefore, a plausible hypothetical scenario might be a situation in which milk with a naturally low level of protein (say 3.0% protein) is diluted with an aqueous solution of melamine that itself appears, to Kjeldahl testing, to contain 3.0% protein (or $3.0\% \div 6.38 = 0.47\%$ of nitrogen). With melamine (Fig. 17.4) containing 67% nitrogen, this would require the water used for dilution to be emulsified with 0.7% by weight of melamine. If adulteration with a melamine emulsion in water occurred at a 3% rate, then the milk would contain 210 ppm melamine. Once dried to a solid powder, the melamine would be concentrated eightfold to 1680 ppm. Surveys of Chinese powdered infant formula found melamine at levels ranging from <0.05 to 4700 ppm, with a median concentration of 1700 ppm (WHO, 2009). Those samples with relatively low levels of melamine probably reflected dilution at the dairy factory, where finished products were made from milk adulterated at intermediate milk collection stations; the samples with higher levels of adulteration probably reflected the increased overconfidence of the adulterators, whose prior illegal activity may have gone uncaught for some time.

Prior to 2007, melamine had generally been thought to be relatively nontoxic. However, in that year, there was an epidemic of animal deaths amongst pets that had been fed on pet food that contained wheat gluten from China. It was later established that the wheat gluten had been adulterated with low-grade "scrap melamine" that contained cyanuric acid as a significant impurity, a compound that is analogous to melamine. Melamine (water solubility 3240 mg/L) in the presence of cyanuric acid (water solubility 2000 mg/L) forms a highly insoluble complex of melamine–cyanurate crystals (water solubility 2 mg/L) (Fig. 17.5). In the acidic stomach environment, melamine would have formed its conjugate acid and dissociated from the melamine–cyanurate complex, allowing the neutral cyanuric acid to become passively absorbed into the body from the stomach while the basic melamine would later have been absorbed from the large intestine. The two compounds would then have recombined in the renal filtrate to form the highly insoluble complex of melamine–cyanurate crystals within the kidney tubules (Dobson et al., 2008). This toxicity model was confirmed in

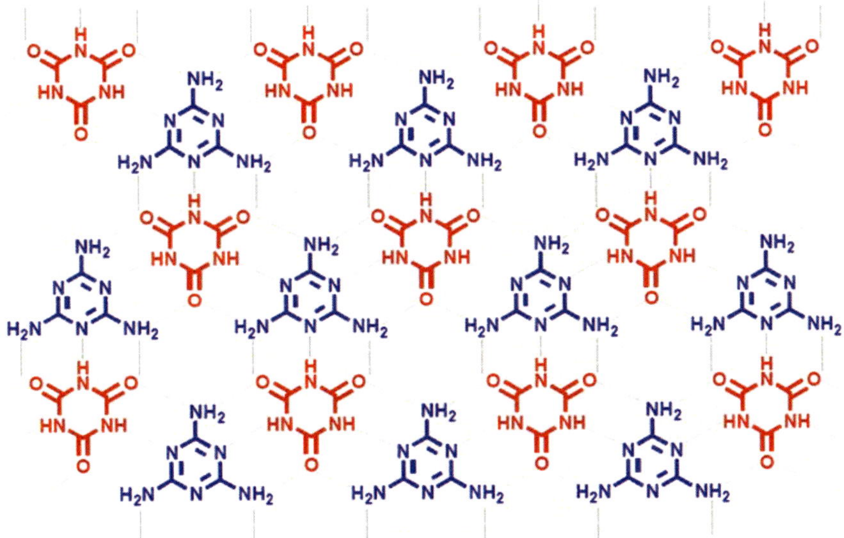

Figure 17.5 Lattice structure of melamine–cyanurate.

experimentally dosed pigs (Reimschuessel et al., 2008), which are a close model animal for human kidney function.

Between 2003 and 2006, the two melamine congeners, ammeline and ammelide, also caused kidney blockages in piglets fed on a protein concentrate, although the cause of their deaths was not established until after the 2007 melamine–cyanurate pet food poisonings, when the stored tissue samples of the piglets were reexamined (González et al., 2009).

Very early literature examining whether melamine might be useful as a dietary source of nitrogen for sheep had found that the sheep would dramatically reduce their food intake and many animals in the trial died (MacKenzie, 1966). It was quickly realized that these sheep deaths were caused by the blockage of kidney tubules with crystallized melamine, a condition termed "crystalluria" (Clark, 1966). Similar deaths of sheep by crystalluria occurred in an early trial with ammeline and ammelide (MacKenzie and van Rensburg, 1968).

The melamine that was used to adulterate milk in 2008 was of a higher purity than had been used to adulterate wheat gluten in 2007, containing only traces of cyanuric acid (WHO, 2009). Nevertheless, the adulterated milk still proved to be toxic, with the symptoms amongst affected infants exposed to melamine-adulterated infant formula including: crystals blocking the kidneys or urethra; restricted passage of urine; passage of blood in urine; rupture of urethra; and vomiting, diarrhea, anorexia, and abdominal distension (Sun et al., 2009). Treatments, in order of increasing invasiveness for increasing severity, consisted of: alkalization of urine; cystoscopy (insertion of a catheter tube into the urethra would sometimes dislodge sand/gravel-like solids); dialysis (peritoneal or hemodialysis); and lithotomy (surgical removal, through either the pelvis or the urethra) (Sun et al., 2009). Unlike the sharp, spiky, needle crystals of melamine–cyanurate complex, which could lodge in the kidneys of animals (Reimschuessel et al., 2008), the material blocking the kidneys and urethra of affected infants was sandy and gravel-like, and consisted mostly of melamine and uric acid in a 1:2 ratio (Jia et al., 2009). Like the melamine–cyanuric crystals that are formed by layers of melamine and cyanuric acid linked by multiple hydrogen bonds (Wang et al., 1990), melamine and uric acid form a similar structurally arranged complex of melamine–urate (Anderson et al., 2008) (Fig. 17.6). The urine of infants is known to contain a larger proportion of uric acid than that of adults, and the solubility of melamine is unfortunately lower in human urine than it would be in water, although melamine–cyanurate complex has a greater solubility in urine (Dominguez-Estevez et al., 2010).

In response to the melamine disaster, the World Health Organization quickly convened a meeting of experts to assess its toxicological and health aspects (WHO, 2009). This meeting established a tolerable daily intake (TDI) for melamine of 0.2 mg/kg body weight per day. Furthermore, the meeting noted that many countries had established their own limits for melamine of 1 ppm in powdered infant formula and 2.5 ppm in other foods, and stated that such limits provided a margin of safety for the TDI.

The International Dairy Federation (IDF) and the International Organization for Standardization (ISO) Methods and Standards Steering Group were proactive in evaluating available analytical methodology and then developing an international test standard for melamine and cyanuric acid. This test standard was published in November

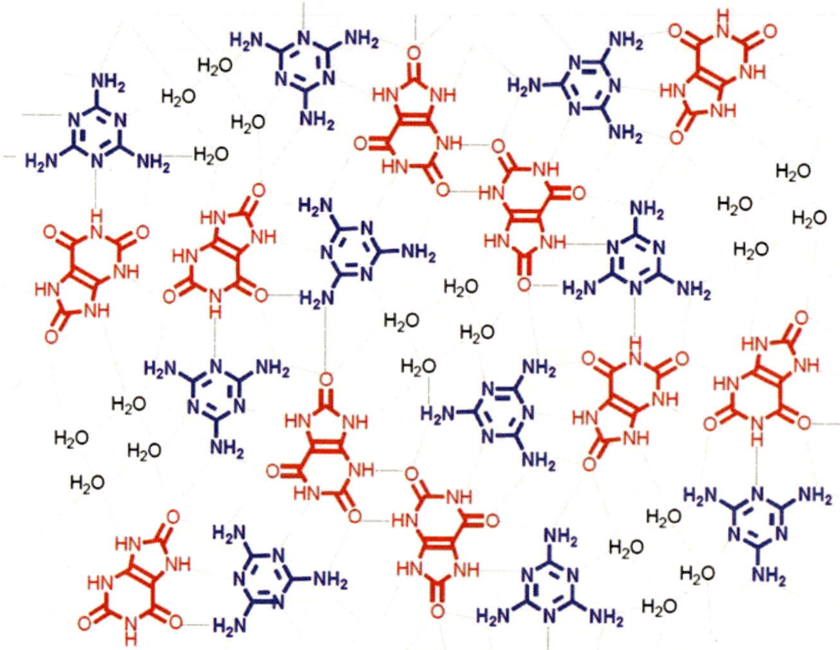

Figure 17.6 Lattice structure of melamine–urate–dihydrate.

2010 (ISO|IDF, 2010b) and was subsequently endorsed by Codex Alimentarius Standard 234-1999 as the recommended method of analysis.

Relevant research questions about melamine in foods do remain to be solved and continue to be addressed by academic researchers. They deal mainly with issues, such as physiological details influencing crystal formation in the kidneys (Poon et al., 2012), possible health effects from melamine that are additional to kidney-related effects (An et al., 2012; An and Zhang, 2014), and the ongoing health monitoring of children who were exposed to melamine as infants (Yang et al., 2013a).

In an effort to combat the economic adulteration of milk, dairy industry researchers have established rapid methods to screen large numbers of milk samples for multiple high-nitrogen-content compounds simultaneously (Abernethy and Higgs, 2013a). This approach would not necessarily achieve the low levels of detection required for compliance with regulatory limits for melamine. However, the underlying intention is different, namely to screen for economic adulteration that could be profitable only if it occurred at significant levels. Compounds screened for include: melamine, ammeline, ammelide, cyanuric acid, allantoin, thiourea, urea, biuret, triuret, semicarbazide, aminotriazine, 3- and 4-aminotriazole, dicyanamide, cyandiamide, guanidine, choline, nitrate, and the amino acids glycine, alanine, serine, proline, valine, threonine, leucine, isoleucine, hydroxyproline, aspartic acid, lysine, glutamic acid, methionine, histidine, phenylalanine, arginine, and tyrosine.

Another important control that the dairy industry used during the crisis stage of the melamine disaster was to permanently dispose of melamine-adulterated dairy products through incineration in cement kilns and steel factories in order to ensure that consumers could never be exposed to them (Reuters, 2008b). Unfortunately, this step was not taken by all affected dairy companies or distributors, and melamine-adulterated Chinese milk powder had made its way to Africa by 2010, where it was being sold on the black market (Schoder, 2010). South Africa had previously suffered from black market—sourced adulterated Chinese wheat protein from the 2007 pet food incident being used as a feed for cattle; melamine consequently passed through to the milk and created a second scare around melamine-contaminated milk in late 2008. Melamine ingested by pregnant cows transferred to the fetus, where it caused kidney damage and abortion. Milk from cows fed unusually high quantities of melamine-adulterated feed contained up to 1 ppm of melamine, although milk from cows fed on normal amounts of the feed contained only 0.4 ppm of melamine (Reyers, 2008a,b). The transfer of melamine from cattle feed to milk was confirmed experimentally (Cruywagen et al., 2009), and transfer rates from feed to milk have been established both for a single oral dose (Battaglia et al., 2010) and for continuous oral dosing (Shen et al., 2010).

17.2.7 Synthetic Milk

An issue that threatens milk supplies in India is the extension of milk between 5% and 10% with so-called "synthetic milk." In 2004, surveys indicated that about 30% of milk in north India was adulterated in this manner (Arora et al., 2004). "Synthetic milk" is a mixture that is designed to resemble milk and to provide no obvious changes to taste, color, or consistency, which would otherwise alert customers when synthetic milk is incorporated at low levels. Its components are urea (to contribute to the nitrogen), vegetable oil (to replace milk fat), salt (to adjust lactometer readings), baking soda (to adjust alkalinity and also lactometer readings), and detergent (to emulsify).

Another reason for adding urea to milk is to increase its heat stability. Straightforward analytical methods have been developed for the detection of each of these components. Viscosity measurements at low shear rate were found to be a simple and sensitive technique for detecting such adulteration (Paradkar et al., 2000a,b, 2001a,b; Barui et al., 2012).

Although urea is a natural component of milk and of many other protein-containing foods, too much urea can be toxic to both humans (Hewlett et al., 1916) and cattle (Villar et al., 2003). It has been shown that urea-adulterated milk can also be harmful to the liver and kidneys of experimental mice (Kommadath et al., 2001).

17.2.8 Counterfeit Branded Dairy Products

Counterfeiting of dairy product brands occurs when a nongenuine food item is packaged in such a way as to mimic a specific brand of product. This is a problem that has increased globally over the last decade (Stuff.co.nz, 2014). A counterfeiter may either replicate a brand's packaging entirely or "recycle" discarded genuine packaging materials and refill them with a nongenuine product. In most instances, the nongenuine product will have either an inferior flavor or an inferior functionality, such as poor solubility or dispersibility of the powder, poor appearance, and perhaps a different color or flowability of the powder. This will make such counterfeiting obvious to a consumer who has prior experience with the genuine product and who is then likely to bring the defective product to the manufacturer as a complaint. In such instances, comparison of the composition of the complaint sample (fat, protein, minerals) against a retention sample of the genuine product, manufactured at the same date as claimed for the complaint sample, is sufficient to quickly demonstrate whether the sample is nongenuine.

Because milk is a naturally produced food, there will be small natural variations in the relative compositions of fat, protein, and minerals, all of which are dependent upon the season and the stage of lactation of the cow, as well as on other factors, such as weather conditions (drought, temperature). This makes a library of small retention samples held under stable conditions by the dairy manufacturer from each batch of its manufacture and used in conjunction with compositional analysis a powerful tool in the detection of counterfeit product.

Counterfeit branded dairy products can be either adulterated products, such as those described earlier, or dairy products that were previously deemed to be unfit for sale (perhaps for a quality problem or for containing an unacceptable amount of a pesticide or veterinary drug residue). This reinforces the need for manufacturers to ensure the proper destruction of any dairy materials that are unfit for human consumption, lest they reappear via the black market in another location.

Such counterfeiting is also combated by using packaging designs and materials that are both difficult to replicate and tamper evident.

17.2.9 Extortion

In 1995, five British dairies were blackmailed for £250,000 by a university-trained microbiologist who had procured a supply of *Yersinia enterocolitica* and who sent the dairies cartons of their milk tampered with blue dye without any outward appearance of tampering, along with vials of *Y. enterocolitica* cultures. He was caught by authorities upon attempting to withdraw money from an anonymous Austrian bank account into which the dairies had deposited funds (Carus, 2001). The threat of a microbiological or chemical threat to the food supply, including milk, was considered by the US Food and Drug Administration in its 2003 risk assessment for food terrorism (US FDA, 2003). Since then, hypothetical risks to milk have been considered and these include: botulinum (Alberts, 2005; Wein and Liu, 2005); strychnine, aconitine, and nicotine (Jablonski et al., 2006); ricin (He et al., 2007); abrine (Owens and Koester, 2008); picrotoxin (Jablonski and Jackson, 2008); the chemical warfare agents methylphosphonic acid (MPA), ethyl-MPA, isopropyl-MPA, cyclohexyl-MPA, and pinacolyl-MPA (Owens and Koester, 2009), and saxitoxin (Lumor et al., 2012).

The testing approach to mitigate an extortion threat has very different requirements from a testing regime for environmental contaminants or veterinary drug residues. With contaminants, a statistically based sampling and testing approach provides a measure of the range of concentrations in which a contaminant may occur for an agricultural product, which then provides a calculable degree of confidence that those agricultural products conform to their regulatory requirements. However, with an extortion threat, only a single batch of product would need to be poisoned for the threat to be accomplished.

17.2.10 Authenticity of Geographical Region

As noted previously, "authenticity" is the certainty of knowing that a product is really what it claims to be on the label. The preeminent dairy food example of analytical techniques being used to establish authenticity is the case of "Emmentaler Switzerland" cheese, which has "Appellation d'Origine Protegée" status that guarantees that the product is manufactured and processed in a specified geographic region. "Emmental" cheese, as a cheese variety, is made in France, Germany, and Finland with only about 10% of the Emmental cheese sold in Europe being made in Switzerland. Because Emmentaler Switzerland cheese is expensive to produce from alpine regions that are difficult to farm, is made in small village dairies in small production sizes, it attracts a considerable price premium over Emmental cheese made elsewhere. Therefore, it is important that Emmentaler Switzerland cheese can be differentiated from other Emmental cheeses. A major analytical project explored which analytical techniques were feasible or nonfeasible for such differentiation (Pillonel et al., 2002a,b; Pillonel et al., 2003a). Infrared spectroscopy was found to be one of the most useful techniques for distinguishing between the regions of origin of Emmental cheeses, with mid-infrared transmission spectra being particularly useful (Pillonel et al., 2003b); the distinction between the regions of cheese origin was improved when mid-infrared spectroscopy was combined with fluorescence spectroscopy (Karoui et al., 2004,

2005a,b). Complete differentiation of Emmentaler Switzerland cheese from other Emmental cheeses could be achieved in the most cost-effective manner by applying discriminant analysis to measurements of the following 15 factors: acetic acid, propionic acid, pH, total nitrogen, obligately heterofermentative lactobacilli, enterococci, D- and L-lactate, succinate, pyruvate, L-leucine-aminopeptidase, and the ‰ ratios of heavier stable isotopes relative to international standards for δ^2H, $\delta^{13}C$, $\delta^{15}N$, and $\delta^{34}S$ (Pillonel et al., 2005).

17.2.11 Authenticity of Species

Another form of authenticity deception is to substitute the milk of one species with the milk of another. Because cow's milk is the cheapest source, it is usually used as the adulterant. For example, cheeses that are made from ewe's milk, goat's milk, or buffalo's milk in Europe have high value because of their low production volumes and must not contain cow's milk (EU, 2008). The reference method for detection of cow's milk in cheeses uses gel electrophoresis and has a detection limit of less than 0.5% (v/v) (EU, 2008). More recently, the analysis of mitochondrial DNA targets has been used to detect 1% (v/v) cows' milk in binary mixtures of ewe's milk, goat's milk, or buffalo's milk used to make fresh milk, yogurt, cheese, and butter (Goncalves et al., 2012). That study found that 12 out of 96 commercial samples from the European market failed to conform to their species labeling, either through the presence of cow's milk in a product that should not have contained any or by the absence of sheep's or goat's milk in products in which they were claimed to be present. Advances in the fatty acid analysis of triglycerides, and particularly in the stereospecific positioning of the various fatty acids at the *sn*-1-, *sn*-2-, and *sn*-3- positions on the glycerol backbone, have also made it possible to identify 1% of cow's milk in sheep's milk (Blasi et al., 2013).

The presence of cow's milk in sheep's or goat's milk products is widely known as a potential food safety risk because of cow's milk allergenicity. What is less widely known is that people can be allergic to either sheep's or goat's milk without necessarily being allergic to cow's milk (Paty et al., 2003; Ah-Leung et al., 2006) and that the undeclared presence of either of these milk can cause life-threatening anaphylaxis (Calvani and Alessandri, 1998).

17.3 Chemical Methods to Combat Nonauthenticity

As reviewed so comprehensively a decade ago, there are many different ways of adulterating milk and many different analytical techniques to detect each of those adulteration methods (de la Fuente and Juárez, 2005). From a commercial perspective, rather than to revisit those techniques, there is more benefit in asking the question: what are the practical means for combating such adulteration practices?

Confidence in food safety comes primarily from knowing that a process is under control with regard to microbiological, chemical, and physical hazards, and that the correct controls are in place. Testing alone—even at an intensive sampling rate—cannot provide confidence that all the risks posed by microbiological, chemical, and physical hazards have been adequately mitigated. For this reason, commercial dairy product manufacture depends upon having reliable quality systems in place. In-process and final product testing, at an appropriate statistically based sampling rate, serve as means to confirm that the controls are working as intended.

Faced with a situation of being presented with a dairy product of uncertain pedigree, such as a complaint from a customer or consumer with whom there is no established prior relationship, a dairy product manufacturer is placed in a difficult position. The product that is being complained about may indeed be defective; however, unless it can first be established that it is actually a product that the manufacturer supplied to market, there is a potentially damaging business risk to the manufacturer.

For this reason, it is prudent for a dairy product manufacturer to retain small samples of each batch of its products for a time period that is at least equal to the stated shelf life of the product. As noted previously, the "retention sample" manufactured on the same date as claimed for the complaint sample can then have its composition (fat, protein, and minerals) compared against the composition of any complaint sample to ensure that the latter is a genuine product. Natural variations in milk composition throughout the season and lactation stages serve to provide a "moving target" that makes the exact matching of any counterfeit product to a specific date of genuine product both difficult and less economically viable to an adulterator.

Dairy companies can assist in making business difficult for adulterators by properly disposing of any downgraded dairy materials that might otherwise find their way back into the human food chain by means of the black market. For example, in the case of 2200 tons of chloramphenicol-contaminated skim milk powder, that would have passed all tests for being genuine, the product was best disposed of by incineration and conversion into cement (Dairy Industry Newsletter, 2003).

Tamper-evident packaging is another critical means that a dairy product manufacturer can use to protect against this type of fraud. If a complaint sample turns out not to have genuine packaging, then the issue can be handed over to be dealt with as a criminal matter more quickly.

The types of chemical testing that are required for composition work have been validated internationally and are readily available to competent dairy laboratories. Chief amongst them would be the analysis of fatty acids from milk fat. Triglycerides are *trans*-esterified with sodium methoxide to form fatty acid methyl esters (FAMEs) (ISO|IDF, 2002b), which are then quantified by gas chromatography (ISO|IDF, 2002a). Although work on the authenticity of Emmental cheese found that lipid composition had too broad a range to distinguish between all geographical production regions for all cases of Emmental cheese (Pillonel et al., 2002b), in commercial reality, when dealing with a case in which a sample has a suspect origin, the labeling information on the packaging will provide a specific claimed date of manufacture from a specific claimed factory, which can then be matched against a specific retention sample. Ironically, the broad natural range of lipid composition from seasonal and feeding variation then serves as an advantage against the counterfeiter.

However, because of the need for adulteration to be economically profitable, the most common cases of adulteration still use cheaper fats, such as tallow, lard, or vegetable oils. Small percentages of these oils mixed in with milk fat are readily identifiable by examining both saturated and unsaturated C_{18} fatty acids (Ulberth, 1994); even simple fat (ISO|IDF, 2008, 2010c) or nitrogen (ISO|IDF, 2014) measurements will be sufficient to identify most cases of fraud. In cases for which more sophisticated analysis is required, analysis of the intact triglycerides is a powerful tool (Molkentin, 2007; ISO-|IDF, 2010a).

17.4 Spectroscopic Methods to Determine Adulteration

Given that methods for testing food should be rapid and easy to apply, there has been a trend toward the use of spectroscopic methods for food testing over the past 10 years. Published spectroscopic methods that have been applied to milk and milk products can be divided into four areas, depending on the technology employed: vibrational spectroscopy [including mid-infrared (MIR), near-infrared (NIR), visible, and Raman spectroscopy]; nuclear magnetic resonance (NMR) spectroscopy; fluorescence spectroscopy and a range of mass spectroscopic techniques.

Use of spectroscopy to detect the adulteration of foods via fingerprinting was the subject of a 2012 review (Ellis et al., 2012) that covered a wide range of foods, including liquid milk and milk products, such as milk powder, cheese, and butter. Similarly, Brandt et al. (2010) reviewed a wide range of technical solutions for the analysis of milk constituents and abnormal milk, including some spectroscopic techniques. Here, we cover more recent work, with a focus on work that has been aimed at rapidly gathering a "fingerprint" of the sample using a spectroscopic technique and, from that, detecting noncompliance with standard product. In addition, we cover techniques that are aimed at more qualitative analysis of adulterants using molecular spectroscopy.

We also suggest that many of the references cited in this section rely on the distinction between targeted and nontargeted analyses. A targeted method seeks to detect and quantify a specific analyte or a range of analytes with established limits of detection. In contrast, a nontargeted method has the ability to detect an abnormality in a single sample when comparing it with a range of samples that have been established as normal in the context of the spectroscopic technique in question. Very recently, as more focus is put on fingerprinting-type assays, the distinction is important and considerations on method development and validation have become more important (Botelho et al., 2015).

Traditional MIR spectroscopy on milk uses a thin transmission cell to optimize the signal-to-noise ratio. Current Fourier transform infrared (FTIR) spectrometers can rapidly and reliably measure the spectra of liquid milk samples, as shown in Fig. 17.7.

Using this technology, commercial MIR instruments from a number of sources have been available for over 20 years. In March 2013, a commercial application utilizing both targeted and nontargeted methods on currently available FTIR liquid milk analyzers was released (www.foss.dk). The targeted aspect of these applications across several instrument platforms focused on melamine, cyanuric acid, maltodextrin,

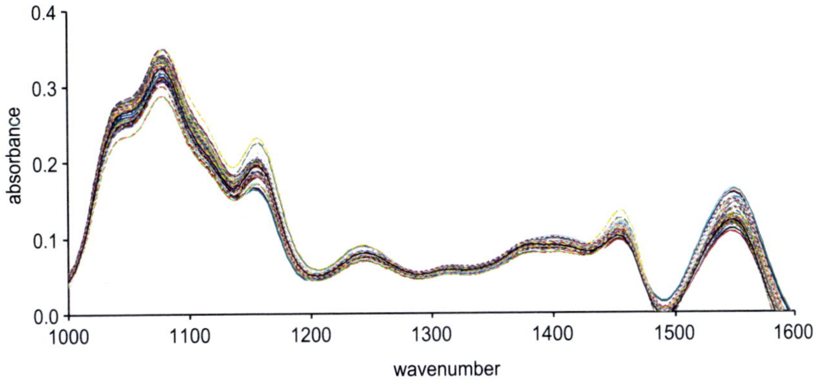

Figure 17.7 Mid-infrared transmission absorbance spectra of liquid milk across wavelength range 1000–1600/cm.

sodium and potassium nitrite, hydroxyproline (as a surrogate marker for hydrolyzed leather protein), urea, sucrose, sodium bicarbonate, and formaldehyde. The nontargeted application utilizes a package that has the abnormal spectrum module and uses a principal components statistical approach coupled with examination of spectral residuals to detect the presence of adulteration down to levels of 100–500 ppm. Several other authors have explored the utility of attenuated total reflectance (ATR) attachments on MIR instruments for milk analysis. Jawaid et al. (2013) showed that melamine in liquid milk could be detected at levels as low as 2.5 ppm using single-bounce ATR. The technique relies on samples of liquid milk being freeze-dried and spiked with a known quantity of melamine, or on samples of powdered milk being spiked. These techniques assume that the sample being assessed on the surface of the ATR crystal is representative of the whole, and that mixing of the spiked material is uniform. Santos et al.(2013) spiked liquid milk with whey, hydrogen peroxide, synthetic urine, and synthetic milk (a combination of emulsifying vegetable oils, detergents, and urea) and used the liquids directly on the single-bounce ATR crystal surface. Partial least squares regression produced prediction errors of between 14 and 2330 ppm for these analytes. Fadzlillah et al. (2013) used horizontal ATR to estimate the adulteration of butter with other animal fat. Validation using an independent test set showed that a level as low as 1.7% on a weight/weight basis could be detected. Yang et al. (2013b) used MIR spectroscopy and a transflectance technique to record the spectra of milk that was deliberately adulterated with melamine, urea, and glucose. Novel data treatment comprising two-dimensional correlation spectroscopy with least squares support vector machines suggested that over 90% of the adulterated samples could be distinguished from nonadulterated samples.

NIR spectroscopy has been applied frequently to a wide variety of foodstuffs but, given its ease of use, is more typically applied to solid and semisolid dairy products than to liquids. Yogurt has been analyzed for adulterants by NIR spectroscopy (Xu et al., 2013) using a nontargeted technique to detect the presence of nondairy proteins and gelatin. The use of NIR spectroscopy for the determination of the adulteration and contamination of milk and milk powder has been reviewed recently (Cattaneo and Holroyd, 2013). Although that review cites numerous publications since 2002, it cautions that NIR spectroscopy is not a particularly sensitive technique because of the different sources of noise relative to the signal strength. Hence, it is often best applied for quantification of the major constituents in a sample, typically has a lower detection limit of 0.1% (v/v), and is thus unsuitable for detecting low concentrations of adulterants.

Image analysis using the visible region (380–700 nm) has been used recently by two research groups (Santos et al., 2012; dos Santos and Pereira-Filho, 2013; Yang et al., 2013c). Both focused on rapid, simple, low-cost sensor arrays that were able to detect the addition of water, sodium hydroxide, whey, hydrogen peroxide, synthetic milk, synthetic urine, and melamine and its chemical analogs in liquid milk at concentrations of 5–50% (w/w) for water and 1–20 ppm for melamine. They noted that the techniques could be useful for the in situ screening of milk because of their portability.

Raman spectroscopy is less widely established than either MIR- and NIR-based techniques in the dairy industry. Nevertheless, a number of authors have shown proof-of-concept studies that have detected different types of adulteration in milk, milk powder, and butter. Two of the studies also used imaging methods. Qin et al. (2013) were able to detect melamine, cyanuric acid, urea, and ammonium sulfate across a range of 0.1–5% (w/w) in milk powder using macroscale Raman imaging. Similarly, de Alemida et al. (2012) detected the addition of whey and starch to milk powders at concentrations of 1.6–2.3% (w/w). da Rocha et al. (2015) used Raman microscopy to detect whey added to milk across the range 0–100% (w/w). Sample preparation in this case included air-drying. Khan et al. (2015) also studied milk but used a cuvette with a 10-mL path length to quantify urea across the range 1–1000 ppm. Üçüncüoğlu et al. (2013) used both Raman and NIR spectroscopy to examine butter and margarine in bakery products for adulteration. Raman spectroscopy was found to be superior to NIR spectroscopy in this instance.

NMR spectroscopy has been applied to dairy products for many years (Belloque and Ramos, 1999) but applications with reference to the detection of adulteration are rare. A review by Karoui and de Baerdemacker (2007) suggested that NMR spectroscopy was a sensitive probe for dairy matrices, given that the decay of a signal from a given proton is heavily influenced by its electronic surroundings. As NMR spectroscopy also examines a larger sample volume, it is potentially useful for more heterogeneous samples. Therefore, NMR can gather information that is not available from other forms of spectroscopy. In particular, NMR can be useful for a nontargeted approach to screening for adulterants (Lachenmeier et al., 2009).

The use of high-field NMR spectroscopy for the quantification of milk constituents in detail suggests that there is scope for its application (Picariello et al., 2013; Prema et al., 2013) to adulteration detection. This, coupled with the recent advent of reliable low-field instruments with relatively good signal-to-noise ratio and resolution, promises further scope for the development of NMR spectroscopy in this area. Jiang et al. (2010) indicated that milk adulterated with water, salt, urea, soybean milk, or reconstituted milk could be detected with low-field NMR spectroscopy.

Fluorescence spectroscopy is a widely used and very sensitive technique. Liu et al. (2014) have reported the application of fluorescence spectroscopy to detect adulteration of pure milk fat with various levels of vegetable fat. Similarly, Dankowska et al. (2014) have used synchronous fluorescence spectroscopy to detect the adulteration of butter with palm and coconut oils, with a limit of detection of 5.5% (w/w). With reference to liquid milk, Ntakatsane et al. (2013) examined both targeted and nontargeted applications for assessing the level of milk reconstituted from milk powder as an adulterant in raw and pasteurized milk using fluorescence spectroscopy. Neelima et al. (2012) used a fluorimetric assay to quantify sialic acid in milk and thus to detect the addition of whey to a level as low as 5% (w/w).

Overall, spectroscopy has been shown to be a versatile tool for detecting the adulteration of milk and milk products. Its ability to be applied rapidly and thus to cope with a high volume of samples is clearly a major advantage. The predominance of MIR and NIR techniques for the current routine analysis of milk and milk products suggests that there is a major opportunity to leverage the existing instrument networks for further developments of assays that are aimed at the detection of adulterants and contaminants. This is provided that there is an appreciation of the inherent limitation of the sensitivity of these and other techniques covered in this review.

Techniques based on liquid chromatography with mass spectroscopic (LC−MS) detection are advantageous in terms of high selectivity and offer low-level quantification; many LC−MS analysis methods for the detection of individual or groups of nitrogen-based economically motivated adulterants, including melamine and cyanuric acid in milk and infant formula (Turnipseed et al., 2008; Desmarchelier et al., 2009), the latter compounds plus dicyandiamide, urea, biuret, cyromazine, triuret and amidinourea (MacMahon et al., 2012), and ammeline and ammelide along with the addition of isotope-labeled compounds for accurate quantification (Draher et al., 2014), have become available. However, the multitude of possible adulterant compounds combined with the relatively low speed of analysis of quantitative LC−MS methods means that it is difficult to envisage using single- or even multiple-compound LC−MS methods for the routine screening of large sample numbers, although the utility of LC−MS in the confirmation and quantification of tentative detections is without doubt.

Dairy researchers have established rapid LC−MS methodology to screen large numbers of milk samples for multiple high-nitrogen-content compounds simultaneously. A complementary spectroscopic prescreen using, eg, Fourier-transform infrared spectroscopy is used to identify likely nonconforming samples, and then a fast, qualitative, multiple-compound LC−MS screening method is used to either clear the sample or further refine the identity of a likely adulterant (Abernethy and Higgs, 2013a). As noted previously, such an approach would not necessarily achieve the quantification performance required for compliance with regulatory guidelines, but the underlying intention is different, namely to quickly filter already suspect samples for economic adulteration and to provide direction for the evidential testing of single analytes. Compounds screened for include: melamine, ammeline, ammelide, cyanuric acid, allantoin, thiourea, urea, biuret, triuret, semicarbazide, aminotriazine, 3- and

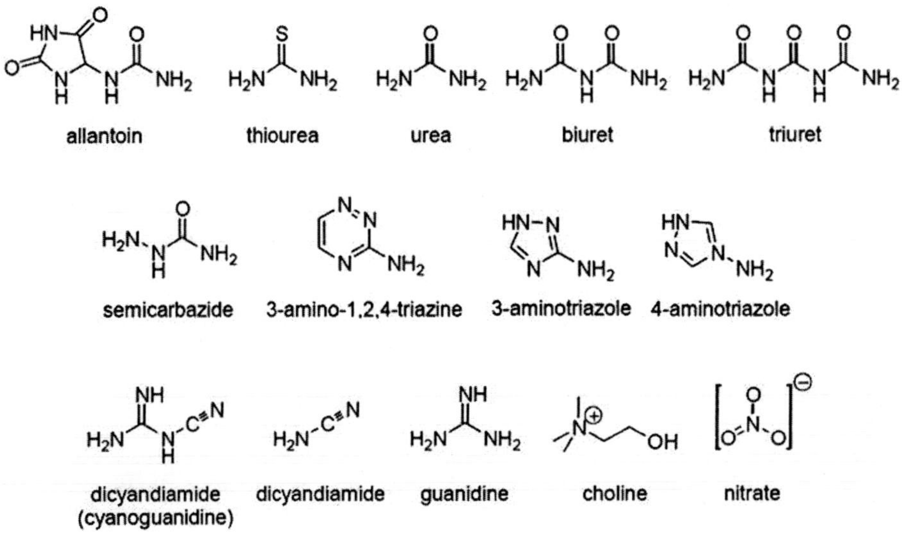

Figure 17.8 Structures of allantoin, thiourea, urea, biuret, triuret, semicarbazide, aminotriazine, 3- and 4-aminotriazole, dicyandiamide, cyanamide, guanidine, choline, and nitrate.

4-aminotriazole, dicyanamide, cyandiamide, guanidine, choline, nitrate, and the amino acids glycine, alanine, serine, proline, valine, threonine, leucine, isoleucine, hydroxyproline, aspartic acid, lysine, glutamic acid, methionine, histidine, phenylalanine, arginine, and tyrosine (Fig. 17.8).

When examining milk for potential adulterants, it should be noted that several compounds that react and therefore change identity with the milk matrix have so far been identified. Both melamine (unpublished data) and semicarbazide have been shown to combine with lactose in solution (Abernethy and Higgs, 2013b) and aminotriazine appears to undergo rapid oxidation to aminotriazin-5-one in the milk matrix (Abernethy and Higgs, 2013c). Urea is detectable by mass spectroscopy but is also a natural compound that is present in milk at levels similar to those added as a potential adulterant. An effective means to detect the addition of synthetic urea has been proposed; it involves looking for by-products of the commercial manufacture of urea, namely biuret, triuret, and methylenediurea, as markers (Abernethy and Higgs, 2013a). These marker compounds are present in synthetic urea at levels that are sufficient for detection if a commercially relevant adulteration of milk with urea has taken place.

17.5 Future Developments

As the risks to brand damage and international trade increase with faster-paced and more widespread media coverage of food scandals, the pressure on dairy companies to confirm the identity of their products in market, especially in situations where there is doubt, will continue unabated. Increasingly sophisticated analytical techniques continue to be developed, such as the ‰ ratios for δ^2H and $\delta^{13}C$ stable isotopes of individual fatty acids (Ehtesham et al., 2013, 2015). However, dairy manufacturers must not lose sight of the fact that testing, alone, can never reinstate confidence in the food safety of a product the pedigree of which is in doubt. Such confidence can be achieved only through a process that ensures that microbiological, chemical, and physical hazards are correctly controlled, in combination with a supply chain the integrity of which is maintained from end to end. The task of dairy processors is to be able to differentiate any fraudulent dairy products in the marketplace from their genuine products, after which it becomes the task of law enforcement agencies to understand the supply routes of nongenuine dairy products. The dairy industry can then assist in making business difficult for adulterators by properly disposing of any downgraded dairy materials that might otherwise find their way back into the human food chain by means of the black market. The wide range of analytical testing methodologies reviewed here are tools that have an important place in protecting the reputation of milk and milk products as important and safe sources of nutrition globally. The continuing evolution of both these tools and the threats to food safety require ongoing vigilance from dedicated analytical scientists and food safety professionals.

Acknowledgment

We are grateful to Peter Varelis for sharing his insightful knowledge and for reviewing this chapter.

References

Abernethy, G., Higgs, K., 2013a. Rapid detection of economic adulterants in fresh milk by liquid chromatography—tandem mass spectrometry. Journal of Chromatography A 1288, 10—20.

Abernethy, G., Higgs, K., 2013b. Lactose semicarbazone as a marker for semicarbazide adulteration in milk. Journal of Chromatography A 1295, 152—155.

Abernethy, G., Higgs, K., 2013c. Detection of 3-amino-1,2,4-triazine adulteration in milk using an oxidation product 3-amino-1,2,4-triazin-5(2H)-one. Journal of Chromatography A 1285, 165—167.

Ah-Leung, S., Bernard, H., Bidat, E., Paty, E., Rancé, F., Scheinmann, P., Wal, J.M., 2006. Allergy to goat and sheep milk without allergy to cow's milk. Allergy 61, 1358—1365.

Alberts, B., 2005. Modeling attacks on the food supply. Proceedings of the National Academy of Sciences of the United States of America 102, 9737—9738.

An, L., Zhang, T., 2014. Prenatal melamine exposure induces impairments of spatial cognition and hippocampal synaptic plasticity in male adolescent rats. Reproductive Toxicology 49, 78—85.

An, L., Li, Z., Yang, Z., Zhang, T., 2012. Melamine induced cognitive impairment associated with oxidative damage in rat's hippocampus. Pharmacology, Biochemistry, and Behavior 102, 196—202.

Anderson, K.M., Day, G.M., Paterson, M.J., Byrne, P., Clarke, N., Steed, J.W., 2008. Structure calculation of an elastic hydrogel from sonication of rigid small molecule components. Angewandte Chemie International Edition 47, 1058—1062.

Arora, S., Sharma, V., Raj, D., Ram, M., Kishmore, K., 2004. Status of milk adulteration in some states of North India. Indian Journal of Dairy Science 57, 65—66.

Auldist, M.J., Walsh, B.J., Thomson, N.A., 1998. Seasonal and lactational influences on bovine milk composition in New Zealand. Journal of Dairy Research 65, 401–411.

Aziz, T., Khan, H., 2013. A survey on milk adulteration at retail outlets of Islamabad, Pakistan. Carpathian Journal of Food Science & Technology 6, 44–52.

Ballin, N.Z., 2006. Estimation of whey protein in casein coprecipitate and milk powder by high-performance liquid chromatography quantification of cysteine. Journal of Agricultural and Food Chemistry 54, 4131–4135.

Barui, A.K., Sharma, R., Rajput, Y.S., 2012. Detection of non-dairy fat in milk based on quantitative assay of anionic detergent using azure A dye. International Dairy Journal 24, 44–47.

Battaglia, M., Cruywagen, C.W., Bertuzzi, T., Gallo, A., Moschini, M., Piva, G., Masoero, F., 2010. Transfer of melamine from feed to milk and from milk to cheese and whey in lactating dairy cows fed single oral doses. Journal of Dairy Science 93, 5338–5347.

Belitz, H.-D., Grosch, W., Schieberle, P., 2004. Food Chemistry, third ed. Springer, Berlin, p. 509.

Belloque, J., Ramos, M., 1999. Application of NMR spectroscopy to milk and dairy products. Trends in Food Science & Technology 10, 313–320.

Blasi, F., Lombardi, G., Damiani, P., Simonetti, M.S., Giua, L., Cossignani, L., 2013. Triacylglycerol stereospecific analysis and linear discriminant analysis for milk speciation. Journal of Dairy Research 80, 144–151.

Botelho, B.G., Reis, N., Oliveira, L.S., Sena, M.M., 2015. Development and analytical validation of a screening method for simultaneous detection of five adulterants in raw milk using mid-infrared spectroscopy and PLS-DA. Food Chemistry 181, 31–37.

Brandt, M., Haeussermann, A., Hartung, E., 2010. Invited review: technical solutions for analysis of milk constituents and abnormal milk. Journal of Dairy Science 93, 427–436.

Calvani Jr., M., Alessandri, C., 1998. Anaphylaxis to sheep's milk cheese in a child unaffected by cow's milk protein allergy. European Journal of Pediatrics 157, 17–19.

Calvano, C.D., Monopoli, A., Loizzo, P., Faccia, M., Zambonin, C., 2013. Proteomic approach based on MALDI-TOF MS to detect powdered milk in fresh cow's milk. Journal of Agricultural and Food Chemistry 61, 1609–1617.

Capuano, E., Boerrigter-Eenling, R., Koot, A., van Ruth, S.M., 2015. Targeted and untargeted detection of skim milk powder adulteration by near-infrared spectroscopy. Food Analytical Methods 8, 2125–2134.

Carus, W.S., 2001. Bioterrorism and Biocrimes. The Illicit Use of Biological Agents Since 1900. Center for Counterproliferation Research, National Defense University, Washington, DC, 2001 revision, 219 pages.

Cattaneo, T.M.P., Holroyd, S.E., 2013. Review: the use of near infrared spectroscopy for determination of adulteration and contamination in milk and milk powder: updating knowledge. Journal of Near Infrared Spectroscopy 21, 341–349.

Cheese Reporter, 7 January 2005. Criminal Complaint Charges Dairy Farmers With Adding Water to Milk in 2003–04. Cheese Reporter, p. 11.

China Daily, 29 July 2004. 47 Detained for Selling Baby-killer Milk. China Daily. Available from: http://www.chinadaily.com.cn/english/doc/2004-05/10/content_329449.htm.

China Daily, 18 February 2011. Ministry Says No Leather Protein Tested in Milk. China Daily. Available from: http://www.chinadaily.com.cn/china/2011-02/18/content_12037151.htm.

China Daily, 14 March 2012. Dextrin in Baby Food Safe: Authority. China Daily. Available from: http://www.chinadaily.com.cn/china/2012-03/14/content_14836758.htm.

Clark, R., 1966. Melamine crystalluria in sheep. Journal of the South African Veterinary Medical Association 37, 349–351.

Cruywagen, C.W., Stander, M.A., Adonis, M., Calitz, T., 2009. Hot topic: pathway confirmed for the transmission of melamine from feed to cow's milk. Journal of Dairy Science 92, 2046–2050.

da Rocha, R.A., Paiva, I.M., Anjos, V., Furtado, M.A.M., Bell, M.J.V., 2015. Quantification of whey in fluid milk using confocal Raman microscopy and artificial neural network. Journal of Dairy Science 98, 3559–3567.

Dairy Industry Newsletter, 7 October 2003. Contaminated SMP turned into cement. Barry Wilson's Dairy Industry Newsletter 15 (12), 1.

Dairy Markets, 15 July 2004. Major Milk Fraud Uncovered in the North. Dairy Markets. Available from: https://www.agra-net.net/agra/dairy-markets/major-milk-fraud-uncovered-in-the-north%5f1.htm.

Dairy Markets, 9 March 2005. Six Arrested in Italian Milk Tainting Scandal. Dairy Markets. Available from: https://www.agra-net.net/agra/dairy-markets/six-arrested-in-italian-milk-tainting-scandal%5f1.htm.

Dairy Markets, 21 February 2008. Milk Prices Down 15% After Adulteration Scandal. Dairy Markets. Available from: https://www.agra-net.net/agra/dairy-markets/milk-prices-down-15-after-adulteration-scandal%5f1.htm.

Dairy Markets, 12 February 2009. Consumer Scare Over Parmalat Tainted Milk in Colombia. Dairy Markets. Available from: https://www.agra-net.net/agra/dairy-markets/analysis/company/consumer-scare-over-parmalat-tainted-milk-in-colombia%5f1.htm.

Dankowska, A., Małecka, M., Kowalewski, W., 2014. Application of synchronous fluorescence spectroscopy with multivariate data analysis for determination of butter adulteration. International Journal of Food Science & Technology 49, 2628–2634.

de Almeida, M.R., de Sá Oliveira, K., Stephani, R., de Oliveira, L.F.C., 2012. Application of FT-Raman spectroscopy and chemometric analysis for determination of adulteration in milk powder. Analytical Letters 45, 2589–2602.

de la Fuente, M.A., Juárez, M., 2005. Authenticity assessment of dairy products. Critical Reviews in Food Science & Nutrition 45, 563–585.

Demeter, K.J., Kundrat, W., Faber, A.-G., Schellner, H., Hahn, H., 1959. Bacterial destruction in cheese milk treated by the H_2O_2-catalase method. Part I. Saprophytic bacteria. Part II. Pathogenic bacteria. Proceedings of the XV International Dairy Congress 2, 538–546 (Article in German).

Desmarchelier, A., Cuadra, M.G., Delatour, T., Mottier, P., 2009. Simultaneous quantitative determination of melamine and cyanuric acid in cow's milk and milk-based infant formula by liquid chromatography-electrospray ionization tandem mass spectrometry. Journal of Agricultural and Food Chemistry 57, 7186–7193.

Dobson, R.L.M., Motlagh, S., Quijano, M., Cambron, R.T., Baker, T.R., Pullen, A.M., Regg, B.T., Bigalow-Kern, A.S., Vennard, T., Fix, A., Reimschuessel, R., Overmann, G., Shan, Y., Daston, G.P., 2008. Identification and characterization of toxicity of contaminants in pet food leading to an outbreak of renal toxicity in cats and dogs. Toxicological Sciences 106, 251–262.

Dominguez-Estevez, M., Constable, A., Mazzatorta, P., Renwick, A.G., Schilter, B., 2010. Using urinary solubility data to estimate the level of safety concern of low levels of melamine (MEL) and cyanuric acid (CYA) present simultaneously in infant formulas. Regulatory Toxicology and Pharmacology 57, 247–255.

dos Santos, P.M., Pereira-Filho, E.R., 2013. Digital image analysis — an alternative tool for monitoring milk authenticity. Analytical Methods 5, 3669–3674.

Draher, J., Pound, V., Reddy, T.M., 2014. Validation of a rapid method of analysis using ultrahigh-performance liquid chromatography – tandem mass spectrometry for nitrogen-rich adulterants in nutritional food ingredients. Journal of Chromatography A 1373, 106–113.

Ehtesham, E., Hayman, A.R., McComb, K.A., Van Hale, R., Frew, R.D., 2013. Correlation of geographical location with stable isotope values of hydrogen and carbon of fatty acids from New Zealand milk and bulk milk powder. Journal of Agricultural and Food Chemistry 61, 8914–8923.

Ehtesham, E., Hayman, A., Van Hale, R., Frew, R., 2015. Influence of feed and water on the stable isotopic composition of dairy milk. International Dairy Journal 47, 37–45.

Ellis, D.I., Brewster, V.L., Dunn, W.B., Allwood, J.W., Golovanov, A.P., Goodacre, R., 2012. Fingerprinting food: current technologies for the detection of food adulteration and contamination. Chemical Society Reviews 41, 5706–5727.

EU, 2000. Special Report No. 8/2000 on the Community measures for the disposal of butterfat accompanied by the Commission's replies. Official Journal of the European Union C 132, 1–32, 12/5/2000.

EU, 2008. Commission Regulation (EC) No 273/2008 of 5 March 2008 laying down detailed rules for the application of Council Regulation (EC) No 1255/1999 as regards methods for the analysis and quality evaluation of milk and milk products. Official Journal of the European Union L 88, 1–115, 29/3/2008.

EU, 2009. Commission regulation (EU) No 1272/2009 of 11 December 2009 laying down common detailed rules for the implementation of Council Regulation (EC) No 1234/2007 as regards buying-in and selling of agricultural products under public intervention. Official Journal of the European Union L 349, 1–68, 29/12/2009.

Fadzlillah, N.A., Rohman, A., Ismail, A., Mustafa, S., Khatib, A., 2013. Application of FTIR-ATR spectroscopy coupled with multivariate analysis for rapid estimation of butter adulteration. Journal of Oleo Science 62, 555–562.

Fay, L., Richli, U., Liardon, R., 1991. Evidence for the absence of amino acid isomerization in microwave-heated milk and infant formulas. Journal of Agricultural and Food Chemistry 39, 1857–1859.

Food News, 3 February 2009. Parmalat Milk Found to Contain Hydrogen Peroxide in Colombia. Food News. Available from: https://www.agra-net.net/agra/foodnews/parmalat-milk-found-to-contain-hydrogen-peroxide-in-colombia%5f1.htm.

Gem, H., 1857. The adulteration of milk. Lancet 69, 156.

Goncalves, J., Pereira, F., Amorim, A., van Asch, B., 2012. New method for the simultaneous identification of cow, sheep, goat, and water buffalo in dairy products by analysis of short species-specific mitochondrial DNA targets. Journal of Agricultural and Food Chemistry 60, 10480–10485.

González, J., Puschner, B., Pérez, V., Ferreras, M.C., Delgado, L., Muñoz, M., Pérez, C., Reyes, L.E., Velasco, J., Fernández, V., García-Marín, J.F., 2009. Nephrotoxicosis in Iberian piglets subsequent to exposure to melamine and derivatives in Spain between 2003 and 2006. Journal of Veterinary Diagnostic Investigation 21, 558–563.

He, X., Carter, J.M., Brandon, D.L., Cheng, L.W., McKeon, T.A., 2007. Application of a real time polymerase chain reaction method to detect castor toxin contamination in fluid milk and eggs. Journal of Agricultural and Food Chemistry 55, 6897–6902.

Hewlett, A.W., Gilbert, Q.O., Wickett, A.D., 1916. The toxic effects of urea on normal individuals. Archives of Internal Medicine (Chicago) 18, 636–651.

IDF, 2006. Comprehensive review of scientific literature pertaining to nitrogen protein conversion factors. Bulletin of the International Dairy Federation, 405/2006. Available from: http://www.fil-idf.org/Public/Download.php?media=28573.

ISO|IDF, 2002a. Milkfat — Determination of the Fatty Acid Composition by Gas-liquid Chromatography. ISO 15885|IDF 184:2002. Available from: http://www.fil-idf.org/Public/Publication.php?ID=28140&ajax=true.

ISO|IDF, 2002b. Milkfat — Preparation of Fatty Acid Methyl Esters. ISO 15884|IDF 182:2002. Available from: http://www.fil-idf.org/Public/Publication.php?ID=28138&ajax=true.

ISO|IDF, 2006. Milk Powder — Determination of Soy and Pea Proteins Using Capillary Electrophoresis in the Presence of Sodium Dodecyl Sulfate (SDS-ce) — Screening Method. ISO 17129|IDF 206:2006. Available from: http://www.fil-idf.org/Public/Publication.php?ID=28080&ajax=true.

ISO|IDF, 2008. Dried Milk and Dried Milk Products — Determination of Fat Content — Gravimetric Method (Reference Method). ISO 1736|IDF 009:2008. Available from: http://www.fil-idf.org/Public/Publication.php?ID=28157&ajax=true.

ISO|IDF, 2009. Milk — Determination of Freezing Point — Thermistor Cryoscope Method (Reference Method). ISO 5764|IDF 108:2009. Available from: http://www.fil-idf.org/Public/Publication.php?ID=28180&ajax=true.

ISO|IDF, 2010a. Milk and Milk Products — Determination of Milk Fat Purity by Gas Chromatographic Analysis of Triglycerides (Reference Method). ISO 17678|IDF 202:2010. Available from: http://www.fil-idf.org/Public/Publication.php?ID=28107&ajax=true.

ISO|IDF, 2010b. Milk, Milk Products and Infant Formulae — Guidelines for the Quantitative Determination of Melamine and Cyanuric Acid by LC-MS/MS. ISO/TS 15495|IDF/RM 230: 2010. Available from: http://www.fil-idf.org/Public/Publication.php?ID=38121&ajax=true.

ISO|IDF, 2010c. Milk — Determination of Fat Content — Gravimetric Method (Reference Method). ISO 1211|IDF 001:2010. Available from: http://www.fil-idf.org/Public/Publication.php?ID=28144&ajax=true.

ISO|IDF, 2014. Milk and Milk Products — Determination of Nitrogen Content — Part 1: Kjeldahl Principle and Crude Protein Calculation. ISO 8968-12|IDF 020-1:2014. Available from: http://www.fil-idf.org/Public/Publication.php?ID=28164&ajax=true.

Jablonski, J.E., Jackson, L.S., 2008. Stability of picrotoxin during yogurt manufacture and storage. Journal of Food Science 73, T121–T128.

Jablonski, J.E., Schlesser, J.E., Mariappagoudar, P., 2006. HPLC-UV method for nicotine, strychnine, and aconitine in dairy products. Journal of Agricultural and Food Chemistry 54, 7460–7465.

Jackson, L.S., 2009. Chemical food safety issues in the United States: past, present, and future. Journal of Agricultural and Food Chemistry 57, 8161–8170.

Jawaid, S., Talpur, F.N., Sherazi, S.T.H., Nizamani, S.M., Khaskheli, A.A., 2013. Rapid detection of melamine adulteration in dairy milk by SB-ATR-Fourier transform infrared spectroscopy. Food Chemistry 141, 3066–3071.

Jia, L.-Q., Shen, Y., Wang, X.-M., He, L.-J., Xin, Y., Hu, Y.-X., 2009. Ultrasonographic diagnosis of urinary calculus caused by melamine in children. Chinese Medical Journal 122, 252–256.

Jiang, C., Han, J., Fan, J., Tian, S., 2010. Rapid detection of adulterated milk by low field-nuclear magnetic resonance coupled with PCA method. Transactions of the Chinese Society of Agricultural Engineering 26, 340–344.

Jin, S.-Y., Lin, X.-R., Zhao, Z.-H., Zhu, H., Shi, W.-R., 2009. Determination of hydroxyproline in milk powder and other dairy products by HPLC. Beverage Industry 12, 28–30 (Article in Chinese).

Karoui, R., de Baerdemaeker, J., 2007. A review of the analytical methods coupled with chemometric tools for the determination of the quality and identity of dairy products. Food Chemistry 102, 621–640.

Karoui, R., Dufour, E., Pillonel, L., Picque, D., Cattenoz, T., Bosset, J.-O., 2004. Determining the geographic origin of Emmental cheeses produced during winter and summer using a technique based on the concatenation of MIR and fluorescence spectroscopic data. European Food Research and Technology 219, 184–189.

Karoui, R., Bosset, J.-O., Mazerolles, G., Kulmyzaev, A., Dufour, E., 2005a. Monitoring the geographic origin of both experimental French Jura hard cheeses and Swiss Gruyère and L'Etivaz PDO cheeses using mid-infrared and fluorescence spectroscopies: a preliminary investigation. International Dairy Journal 15, 275–286.

Karoui, R., Dufour, E., Pillonel, L., Schaller, E., Picque, D., Cattenoz, T., Bosset, J.-O., 2005b. The potential of combined infrared and fluorescence spectroscopies as a method of determination of the geographic origin of Emmental cheeses. International Dairy Journal 15, 287–298.

Kenny, M., 2013. Safety and quality. In: Muehlhoff, E., Bennett, A., McMahon, D. (Eds.), Milk and Dairy Products in Human Nutrition. Food and Agriculture Organization of the United Nations, Rome, pp. 243–273.

Khan, K.M., Krishna, H., Majumder, S.K., Gupta, P.K., 2015. Detection of urea adulteration in milk using near-infrared Raman spectroscopy. Food Analytical Methods 8, 93–102.

Kommadath, A., Sharma, A., Jakhar, K.K., 2001. Hepatotoxic, nephrotoxic and genotoxic effects in mice fed urea adulterated milk. Indian Journal of Dairy Science 54, 316–321.

Lachenmeier, D.W., Humpfer, E., Fang, F., Schütz, B., Dvortsak, P., Sproll, C., Spraul, M., 2009. NMR-Spectroscopy for nontargeted screening and simultaneous quantification of health-relevant compounds in foods: the example of melamine. Journal of Agricultural and Food Chemistry 57, 7149–7199.

Lancet, 1857. Medical annotations. Lancet 69, 98.

Li, J.-H., Meng, X.-C., 2008. Detection of hydrolyzed animal collagen proteins in milk by HPLC. China Dairy Industry 36, 56–59.

Li, X., Rezaei, R., Li, P., Wu, G., 2011. Composition of amino acids in feed ingredients for animal diets. Amino Acids 40, 1159–1168.

Liu, H., Han, D.H., Wang, S.P., 2014. Potentiality of synchronous fluorescence technology for determination of reconstituted milk adulteration in fresh milk. Spectroscopy & Spectral Analysis 34, 2685–2689 (Article in Chinese).

Lück, H., 1956. The use of hydrogen peroxide as a dairy preservative. Dairy Science Abstracts 18, 363–386.

Lumor, S.E., Deen, B.D., Ronningen, I., Smith, K., Fredrickson, N.R., Diez-Gonzalez, F., Labuza, T.P., 2012. Detection and inactivation of saxitoxin in skim milk. Journal of Food Protection 75, 1113–1116.

MacKenzie, H.I., 1966. Melamine for sheep. Journal of the South African Veterinary Medical Association 37, 153–157.

MacKenzie, H.I., van Rensburg, I.B.J., 1968. Ammelide and ammeline as nonprotein nitrogen supplements for sheep. Journal of the South African Veterinary Medical Association 39 (2), 41–45.

MacMahon, S., Begley, T.H., Diachenko, G.W., Stromgren, S.A., 2012. A liquid chromatography–tandem mass spectrometry method for the detection of economically motivated adulteration in protein-containing foods. Journal of Chromatography A 1220, 101–107.

McCarron, D.A., 2011. Healthcare Savings From Adequate Dairy Food Consumption. An Estimate Based on the Medical Literature in 2011. Presentation. Available from: http://www.wds2011.com/Files/media/PrivateSpace/Presentations/IDFnutritioneconomics/14.30%5f-15.00%5f-David-McCarron%5f-Heathcare-....pdf.

McCarron, D.A., Heaney, R.P., 2004. Estimated healthcare savings associated with adequate dairy food intake. American Journal of Hypertension 17, 88–97.

McCarthy, M.J., Kuksis, A., Beveridge, J.M.R., 1964. Composition of molecular distillates of butter oil: isolation and identification of components other than glycerides. Journal of Lipid Research 5, 609–615.

McConnell, P., 18 December 1908. London milk supply from a farmer's point of view. Journal of the Royal Society of Arts 57, 84–93.

McDonald, H.B., 2008. Dairy nutrition: what we knew then to what we know now. International Dairy Journal 18, 774–777.

Molkentin, J., 2007. Detection of foreign fat in milk fat from different continents by triacylglycerol analysis. European Journal of Lipid Science and Technology 109, 505–510.

Mollé, D., Léonil, J., 2005. Quantitative determination of bovine κ-casein macropeptide in dairy products by liquid chromatography/electrospray coupled to mass spectrometry (LC-ESI/MS) and liquid chromatography/electrospray coupled to tandem mass spectrometry (LC-ESI/MS/MS). International Dairy Journal 15, 419–428.

Moore, J.C., Spink, J., Lipp, M., 2012. Development and application of a database of food ingredient fraud and economically motivated adulteration from 1980 to 2010. Journal of Food Science 77 (4), R108–R116.

Nakano, T., Ozimek, L., 2003. Analysis of hydroxyproline in yogurt with and without gelatin. Milchwissenschaft 58, 517–519.

Neelima, R.P.S., Sharma, R., Rajput, Y.S., 2012. Direct estimation of sialic acid in milk and milk products by fluorimetry and its application in detection of sweet whey adulteration in milk. Journal of Dairy Research 79, 495–501.

New York Times, 8 October 2008. Milk Scandal Pushes China to Set Limits on Melamine. New York Times. Available from: http://www.nytimes.com/2008/10/09/world/asia/09milk.html?_r=0.

Ntakatsane, M.P., Liu, X.M., Zhou, P., 2013. Short communication: rapid detection of milk fat adulteration with vegetable oil by fluorescence spectroscopy. Journal of Dairy Science 96, 2130–2136.

Ohta, T., Yoshida, T., Kanzaki, B., Hosono, A., Suyama, K., 2002. Quantitative determination of furosine in cow's milk containing reconstituted skim milk. Milchwissenschaft 57, 70–73.

Owens, J., Koester, C., 2008. Quantitation of abrine, an indole alkaloid marker of the toxic glycoproteins abrin, by liquid chromatography/tandem mass spectrometry when spiked into various beverages. Journal of Agricultural and Food Chemistry 56, 11139–11143.

Owens, J., Koester, C., 2009. Quantitative analysis of chemical warfare agent degradation products in beverages by liquid chromatography tandem mass spectrometry. Journal of Agricultural and Food Chemistry 57, 8227–8235.

Paradkar, M.M., Singhal, R.S., Kulkarni, P.R., 2000a. An approach to the detection of synthetic milk in dairy milk: 1. Detection of urea. International Journal of Dairy Technology 53, 87–91.

Paradkar, M.M., Singhal, R.S., Kulkarni, P.R., 2000b. An approach to the detection of synthetic milk in dairy milk: 2. Detection of detergents. International Journal of Dairy Technology 53, 92–95.

Paradkar, M.M., Singhal, R.S., Kulkarni, P.R., 2001a. An approach to the detection of synthetic milk in dairy milk: 3. Detection of vegetable oil and sodium bicarbonate. International Journal of Dairy Technology 54, 34–35.

Paradkar, M.M., Singhal, R.S., Kulkarni, P.R., 2001b. An approach to the detection of synthetic milk in dairy milk: 4. Effect of the addition of synthetic milk on the flow behaviour of pure cow milk. International Journal of Dairy Technology 54, 36–37.

Parmar, S.C., Sofia, Z.P., Jain, A.K., Nath, B.S., 2010. Quality of ghee from Bangalore market. Indian Journal of Dairy Science 65, 364–370.

Paty, E., Chedevergne, F., Scheinmann, P., Wal, J.-M., Bernard, H., 2003. Allergie au lait de chèvre et de brebis sans allergie associée au lait de vache. Allergy to goat's milk and sheep's milk without allergy to cow's milk. Revue Française d'Allergologie et d'Immunologie Clinique 43, 455–462 (Article in French).

People's Daily Online, 26 October 2008. Survey: 25% Beijing Babies Consumed Tainted Milk Powder. People's Daily Online. Available from: http://en.people.cn/90001/90776/90882/6521481.html.

Picariello, G., Sacchi, R., Fierro, O., Melck, D., Romano, R., Paduano, A., Motta, A., Addeo, F., 2013. High resolution ^{13}C NMR detection of short- and medium-chain synthetic triacylglycerols used in butterfat adulteration. European Journal of Lipid Science & Technology 115, 858–864.

Pillonel, L., Badertscher, R., Bütikofer, U., Casey, M., Dalle Torre, M., Lavanchy, P., Meyer, J., Tabacchi, R., Bosset, J.O., 2002a. Analytical methods for the determination of the geographic origin of Emmentaler cheese. Main framework of the project; chemical, biochemical, microbiological, colour and sensory analyses. European Food Research and Technology 215, 260–267.

Pillonel, L., Collomb, M., Tabacchi, R., Bosset, J.-O., 2002b. Analytical methods for the determination of the geographic origin of Emmental cheese. Free fatty acids, triglycerides and fatty acid composition of cheese fat. Mitteilungen aus Lebensmitteluntersuchung und Hygiene 93, 217–231.

Pillonel, L., Tabacchi, R., Bosset, J.-O., 2003a. Analytical methods for the determination of the geographic origin of Emmental cheese. Summary of a screening study. Mitteilungen aus Lebensmitteluntersuchung und Hygiene 94, 60–69.

Pillonel, L., Luginbühl, W., Picque, D., Schaller, E., Tabacchi, R., Bosset, J.O., 2003b. Analytical methods for the determination of the geographic origin of Emmental cheese: mid- and near-infrared spectroscopy. European Food Research and Technology 216, 174–178.

Pillonel, L., Badertscher, R., Casey, M., Meyer, J., Rossmann, A., Schlichtherle-Cerny, H., Tabacchi, R., Bosset, J.O., 2005. Geographic origin of European Emmental cheese: characterisation and descriptive statistics. International Dairy Journal 15, 547–556.

Poon, N.-W., Gohel, M.D.I., Lau, C., Hon, E.K.-L., Leung, P.-C., Ng, C.-F., 2012. Melamine crystallization: physicochemical properties, interactions with other lithogenic salts and response to therapeutic agents. Journal of Urology 187, 1483–1490.

Povolo, M., Pelizzola, V., Ravera, D., Contarini, G., 2009. Significance of the nonvolatile minor compounds of the neutral lipid fraction as markers of the origin of dairy products. Journal of Agricultural and Food Chemistry 57, 7387–7394.

Prema, D., Pilfold, J.L., Krauchi, J., Church, J.S., Donkor, K.K., Cinel, B., 2013. Rapid determination of total conjugated linoleic acid content in select Canadian cheeses by ^{1}H NMR spectroscopy. Journal of Agricultural and Food Chemistry 61, 9915–9921.

Punch, 4 August 1855. What to Eat, Drink, and Avoid. Punch, 45, 47.

Qin, J., Chao, K., Kim, M.S., 2013. Simultaneous detection of multiple adulterants in dry milk using macro-scale Raman chemical imaging. Food Chemistry 138, 998–1007.

Reimschuessel, R., Gieseker, C.M., Miller, R.A., Ward, J., Boehmer, J., Rummel, N., Heller, D.N., Nochetto, C., de Alwis, G.K.H., Bataller, N., Andersen, W.C., Turnipseed, S.B., Karbiwnyk, C.M., Satzger, R.D., Crowe, J.B., Wilber, N.R., Reinhard, M.K., Roberts, J.F., Witkowski, M.R., 2008. Evaluation of the renal effects of experimental feeding of melamine and cyanuric acid to fish and pigs. American Journal of Veterinary Research 69, 1217–1228.

Reuters, 11 September 2008a. Baby Dies as New Milk Powder Scare Spreads Across China. Available from: http://www.reuters.com/article/2008/09/11/us-china-babies-idUSPEK34255620080911.

Reuters, 25 October 2008b. China Burns Milk Prodcuts [sic] in Giant Furnaces. Available from: http://in.reuters.com/article/2008/10/25/idINIndia-36148820081025.

Reyers, F., 2008a. Alert (heads up) message for South African Veterinary Livestock Health and Production Group. Melamine contamination of fresh milk in South Africa – dairy meal adulteration. Livestock Health and Production Review 8, 4–5.

Reyers, F., December 2008b. Melamine Is Back. In Milk and in South Africa. A Veterinary Perspective. Veterinary News, pp. 14–15.

Rutherfurd, S.M., Fanning, A.C., Miller, B.J., Moughan, P.J., 2015. Protein digestibility-corrected amino acid scores and digestible indispensable amino acid scores differentially describe protein quality in growing male rats. Journal of Nutrition 145, 372–379.

Santos, P.M., Wentzell, P.D., Pereira-Filho, E.R., 2012. Scanner digital images combined with colour parameters: a case study to detect adulterations in liquid cow's milk. Food Analytical Methods 5, 89–95.

Santos, P.M., Pereira-Filho, E.R., Rodriguez-Saona, L.E., 2013. Rapid detection and quantification of milk adulteration using infrared microspectroscopy and chemometrics analysis. Food Chemistry 138, 19–24.

Sanvido, G.B., Garcia, J.S., Corilo, Y.E., Vaz, B.G., Zacca, J.J., Cosso, R.G., Eberlin, M.N., Peter, M.G., 2010. Fast screening and secure confirmation of milk powder adulteration with maltodextrin via electrospray ionization-mass spectrometry [ESI(+)-MS] and selective enzymatic hydrolysis. Journal of Agricultural and Food Chemistry 58, 9407–9412.

Schoder, D., 2010. Melamine milk powder and infant formula sold in East Africa. Journal of Food Protection 73, 1709–1714.

Shen, J.S., Wang, J.Q., Wei, H.Y., Bu, D.P., Sun, P., Zhou, L.Y., 2010. Transfer efficiency of melamine from feed to milk in lactating dairy cows fed with different doses of melamine. Journal of Dairy Science 93, 2060–2066.

Smedman, A., Lindmark-Månsson, H., Drewnowski, A., Edman, A.-K.M., 2010. Nutrient density of beverages in relation to climate impact. Food & Nutrition Research 54, 5170–5177.

Stuff.co.nz, 10 June 2014. Fonterra Increases Fight Against Food Fraud. Stuff.co.nz. Available from: http://www.stuff.co.nz/business/10134345/Fonterra-increases-fight-against-food-fraud.

Sun, N., Shen, Y., Sun, Q., Li, X.-R., Jia, L.-Q., Zhang, G.-J., Zhang, W.-P., Chen, Z., Fan, J.-F., Jiang, Y.-P., Feng, D.-C., Zhang, R.-F., Zhu, X.-Y., Xiao, H.-Z., 2009. Diagnosis and treatment of melamine-associated urinary calculus complicated with acute renal failure in infants and young children. Chinese Medical Journal 122, 245–251.

Tunick, M.H., 2009. Dairy innovations over the past 100 years. Journal of Agricultural and Food Chemistry 57, 8093–8097.

Turnipseed, S., Casey, C., Nochetto, C., Heller, D.N., 2008. Determination of melamine and cyanuric acid residues in infant formula using LC-MS/MS. US FDA Laboratory Information Bulletin 24. LIB No. 4421. Available from: http://www.fda.gov/Food/FoodScienceResearch/LaboratoryMethods/ucm071637.htm.

Üçüncüoğlu, D., İlaslan, K., Boyacı, İ.H., Özay, D.S., 2013. Rapid detection of fat adulteration in bakery products using Raman and near-infrared spectroscopies. European Food Research and Technology 237, 703–710.

Ulberth, F., 1994. Detection of milk fat adulteration by linear discriminant analysis of fatty acid data. Journal of AOAC International 77, 1326–1334.

US FDA, 2003. Risk assessment for food terrorism and other food safety concerns. CFSAN/Office of Regulations and Policy. No longer available at the original site, but a cached copy available from: http://seafood.oregonstate.edu/.pdf%20Links/Risk%20Assessment%20for%20Food%20Terrorism%20and%20Other%20Food%20Safety%20Concerns.pdf.

Villar, D., Schwartz, K.J., Carson, T.L., Kinker, J.A., Barker, J., 2003. Acute poisoning of cattle by fertilizer-contaminated water. Veterinary and Human Toxicology 45, 88–90.

Wang, Y., Wei, B., Wang, Q., 1990. Crystal structure of melamine cyanuric acid complex (1:1) trihydrochloride, MCA·3HCl. Journal of Crystallographic and Spectroscopic Research 20, 79–84.

Wang, Y.-H., Li, P.-B., Deng, B.-N., Nan, W.-K., Jin, H., 2009. Detection of hydrolyzed animal proteins in milk by Hitachi L-8800 high speed amino acid analyzer. Chinese Journal of Health Laboratory Technology 19, 2547–2548.

Wein, L.M., Liu, Y., 2005. Analyzing a bioterror attack on the food supply: the case of botulinum toxin in milk. Proceedings of the National Academy of Sciences of the United States of America 102, 9984–9989.

Weinstein, I., 1947. Eighty years of public health in New York City. Bulletin of the New York Academy of Medicine 23, 221–237.

WHO, 1980. Evaluation of Certain Food Additives and Contaminants. Twenty-fourth report of the Joint FAO/WHO Expert Committee on Food Additives. WHO Technical Report Series 653. World Health Organisation, Geneva, pp. 12–14.

WHO, 2008. Expert Meeting to Review Toxicological Aspects of Melamine and Cyanuric Acid. Available from: http://www.who.int/foodsafety/fs_management/Exec_Summary_melamine.pdf.

WHO, 2009. Toxicological and Health Aspects of Melamine and Cyanuric Acid. Available from: http://apps.who.int/iris/bitstream/10665/44106/1/9789241597951_eng.pdf?ua=1.

Wiles, P.G., Gray, I.K., Kissling, R.C., 1998. Routine analysis of proteins by Kjeldahl and Dumas methods: review and interlaboratory study using dairy products. Journal of AOAC International 81, 620–632.

Woods, R.I., Watterson, P.A., Woodward, J.H., 1989. The causes of rapid infant mortality decline in England and Wales, 1861–1921. Part II. Population Studies 43, 113–132.

Xin, H., Stone, R., 2008. Chinese probe unmasks high-tech adulteration with melamine. Science 322, 1310–1311.

Xu, L., Yan, S.-M., Cai, C.-B., Wang, Z.-J., Yu, X.-P., 2013. The feasibility of using near-infrared spectroscopy and chemometrics for untargeted detection of protein adulteration in yogurt: removing unwanted variations in pure yogurt. Journal of Analytical Methods in Chemistry. Article ID 201873, 9 pages.

Yang, L., Wen, J.G., Wen, J.J., Su, Z.Q., Zhu, W., Huang, C.X., Yu, S.L., Guo, Z., 2013a. Four years follow-up of 101 children with melamine-related urinary stones. Urolithiasis 41, 265–266.

Yang, R., Liu, R., Xu, K., Yang, Y., Dong, G., Zhang, W., 2013b. Classification of adulterated milk with the parameterization of 2D correlation spectroscopy and least squares support vector machines. Analytical Methods 5, 5949–5953.

Yang, L., Huo, D., Jiang, Y., Hou, C., Zhang, S., 2013c. Monitoring the adulteration of milk with melamine: a visualised sensor array approach. Food Additives & Contaminants: Part A 30, 786–795.

Advances in the Identification of Adulterated Cereals and Cereal Products

18

S.R. Delwiche
USDA, Agricultural Research Service, Beltsville, MD, United States

Chapter Outline

18.1 Introduction

> *Whatever the British consumer may feel inclination to devour, let him devour it at his peril; he will himself be thereby preyed upon, devoured, consumed. Every warm-blooded animal expresses indignation if its food be meddled with. The food of the British consumer is meddled with, and he is warm-blooded; he is, therefore, irritable and suspicious on the subject of provisions.*
> *Page 423 of Household Words: A Weekly Journal: Conducted by Charles Dickens, Vol. 5, 1852*

Adulteration of cereal grains is not a new occurrence. In fact, in earlier pages of the Dickens' journal, he describes the widespread cheating by bakers through the use of alum, which served the dual purpose of whitening the flour and permitting more water to be added to the dough, thus producing 94–100 loaves in a batch that would normally yield 80. With the simultaneous increased reliance on international trade of food ingredients and the increased industrialization of food processing, the opportunity for food fraud today is ever present (Scally, 2013). Cereals have the benefit of being less affected by adulteration because of their relative low cost. A material of even lesser value or whose active ingredient is of lesser value than the targeted commodity would be needed to justify the necessary financial incentive.

This chapter is divided into several small sections, with the first section addressing legislation in the European Union and United States on food adulteration with respect to the cereals. Next, some of the common methods of measurement are described, including enzyme-linked immunosorbent assay (ELISA), polymerase chain reaction (PCR), and spectroscopy. The bulk of the chapter discusses some of the most common occurrences of cereals adulteration, namely, in wheat flour or gluten adulterated with melamine, durum wheat semolina or flour adulterated with common wheat flour, and Basmati rice adulterated with Basmati-like rice. Included among these topics are the author's own trials of detection and measurement of common wheat in waxy wheat using near-infrared spectroscopy (NIR). Finally, attention is given to the circumstance when the cereal (wheat, barley, or rye) itself is the adulterant in foods that are labeled as gluten-free. Emphasis is placed on cereals adulteration activity of the past decade (2005–2014), with adulteration summarized in Table 18.1 by cereal, adulterant, and method. No coverage is given to the detection and measurement of genetically

Table 18.1 Cereal Adulteration Research 2007 to Present

Cereal or Cereal Product	Adulterant	Method of Analysis	References
Durum wheat for pasta	Common wheat	DNA microsatellite	Sonnante et al. (2009)
Durum wheat for bread	Common wheat	DNA microsatellite	Pasqualone et al. (2007, 2010)
Durum wheat	Common wheat	DNA tubulin-based polymorphism	Casazza et al., 2012
Durum wheat	Common wheat	Mass spectrometry	Russo et al. (2014)
Durum wheat	Common wheat	NIR reflectance	Cocchi et al. (2006)
Wheat-based products (crackers, flour, bread, noodles, breakfast cereal, cakes, snacks, soups)	Melamine	ELISA	Garber and Brewer (2010)

Table 18.1 Cereal Adulteration Research 2007 to Present—cont'd

Cereal or Cereal Product	Adulterant	Method of Analysis	References
Wheat flour, corn flour, rice flour	Melamine	HPLC	Ehling et al. (2007)
Wheat flour	Peanut flour	NIR HSI	Mishra et al. (2015)
Wheat and rye	Ergot bodies	NIR HSI	Vermeulen et al. (2012, 2013)
Basmati rice	Non-Basmati	DNA microsatellite	Archak et al. (2007), Vemireddy et al. (2007) and Colyer et al. (2008)
Basmati rice	Non-Basmati	Real-time PCR	Ganopoulos et al. (2011)
Basmati rice	Non-Basmati	SSR markers	Kaur et al. (2015)
Koshihikari rice	Non-Koshihikari	$\delta^{13}C$, $\delta^{15}N$, and $\delta^{18}O$ isotopes	Suzuki et al. (2008)
Waxy common wheat	Common wheat	NIR reflectance	Delwiche and Graybosch (2014)
Gluten-free food	Gluten	ELISA	Rosell et al. (2014)
Gluten-free food	Gluten	PCR	Mujico et al. (2011) and Mustorp et al. (2011)

ELISA, enzyme-linked immunosorbent assay; *HPLC*, high-performance liquid chromatography; *HSI*, hyperspectral imaging; *NIR*, near infrared; *PCR*, polymer chain reaction; *SSR*, simple sequence repeat.

modified cereal grains. Finally, naturally occurring contamination from molds, insects, or other sources that are not the product of mankind's deliberate actions is beyond the scope of this chapter.

18.2 Legislation

Cereals adulteration and food adulteration in general is of continued concern worldwide for reasons of safety and economics. The structure of regulation of food adulterants in the worldwide market was described by Manning and Soon (2014), which laid out the economic and criminal motivation of adulteration as well as describing new strategies for countering adulterated products and ingredients in international trade. An underlying fallibility of the traditional approach to screening for adulteration is that the adulterant must often be known beforehand. An alternative approach is to examine the product's integrity without regard to whatever may be mixed in so long as the purity of the product is measured to the limits of detection. This opposite approach relieves the overseer of the need to develop multiple procedures. Zhang et al. (2011) describe this approach as "fingerprinting," in which the data collected on the evaluated food sample are compared with the corresponding trace from the database of foods or ingredients that are known to be pure. Through a comprehensive search of a Chinese national database, these authors reviewed the literature of articles written in Chinese on the topic of instrumental methods for food authentication and divided these into categories of electrophoresis, spectroscopy (vibrational and mass), and chromatography [gas, liquid, and high-performance liquid chromatography (HPLC)], along with providing the advantages and drawbacks of each. For example, while chromatography fingerprinting is the most expensive, they claimed that the precision is better than electrophoresis fingerprinting, with the latter being limited in terms of quantification. Despite the search of nearly 500 articles, very few dealt with the cereals directly.

18.2.1 Europe

In Europe, EC Regulation 178/2002 established some general principles of food law. In the regulation, the European Food Safety Authority was established as an entity that operates independently of the European Commission, European Parliament, and the EU Member States. In its own words, EC Regulation 178/2002 provided "the basis for the assurance of a high level of protection of human health and consumers' interest in relation to food, taking into account in particular the diversity in the supply of food including traditional products, whilst ensuring the effective functioning of the internal market" (EC, 2002). With regard to the protection of the consumer, Article 8 of the legislation described the aim of food law as being to prevent fraudulent or deceptive practices, food adulteration, and any practices designed to mislead the consumer. In the United Kingdom, for example, the Food Standards Agency has the responsibility to carry out the spirit of the EC regulations.

The UK's Food Standards Agency is primarily responsible for developing methods to verify food authenticity, including the names given to foods, the names and amounts of ingredients, the types of processing and treatments, and claims of production and geographical source (Primrose et al., 2010). Primrose et al. listed various types of adulteration, which they call "misdescription," these being (1) substitution of one ingredient by a similar but cheaper one; (2) extending or adulterating food with a cheaper or base material; (3) the presence of undeclared ingredients; (4) extending or adulterating food to increase value; (5) nondeclaration or false declaration of processes; (6) overdeclaration of a quantitative ingredient; and (7) false claims regarding geographical or production origin. They describe the types of analytical methods that can be used for authentication, including quantitative DNA methods, such as real-time PCR for measuring the level of common wheat mixed in with durum wheat, mass spectrometry of protein fragments (particularly myofibrillar peptides), which are not significantly affected by cooking or heat treatment, and, finally, stable isotopes ($^{2}H/^{1}H$, $^{13}C/^{12}C$, $^{15}N/^{14}N$, and $^{18}O^{16}O$, described later) for distinguishing plant substances originating from C3 versus C4 plants and from different geographical regions.

Throughout the European Union, Regulation 882/2004 describes the manner of feed and food law that Member States must adopt on their own to be in compliance with the entire Union. This took effect on January 1, 2006, with later incorporation of financing aspects in 2007 and refinement of "high-risk" feed and food whose ingredients do not include Products of Animal Origin (POAO).

18.2.2 United States

In the United States, food safety falls under the control of two agencies primarily, these being the Department of Agriculture's Food Safety and Inspection Service and the Department of Health and Human Service's Food and Drug Administration (FDA), with the former being in charge of meat, poultry, and egg safety and the latter being in charge of the balance of the country's food supply. The FDA categorizes food adulterants into four broad classes: poisonous or deleterious substances; filth or foreign matter; economically motivated adulteration; and microbiological contamination and adulteration. The laws that govern the FDA are derived from the Federal Food, Drug, and Cosmetic Act, abbreviated as FFDCA (21 USC 301), the Public Health Service Act (42 USC 201), and the Packaging and Labeling Act (15 USC 1451). The two basic statuary components of the FFDCA are "adulteration" and "misbranding." While Section 342 of this Act describes adulteration in nine broad categories (including poisonous or insanitary ingredients; color additives; ingredients in confectionaries and dietary supplements; reoffering of previously denied foods; and noncompliance with sanitary transportation practices) the category that is most applicable to cereals is that defined as the "Absence, substitution, or addition of constituents." Such constituents may arise from (1) omission or abstraction of a constituent, in whole or part, (2) the substitution of a constituent, in whole or part, (3) the concealment of a damaged or inferior constituent, or (4) the addition of a substance so as to increase the bulk or weight of the substance, or make it appear better or be of higher value than it actually is. The penalty for violating the adulteration aspect of the FFDCA, as stated in Section 333 of the Act, may be imprisonment for 1 year for a first-time offense and 3 years for a second offense.

The Food Safety Modernization Act (FSMA) was enacted on January 4, 2011. Its purpose was to better protect the health, safety, and security of humans and animals with respect to their food supplies. An emphasis was placed on the prevention of food safety problems both domestically and overseas as it is estimated that of the 200,000 food supply facilities in use for Americans, more than half are based outside the United States. Although the Act was passed in 2011, it was envisaged that various components, or rules, of the Act would be phased in over a 5-year period. One of these has to do with the intentional adulteration of foods. Comments for this rule were due on March 31, 2014. According to the FDA (2014a) in their writing of FSMA, adulteration may be the response of those wanting to cause large-scale public health harm, acts of disgruntled employees, consumers, or competitors. Alternatively, adulteration may be motivated by economic reasons without the intention of doing harm. Instead of focusing on certain foods or hazards as culprits for adulteration and remediation, the FDA proposes to focus on vulnerable processes within a facility. The four processes that the FDA identifies of greatest concern with respect to foods vulnerable to large-scale public harm through intentional adulteration are (1) bulk liquid receiving and loading, (2) liquid storage and handling, (3) secondary ingredient handling, that is, that stage at which secondary ingredients are combined before they are added to the primary ingredient, and (4) mixing and similar activities. For cereals it would seem that the third and fourth processes apply. Once a process or step is identified as a potential target for intentional adulteration, the processor will be required to establish a plan to mitigate the risk of intentional adulteration. This will entail drafting a food defense plan that includes seven aspects: (1) actionable process steps, (2) focused mitigation strategies, (3) monitoring, (4) corrective actions, (5) verification, (6) training, and (7) record keeping.

One other organization with interest in the management of adulteration is the US Pharmacopeial Convention (USP), a nongovernment nonprofit body that sets standards (enforced by the FDA) for identity, strength, quality, and purity of medicines, food ingredients, and dietary supplements. Out of concern for adulteration, the USP assembled a database on food ingredient adulterants using literature searches of peer-reviewed publications from 1980 to 2010. The searches were conducted within Google Scholar, Web of Science, and PubMed (Moore et al., 2012). Articles in English from media and nonpeer-reviewed sources were included in the search. Of the scholarly records, 575 publications were found covering 250 different ingredients. An additional 111 ingredients were identified in the latter sources. They also identified the analytical methodologies for measuring and detecting food fraud. Sixteen commonly used technologies were found, these being, in order of prevalence (most to least), the following: HPLC, all forms of infrared spectroscopy (IR), gas chromatography (GC), isotope ratio mass spectrometry (IRMS), hyphenated mass spectrometry (-MS), NIR, PCR, capillary electrophoresis, ELISA, thin-layer chromatography, site-specific natural isotope fractionation nuclear magnetic resonance spectroscopy, mid-infrared spectroscopy, Raman spectroscopy (Raman), nuclear magnetic resonance spectroscopy (NMR), high-performance anion exchange chromatography, and differential scanning calorimetry.

18.3 Methodology for Phenotyping and Geography

Several review articles on food adulteration have been published since 2010. The use of DNA markers in the authentication of foods, including detection of common wheat flour in durum wheat semolina, was reviewed by Scarano and Rao (2014). A review of the spectroscopy-based methods for food authentication and adulteration detection and quantification, including the vibrational spectroscopies (near-IR, mid-IR, and Raman), NMR spectroscopy, and mass spectrometry was released by Ellis et al. (2012), though it has only small descriptions on cereals adulteration other than melamine in wheat gluten or screening of fungicides in wheat. Cozzolino (2014) describes in a short review paper the use of NIR and mid-IR coupled with chemometrics [partial least squares (PLS) regression, artificial neural networks, wavelets, and principal component analysis] to distinguish varieties of wheat, barley, corn, and rice within themselves, as well as distinguishing classes, determining geographical source, screening of genotypes of barley for malting characteristics, and identifying transgenic from non-transgenic grains. The author emphasized that the ability of NIR methods to authenticate samples is not self-explanatory and needs to be backed up with analytical techniques, such as GC-MS; however, the authors did not directly address the subject of adulteration of cereals.

Fortunately, with the exception of melamine and its derivatives, adulteration of cereals does not impose health risks to consumers. Rather, the occurrences are economically motivated and take the form of either variety substitution in the case of rice or related species substitution in the case of wheat. However, these subtle differences can present a challenge to analytical methodologies needed for their quantification. van Leeuwen et al. (2014) reviewed the research on using the combination of GC-IRMS to authenticate and trace foods and beverages, specifically through examination of aroma compounds, sugars, amino acids, and oils. Briefly, in the GC-IRMS procedure, eluted compounds from the GC column are injected into a combustion system from which gases are then fed into an isotope ratio mass spectrometer. Combustion involves the oxidation of the organic compounds of C, H, and N into CO_2, H_2O, and NO_x followed by the reduction to N_2 and removal of O_2 and H_2O. The dried gases leave the combustion chamber and move to the IRMS detector where they are exposed to electron-impact ionization followed by exposure to an electromagnetic analyzer that separates them according to weight and charge. The ion currents are subsequently related to relative isotope abundances. Isotope ratios, such as $^{13}C/^{12}C$, are determined by integrating the traces of each of the component isotopes, whereupon the ratios are corrected against those from standard reference materials. Small differences in the ratios of $^{13}C/^{12}C$ or $^{15}N/^{14}N$ can be associated with the species or geographical origin of the food's organic compounds. Isotope ratio analysis involves measuring the ratio of the heavier isotope to the lighter and then referencing it to a compound of normal and known ratio. The notation and calculation of relative abundance of the isotope is

$$\delta_{\text{ref}} = 1000\left(\frac{R_{\text{sample}}}{R_{\text{reference}}} - 1\right)$$

where δ_{ref} is the sample isotope ratio in "delta" units, and R_{sample} and $R_{\text{reference}}$ are the absolute isotope ratios of the sample and reference material, respectively, represented in parts per thousand. For carbon, these distinctions can arise because of two different pathways, C3 and C4, for carbon fixation during plant photosynthesis by which $\delta^{13}C$ for C3 plants (wheat and rice) is naturally different from that of C4 plants (corn). So long as the adulterant is derived from a plant source of the opposite pathway, isotope ratio analysis can be effective at discerning the presence and possibly the level of the adulterant. In Europe, the incentive for intentional mislabeling or adulteration is heightened because of the regulation known as the European Union Protected Food Names Schemes, which established categories to designate agricultural products according to geographical region of growth or processing, as well as character in production techniques or composition (Kelly et al., 2005). Cheajesadagul et al. (2013) summarized the applications of stable isotope analysis as follows: $\delta^{2}H$ or $\delta^{18}O$ for evaporation, condensation, and precipitation of water, indicating geographical origin; $\delta^{11}B$ for geochemical processes, indicating geographical origin, $\delta^{13}C$ for C3 versus C4 plants, indicating diet of herbivores, and hence geographical location; $\delta^{87}Sr$ for rock age determination; and $\delta^{20x}Pb$ for anthropogenic sources.

Literature on the application of GC-IRMS to cereals authentication or adulteration is scarce compared to that of higher value food compounds. Mottram et al. (2003) used this technology on $\delta^{13}C$ of corn oil to detect and quantify adulteration with six other oils, including peanut, sunflower, rapeseed, and soybean. This was further broken down to isotope ratio differences of the oil's minor components, sterols and tocopherols. When used in conjunction with conventional fatty acid profiling, the limit of detection of adulteration of corn oil is reduced to 5% (w/w).

Visible or NIR hyperspectral imaging (HSI) is a relatively new technique that was initially popularized in remote sensing but in the past 15 years it has also found utility in food and agriculture applications. As a combination of digital imaging and spectroscopy, HSI is particularly well suited to the imaging of objects that have spatial and spectral heterogeneity. Two broad approaches may be taken. First, spatial regions of interest (ROIs) can be identified either manually or automatically, whereupon individual pixel spectral responses are then averaged to produce a mean spectrum that is representative of the ROI. Conventional quantitative chemometric algorithms may then be applied to develop calibrations for analyte concentrations. Alternatively, the second approach capitalizes on the information within each pixel's spectrum, whereby qualitative algorithms are applied to classify each pixel into one class or another. The proportions of pixels belonging to the respective classes can then be used to determine contamination, defect, or damaged regions of the objects. When used successfully, HSI offers advantages in speed of analysis compared to manual, visual inspection of cereal grain samples for grade determination, which, in the United States, typically means 15 min for a 15 g sample of wheat [and more than 30 min for a 50–100 g sample in Europe as prescribed by EC Regulation 687/2008 (EC, 2008)] to visually examine for impurities including broken kernels, other cereals, sprout, insect damage, frost, discoloration, mottled grain, ergot, decay, live and dead insects, and other damage.

As an example, the use of NIR HSI to measure weight percentages of contaminants (in this case, naturally occurring ones) based on Soft Independent Method of Class Analogy of PCA scores or partial least squares discriminant analysis (PLS-DA), were reported by Vermeulen et al. (2013). Wheat and rye samples were spiked with ergot bodies at levels ranging from 0.02% to 0.52%. Model accuracies were substantially improved when morphological features, such as object size, as measured by the number of pixels, and object roundness were incorporated in the discrimination models. An earlier study by this same team reported that HSI could detect ergot at mass concentrations as low as 145 mg/kg, thus meeting the EC regulatory limit of 0.1% for feedstuffs containing unground cereals and 0.05% in foods for human consumption (EC, 2008). Their work demonstrated that, with inspection using a conveyor belt configuration, a sample of 250 g could be analyzed in less than 1 min Mishra et al. (2015) applied principal component analysis to hyperspectral images (1000–2200 nm) of mixtures of ground peanut and wheat flour. Pixels were assigned to either peanut or wheat flour classes based on score values on PCs 1 and 2 of normalized absorbance spectra, whereupon the percentage of peanut pixels was compared to the mass concentration of peanut. They were able to achieve a coefficient of determination (R^2) of 0.946 for a peanut concentration range of 0.1–10%, with a level of detection down to 0.01%. Similar analysis was developed by Pierna et al. (2014) in which PLS-DA scores of pixel spectra in hyperspectral images (1100–2400 nm) were used to determine mixture levels of melamine in soybean meal at concentrations from 0.5% to 5%. Perhaps more critical than in other analytical procedures, successful results using HSI are dependent on the sampling scheme, especially in applications of online imaging. This is because the material, seeds in this case, is typically intact so that the analyst is confronted with a more acute sampling challenge than in other analytical procedures when much of the sampling decisions have already been made before the analyst receives the test sample. Aspects of sampling are covered extensively in Petersen et al. (2005), along with specificity to seed lots for genetically modified organism detection in a series of articles by Esbensen et al. (Esbensen et al., 2012a,b; Minkkinen et al., 2012) and summarized by Freese et al. (2015).

Branch et al. (2003) studied the origin of wheat grown in Europe and North America by stable isotope analysis of ^{13}C and ^{15}N along with elemental isotope analysis of cadmium, selenium, strontium, and lead. Of these six isotopes, $\delta^{13}C$ was sufficient on a limited set of 20 samples for discriminating between the three locations, with speculation that the method could be used to detect levels of European wheat (lesser value) mixed in with North American wheat. Direct isotope measurement of various elements originating in the soil (Be, Na, Mg, Al, K, Ca, V, Mn, Fe, Cu, Zn, Mo, Cd, Ba, and Th) have been shown to be useful in identifying the geographical origin of wheat, though care must be taken to handle variations caused by variety, growing season, and cultivation practices (Zhao et al., 2011). It is unclear, however, whether this form of multi-element isotope analysis would be useful in detection of mixtures arising from more than one geographical location.

Reis et al. (2013) used mid-IR Fourier transform spectroscopy (4000–400 cm^{-1}, subsequently truncated to 3200–700 cm^{-1}) to develop quantitative models for percentage of adulteration, varying from 1% to 66%. The adulterants were spent coffee grounds, coffee husks, barley, and corn. These were mixed together in 20 different formulations, replicated five times, for a total of 100 adulterated samples. These were combined during modeling with 45 samples of pure coffee. PLS with common pretreatments (normalization by max min, standard normal variate (SNV), multiplicative signal (or "scatter") correction (MSC), derivatives, mean centering, etc.) was performed. Typical results showed that a 10 factor model produced an RMSEC (the square root of the mean of the squared residuals of the calibration set samples) of 1.23% (w/w) and an RMSEP (the square root of the mean of the squared residuals of the prediction set samples) of 2.67% after removing 9 of 97 samples from calibration and 4 of 48 samples from validation. Differences in concentrations of components of the ingredients, such as lipids (higher in coffee), caffeine (only in pure coffee), starch (higher in corn and barley), gluten (present in barley), and chlorogenic acids (present in coffee), were reasoned to be the basis for quantification of coffee adulterant levels. Best PLS modeling occurred when the wavenumber region was split into two sections, 3200–2730 cm^{-1} and 1800–700 cm^{-1}. The authors claimed that their method could predict adulteration at levels as low as 1% w/w.

Schmidt et al. (2005) used isotope ratios in conjunction with mass spectrometry to examine $^{15}N/^{14}N$ in wheat as a way to differentiate organic versus conventional (chemical fertilizer) cultivation practices. The expectation was that plants grown organically, which are typically enriched with compost and green manure and fertilized with solid and liquid manure, will be enriched in ^{15}N. They found that, while there was a slight level of enrichment, the overlap between organic and conventional practices was sufficiently large to make identification of unknown samples impractical using this technique. They reasoned that large N losses from NH_3 evaporation that is accompanied by ^{15}N enrichment in the soil make it difficult to determine the source of the isotope.

Use of Fourier transform-IRspectroscopy, inclusive of the mid (4000–400 cm^{-1}) and near-IR (14,000–4000 cm^{-1}), in authentication of agricultural commodities, as well as adulteration of commodities and products was reviewed by Rodriguez-Saona and Allendorf (2011). This includes their own work on the development of calibrations for castor bean meal (CBM) spiked into food matrices, such as wheat flour, bleached flour, and pancake mix. Castor beans contain ricin, a cytotoxin. In that work, these authors (Rodriguez-Saona et al., 2000) developed calibrations for the mass concentration of CBM over a range of 0.5–8%, obtaining a standard error of cross-validation of <0.6% and claiming the ability to distinguish between CBM and other protein sources, such as egg white, soybean meal, tofu, and infant formula. The lower limit for detection of CBM by the Fourier transform-NIR technique with PLS regression was 0.3% in wheat flour.

18.4 Melamine

Melamine (1,3,5-triazine-2,4,6-triamine) is a nitrogen-rich compound that is used in the production of plastics, specifically those in conjunction with formaldehyde to form thermoset resins, the finished products of which include kitchenware, tableware, and laminates for furniture and building materials. Because of its high level of nitrogen (66.6% w/w), unscrupulous processors have used this as an adulterant in foods, such as infant formula and in animal feeds to boost the apparent protein content. A large-scale incident of melamine-tainted (by melamine directly or its by-products, ammeline, ammelide, and cyanuric acid, as depicted in Fig. 18.1) infant formula from a food manufacturing plant affected (by kidney stone induction) more than 50,000 infants in China in the fall of 2008 and caused several deaths (WHO, 2008). This outbreak followed the detection of melamine and its structural analog cyanuric acid adulterants 1 year earlier in pet food ingredients sourced in China and sold in the United States, which caused kidney failure in hundreds of cats and dogs. Because China was and continues to be an exporter of food and feed ingredients, the melamine scare of 2007–08 continues to focus worldwide attention on this substance.

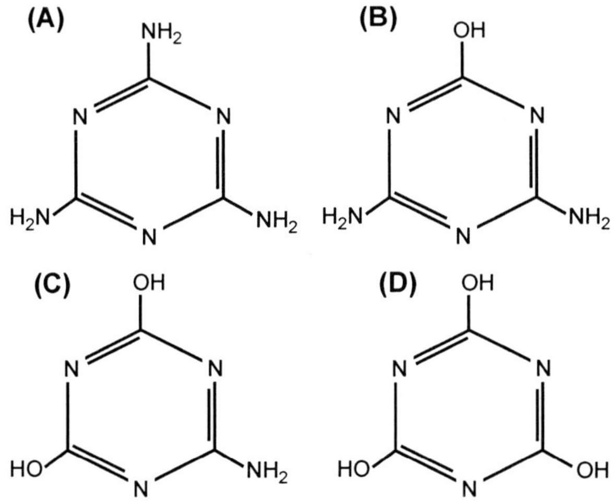

Figure 18.1 Structure of melamine and its derivatives. (A) melamine, (B) ammeline, (C) ammelide, (D) cyanuric acid.

The subject of protein measurement in food is extensively reviewed in Moore et al. (2010) for the purpose of motivating the scientific community to develop an updated method for protein measurement that goes beyond the Kjeldahl and combustion (Dumas) methods, both developed in the 1800s. The traditional methods are reliant on the measurement of mostly organic nitrogen, which is then converted to protein content by a conversion factor, typically around 6.25 (representative of a 16:1 ratio that early researchers assumed to exist between nitrogen and protein), which ignores the complexities of the amino acids that comprise protein and ignores the fact that the nitrogen may be of nonprotein nature, such as in free amino nitrogen, nucleic acids, phospholipids, and nitrogenous glycosides (Mariotti et al., 2008). For Kjeldahl, although the method is applicable to most food matrices and does not suffer from food matrix interference in unadulterated samples, it is susceptible to adulteration with nitrogenous substances, such as aspartic acid or melamine and its derivatives. The combustion method is also susceptible to melamine adulteration.

Tittlemier (2009) reviewed the available methods for melamine detection and quantification in infant formula, animal feeds, or feed ingredients containing, among other ingredients, wheat flour and wheat gluten. Methods of measurement included HPLC-tandem mass spectrometry (Titleemier et al., 2009; Turnipseed et al., 2008; Heller and Nochetto, 2008), GC-MS (Litzau et al., 2008), HPLC-diode array detection (Ehling et al., 2007; Muñiz-Valencia et al., 2008), and ELISA (Garber and Brewer, 2010). Melamine as an adulterant is troubling because the amounts added to a food matrix to boost the apparent protein content by just 1%, for example, raising the protein content in wheat flour from 11% to 12%, as shown in Fig. 18.2, will result in a contamination level more than three orders of magnitude above the common internationally accepted allowable level of 2.5 mg/kg for foods for human consumption (WHO, 2009). Ehling et al. (2007) developed an HPLC-based method that could

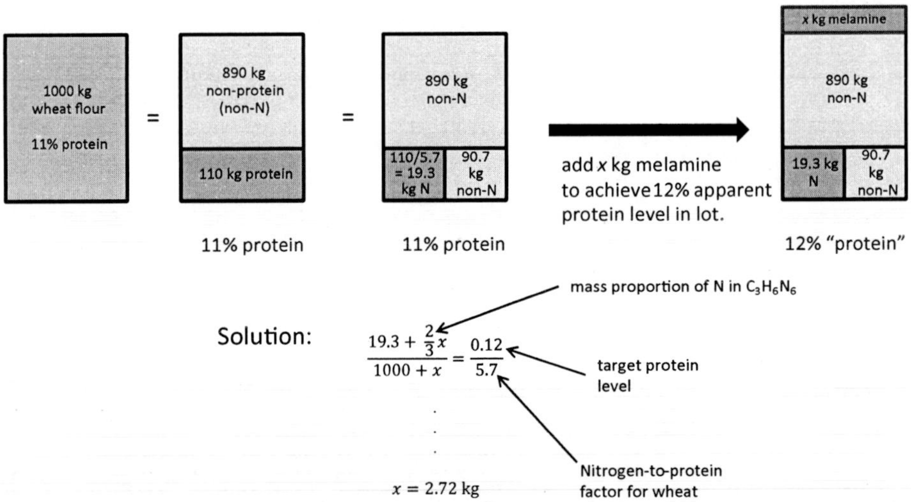

melamine contamination level = 2.72 / (1000. + 2.72) = 2.71 x 10^{-3} kg/kg = 2.71 x 10^{3} mg/kg

melamine industrial unit cost = 1,000 USD/MT= $1.00/kg
at $0.013/kg differential in 11% vs. 12% protein flour,
profit = added value – cost = $0.013/kg x 1000 kg – $1.00/kg x 2.72 kg
= $10 per MT

Figure 18.2 Worked example of amount of melamine adulterant needed to raise wheat flour protein content in a 1 metric ton lot from a natural 11% to an apparent 12% (as measured by Kjeldahl or combustion) and the profit to be gained from adulteration.

simultaneously measure melamine and three by-products (ammeline, ammelide, and cyanuric acid) in spiked samples of wheat flour, corn flour, and rice flour, with limits of detection for melamine and the three respective compounds stated to be 6, 4, 5, and 92 mg/kg with corresponding calibration ranges of 5–500 mg/kg for all except cyanuric acid, the range of which was 70–7000 mg/kg. Animal feed is especially targeted for adulteration by melamine because its complex composition, including cereals, oilseeds, citrus pulp, animal by-products, and vitamins, make it very challenging for an analytical system, such as HPLC, to operate with accuracy (Muñiz-Valencia et al., 2008). For humans, including infants, the tolerable daily intake level, as established by the WHO (2009), is 0.2 mg/kg body weight/day. The toxicological effect in humans is in the formation of intrarenal uric acid crystals brought on by the lowering of pH to less than 5.5, which leads to obstructed tubules, elevated renal pressure, and acute uric acid nephropathy (Conger, 1990; Davidson et al., 2004). Despite worldwide knowledge of the melamine in formula scandal in 2008 in China, the lure of melamine as an adulterant in food products continues, as reported by Hassani et al. (2013), who detected melamine contamination in 13 of 14 samples of powder milk and liquid milk samples purchased at food markets in Iran.

18.5 Durum

The coarse flour obtained from durum wheat (*Triticum durum* L.), called semolina, is the primary ingredient in pasta. From a genetic standpoint, durum wheat differs from common, bread wheat (*Triticum aestivum* L.) in that the former is a tetraploid species consisting of the ancestral A and B genomes whereas the latter is hexaploid and includes the D genome (along with the A and B genomes), with the D genome possessing genes that are largely responsible for imparting the unique dough rheological and bread-making characteristics of common wheat (Gooding, 2009). Early work by McCarthy et al. (1990) demonstrated a measurable inverse relationship between the ratio of two eluted gliadin peaks and the level of adulteration of durum wheat with common wheat as long as the level of adulteration was above 20% (w/w). The newer work of Brenchley et al. (2012) on gene sequencing of common wheat found that between 94,000 and 96,000 genes exist in wheat including those belonging to classes associated with crop productivity. The potential benefit of knowledge of the three genomes of hexaploid wheat is that future breeding activity can be directed at circumventing genetic bottlenecks, starting from when the diploid progenitors of wheat were domesticated about 8000 years ago through the conventional breeding practices of today.

Phenotypically, durum varieties, typically grown in areas of hot and dry conditions (eg, Mediterranean region, north central United States), are generally harder than common wheat and better suited to pasta making. Durum wheat is typically more expensive, although the differential varies from year to year, as demonstrated by the prices of US wheat classes at first point of sale during a 5-year period (2010–14) (Fig. 18.3). Such differentials invite economically motivated adulteration. Italy, France, and Greece have their own national laws that prohibit the blending of common wheat into durum wheat for pasta intended for domestic consumption. As an example, the Italian law on pasta consumed domestically specifies a maximum allowable level of 3% of common wheat in durum wheat through nondeliberate, adventitious contamination for pasta products. Pasta for export may contain intentionally added common wheat so long as the product is labeled with the mixture percentage. In addition, some regions in southern Italy produce breads with ingredients that include durum semolina. The bread "Pane di Altamura" carries the European Union's status protected designation of origin (PDO) as defined in Regulation (EC) No. 1291/2003 (Arvanitoyannis and Tserkezou, 2013). This regulation legally protects the product because of its unique ingredients defined not only by variety (in this case durum varieties "Appulo," "Arcangelo," "Duilio," or "Simeto"), but also by the product being essentially or exclusively produced in a certain geographical location, in this case the region around the town of Altamura in southern Italy.

In the 1990s and earlier, verification of durum was performed by electrophoretic or immunochemical assays of albumins or peroxidase enzymes specific to the D genome, and further extended by electrophoresis of 1D ω-gliadins, reversed phase HPLC of γ-gliadins, and immunoassay of puroindolines (Autran et al., 1994). Legislation in Europe enacted in 1993 loosened restrictions on durum wheat/common wheat mixtures by allowing these, with proper labeling, to be traded between

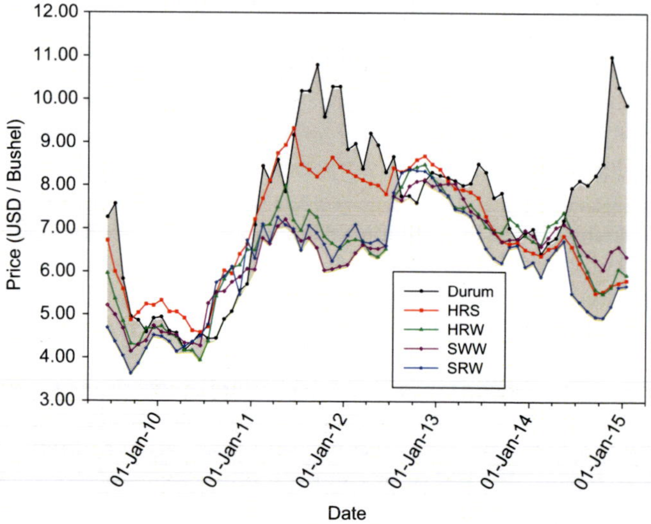

Figure 18.3 Unit prices of various US wheat classes at first point of sale over a 5-year period. *Gray shaded region* represents the incentive to cheat by misrepresenting nondurum wheat as durum for semolina production. *HRS*, hard red spring; *HRW*, hard red winter; *SRW*, soft red winter; SWW, soft white wheat.
Data from USDA Economic Research Service, http://www.ers.usda.gov/data-products/wheat-data.aspx.

countries in Europe. However, with the restriction lifted, the need for an efficient means of measuring mixture levels, especially in the expected concentration range of 0–5% common wheat, became even greater. Further exacerbating the measurement procedure was the need to perform detection and measurement of common wheat in pasta dried at elevated temperature levels or in bread, a product which experiences temperatures during baking that exceed those in pasta processing, with the accompanying potential for protein degradation. Toward the second half of the decade, PCR methods for common wheat measurement became popularized because of greater heat stability and potentially lower levels of detection and better accuracy than protein-based techniques (Bryan et al., 1998; Alary et al., 2002). The specificity of DNA technologies to the detection and quantification of mixtures of small grain cereals, and even beyond to the potential for identification of varieties within a single species mixture, such as in *T. aestivum*, was reviewed and tabulated by Terzi et al. (2005).

Pasqualone et al. (2007) developed a real-time PCR microsatellite procedure using a repetitive DNA D-genome-specific sequence to detect common wheat in semolina and breads from durum flour-based breads. They demonstrated threshold levels of 3% and 5% for common wheat in semolina and durum flour, respectively, which were lowered to 2.5% by real-time PCR. Sonnante et al. (2009) improved the DNA approach with a PCR assay that was based on a dual probe as a means of avoiding the problem of non-DNA-specific binding by SYBR Green dye (the tracer used by Pasqualone et al.). A liability of the SYBR Green approach was that it was sensitive to double-stranded DNA fragments in general and therefore had diminished sensitivity to the D-genome-specific amplicons especially when these were denatured during baking. As an alternative, Sonnante et al. used a dual-labeled probe for quantitative real-time PCR that was able to measure the level of common wheat in pasta and even bread at weight concentrations as low as 1.25%. In related work, Pasqualone et al. (2010) developed a microsatellite method for verifying the presence and individual mass concentration of the four allowable durum cultivars in PDO Altumura bread, the collective inclusion concentration level of which must be at least 80% to receive the PDO designation.

Recent work by Italian researchers addressed the need for a more time efficient method for detection of common wheat in durum wheat. Italy's official methodology is based on gel isoelectric focusing of the water-soluble fraction of wheat protein and how this differs between common and durum wheats. Cocchi et al. (2006) explored the use of NIR reflectance on a limited set of binary mixtures of common and durum wheat. Although both PLS and wavelet regression calibrations demonstrated a reasonably low standard error of 0.3% over a range of 0–7% conventional wheat, the very limited nature of the mixture set makes it difficult to generalize the findings to mixtures encountered in trade. Casaszza et al. (2012) developed a PCR tubulin-based polymorphism procedure that not only has high specificity to *T. aestivum* but is fast in isolating DNA polymorphic sequences, with many other potential applications for species-specific probes. Alternatively, an immunochemical methodology sensitive to an antigen in common wheat may be utilized; however, both of these methodologies are complex and time consuming. As an alternative, Russo et al. (2014) developed a mass spectrometry method that monitors the transitions of tryptic peptide markers from puroindoline-a (Pin-a), a protein found in common wheat but absent in durum wheat, and references these transitions to those of a reference peptide, purothionin A-1, that is common to both species. Using binary mixtures involving four common wheat varieties and four durum wheat varieties at common wheat concentration levels ranging between 1% and 80%, they were able to demonstrate excellent linearity in response ($r > 0.90$), with a limit of detection for Pin-a of 0.01% and a limit of quantification of 0.03%. Extraction times for the puroindolines were reduced from 20 to 1 h.

18.6 Basmati

Basmati rice, a long grain breed, is grown in the Punjab province of India and Pakistan and in the Haryana and Uttar Pradesh regions of these two countries. The traditional varieties of Basmati can fetch more than five times the price of non-Basmati varieties and thus provide an incentive for unscrupulous merchants to mix in non-Basmati rice of similar appearance.

In India, certification of Basmati rice is performed at APEDA-CDFD (Agricultural and Processed Food Products Export Development Authority, Centre for DNA Fingerprinting and Diagnostics), which began operation in 2005 using a protocol developed at the CDFD. As described in a review by Vemireddy et al. (2015), the CDFD receives rice samples from the export inspection agency, export inspection council, or large multinational food companies. The method applied is based on a DNA microsatellite marker procedure followed by capillary electrophoresis in which the percentage of adulterant (non-Basmati rice) is calculated as the peak area, in relative fluorescence units, of a non-Basmati band divided by the sum of peak areas of the non-Basmati band and a band unique to Basmati. A certificate with purity level will then be issued by the government of India, which becomes the basis for other countries to allow or reject Basmati lots. In the United Kingdom the 7% limit is deemed the maximum allowable level of impurity when the product is labeled as "Basmati rice," with nine Indian or Pakistani varieties permissible with zero import duty by EC Regulation 1549/2004, and another six varieties from the same countries that are permissible but presumably with associated import duties (The Rice Association, 2005).

Early work by Osborne et al. (1993) explored Basmati identification by NIR spectroscopy. Principal component analysis followed by linear discriminant analysis was performed on bulk-milled rice as well as averages of single kernel spectra. Although perfect discrimination was realized for identifying the Basmati samples, based on the first three PCs from the bulk sample spectra, the unanswered question was whether the approach would be acceptable for quantification of mixtures. Interestingly, electrophoretic and DNA-based methodologies for Basmati authentication occurred after Osborne's early NIR research, an order that is opposite the usual occurrence of when NIR applications are developed.

A DNA approach to the issue of Basmati rice adulteration was first addressed by Bligh (2000) through the use of fluorescent simple sequence length polymorphisms. Using 12 commercially available primer sets on Basmati rice from India or Pakistan adulterated with Basmati-type rice from the United States, Bligh was able to detect adulteration at relatively high levels (>25% adulterant), though quantification estimates were crude. Other research on the use of microsatellite markers can be found in Archak et al. (2007), Vemireddy et al. (2007), and Colyer et al. (2008).

Vemireddy et al. (2007) compared various fragmentation methods for authentication of Basmati rice, including agarose gel electrophoresis, slab gel electrophoresis, and capillary electrophoresis using eight microsatellite loci. Adulteration, created by mixing a common evolved Basmati variety "Haryana Basmati" at levels ranging from 10% to 90% (w/w), was estimated by measuring the peak area in relative fluorescence units of two informative loci, RM72 and RM348. They found that capillary electrophoresis was superior to the other two electrophoresis techniques by providing better estimations of allele sizes. At that time, researchers did not say whether the countries of India and Pakistan had a threshold limit on the percentage of non-Basmati material mixed in with Basmati rice. Since then, in India a maximum allowable amount of 7% non-Basmati rice has been decided upon as reasonable to account for adventitious mixing that may occur in storage and transport operations.

Ganopoulos et al. (2011) described a real-time PCR technique that was sensitive to the single allele (badh2.1) of the gene that encodes for the enzyme that is responsible for Basmati's distinctly aromatic trait. Operation time (under 2 h) was reduced by the application of high-resolution melting in lieu of gel electrophoresis to quantify the level of adulteration of Basmati rice with other rice cultivars. In high-resolution melting, as described in the review by Druml and Cichna-Markl (2014), a fluorescent dye is used to measure the dissociation of double-stranded DNA, an amplicon, to single-stranded DNA. The rate of dissociation is uniquely related to the DNA product, specifically by guanine-cytosine content, length sequence and heterozygosity. Ganopoulos et al. (2011) developed a calibration that possessed a linear response ($r^2 = 0.957$) between fluorescence level and mixture level over a range of 1−100% adulteration. Simple sequence repeat (SSR) markers in rice, which can be used for genotyping and marker-assisted selection in breeding, were reviewed by Kaur et al. (2015); advantages of these markers compared to other genetic marker types were identified as cost, reliability, reproducibility, and standardization. These markers can be used in traceability and authenticity determination in foods in general.

Japan is confronted with a challenge similar to that faced in India and Pakistan, this being the protection of its premium rice cultivar Koshihikari. Visual or camera-assisted analysis of milled rice is generally inadequate for distinguishing Koshihikari from lookalike rice varieties. Growing location also influences the market value of this cultivar. Suzuki et al. (2008) explored the use of multiple element isotope analysis in which $\delta^{13}C$, $\delta^{15}N$, and $\delta^{18}O$ were measured on samples of this single cultivar grown in 14 separate geographical areas in three continents (Japan, Australia, and the United States). Along with measurements of carbon and nitrogen content, the use of three stable isotopes was successful in identifying geographical origin but with a cautionary remark that because only one sample was tested from each of Australia and the United States, natural variability within these countries in the isotope compositions was uncertain.

18.7 Wheat Gluten as an Adulterant

In a reversal of this chapter's main contents, cereals can also be implicated in being the adulterant. A prominent example for today is the unintended or fraudulent presence of gluten in food, a circumstance that can affect the health of people suffering from celiac disease, an immune reaction that results in the irritation of the lining of the small intestine and degeneration of the villi. Gluten is defined as the protein contained in the endosperm of wheat, barley, rye, or crossbred hybrids of these, such as triticale. It is this compound, consisting of glutelins from glutenin and prolamins from gliadins, that, in conjunction with the complexed starch granules within the endosperm, is responsible for the viscoelastic properties in dough that allow for gas bubble retention during fermentation (proofing) of dough, giving volume to bread and providing its chewy texture. In the United States, the FDA issued a final rule in August 2013 (21 CFR Part 101, page 47154 Federal Register Vol. 78, No. 150, August 5, 2013) that defined the meaning of "gluten-free" in manufactured food products to mean "that the food bearing the claim does not contain an ingredient that is a gluten-containing grain (e.g., spelt wheat); an ingredient that is derived from a gluten-containing grain and that has not been processed to remove gluten (e.g., wheat flour); or an ingredient that is derived from a gluten containing grain and that has been processed to remove gluten (e.g., wheat starch), if the use of that ingredient results in the presence of 20 parts per million (ppm) or more gluten in the food (i.e., 20 milligrams (mg) or more gluten per kilogram (kg) of food); or inherently does not contain gluten; and that any unavoidable presence of gluten in the food is below 20 ppm gluten (i.e., below 20 mg gluten per kg of food)." The same threshold level exists for the European Union through Commission Regulation 41/2009 (EC, 2009), based on Codex Standard 118 (Diaz-Amigo and Popping, 2013), with terminology updated in July 2014 in Regulation 828/2014 (EC, 2014). Although the use of this term in the United States is voluntary, when it is used, the food, whether it is of domestic origin or imported, may not contain gluten at levels exceeding 20 ppm and any detectable amount must not have occurred from deliberate measures. Food manufacturers wishing to use the label "gluten-free" are responsible for ensuring that their products do not contain gluten at levels higher than the 20 ppm threshold and will be held accountable to such claims during periodic inspection by the FDA. Compliance with this regulation has been shown to be high, as documented by a FDA survey of 275 gluten-free labeled commercial foods in which only three had gluten contents in excess of 20 ppm (Sharma et al., 2015).

In Europe, as recommended by the Codex Alimentarius Commission (2006), the sandwich R5 monoclonal antibody ELISA procedure has been widely used for gluten quantification because of its sensitivity in measuring the prolamin fraction at concentrations lower than 2 ppm (Rosell et al., 2014). One of the limitations of the R5 ELISA procedure is in its specificity to gliadin fraction at the expense of the other broad fraction in gluten, the glutenins. Although the gliadins are primarily responsible for the immunological response in gluten-intolerant individuals, this may lead to procedures that overlook the other components and hence deviate from the intention of the Codex Standard, that is, that a test be sensitive to the protein fractions that are toxic to persons intolerant to gluten, be it gliadin or another compound.

In the United States the FDA has supported a more flexible approach to the requirement of a particular analytical method by favoring the allowance of any method as long as the results are comparable. In its August 5, 2014 update of questions and answers about the final rule on gluten-free, the FDA (2014b) identified two sandwich ELISA-based methods by different manufacturers [R-Biopharm: Food & Feed Analysis; Morinaga Institute of Biological Science, Inc.: Wheat Protein ELISA Kit (Gliadin)] that could be used in enforcement of the regulation. Diaz-Amigo and Popping (2013) describe the challenges of establishing reference materials that are suitable for use in checking the accuracy of ELISA-based gluten measurement kits [as described by Diaz-Amigo and Popping (2012) and Haraszi et al. (2011)], in which the single material or more likely a set of materials will be able to additively measure the concentration of gluten from wheat, rye, and barley. Diaz-Amigo and Popping (2013) suggest that in the selection of a reference material for standardizing gluten analytical procedures, the material contains both prolamin and glutelin fractions. Further, the material(s) should originate from not just wheat, but from barley and rye as well and, more realistically, in the form of one reference for each of the three species. Another limitation of ELISA methods for allergenic proteins is in the difficulty of developing antibodies that remain sensitive to the processed (ie, heat denatured) food material. Török et al. (2015) found that, compared to precision, the accuracy of an ELISA-based gluten procedure is more problematic and depends on the type of food matrix, the level of processing, and commercial kit used to perform the analysis.

DNA methodologies have also been developed for gluten identification. The early work of Terzi et al. (2003) identified the amplicons that are useful in detection of *Triticum* species in food by end-point and real-time PCR, as well as the suggestion of applying these procedures to quantifying the level of common wheat in durum wheat, as also reported 1 year earlier by Alary et al. (2002). A quantitative real-time PCR method was reported by Mujico et al. (2011) that utilized fluorescent dye SYBR Green I and a modified sodium dodecyl sulfate (SDS)/guanidine-hydrochloric acid (HCL)/proteinase K extraction procedure. This procedure was sensitive to wheat in general as opposed to prolamins, thus being of use not only to celiac sufferers but also to those possessing allergies to wheat in general. Mustorp et al. (2011) developed a multiplex ligation-dependent probe amplification PCR method for detection of wheat gluten and other allergens, such as sesame, soy, hazelnut, peanut, lupine, mustard, and celery. A TaqMan real-time PCR method was reported by Pegels et al. (2015) that, in binary mixtures of wheat:soy, barley:soy, rye:maize, and even oat:maize, could detect gluten at concentrations of 1, 1, 100, and 0.1 ppm, respectively. The work was performed in response to the EU's legislation on mandatory labeling of ingredients causing allergies or intolerances, and specifically on the ability to detect cereals containing gluten in non-gluten matrices. Four species-specific TaqMan real-time primer/probe systems were designed and utilized on the binary mixtures as well as 270 food and pet food products for the purpose of corroborating whether the cereals were either declared, not declared, or declared as possible trace quantities.

18.8 Application of Using NIR Technology for Mixtures of Nonwaxy (Conventional) and Waxy Wheat

Starch in common bread wheat (*T. aestivum* L.) constitutes 54–72% of the seed mass, of which the linear [α-(1→4)-linked glucan units] macromolecule amylose comprises one-quarter of the starch and the branched [combination of α-(1→4)-linkages and α-(1→6)-linkages] macromolecule amylopectin comprises the balance

(Maningat et al., 2009). The occurrence of null mutations at each of the three genetic loci (*Wx-A1*, *Wx-B1*, and *Wx-D1*) that encode granule-bound starch synthase (GBSS, the enzyme that controls the synthesis of amylose) results in the endosperm starch consisting of only trace amounts of amylose. Through conventional plant-breeding practices it is possible to develop genotypes that possess this "waxy" condition. Beginning with the development of waxy wheat genotypes in Japan in the mid-1990s (Nakamura et al., 1993; Nakamura and Yamamori, 1995), breeding efforts have been ongoing in the United States and elsewhere to develop commercial releases of waxy wheat that have potential uses in baking, shelf-life extension for baked products, ethanol production, and other industrial uses (Graybosch, 1998; Lee et al., 2001; Hung et al., 2006; Zhao et al., 2009). In the United States, Graybosch et al. (2014) released the commercial hard winter waxy wheat cultivar "Mattern." With the release, the need has arisen for an analytical method that could be used at point of sale to verify the level of purity of a waxy lot, given that to the untrained eye, waxy kernels closely resemble conventional kernels. Waxy genotyping is typically conducted by PCR (Nakamura et al., 2002), SDS-PAGE (sodium dodecyl sulfate polyacrylamide gel electrophoresis) (Zhao and Sharp, 1996; Graybosch et al., 1998), or by ELISA on the GBSS isoforms (Rahman et al., 1995). Although these methods are highly accurate, their application at country elevators and sales points downstream is not realistic. NIR spectroscopy for protein and moisture determination is used at all points from field to finished product, thereby making it an ideal method for waxiness measurement provided it has the sensitivity to discern the structural chemical differences between amylose and amylopectin. The possibility of using NIR is alluded to in cursory examination of "difference" spectra, which are formed as the spectrum of conventional waxy wheat subtracted from a spectrum of waxy wheat (Fig. 18.4). The 2100–2400-nm wavelength region offers the greatest promise of discerning the waxy condition. In Delwiche and Graybosch's study (2014), the accuracy of NIR spectroscopy models was established for estimating the mixture levels of conventional hard winter wheat and waxy hard winter wheat. On a set of nine pairings of conventional:waxy mixture sets, with each pairing consisting of 29 mixture levels ranging from 0% to 100%, PLS calibrations utilizing either ground meal or bulk kernels were developed and validated. The results demonstrated good accuracy, with calibration set R^2 values in excess of 0.98 and cross-validation standard errors of 4–7%. Although this level of accuracy is 10 times larger than what could be expected by DNA genotyping, the advantages associated with the rapidity and adaptability of the NIR method may outweigh the superior accuracy of the DNA-based procedures. Earlier research by Delwiche et al. (2011) led to the suggestion that the spectral differences may arise from two situations: first, by changes in the strengths of the C–H bonds and the hydrogen bonds (Miller, 2001) caused by the differing degrees of crystallinity between amylopectin (more crystalline) and amylose (less crystalline), and second, by differences in the prevalence of the amylose–lipid complex, as described for diploid cereal species (Morrison et al., 1984) and later for hexaploid wheat (Yoo and Jane, 2002).

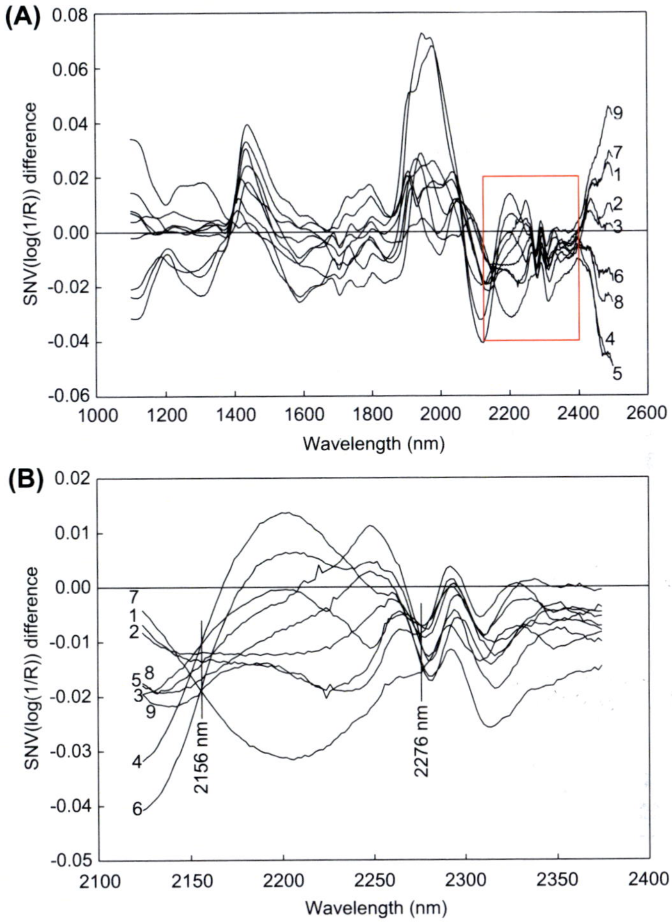

Figure 18.4 Difference (conventional minus waxy) spectra of ground wheat meal. (A) full wavelength range, (B) wavelength range limited to 2124–2374 nm, as identified by the *red box* in graph A, with vertical lines indicating wavelengths with consistent behavior among the nine pairs of nonwaxy:waxy wheat examined.
From Delwiche, S.R., Graybosch, R.A., 2014. Measurement of blend concentrations of conventional and waxy hard wheats using NIR spectroscopy. Cereal Chemistry 91, 358–365.

18.9 Conclusion

Adulteration of cereals, although not as systemic a problem as is the case for commodities of higher unit value (olive oil, milk, honey, etc.), continue to be targeted for economically motivated activity primarily through blending of like species (eg, common wheat in durum wheat) or like varieties within a species (Basmati rice). Detection methodology, with continued refinement of DNA fingerprinting methods, is well advanced, highly accurate, and capable of achieving detection limits in the parts per million range. However, with the exception of the adulterant melamine (and even with this, the targeted compound of concern is more often milk-based infant formula), human health concerns are much less prevalent than economic ones. This generally leaves the industry in the somewhat enviable position of being allowed to devise solutions as tradeoffs between high accuracy (PCR or immunochemical methodologies) and high throughput (optical and spectroscopic methodologies).

Sources of Further Information

1. Basmati rice certification, under the Agricultural and Processed Food Products Export Development Authority (APEDA), Ministry of Commerce and Industry, Government of India. Available at: http://apeda.gov.in/apedawebsite/about_apeda/bas_ex_dev_found.htm.
2. European protected designation of origin (PDO), protected geographical indication (PGI), and traditional specialty guaranteed (TGI) policies, with emphasis on Regulation No. 1151/2012. Available at: http://ec.europa.eu/agriculture/quality/schemes/legislation/index_en.htm.
3. United States Food Safety Modernization Act (FSMA). Available at: http://www.fda.gov/Food/GuidanceRegulation/FSMA.
4. Scientific nonprofit organization in the United States, called the US Pharmacopeial Convention (USP), which sets standards for the identity, strength, quality, and purity of medicines, food ingredients, and dietary supplements, with information on melamine. Available at: http://www.usp.org/usp-nf/key-issues/melamine-contamination.
5. Policies in the United Kingdom on food adulteration, as overseen by the Food Standards Agency. Available at: http://www.food.gov.uk/enforcement/foodfraud.
6. Official standards for grain in the United States. Available at: http://www.gipsa.usda.gov/fgis/usstandards.aspx.
7. Rules in the United States on gluten-free labeling, as administered by the US Food and Drug Administration. Available at: http://www.fda.gov/Food/GuidanceRegulation/GuidanceDocumentsRegulatoryInformation/Allergens/ucm362510.htm.

References

Archak, S., Lakshminarayanaredy, V., Nagaraju, J., 2007. High-throughput multiplex microsatellite marker assay for detection and quantification of adulteration in Basmati rice (*Oryza sativa*). Electrophoresis 28, 2396–2405.

Alary, R., Serin, A., Duviau, M.P., Joudrier, P., Gautier, M.F., 2002. Quantification of common wheat adulteration of durum wheat pasta using real-time quantitative polymerase chain-reaction (PCR). Cereal Chemistry 79, 553–558.

Arvanitoyannis, I.S., Tserkezou, P., 2013. Protected designation of origin (PDO) wheat and corn. In: de la Guardia, M., Gonzálvez, A. (Eds.), Food Protected Designation of Origin: Methodologies and Applications, vol. 60. Elsevier, Amsterdam, pp. 599–621.

Autran, J.C., Bony, M., Landi, A., Lumley, I., Griffin, M., Paraf, A., Resmini, P., Stimson, W., Violle, P., 1994. Determination of Common Wheat in Pasta Products Dried at Elevated Temperatures. European Commission Report EUR 16070 EN.

Bligh, H.F.J., 2000. Detection of adulteration of Basmati rice with non-premium long-grain rice. International Journal of Food Science & Technology 35, 257–265.

Branch, S., Burke, S., Evans, P., Fairman, B., Wolff Briche, C.S.J., 2003. A preliminary study in determining the geographical origin of wheat using isotope ratio inductively coupled plasma spectrometry with 13C, 15N, mass spectrometry. Journal of Analytical Atomic Spectrometry 18, 17–22.

Brenchley, R., Spannagl, M., Pfeifer, M., Barker, G.L.A., D'Amore, R., Allen, A.M., McKenzie, N., Kramer, M., Kerhornou, A., Bolser, D., Kay, S., Waite, D., Trick, M., Bancroft, I., Gu, Y., Huo, N., Luo, M.C., Sehgal, S., Gill, B., Klanian, S., Anderson, O., Kersey, P., Dvorak, J., McGombie, W.R., Hall, A., Mayer, K.F.X., Edwards, K.J., Bevan, M.W., Hall, N., 2012. Analysis of the bread wheat genome using whole-genome shotgun sequencing. Nature 491, 705–710.

Bryan, G.J., Dizon, A., Gale, M.D., Wisemane, G., 1998. A PCR-based method for the detection of hexaploid bread wheat adulteration of durum wheat and pasta. Journal of Cereal Science 28, 135–145.

Casazza, A.P., Morcia, C., Ponzoni, E., Gavazzi, F., Benedettelli, S., Breviario, D., 2012. A reliable assay for the detection of soft wheat adulteration in Italian pasta is based on the use of new DNA molecular markers capable of discriminating between *Triticum aestivum* and *Triticum durum*. Journal of Cereal Science 56, 733–740.

Cheajesadagul, P., Shiwatana, J., Siripinyanond, A., Szpunar, J., 2013. Rice. In: de la Guardia, M., Gonzálvez, A. (Eds.), Food Protected Designation of Origin: Methodologies and Applications, vol. 60. Elsevier, Amsterdam, pp. 623–655.

Cocchi, M., Durante, C., Foca, G., Marchetti, A., Tassi, L., Ulrici, A., 2006. Durum wheat aduleration detection by NIR spectroscopy multivariate calibration. Talanta 68, 1505–1511.

Codex Alimentarius Commission, May 15–19, 2006. Report of the 27th Session of the Codex Committee on Methods of Analysis and Sampling. Hungary, Budapest. ALINORM 06/29/23.

Colyer, A., Macarthur, R., Lloyd, J., Hird, H., 2008. Comparison of calibration methods for the quantification of Basmati and non-Basmati rice using microsatellite analysis. Food Additives & Contaminants, Part A 25, 1189–1194.

Conger, J.D., 1990. Acute uric acid nephropathy. The Medical Clinics of North America 74, 859–871.

Cozzolino, D., 2014. An overview of the use of infrared spectroscopy and chemometrics in authenticity and traceability of cereals. Food Research International 60, 262–265.

Davidson, M.B., Thakkar, S., Hix, J.K., Bhandarkar, N.D., Wong, A., Schreiber, M.J., 2004. Pathophysiology, clinical consequences, and treatment of tumor lysis syndrome. American Journal of Medicine 116, 546–554.

Delwiche, S.R., Graybosch, R.A., St Amand, P., Bai, G., 2011. Starch waxiness in hexaploid wheat (*Triticum aestivum* L.) by NIR reflectance spectroscopy. Journal of Agricultural and Food Chemistry 59, 4002–4008.

Delwiche, S.R., Graybosch, R.A., 2014. Measurement of blend concentrations of conventional and waxy hard wheats using NIR spectroscopy. Cereal Chemistry 91, 358–365.

Diaz-Amigo, C., Popping, B., 2012. Gluten and gluten-free: issues and considerations of labeling regulations, detection methods, and assay validation. Journal of AOAC International 95, 337–348.

Diaz-Amigo, C., Popping, B., 2013. Accuracy of ELISA detection methods for gluten and reference materials: a realistic assessment. Journal of Agricultural and Food Chemistry 71, 5681–5688.

Druml, B., Cichna-Markl, M., 2014. High resolution melting (HRM) analysis of DNA – its role and potential in food analysis. Food Chemistry 158, 245–254.

EC, 2002. Laying Down the General Principles and Requirements of Food Law, Establishing the European Food Safety Authority and Laying Down Procedures in Matters of Food Safety. No 178/2002, European Parliament and of the Council of 28 January 2002.

EC, 2008. Regulation (EC) No. 687/2008 of 18 July 2008 establishing procedures for the taking-over of cereals by intervention agencies or paying agencies and laying down methods of analysis for determining the quality of cereals. Official Journal of the European Communities L192, 20–48.

EC, 2009. Commission regulation (EC) no 41/2009 of 20 January 2009 concerning the composition and labeling of foodstuffs suitable for people intolerant to gluten. Official Journal of the European Union 16, 13–16/15.

EC, 2014. Commission implementing regulation (EU) No. 828/2014 of 30 July 2014 on the requirements for the provision of information to consumers on the absence or reduced presence of gluten in food. Official Journal of the European Union. L 228/5.

Ehling, S., Tefera, S., Ho, I.P., 2007. High-performance liquid chromatographic method for the simultaneous detection of the adulteration of cereal flours with melamine and related triazine by-products ammeline, ammelide, and cyanuric acid. Food Additives and Contaminants 24, 1319–1325.

Ellis, D.I., Brewster, V.L., Dunn, W.B., Allwood, J.W., Golovanov, A.P., Goodacre, R., 2012. Fingerprinting food: current technologies for the detection of food adulteration and contamination. Chemical Society Reviews 41, 5706–5727.

Esbensen, K.H., Paoletti, C., Minkkinen, P., 2012a. Representative sampling of large kernel lots I. Theory of sampling and variographic analysis. Trends in Analytical Chemistry 32, 154–164.

Esbensen, K.H., Paoletti, C., Minkkinen, P., 2012b. Representative sampling of large kernel lots III. General considerations on sampling heterogeneous foods. Trends in Analytical Chemistry 32, 178–184.

FDA, 2014a. FSMA Proposed Rule for Focused Mitigation Strategies to Protect Food Against Intentional Adulteration. Available from: http://www.fda.gov/Food/GuidanceRegulation/FSMA/ucm378628.htm.

FDA, 2014b. Questions and Answers: Gluten-Free Food Labeling Final Rule. Available from. http://www.fda.gov/Food/GuidanceRegulation/GuidanceDocumentsRegulatoryInformation/Allergens/ucm362880.htm.

Freese, L., Chen, J.W., Shillito, R.D., 2015. Sampling of grain and seed to estimate the adventitious presence of biotechnology-derived seeds in a lot. Cereal Foods World 60, 9–15.

Ganapoulos, I., Argiriou, A., Tsaftaris, A., 2011. Adulterations in Basmati rice detected quantitatively by combined use of microsatellite and fragrance typing with high resolution melting (HRM) analysis. Food Chemistry 652–659.

Garber, E.A., Brewer, V.A., 2010. Enzyme-linked immunosorbent assay detection of melamine in infant formula and wheat food products. Journal of Food Protection® 73 (4), 701–707.

Gooding, M.J., 2009. The wheat crop. In: Khan, K., Shewry, P.R. (Eds.), Wheat: Chemistry and Technology, fourth ed. AACC International, St. Paul, pp. 19–49.

Graybosch, R.A., 1998. Waxy wheats: origin, properties, and prospects. Trends in Food Science & Technology 9, 135–142.

Graybosch, R.A., Peterson, C.J., Hansen, L.E., Rahman, S., Hill, A., Skerritt, J.H., 1998. Identification and characterization of U.S. Wheats carrying null alleles at the *wx* loci. Cereal Chemistry 75, 162–165.

Graybosch, R.A., Baenziger, P.S., Santra, D.K., Regassa, T., Jin, Y., Kolmer, J., Wegulo, S., Bai, G., St Amand, P., Chen, X., Seabourn, B., Dowell, F., Bowden, R., Marshall, D.M., 2014. Registration of 'Mattern' waxy (amylose-free) winter wheat. Journal of Plant Registrations 8, 43–48.

Haraszi, R., Chassaigne, H., Maquet, A., Ulberth, F., 2011. Analytical methods for detection of gluten in food – method developments in support of food labeling legislation. Journal of AOAC International 94, 1006–1025.

Hassani, S., Tavakoli, F., Amini, M., Kobarfard, F., Nili-Ahamadabadi, A., Sabzevari, O., 2013. Occurrence of melamine contamination in powder and liquid milk in market of Iran. Food Additives & Contaminants, Part A 30, 413–420.

Heller, D.N., Nochetto, C.B., 2008. Simultaneous determination and confirmation of melamine and cyanuric acid in animal feed by zwitterionic hydrophilic interaction chromatography and tandem mass spectrometry. Rapid Communications in Mass Spectrometry 22, 3624–3632.

Hung, P.V., Maeda, T., Morita, N., 2006. Waxy and high-amylose wheat starches and flours–characteristics, functionality and application. Trends in Food Science & Technology 17, 448–456.

Kaur, S., Panesar, P.S., Bera, M.B., Kaur, V., 2015. Simple sequence repeat markers in genetic divergence and marker-assisted selection of rice cultivars: a review. Critical Reviews in Food Science and Nutrition 55, 41–49.

Kelly, S., Heaton, K., Hoogewerff, J., 2005. Tracing the geographical origin of food: the application of multi-element and multi-isotope analysis. Food Science and Technology 16, 555–567.

Lee, M.R., Swanson, B.G., Baik, B.K., 2001. Influence of amylose content on properties of wheat starch and breadmaking quality of starch and gluten blends. Cereal Chemistry 78, 701–706.

Litzau, J.J., Mercer, G.E., Mulligan, K.J., 2008. GC-MS screen for the presence of melamine, ammeline, ammelide, and cyanuric acid. US FDA Laboratory Information Bulletin 4423.

Maningat, C.C., Seib, P.A., Bassi, S.D., Woo, K.S., Lasater, G.D., 2009. Wheat starch: production, properties, modification and uses. In: BeMiller, J.N., Whistler, R.L. (Eds.), Starch: Chemistry and Technology, third ed. Academic Press, New York, pp. 441–510.

Manning, L., Soon, J.M., 2014. Developing systems to control food adulteration. Food Policy 49, 23–32.

Mariotti, F., Tomé, D., Mirand, P.P., 2008. Converting nitrogen into protein-beyond 6.25 and Jones' factors. Critical Reviews in Food Science and Nutrition 48, 177–184.

McCarthy, P.K., Scanlon, B.F., Lumley, I.D., Griffin, M., 1990. Detection and quantification of adulteration of Durum wheat flour by flour from common wheat using reverse phase HPLC. Journal of the Science of Food and Agriculture 50, 211–226.

Miller, C.E., 2001. Chemical principles of near-infrared technology. In: Williams, P., Norris, K. (Eds.), Near-infrared Technology in the Agricultural and Food Industries, second ed. American Association of Cereal Chemists, St. Paul, pp. 19–37.

Minkkinen, P., Esbensen, K.H., Paoletti, C., 2012. Representative sampling of large kernel lots II. Application to soybean sampling for GMO control. Trends in Analytical Chemistry 32, 165–177.

Mishra, P., Herrero-Langreo, A., Barreiro, P., Roger, J., Diezma, B., Gorretta, N., Lleó, L., 2015. Detection and quantification of peanut traces in wheat flour by near infrared hyperspectral imaging spectroscopy using principal-component analysis. Journal of Near Infrared Spectroscopy 23, 15–22.

Moore, J.C., DeVries, J.W., Lipp, M., Griffiths, J.C., Abernethy, D.R., 2010. Total protein methods and their potential utility to reduce the risk of food protein adulteration. Comprehensive Reviews in Food Science and Food Safety 9, 330–357.

Moore, J.C., Spink, J., Lipp, M., 2012. Development and application of a database of food ingredient fraud and economically motivated adulteration from 1980 to 2010. Journal of Food Science 77, R118–R126.

Morrison, W.R., Milligan, T.P., Azudin, M.N., 1984. A relationship between the amylose and lipid contents of starches from diploid cereals. Journal of Cereal Science 2, 257–271.

Mottram, H.R., Woodbury, S.E., Rossell, J.B., Evershed, R.P., 2003. High-resolution detection of adulteration of maize oil using multi-component compound-specific $\delta^{13}C$ values of major and minor components and discriminant analysis. Rapid Communications in Mass Spectrometry 17, 706–712.

Muñiz-Valencia, R., Ceballos, M., Rosales-Martinez, D., Gonzalo-Lumbreras, R., Santos-Montes, A., Cubedo-Fernandez-Trapiella, A., Izquierdo-Homillos, C., 2008. Method development and validation for melamine and its derivatives in rice concentrates by liquid chromatography. Application to animal feed samples. Analytical and Bionanalytical Chemistry 392, 523–531.

Mujico, J.R., Lombardia, M., Mena, M.C., Méndez, E., Albar, J.P., 2011. A highly sensitive real-time PCR system for quantification of wheat contamination in gluten-free food for celiac patients. Food Chemistry 128, 795–801.

Mustorp, S.L., Dromtorp, S.M., Holck, A.L., 2011. Multiplex, quantitative, ligation-dependent probe amplification for determination of allergens in food. Journal of Agricultural and Food Chemistry 59, 5231–5239.

Nakamura, T., Yamamori, M., Hirano, H., Hidaka, S., 1993. Identification of three *wx* proteins in wheat. Biochemical Genetics 31, 75–86.

Nakamura, T., Yamamori, M., 1995. Production of waxy (amylose-free) wheats. Molecular and General Genetics 248, 253–259.

Nakamura, T., Vrinten, P., Saito, M., Konda, M., 2002. Rapid classification of partial waxy wheats using PCR-based markers. Genome 45, 1150–1156.

Osborne, B., Mertens, B., Thompson, M., Fearn, T., 1993. The authentication of Basmati rice using near infrared spectroscopy. Journal of Near Infrared Spectroscopy 1, 77–83.

Pasqualone, A., Montemurro, C., Grinn-Gofron, A., Sonnante, G., Blanco, A., 2007. Detection of soft wheat in semolina and durum wheat bread by analysis of DNA microsatellites. Journal of Agricultural and Food Chemistry 55, 3312–3318.

Pasqualone, A., Alba, V., Mangini, G., Blanco, A., Montemurro, C., 2010. Durum wheat cultivar traceability in PDO Altamura bread by analysis of DNA microsatellites. European Food Research and Technology 230, 723–729.

Pegels, N., González, I., García, T., Martin, R., 2015. Authenticity testing of wheat, barley, rye, and oats in food and feed market samples by real-time PCR assays. LWT – Food Science and Technology 60, 867–875.

Petersen, L., Minkkinen, P., Esbensen, K.H., 2005. Representative sampling for reliable data analysis: theory of sampling. Chemometrics and Intelligent Laboratory Systems 77, 261–277.

Pierna, J.A.F., Vincke, D., Dardenne, P., Yang, Z., Han, L., Baeten, V., 2014. Line scan hyperspectral imaging spectroscopy for the early detection of melamine and cyanuric acid in feed. Journal of Near Infrared Spectroscopy 22, 103–112.

Primrose, S., Woolfe, M., Rollinson, S., 2010. Food forensics: methods for determining the authenticity of foodstuffs. Food Science and Technology 21, 582–590.

Rahman, S., Kosarhashemi, B., Samuel, M.S., Hill, A., Abbott, D.C., Skerritt, J.H., Preiss, J., Appels, R., Morell, M.K., 1995. The major proteins of wheat endosperm starch granules. Australian Journal of Plant Physiology 22, 793–803.

Reis, N., Franca, A.S., Oliveira, L.S., 2013. Quantitative evaluation of multiple adulterants in roasted coffee by diffuse reflectance infrared Fourier transform spectroscopy (DRIFTS) and chemometrics. Talanta 115, 563–568.

Rodriguez-Saona, L.E., Allendorf, M.E., 2011. Use of FTIR for rapid authentication and detection of adulteration of food. Annual Review of Food Science and Technology 2, 467–483.

Rodriguez-Saona, L.E., Fry, F.S., Calvey, E.M., 2000. Use of Fourier transform near-infrared reflectance spectroscopy for rapid quantification of castor bean meal in a selection of flour-based products. Journal of Agricultural and Food Chemistry 48, 5169–5177.

Rosell, C.M., Barro, F., Sousa, C., Mena, M.C., 2014. Cereals for developing gluten-free products and analytical tools for gluten detection. Journal of Cereal Science 59, 354–364.

Russo, R., Cusano, E., Perissi, A., Ferron, F., Severino, V., Parente, A., Chambery, A., 2014. Ultra-high performance liquid chromatography tandem mass spectrometry for the detection of durum wheat contamination or adulteration. Journal of Mass Spectrometry 49, 1239–1246.

Scally, G., 2013. Adulteration of food: what it doesn't say on the tin. British Medical Journal 346, f1463.

Scarano, D., Rao, R., 2014. DNA markers for food products authentication. Diversity 6, 579–596.

Schmidt, H.L., Rossman, A., Voerkelius, S., Schnitzler, W.H., Georgi, M., Grassmann, J., Zimmermann, G., Winkler, R., 2005. Isotope characteristics of vegetables and wheat from conventional and organic production. Isotopes in Environmental and Health Studies 41, 223–228.

Sharma, G.M., Pereira, M., Williams, K.M., 2015. Gluten detection in foods available in the United States – a market survey. Food Chemistry 169, 120–126.

Sonnante, G., Montemurro, C., Morgese, A., Sabetta, W., Blanco, A., Pasqualone, A., 2009. DNA microsatellite region for a reliable quantification of soft wheat adulteration in Durum wheat-based foodstuffs by real-time PCR. Journal of Agricultural and Food Chemistry 57, 10199–10204.

Suzuki, Y., Chikaraishi, Y., Ogawa, N.O., Ohkouchi, N., Korenaga, T., 2008. Geographical origin of polished rice based on multiple element and stable isotope analyses. Food Chemistry 109, 470–475.

The Rice Association, 2005. Code of Practice on Basmati Rice. Available from: http://www.riceassociation.org.uk/content/1/4/documents.html.

Terzi, V., Malnati, M., Barbanera, M., Stanca, A.M., Faccioli, P., 2003. Development of analytical systems based on real-time PCR for *Triticum* species-specific detection and quantitation of bread wheat contamination in semolina and pasta. Journal of Cereal Science 38, 87–94.

Terzi, V., Morcia, C., Gorrini, A., Stanca, A.M., Shewry, P.R., Faccioli, P., 2005. DNA-based methods for identification and quantification of small grain cereal mixtures and fingerprinting of varieties. Journal of Cereal Science 41, 213–220.

Tittlemier, S.A., Lau, B.P.Y., Ménard, C., Corrigan, C., Sparling, M., Gaertner, D., Pepper, K., Feeley, M., 2009. Melamine in infant formula sold in Canada: occurrence and risk assessment. Journal of Agricultural and Food Chemistry 57, 5340–5344.

Török, K., Hajas, L., Horváth, V., Schall, E., Bugyi, Z., Kemény, S., Tömösközi, S., 2015. Identification of the factors affecting the analytical results of food allergen ELISA methods. European Food Research and Technology. http://dx.doi.org/10.1007/s00217-015-2441-y.

Turnipseed, S., Casey, C., Nochetto, C., Heller, D.N., 2008. Determination of Melamine and Cyanuric Acid Residues in Infant Formula Using LC-MS/MS. US FDA Laboratory Information Bulletin 4421.

van Leeuwen, K.A., Prenzler, P.D., Ryan, D., Camin, F., 2014. Gas chromatography-combustion-isotope ratio mass spectrometry for traceability and authenticity in foods and beverages. Comprehensive Reviews in Food Science and Food Safety 13, 814–837.

Vemireddy, L.R., Abchak, S., Nagaraju, J., 2007. Capillary electrophoresis is essential for microsatellite marker based detection and quantification of adulteration of Basmati rice (*Oryza sativa*). Journal of Agricultural and Food Chemistry 55, 8112–8117.

Vemireddy, L.R., Satyavathi, V.V., Siddiq, E.A., Nagaraju, J., 2015. Review of methods for the detection and quantification of adulteration of rice: Basmati as a case study. Journal of Food Science and Technology 52, 3187–3202.

Vermeulen, P., Pierna, J.A.F., van Egmond, H.P., Dardenne, P., Baeten, V., 2012. Online detection and quantification of ergot bodies in cereals using near infrared hyperspectral imaging. Food Additives and Contaminants 29, 232–240.

Vermeulen, P., Pierna, J.A.F., van Egmond, H.P., Zegers, J., Dardenne, P., Baeten, V., 2013. Validation and transferability study of a method based on near-infrared hyperspectral imaging for the detection and quantification of ergot bodies in cereals. Analytical and Bioanalytical Chemistry 405, 7765–7772.

WHO, 2008. Melamine-Contaminated Powdered Infant Formula in China – Update 2. World Health Organization. Available from: http://www.who.int/csr/don/2008_09_29a/en/.

WHO, 2009. Toxicological and Health Aspects of Melamine and Cyanuric Acid. World Health Organization. Available from: http://apps.who.int/iris/bitstream/10665/44106/1/9789241597951_eng.pdf?ua=1.

Yoo, S.H., Jane, J.L., 2002. Structural and physical characteristics of waxy and other wheat starches. Carbohydrate Polymers 49, 297–305.

Zhang, J., Zhang, X., Dediu, L., Victor, C., 2011. Review of the current application of fingerprinting allowing detection of food adulteration and fraud in China. Food Control 22, 1126–1135.

Zhao, H., Guo, B., Wei, Y., Zhang, B., Sun, S., Zhang, L., Yan, J., 2011. Determining the geographical origin of wheat using multielement analysis and multivariate statistics. Journal of Agricultural and Food Chemistry 59, 4397–4402.

Zhao, R., Wu, X., Seabourn, B.W., Bean, S.R., Guan, L., Shi, L., Wilson, J.D., Madl, R., Wang, D., 2009. Comparison of waxy vs. nonwaxy wheats in fuel ethanol fermentation. Cereal Chemistry 86, 145–156.

Zhao, X.C., Sharp, P.J., 1996. An improved 1-D SDS-PAGE method for the identification of three bread wheat 'waxy' proteins. Journal of Cereal Science 23, 191–193.

Advances in the Identification of Adulterated Vegetable Oils

19

O. Abbas, V. Baeten
Walloon Agricultural Research Centre (CRA-W), Gembloux, Belgium

Chapter Outline

19.1 Introduction

Increased consumer income, innovations in production, international trade, and other factors have led to a transformation in the food marketplace from product oriented to consumer driven (Siskos et al., 2001). In recent years, the production, marketing, and consumption of vegetable oil have attracted public attention because of health concerns about *trans* fatty acids and changes in industrial use. Vegetable oils are some of the most widely traded agricultural products in the world. There is a great variety of vegetable oils that contribute significantly to the human diet. They are used in cooking, frying, and salad dressing and are popular because they add flavor to food and have health and nutritional benefits. In Europe, they are seen as an essential source of energy in the human diet. A survey conducted for the European Union (EU) Centre for the Promotion of Imports from Developing Countries (CBI, 2014) showed that, in the 2008–12 period, vegetable oil consumption in EU countries increased by 7%, reaching 6.6 million t in 2012 (http://www.cbi.eu/sites/default/files/study/trade-statistics-europe-vegetable-oils-2014.pdf). In addition, greater demand from emerging economies and the growing biofuel industry have increased the pressure on supplies, which is likely to result in high prices in future years. In 2013, European exports of vegetable oils amounted to 2.4 million t, equivalent to €2.3 billion. In the 2009–13 period, total European exports increased significantly in terms of both value (+13%) and volume (+7%) (http://www.cbi.eu/sites/default/files/study/trade-statistics-europe-vegetable-oils-2014.pdf). It is worth noting that most European vegetable oil exports go to destinations within Europe, including the developing eastern European countries. At the same time, Europe imports significant quantities of special vegetable oils, such as toasted sesame oil, virgin coconut oil, and walnut oil. Consumption of these oils continues to grow, despite current global economic problems. The Philippines is the largest coconut producer worldwide, making it the leading coconut oil supplier, while Brazil and Argentina are the largest suppliers of groundnut oil. Sesame oil is produced mainly in Mexico, but China and India are also important suppliers. Other oils involved in the food industry, such as palm oil, are supplied mainly by Malaysia and Indonesia, which account for 66% of the total palm oil supplies to Europe. In the 2009–13 period, there was an annual decline of 9.1% in palm oil imports due to sustainability issues around palm oil production and a saturated market (http://www.cbi.eu/sites/default/files/study/trade-statistics-europe-vegetable-oils-2014.pdf). The CBI reported on the global distribution of edible oil production in 2009 (http://www.cbi.eu/sites/default/files/study/trade-statistics-europe-vegetable-oils-2014.pdf). As the CBI document shows, two edible oils—soybean oil and palm oil—account for about 61% of total edible oil production worldwide, whereas sunflower seed, coconut, cottonseed, olive, palm kernel, peanut, and rapeseed oils account for 8%, 3%, 3%, 2%, 4%, 3%, and 16%, respectively.

Fig. 19.1 shows the production, import, and export figures for the five top-selling vegetable oils in Europe in 2010: refined rape, colza, or refined mustard oil; refined palm oil; refined sunflower seed and safflower oil; virgin olive oil; and crude rape, colza, or mustard oil. The graph is based on statistics published on the Eurostat Website on vegetable oil production (Martinez-Palou and Rohner-Thielen, 2011).

Fig. 19.1 gives an idea of the vegetable oil trade in Europe and the size of that market, with refined rape, colza, and mustard oil showing the highest production figures, virgin olive oil the highest export figures, and refined palm oil the highest import figures.

Olive oil is particularly important in the Mediterranean diet (Nestle, 1995; Ness, 2002) but for a long time consumption was limited to the producing countries in Europe (Ramon-Muñoz, 2000). Since the 1970s, however, olive oil production, trade, and consumption in non-producing European countries have increased significantly (Scheidel and Krausmann, 2011) due to major modifications in land use and land cover patterns in these regions. Several studies have been conducted on the agro-economic, historical, and current dynamics of the olive oil market (Mili and Rodríguez-Zuñiga, 2001; Tasdogan et al., 2005). The Mediterranean basin is the center of most of the world's olive oil marketing activities. Torrecilla (2010) reported that in the

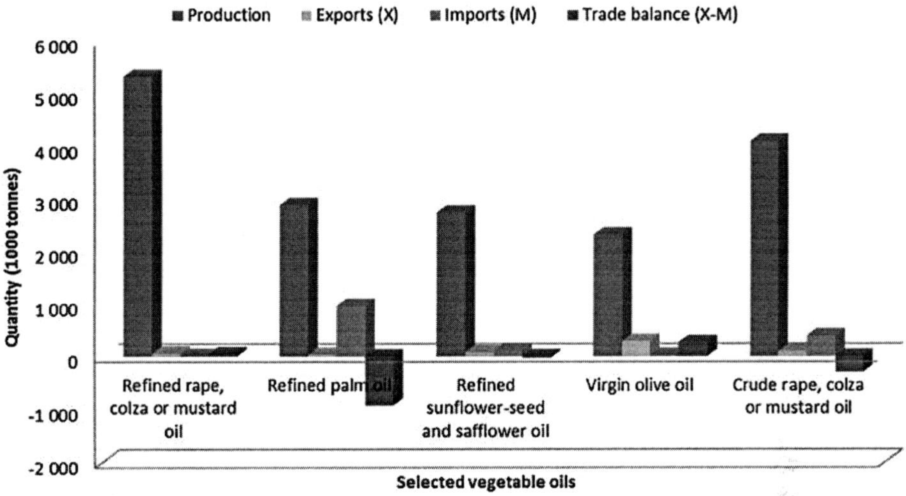

Figure 19.1 Production quantities and trade indicators for selected vegetable oils in Europe in 2010.

2008–09 season, more than 2.8×10^6 t of extra virgin olive oil was produced globally, with more than 75% originating within the European Community (EC).

Trade globalization has led to increased demand for vegetable oils, an increase in products with different sensory and nutritional characteristics, and greater use of vegetable oils as biofuels, which in turn has increased the risk of counterfeit products appearing on the market. Adulterated products are sold to increase profits, but this leads, at the very least, to a loss in consumer confidence. It is therefore necessary to guarantee food authenticity by developing analytical tools that address current market issues and challenges. Authenticity assessment is necessary to detect the replacement of a given costly and high-quality ingredient or product by cheaper and similar ingredients, the addition of adulterant(s) to food, the use of an undeclared process, and the falsification of the origin of a product (Esslinger et al., 2014). In essence, authentication of food refers to the need for all requirements regarding legal product description to be respected and the absence of any fraudulent substance to be confirmed (Gary et al., 2011; Lees, 2003; MoniQA, 2013). This chapter focuses mainly on the latter issue. Food adulteration can be defined as the addition of cheaper, inferior, harmful, or unnecessary substance(s) to food that could affect the nature and quality of the original food (Bell and Gillatt, 2004). Aparicio et al. (2013) reported that adulteration was one of the main authenticity issues. It can take the form of the addition of cheap oil to expensive oils, as in the case of adding refined oils to virgin olive oil, or the addition of low- to high-quality olive oils. Adulteration can also affect health, as illustrated by the following examples: the addition of orthocresyl phosphate to oil sold as suitable for human consumption in Morocco (Torrecilla et al., 2011a,b); the accidental contamination of rice oil with polychlorinated biphenyls in Japan (Lees, 2003); olive oil spiked with toxic aniline-denatured rapeseed oil, affecting more than 20,000 people

(Abaitua and Posada, 1992); the sale of non-edible rapeseed oil as an edible oil or as an olive oil in Spain, causing toxic oil syndrome (Posada de la Paz et al., 1996); the adulteration of mustard oil with poisonous Argemone oil in India (Clemente and Cahoon, 2009), causing a disease known as "epidemic dropsy."

Although adulteration can occur accidentally during the production process, in most cases it involves vegetable oils that are expensive and are important in human nutrition. Such oils are more susceptible to adulteration. Jee (2002) defined two major types of adulteration: admixing cold pressed oil with a refined oil; and replacing more expensive oils and fats with cheaper varieties (eg, mixing costly sunflower and soybean oils with cheap oils such as cotton seed or castor oil, as reported by Naveen et al. (2013)). Adulteration has become even more sophisticated now, making its detection in vegetable oils difficult and reinforcing the need for advanced analytical methods (Elbashbashy and Ibrahim, 1993). It is important to be aware of the challenges posed by fraudsters and to continue to develop new techniques and to revise and upgrade official methods. In the case of olive oil, adulterant oil is chosen for its chemical similarity to extra virgin olive oil. Such oils include refined olive oil, refined olive pomace oil, and hazelnut oil. These adulterations are difficult to detect, especially at percentages below 10% (v/v) (Mildner-Szkudlarz and Jelen, 2008; Peña et al., 2005). Olive oil adulteration has always been a problem and has never been confined to one region or country (Torrecilla et al., 2011a,b). These examples illustrate the dangers of the adulteration of vegetable oils. Several international institutions, such as the International Olive Council (IOC) and the Antifraud Unit of the European Union (OLAF) are focusing on drafting antifraud legislation aimed at improving the control of the trade of olive oil. They are also working on detecting fraud through the development of rapid, simple, sensitive, and accurate analytical methods.

The development of analytical techniques for the authentication of vegetable oils is an ongoing requirement because fraudsters continue to find new ways of adulterating oils that appear to remain within the normal compositional ranges and criteria (absence/presence) established by regulations. These techniques include combining chromatographic and spectroscopic methods, using chemometric data analysis, and developing large databases of authentic vegetable oils. Other biomolecular, physical, and thermal techniques are beginning to be investigated to detect the adulteration of vegetable oils. The purpose of this chapter is to review recent publications on developments and trends in the detection of the adulteration of vegetable oils. The selected vegetable oils are olive oil, hazelnut oil, palm oil, sunflower oil, soybean oil, argan oil, coconut oil, sesame oil, pumpkin seed oil, and peanut oil. Most official methods for assessing vegetable oil adulteration are based on chromatographic techniques, but the increased sophistication in methods used by fraudsters makes it necessary to consider alternative or complementary methods, such as spectroscopy. Analytical methods can be classified as targeted or nontargeted/profiling methods. Targeted methods have the ability to separate, identify, and quantify the components of oils, whereas nontargeted/profiling methods provide overall information about a sample.

This chapter outlines work on the application of targeted, nontargeted, and other analytical methods to the analysis of olive and other edible oils, with the main focus on simplicity and speed of analysis, interpretation of data obtained, calculation of an adulteration LOD and qualitative and/or quantitative aspects, as well as the validation and general applicability of these methods. The chapter closes with the conclusions drawn from the review and a look at future trends in this field.

19.2 Authenticity Testing of Adulterated Vegetable Oils, Including Case Studies

19.2.1 Targeted Methods: Chromatographic Techniques for Assessing Vegetable Oil Adulteration

Most reports on the detection of vegetable oil adulteration focus on the use of liquid and gas chromatographic analysis to identify and quantify fatty acids, triglycerols, sterols, tocopherols, and hydrocarbons (Eisner et al., 1965). A gas–liquid chromatographic technique for detecting adulteration was described by the Codex Committee on Fats and Oils (Codex Alimentarius Commission, 1987), which set the fatty acid distributional ranges for various edible oils and fats. Subsequently, this became the international basis for establishing the authenticity of oils and fats (Rossell, 1998), with Aparicio and Aparicio-Ruiz (2000) publishing an overview of chromatographic methods used in vegetable oil authentication for that purpose.

19.2.1.1 Olive Oil

Olive oil is one of the most adulterated vegetable oils because of its low production and high price compared with some other oils. The IOC has defined the criteria for classifying olive oil according to chemical, sensory, and organoleptic properties (Gonzalez and Aparicio, 2002; Oliveros et al., 2002; International Olive Council). Olive oils fall into four categories (Piravi Vanak et al., 2010) depending on the extent to which their free acidity is expressed as oleic acid; this should not exceed 0.8 g/100 g for extra virgin olive oil, 2 g/100 g for virgin olive oil, 3.3 g/100 g for ordinary virgin olive oil, and 0.3 g/100 g for refined olive oil. Extra virgin olive oil can be adulterated with olive oil of lower-quality (eg, olive-pomace olive oil, virgin olive oil, and gently deodorized olive oil) or with seed oils such as corn, soybean, or palm oils, although there is now increasing use of hazelnut oil because of its similar triacylglycerol content, total sterol and fatty acid profile, in addition to its high oleic and linoleic fatty acid content (Patricio et al., 1997). The EC has amended its regulations concerning the quality control of olive oil, particularly with regard to adulteration with hazelnut oil (European Union Commission Regulation 1513/2001).

Several studies have reported the development of chromatographic techniques for detecting adulteration of olive oil with hazelnut oil, and some solutions have been proposed. Flores et al. (2006), for example, based their analysis on the detection of filbertone, a specific flavor compound of hazelnut, in order to detect the adulteration of olive oil by virgin hazelnut oil. Filbertone was determined using solid-phase microextraction and multidimensional gas chromatography (SPME–MDGC), which can detect an adulteration level of up to 7%. Capote et al. (2007) proposed a step-by-step method using chromatographic peak areas for the detection, identification, and quantification of the adulteration of extra virgin olive oil. Data from the application of gas chromatography-mass spectrometry (GC–MS) on the lipid fraction of a set of 566 samples were used to establish chemometric models based on a soft independent modeling of class analogy (SIMCA) and K-nearest neighbors analysis. Both approaches demonstrated prediction abilities that were always higher than 91% for adulterant detection and 88% for the identification of type of adulterant. Quantitative analysis using a partial least squares regression (PLSR) model yielded R^2 values of >0.90. Calvano et al. (2010) measured polar components and the phospholipid fraction usually present in seed oils at a concentration range of 10–20 g/kg, and showed that phospholipid quantities in virgin olive oil are 300–400 times lower. The analysis of phospholipids using an ionic liquid matrix and solvent extraction, followed by the application of MALDI-TOF mass spectrometry (MS), allowed adulteration of extra virgin oil with hazelnut oil to be detected (Calvano et al., 2012) down to a level of 1% (v/v) contamination. Bakre et al. (2015) proposed using alpha-tocopherol content as a discriminating parameter in the detection of olive oil adulteration by sunflower oil. Determining this content by coupling reversed-phase high-pressure liquid chromatography (HPLC) to a fluorescence detector with excitation and emission wavelengths at 290 and 330 nm, respectively, allowed 5% (v/v) sunflower oil in olive oil to be detected. This method was shown to be selective, sensitive, and precise (relative standard deviation = 2.65%).

19.2.1.2 Other Oils

Zhao et al. (2015) proposed analyzing some minor constituents for the authentication of vegetable oils. Isoflavones and resveratrol, found only in soybean and peanut oils (Eisenbrand, 2007; Sobolev and Cole, 1999), are considered to be biomarker constituents in the detection of the adulteration of soybean and peanut oils with other vegetable oils. Soybean oil is the most heavily consumed vegetable oil in the United States, and palm oil is the lowest priced one (Kojima, 2014). The analytical method was based on solid-phase extraction coupled with liquid chromatography tandem MS (SPE LC–MS/MS), a method that was successfully tested in 13 vegetable oils obtained from retailers. Liquid chromatography has also been applied to Brazil nut oil (*Bertholletia excelsa* Bonpl., Lecythidaceae), which originates in the Amazon region and is highly valued in food markets because of its composition and health benefits (Yang, 2009). Funasaki et al. (2012) assessed the applicability of liquid chromatography coupled with easy ambient sonic-spray ionization MS (EASI-MS) for the quality control of Amazonian Brazil nut oil. This method allowed authentic, commercial, and adulterated oils (5% soybean oil) to be characterized in a few minutes and without any sample preparation. Quality control is important, but in some cases religious prohibitions also come into play (eg, the use of lard as an adulterant in the food system). Marikkar et al. (2005) used gas–liquid chromatography to identify lard contamination in palm, palm kernel, and canola oils. Adulteration by animal fats such as lard, beef tallow, and chicken fat in proportions ranging from 2% to 20% (w/w) was assessed. Gas–liquid chromatography analyses of fatty acid methyl esters were conducted on

2-monoacylglycerol and neutral triacylglycerol isolated from each sample. Canonical discriminant analysis of the resulting data enabled oil samples contaminated with as little as 2% (w/w) of lard to be detected. Later, Bonvehi and Col (2009) developed a chromatographic method for detecting the refined vegetable oils (peanut, high oleic acid sunflower, corn, and soybean) most often added to hazelnut oil. Hazelnut oil is very rich in polyunsaturated fatty acids, including monounsaturated (92% of total fatty acids), vitamin E, and natural antioxidants (Cuvelier et al., 2003). Found in the market as either crude or refined oil, its price depends mainly on the quality of the hazelnut variety used to produce the oil and can be as high as the price of virgin olive oil, thus making it a target for adulteration. Only a few studies have focused on the need to develop analytical methods to verify its quality and safety. Adulteration occurs at the level of hazelnut paste. Results obtained by Bonvehi and Col (2009) showed that fatty acid and triacylglycerol content were the best indicators of adulteration between 5% and 30% (w/w), except for high oleic-sunflower oil, which was not possible to detect. Other variants of liquid chromatography continue to be developed in an effort to enhance its performance. An analytical procedure was developed by Deineka and Deineka (2004) for characterizing some vegetable oils (linseed, corn, olive, sunflower, and pumpkin) and detecting adulterated oils (using olive oil as an example). The procedure was based on the use of microcolumn reversed-phase HPLC coupled with ultraviolet (UV) detection to determine triglycerides and the degree of unsaturation in vegetable oils.

Gas chromatography has also been widely studied for its ability to assess vegetable oil adulteration. Yu et al. (2013) used it to rapidly detect and quantify the adulteration of rice bran oil with palm oil. Rice bran oil is used in cooking because of its high level of linoleic acid, vitamin E, unsaponifiable matter, and gamma-oryzanol content (Gopala Krishna, 2008; Yu et al., 2012; Crevel et al., 2000). Based on calculations using gas chromatographic data and mathematical tools, a linear model of characteristic fatty acid content and level of palm oil adulteration was established. This model was suitable for detecting adulteration levels 10—20% (w/w). A vectorial angle method was used to calculate the similarity of the chromatographic fingerprints of adulterated and unadulterated oil. The fitted model provided a low LOD of 2% (w/w) and an average relative error of 2.22%. Hilali et al. (2007) used gas chromatography analysis to define campesterol as an adulteration marker in the analysis of argan oil purity. Campesterol, a sterol found in seed oils, represents less than 0.4% of argan oil total sterol content, but in other vegetable oils it can account for between 2% and more than 10% of the total sterol content. Determining the campesterol level in argan oil (or oil presented as argan oil) could be an efficient way of assessing argan oil purity up to 98%. Ourrach et al. (2012) identified 3,5-stigmastadiene (a steroidal compound used as a marker for virgin olive oil authentication), kaurene hydrocarbon, and pheophytin (a pigment) as possible new markers for argan oil adulterated by up to 5% with refined sunflower oil and virgin olive oil. After extraction, markers were identified using gas or liquid chromatography, but with an LOD higher than 10% because of the similarity in fatty acid composition between the adulterating edible oils studied and argan oil. Argan oil is produced from the fruits of the argan tree (*Argania spinosa*), which is endemic to southwestern Morocco and protected by UNESCO (2007).

The oil is extracted from the fruit pip using a traditional method or press or solvent extraction. Because of its restricted source and the health benefits of its bactericidal and fungicidal properties, it is considered a luxury item and is expensive (about €100/L in Europe) (Cherki et al., 2006). Its high price makes it a target for fraudsters, who add cheaper oils (eg, olive or sunflower oil) colored with paprika or other substances (Gonzálvez et al., 2010). Another example of a less well-known vegetable oil is Styrian pumpkin seed oil, which has become a target of adulteration although it has been protected under the EU Protected Geographical Indication scheme since 1995, which should guarantee its origin and purity. It is consumed mainly in southern Austria and adjacent regions in Slovenia and Hungary, where it is cultivated. The oil is used in some therapies and is favored for its antioxidant properties (Al Zhair et al., 2000; Schiebel-Schlosser and Friederich, 1998). Cultivating the pumpkins and extracting the oil is manually laborious, making the oil expensive. Unlike other edible oils, its D5-sterol content is very low, whereas its D7-sterol content is higher than in other oils. The procedure used by Wenzl et al. (2002) to detect foreign oils in pumpkin seed oil included the saponification of the triglycerides as a first step, followed by separation of the potassium salts in the fatty acids from the unsaponifiable fraction using adsorption chromatography. The analytes were then separated on a capillary column of medium polarity and detected using flame ionization.

19.2.2 Nontargeted: Spectroscopic Techniques for Assessing Vegetable Oil Adulteration

Esslinger et al. (2014) published a review of the nontargeted or so-called "fingerprinting" spectroscopic methods used for characterizing and verifying food matrices such as olive oil. They discussed the challenges encountered in the use of food fingerprinting in official food control. Here we outline work based on using fluorescence, UV, near and mid-infrared (NIR, MIR), and Raman and nuclear magnetic resonance (NMR) spectroscopies to detect vegetable oil adulteration.

19.2.2.1 Olive Oil

The rapidity, simplicity, and lack of any need for solvents make spectroscopic methods attractive for vegetable oil authentication and quality control. Fluorescence spectroscopy has been used for the detection of virgin olive oil adulteration. Sayago et al. (2004) analyzed virgin olive oil adulterated with hazelnut oil in percentages varying between 5% and 30% (w/w) at $\lambda_{ex} = 350$ nm (Sayago et al., 2004). Chemometric analysis of the collected spectral data, such as stepwise linear discriminant analysis (SLDA), gave a 100% correct classification of samples as either authentic or adulterated. Poulli et al. (2006) also tried to differentiate virgin olive oil from sunflower oil using synchronous fluorescence and succeeded in detecting adulteration at 3.4% (w/v). The method was also used successfully to detect the adulteration of extra virgin olive oil by olive pomace oil (Guimet et al., 2005). Excitation−emission fluorescence spectroscopy combined with three-way data analysis allowed levels of adulteration as low as 5% (w/w) to be detected.

Ultraviolet spectroscopy can provide information on the quality of oil. Absorption in this wavelength range is due to the presence of conjugated diene and triene systems. A study of the adulteration of olive oils from the northern governorates of Palestine by sunflower, corn, and soybean oils at levels between 5% and 40% was undertaken by Houshia et al. (2014). UV−Vis spectroscopic measurements showed that absorbance at 232 nm could be used to detect olive oil adulteration, whereas measuring absorbance at 266, 270, and 274 nm to calculate the "Delta-K" formula was useful in detecting oil adulteration, but only at percentages above 5%. Sometimes virgin olive oil is adulterated with refined oils. Aued-Pimentel et al. (2013) succeeded in detecting such adulteration by measuring UV absorbance (specific extinction) at 270 nm and the stigmastadiene content. These parameters were chosen because, during the vegetable oil refining process, compounds with conjugated double bonds, such as stigmasta-3,5-diene, are generated from unsaturated fatty acids that absorb at 270 nm and from sterol. Extra virgin olive oil can also be mixed with refined olive or refined olive pomace oils. Torrecilla et al. (2010) developed a method based on calculating the so-called "chaotic parameters" (CPs; Lyapunov exponent, autocorrelation coefficients, and two fractal dimensions) in order to quantify the adulteration of extra virgin olive oil with low-grade olive oils from UV−Vis scans of 396 adulterated extra virgin olive oil samples. For external validation, when the adulterating agent concentration was less than 10%, the integrated CPs/UV−Vis model estimated the adulterant agent concentration with a mean correlation coefficient (estimated versus real concentration of low-grade olive oil) greater than 0.97 and a mean square error of less than 1%. The feasibility of quantifying the adulteration of extra virgin olive oil with low-grade olive oils is therefore possible.

NIR spectroscopy has been widely used to detect the adulteration of olive oil by sunflower, corn, walnut, and hazelnut oils (Christy et al., 2004). The adulteration of extra virgin olive oil by lower-grade olive oils (varying concentrations of olive pomace, refined olive, deodorized olive, and refined olive pomace oils) was studied by Mignani et al. (2011), who developed an original approach based on diffuse-light absorption spectroscopy in the 400−1700 nm spectral range. Principal component analysis (PCA) and SLDA were successfully applied to the data collected and enabled adulteration concentration and type to be predicted.

Fourier-transform MIR (FT-MIR) spectroscopy has been used to detect the adulteration of extra virgin olive oil with a corn-sunflower binary mixture (5% (v/v)), cottonseed and rapeseed oils (5% (v/v)) (Gurdeniz and Ozen, 2009), sunflower, corn, soybean, and hazelnut oils (5% (w/w)) (Lerma-Garcia et al., 2010), palm oil (1% (w/w)) (Rohman and Man, 2010), lard (1% (v/v)) (Rohman et al., 2011), and rice bran oil (5% (v/v)) (Rohman and Man, 2012). Baeten et al. (2005) proposed using FT-MIR spectroscopy in combination with FT-Raman spectroscopy to determine the presence of hazelnut oil in olive oil. Spectroscopic analysis has been used for the entire oil as well as with its unsaponifiable fraction. SLDA was designed for differentiation purposes. Fig. 19.2 shows the application of the SLDA model to the FT-MIR spectra of the unsaponifiable matter.

The figure shows that the FT-MIR spectra of the unsaponifiable samples enable the pure olive oil samples to be differentiated from most of the adulterated samples.

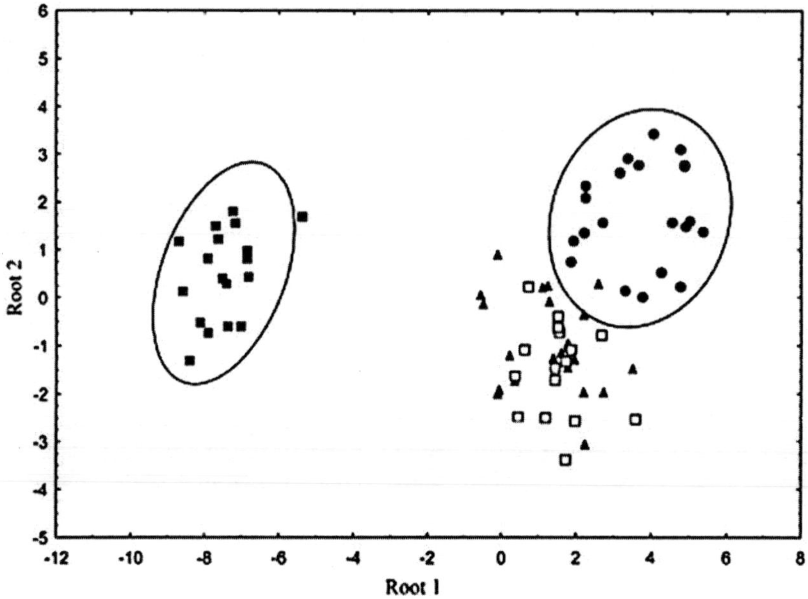

Figure 19.2 FT-MIR spectra of the unsaponifiable matter of the test samples: classification of genuine olive oil (●) and hazelnut oil (■) and their mixtures [>10% (□) and <10% (▲)] using SLDA. Genuine edible oils are delimited by ellipses of confidence at $\alpha = 0.90$ (Baeten et al., 2005).

FT-MIR spectroscopy has also been used to assess the quality of groundnut oil, another target of adulteration by cheaper oils such as palm or rice bran oil (Pandurangan et al., 2014). The percentages of adulteration found were between 5% and 15% (v/v). FT-MIR spectra collected for pure oils and prepared mixtures were interpreted in order to highlight changes in the spectra of groundnut oil after adulteration; the changes included a band shift at about 3011 cm^{-1} due to the C-H stretching vibration of *cis*-double bonds and indirectly via an absorbance change at about 1753 cm^{-1}, which is characteristic of oils with a saturated fatty acid content and a short carbohydrate chain. Even if the spectral differences were subtle, they enabled the adulteration of virgin groundnut oil by palm and rice bran oils to be detected.

Several studies have also described the use of Raman spectroscopy for detecting and quantifying the adulteration of olive oil (Baeten et al., 1996). The method is suitable for the analysis of compounds rich in unsaturated functional groups and has proved to be useful in studies involving olive oil. As applied by Zou et al. (2009), it is based on the intensity ratio of the *cis* (=C—H) and *cis* (C=C) bonds normalized by the band at 1441 cm^{-1} (CH_2) and applied for authentication or the detection of fake olive oil. It is then possible to differentiate genuine olive oils from olive oils with 5% (v/v) or more of other edible oils, such as soybean, rapeseed, sunflower seed, or corn oils. Although the excitation wavelength in that study was set at 785 nm (portable Raman), El-Abassy et al. (2009) tested a dispersive Raman system using a 514-nm laser to discriminate olive oils from different types of sunflower oils and claimed to be able to detect adulteration at low concentrations (eg, 1% (v/v)) using a measurement that required only a few seconds. Researchers constantly strive to improve the quantitative spectroscopic analysis of adulteration by developing more powerful chemometric tools, such as Bayesian framework least squares support vector machines (SVMs), in order to predict the adulteration of extra virgin olive oils more accurately based on their Raman spectra (Dong et al., 2012).

NMR spectroscopy offers qualitative and quantitative information by identifying the atoms in a given sample and the intensities of specific peaks, respectively (Hidalgo and Zamora, 2003). NMR data from the olefin group have enabled olive oil adulteration to be detected (Alonso-Salces et al., 2010; Smejkalova and Piccolo, 2010). Similarly, the adulteration of original olive oil by hazelnut oil (5%) can be detected based on the whole NMR spectrum or 1H NMR data (Zamora et al., 2001; Mannina et al., 2009). García-González et al. (2004) used 1H and 13C NMR techniques. 1H NMR spectra provide information on several compounds, including fatty acids and minor compounds such as aldehydes, terpenes, and sterols. 13C NMR provides information on the acyl positional distribution in a glycerol moiety. These methods can detect olive oil adulteration by hazelnut oil at a level of 8%, but with some limitations. The detection of seed oil adulteration of virgin oil at 5%, using 31P and 1H NMR spectroscopy combined with chemometric data analysis, was shown to be feasible through the quantitative determination of 1,2-diacyloglycerol concentrations (Vigli et al., 2003).

Lizhi et al. (2010) proposed using dielectric spectroscopy for discriminating olive oil from adulterating vegetable oils such as soy, corn, canola, sesame, and perilla oils. A PCA scores plot showed a clear differentiation of samples, depending on the different concentrations of the adulterant (varying from 0% to 100% (w/w)), whereas a PLS regression model showed good prediction performance and the possibility of being able to detect adulterant oils at levels below 5%. An analytical strategy based on a direct sample analysis time-of-flight (DSA/TOF) MS system has also been proposed as a rapid method for screening for the adulteration of olive oil with soybean oil (Dalmia and Perkins, 2013). The ratio of linoleic acid to oleic acid in the olive oil was used to detect its adulteration with a mass accuracy of less than 5 ppm.

19.2.2.2 Other Oils

MIR and NIR spectroscopies were studied in order to develop rapid qualitative and quantitative analysis for the authentication of Chinese sesame oils. Sesame oil is a high-quality vegetable oil derived from sesame seeds (*Sesamum indicum* L.) and is one of the oldest oilseed crops (Tashiro et al., 1990). It is grown in tropical and subtropical areas on 7.54 million ha worldwide, yielding 3.3 million t of seed (Jyothi et al., 2011). China is one of the most important producers of sesame, accounting for about 25% of total global output (Salunkhe et al., 1992). It is traditionally used for cooking in China, Korea, and elsewhere in Asia, is reported to provide many health benefits, and is a good source of antioxidants and polyunsaturated fatty acids (Liu et al., 2013; Alipoor et al., 2012). Sesame oil is 5–6 times more expensive than other vegetable oils, and the risk of adulteration with lower-quality oils (eg, corn, soybean, perilla, canola, corn, rapeseed, and palm oils) is increasing. Deng et al. (2012) analyzed a variety of sesame oils from the six most important sesame-producing areas of China, in addition to samples adulterated at levels of 2%, 3%, 4%, 5%, 8%, 10%, and 20% (w/w). SIMCA and PLS class model (PLSCM) were shown to be able to detect a 3% adulteration of sesame oils with cheaper oils (rapeseed, soybean, palm, and peanut oils). The best performance was obtained using SIMCA on second-derivative spectra (0.91 sensitivity and 0.94 specificity) and PLSCM (0.95 sensitivity and 0.94 specificity). Ding et al. (2014) also used FTIR analysis to authenticate sesame oils. They collected the spectra of sesame, soybean, and sunflower seed oils and observed the region between 1800 and 650 cm^{-1}, where they identified slight spectral differences because of differences in fatty acid composition between the oils. PCA and SIMCA models were then developed on sesame samples adulterated with soybean and sunflower seed oils, leading to a 100% correct recognition rate for samples adulterated at levels higher than 10%. Partial least squares (PLS) processing was used to develop the model of a binary system of sesame oil mixed with soybean or sunflower oil. The predicted adulterant values correlated well with the reference values, and the relative error of prediction was between 6.9% and 8.1%. Similarly, Xuebao (2012) investigated the adulteration of sesame oils with soybean, corn, and peanut oils using NIR spectroscopy by analyzing samples in transmission mode and establishing an interval PLS (iPLS) model. Important relevant wavelength bands could be selected by iPLS, which helped in developing the final quantitative PLS models. The performances of calibration models for the soybean, corn, and peanut oils showed coefficients of correlation of 0.99, 0.99, and 0.99, respectively, and the root mean square error (RMSE) of prediction was 0.24%, 0.24%, and 0.19%, respectively, indicating a high level of predictive accuracy.

These studies on infrared techniques show their potential for the rapid detection and determination of the adulteration of sesame oils. Likewise, with virgin coconut oil becoming almost as valuable as virgin olive oil because of its high-therapeutic value, it has become important to verify its purity and protect it from adulteration. Coconut oil is one of the most important oils in the tropical regions. It is used mainly for edible and industrial purposes, as well as in cooking. It can be consumed without refining, thereby retaining its natural flavor and aroma (Man et al., 1997). It is rich in medium-chain fatty acids and exhibits good digestibility (Odl, 1997), it protects low-density lipoprotein against oxidation, and has been reported to reduce lipid levels in serum and tissues (Nevin and Rajamohan, 2004). Unlike commercial coconut oil, virgin coconut oil is obtained from fresh coconut milk by wet processing without exposure to chemical or high-heat treatment (Marina et al., 2010). Some studies have used FT-MIR spectroscopy to analyze the adulteration of virgin coconut oil by palm kernel olein (Marina et al., 2007) and lard (Mansor et al., 2011). Palm kernel olein has a very similar chemical composition to virgin coconut oil, and lard has a transparent to yellowish color and is solid at room temperature, as is virgin coconut oil. Binary mixtures of virgin coconut oil and an adulterant varying from 1% to 50% (v/v) were analyzed using an MIR spectrometer equipped with a horizontal attenuated total reflectance accessory. It was possible to detect adulteration at levels as low as 1%. SLDA made it possible to distinguish adulterated oils from pure samples. A PLS model developed between FT-MIR spectra and actual values of adulteration produced coefficients of determination (R^2) of 0.99 and 0.99 and RMSE cross-validation (RMSECV) values of 1.70 and 1.54 for palm kernel and lard, respectively. When gas chromatography was used with a surface acoustic wave (SAW) detector (GC-SAW) and FT-MIR spectroscopy to determine lard adulteration, one of chromatographic peaks identified as an adulterant peak enabled a model with a coefficient of determination R^2 value of 0.93 to be obtained.

Another type of adulteration concerns the use of used frying oils. The disposal of these oils is a major problem for the catering industry, with some fraudsters adding it to edible vegetable oils in order to increase profits. Rapid detection methods for this kind of adulteration are needed urgently, but only a few articles on this kind of adulteration have been published. Zhang et al. (2012) used FT-MIR spectroscopy to show that edible vegetable oils (corn, peanut, rapeseed, and soybean oils) had been adulterated with used frying oil at levels between 1% and 90%. The FTIR spectra collected were interpreted and then split into 22 regions related to the different chemical component structures of the vegetable oils studied. One band was used as a divisor and produced 21 area ratios, which were then used as parameters for cluster analysis. The area ratio between bands 19 and 20 and the wavenumber of band 19 were used to construct linear regression equations; the limits of detection (LODs) of the corn, peanut, rapeseed, and soybean oils adulterated with used frying oil were 6.6%, 7.2%, 5.5%, and 3.6%, based on the area ratio, and 8.1%, 9.0%, 6.9%, and 5.6% when using the wavenumber band, respectively. This suggests that the combination of FT-MIR spectroscopy with chemometrics can be used to detect the adulteration of edible vegetable oils by used frying oils. Other solutions have been proposed to determine the adulteration of vegetable cooking oils with inedible used oils, a practice recently reported in China (Cao et al., 2012; Huang et al., 2008). Xu et al. (2014) developed a sensitive optical sensing method based on the fluorescence quenching of CdSe/ZnS quantum dots (QDs) for identifying adulterated vegetable cooking oils. High-quality hydrophilic photoluminescent nanoparticles were synthesized by encapsulating hydrophobic QDs into the micellar structure of an amphiphilic surfactant (cetyltrimethyl ammonium bromide, CTAB) via a phase transfer method. Transmission electron microscopy, atomic force microscopy, and fluorescence spectroscopy were used to characterize the prepared CTAB-coated QDs. Oil samples were initially captured in the core of the two-layer-structural micelle and then the fluorescence of the CTAB-coated QDs, working as fluorescence probes, was selectively quenched by components of the adulterated oils, such as heavy metal ions and free radicals. The authors reported a high correlation between quenching percentage and adulteration concentration ($R^2 = 0.94$). This sensitive, simple, and low-cost sensing method did not require sample pretreatment and could detect refined used oils at levels as low as 0.4% (v/v). The method needs to be applied to a much larger number of vegetable oils, however, before it can be considered validated.

Ensuring good vegetable oil quality is challenging because of the growing problem of adulteration motivated by the prospect of high profits. It is therefore important to define the fatty acid composition of vegetable oils and develop accurate analytical methods to use in quality control. Dong et al. (2013) proposed Raman spectroscopy combined with chemometric treatment as a rapid analytical solution. A set of vegetable oils and their binary mixtures were characterized by Raman spectra in the region of 800–2000 cm^{-1}. A model for predicting fatty acid content based on least squares SVM (LS-SVM) was established between the Raman spectral data and gas chromatographic data (reference method). The correlation coefficients for the prediction of oleic, linoleic, and α-linolenic acids were 0.99, 0.99, and 0.98, respectively. The simplicity and rapidity of Raman spectroscopy based on LS-SVM make it a promising technique for predicting the fatty acid composition of vegetable oils.

Aparicio and Baeten (1998) assessed the relative potential of NIR, MIR, and Raman spectroscopies using seven types of vegetable oils (corn, soybean, rapeseed, peanut, sunflower, high oleic sunflower, and virgin olive oils). The Fischer coefficient was used to highlight spectral signals responsible for the discrimination of these oils. NIR identified signals corresponding to the C–H vibration of unsaturated groups, MIR wavenumbers characterized the C–H and C–C vibrations of the carbon skeleton and the C–O of ester groups while Raman wavenumbers selected corresponded to the C–H vibration of unsaturated groups. The other wavenumbers were characteristic of C–H and C=C vibrations. These techniques can also be combined to achieve a more accurate characterization of vegetable oils.

A final example is a simple NMR method used for authenticating sesame oil (Nam et al., 2014). The proton signal of sesame is well resolved at about 5.95 ppm and highly correlated with the quantities of other types of vegetable oils present in adulterated sesame oil ($R^2 = 0.99$). It can be considered as a marker with which to determine the authenticity of sesame oil and the adulterants in that oil. HPLC was used to confirm the validity of these results obtained by NMR.

19.2.3 Other Analytical Techniques for Assessing Vegetable Oil Adulteration

19.2.3.1 Olive Oil

Using classical methods, the LOD of vegetable oil adulteration was estimated to be about 5% (Giménez et al., 2010). A new method for detecting olive oil adulteration of olive oil recently has been proposed by a group of Swiss researchers (FAO-Trade and Markets Division, Oilseeds, 2014). It involves adding a miniscule amount of synthetic DNA to oil products in order to trace the oil by recording its origin and other specific information. This marker can then be extracted and analyzed. When the DNA concentration does not match the original value, this means that the oil has been adulterated with other oils. The method is safe, simple, and cost effective and could be applied to any edible oil. DNA-based technologies have been able to detect the adulteration of olive oil by hazelnut oil at levels lower than 10% (Kumar et al., 2011).

Chiavaro et al. (2008) assessed thermophysical analyses and suggested using differential scanning calorimetry (DSC) analyses to detect the adulteration of extra virgin olive oil by refined hazelnut oil. These two oils have different cooling and heating DSC thermal profiles. The heating thermogram profiles of extra virgin olive oil were significantly altered by the addition of hazelnut oil. Torrecilla et al. (2011a,b) tried to quantify adulterant agents in extra virgin olive oil using models based on its thermophysical properties. A linear correlation between density and refractive indices (RIs) ($R^2 = 0.93$ and RMSECV less than 8.9%) allowed the adulteration of extra virgin olive oil by sunflower or corn oils to be detected. Models based on combining DSC and a chaotic parameter CP (lag-k autocorrelation coefficients, LCCs) (R^2 greater than 0.921 and RMSEP less than 4.9%) allowed the adulteration of extra virgin olive oil by refined olive, refined olive pomace, sunflower, and corn oils to be detected.

19.2.3.2 Other Oils

Techniques other than chromatography have been proposed for simplifying and improving the sensitivity and rapidity of detecting vegetable oil adulteration. Real-time PCR has been used to detect genetically modified soybean DNA in refined vegetable oils (Costa et al., 2010). The method is rapid, but it is still expensive. In order to address this problem and working with the specific-species genes of eight vegetable oils, Bai et al. (2011) demonstrated that an optical thin-film biosensor chip could be used as a simple, rapid, and sensitive way of specifically detecting trace amounts of DNA. Zougagh et al. (2011) proposed a colorimetric method based on the formation of gold nanoparticles (AuNPs) as a result of the redox reaction caused by phenolic compounds in virgin argan oils. The method is rapid, needs only a small amount of test material, and does not use toxic solvents (Tan et al., 1999). The objective in this study was to evaluate the adulteration of argan oil samples with olive and sunflower oils, using ferulic acid as a marker present in high concentrations in these oils in contrast to the other common oils in the marketplace. The formation of AuNPs resulted in color changes and strong absorption signals at about 555 nm. These results were confirmed using an HPLC-diode-array detector/fluorimetric detection method. This enabled samples to be classified as either adulterated or nonadulterated, but also provided quantitative information, albeit with low accuracy. This approach is characterized by simplicity, rapidity, and low cost. Karthik et al. (2014) investigated using a colorimetric method for detecting sunflower oil adulteration based on a change in absorption. They found that, even in combination with chemometrics, the detection of paraffin oil very light oil is not possible with a colorimeter, in contrast to the success of this method in detecting adulteration with palm oil. Palm oil is the main constituent of edible oils, contributing to 30% of world oil and fat production in 2012 (Mielke, 2013); it is dark yellow and is denser than sunflower oil. Sunflower is a fast-growing crop and its oil is very rich in linoleic acid, it is therapeutically very useful against high serum cholesterol and it has a good aroma. With the increase in demand, there has been a growth in the adulteration of sunflower oil, usually with cheaper saturated oils. Viscosity is an important property of edible oils that depends on molecular size, length, and temperature. The variation in viscosity and density between pure and adulterated edible oil products was used by Ebong et al. (2014) to detect adulteration, and results obtained showed sensitivity depending on the type of adulterant; variation tended to be detected above a 30% adulterant level. The density and viscosity values of pure and adulterated oil samples are very close, making the detection of adulteration using this method almost impossible. Other physical properties (such as refractive index, melting point, saponification, and iodine value) also appear not to be useful in the detection of adulteration (Azadmard-Damirchi and Torbati, 2015). As in the case of olive oil, thermophysical properties were used in the analysis of other vegetable oils. DSC is rapid, does not require sample preparation, and does not involve the use of solvents or toxic chemicals. It has been used in several studies reported by Marikkar et al. (2002a,b, 2003) for detecting animal fat in canola and palm olein, as well as for detecting enzymatically randomized lard in palm oil. Marina et al. (2009) used the technique for monitoring the adulteration of virgin coconut oil by palm kernel and soybean oils. The adulteration of virgin coconut oil with added oils ranged from 2% to 40% (w/w) of added oils; DSC cooling and heating thermograms were then used to monitor the adulteration. Regression analyses using stepwise multiple linear regression were used to predict the percentage of the adulterant. For added soybean oil, the quantification was based on a peak of melting curves, whereas for palm kernel oil (which did not show any adulteration peak) there was a good relationship between its main exothermic peak height (showing a gradual decrease) and the percentage of adulteration.

Marina et al. (2010) tested a SAW electronic nose for detecting the adulteration of virgin coconut oil by refined, bleached, and deodorized palm kernel olein at concentrations between 1% and 20% (w/w). The electronic nose was based on an SAW sensor used to generate a pattern of volatile compounds present in the sample. A linear regression model was then established between the chromatographic peak identified as methyl dodecanoate and the percentage of adulteration, showing a correlation coefficient of 0.91. A PCA score plot (which explained 74% of the variation in the data) revealed a distinction between adulterated and nonadulterated virgin coconut oil.

A new approach has recently been developed for detecting the presence of animal oil in food. This can be a problem for some communities for religious reasons, but it is also an economic problem, with vegetable oils being adulterated with animal oils in order to reduce production costs. He et al. (2014) proposed combining standard chemical methods with image texture analysis technology for detecting the adulteration of vegetable oils (soybean, corn germ, and sunflower seed oils) by animal fats (fresh lard, beef tallow, and chicken oil) (He et al., 2014). As the selected vegetable oils are free from cholesterol, this method was used to estimate animal oil content in vegetable oil. The comparison of the cholesterol content of adulterated oil samples using the proposed and standard chemical methods revealed a maximum relative error of cholesterol content of 3.5% (w/w); a significant correlation between the image texture feature parameters and cholesterol content ($R^2 = 0.99$) with an LOD of 6.5% was calculated. It was then possible, with image texture analysis technology, to detect vegetable oil adulteration using this application.

19.3 Conclusions and Future Trends

This chapter has provided an overview of analytical methods used to detect the adulteration of vegetable oils. The literature shows the continual development of methods to meet this analytical challenge. The methods can be seen as complementary. Chromatography, as a targeted technique, makes it possible to identify foreign molecules, but it destroys samples and uses solvents. Spectroscopy, as a nontargeted technique, preserves the sample, is environmentally friendly, detects changes in the overall complex of the pure oils matrix, and then detects adulteration. Other biomolecular (eg, PCR) or physical (eg, calorimetry or DSC) techniques are starting to be proposed as simple and rapid ways of detecting the adulteration of vegetable oils.

These studies are useful in understanding the methods and techniques used in adulteration analysis. They show the usefulness of a multicriterion approach for the analysis of vegetable oils and to address marketing and production issues in agribusiness. It is important that further work on the detection of vegetable oil adulteration is conducted with reference to the advances already achieved in order to find an efficient way of fighting against this fraud.

References

Abaitua, I., Posada, M., 1992. Toxic Oil Syndrome: Current Knowledge and Future Perspectives. In: European Series, vol. 42. WHO Regional Publication, Copenhagen, p. 27.

Al Zhair, H., Abd El-Fattah, A.A., Ibrahim El-Sayed, M., 2000. Pumpkin-seed oil modulates the effect of felodipine and captopril in spontaneously hypertensive rats. Pharmacological Research 41, 555–563.

Alipoor, B., Haghighian, M.K., Sadat, B.E., Asghari, M., 2012. Effect of sesame seed on lipid profile and redox status in hyperlipidemic patients. International Journal of Food Sciences and Nutrition 63, 674–678.

Alonso-Salces, R.M., Heberger, K., Holland, M.V., Moreno-Rojas, J.M., Mariani, C., Bellan, G., Reniero, F., Guillou, C., 2010. Multivariate analysis of NMR fingerprint of the unsaponifiable fraction of virgin olive oils for authentication purposes. Food Chemistry 118, 956–965.

Aparicio, R., Aparicio-Ruiz, R., 2000. Authentication of vegetable oils by chromatographic techniques. Journal of Chromatography 881, 93–104.

Aparicio, R., Baeten, V., 1998. Authentication of olive oil by FT-Raman. OCL 5, 14–16.

Aparicio-Ruiz, R., Harwood, J., 2013. Handbook of Olive Oil: Analysis and Properties, second ed. ISBN:978-1-4614-7776.

Aued-Pimentel, S., Alves Da Silva, S., Takemoto, E., Bonaldi Cano, C., 2013. Stigmastadiene and specific extinction (270 nm) to evaluate the presence of refined oils in virgin olive oil commercialized in Brazil. Food Science and Technology (Campinas) 33 (3).

Azadmard-Damirchi, S., Torbati, M., 2015. Adulterations in some edible oils and fats and their detection methods. Journal of Food Quality and Hazards Control 2, 38–44.

Baeten, V., Fernandez-Pierna, J.A., Dardenne, P., Meurens, M., Garcia-Gonzalez, D.L., Aparicio-Ruiz, R., 2005. Detection of the presence of hazelnut oil in olive oil by FT-Raman and FT-MIR spectroscopy. Journal of Agricultural and Food Chemistry 53, 6201–6206.

Baeten, V., Meurens, M., 1996. Detection of virgin olive oil adulteration by Fourier transform Raman spectroscopy. Journal of Agricultural and Food Chemistry 44 (8), 2225–2230.

Bai, S., Li, S., Yao, T., Hu, Y., Bao, F., Zhang, J., Zhang, Y., Zhu, S., He, Y., 2011. Rapid detection of eight vegetable oils on optical thin-film biosensor chips. Food Control 22, 1624–1628.

Bakre, S.M., Gadmale, D.K., Toche, R.B., Gaikwad, V.B., 2015. Rapid determination of alpha tocopherol in olive oil adulterated with sunflower oil by reversed phase high-performance liquid chromatography. Journal of Food Science and Technology 52 (5), 3093–3098.

Bell, J.R., Gillatt, P.N., 2004. Standards to Ensure the Authenticity of Edible Oil and Fats. FAO Corporate Document Repository. Online: http://www.fao.org/docrep/t4660t/t4660t0e.htm/.

Bonvehi, J.S., Col, F.V., 2009. Detecting vegetable oil adulteration in hazelnut paste (*Corylus avellana* L.). International Journal of Food Science & Technology 44 (3), 456–466.

Calvano, C.D., Aresta, A., Zambonin, C.G., 2010. Detection of hazelnut oil in extra-virgin olive oil by analysis of polar components by micro-solid phase extraction based on hydrophilic liquid chromatography and MALDI-ToF mass spectrometry. Journal of Mass Spectrometry 45 (9), 981–988.

Calvano, C.D., De Ceglie, C., D'accolti, L., Zambonin, C.G., 2012. MALDI-TOF mass spectrometry detection of extra-virgin olive oil adulteration with hazelnut oil by analysis of phospholipids using an ionic liquid as matrix and extraction solvent. Food Chemistry 134 (2), 1192–1198.

Cao, W., Sun, X., Chen, F., Xue, B., Chen, W., Jin, Q., Wang, X., 2012. China Oils and Fats 37, 1–5 (in Chinese).

Capote, F.P., Jiménez, J.R., De Castro, M.D., 2007. Sequential (step-by-step) detection, identification and quantitation of extra virgin olive oil adulteration by chemometric treatment of chromatographic profiles. Analytical and Bioanalytical Chemistry 388 (8), 1859–1865.

CBI Trade Statistics for Vegetable Oils, 2014. Online: http://www.cbi.eu/sites/default/files/study/trade-statistics-europe-vegetable-oils-2014.pdf/.

Cherki, M., Berrougui, H., Drissi, A., Adlouni, A., Khalil, A., 2006. Argan oil: which benefits on cardiovascular diseases? Pharmacological Research 54 (1), 5.

Chiavaro, E., Vittadini, E., Rodriguez-Estrada, M.T., Cerretani, L., Bendini, A., 2008. Differential scanning calorimeter application to the detection of refined hazelnut oil in extra virgin olive oil. Food Chemistry 110, 248–256.

Christy, A.A., Kasemsumran, S., Du, Y., Ozaki, Y., 2004. The detection and quantification of adulteration in olive oil by near-infrared spectroscopy and chemometrics. Analytical Sciences 20, 935–940.

Clemente, T.E., Cahoon, E.B., 2009. Soybean oil: genetic approaches for modification of functionality and total content. Plant Physiology 151, 1030–1040.

Codex Alimentarius Commission, 1987. Report of the Thirteenth Session of the Codex Committee on Fats and Oils (London).

Costa, J., Mafra, I., Amaral, J.S., Oliveira, M.B., 2010. Detection of genetically modified soybean DNA in refined vegetable oils. European Food Research and Technology 230, 915–923.

Crevel, R.W., Kerkhoff, M.A., Koning, M.M., 2000. Allergenicity of refined vegetable oils. Food and Chemical Toxicology 38 (4), 385–387.

Cuvelier, C., Dotreppe, O., Istasse, L., 2003. Chimie, sources alimentaires et dosage de la vitamine E. Annales de Médecine Vétérinaire 147 (5), 315–324.

Dalmia, A., Perkins, G.L., 2013. Shelton, CT USA, Application Note. Rapid Measurement of Olive Oil Adulteration With Soybean Oil With Minimal Sample Preparation Using DSA/TOF, Copyright ©2013. PerkinElmer, Inc. (All rights reserved).

Deineka, V.I., Deineka, L.A., 2004. Analysis of vegetable oils by microcolumn high-performance liquid chromatography. Journal of Analytical Chemistry 59 (9), 895–898.

Deng, D.H., Xu, L., Ye, Z.H., Cui, H.F., Cai, C.B., Yu, X.P., 2012. FTIR spectroscopy and chemometric class modeling techniques for authentication of Chinese sesame oil. Journal of the American Oil Chemists' Society 89, 1003–1009.

Ding, Q.Z., Liu, L.L., Wu, Y.W., Li, B.N., Ouyang, J., 2014. Authentication and adulteration analysis of sesame oil by FTIR spectroscopy. Guang Pu Xue Yu Guang Pu Fen Xi (Article in Chinese) 34 (10), 2690–2695.

Dong, W., Zhang, Y., Zhanga, B., Wang, X., 2012. Quantitative analysis of adulteration of extra virgin olive oil using Raman spectroscopy improved by Bayesian framework least squares support vector machines. Analytical Methods 4, 2772–2777.

Dong, W., Zhang, Y., Zhang, B., Wang, X., 2013. Rapid prediction of fatty acid composition of vegetable oil by Raman spectroscopy coupled with least squares support vector machines. Journal of Raman Spectroscopy 44, 1739–1745.

Ebong, S.T., Akpabio, G.T., Attai, E.S., Oji, H.E., 2014. Adulteration detection in some edible oil products in Nigeria. International Journal of Research Studies in Science, Engineering and Technology 1 (4), 68–72.

Eisenbrand, G., 2007. Isoflavones as phytoestrogens in food supplements and dietary foods for special medical purposes. Molecular Nutrition & Food Research 51, 1305–1312.

Eisner, J., Iverson, J.L., Mozingo, A.K., Firestone, D., 1965. Gas chromatography of unsaponifiable matter. III. Identification of hydrocarbons, aliphatic alcohols, tocopherols, triterpenoid alcohols, and sterols present in olive oils. Journal of AOAC International 48, 417–433.

El-Abassy, R.M., Donfack, P., Materny, A., 2009. Visible Raman spectroscopy for the discrimination of olive oils from different vegetable oils and the detection of adulteration. Journal of Raman Spectroscopy 40 (9), 1284–1289.

Elbashbashy, E.M.A., Ibrahim, F.N., 1993. Steady free convention flow with variable viscosity and thermal diffusivity along a vertical plate. Journal of Physics and Applied Physics 26, 2137–2143.

Esslinger, S., Riedl, J., Fauhl-Hassek, C., 2014. Potential and limitations of non-targeted fingerprinting for authentication of food in official control. Food Research International 60, 189–204.

European Community, 2001. Commission regulation No. 1513/2001 of 23 July 2001 amending regulations No. 136/66/EEC. Official Journal of the European Communities L201, 4–7.

Flores, G., Ruiz-Del Castillo, M.L., Blanch, G.P., Herraiz, M., 2006. Detection of the adulteration of olive oils by solid phase microextraction and multidimensional gas chromatography. Food Chemistry 97, 336–342.

Funasaki, M., Oliveira, R.S., Zanotto, S.P., Carioca, C.R.F., Simas, R.C., Eberlin, M.N., Alberici, R.M., 2012. Brazil nut oil: quality control via triacylglycerol profiles provided by easy ambient sonic-spray ionization mass spectrometry. Journal of Agricultural and Food Chemistry 60, 11263–11267.

García-González, D., Mannia, L., D'imperio, M., Segre, A.L., Aparicio, R., 2004. Using 1H and 13C NMR techniques and artificial neural networks to detect the adulteration of olive oil with hazelnut. European Food Research and Technology 219, 545–548.

Gary, R.T., Ebeler, S.E., 2011. Progress in authentication of food and wine. In: Gary, R.T., Ebeler, S.E., Winterhalter, P. (Eds.), Progress in Authentication of Food and Wine. American Chemical Society.

Giménez, M.J., Pistón, F., Martín, A., Atienza, S.G., 2010. Application of real-time PCR on the development of molecular markers and to evaluate critical aspects for olive oil authentication. Food Chemistry 118, 482–487.

Gonzalez, D.R., Aparicio, R., 2002. Detection of defective virgin oils by metal oxide sensors. Journal of Agricultural and Food Chemistry 50 (7), 1809–1814.

Gonzálvez, A., Armenta, S., Guardia, M., 2010. Adulteration detection of argan oil by inductively coupled plasma optical emission spectrometry. Food Chemistry 121, 878–886.

Gopala Krishna, A.G., 2008. Nutritional components of rice bran oil in relation to processing. Lipid Technology 14, 80–84.

Guimet, F., Ferré, J., Boqué, R., 2005. Rapid detection of olive-pomace oil adulteration in extra virgin olive oils from the protected denomination of origin 'Siurana' using excitation-emission fluorescence spectroscopy and three way methods of analysis. Analytica Chimica Acta 544, 143–152.

Gurdeniz, G., Ozen, B., 2009. Detection of adulteration of extra-virgin olive oil by chemometric analysis of mid-infrared spectral data. Food Chemistry 116, 519–525.

He, P., Wan, X., Wang, C., Jiao, Y., 2014. Determination of animal oil added in vegetable oil by standard chemical method coupled with image texture analysis technology. International Journal of Innovative Computing, Information and Control 10 (1), 67–80.

Hidalgo, F.J., Zamora, R., 2003. Edible oil analysis by high-resolution nuclear magnetic resonance spectroscopy: recent advances and future perspectives. Trends in Food Science & Technology 14, 499–506.

Hilali, H., Charrouf, Z., Soulhi, A., Hachimi, L., Guillaume, D., 2007. Detection of argan oil adulteration using quantitative campesterol GC-analysis. Journal of the American Oil Chemists' Society 84, 761–764.

Houshia, O.J.R., Zaid, O., Shqair, H., Zaid, M., Fashafsheh, N., Bzoor, R., 2014. Effect of olive oil adulteration on peroxide value, Delta-K and on the acidity Nabali-Baladi olive oil quality. Advances in Life Sciences 4 (5), 235–244.

Huang, J., Xiong, H., Li, L., Luo, C., 2008. China Oils and Fats 33, 70–74 (in Chinese).

Jee, M., 2002. Adulteration and authentication of oils and fats: an overview. In: Jee, M. (Ed.), Oils and Fats Authentication. CRC Press.

Jyothi, B., Ansari, N.A., Vijay, Y., Anuradha, G., Sarkar, A., Sudhakar, R., Siddiq, E.A., 2011. Assessment of resistance to Fusarium wilt disease in sesame (*Sesamum indicum* L.) germplasm. Australasian Plant Pathology 40, 471–475.

Karthik, D., Vijayarekha, K., Manickkam, V., 2014. A simple method for detecting adulteration in sunflower oil using chemometry. Rasayan Journal of Chemistry 7 (1), 99–103.

Kojima, Y., Parcell, J.L., Cain, J.S., 2014. A demand model of the wholescale vegetable oils market in the Usa. In: Southern Agricultural Economics Association (SAEA) Annual Meeting, Dallas, Texas, 1–4 February.

Kumar, S., Kahlon, T., Chaudhary, S., 2011. A rapid screening for adulterants in olive oil using DNA barcodes. Food Chemistry 127, 1335–1341.

Lees, M., 2003. In: Lees, M. (Ed.), Food Authenticity and Traceability. Woodhead Publishing, France. Eurofins.

Lerma-Garcia, M.J., Ramis-Ramos, G., Herrero-Martinez, J.M., Simon-Alfonso, E.F., 2010. Authentication of extra virgin olive oils by Fourier-transform infrared spectroscopy. Food Chemistry 118, 78–83.

Liu, C.M., Zheng, G.H., Ming, Q.L., Chao, C., Sun, J.M., 2013. Sesamin protects mouse liver against nickel-Induced oxidative DNA damage and apoptosis by the PI3K-Akt pathway. Journal of Agricultural and Food Chemistry 61, 1146–1154.

Lizhi, H., Toyoda, K., Ihara, I., 2010. Discrimination of olive oil adulterated with vegetable oils using dielectric spectroscopy. Journal of Food Engineering 96 (2), 167–171.

Che Man, Y.B., Abdul Karim, M.I.B., Teng, C.T., 1997. Extraction of coconut oil with *Lactobacillus plantarum* 1041 IAM. Journal of the American Oil Chemists' Society 74, 1115–1119.

Mannina, L., D'imperio, M., Capitani, D., Rezzi, S., Guillou, C., Mavromoustakos, T., Vilchez, M.D.M., Fernandez, A.H., Thomas, F., Aparicio, R., 2009. 1H NMR-based protocol for the detection of adulterations of refined olive oil with refined hazelnut oil. Journal of Agricultural and Food Chemistry 57, 11550–11556.

Mansor, T.S.T., Che Man, Y.B., Rohman, A., 2011. Application of fast gas chromatography and Fourier transform infrared spectroscopy for analysis of lard adulteration in virgin coconut oil. Food Analytical Methods 4 (3), 365–372.

Marikkar, J.M.N., Ghazali, H.M., Che Man, Y.B., Lai, O.M., 2003. Differential scanning calorimetric analysis for determination of some animal fats as adulterants in palm olein. Journal of Food Lipids 10, 63–79.

Marikkar, J.M.N., Lai, O.M., Ghazali, H.M., Che Man, Y.B., 2002a. Compositional and thermal analysis of RBD palm oil adulterated with lipase-catalyzed inter-esterified lard. Food Chemistry 76, 249–258.

Marikkar, J.M.N., Ghazali, H.M., Che Man, Y.B., Lai, O.M., 2002b. The use of cooling and heating thermograms for monitoring of tallow, lard, and chicken fat adulterations in canola oil. Food Research International 35, 1007–1014.

Marikkar, J.M.N., Ghazali, H.M., Che Man, Y.B., Peiris, T.S.G., Lai, O.M., 2005. Use of gas liquid chromatography in combination with pancreatic lipolysis and multivariate data analysis techniques for identification of lard contamination in some vegetable oils. Food Chemistry 90, 23–30.

Marina, A.M., Che Man, Y.B., Amin, I., 2010. Use of the SAW sensor electronic nose for detecting the adulteration of virgin coconut oil with RBD palm kernel olein. Journal of Oil & Fat Industries 87 (3), 263–270.

Marina, A.M., Che Man, Y.B., Nazimah, S.A.H., Amin, I., 2009. Monitoring the adulteration of virgin coconut oil by selected vegetable oils using differential scanning calorimetry. Journal of Food Lipids 16, 50–61.

Marina, A.M., Che Man, Y.B., Nazimah, S.A.H., Amin, I., Syahariza, Z.A., 2007. Analysis of adulteration of virgin coconut oil by palm kernel olein using Fourier transform infrared spectroscopy. Journal of Food Lipids 14, 111–121.

Martinez-Palou, A., Rohner-Thielen, E., 2011. Statistics in Focus 62/2011. Online: Eurostat Website: http://ec.europa.eu/eurostat/.

Method of analysis spectrophotometric investigation in the ultraviolet. In: International Olive Council, COI/T20/Doc. No. 19/Rev. 3, 2010. Online: http://www.internationaloliveoil.org/.

Mielke, T., 2013. Palm oil the leader in global oils and fats supply. In: Paper Presented at the Malaysia/Myanmar Palm Oil Trade Fair and Seminar. Yangoon, Myanmar, June 28, 2014. Online: http://www.mpoc.org.my/upload/Plenary_Paper-Thomas-Mielke.pdf.

Mignani, A.G., Ciaccheri, L., Ottevaere, H., Thienpont, H., Conte, L., Marega, M., Cichelli, A., Attilio, C., Cimato, A., 2011. Visible and near-infrared absorption spectroscopy by an integrating sphere and optical fibers for quantifying and discriminating the adulteration of extra virgin olive oil from Tuscany. Analytical and Bioanalytical Chemistry 399 (3), 1315–1324.

Mildner-Szkudlarz, S., Jelen, H.H., 2008. The potential of different techniques for volatile compounds analysis coupled with PCA for the detection of the adulteration of olive oil with hazelnut oil. Food Chemistry 110, 751–761.

Mili, S., Rodríguez-Zuñiga, M., 2001. Exploring future developments in international olive oil trade and marketing: a Spanish perspective. Agribusiness: An International Journal 17 (3), 397–415.

MoniQA, 2013. Food Authenticity d General Considerations. Online: http://www.moniqa.eu/authenticity/.

Nam, Y.S., Noh, K.C., Roh, E.J., Keum, G., Lee, Y., Lee, K.B., 2014. Determination of edible vegetable oil adulterants in sesame oil using 1H nuclear magnetic resonance spectroscopy. Analytical Letters 47 (7), 1190–1200.

Naveen, R.E., Pavan, A., Bindu, G., Thejaswi, S., Sunitha, G., 2013. Edible oil scenario in India-demand-supply gap, dietary needs and adulteration menace. Antharmukha 23–27.

Ness, A., 2002. Commentary: is olive oil a key ingredient in the Mediterranean recipe for health? International Journal of Epidemiology 31 (2), 481–482.

Nestle, M., 1995. Mediterranean diets: historical and research overview. The American Journal of Clinical Nutrition 61 (6), 1313–1320.

Nevin, K.G., Rajamohan, T., 2004. Beneficial effects of virgin coconut oil on lipid parameters and in vitro LDL oxidation. Clinical Biochemistry 37 (9), 830–835.

Odl, J., 1997. New insight into the utilization of medium-chain triglycerides by the neonate: observation from a piglet model. Journal of Nutrition 127, 1061–1067.

Oilseeds, 2014. Oilseeds, Oils & Meals-Monthly Price and Policy Update, FAO-Trade and-Markets Division, vol. 59, pp. 1–12. Online: http://www.fao.org/fileadmin/templates/est/COMM_MARKETS_MONITORING/Oilcrops/Documents/MPPU_May__14.pdf.

Oliveros, C.M., Pavon, J.L., Pinto, C.G., Laespada, F.M.E., Cordero, B.M., Forina, M., 2002. Electronic nose based on metal oxide semiconductor sensors as a fast alternative for the detection of adulteration of virgin olive oils. Analytica Chimica Acta 459 (2), 219–228.

Ourracha, I., Radab, M., Pérez-Caminob, M.C., Benaissaa, M., Guinda, Á., 2012. Detection of argan oil adulterated with vegetable oils: new markers. Grasas Y Aceites 63 (4), 355–364.

Pandurangan, M.K., Murugesan, S., Gajivaradhan, P., 2014. Application of FTIR spectroscopy to assess the groundnut oil adulteration. Journal of Chemical and Pharmaceutical Research 6 (8), 553–560.

Patricio, J., Richardson, D.G., Rafecas, M., Codony, R., Boatella, J., 1997. Fatty acid distribution in polar and non-polar lipid classes of classes of hazelnut (*Corylus avellana* L.). Journal of Agricultural and Food Chemistry 45, 3887.

Peña, F., Cárdenas, S., Gallego, M., Valcárcel, M., 2005. Direct olive oil authentication: detection of adulteration of olive oil with hazelnut oil by direct coupling of headspace and mass spectrometry, and multi-variate techniques. Journal of Chromatography 1074, 215–221.

Piravi Vanak, Z., Ghasemi, J.B., Ghavami, M., Ezzatpanah, H., 2010. Detection and quantification of adulteration in olive oils by global method and extinction coefficient. Australian Journal of Basic and Applied Sciences 4 (12), 6254–6259.

Posada De La Paz, M., Philen, R.M., Abaitua Borda, I., Sicilia Socias, J.M., Gomez De La Camara, A., Kilbourne, E.M., 1996. Toxic oil syndrome: trace back of the toxic oil and evidence for a point source epidemic. Food Chemistry and Toxicology 34, 251–257.

Poulli, K.I., Mousdi, G.A., Georgiou, C.A., 2006. Synchronous fluorescence spectroscopy for quantitative determination of virgin olive oil adulteration with sunflower oil. Analytical and Bioanalytical Chemistry 386, 1571–1575.

Ramon-Muñoz, R., 2000. Specialization in the international market for olive oil before World War II. In: Pamuk, S., Williamson, J.G. (Eds.), The Mediterranean Response to Globalization Before 1950. Routledge, London/New York, pp. 159–198.

Rohman, A., Che Man, Y.B., Hashim, P., Ismail, A., 2011. FTIR spectroscopy combined with chemometrics for analysis of lard adulteration in some vegetable oils. CyTA Journal of Food 9, 96–101.

Rohman, A., Man, Y.B.C., 2010. Fourier transform infrared (FTIR) spectroscopy for analysis of extra virgin olive oil adulterated with palm oil. Food Research International 43, 886–892.

Rohman, A., Man, Y.B.C., 2012. The chemometrics approach applied to FTIR spectral data for the analysis of rice bran oil in extra virgin olive oil. Chemometrics and Intelligent Laboratory Systems 110, 129–134.

Rossell, J.B., 1998. Development of purity criteria for edible vegetable oils. In: Hamilton, R.J. (Ed.), Lipid Analysis in Oils and Fats London. Blackie Academic and Professional, pp. 265–289.

Salunkhe, D.K., Chavan, J.K., Adsule, R.N., Kadam, S.S., 1992. World Oilseeds: Chemistry Technology and Utilization. Van Nostrand Reinhold, New York.

Sayago, A., Morales, M.T., Aparicio, R., 2004. Detection of hazelnut oil in virgin olive oil by a spectrofluorimetric method. European Food Research and Technology 218, 480–483.

Scheidel, A., Krausmann, F., 2011. Diet, trade and land use: a socio-ecological analysis of the transformation of the olive oil system. Land Use Policy 28, 47–56.

Schiebel-Schlosser, G., Friederich, M., 1998. Phytotherapy of BPH with pumpkin seeds – a multicentric clinical trial. zeitschrift-fur-Phytotherapie 19, 71–76.

Siskos, Y., Matsatsinis, N.F., Baourakis, G., 2001. Multicriteria analysis in agricultural marketing: the case of French olive oil market. European Journal of Operational Research 130, 315–331.

Smejkalova, D., Piccolo, A., 2010. High-power gradient diffusion NMR spectroscopy for the rapid assessment of extra-virgin olive oil adulteration. Food Chemistry 118, 153–158.

Sobolev, V.S., Cole, R.J., 1999. Trans-resveratrol content in commercial peanuts and peanut products. Journal of Agricultural Food Chemistry 47, 1435–1439.

Tan, C.P., Che Man, Y.B., 1999. Differential scanning calorimetric analysis for monitoring the oxidation of heated oils. Food Chemistry 67, 177–184.

Tasdogan, C., Tsakiridou, E., Mattas, K., 2005. Country market power in EU olive oil trade. South-Eastern Europe Journal of Economics 2, 211–219.

Tashiro, T., Fukuda, Y., Osawa, T., Namiki, M., 1990. Oil and minor components of sesame (*Sesamum indicum* L.) strains. Journal of the American Oil Chemists' Society 67, 508–511.

Torrecilla, J.S., 2010. The Olive – Its Processing and Waste Management. Nova Publishers, New York.

Torrecilla, J.S., García, J., García, S., Rodríguez, F., 2011a. Quantification of adulterant agents in extra virgin olive oil by models based on its thermophysical properties. Journal of Food Engineering 103 (2), 211–218.

Torrecilla, J.S., Rojo, E., Domínguez, J.C., Rodríguez, F., 2010. A novel method to quantify the adulteration of extra virgin olive oil with low-grade olive oils by UV-vis. Journal of Agricultural and Food Chemistry 58 (3), 1679–1684.

Torrecilla, J.S., García, J., García, S., Rodríguez, F., 2011b. Application of lag-k autocorrelation coefficient and the TGA signals approach to detecting and quantifying adulterations of extra virgin olive oil with inferior edible oils. Analytical Chimica Acta 688 (2), 140–145.

Unesco, 2007. Biosphere Reserve Information. MAB Programme.

Vigli, G., Philippidis, A., Spyros, A., Dais, P., 2003. Classification of edible oils by employing 31P and 1H NMR spectroscopy in combination with multivariate statistical analysis. A proposal for the detection of seed oil adulteration in virgin olive oils. Journal of Agricultural and Food Chemistry 51, 5715–5722.

Wenzl, T., Prettner, E., Schweiger, K., Wagner, F.S., 2002. An improved method to discover adulteration of Styrian pumpkin seed oil. Journal of Biochemical and Biophysical Methods 53, 193–202.

Xu, L., Xu, X., Xiong, H., Chen, L., Li, Y., 2014. Rapid detection of vegetable cooking oils adulterated with inedible used oil using fluorescence quenching method with aqueous CTAB-coated quantum dots. Sensors and Actuators B Chemical 203, 697–704.

Xuebao, N.J., 2012. Analysis of sesame oil adulteration using near infrared transmission spectroscopy. Transactions of the Chinese Society of Agricultural Machinery 43 (7).

Yang, J., 2009. Brazil nuts and associated health benefits: a review. LWT – Food Science and Technology 42, 1573–1580.

Yu, F., Chen, X., Lin, Q., Tan, J., Xiao, H., Xiaojun, W., 2013. Determination of rice bran oil adulterated with palm oil. Advances in Information Sciences and Service Sciences (AISS) 5, 5.

Yu, F.-X., Lin, Q.-L., Chen, X., et al., 2012. Analysis on fatty acids of crude rice bran oil from main rice region in China. Food Industry 33 (8), 156–158.

Zamora, R., Alba, V., Hidalgo, F.J., 2001. Use of high-resolution 13C nuclear magnetic resonance spectroscopy for the screening of virgin olive oils. Journal of the American Oil Chemists' Society 78, 89–94.

Zhang, Q., Liu, C., Sun, Z., Hu, X., Shen, Q., Wu, J., 2012. Authentication of edible vegetable oils adulterated with used frying oil by Fourier transform infrared spectroscopy. Food Chemistry 132, 1607–1613.

Zhao, X., Maa, F., Li, P., Li, G., Zhang, L., Zhang, Q., Zhang, W., Wanga, X., 2015. Simultaneous determination of isoflavones and resveratrols for adulteration detection of soybean and peanut oils by mixed-mode SPE LC–MS/MS. Food Chemistry 176, 465–471.

Zou, M., Zhang, X., Qi, X., Ma, H., Dong, Y., Liu, C., Guo, X., Wang, H., 2009. Rapid authentication of olive oil adulteration by Raman spectrometry. Journal of Agricultural and Food Chemistry 57, 6001–6006.

Zougagh, M., Salghi, R., Dhair, S., Rios, A., 2011. Nanoparticle-based assay for the detection of virgin argan oil adulteration and its rapid quality evaluation. Analytical and Bioanalytical Chemistry 399, 2395–2405.

Advances in the Identification of Genetically Modified Foods

20

M.-A. Fraiture [1], *S. Broeders* [1], *P. Herman* [1], *I. Taverniers* [2], *M. De Loose* [2], *D. Deforce* [3], *N.H. Roosens* [1]
[1]Scientific Institute of Public Health, Brussels, Belgium; [2]Institute for Agricultural and Fisheries Research (ILVO), Merelbeke, Belgium; [3]Ghent University, Ghent, Belgium

Chapter Outline

20.1 Introduction

In 2014, the planting of 181.5 million hectares of genetically modified organisms (GMOs) by 18 million farmers in 28 countries was reported (James, 2014). To guarantee the traceability of the food/feed chain and the freedom of choice for the consumer, legislations concerning the detection and quantification of GMOs have been established by the relevant competent authorities worldwide (Kamle et al., 2013). In this respect, several strategies, classified as indirect (protein-based methods) or direct (DNA-based methods), have been developed (Mazzara et al., 2013; Morisset et al., 2008a). DNA-based methods, especially the real-time polymerase chain reaction (qPCR) technology, are generally favored because of their higher sensitivity and more exact quantification. The qPCR technique allows the analyst not only to screen for genetically modified (GM) elements but also to identify the integrated transgenic cassette as well as to quantify the GM event (Broeders et al., 2012a).

However, with the increasing amount of GMOs brought to the market, the necessity to identify GMOs present at trace levels (EC/619/2011 on low level presence (LLP) of GMO in feed) and the growing possible presence of GMOs that are authorized in one country but not in another, the herein-mentioned methods are no longer sufficient (Commission Regulation (EC) No. 619/2011). In order to strengthen the qPCR analysis in GMO routine analysis, a DNA walking strategy was recently developed to unequivocally prove the presence of GMOs in food and feed samples via the identification and characterization of sequences of the transgene flanking regions and unnatural element combinations (Fraiture et al., 2014, 2015a,b).

Here, the use of qPCR for GMO identification as currently performed is described and different theoretical outcomes typically encountered by the enforcement laboratories are reported. In addition, alternative DNA-based approaches for the identification of GMOs that may be used in combination with qPCR are illustrated. Furthermore, we discuss the potential application, including advantages and disadvantages in routine GMO analysis, of several other technologies, such as loop-mediated isothermal amplification (LAMP), PCR capillary gel electrophoresis (CGE), microarray, Luminex, digital PCR (dPCR), and next-generation sequencing (NGS) (Fraiture et al., 2015c).

20.2 Processes Used for Identification of Genetically Modified Foods

Classically, GMO routine analysis is performed using qPCR technology to detect, identify, and quantify GM events (Fig. 20.1) (Angers-Loustau et al., 2014). With the help of a specific primer pair, the sequence of interest is amplified and the corresponding fluorescence, emitted by using either the asymmetrical cyanine dye binding to double-stranded DNA (SYBRGreen chemistry) or a fluorogenic probe specific to the targeted sequence (TaqMan chemistry), is recorded in real time (Navarro et al., 2015). GMO routine analysis is commonly composed of three successive steps (Broeders et al., 2012a). The potential presence of GMOs is first determined by qPCR screening. To this end, sequences recurrently found in GMOs, eg, 35S promoter (p35S) from the *Cauliflower Mosaic Virus* and nopaline synthase terminator (tNOS) from *Agrobacterium tumefaciens*, are employed. The additional use of taxon-specific targets as well as more discriminating markers targeting single transgenic regions (less frequent elements or specific constructs) permit a reduction in the number of subsequent analysis required (Angers-Loustau et al., 2014; Broeders et al., 2012a, 2015; Fraiture et al., 2014). The outcome of this analysis, based on the positive and negative signals observed, is a list of all GM events potentially present in the sample being tested. Next, in order to identify the GM events truly present in the sample under investigation, the related event-specific methods, targeting the junction between the transgenic cassette and the plant genome, are applied (Broeders et al., 2012a). Finally, identified GM events are quantified using the corresponding event-specific and taxon-specific methods (Broeders et al., 2012a). In the European Union (EU), the

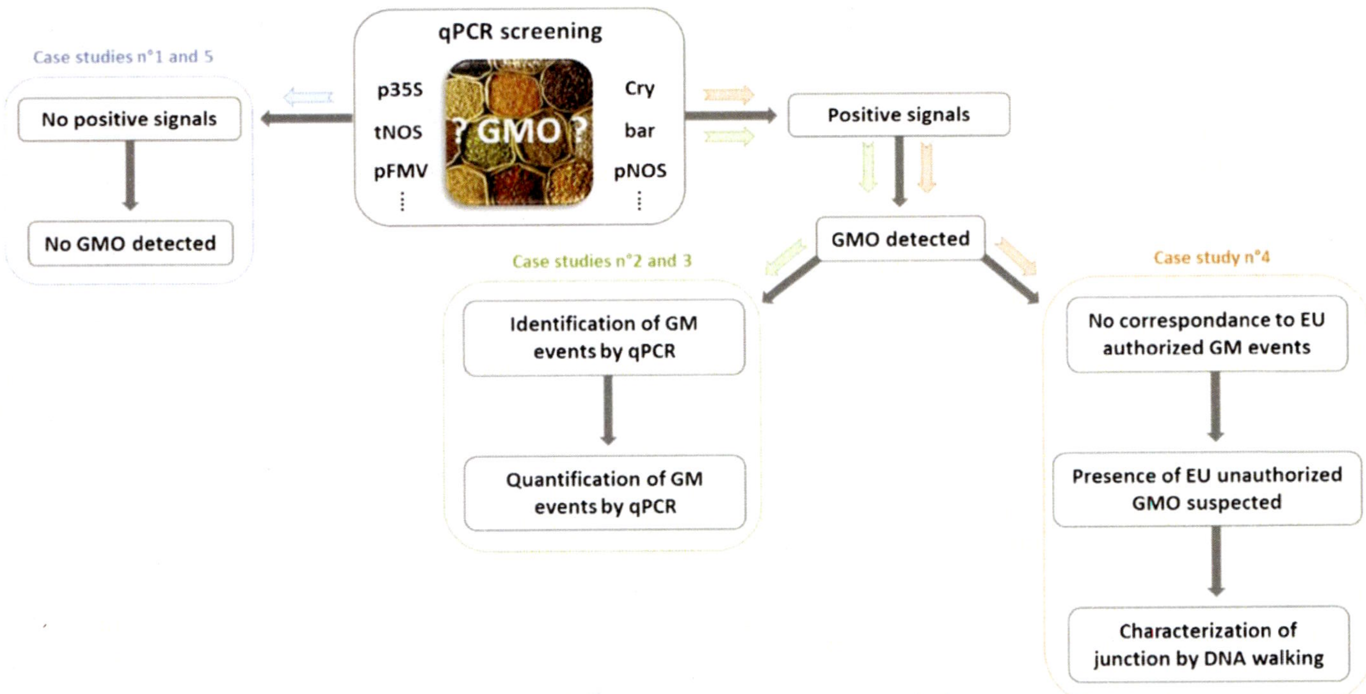

Figure 20.1 Traditional GMO routine analysis workflow. The case studies described in Section 20.3 are indicated in blue (n°1 and 5), green (n°2 and 3) and orange (n°4).

event-specific qPCR methods used by enforcement laboratories have been validated at EU level in agreement with the established document "Minimum Performance Requirements for Analytical Methods of GMO Testing" and are reported in the Compendium of reference methods for GMO analysis (ENGL, 2015; JCR GMOMETHODS). To facilitate the application of this workflow and to reduce the time frame of the analysis, a 96-well, prespotted plate, including several taxon-specific, event-specific, and construct-specific TaqMan methods, was developed by the EU Reference Laboratory for GM Food and Feed allowing the simultaneous identification of 39 GM events (Querci et al., 2010).

Besides the fact that the rising number of GMOs to be identified renders the laboratory work more time consuming, analysis of the qPCR data is also intensified. This can be simplified by using analytical tools simultaneously integrating the results of several methods. For instance, Combinatory SYBRGreen qPCR Screening (CoSYPS) is a practical decision support system that allows the analyst to quickly determine which GMO is potentially present in a sample and should thus further be identified and eventually quantified. This system is based on the introduction of the experimentally obtained C_q and, in case of SYBRGreen chemistry, T_m values that are then compared to the corresponding data obtained during in-house validation (screening) and verification (event-specific methods) of the methods. Currently, CoSYPS includes data for the 20 SYBRGreen taxon-, element-, and construct-specific screening methods developed by the Scientific Institute of Public Health in Belgium (WIV-ISP) as well as for all EU-authorized GMO and LLP cases (Broeders et al., 2012a; Commission Regulation (EC) No. 619/2011; Van den Bulcke et al., 2010). Alternatively, systems, such as GMOseek and GMOfinder databases, allow, on the basis of name of the positive elements observed, giving rise to a theoretical list of the GM events potentially present in the sample. These results have, however, to be analyzed with prudence since dissimilar sequences are sometimes named identically (Block et al., 2013; Gerdes et al., 2012). Recently, the JRC-GMO-Matrix has been developed to generate the list of GM events potentially present by integrating experimental positive and negative signals from EU-validated methods (Angers-Loustau et al., 2014; JRC-GMO-Matrix).

Nevertheless, the approach described herein still presents certain limitations. First, taking into account that usually only one method per reaction is used, the laboratory work could become quite laborious and complex, especially due to the growing number of GMOs (Broeders et al., 2012b). Second, as the qPCR strategy is based on knowledge of the targeted sequences, the presence and quantity of only GMOs for which the elements of the transgenic cassette (screening) and the junction sequence (identification and quantification) are known can be assessed. In addition, the validated EU-event-specific methods are only available for EU authorized GM events. This implicates that when the observed screening signals cannot be explained by the presence of EU-authorized GM events, the presence of unknown/unauthorized GMO can only be suspected (Fraiture et al., 2014). Third, certified reference materials (CRMs), mandatory for the quantification step, are also only available for the EU-authorized GM events (Broeders et al., 2012a; Fraiture et al., 2014; Holst-Jensen et al., 2012). Finally, due to the sensitivity of qPCR to inhibitors that may negatively affect its efficiency (eg, polysaccharides, polyphenols, pectin, xylan, or fat), the quantity of GMO may be underestimated or even remain undetected (Demeke et al., 2010; Opel et al., 2010; Schrader et al., 2012). There is thus a need for several complementary and alternative methods to circumvent these drawbacks of singleplex qPCR methods and render GMO analysis more efficient and effective.

20.2.1 Multiplex qPCR Strategy

To deal with the growing number of GMOs and the established one-by-one detection strategy, multiplex qPCR TaqMan methods were developed that allow the detection of several targets in one reaction. Even if most of them combine only two or three markers, tetraplex, pentaplex, and even hexaplex qPCR have also been elaborated (eg, Bahrdt et al., 2010; Chaouachi et al., 2014; Cottenet et al., 2013; Dörries et al., 2010; Huber et al., 2013; Köppel et al., 2014, 2015; Park et al., 2015; Samson et al., 2013; Waiblinger et al., 2008). However, the development of multiplex qPCR assays is not straightforward and several factors should be taken into account. In addition, the establishment of multiplex assays with similar performance (eg, sensitivity and specificity) to singleplex qPCR assays could be complicated. Moreover, the throughput of this strategy is limited by the inherent properties of the qPCR technology, which implies that fluorescence emitted by the dyes coupled to each marker should be sufficiently distinct, a factor that is also restrained by the current brand of qPCR instruments (Bahrdt et al., 2010; JCR GMOMETHODS).

20.2.2 DNA Walking

In the case that positive signals obtained in the qPCR screening step cannot be explained by EU-authorized events, the presence of unknown/unauthorized GM events can be determined by the DNA walking technique (Fraiture et al. (2014, 2015a) and references therein; Fraiture et al. (2015b) and references therein). Indeed, this technique allows characterization of unknown nucleotide sequences adjacent to already known DNA regions in any given genome. Even though several DNA walking methods have already been suggested to characterize transgenic plants, most of them could not easily be implemented in GMO routine analysis due to their experimental complexity as well as insufficient specificity, sensitivity, or yield. A rapid, simple, and cost-effective DNA walking strategy was thus developed and validated on both processed and unprocessed food matrices containing minute amounts of GM targets (Fraiture et al. (2014, 2015a) and references therein; Fraiture et al. (2015b) and references therein). Following qPCR screening, a PCR amplification is carried out using primers specific to the known sequence of the detected transgenic element(s) combined with degenerated random primers. With the aim of increasing the yield and specificity of the GM targets, two successive seminested PCR analyses are then performed. The purified final PCR products are subsequently sequenced using Sanger or NGS platforms and analyzed using available databases (eg, NCBI and JRC GMO-Amplicons) (Fraiture et al. (2014) and references therein; JRC GMO-Amplicons). The characterized transgene flanking regions and unnatural combinations of transgenic elements will prove the presence of GMO in the tested food/feed matrix beyond any doubt. Subsequently, these sequences can also be used to develop new event-specific qPCR methods. Moreover, as the same primers are used for the qPCR screening (potential detection of GMO) and the DNA walking (GMO identification), the present DNA walking system can be fully integrated into routine GMO analysis. Nowadays, in order to cover a broad range of GMOs, this DNA walking strategy has been developed to target the t35S sequence as found in the pCAMBIA vectors, frequently observed in EU-unauthorized GMOs, as well as the p35S and tNOS sequences, commonly used in EU-authorized and EU-unauthorized GMOs (Fraiture et al. (2014, 2015a) and references therein; Fraiture et al. (2015b) and references therein).

20.3 Case Studies

On the basis of results obtained in the qPCR screening step, subsequent analysis can present some variations (Fig. 20.1). To illustrate this, theoretical case studies of typical outcomes observed in GMO routine analysis are described next.

First, the simplest situation is encountered when only taxon-specific markers give a positive and specific amplification signal with none of the transgenic screening markers tested, designed to cover at least all EU-authorized GM events and LLP cases, being detected (Case study n°1 in Fig. 20.1). This means that no GM events containing the targeted sequences are present at a reliable detection level and no further analysis is thus undertaken. This case study highlights here the importance of the screening step, composed of markers targeting a broad spectrum of GMOs, to determine their presence or absence in any given sample.

Second, matrices like raw and unprocessed materials are usually composed of only one plant species, indicated by the observation of only one positive taxon-specific marker. Similarly to case study n°1, screening methods that cover a broad range of GMOs are applied to the tested sample to determine the presence of GMOs. When positive signals corresponding to transgenic elements are found, all the event-specific methods targeting EU-authorized GM events and LLP cases potentially present for the identified species are tested in a subsequent identification step (Case study n°2 in Fig. 20.1). However, depending on the identified species, this list may vary currently from one (eg, rice species that includes only the LLRICE62 event) to 18 (eg, maize species) required identifications. Therefore, more discriminative screening methods are further used to decrease the number of reactions needed to be carried out downstream (Fig. 20.2A). For instance, when the rapeseed species is detected, 10 EU-authorized GM events or LLP cases can be suspected. In the situation where only p35S and tNOS screening methods, known to target a broad spectrum of GMOs, are applied, seven GM events are still required to be identified. With the help of more discriminative screening methods, this list of GM rapeseed events can be reduced. If, among the panel of screening methods, a positive signal is only observed for the gat-tpinII method, the list of 10 GM rapeseed events potentially present is

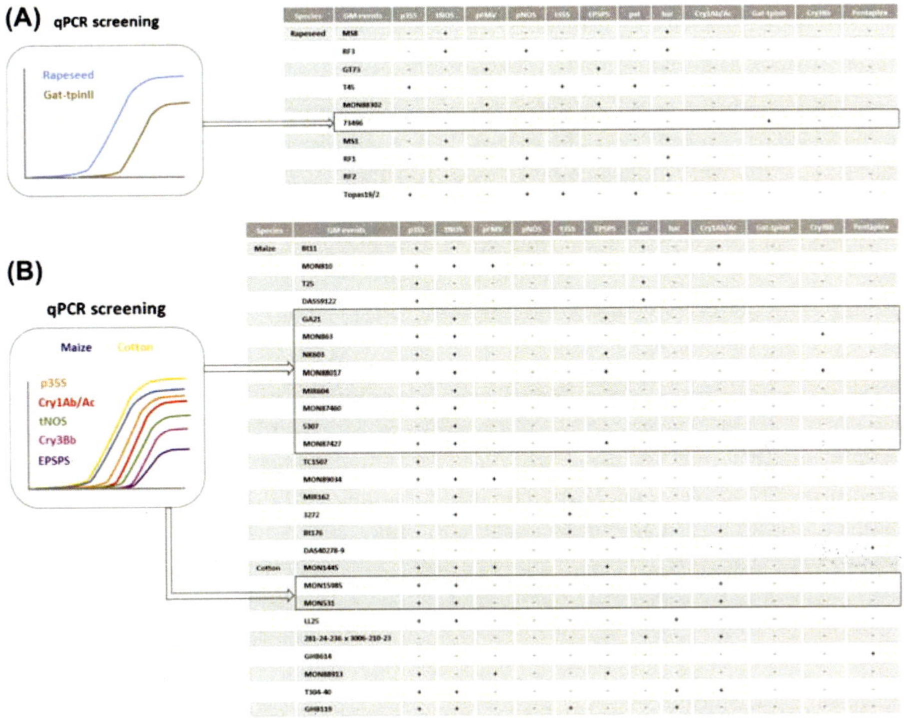

Figure 20.2 Examples of results encountered with EU-authorized GM events and LLP cases in routine GMO analysis: Case studies n°2 (A) and n°3 (B). For each matrix tested, positive signals observed in qPCR screening analysis for rapeseed species (light-blue), cotton species (yellow), maize species (dark-blue), gat-tpinII (brown), p35S (orange), tNOS (green), Cry1Ab/Ac (red), Cry3Bb (dark-pink), and EPSPS (purple) methods are represented by schematic amplification curves. In the tables, all positive (+) and negative (−) signals expected with the screening methods tested are indicated for each GM event. The current panel of screening methods includes p35S, tNOS, pFMV, pNOS, t35S, EPSPS, pat, bar, Cry1Ab/Ac, gat-tpinII, Cry3Bb, and a pentaplex (Barbau-Piednoir et al., 2010, 2014; Broeders et al., 2013, 2015; in-house).

reduced to only one (73496) (Fig. 20.2A). The presence of this event will be then confirmed with the corresponding event-specific method in the identification step and subsequently quantified to determine the amount of this GM event present in the sample under test. Thus, this case study illustrates the usefulness of taxon-specific methods and the diverse panel of GM-screening methods, allowing coverage of a broad range of GM events as well as indication of a limited number of GM events to be analyzed in further steps.

Third, the benefit of using a panel of screening methods is even more apparent in the case of more complex matrices, such as feed, that may contain several GM events of different plant species. qPCR screening of this kind of sample will thus result in several detected taxon- and element-specific markers, providing a long list of GM events that are potentially present (Case study n°3 in Fig. 20.1). In such samples, identification of numerous GMOs in different amounts is usual, from which several need to be quantified using the corresponding taxon-specific and event-specific methods. As an example, suppose that the qPCR screening results indicate that ingredients from the tested food/feed matrix belong to maize and cotton species; 27 EU-authorized GM events or LLP cases are then to be suspected as present (Fig. 20.2B). According to the positive signals for the p35S and tNOS methods, 24 GM events must still be investigated during the identification step. However, using the panel of screening methods, this list could be reduced. Indeed, if negative signals are additionally observed with pFMV, pNOS, t35S, pat, bar, gat-tpinII, and the pentaplex methods while the EPSPS, Cry1Ab/Ac, and Cry3Bb methods are positive, 10 GM events (GA21, MON 863, NK603, MON 88017, MIR604, MON 87460, 5307, MON 87427, MON 15985, and MON 531), instead of 34, are finally designated for the identification step. Event-specific methods of these suspected 10 GM events will thus be applied to determine which GM events are truly present. Next, the GM amount of identified GM events in the matrix tested will be quantified. In this case study, the importance of using a combination of screening markers targeting sequences from both elements present at high and low frequency in GMOs is demonstrated. Moreover, the use of a decision support system is crucial to simplify the analysis of the correspondence between all signals observed within the screening phase and the numerous EU-authorized GM events and LLP cases that exist.

Fourth, food or feed matrices can also contain unknown or unauthorized GM events (Case study n°4 in Fig. 20.1). For instance, if the specific amplification signals from the qPCR screening cannot be related to any authorized GM event, the presence of unknown or unauthorized GMOs is suspected. To reveal the truth of this hypothesis, a DNA walking strategy can be applied starting from one of the detected transgenic screening elements. This technique permits further characterization of the GM event through sequences of the transgene flanking regions and the unnatural combination of elements. Based on this sequence information, qPCR event-specific methods can be developed thereafter to allow not only identification but also, in combination with taxon-specific methods, quantification of these GMOs. To illustrate this case study, two examples are given. On the one hand, the presence of an unknown/unauthorized GMO can be detected using the t35S pCAMBIA screening method targeting a sequence observed only in EU-unauthorized GM events at a frequency of approximately 30% (Fraiture et al., 2014). A positive signal for this screening method automatically triggers application of the DNA walking strategy (Fig. 20.3A). On the other hand, positive signals are observed for taxon-specific methods targeting rapeseed and cotton species as well as for the p35S method while all other screening methods tested show no amplification (Fig. 20.3B). No correspondence can be established between the observed qPCR signals and all existing EU-authorized GM events and LLP cases. Indeed, among the cotton and rapeseed species, nine GM events possess the p35S element in their transgenic cassettes. However, this marker is always present in combination with other elements that were not detected in the analysis. Therefore, the presence of unknown/unauthorized GMO is highly probable. The same

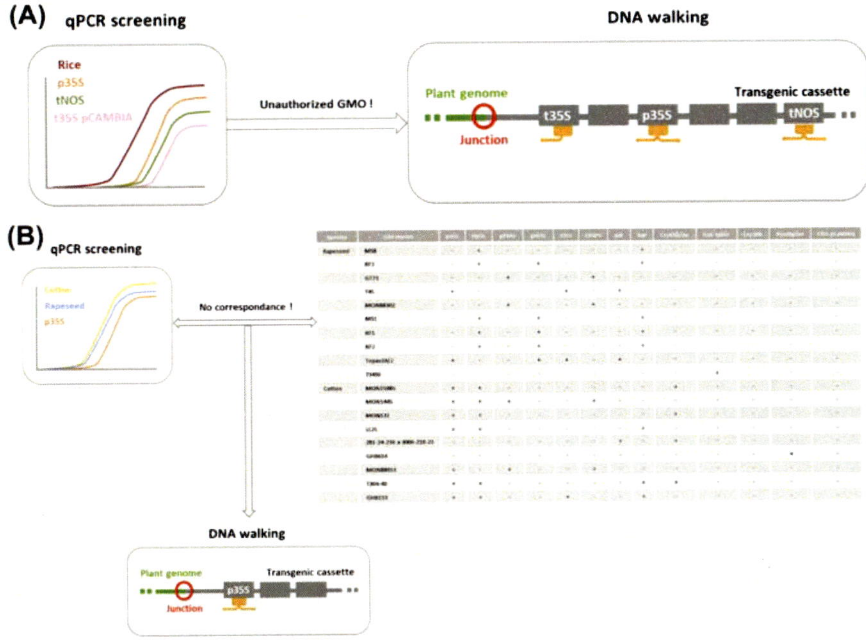

Figure 20.3 Examples of results encountered with EU-unauthorized GM events in routine GMO analysis (A and B). For each matrix tested, positive signals observed in qPCR screening analysis for the rapeseed species (light-blue), cotton species (yellow), rice species (burgundy), p35S (orange), tNOS (green), and t35S pCAMBIA (light-pink) methods are represented by schematic amplification curves. In the table, all positive (+) and negative (−) signals expected with the screening methods tested are indicated for each GM event. The current panel of screening methods includes p35S, tNOS, pFMV, pNOS, t35S, EPSPS, pat, bar, Cry1Ab/Ac, gat-tpinII, Cry3Bb, a pentaplex, and t35S pCAMBIA (Barbau-Piednoir et al., 2010, 2014; Broeders et al., 2013, 2015; Fraiture et al., 2014; in-house).

supposition is also made when no GM events, potentially suspected in the tested sample based on the outcome of the screening, are identified using the corresponding event-specific methods. To confirm this hypothesis, the DNA walking strategy must be applied to characterize sequences surrounding the detected p35S element in order to get transgene flanking regions and/or unnatural combinations of transgenic elements. With the aim of detecting the entire population of GMOs present in the tested sample, all sequences generated by the DNA walking approach have to be analyzed. However, this step could be quite time-consuming and laborious, especially in case of food/feed matrices composed of several GMOs harboring the same transgenic element. Use of NGS technology in the sequencing step instead of the Sanger method could be highly helpful in this case (Fraiture et al., 2015b). However, when unknown GMOs, composed only of transgenic elements not targeted in the qPCR screening step, are present, the DNA walking strategy is not applicable (Case study n°5 in Fig. 20.1). The absence of positive signals with the panel of screening methods cannot exclude the possible presence of unknown/unauthorized GMO in the sample under test. For these GMOs, detection still represents a real challenge.

Although advances in GMO detection using additional techniques and strategies continue, there is still room for improvement to reach the ideal GMO analysis, able to deal in a time- and cost-effective way with the increasing number and diversity of GMOs, mixtures of several GMOs and the potential presence of unauthorized/unknown GMOs. Moreover, the problems of the current need for CRM and qPCR quantification drawbacks should be taken into account when developing new methodologies for routine analysis. To this end, alternative strategies are further proposed.

20.4 Future Trends

20.4.1 Alternative Multiplex Strategies

To enable increased throughput of analysis, non-qPCR based multiplex assays have been investigated. While GMOs may be present at trace levels, the targets still need to be initially amplified by PCR to permit their analysis using CGE, microarray, and Luminex technologies. However, inherent properties linked to the necessary PCR step limit the multiplexing level in general to 10 targets per PCR assay (Pla et al., 2013; Vega and Marina, 2014).

With the CGE system, multiple GM targets, previously amplified with fluorescently labeled primers, are easily discriminated even if the size range of the generated amplicons is similar. It also allows higher multiplexing than qPCR since tetraplex, pentaplex, hexaplex, octaplex, and nonaplex PCR assays have already been developed to detect GMOs (Basak et al., 2014; Guo et al., 2011; Heide et al., 2008a,b; Holck et al., 2010; Holck and Pedersen, 2011; Nadal et al., 2006, 2009). However, compared to the qPCR technology, the sensitivity of the CGE system is slightly lower (Milavec et al., 2014).

Regarding microarray technology, more than 250,000 targets, initially amplified by PCR using target-specific and/or universal primers, can be simultaneously detected, resulting in a much higher throughput than the current analyses. In the field of GMO detection, several multiplex PCR assays, from duplex to dodecaplex, have been established (Dobnik et al., 2010; Hamels et al., 2009; Leimanis et al., 2006, 2008; Morisset et al., 2008b; Pla et al., 2013; Prins et al., 2008; Rudi et al., 2003; Shao et al., 2014; Von Götz, 2010). Recently, with the help of constant improvements in the technology, one approach has allowed detection of unamplified GM DNA from three GM soybean and nine GM maize events at levels as low as or equal to 1% using a comparative genomic hybridization microarray platform (Turkec et al., 2016). However, as is the case for the GCE approach, microarray technology never reaches the sensitivity obtained by qPCR.

Using Luminex technology, up to 500 different targets can be identified. To this end, the target-specific amplicons are generated in a biotinylated form by PCR and subsequently hybridized to nucleic acid probes specific for the targets under investigation, which are then independently coupled to spectrally distinct sets of beads. The fact that the beads are composed of different amounts of red and infrared color facilitates the high multiplexing property. Compared to the microarray system, this liquid bead array technology is potentially more sensitive and faster. Utilizing singleplex, triplex, tetraplex, pentaplex, or hexaplex PCR assays, several GMOs have already been detected by this technology (Choi et al., 2010, Choi, 2011; Fantozzi et al., 2008; Fu et al., 2015a; Han et al., 2013; Luminex®).

20.4.2 Digital PCR Technology

Digital PCR (dPCR) technology, based on binomial Poisson statistics, allows absolute quantification, in contrast to the relative quantification with qPCR, of the number of nucleic acid targets present in the tested sample. Contrary to qPCR, this end-point PCR system is efficient even if the copy number of the target is low and/or PCR inhibitors are present. Moreover, no calibration curves are needed for the measurement, thus reducing drastically the need for a high amount of CRM. The fact that this technology is based on a stand-alone PCR would simplify its introduction for routine use especially if the current validated event-specific qPCR methods could be transferred. However, this process may require some optimization. Nowadays, several GMOs have been quantified using the chamber dPCR approach or the droplet dPCR approach, in which samples are partitioned either into thousands of microfluidic chambers or thousands of droplets generated by a water—oil emulsion (eg, Bhat et al., 2009; Brod et al., 2014; Burns et al., 2010; Corbisier et al., 2010; Fu et al., 2015b; Köppel et al., 2015; Köppel and Bucher, 2015; Li et al., 2015; Morisset et al., 2013; Strain et al., 2013). To specifically identify the target, the throughput level of this dPCR technology is nonetheless limited to one singleplex or one duplex PCR assay per reaction. However, if the aim is to analyze the GMO content per type of ingredient, this throughput could be increased. As such, 12 EU-authorized GMOs were recently targeted by combining one tetraplex dPCR assay with one decaplex dPCR assay (Dobnik et al., 2015).

20.4.3 Loop-Mediated Isothermal Amplification

With the LAMP approach, sequences of interest are first amplified under isothermal conditions using four primers specific to six distinct regions of the target and then visualized with the help of color indicators, fluorescent dyes, or precipitation processes. As no sophisticated equipment is necessary, this analysis can also be carried out on field. In addition, a tolerance to PCR inhibitors has been observed with this technology (Morisset et al., 2008a; Zhang et al., 2013). In GMO detection, several specific and sensitive element-specific, construct-specific, event-specific, and taxon-specific methods have been successfully developed (eg, Chen et al., 2011, 2012, 2014; Di et al., 2014; Fukuta et al., 2004; Guan et al., 2010; Huang et al., 2014; Kiddle et al., 2012; Lee et al., 2009; Li et al., 2013, 2014; Liu et al., 2009; Randhawa et al., 2013; Wang et al., 2015; Xu et al., 2013; Zahradnik et al., 2014; Zhang et al., 2013). Use of the LAMP system does, however, present some difficulties around the design of four primers per target as well as the impossibility to individually identify targets within a multiplex PCR assay (Morisset et al., 2008a; Zhang et al., 2013).

20.4.4 High-Throughput Sequencing Technologies

Given the fact that characterization of the GM junction sequences is an incontrovertible proof of GMO presence in a given sample, application of NGS technology in GMO detection has been investigated. Due to the possibility of barcoding individually different targets, this technology potentially offers a high throughput. Among all NGS strategies, two main approaches are distinguished, namely targeted sequencing and whole-genome sequencing (WGS) (Buermans et al., 2014; Liang et al., 2014; Willems et al., 2016).

For the targeted-sequencing strategy, sequences of interest are first selected to be then sequenced, thus requiring some prior knowledge.

On the one hand, sequences of interest can be enriched by PCR (amplicon sequencing) to compose a DNA library of final PCR products that are subsequently sequenced. Using a pyrosequencing device, this approach was used to characterize amplicons generated by GM-specific methods from samples presenting a low amount of GM soybean and GM maize targets (Song et al., 2014; Wu et al., 2011). Instead of C_q values with qPCR technology, the sequence of each targeted region is thus directly known. Moreover, the sequencing of amplicons from event-specific PCR methods using the Ion Torrent platform has allowed determination of the zygosity of transgenic maize lines, providing crucial information for the conversion between GM mass percentages and GM copy numbers (Fritsch et al., 2015). With the aim of characterizing unknown regions, PCR products from a DNA walking approach targeting the vip3Aa20 element, notably found in the GM MIR162 maize, have also been sequenced on the Illumina and Pacific Biosciences platforms (Liang et al., 2014).

On the other hand, a DNA library can also be prepared from the whole genome followed by sequencing of selected sequences of interest (target enrichment sequencing). To this end, appropriate hybridizations to specific probes are carried out via magnetic beads or microarrays. However, to our knowledge, this approach has not yet been applied to GMO detection although successfully used in other fields (Clarke et al., 2013; Dasgupta et al., 2015; DuBose et al., 2013; Zhou and Holliday, 2012).

Taking into account the expected improvements in terms of cost and bioinformatics tools, this targeted NGS strategy therefore represents a promising alternative for enforcement laboratories.

Regarding the WGS strategy, the DNA library contains the entire genome that is fully sequenced. The generated reads can then be treated with bioinformatics, eventually using knowledge available on the tested GMO.

For entirely unknown GMOs, the insert is characterized via all inferred contigs from reads that partially match or unmatch the reference genome of the plant species (Yang et al., 2013). In this way, LLRICE62, TT51-1, T1c-19, and FP967 events were identified (Wahler et al., 2013; Yang et al., 2013;

Young et al., 2015). However, if no appropriate reference genome is available, a strategy of de novo assembly needs to be carried out. To this end, all generated reads are analyzed to find overlaps between each other; this can be difficult due notably to the large size and complexity of plant genomes as well as the possible presence of several different GMOs in the tested sample (Kovalic et al., 2012; Schatz et al., 2012). In order to deal with some of these issues, long reads generated by the PacBio technology could constitute an alternative to the unavailability of reference genomes of the plant species concerned to which short reads from the Illumina technology can then be aligned (Au et al., 2012).

When the sequence of the transgenic insert is partially known, the generated reads can be compared to a DNA transgene sequence database containing transgenic elements commonly found in GMOs. The TT51-1 and T1c-19 events were, for instance, identified by this approach (Yang et al., 2013).

If the sequence of the insert is entirely known, two main bioinformatics analyses have been proposed. On the one hand, as tested with TT51-1, T1c-19, MON 17903, and MON 87704 events, the obtained reads, which present only a partial similarity to the reference genome of the investigated plant species, are subsequently aligned to the sequence of the transgenic insert to locate and characterize the transgene flanking regions (Kovalic et al., 2012; Yang et al., 2013). On the other hand, the generated reads can also be analyzed according to an analytical workflow composed of three steps. Firstly, the presence of GMO(s) is demonstrated if reads corresponding to the transgenic insert sequence are found. Next, these reads are compared to the plant-species genome to roughly locate the transgene flanking regions. Finally, characterization of the transgenic insert with its precise localization is determined by simultaneous aligning these selected reads to the plant reference genome and the sequence of the transgenic insert. This WGS strategy was successfully applied on pure GM rice, GM/non-GM rice mixtures, and processed GM rice (Willems et al., 2016).

Although its implementation by enforcement laboratories is nowadays still difficult in terms of cost, staff training, and bioinformatics analysis, the WGS strategy represents a promising support for routine GMO analysis, especially for totally unknown GMOs (Buermans and den Dunnen, 2014; Liang et al., 2014; Willems et al., 2016).

Sources of Further Information

See references Broeders et al. (2012a), and Fraiture et al. (2015b,c).

Acknowledgments

The research that yielded these results was funded by the Belgian Federal Public Service of Health, Food Chain Safety and Environment through the contact UGMMONITOR (convention RF 11/6242).

References

Au, K.F., Underwood, J.G., Lee, L., Wong, W.H., 2012. Improving PacBio long read accuracy by short read alignment. PLoS One 7 (10), e46679.

Angers-Loustau, A., Petrillo, M., Bonfini, L., Gatto, F., Rosa, S., Patak, A., Kreysa, J., 2014. JRC GMO-matrix: a web application to support genetically modified organisms detection strategies. BMC Bioinformatics 5 (1), 417.

Bahrdt, C., Krech, A.B., Wurz, A., Wulff, D., 2010. Validation of a newly developed hexaplex real-time PCR assay for screening for presence of GMOs in food, feed and seed. Analytical and Bioanalytical Chemistry 396 (6), 2103–2112.

Barbau-Piednoir, E., Lievens, A., Mbongolo-Mbella, G., Roosens, N., Sneyers, M., Leunda-Casi, A., Van den Bulcke, M., 2010. SYBR®Green qPCR screening methods for the presence of "35S promoter" and "NOS terminator" elements in food and feed products. European Food Research and Technology 230 (3), 383–393.

Barbau-Piednoir, E., Stragier, P., Roosens, N., et al., 2014. Interlaboratory testing of GMO detection by combinatory SYBRGreen PCR screening (CoSYPS). Food Analytical Methods 7 (8), 1719–1728.

Basak, S., Ehtesham, N.Z., Sesikeran, B., Ghosh, S., 2014. Detection and identification of transgenic elements by fluorescent-PCR-based capillary gel electrophoresis in genetically modified cotton and soybean. Journal of AOAC International 97 (1), 159–165.

Bhat, S., Herrmann, J., Armishaw, P., Corbisier, P., Emslie, K.R., 2009. Single molecule detection in nanofluidic digital array enables accurate measurement of DNA copy number. Analytical and Bioanalytical Chemistry 394 (2), 457–467.

Block, A., Debode, F., Grohmann, L., Hulin, J., Taverniers, I., Kluga, L., Barbau-Piednoir, E., Broeders, S., Huber, I., Van den Bulcke, M., Heinze, P., Berben, G., Busch, U., Roosens, N., Janssen, E., Žel, J., Gruden, K., Morisset, D., 2013. The GMOseek matrix: a decision support tool for optimizing the detection of genetically modified plants. BMC Bioinformatics 14, 259.

Brod, F.C.A., van Dijk, J.P., Voorhuijzen, M.M., Dinon, A.Z., Guimarães, L.H., Scholtens, I.M., Arisi, A.C., Kok, E.J., 2014. A high-throughput method for GMO multi-detection using a microfluidic dynamic array. Analytical and Bioanalytical Chemistry 406 (5), 1397–1410.

Broeders, S., Barbau-Piednoir, E., Vandermassen, E., Debode, F., Mazzara, M., Roosens, N., 2013. New SYBRGreen methods targeting promoter sequences used for screening of several GM events pending for authorisation in Europe. European Food Research and Technology 236 (3), 537–547.

Broeders, S., Fraiture, M.A., Vandermassen, E., Delvoye, M., Barbau-Piednoir, E., Lievens, A., Roosens, N., 2015. New trait-specific qualitative SYBR®Green qPCR methods to expand the panel of GMO screening methods used in the CoSYPS. European Food Research and Technology 241 (2), 275–287.

Broeders, S., Papazova, N., Van den Bulcke, M., Roosens, N., 2012a. Development of a Molecular Platform for GMO Detection in Food and Feed on the Basis of "combinatory qPCR" Technology", in Polymerase Chain Reaction, pp. 363–404. Rijeka, Croatia.

Broeders, S.R.M., De Keersmaecker, S.C.J., Roosens, N.H.C., 2012b. How to deal with the upcoming challenges in GMO detection in food and feed. Journal of Biomedicine and Biotechnology 2012, 275–287.

Buermans, H.P.J., den Dunnen, J.T., 2014. Next generation sequencing technology: advances and applications. Biochimica et Biophysica Acta 1842, 1932–1941.

Burns, M.J., Burrell, A.M., Foy, C.A., 2010. The applicability of digital PCR for the assessment of detection limits in GMO analysis. European Food Research and Technology 231 (3), 353–362.

Chaouachi, M., Zellama, M.S., Nabi, N., Ben Hafsa, A., Saïd, K., 2014. Molecular identification of four genetically modified maize (Bt11, Bt176, Mon810 and T25) by duplex quantitative real-time PCR. Food Analytical Methods 7 (1), 224–233.

Chen, L., Guo, J., Wang, Q., Kai, G., Yang, L., 2011. Development of the visual loop-mediated isothermal amplification assays for seven genetically modified maize events and their application in practical samples analysis. Journal of Agricultural and Food Chemistry 59 (11), 5914–5918.

Chen, X., Wang, X., Jin, N., Zhou, Y., Huang, S., Miao, Q., Zhu, Q., Xu, J., 2012. Endpoint visual detection of three genetically modified rice events by loop-mediated isothermal amplification. International Journal of Molecular Sciences 13 (11), 14421–14433.

Clarke, W.E., Parkin, I.A., Gajardo, H.A., Gerhardt, D.J., Higgins, E., Sidebottom, C., Sharpe, A.G., Snowdon, R.J., Federico, M.L., Iniguez-Luy, F.L., 2013. Genomic DNA enrichment using sequence capture microarrays: a novel approach to discover sequence nucleotide polymorphisms (SNP) in *Brassica napus* L. PLoS One 8 (12), e81992.

Cheng, Y., Zhang, M., Hu, K., Sun, F., Tao, R., Gao, X., Luan, F., 2014. Loop-Mediated isothermal amplification for the event-specific detection of wheat B73-6-1. Food Analytical Methods 7 (2), 500–505.

Choi, S.H., 2011. Hexaplex PCR assay and liquid bead array for detection of stacked genetically modified cotton event 281-24-236×3006-210-23. Analytical and Bioanalytical Chemistry 401 (2), 647–655.

Choi, S.H., Oh, Y.T., Kwon, J.Y., Lee, S.N., Han, B.D., Ryu, K.H., 2010. Development of detection system using multiplex PCR and liquid beadarray for stacked genetically modified rice event (LS28×Cry1Ac). Journal of the Korean Society for Applied Biological Chemistry 53 (5), 639–646.

Commission Regulation (EC) No 619/2011 of 24 June 2011 laying down the methods of sampling and analysis for the official control of feed as regards presence of genetically modified material for which an authorisation procedure is pending or the authorisation of which has expired.2011 Official Journal of the European Union L166 9–15.

Corbisier, P., Bhat, S., Partis, L., Rui, V., Xie, D., Emslie, K.R., 2010. Absolute quantification of genetically modified MON810 maize (*Zea mays* L.) by digital polymerase chain reaction. Analytical and Bioanalytical Chemistry 396 (6), 2143–2150.

Cottenet, G., Blancpain, C., Sonnard, V., Chuah, P.F., 2013. Development and validation of a multiplex real-time PCR method to simultaneously detect 47 targets for the identification of genetically modified organisms. Analytical and Bioanalytical Chemistry 405 (21), 6831–6844.

Dasgupta, M.G., Dharanishanthi, V., Agarwal, I., Krutovsky, K.V., 2015. Development of genetic markers in Eucalyptus species by target enrichment and exome sequencing. PLoS One 10 (1), e0116528.

Demeke, T., Jenkins, G.R., 2010. Influence of DNA extraction methods, PCR inhibitors and quantification methods on real-time PCR assay of biotechnology-derived traits. Analytical and Bioanalytical Chemistry 396 (6), 1977–1990.

Di, H., Shi, L., Shen, H., Yan, H., Meng, H., Li, L., Alam, M.J., Yamasaki, S., Ye, L., 2014. Rapid detection of genetically modified ingredients in soybean products by real-time loop-mediated isothermal amplification. Journal of Food and Nutrition Research 2 (7), 363–368.

Dobnik, D., Morisset, D., Gruden, K., 2010. NAIMA as a solution for future GMO diagnostics challenges. Analytical and Bioanalytical Chemistry 396 (6), 2229–2233.

Dobnik, D., Spilsberg, B., Bogožalec, A., Holst-Jensen, A., Žel, J., 2015. Multiplex quantification of 12 European union authorized genetically modified maize lines with droplet digital polymerase chain reaction. Analytical Chemistry 87 (16), 8218–8226.

Dörries, H.H., Remus, I., Grönewald, A., Grönewald, C., Berghof-Jäger, K., 2010. Development of a qualitative, multiplex real-time PCR kit for screening of genetically modified organisms (GMOs). Analytical and Bioanalytical Chemistry 396 (6), 2043–2054.

DuBose, A., Lichtenstein, S.T., Narisu, N., Bonnycastle, L.L., Swift, A.J., Chines, P.S., Collins, F.S., 2013. Use of microarray hybrid capture and next-generation sequencing to identify the anatomy of a transgene. Nucleic Acids Research 41 (6), e70.

European Network of GMO Laboratories (ENGL). (2015). Definition of minimum performance requirements for analytical methods of GMO testing. URL < http://www.iss.it/binary/rogm/cont/MPR_Report_Application_20_10_2015.pdf >.

Fantozzi, A., Ermolli, M., Marini, M., Balla, B., Querci, M., Van den Eede, G., 2008. Innovative application of fluorescent microsphere based assay for multiple GMO detection. Food Analytical Methods 1 (1), 10–17.

Fraiture, M.A., Herman, P., Taverniers, I., De Loose, M., Deforce, D., Roosens, N.H., 2014. An innovative and integrated approach based on DNA walking to identify unauthorised GMOs. Food Chemistry 147, 60–69.

Fraiture, M.A., Herman, P., Taverniers, I., De Loose, M., Van Nieuwerburgh, F., Deforce, D., Roosens, N.H., 2015a. Validation of a sensitive DNA walking strategy to characterize unauthorised GMOs using model food matrices mimicking common rice products. Food Chemistry 173, 1259–1265.

Fraiture, M.A., Herman, P., Lefèvre, L., Taverniers, I., De Loose, M., Deforce, D., Roosens Nancy, N., 2015b. Integrated DNA walking system to characterize a broad spectrum of GMOs in food/feed matrices. BMC Biotechnology 2015, 1–11.

Fraiture, M.A., Herman, P., Taverniers, I., De Loose, M., Deforce, D., Roosens, N.H., 2015c. Current and new approaches in GMO detection: challenges and solutions. BioMed Research International 2015, 1–22.

Fritsch, L., Fischer, R., Wambach, C., Dudek, M., Schillberg, S., Schröper, F., 2015. Next-generation sequencing is a robust strategy for the high-throughput detection of zygosity in transgenic maize. Transgenic Research 24 (4), 615–623.

Fu, K., Huang, W., Deng, T., Li, F., Liu, H., Chen, Y., 2015a. Multiplex PCR assay and liquid bead array for detection of 13 lines genetically modified maize. Journal of Chinese Institute of Food Science and Technology 15 (1), 188–197.

Fu, W., Zhu, P., Wang, C., Huang, K., Du, Z., Tian, W., Wang, Q., Wang, H., Xu, W., Zhu, S., 2015b. A highly sensitive and specific method for the screening detection of genetically modified organisms based on digital PCR without pretreatment. Scientific Reports 5, 12715.

Fukuta, S., Mizukami, Y., Ishida, A., Ueda, J., Hasegawa, M., Hayashi, I., Hashimoto, M., Kanbe, M., 2004. Real-time loop-mediated isothermal amplification for the CaMV-35S promoter as a screening method for genetically modified organisms. European Food Research and Technology 218 (5), 496–500.

Gerdes, L., Busch, U., Pecoraro, S., 2012. GMOfinder-a GMO screening database. Food Analytical Methods 5 (6), 1368–1376.

Guan, X., Guo, J., Shen, P., Yang, L., Zhang, D., 2010. Visual and rapid detection of two genetically modified soybean events using loop mediated isothermal amplification method. Food Analytical Methods 3 (4), 313–320.

Guo, J., Yang, L., Chen, L., Morisset, D., Li, X., Pan, L., Zhang, D., 2011. MPIC: a high-throughput analytical method for multiple DNA targets. Analytical Chemistry 83 (5), 1579–1586.

Hamels, S., Glouden, T., Gillard, K., Mazzara, M., Debode, F., Foti, N., Sneyers, M., Nuez, T.E., Pla, M., Berben, G., Moens, W., Bertheau, Y., Audéon, C., Van den Eede, G., Remacle, J., 2009. A PCR-microarray method for the screening of genetically modified organisms. European Food Research and Technology 228 (4), 531–541.

Han, X., Wang, H., Chen, H., Mei, L., Wu, S., Jia, G., Cheng, T., Zhu, S., Lin, X., 2013. Development and primary application of a fluorescent liquid bead array for the simultaneous identification of multiple genetically modified maize. Biosensors and Bioelectronics 49, 360–366.

Heide, B.R., Drømtorp, S.M., Rudi, K., Heir, E., Holck, A.L., 2008a. Determination of eight genetically modiWed maize events by quantitative, multiplex PCR and Xuorescence capillary gel electrophoresis. European Food Research and Technology 227 (4), 1125–1137.

Heide, B.R., Heir, E., Holck, A., 2008b. Detection of eight GMO maize events by qualitative, multiplex PCR and Xuorescence capillary gel electrophoresis. European Food Research and Technology 227 (2), 527–535.

Holck, A.L., Pedersen, B.O., 2011. Simple, sensitive, accurate multiplex quantitative competitive PCR with capillary electrophoresis detection for the determination of genetically modified maize. European Food Research and Technology 233 (6), 951–961.

Holck, A.L., Pedersen, B.O., Heir, E., 2010. Detection of five novel GMO maize events by qualitative, multiplex PCR and fluorescence capillary gel electrophoresis. European Food Research and Technology 231 (3), 475–483.

Holst-Jensen, A., Bertheau, Y., De Loose, M., Grohmann, L., Hamels, S., Hougs, L., Morisset, D., Pecoraro, S., Pla, M., Van Den Bulcke, M., Wulff, D., 2012. Detecting unauthorized genetically modified organisms (GMOs) and derived materials. Biotechnology Advances 30 (6), 1318–1335.

Huang, X., Chen, L., Xu, J., Ji, H.F., Zhu, S., Chen, H., 2014. Rapid visual detection of phytase gene in genetically modified maize using loop-mediated isothermal amplification method. Food Chemistry 156, 184–189.

Huber, A., Block, D., Sebah, F., Debode, D., Morisset, L., Grohmann, G., Berben, G., Štebih, D., Milavec, M., Žel, J., Busch, U., 2013. Development and validation of duplex, triplex, and pentaplex real-time PCR screening assays for the detection of genetically modified organisms in food and feed. Journal of Agricultural and Food Chemistry 61 (43), 10293–10301.

James, C., 2014. Global Status of Commercialized Biotech/GM Crops: 2014. ISAAA Brief 49. Ithaca, NY, USA: ISAAA. ISBN:978-1-892456-59-1. http://www.isaaa.org/resources/publications/briefs/49/ (pp. 8, 50, 88, 92, 150).

JRC GMO-Amplicons. URL <http://gmo-crl.jrc.ec.europa.eu/jrcgmoamplicons/>.

JRC GMO-Matrix. URL <http://gmo-crl.jrc.ec.europa.eu/jrcgmomatrix/>.

JCR GMOMETHODS. URL <http://gmo-crl.jrc.ec.europa.eu/gmomethods/>.

Kamle, S., Ali, S., 2013. Genetically modified crops: detection strategies and biosafety issues. Gene 522 (2), 123–132.

Kiddle, G., Hardinge, P., Buttigieg, N., 2012. GMO detection using a bioluminescent real time reporter (BART) of loop mediated isothermal amplification (LAMP) suitable for field use. BMC Biotechnology 12, 15.

Köppel, R., Bucher, T., Frei, A., Waiblinger, H.U., 2015. Droplet digital PCR versus multiplex real-time PCR method for the detection and quantification of DNA from the four transgenic soy traits MON87769, MON87708, MON87705 and FG72, and lectin. European Food Research and Technology 241, 521–527.

Köppel, R., Bucher, T., 2015. Rapid establishment of droplet digital PCR for quantitative GMO analysis. European Food Research and Technology 241, 427–439.

Köppel, R., Sendic, A., Waiblinger, H.U., 2014. Two quantitative multiplex real-time PCR systems for the efficient GMO screening of food products. European Food Research and Technology 239 (4), 653–659.

Kovalic, D., Garnaat, C., Guo, L., Yan, Y., Groat, J., Silvanovich, A., Ralston, L., Huang, M., Tian, Q., Christian, A., Cheikh, N., Hjelle, J., Padgette, S., Bannon, G., 2012. The use of next generation sequencing and junction sequence analysis bioinformatics to achieve molecular characterization of crops improved through modern biotechnology. The Plant Genome 5, 149–163.

Lee, D., La Mura, M., Allnutt, T.R., Powell, W., 2009. Detection of genetically modified organisms (GMOs) using isothermal amplification of target sequences. BMC Biotechnology 9, 7.

Leimanis, S., Hamels, S., Nazé, F., Mbongolo Mbella, G., Sneyers, M., Hochegger, R., Broll, H., Roth, L., Dallmann, K., Micsinai, A., La Paz, J.L., Pla, M., Brünen-Nieweler, C., Papazova, N., Taverniers, I., Hess, N., Kirschneit, B., Bertheau, Y., Audeon, C., Laval, V., Busch, U., Pecoraro, S., Neumann, K., Rösel, S., van Dijk, J., Kok, E., Bellocchi, G., Foti, N., Mazzara, M., Moens, W., Remacle, J., Van Den Eede, G., 2008. Validation of the performance of a GMO multiplex screening assay based on microarray detection. European Food Research and Technology 227 (6), 1621–1632.

Leimanis, S., Hernandez, M., Fernandez, S., Boyer, F., Burns, M., Bruderer, S., Glouden, T., Harris, N., Kaeppeli, O., Philipp, P., Pla, M., Puigdomènech, P., Vaitilingom, M., Bertheau, Y., Remacle, J., 2006. Microarray-based detection system for genetically modified (GM) food ingredients. Plant Molecular Biology 61 (1–2), 123–139.

Li, Q., Fang, J., Liu, X., Xi, X., Li, M., Gong, Y., Zhang, M., 2013. Loop-mediated isothermal amplification (LAMP) method for rapid detection of cry1Ab gene in transgenic rice (*Oryza sativa* L.). European Food Research and Technology 236 (4), 589–598.

Li, F., Yan, W., Long, L., Qi, X., Li, C., Zhang, S., 2014. Development and application of loop-mediated isothermal amplification assays for rapid visual detection of cry2Ab and cry3A genes in genetically-modified crops. International Journal of Molecular Sciences 15 (9), 15109–15121.

Li, X., Wu, Y., Li, J., Li, Y., Long, L., Li, F., Wu, G., 2015. Development and validation of a 48-target analytical method for high-throughput monitoring of genetically modified organisms. Scientific Reports 5, 7616.

Liang, C., van Dijk, J.P., Scholtens, I.M., Staats, M., Prins, T.W., Voorhuijzen, M.M., da Silva, A.M., Arisi, A.C.M., den Dunnen, J.T., Kok, E.J., 2014. Detecting authorized and unauthorized genetically modified organisms containing vip3A by real-time PCR and next-generation sequencing. Analytical and Bioanalytical Chemistry 406 (11), 2603–2611.

Liu, M., Luo, Y., Tao, R., He, R., Jiang, K., Wang, B., Wang, L., 2009. Sensitive and rapid detection of genetic modified soybean (Roundup Ready) by loop-mediated isothermal amplification. Bioscience Biotechnology and Biochemistry 73 (11), 2365–2369.

Luminex ®. URL < https://www.luminexcorp.com/>.

Mazzara, M., Paoletti, C., Corbisier, P., Grazioli, E., Larcher, S., Berben, G., De Loose, M., Folch, I., Henry, C., Hess, N., Hougs, L., Janssen, E., Moran, G., Onori, R., Van den Eede, G., 2013. Kernel lot distribution assessment (KeLDA): a comparative study of protein and dna-based detection methods for GMO testing. Food Analytical Methods 6 (1), 210–220.

Milavec, M., Dobnik, D., Yang, L., Zhang, D., K.Gruden, Zel, J., 2014. GMO quantification: valuable experience and insights for the future. Analytical and Bioanalytical Chemistry 406 (26), 6485–6497.

Morisset, D., Stebih, D., Cankar, K., Zel, J., Gruden, K., 2008a. Alternative DNA amplification methods to PCR and their application in GMO detection: a review. European Food Research and Technology 227 (5), 1287–1297.

Morisset, D., Dobnik, D., Hamels, S., Že, J., Gruden, K., 2008b. NAIMA: target amplification strategy allowing quantitative on-chip detection of GMOs. Nucleic Acids Research 36 (18), e118.

Morisset, D., Štebih, D., Milavec, M., Gruden, K., Žel, J., 2013. Quantitative analysis of food and feed samples with droplet digital PCR. PLoS One 8 (5s), e62583.

Nadal, A., Coll, A., La Paz, J.L., Esteve, T., Pla, M., 2006. A new PCR-CGE (size and color) method for simultaneous detection of genetically modified maize events. Electrophoresis 27 (19), 3879–3888.

Nadal, A., Esteve, T., Pla, M., 2009. Multiplex polymerase chain reaction-capillary gel electrophoresis: a promising tool for GMO screening-assay for simultaneous detection of five genetically modified cotton events and species. Journal of AOAC International 92 (3), 765–772.

Navarro, E., Serrano-Heras, G., Castañoa, M.J., Solera, J., 2015. Real-time PCR detection chemistry. Clinica Chimica Acta 439, 231–250.

Opel, K.L., Chung, D., McCord, B.R., 2010. A study of PCR inhibition mechanisms using real time PCR. Journal of Forensic Sciences 55 (1), 25–33.

Park, S.B., Kim, H.Y., Kim, J.H., 2015. Multiplex PCR system to track authorized and unauthorized genetically modified soybean events in food and feed. Food Control 54, 47–52.

Pla, M., Nadal, A., Baeten, V., Bahrdt, C., Berben, G., Bertheau, Y., Coll, A., van Dijk, J.P., Dobnik, D., Fernandez Pierna, J.A., Gruden, K., Hamels, S., Holck, A., Holst-Jensen, A., Janssen, E., Kok, E.J., La Paz, J.L., Laval, V., Leimanis, S., Malcevschi, A., Marmiroli, N., Morisset, D., Prins, T.W., Remacle, J., Ujhelyi, G., Wulff, D., 2013. New multiplexing tools for reliable GMO detection. In: Genetically Modified and Non-genetically Modified Food Supply Chains: Co-existence and Traceability. Oxford, UK, pp. 333–366.

Prins, T.W., van Dijk, J.P., Beenen, H.G., Van Hoef, A.M.A., Voorhuijzen, M.M., Schoen, C.D., Aarts, H.J.M., Kok, E.J., 2008. Optimised padlock probe ligation and microarray detection of multiple (non-authorised) GMOs in a single reaction. BMC Genomics 9, 584.

Querci, M., Van den Bulcke, M., Žel, J., Van den Eede, G., Broll, H., 2010. New approaches in GMO detection. Analytical and Bioanalytical Chemistry 396 (6), 1991–2002.

Randhawa, G.J., Singh, M., Morisset, D., Sood, P., Zel, J., 2013. Loop-Mediated isothermal amplification: rapid visual and real-time methods for detection of genetically modified crops. Journal of Agricultural and Food Chemistry 61 (47), 11338–11346.

Rudi, K., Rud, I., Holck, A., 2003. A novel multiplex quantitative DNA array based PCR (MQDA-PCR) for quantification of transgenic maize in food and feed. Nucleic Acids Research 31 (11), e62.

Samson, M.C., Gullí, M., Marmiroli, N., 2013. Multiplex real-time PCR assays for simultaneous detection of maize MON810 and GA21 in food samples. Food Control 30, 518–525.

Schatz, M.C., Witkowski, J., McCombie, W.R., 2012. Current challenges in de novo plant genome sequencing and assembly. Genome Biology 13 (4), 243.

Schrader, C., Schielke, A., Ellerbroek, L., Johne, R., 2012. PCR inhibitors – occurrence, properties and removal. Journal of Applied Microbiology 113 (5), 1014–1026.

Shao, N., Jiang, S.M., Zhang, M., Wang, J., Guo, S.J., Li, Y., Jiang, H.W., Liu, C.X., Zhang, D.B., Yang, L.T., Tao, S.C., 2014. MACRO: a combined microchip-PCR and microarray system for high-throughput monitoring of genetically modified organisms. Analytical Chemistry 86 (2), 1269–1276.

Song, Q., Wei, G., Zhou, G., 2014. Analysis of genetically modified organisms by pyrosequencing on a portable photodiode-based bioluminescence sequencer. Food Chemistry 154, 78–83.

Strain, M.C., Lada, S.M., Luong, T., Rought, S.E., Gianella, S., Terry, V.H., Spina, C.A., Woelk, C.H., Richman, D.D., 2013. Highly precise measurement of HIV DNA by droplet digital PCR. PLoS One 8 (4), e55943.

Turkec, A., Lucas, S.J., Karacanli, B., Baykut, A., Yuksel, H., 2016. Assessment of a direct hybridization microarray strategy for comprehensive monitoring of genetically modified organisms (GMOs). Food Chemistry 194, 399–409.

Van den Bulcke, M., Lievens, A., Barbau-Piednoir, E., bongoloMbella, G., Roosens, N., Sneyers, M., Leunda Casi, A., 2010. A theoretical introduction to "combinatory SYBR Green qPCR Screening", a matrix-based approach for the detection of materials derived from genetically modified plants. Analytical and Bioanalytical Chemistry 396 (6), 2113–2123.

Vega, E.D., Marina, M.L., 2014. Characterization and study of transgenic cultivars by capillary and microchip electrophoresis. International Journal of Molecular Sciences 15 (12), 23851–23877. http://dx.doi.org/10.3390/ijms151223851 (pp. 20, 62).

Von Götz, F., 2010. See what you eat—broad GMO screening with microarrays. Analytical and Bioanalytical Chemistry 396 (6), 1961–1967.

Wahler, D., Schauser, L., Bendiek, J., Grohmann, L., 2013. Next-Generation sequencing as a tool for detailed molecular characterisation of genomic insertions and flanking regions in genetically modified plants: a pilot study using a rice event unauthorised in the EU. Food Analytical Methods 6 (6), 1718–1727.

Waiblinger, H.U., Ernst, B., Anderson, A., Pietsch, K., 2008. Validation and collaborative study of a P35S and T-nos duplex real-time PCR screening method to detect genetically modified organisms in food products. European Food Research and Technology 226 (5), 1221–1228.

Wang, R., Li, S., Quan, P., Shen, D., Zhang, J., Shi, J., Yang, L., 2015. GMO detection in food and feed through screening by visual loop-mediated isothermal amplification assays. Analytical and Bioanalytical Chemistry 407 (16), 4829–4834.

Willems, S., Fraiture, M.A., Deforce, D., De Keersmaecker, S., Herman, P., De Loose, M., Ruttink, T., Van Nieuwerburgh, F., Roosens, N.H., 2016. Statistical framework for detection of genetically modified organisms based on next generation sequencing. Food Chemistry 192, 788–798.

Wu, A., Wu, W., Chen, Z., Wang, W., Zhou, G., Kajiyama, T., Kambara, H., 2011. Highly sensitive pyrosequencing based on the capture of free adenosine 5′ phosphosulfate with adenosine triphosphate sulfurylase. Analytical Chemistry 83 (9), 3600–3605.

Xu, J., Zheng, Q., Yu, L., Liu, R., Zhao, X., Wang, G., Wang, Q., Cao, J., 2013. Loop-mediated isothermal amplification (LAMP) method for detection of genetically modified maize T25. Food Science & Nutrition 1 (6), 432–438.

Yang, L., Wang, C., Holst-Jensen, A., Morisset, D., Lin, Y., Zhang, D., 2013. Characterization of GM events by insert knowledge adapted re-sequencing approaches. Scientific Reports 3, 2839.

Young, L., Hammerlindl, J., Babic, V., McLeod, J., Sharpe, A., Matsalla, C., Bekkaoui, F., Marquess, L., Booker, H.M., 2015. Genetics, structure, and prevalence of FP967 (CDC Triffid) T-DNA in flax. SpringerPlus 4, 146.

Zahradnik, C., Kolm, R., Martzy, R.L., Mach, R., Krska, A.H., Farnleitner, Brunner, K., 2014. Detection of the 35S promoter in transgenic maize via various isothermal amplification techniques: a practical approach. Analytical and Bioanalytical Chemistry 406 (27), 6835–6842.

Zhang, M., Liu, Y., Chen, L., Quan, S., Jiang, S., Zhang, D.B., Yang, L.T., 2013. One simple DNA extraction device and its combination with modified visual loop-mediated isothermal amplification for rapid on-field detection of genetically modified organisms. Analytical Chemistry 85 (1), 75–82.

Zhou, L., Holliday, J.A., 2012. Targeted enrichment of the black cottonwood (*Populus trichocarpa*) gene space using sequence capture. BMC Genomics 13, 703.

Advances in the Detection of the Adulteration of Alcoholic Beverages Including Unrecorded Alcohol

21

D.W. Lachenmeier
Chemisches und Veterinäruntersuchungsamt (CVUA) Karlsruhe, Karlsruhe, Germany

Chapter Outline

21.1 Introduction

The adulteration of alcoholic beverages may not only be conducted to increase the alcoholic strength by using cheaper sources of sugar and starch besides grapes or fruit (so-called chaptalization), sometimes combined with watering-down, but also to increase the presumed or apparent quality of the product (see Lachenmeier and Rehm, 2013 for general remarks on alcohol quality), such as in the case of the 1985 scandal in Austria, when diethylene glycol was added to wine to increase sweetness (Tagliabue, 1985). This is a case very similar to the melamine addition to increase the apparent protein content of milk (Lachenmeier et al., 2009a). Melamine and diethylene glycol were chosen as adulterants because they were not included in the spectrum of compounds for which foods were tested. Unlike melamine, diethylene glycol is of comparably low toxicity, so that this wine scandal was a case of deception rather than public health infringement. Nevertheless, the reputation of Austrian wine was damaged for years to come.

Another agent to sweeten wine that has been historically applied is lead acetate, which was documented at Greco-Roman times (Lessler, 1988), and chronic lead-poisoning outbreaks have been frequently recorded over history (Eisinger, 1982). The causality with wine adulteration was also recognized early and lead addition was prohibited, for example, in 1427 in France and Spain and in 1478 in Germany (Lessler, 1988).

Another early food law intended to tackle adulteration of alcoholic beverages was the German beer law of 1516, which is still in force today (Narziss, 1984). The law only allows certain ingredients for beer making (water, barley malt, hops, and yeast for bottom-fermented beers), due to the previously common adulteration with various ingredients such as cheaper oat malt and poisonous plants instead of hops.

Interestingly, the frequent adulteration of alcoholic beverages in the 19th century, which mostly could not be detected, was used by the temperance movement to warn against the consumption of alcoholic beverages. In his 1869 essay, Dunn (1869) claims that most of the wines and spirits imported into the United States were counterfeited at this time. Another historic, but more scientific, overview of the adulteration of beer during the 19th century was provided by Cornwall (1884). The major problems described were the substitution of hops with other bitter plants such as aloe or wormwood, but also with bitter chemicals such as picrotoxin.

This chapter reviews the authentication of alcoholic beverages. The literature research was conducted in December 2014 using Google Scholar, ISI Web-of-Knowledge, and Scopus using keyword combinations (authentication/identification and wine/beer/spirits/unrecorded/vodka/brandy/whiskey/rum/tequila). Additionally, the extensive literature archive of the author (>10,000 papers on alcoholic beverages) was hand searched for the keywords. Inclusion criteria were novelty, interest, generalizability, and appropriateness for routine analysis.

21.2 Processes Used in the Detection of Alcoholic Beverage Adulteration

21.2.1 Wine

"It is sufficiently obvious that few of those commodities, which are the objects of commerce, are adulterated to a greater extent than wine" (Accum, 1820). This citation from one of the earliest systematic monographs of the detection of food adulteration has been probably as true during the last decades as in 1820. In the 19th century, aluminum salts were added for brightening the wine color, or berry extracts to improve the purple color of red wine. Cask aging was simulated using oakwood sawdust, which may have been a predecessor to today's legalized technique of oak chips addition. More hazardous adulterations were the addition of lead salts for clarification and sweetening (Accum, 1820). Watering-down and addition of sugars (chaptalization) were the most common practices of wine adulteration in 19th century France (Stanziani, 2007, 2009). In more recent years, adulterations became more refined when analytical chemistry was able to easily detect these cruder forms of adulteration (see Table 21.1 for overview of common forms of wine adulteration). The 1980s wine scandal surrounding diethylene glycol was already mentioned in the introduction. More recent examples are the Brunello wine scandal, which was adulteration by cutting of 100% Sangiovese grapes with other low-quality wines from other origins (Cavicchi and Santini, 2011). It has been speculated that approximately 10% of wine on the European market is of lesser quality than touted on the label (Holmberg, 2010) but that most consumers will not detect the fraud because the products cannot be organoleptically differentiated, even by wine experts (Holmberg, 2010). Wine authentication including classical methods have been comprehensively reviewed by Arvanitoyannis (1999), Medina (1997), and Jackson (2000), and the following discussion will focus on new developments since these reviews.

The detection of the geographical origin of wine is a central question of wine authentication. Several methods were suggested, which are typically based on the multivariate analysis of data from instrumental methods (sometimes including combined data from several different methodologies) and the comparison with a collective of authentic samples.

The most common methods for wine authentication are based on ratios of stable isotopes. The Organisation Internationale de la Vigne et du Vin (OIV) has published

Table 21.1 The Types of Wine Fraud

Type	Description	Risk for Consumer
Mislabeling regarding origin, classification, or vintage	Most common type of wine fraud. Often facilitated by a "chain of bills," when wine is sold in a chain of retailers with a stepwise "quality enhancement."	Typically no health risk because potable cheap wine is misrepresented as being of better quality. Deception and fraud of the consumer.
Artificial wine	Wine based solely on additives and water. Occurs very seldom today.	Health risk such as allergenic risk dependent on the (unlabeled) additives.
Wine enhancement	Enhancement, most often accomplished by adding sugar, glycerol, diethylene glycol, or other sweeteners and/or other flavor compounds to the wine, or through blending with sweeter, foreign wine.	Typically no health risk except cases of addition of toxic compounds (eg, methanol). Deception and fraud of the consumer.

Summary based on Holmberg, L., 2010. Wine fraud. International Journal of Wine Research 2010, 105–113.

several methods in its compendium of international methods of analysis of wines and musts, such as the use of site-specific natural isotope fractionation nuclear magnetic resonance (SNIF-NMR) for determination of the deuterium distribution in ethanol, as well as the isotopic ratio of $^{18}O/^{16}O$ of water, of $^{13}C/^{12}C$ of ethanol, and of $^{13}C/^{12}C$ of glycerol. For details on methodology see Martin et al. (1988), Roßmann et al. (1998, 1999), Guillou et al. (2001), Fauhl and Wittkowski (2000), and Calderone and Guillou (2008). The methods were described as "cumbersome and expensive" (Medina, 1997), but still are most practical for the purpose. This is evident by the large number of applications that have been published on wine authentication using isotopic ratio determination. The differentiation of wines from different Italian (Versini et al., 1997) and Spanish (Giménez-Miralles et al., 1999) regions was possible. The addition of C4-plant sugar to wine can be detected (Versini et al., 2006). The determination of chaptalization, vintage, and geographical origin of Slovenian wines was possible (Kosir et al., 2001; Ogrinc et al., 2001). Long-term studies of isotopic ratios in German wines were presented by Hermann (2003) and Christoph et al. (2003).

The European Union (EU) has established a wine databank that contains the isotope ratios of authentic wine from all regions, which can be used for comparison in cases of suspect wine (Roßmann et al., 1999; Wachter, 2009).

Results from a large European project, which included a database of 600 wines from four countries, were published in a series of papers (Römisch et al., 2009; Schlesier et al., 2009; Smeyers-Verbeke et al., 2009). Using a combination of 63 chemical parameters, the investigators were able to distinguish South African from Eastern European wines. However, it was not possible to distinguish regions within the investigated countries. Other methods for geographical classification of wines include mass spectrometry—based electronic noses (Cynkar et al., 2010).

A completely different approach than the chemical methods is the extraction of residual DNA, which would allow the authentication of varietal wines. However, the DNA concentration in finished wine is quite low, so that amplification was not reproducible and even impossible in some samples. Improvements of the DNA technique are still required and its routine use is currently not possible (Siret et al., 2000).

The newest approach for wine authentication is the use of nontargeted ^{1}H NMR analysis. This technique treats the complete NMR spectrum as fingerprint and provides a multivariate comparison to a database of authentic spectra. The technique has been commercialized by Bruker as "Wine Screener" (Bruker, 2015; Spraul et al., 2013). The sensitivity of the method has been considerably improved during the last decade by advances in spectrometer technology and solvent suppression techniques, which now allow the determination of minor compounds in alcoholic beverages down to the lower ppm range (Monakhova et al., 2011b). Besides the geographical origin, ^{1}H NMR is the first method to provide a comprehensive prediction of the grape variety. In a sample of more than 600 German wines, it was shown that several grape types including Pinot Noir, Müller-Thurgau, Riesling, and Gewürztraminer could be distinguished with high accuracy (95% correct predictions) (Godelmann et al., 2013). Besides the classification, ^{1}H NMR allows the simultaneous quantitative determination of 56 compounds from the same spectrum (Bruker, 2015; Godelmann et al., 2013; Spraul et al., 2013) (Fig. 21.1). Besides a general nontargeted verification of sample

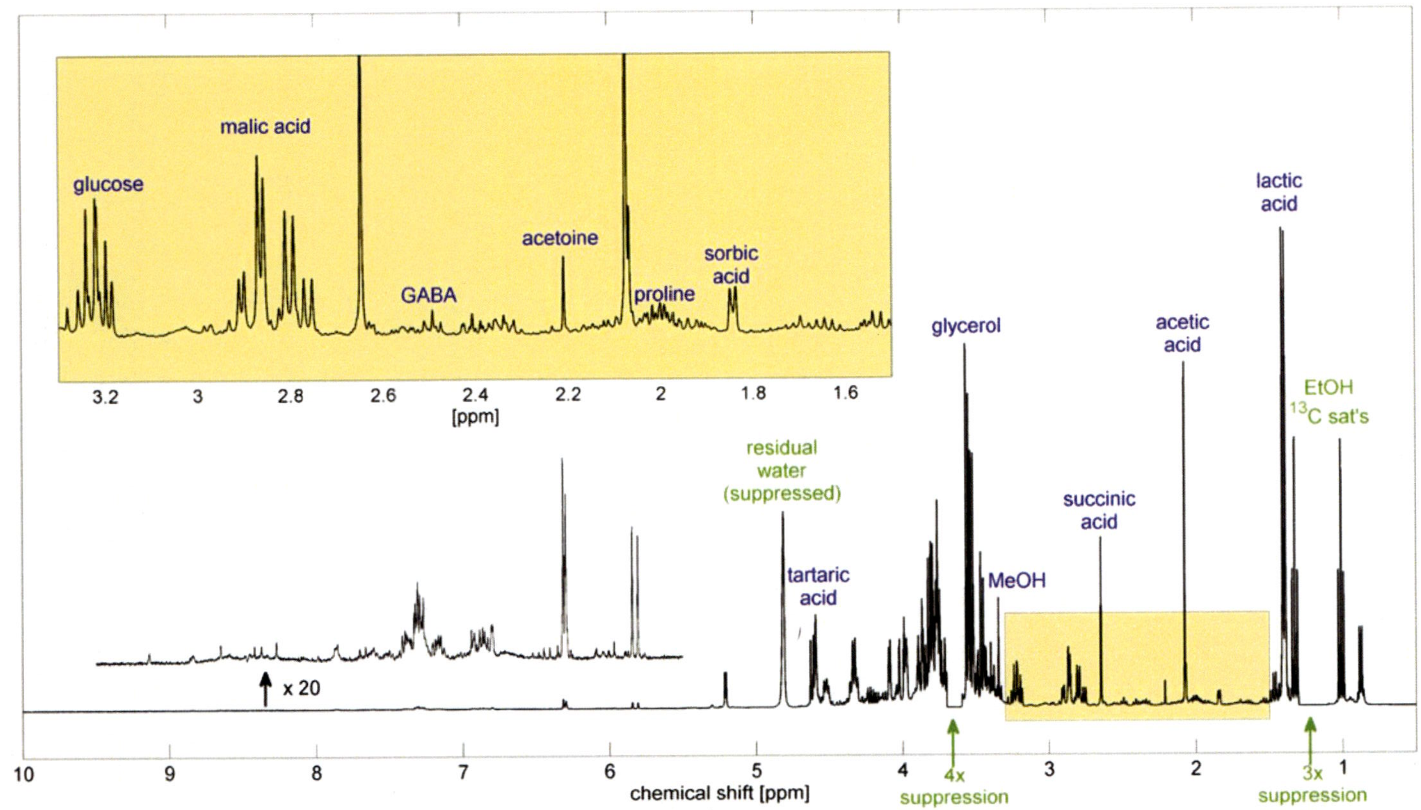

Figure 21.1 Proton NMR spectrum with eight-band suppression of a wine sample with compound assignment (details in magnification). Reprinted with permission from Godelmann, R., Fang, F., Humpfer, E., Schütz, B., Bansbach, M., Schäfer, H., Spraul, M., 2013. Targeted and nontargeted wine analysis by ^{1}H NMR spectroscopy combined with multivariate statistical analysis. Differentiation of important parameters: grape variety, geographical origin, year of vintage. Journal of Agricultural and Food Chemistry 61, 5610–5619. Copyright 2013, American Chemical Society.

conformity by comparison to authentic reference data, the wine profiling database maintained by Bruker currently allows a geographical origin verification of the major European wine-growing countries, including regional origin verification of some regions in France, Italy, and Spain. Twenty-two different grape varieties can be detected, including detection of water addition for some of the grape varieties (Bruker, 2015). A combination of stable isotope data and ^{1}H NMR spectra may be used in cases where the single methods lead to inconclusive results (Monakhova et al., 2014).

21.2.2 Beer

From a quantitative standpoint, there is considerably less literature on the authentication of beer than on the authentication of wine. This may have several reasons. Most probably, the economic benefit in adulterating beer is not so large as in the wine sector, where bottles can regularly reach prices beyond 10 EUR/l, which is seldom the case for beer. Beer is also produced with the aim to generate a consistent product quality, which unlike wine is mostly independent of vintage and origin (eg, Pilsner beer may be brewed everywhere with quite similar results). In contrast to the constant wine scandals, there also has not been a widespread beer adulteration scandal, which might have led interest and resources to the field of wine rather than beer. Nevertheless, there have been some approaches to verify the geographical origin of beer or to assign a specific brewery. Similar to wine analysis, the SNIF-NMR analysis is also able to analyze the deuterium distribution in ethanol extracted from beers. The D/H ratio allowed a rough geographical distinction of beers brewed in Germany, France, and Belgium (Martin et al., 1985b); but besides this publication of proof of concept, the routine application and validation of SNIF-NMR in the beer field has never been shown. According to the author's knowledge, comprehensive isotopic ratio databases for beer have not been established, and the method must be treated as obsolete. More modern approaches applied chromatographic or spectroscopic data as fingerprints for beer authentication. LC-MS was applied to differentiate Belgian Trappist beers (Mattarucchi et al., 2010). ^{1}H NMR was used to allocate the brewing site of German breweries as well as to differentiate between malt types (Fig. 21.2) (Lachenmeier et al., 2004). Finally, FTIR has been suggested to distinguish beer types and to detect outlying samples (Lachenmeier, 2007). NMR or FTIR could also be used to detect brand fraud, eg, in cases of draft beer not corresponding to the menu offering.

None of these nontargeted approaches has gained a wider application range over the single laboratories in which they have been developed. A commercial NMR-beer-screener (eg, similar to Bruker's fruit juice or wine screener systems) is also unavailable. Currently, beer analysis is quite traditional and mostly relies on classical physicochemical parameters (such as alcoholic strength, original gravity, extract, etc.), which are used to verify legal requirements and the consistency of the batches. Because of the lesser risk for adulteration of beer compared to other alcoholic beverages, it remains questionable if this situation will change in the near future, as resources are probably first given to the more relevant field of wine and spirits authenticity.

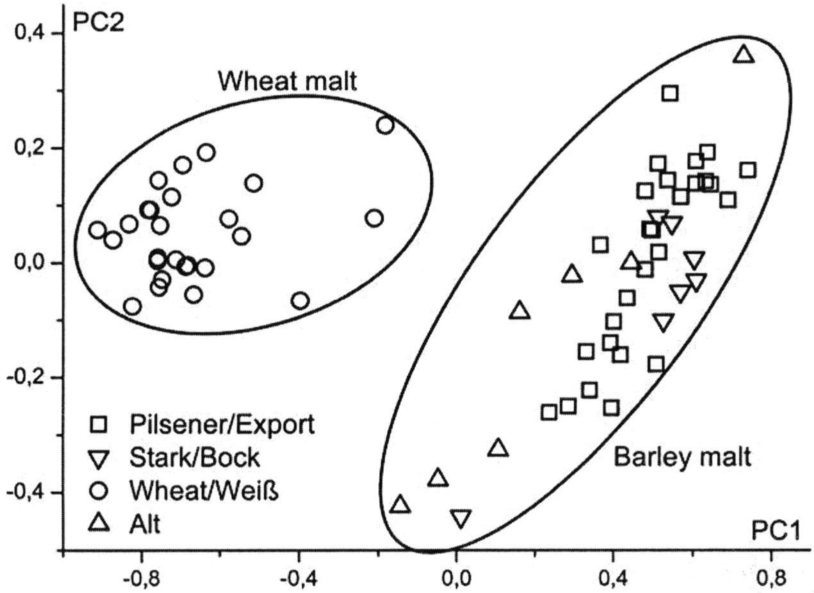

Figure 21.2 Differentiation of beers manufactured exclusively with barley malt according to the German beer purity law from beers manufactured with wheat malt. Principal component analysis (PCA) scores scatter plot for the aromatic region (7.6–6.7 ppm) of ^{1}H NMR spectra. Reprinted from Lachenmeier, D.W., Frank, W., Humpfer, E., Schäfer, H., Keller, S., Mörtter, M., Spraul, M., 2004. Quality control of beer using high-resolution nuclear magnetic resonance spectroscopy and multivariate analysis. European Food Research and Technology 220, 215–221 with kind permission from Springer Science and Business Media.

21.2.3 Spirits

The authentication of spirits is a quite diverse field because the composition of spirits has a considerably higher variation than the one of beer or wine, since numerous raw materials are allowed for production of spirits. Therefore, most authentication methods were conducted for certain subtypes of spirits (such as brandy, whiskey, or tequila). Unlike wine, for which reference procedures for isotopic ratio measurement are available, including international databases, such information is unavailable for spirits. For wine-based spirits, some of the mentioned OIV methods developed for wine analysis (see Section 21.2.1) may be suitable. Additionally, it must be mentioned that most of the procedures for spirits reviewed in the following text are scientific studies typically conducted with a restricted number of samples, and beyond the proof of concept, the applicability for routine analysis had not been investigated.

An overview of chromatographic and spectroscopic methods to the authentication of spirits was provided by Savchuk and Vlasov (2001). Classically, the gas chromatography (GC) analysis of minor components of alcoholic fermentation (so-called congeners including fusel alcohols) may be used to provide a rough assignment of the type of spirit (Simpkins, 1985). For example, fake cognacs may be detected by GC analysis alone (Schee et al., 1989), several different types of whiskey (Scotch, Bourbon, Canadian) can be differentiated (Headley and Hardy, 1989), as well as mixto-tequila (ie, tequila with added cane sugar) from 100% agave tequila (Lachenmeier et al., 2006). However, due to the large natural variation of these compounds these methods often provide only a hint rather than proof.

Similar to wine adulteration, there is the possibility of the addition of cheaper sources of sugar instead of the actually labeled raw materials. In Europe, such a practice is not allowed (ie, brandy, whiskey, rum, or fruit spirits must be exclusively produced from the pure raw materials). The isotopic ratios of deuterium/hydrogen and $^{13}C/^{12}C$ often allow to detect the illegal addition of foreign sugar (such as root or cane sugar) (Fig. 21.3) (Bauer-Christoph, 2010) and the assignment of raw materials (Bauer-Christoph et al., 1997). Stable isotope analysis also allowed the differentiation of European and Australasian ciders (Carter et al., 2015). The addition of cane or beet ethanol to whiskey may also be detected by differences in the $^{13}C/^{12}C$ ratios (Goodall et al., 2004). The measurement techniques of SNIF-NMR and IRMS in the field of spirits was reviewed by Guillou et al. (1992). Further applications include authentication of tequila (Aguilar-Cisneros et al., 2002; Bauer-Christoph et al., 2003) and fruit spirits (Baudler et al., 2006).

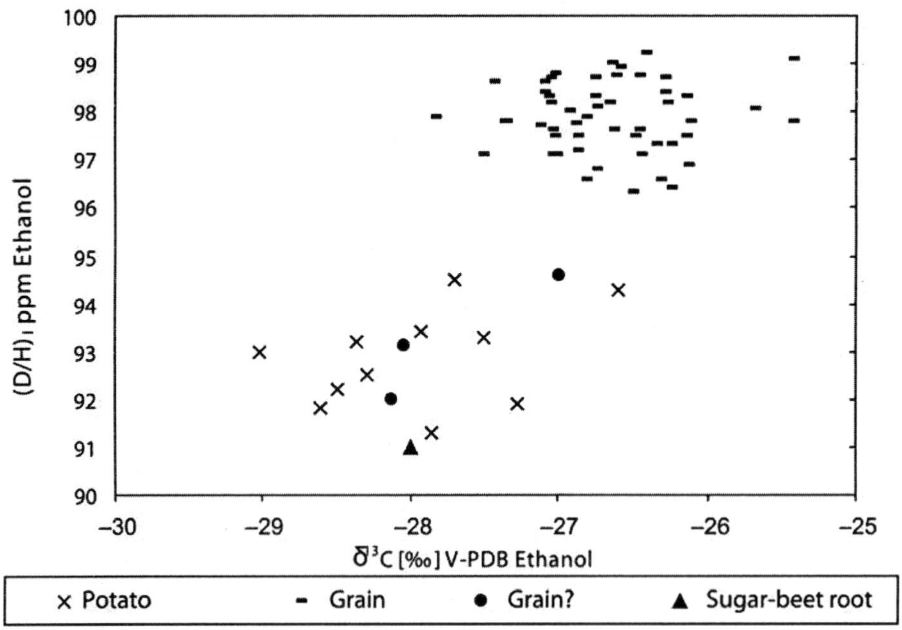

Figure 21.3 Detection of adulterated spirits incorrectly labeled as deriving from grain cereals by comparing the isotopic ratios of ethanol with those of authentic samples.
Reprinted from Bauer-Christoph, C., 2010. Spirituosen und spirituosenhaltige Getränke. In: Frede, W. (Ed.), Handbuch für Lebensmittelchemiker, Berlin, Heidelberg, Germany, Springer, pp. 719–735 with kind permission from Springer Science and Business Media.

Besides isotopic ratio analysis, spectroscopic techniques were often suggested as complementary techniques for differentiation of spirits. FTIR was used by Palma and Barroso (2002) to distinguish cognac and armagnac from brandies of Spanish and South African origin. The appropriateness of the method for discrimination of cognac from other distilled spirits was confirmed by Picque et al. (2006). A similar FTIR method was able to distinguish mixto-tequila from 100% agave tequila (Lachenmeier et al., 2005). Methanol adulteration in Turkish raki is also detectable using FTIR spectroscopy (Yucesoy and Ozen, 2013). FTIR allowed to authenticate fruit spirits; specifically it was possible to distinguish fruit spirits that have been produced from microbiologically spoiled mashes (Lachenmeier, 2007).

A special question for cask-aged spirits may be the confirmation of the storage time. For this purpose, HPLC analysis of oakwood related compounds such as 2-furaldehyde or 5-hydroxymethylfurfural has been suggested (Jaganathan and Dugar, 1999). Finally, the most promising method of the coming years will probably be ^{1}H NMR analysis for spirits similar to the NMR wine screener. First applications have been reported (Petrakis et al., 2005).

21.2.4 Unrecorded Alcohol

Unrecorded alcohol may be any alcohol discussed previously (ie, wine, beer, and spirits), with the difference that its production was not officially registered in the jurisdiction where the alcohol was consumed, either by illegal production, by home production (which may be licit in some legislations), or by cross-border trade. Besides these groups of beverage-type unrecorded alcohol, other forms of alcohol may be illicitly brought into the food chain (so-called surrogate alcohols), which were not produced as intended for human consumption (such as cosmetics alcohol, medicinal alcohol, disinfectant alcohol, denatured alcohol, synthetic alcohol, or other forms of industrial alcohol). For more details on definition of unrecorded alcohol, see Lachenmeier et al. (2007a, 2009b).

Besides targeted analysis for toxic constituents and adulterants (see review in Lachenmeier et al., 2011), the major question in the authentication of unrecorded alcohol is therefore the differentiation from recorded types of alcohol. This may be difficult when normal alcohol producers may illegally sell part of their alcohol without paying taxes, or when alcohol is smuggled from a low-tax state to a high-tax state (diversion fraud, which was described as common in the EU (WHO Regional Office for Europe, 2009)). Such types of alcohol may be absolutely identical to the conventional, taxed products and therefore not distinguishable by any of the previously mentioned methodologies. Such cases can only be resolved by other means (eg, different labeling or bottle types, or missing or forged tax labels, where required). The computerization of the movement and surveillance system of excisable products and improved enforcement was suggested in the EU as an effective tool against these forms of unrecorded alcohol (Commission of the European Communities, 2004; WHO Regional Office for Europe, 2009).

In cases where no prior information about composition of the unrecorded alcohol is available, a nontargeted analysis may be most preferable. Currently, only NMR has been suggested for this purpose to detect hazardous samples in a collection of unrecorded alcohol samples (Monakhova et al., 2012). This method was able to select samples that contained high concentrations of contaminants or denaturants, such as methanol, ethyl carbamate, diethyl phthalate, or polyhexamethyleneguanidine (Fig. 21.4).

The differentiation of surrogate alcohol from beverage alcohol is sometimes possible, especially when denatured alcohol is sold in pure form or admixed to beverage alcohol. Several methods were suggested in the literature to detect denaturants including diethyl phthalate typically with GC/MS (Leitz et al., 2009; Monakhova et al., 2011a). Denatonium benzoate (bitrex) can be detected using a portable Raman spectrometer (Kwiatkowski et al., 2014) or by liquid chromatography (Daunoravicius et al., 2006; Faulkner and DeMontigny, 1995; Henderson et al., 1998; Kovar and Loyer, 1984), GC/MS (Ng et al., 1998), or UV/VIS spectrophotometry (Bucci et al., 2006). The compound polyhexamethyleneguanidine, which was observed in some surrogate alcohols based on disinfectant solutions, may be detected by spectrophotometry (Solodun et al., 2011).

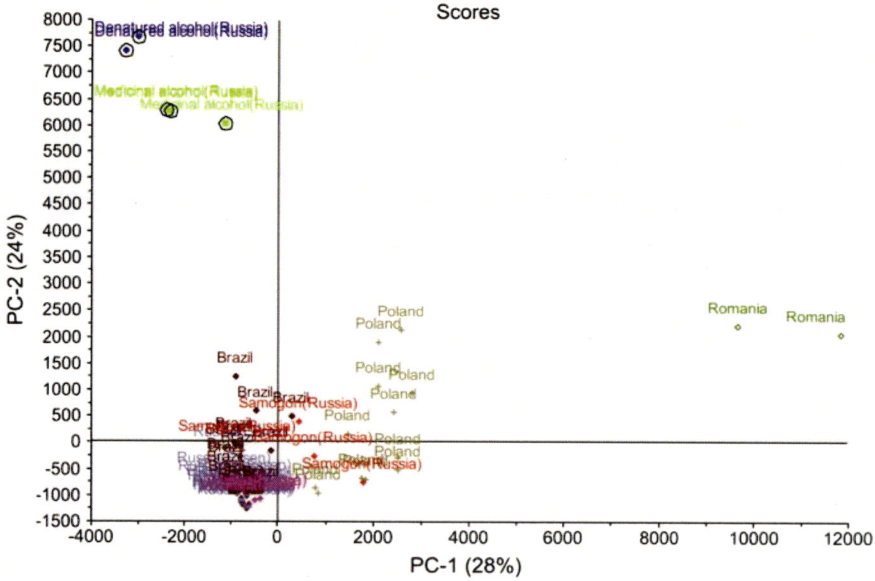

Figure 21.4 Nontargeted analysis of unrecorded alcohol to detect hazardous samples. A scatter plot of the principal component analysis (PCA) scores (10−0.25 ppm) of ^{1}H NMR spectra of 304 samples of international unrecorded alcohols is shown. The outlying samples include denatured and medicinal alcohols from Russia and two samples with extreme concentrations of ethyl carbamate from Romania.

Reprinted from Monakhova, Y.B., Kuballa, T., Lachenmeier, D.W., 2012. Nontargeted NMR analysis to rapidly detect hazardous substances in alcoholic beverages. Applied Magnetic Resonance 42, 343−352 with kind permission from Springer Science and Business Media.

21.3 Case Studies

21.3.1 Falsification of Brand Spirits

An important question in the field is not only the authentication of a type of spirit (see Section 21.2.3), but to verify a specific brand (Aylott, 2010). This may be the case in large-scale counterfeiting (eg, relabeling of cheap alcohol types, sometimes including unrecorded alcohol types), but brand fraud has also been observed in gastronomy (especially in establishments that very cheaply sell alcohol such as discotheques with flat-rate drinking). In such cases, the bar operator may refill the bottles of brand spirits with cheaper brands of the same type of spirit (in Germany often from so-called discount stores) (Lachenmeier et al., 2003). Additionally, dilution of the brand spirits or cheaper spirits with some quantities of water may occur. Such brand fraud can often be quite easily detected, especially in cases where the alcohol content of the fraudulent product is considerably lower than the one of the brand product. Portable alcohol sensors are available for field testing (Lachenmeier et al., 2010).

Another rapid and easy indicator is the conductivity of the spirit, which may be measured with cheap, hand-held devices. In the case of vodka it was shown that the brand products had significantly lower conductivity than the discount products (Fig. 21.5) (Lachenmeier et al., 2007b). The conductivity analyses can be confirmed in the laboratory using ion chromatography, as has been shown for brand confirmation in vodka and rum (Lachenmeier et al., 2003) or brandy (Lachenmeier and Attig, 2005).

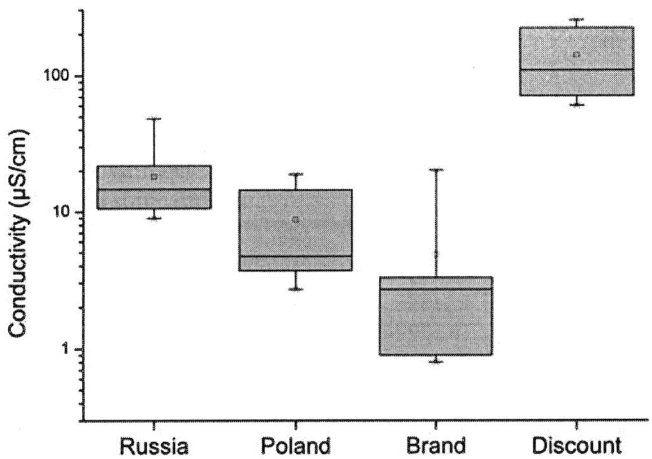

Figure 21.5 Brand authentication of vodka using portable conductivity measurement. The box charts of vodka ($n = 60$) show that products from so-called discount shops have significantly higher conductivities than Russian, Polish, or other premium-brand products.
Reprinted from Lachenmeier, D.W., Schmidt, B., Bretschneider, T., 2007b. Rapid and mobile brand authentication of vodka using conductivity measurement. Microchim Acta 160, 283–289 with kind permission from Springer Science and Business Media.

The anion–cation composition of vodkas from the same distillery were found to be quite stable and may serve as an identification feature (Arbuzov and Savchuk, 2002).

Field testing using a portable UV/VIS spectrometer (a so-called "brand authenticator") may also be conducted for Scotch whiskey (Aylott, 2010; MacKenzie and Aylott, 2004). The instrument compares the spectrum to a database of authentic whiskey spectra and indicates a binary result similar to a traffic light. The confirmation of suspicious whiskey samples may then be conducted using various techniques such as GC or GC/MS analysis (Aylott et al., 1994).

For the reason that brand authentication may be still difficult when the products are quite similar (such as in cases of white spirits), the industry may add so-called "brand indicators" to its products. The indicators can be unique flavorings, sugars, or trace additives (which must be permitted for use in foodstuffs). However, some spirits categories do not allow any additives (such as Scotch whiskey) (Aylott, 2010).

21.3.2 Authentication of Vintage Wines and Spirits

During the last decades, the market for old and rare wines and spirits has been considerably expanded and the products are often bought as an investment rather than for drinking purposes (Holmberg, 2010). The collector fraud, which is a subtype of mislabeling mentioned in Section 21.2.1, has been recently acknowledged as major problem (Holmberg, 2010).

Several radioactive nuclei have been suggested for authentication of wine of vintages between the 1950s and 1990s. The atmospheric concentrations of the radioactive nuclei of several elements, which also are incorporated into the grapes and finally the wine, were increased due to nuclear weapon tests in the late 1950s, with highest levels in the mid-1960s, and decreased to background levels in the 1990s (Hubert et al., 2009). The most commonly applied method is ^{14}C analysis (Baxter and Walton, 1971; Burchuladze et al., 1989; Kostadinov and Yanev, 1986; Martin et al., 1995; Schönhofer, 1989, 1992; Zoppi et al., 2004) and ^{3}H analysis (Fischer et al., 1980; Scherer et al., 2009). The ^{14}C method is also able to distinguish synthetic ethanol addition and artificial carbonation, because ethanol and CO_2 from fossil sources have much lower ^{14}C activities (Martin et al., 1981, 1985a). A more recent approach for dating of old wines is the measurement of ^{137}Cs, which can be facilitated nondestructively through the glass bottle without opening (Hubert et al., 2009; Hubert, 2005).

Because the chemical detection and differentiation of collector wines is typically impossible beyond 1990, producers are currently experimenting with a number of security measures, such as UV-marked labels or proof tags that allow the traceability of the product (Holmberg, 2010).

A novel approach for dating wine may be the use of ^{1}H NMR and multivariate analysis. In a first application of this approach, a differentiation of German wines from 2008 to 2009 has been possible (Godelmann et al., 2013). The drawback of this technique is the requirement of large databases of each vintage and each wine-growing region.

21.3.3 Methanol Crisis in the Czech Republic

Major hazards from other compounds besides ethanol are predominantly restricted to methanol (Lachenmeier et al., 2007a). Pure methanol can be bought from chemical suppliers and used in criminal intent or in pure stupidity in pure form or admixed to other alcohols. Most cases of methanol poisoning in the last decades stemmed from the illegal admixture of methanol rather than from the use of methanol-denatured alcohol (which was prohibited in most jurisdictions). For example, the 1986 methanol scandal in Italy occurred when prices for methanol plummeted due to a tax exemption for this alcohol (MacKenzie, 1986).

A more recent example of this was in early September 2012, when the Czech food safety authority informed the public of persons suffering from methanol poisoning after having consumed "on tap" spirits. The product was unlabeled and supplied "in bulk" in plastic barrels. The public was immediately warned by the media and by local municipal offices. The levels of methanol were so high that they were caused by deliberate adulteration. The public was urged not to consume any spirits as a precaution and to dispose of any spirit that could be contaminated. When more cases were reported, Czech authorities decided to take more drastic measures. Consumption of spirits with more than 20% alcohol was forbidden. Existing stocks of spirits were destroyed and replaced by new productions bearing a new tax seal. Investigations into traceability of the adulterated spirits showed that fortunately they were not widespread outside of the Czech Republic. Only in Poland and Slovakia cases were reported though sometimes after having traveled to the Czech Republic. By early December 2012, the total number of deaths related to this incident was 36 (European Commission, 2013). The epidemiology of this poisoning crisis was reviewed by Zakharov et al. (2014). Such crises present analytical chemistry with special demands, as many samples have to be analyzed in a short time. Nearly 4000 samples had to be analyzed for methanol in a four-month period (Vaskova et al., 2014). To achieve a rapid and easy analysis, portable Raman spectrometers were applied in the Czech Republic, which also allow the analysis without opening the bottle. It was noted that the sensitivity of such spectrometers is not enough to control the normal trace-methanol levels in spirits, but it was sufficient to control for the health-relevant concentrations in the adulterated alcohol, which was in the percent range (Vaskova et al., 2014). Another suitable method for laboratory analysis might be FTIR spectroscopy, which allows to analyse samples for methanol within 1 min (Lachenmeier, 2007).

21.4 Future Trends

The case of diethylene glycol in wine, which went undetected for a time because of not being included in the list of tested compounds, is an excellent reminder of the limitation of targeted analysis, which is still predominant in private and governmental food-testing laboratories. There are only first approaches into the use of nontargeted analysis, which may have the capability to detect novel or unusual compounds, or may just provide a "fingerprint" of the beverage that can be compared against a database of authentic beverages (see, eg, Monakhova et al., 2013 or Le Gall and Colquhoun, 2003 for introductory reviews). Various techniques may be suitable for such a nontargeted analysis, including UV/VIS or IR spectroscopy, but specifically NMR spectroscopy, for which several promising approaches were published (Lachenmeier et al., 2009a). The wine screening using targeted and nontargeted NMR spectroscopy has become the first method in the field of alcoholic beverages that is applied in a routine fashion (Godelmann et al., 2013). It would be important to establish publicly available databases with spectra of authentic alcoholic beverages similar to the EU wine databases of isotopic ratios.

From a standpoint of production technology, a tighter implementation of the hazard analysis critical control point (HACCP) system was suggested to avoid adulteration (Kourtis and Arvanitoyannis, 2001). Indeed, this may detect crude forms of adulteration (eg, methanol addition) along the supply chain, if regular sampling and analysis is implemented. However, HACCP would probably not be able to prevent intentional fraud on the last steps of thc supply chain, similar to what occurred in the Czech Republic.

Another trend may be so-called electronic noses, which may have potential in fingerprinting alcoholic beverages similar to NMR spectroscopy. Some first applications were described (Marti et al., 2005; Novakowski et al., 2011), but currently the technique does not appear as being robust for routine analysis.

Sources of Further Information

1. Excellent reviews about the topic are available by Arvanitoyannis (1999), Medina (1997), Jackson (2000), and Aylott (2013).
2. The Joint Research Centre of the European Commission has published a report on the analysis and characterization of alcoholic products (Segebarth et al., 2008).
3. The currently ongoing project "Food Integrity" in the EU's Seventh Framework Programme (www.foodintegrity.eu) contains a work package on spirit drinks authentication. Among the key objectives are the development of field devices to detect harmful and nonpotable constituents in spirits as well as to authenticate branded spirits.

References

Accum, F.C.A., 1820. A Treatise on Adulterations of Food, and Culinary Poisons. Longman, Hurst, Rees, Orme, and Brown, London, UK.

Aguilar-Cisneros, B.O., López, M.G., Richling, E., Heckel, F., Schreier, P., 2002. Tequila authenticity assessment by headspace SPME-HRGC-IRMS analysis of $^{13}C/^{12}C$ and $^{18}O/^{16}O$ ratios of ethanol. Journal of Agricultural and Food Chemistry 50, 7520–7523.

Arbuzov, V.N., Savchuk, S.A., 2002. Identification of vodkas by ion chromatography and gas chromatography. Journal of Analytical Chemistry 57, 428–433.

Arvanitoyannis, I.S., 1999. Application of quality control methods for assessing wine authenticity: use of multivariate analysis (chemometrics). Trends in Food Science & Technology 10, 321–336.

Aylott, R.I., Clyne, A.H., Fox, A.P., Walker, D.A., 1994. Analytical strategies to confirm Scotch whisky authenticity. Analyst 11, 1741–1746.

Aylott, R., 2010. Assuring brand integrity. Brewer and Distiller International April 50–52.

Aylott, R., 2013. Analytical strategies supporting protected designations of origin for alcoholic beverages. Comprehensive Analytical Chemistry 60, 409–437.

Baudler, R., Adam, L., Rossmann, A., Versini, G., Engel, K.H., 2006. Influence of the distillation step on the ratios of stable isotopes of ethanol in cherry brandies. Journal of Agricultural and Food Chemistry 54, 864–869.

Bauer-Christoph, C., Christoph, N., Aguilar-Cisneros, B.O., López, M.G., Richling, E., Rossmann, A., Schreier, P., 2003. Authentication of tequila by gas chromatography and stable isotope ratio analyses. European Food Research and Technology 217, 438–443.

Bauer-Christoph, C., 2010. Spirituosen und spirituosenhaltige Getränke. In: Frede, W. (Ed.), Handbuch für Lebensmittelchemiker. Springer, Berlin, Heidelberg, Germany, pp. 719–735.

Bauer-Christoph, C., Wachter, H., Christoph, N., Rßmann, A., Adam, L., 1997. Assignment of raw material and authentication of spirits by gas chromatography, hydrogen-and carbon-isotope ratio measurements I. Analytical methods and results of a study of commercial products. Zeitschrift für Lebensmittel-Untersuchung und -Forschung A 204, 445–452.

Baxter, M.S., Walton, A., 1971. Carbon-14 concentrations in recent wines and spirits. Journal of Food Science 36, 540–541.

Bruker, 2015. Wine Profiling. A New Generation of Wine Analysis Has Arrived. Bruker Corporation, Rheinstetten, Germany.

Bucci, R., Balestrieri, F., Magri, A.D., Magri, A.L., Marini, F., 2006. UV-vis spectrophotometric method for the quantitation of all the components of Italian general denaturant and its application to check the conformity of alcohol samples. Talanta 68, 781–790.

Burchuladze, A.A., Chudy, M., Eristavi, I.V., Pagava, S.V., Povinec, P., Sivo, A., Togonidze, G.I., 1989. Anthropogenic ^{14}C variations in atmospheric CO_2 and wines. Radiocarbon 31, 771–776.

Calderone, G., Guillou, C., 2008. Analysis of isotopic ratios for the detection of illegal watering of beverages. Food Chemistry 106, 1399–1405.

Carter, J.F., Yates, H.S., Tinggi, U., 2015. Stable isotope and chemical compositions of European and Australasian ciders as a guide to authenticity. Journal of Agricultural and Food Chemistry 63, 975–982.

Cavicchi, A., Santini, C., 2011. Brunellopoli: a wine scandal under the tuscan sun. Tourism Reviews International 15, 253–267.

Christoph, N., Rossmann, A., Voerkelius, S., 2003. Possibilities and limitations of wine authentication using stable isotope and meteorological data, data banks and statistical tests. Part 1: wines from Franconia. Mitteilungen Klosterneuburg 53, 23–40.

Commission of the European Communities, 2004. Report from the Commission to the Council, the European Parliament and the European Economic and Social Committee on the Rates of Excise Duty Applied on Alcohol and Alcoholic Beverages (Presented Pursuant to Article 8 of Council Directive 92/84/EEC on the Approximation of Excise Duty on Alcohol and Alcoholic Beverages). COM(2004) 223 Final. Commission of the European Communities, Brussels, Belgium.

Cornwall, H.B., 1884. Adulteration of beer. Public Health Papers and Reports 10, 106–115.

Cynkar, W., Dambergs, R., Smith, P., Cozzolino, D., 2010. Classification of Tempranillo wines according to geographic origin: combination of mass spectrometry based electronic nose and chemometrics. Analytica Chimica Acta 660, 227–231.

Daunoravicius, Z., Juknaite, I., Naujalis, E., Padarauskas, A., 2006. Simple and rapid determination of denaturants in alcohol formulations by hydrophilic interaction chromatography. Chromatographia 63, 373–377.

Dunn, J.B., 1869. The Adulteration of Liquors With a Description of the Poisons Used in Their Manufacture. National Temperance Society and Publication House, New York, USA.

Eisinger, J., 1982. Lead and wine. Eberhard Gockel and the colica Pictonum. Medical History 26, 279–302.

European Commission, 2013. RASFF. The Rapid Alert System for Food and Feed. 2012 Annual Report. Publications Office of the European Union, Luxembourg.

Fauhl, C., Wittkowski, R., 2000. Oenological influences on the D/H ratios of wine ethanol. Journal of Agricultural and Food Chemistry 48, 3979–3984.

Faulkner, A., DeMontigny, P., 1995. High-performance liquid chromatographic determination of denatonium benzoate in ethanol with 5% polyvinylpyrrolidone. Journal of Chromatography A 715, 189–194.

Fischer, E., Müller, H., Rapp, A., Steffan, H., 1980. Tritium- und Kohlenstoff-14-Gehalte von Weinen verschiedener Jahrgänge der nördlichen und südlichen Hemisphäre. Zeitschrift fuer Lebensmittel-Untersuchung und -Forschung 171, 269–271.

Giménez-Miralles, J.E., Salazar, D.M., Solana, I., 1999. Regional origin assignment of red wines from Valencia (Spain) by ^{2}H NMR and ^{13}C IRMS stable isotope analysis of fermentative ethanol. Journal of Agricultural and Food Chemistry 47, 2645–2652.

Godelmann, R., Fang, F., Humpfer, E., Schütz, B., Bansbach, M., Schäfer, H., Spraul, M., 2013. Targeted and nontargeted wine analysis by ^{1}H NMR spectroscopy combined with multivariate statistical analysis. Differentiation of important parameters: grape variety, geographical origin, year of vintage. Journal of Agricultural and Food Chemistry 61, 5610–5619.

Goodall, I.C., Reid, K.J.G., Brereton, P.A., Rhodes, C., Heaton, K., 2004. The application of stable carbon isotope ratios to the authentication of Scotch whisky. In: Bryce, J.H., Stewart, G.G. (Eds.), Distilled Spirits. Nottingham University Press, Nottingham, UK, pp. 41–45.

Guillou, C., Jamin, E., Martin, G.J., Reniero, F., 2001. Isotopic analyses of wine and of products derived from grape. Bulletin de l'OIV 74, 839–840.

Guillou, C., Martin, G.J., Vidal, J.P., Cantagrel, R., 1992. The applications of deuterium nuclear magnetic resonance to the analysis of spirits. In: Cantagrel, R. (Ed.), 1er Symposium Scientifique Inernational de Cognac, Paris, France, Lavoisier-Tec & Doc, pp. 417–424.

Headley, L.M., Hardy, J.K., 1989. Classification of whiskies by principal component analysis. Journal of Food Science 54, 1351.

Henderson, M.C., Neumann, C.M., Buhler, D.R., 1998. Analysis of denatonium benzoate in Oregon consumer products by HPLC. Chemosphere 36, 203–210.

Hermann, A., 2003. Isotopic analysis: D/H-ratios in the ethanol of German wines. Mitteilungen Klosterneuburg 53, 132–138.

Holmberg, L., 2010. Wine fraud. International Journal of Wine Research 2010, 105–113.

Hubert, P., Perrot, F., Gaye, J., Médina, B., Pravikoff, M.S., 2009. Radioactivity measurements applied to the dating and authentication of old wines. Comptes Rendus Physique 10, 622–629.

Hubert, P., 2005. Neutrino mass, radioactivity and the dating of wine. Europhysics News 36, 21–23.

Jackson, R.S., 2000. Wine laws, authentication and geography. In: Jackson, R.S. (Ed.), Wine Science, second ed. Academic Press, San Diego, USA, pp. 482–543.

Jaganathan, J., Dugar, S.M., 1999. Authentication of straight whiskey by determination of the ratio of furfural to 5-hydroxymethyl-2-furaldehyde. Journal of AOAC International 82, 997–1001.

Kosir, I.J., Kocjanic, M., Ogrinc, N., Kidric, J., 2001. Use of SNIF-NMR and IRMS in combination with chemometric methods for the determination of chaptalisation and geographical origin of wines (the example of Slovenian wines). Analytica Chimica Acta 429, 195–206.

Kostadinov, K.N., Yanev, Y.L., 1986. Liquid scintillation measurement of ^{14}C in ethanol extracted from Bulgarian wines. Nuclear Instruments & Methods in Physics Research, Section B 17, 511–514.

Kourtis, L.K., Arvanitoyannis, I.S., 2001. Implementation of hazard analysis critical control point (HACCP) system to the alcoholic beverages industry. Food Reviews International 17, 1–44.

Kovar, J., Loyer, M., 1984. Determination of bitrex, quassia powder and sucrose octaacetate next to diethyl phthalate and camphor in specially denatured alcohols by liquid chromatography. Journal of Liquid Chromatography 7, 2163–2177.

Kwiatkowski, A., Czerwicka, M., Smulko, J., Stepnowski, P., 2014. Detection of denatonium benzoate (bitrex) remnants in noncommercial alcoholic beverages by Raman spectroscopy. Journal of Forensic Sciences 59, 1358–1363.

Lachenmeier, D.W., Attig, R., 2005. Authentizitätsprüfung von Weinbrand mittels Ionenchromatographie. In: Eckert, F. (Ed.), Alkohol Jahrbuch 2005. Zimmermann Druck + Verlag, Balve, Germany, pp. 112–117.

Lachenmeier, D.W., Humpfer, E., Fang, F., Schütz, B., Dvortsak, P., Sproll, C., Spraul, M., 2009a. NMR-spectroscopy for nontargeted screening and simultaneous quantification of health-relevant compounds in foods: the example of melamine. Journal of Agricultural and Food Chemistry 57, 7194–7199.

Lachenmeier, D.W., Rehm, J., 2013. Is there a relationship between alcohol quality and health? Alcohol and Alcoholism 48, 127–129.

Lachenmeier, D.W., Rehm, J., Gmel, G., 2007a. Surrogate alcohol: what do we know and where do we go? Alcoholism Clinical and Experimental Research 31, 1613–1624.

Lachenmeier, D.W., Sarsh, B., Rehm, J., 2009b. The composition of alcohol products from markets in Lithuania and Hungary, and potential health consequences: a pilot study. Alcohol and Alcoholism 44, 93–102.

Lachenmeier, D.W., 2007. Rapid quality control of spirit drinks and beer using multivariate data analysis of Fourier transform infrared spectra. Food Chemistry 101, 825–832.

Lachenmeier, D.W., Attig, R., Frank, W., Athanasakis, C., 2003. The use of ion chromatography to detect adulteration of vodka and rum. European Food Research and Technology 218, 105–110.

Lachenmeier, D.W., Frank, W., Humpfer, E., Schäfer, H., Keller, S., Mörtter, M., Spraul, M., 2004. Quality control of beer using high-resolution nuclear magnetic resonance spectroscopy and multivariate analysis. European Food Research and Technology 220, 215–221.

Lachenmeier, D.W., Godelmann, R., Steiner, M., Ansay, B., Weigel, J., Krieg, G., 2010. Rapid and mobile determination of alcoholic strength in wine, beer and spirits using a flow-through infrared sensor. Chemistry Central Journal 4, 5.

Lachenmeier, D.W., Richling, E., López, M.G., Frank, W., Schreier, P., 2005. Multivariate analysis of FTIR and ion chromatographic data for the quality control of tequila. Journal of Agricultural and Food Chemistry 53, 2151–2157.

Lachenmeier, D.W., Schmidt, B., Bretschneider, T., 2007b. Rapid and mobile brand authentication of vodka using conductivity measurement. Microchim Acta 160, 283–289.

Lachenmeier, D.W., Schoeberl, K., Kanteres, F., Kuballa, T., Sohnius, E.M., Rehm, J., 2011. Is contaminated unrecorded alcohol a health problem in the European Union? A review of existing and methodological outline for future studies. Addiction 106 (Suppl), 20–30.

Lachenmeier, D.W., Sohnius, E.M., Attig, R., López, M.G., 2006. Quantification of selected volatile constituents and anions in Mexican Agave spirits (Tequila, Mezcal, Sotol, Bacanora). Journal of Agricultural and Food Chemistry 54, 3911–3915.

Le Gall, G., Colquhoun, I.J., 2003. NMR spectroscopy in food authentication. In: Lees, M. (Ed.), Food Authenticity and Traceability. Woodhead Publishing Ltd, Cambridge, UK, pp. 131–155.

Leitz, J., Kuballa, T., Rehm, J., Lachenmeier, D.W., 2009. Chemical analysis and risk assessment of diethyl phthalate in alcoholic beverages with special regard to unrecorded alcohol. PLoS One 4, e8127.

Lessler, M.A., 1988. Lead and lead poisoning from antiquity to modern times. Ohio Journal of Science 88, 78–84.

MacKenzie, D., 1986. Italy's poisoned wine scandal unfolds. New Scientist 110, 22.

MacKenzie, W.M., Aylott, R.I., 2004. Analytical strategies to confirm Scotch whisky authenticity. Part II: mobile brand authentication. Analyst 129, 607–612.

Marti, M.P., Boque, R., Busto, O., Guasch, J., 2005. Electronic noses in the quality control of alcoholic beverages. Trends in Analytical Chemistry 24, 57–66.

Martin, G.E., Krueger, H.W., Burggraff, J.M., 1985a. Radiocarbon ^{14}C differentiation of sparkling and carbonated wines. Journal of AOAC 68, 440–443.

Martin, G.J., Benbernou, M., Lantier, F., 1985b. Application of site-specific natural isotope fractionation (SNIF-NMR) of hydrogen to the characterization of European beers. Journal of the Institute of Brewing 91, 242–249.

Martin, G.J., Thibault, J.N., Bertrand, M.J., 1995. Spatial and temporal dependence of the ^{13}C and ^{14}C isotopes of wine ethanols. Radiocarbon 37, 943–954.

Martin, G.J., Guillou, C., Martin, M.L., Cabanis, M.T., Tep, Y., Aerny, J., 1988. Natural factors of isotope fractionation and the characterization of wines. Journal of Agricultural and Food Chemistry 36, 316–322.

Martin, G.E., Noakes, J.E., Alfonso, F.C., Figert, D.M., 1981. Liquid scintillation counting of ^{14}C for differentiation of synthetic ethanol from ethanol of fermentation. Journal of AOAC 64, 1142–1144.

Mattarucchi, E., Stocchero, M., Moreno-Rojas, J.M., Giordano, G., Reniero, F., Guillou, C., 2010. Authentication of Trappist beers by LC-MS fingerprints and multivariate data analysis. Journal of Agricultural and Food Chemistry 58, 12089–12095.

Medina, B., 1997. In: Ashurst, P.R., Dennis, M.J. (Eds.), Wine Authenticity. Springer US, Boston, MA, pp. 60–107.

Monakhova, Y.B., Kuballa, T., Leitz, J., Lachenmeier, D.W., 2011a. Determination of diethyl phthalate and polyhexamethylene guanidine in surrogate alcohol from Russia. International Journal of Analytical Chemistry 2011. Article ID 704795.

Monakhova, Y., Kuballa, T., Lachenmeier, D.W., 2013. Chemometric methods in NMR spectroscopic analysis of food products. Journal of Analytical Chemistry 68, 755–766.

Monakhova, Y.B., Godelmann, R., Hermann, A., Kuballa, T., Cannet, C., Schäfer, H., Spraul, M., Rutledge, D.N., 2014. Synergistic effect of the simultaneous chemometric analysis of ^{1}H NMR spectroscopic and stable isotope (SNIF-NMR, ^{18}O, ^{13}C) data: application to wine analysis. Analytica Chimica Acta 833, 29–39.

Monakhova, Y.B., Kuballa, T., Lachenmeier, D.W., 2012. Nontargeted NMR analysis to rapidly detect hazardous substances in alcoholic beverages. Applied Magnetic Resonance 42, 343–352.

Monakhova, Y.B., Schäfer, H., Humpfer, E., Spraul, M., Kuballa, T., Lachenmeier, D.W., 2011b. Application of automated eightfold suppression of water and ethanol signals in (1) H NMR to provide sensitivity for analyzing alcoholic beverages. Magnetic Resonance in Chemistry 49, 734–739.

Narziss, L., 1984. The German beer law. Journal of the Institute of Brewing 90, 351–358.

Ng, L.K., Hupé, M., Harnois, J., Lawrence, A.H., 1998. Direct injection gas chromatographic/mass spectrometric analysis for denatonium benzoate in specific denatured alcohol formulations. Analytical Chemistry 70, 4389–4393.

Novakowski, W., Bertotti, M., Paixao, T.R.L.C., 2011. Use of copper and gold electrodes as sensitive elements for fabrication of an electronic tongue: discrimination of wines and whiskies. Microchemical Journal 99, 145–151.

Ogrinc, N., Kosir, I.J., Kocjancic, M., Kidric, J., 2001. Determination of authenticity, regional origin, and vintage of Slovenian wines using a combination of IRMS and SNIF-NMR analyses. Journal of Agricultural and Food Chemistry 49, 1432–1440.

Palma, M., Barroso, C.G., 2002. Application of FT-IR spectroscopy to the characterisation and classification of wines, brandies and other distilled drinks. Talanta 58, 265–271.

Petrakis, P., Touris, I., Liouni, M., Zervou, M., Kyrikou, I., Kokkinofta, R., Theocharis, C.R., Mavromoustakos, T.M., 2005. Authenticity of the traditional cypriot spirit "Zivania" on the basis of ^{1}H NMR spectroscopy diagnostic parameters and statistical analysis. Journal of Agricultural and Food Chemistry 53, 5293–5303.

Picque, D., Lieben, P., Corrieu, G., Cantagrel, R., Lablanquie, O., Snakkers, G., 2006. Discrimination of Cognacs and other distilled drinks by mid-infrared spectroscopy. Journal of Agricultural and Food Chemistry 54, 5220–5226.

Römisch, U., Jäger, H., Capron, X., Lanteri, S., Forina, M., Smeyers-Verbeke, J., 2009. Characterization and determination of the geographical origin of wines. Part III: multivariate discrimination and classification methods. European Food Research and Technology 230, 31–45.

Roßmann, A., Reniero, F., Moussa, I., Schmidt, H.L., Versini, G., Merle, M.H., 1999. Stable oxygen isotope content of water of EU data-bank wines from Italy, France and Germany. Zeitschrift fuer Lebensmittel-Untersuchung und -Forschung A 208, 400–407.

Roßmann, A., Schmidt, H.L., Hermann, A., Ristow, R., 1998. Multielement stable isotope ratio analysis of glycerol to determine its origin in wine. Zeitschrift fuer Lebensmittel-Untersuchung und -Forschung A 207, 237–243.

Savchuk, S.A., Vlasov, V.N., 2001. Application of chromatography and spectrometry to the authentication of alcoholic beverages. Journal of Analytical Chemistry 56, 214–231.

Schee, H.A., Kennedy, W.B.H., Bouwknegt, J.P., Hittenhausen-Gelderblom, R., 1989. A case of cognac adulteration. Zeitschrift fuer Lebensmittel-Untersuchung und -Forschung 188, 11–15.

Scherer, U.W., Jacobi, M., Castillo, J., Förstel, D.H., 2009. Ultra-low-level measurements of ^{3}H and ^{14}C in wines and champagne. Radiation Effects and Defects in Solids 164, 382–385.

Schlesier, K., Fauhl-Hassek, C., Forina, M., Cotea, V., Kocsi, E., Schoula, R., van Jaarsveld, F., Wittkowski, R., 2009. Characterisation and determination of the geographical origin of wines. Part I: overview. European Food Research and Technology 230, 1–13.

Schönhofer, F., 1989. Determination of ^{14}C in alcoholic beverages. Radiocarbon 31, 777–784.

Schönhofer, F., 1992. ^{14}C in Austrian wine and vinegar. Radiocarbon 34, 768–771.

Segebarth, N., Alonso-Salces, R.M., Skordi, E., Guillou, C., 2008. Analysis and Characterisation of Alcoholic Products (ACAP). Office for Official Publications of the European Communities, Luxembourg.

Simpkins, W.A., 1985. Congener profiles in the detection of illicit spirits. Journal of the Science of Food and Agriculture 36, 367–376.

Siret, R., Boursiquot, J.M., Merle, M.H., Cabanis, J.C., This, P., 2000. Toward the authentication of varietal wines by the analysis of grape (*Vitis vinifera* L.) residual DNA in must and wine using microsatellite markers. Journal of Agricultural and Food Chemistry 48, 5035–5040.

Smeyers-Verbeke, J., Jäger, H., Lanteri, S., Brereton, P., Jamin, E., Fauhl-Hassek, C., Forina, M., Römisch, U., 2009. Characterization and determination of the geographical origin of wines. Part II: descriptive and inductive univariate statistics. European Food Research and Technology 230, 15–29.

Solodun, Y.V., Monakhova, Y.B., Kuballa, T., Samokhvalov, A.V., Rehm, J., Lachenmeier, D.W., 2011. Unrecorded alcohol consumption in Russia: toxic denaturants and disinfectants pose additional risks. Interdisciplinary Toxicology 4, 198–205.

Spraul, M., Schäfer, H., Schütz, B., Krings, D., Cannet, C., 2013. Improved NMR Wine Screening Heralds New Era of Wine Quality Control. Bruker Corporation, Rheinstetten, Germany.

Stanziani, A., 2007. Negotiating innovation in a market economy: foodstuffs and beverages adulteration in nineteenth-century France. Enterprise & Society 8, 375–412.

Stanziani, A., 2009. Information, quality and legal rules: wine adulteration in nineteenth century France. Business History 51, 268–291.

Tagliabue, J., 1985. Scandal Over Poisoned Wine Embitters Village in Austria. NY Times. August 2.

Vaskova, M., Hrdlicka, J., Mika, O.J., Barta, J., Clemensova, G., 2014. Civil protection in mass methanol poisoning in the Czech Republic. International Journal of Medical, Health, Biomedical, and Pharmaceutical Engineering 8, 738–742.

Versini, G., Camin, F., Ramponi, M., Dellacassa, E., 2006. Stable isotope analysis in grape products: ^{13}C-based internal standardisation methods to improve the detection of some types of adulterations. Analytica Chimica Acta 563, 325–330.

Versini, G., Monetti, A., Reniero, F., 1997. Monitoring authenticity and regional origin of wines by natural stable isotope ratios analysis. ACS Symposium Series 661, 113–130.

Wachter, H., 2009. Verifying authenticity of wine by Mahalanobis distance and hypothesis testing of stable isotope pattern – a case study using the EU Wine Databank. Mitteilungen Klosterneuburg 59, 237–249.

WHO Regional Office for Europe, 2009. Evidence for the Effectiveness and Cost-Effectiveness of Interventions to Reduce Alcohol-related Harm. WHO Regional Office for Europe, Copenhagen, Denmark.

Yucesoy, D., Ozen, B., 2013. Authentication of a Turkish traditional aniseed flavoured distilled spirit, raki. Food Chemistry 141, 1461–1465.

Zakharov, S., Pelclova, D., Urban, P., Navratil, T., Diblik, P., Kuthan, P., Hubacek, J., Miovsky, M., Klempir, J., Vaneckova, M., Seidl, Z., Pilin, A., Fenclova, Z., Petrik, V., Kotikova, K., Nurieva, O., Ridzon, P., Rulisek, J., Komarc, M., Hovda, K.E., 2014. Czech mass methanol outbreak 2012: epidemiology, challenges and clinical features. Clinical Toxicology 52, 1013–1024.

Zoppi, U., Skopec, Z., Skopec, J., Jones, G., Fink, D., Hua, Q., Jacobsen, G., Tuniz, C., Williams, A., 2004. Forensic applications of ^{14}C bomb-pulse dating. Nuclear Instruments and Methods in Physics Research Section B 223–224, 770–775.

Advances in Adulteration and Authenticity Testing of Herbs and Spices

22

B. Sasikumar, V.P. Swetha, V.A. Parvathy, T.E. Sheeja
ICAR-Indian Institute of Spices Research, Kozhikode, Kerala, India

Chapter Outline

22.1 Introduction

Herbs and spices are high-value, export-oriented commodities and are extensively used for flavoring food and beverages as well as in medicine, cosmetics, and perfumery. Traded forms of herbs and spices include dried or fresh whole commodity, powdered forms, pastes, dehydrated material, oils, oleoresin, and extractives. Good quality herbs and spices are very relevant for the perceived biological efficiency of these commodities, their flavor, or aroma. The health-conscious public all over the world is increasingly looking for quality herbs and spices, be it for health, culinary, or cosmetic uses. However, spices and herbs are often adulterated with inferior, similar-looking entities leading to erosion of the perceived biological value and public faith in these products.

International organizations like the International Organization for Standardization (ISO), American Spice Trade Association, The Food Safety and Standards Authority, India, etc. impose strict regulations on the quality of spices and herbs imported and exported. Globalization of food trade requires the development of integrated approaches, such as traceability of origin, quality, and authenticity to ensure food safety and quality (Barbuto et al., 2010). In the post-World Trade Organization era, importing countries as well as the consumers pay more and more attention to food quality, demanding clearer product traceability as well as the use of detailed and accurate product labels.

Being low-volume, high-value commodities, spices and herbs are reported to be adulterated with plant-based as well as synthetic adulterants (Singhal et al., 1997; Dhanya and Sasikumar, 2010). Processed foods including spices and herbs, such as powdered forms, often result in the loss of any morphological diagnostic features of the species, increasing the possibility of fraudulent substitutions or adulteration. Conventional analytical tools like thin layer chromatography (TLC), gas chromatography (GC), and high-performance liquid chromatography (HPLC) are ineffective in this regard. Detection of adulteration and determination of authenticity and quality of foods and food ingredients, including herbs and spices, are major challenges for the agricultural and food industry, challenges that have become increasingly important in recent years (Mafra et al., 2008). Regulatory agencies, food processors, and consumers are all interested in detecting adulterants or authenticating raw materials of food products in order to satisfy food quality and safety requirements (Che Man et al., 2005). With globalization of trade, the role of standards and conformity assessment are of paramount importance especially in herbs and spices and their value-added products because non-tariff agreements such as sanitary and phytosanitary as well as preshipment inspection agreements insist that the product(s) is safe, free from adulterants, and has the desired quality. Though acceptable levels of many of the synthetic adulterants and their detection methods are available, there is a paucity of faster and efficient methods to detect the plant-based adulterants in herbs and spices, especially in value-added items.

Adulteration detection and authenticity testing of food and agricultural commodities of plant origin including cereals, legumes, beverages, olive oil, fruit products, spices, and traded medicinal plant materials are important for value assessment in order to stop unfair competition and ensure consumer protection against fraudulent practices commonly observed in unscrupulous trade. Additionally, deceitful adulteration of these products containing undeclared constituents may cause health problems such as allergy in sensitive individuals (Asensio et al., 2008; Marcus and Grollman, 2002).

22.2 Uses of Spices and Herbs

Herbs and spices are plant parts valued for their medicinal and aromatic properties. Herbs are the leafy parts while spices are the nonleafy parts of plants such as seeds, root, stem, bulb, bark, etc. The ISO has categorized 112 plant species as spices and herbs, of which 38 are leafy spices (ISO, 1995).

The value of spices and herbs has been realized from time immemorial. The earliest evidence of spice use comes from the hieroglyphic writings on the wall of the Pyramid of Giza, Egypt (Srinivasan, 2000). The ancient Ayurvedic treatises such as Charaka samhita and Susrutha samhita have also shed light on the medicinal uses of herbs and spices from early ages. During ancient times, they were used as ingredients of incense, embalming, preservatives, ointments, antidotes against poison, cosmetics, perfumes, etc. In addition to their use as flavorants, herbs and spices are also valued for their nutritional, antioxidant, antimicrobial, insect repellant, and medicinal properties. Based on their use, they are classified as culinary, cosmetic, or pharmaceutical and are used in their fresh or dried forms or as value-added items like powders, oils, and oleoresins. Flavor, pungency, and medicinal properties of the herbs and spices result from the chemical constituents of the essential oils and oleoresins present in them.

Spices are used as flavorants in foods in the form of whole spices, ground spices, and spice extracts. They also serve as sources of natural food colors. β-carotene, cryptoxanthin, lutein, and crocin are some of the color components present in them. Owing to their antioxidant properties, they can be added to prevent lipid degradation and food rancidity. Nutritional properties of herbs and spices are also well described: they serve as a rich source of proteins, vitamins, and minerals like calcium, sodium, etc.

Herbs and spices occupy a pivotal position in traditional systems of medicine like Ayurveda, Sidha, Unani, Chinese, etc. owing to their therapeutic function and their ability to act as a bioavailability booster. Extracts of spices and herbs are being used in the preparation of infusions, decoctions, macerations, tinctures, nutraceuticals, fluid extracts, etc. due to their medicinal properties including carminative, diuretic, digestive stimulant, anti-inflammatory, appetizer, cholesterol lowering, etc.

22.3 Adulterants in Spices and Herbs

Adulteration may be defined as mixing or substituting the original material with other spurious, inferior, defective, spoiled, useless parts of the same or different plant, harmful substances or synthetic chemicals that do not conform with official standards. Adulteration can be in two ways: direct/intentional adulteration and indirect/unintentional adulteration. Direct/intentional adulteration includes practices of substitution partially or fully with inferior materials owing to their morphological resemblance or chemicals or inert materials in order to attain financial gain. Unintentional adulteration results mainly from the absence of a proper evaluation method (Preethi et al., 2014), clerical errors (Zhao et al., 2006), etc.

Spices and herbs are reported to be adulterated with plant-based and known synthetic adulterants (Table 22.1). Microbial contamination, insect filth contamination, and addition of adulterants like dyes are the common quality-related issues of spices and herbs. Adulteration is also related to fraud concerning botanical or geographical origin. Some of these adulterants are related botanical species of the target species

Table 22.1 Common Adulterants in Traded Spices and Herbs

Commodity	Chemical and Non-Chemical Adulterant	Biological Adulterant
Ajwain (*Trachyspermum ammi*)	Earthy materials	Spent ajwain seeds, excess stem and chaff
Allspice powder (*Pimenta dioica*)	–	Powdered clove stem, berries of *Myrtus tobasco* and *Lindera benzoin*
Aniseed (*Pimpinella anisum*)	Fine earth materials	Hemlock fruit, parsley, dill fruit
Aniseed powder	–	Fennel
Asafoetida (*Ferula assa-foetida*)	Coal tar dyes, gypsum, red clay, chalk	Foreign resin– Gum arabic, gum resin, resin, barley, wheat or rice flour, slices of potato
Basil (*Ocimum basilicum*)	–	*Ocimum sanctum*
Indian Bay leaf (*Cinnamomum tamala*)	–	*Cinnamomum malabatrum*
Bharangi (*Clerodendrum serratum*)	–	*Solanum xanthocarpum*
Black pepper berries (*Piper nigrum*)	Mineral oil	Dried papaya seed, wild *Piper* spp. (*Piper attenuatum* and *Piper galeatum*), fruits of *Lantana camara* and *Embelia ribes*, seeds of *Mirabilis jalapa*, berries of *Schinus molle*, spent black pepper, light berries, stems and chaff of black pepper
Black pepper powder	Dye	Powdered papaya seed, wild *Piper* berries, *L. camara* and *Embelia ribes*, seeds of *M. jalapa*, berries of *S. molle*, spent black pepper; light berries, starch from cheaper source, chilli

Brahmi (*Bacopa monnieri*)	–	*Centella asiatica*
Camphor (*Cinnamomum camphora*)	–	*Leonotis nepetifolia*
Cardamom fruits (*Elettaria cardamomum*)	Small pebbles	Orange seeds, unroasted coffee seeds
Cardamom seeds	–	Seeds of *Amomum aromaticum, Amomum subulatum*
Cardamom seed powder	–	Powdered cardamom hulls
Caraway (*Carum carvi*)	Gravel and earth	Spent caraway seeds, cumin seeds, carum stems
Chilli fruits (*Capsicum annuum*)	Dye, mineral oil	–
Chilli powder	Dye, coal tar, Sudan red, para red, n-vanilylnonamide, mineral oil, talc powder, brick powder, salt powder	Powdered fruits of "choti ber" (*Ziziphus nummularia)*, red beet pulp, almond shell dust, extra amounts of bleached pericarp, seeds, calyx and peduncles of chilli, starch of cheap source, tomato wastes
Chitrak (*Plumbago zeylanica*)	–	*Baliospermum montanum*
Cinnamon bark (*Cinnamomum verum*)	–	Cassia (*Cinnamomum cassia*)
Cinnamon powder	Eugenol, ceylon oil, yellow brown dye	Aromatized and powdered beechnut husk, hazelnut, almond shell dust
Cinchona bark (*Cinchona officinalis*)	–	Cuprea bark

Continued

Table 22.1 Common Adulterants in Traded Spices and Herbs—cont'd

Commodity	Chemical and Non-Chemical Adulterant	Biological Adulterant
Clove (*Syzygium aromaticum*)	Magnesium salt, sand, earth	Exhausted clove, stem and fruits of clove
Cobra saffron (*Mesua ferrea*)	–	*Nelumbo nucifera*
Coriander (*Coriandrum sativum*)	–	Bombay coriander fruits
Cumin seeds (*Cuminum cyminum*)		Grass seeds covered with charcoal dust
Devil's snare (*Datura stramonium*)	–	*Solanum nigrum* leaves
Durlabha (*Fagonia cretica*)	–	*Alhagi pseudalhagi*
European dill (*Anethum graveolens*)	Terpenes	Indian dill
Fennel (*Foeniculum vulgare*)	Sand, dirt	Exhausted or partially exhausted fennel fruits, stem tissue and stalks of fennel, umbelliferous seeds
Foxglove (*Digitalis purpurea*)	–	Primrose leaves, comfrey leaves
Ginger (*Zingiber officinale*)	Lime, capsaicin	Exhausted ginger (volatile oil extracted)
Ginger powder	Lime	Capsicum, grains of paradise, turmeric, exhausted ginger fortified with flavors, Japanese ginger

Gokhru (*Tribulus terrestris*)	–	*Pedalium murex*
Holy basil (*Ocimum sanctum*)	–	*Vitex negundo*
Indian bdellium (*Commiphora wightii*)	–	*Acacia nilotica*
Indian caper (*Capparis sepiaria*)	–	*Alocasia indica*
Indian crocus (*Kaempferia rotunda*)	–	*Lagenandra toxicana*
Indian elecampane (*Inula racemosa*)	–	*Saussurea lappa*
Indian jalap (*Operculina turpethum*)	–	*Marsdenia tenacissima*
Long pepper (*Piper longum*)	–	*Piper retrofractum*
Mangosteen (*Garcinia mangostana*)	–	*Garcinia indica*
Mediterranean oregano (*Origanum vulgare*)		*Origanum majorana*, *Origanum syriacum*, *Satureja montana*
Mustard seed (*Brassica nigra*)		Argemone seeds (*Argemone mexicana*), rape seed, ragi
Mustard seed powder		Added starch, turmeric

Continued

Table 22.1 Common Adulterants in Traded Spices and Herbs—cont'd

Commodity	Chemical and Non-Chemical Adulterant	Biological Adulterant
Neem (*Azadirachta indica*)	–	*Melia azedarach*
Nigella seeds (*Nigella sativa*)		Onion seeds
Nutmeg (*Myristica fragrans*)	Pieces of clay for repairing broken nutmeg	Wild species – Macassar (*Myristica argentea*), Bombay nutmeg (*Myristica malabarica*), *Myristica otoba*
Peppermint (*Mentha piperita*)	–	*Mentha arvensis*
Poppy seed (*Papaver somniferum*)		Rajgira seeds (*Amaranthus paniculatus*)
Rajmahal hemp (*Marsdenia tenacissima*)	–	*Lannea coromandelica*
Rue (*Ruta graveolens*)	–	*Euphorbia dracunculoides*
Saffron (*Crocus sativus*)	Synthetic dyes – tartrazine, Ponceau 2R, Sunset yellow, amaranth, orange GG, methyl orange, eosin and erythrosine, oil, honey, glycerine, solutions of potassium or ammonium nitrate, sodium sulphate, magnesium sulphate, barium sulphate, borax	Different parts of the saffron flower like styles, stamen, strips of the corolla, dried petals of safflower and scotch marigold, calendula, poppy, arnica, onion skins, turmeric, annatto, stigmata from other species of *Crocus*, pomegranate, Spanish oyster and maize, dyed corn silk, meat fiber, red sandal wood, turmeric powder, paprika powder
Sage (*Salvia officinalis*)	–	Clary sage (*Salvia sclarea*)

Sita Ashok (*Saraca asoca*) (Asoka bark)	–	Barks of *Saraca declinata* and *Polyalthia longifolia*
Star anise (*Illicium verum*)	–	*Illicium anisatum* fruit
Star anise powder		*I. anisatum* powder
Thyme (*Thymus vulgaris*)	–	*Thymus, Satureja, Origanum* spp.
Turmeric powder (*Curcuma longa*)	Dye, Metanil yellow, orange II lead chromate, chalk powder, yellow soap stone powder	Wild *Curcuma* spp. (*Curcuma zedoaria* or *Curcuma malabarica*), starch from cheaper source, sawdust
Vanilla beans (*Vanilla planifolia*)	–	Tonka beans (*Dipteryx odorata*), *Dipteryx oppositifolia,* vanillin (*Vanilla pampona*), little vanilla (*Selenipedium chica*), leaves of orchid *Angreacum fragrans* and *Orchis fusca*, ladies' tresses (*Spiranthes cernua*), "vanilla-plant" (*Trilisa odoratissima*), "herb vanilla" (*Nigritella angustifolia*) and common sweet clovers (*Melilotus* spp.)
Vanilla extract	Synthetic vanillin, ethyl vanillin, veratraldehyde, piperonal, vanitrope, and coumarin	–

Compiled from Al-Qurainy, F., Khan, S., Tarroum, M., Al-Hemaid, F.M., Ali, M.A., 2011. Molecular authentication of the medicinal herb *Ruta graveolens* (Rutaceae) and an adulterant using nuclear and chloroplast DNA markers. Genetics and Molecular Research 10, 2806–2816; Dhanya, K., Sasikumar, B., 2010. Molecular marker based adulteration detection in traded food and agricultural commodities of plant origin with special reference to spices. Current Trends in Biotechnology and Pharmacy 4, 454–489; Khatoon, S., Singh, N., Kumar, S., Srivastava, N., Rathi, A., Mehrotha, S., 2009. Authentication and quality evaluation of an important Ayurvedic drug – Asoka bark. Journal of Scientific and Industrial Research 68, 393–400; Kolhe, R., Acharya, R., Haricha, C.R., 2015. Application of random amplified polymorphic DNA markers for authentication of three different available source plant of a frequently used Ayurvedic drug Trivrut. European Journal of Biomedical and Pharmaceutical Sciences 2, 971–980; Kumar, S.P., 2014. Adulteration and substitution in endangered ASU medicinal plants of India: a Review. International Journal of Medicinal and Aromatic Plants 4, 56–73; Preethi P.J., Padmini, K., Lohitha, M., Swetha, K., Priyanka, K., Rao, V.P., 2014. Adulterants and substitutes of foods and herbs: a review. International Journal of Analytical Chemistry 4, 213–217; Sereena, K., Kumar, U.P., Remashree, B., 2011. Histochemical and phytochemical markers for the authentication of the Ayurvedic raw drug Hallakam (Kaempferia rotunda) and its marketed adulterant. International Journal of Pharmaceutical Sciences and Research 2, 2952–2958.

while others are unrelated species bearing physical resemblance with the target commodity in attributes such as shape, color, aroma, etc. However, in comparison to the whole commodity, value-added items such as powder or paste are more vulnerable to adulteration.

22.4 Techniques for Adulterant Detection

Numerous techniques have been developed to counter adulteration owing to the increased consumer awareness of food safety and quality control.

Adulteration determination is mainly accomplished by comparing measured analytical data with a proper reference set of historical or control data (Wilhelmsen, 2004). Three strategies are employed for demonstrating admixture in agricultural commodities: demonstrating the presence of a foreign substance in the commodity, demonstrating that a component is present at a concentration that deviates significantly from its normal level, and checking the chemical profile of the sample of which the first strategy is considered as the simplest and efficient (Dhanya and Sasikumar, 2010). Authentication tools utilized vary widely depending on the plant and processes involved varying from structural evaluation using physical methods, chemical profiling-based analytical methods, and the most advanced biotechnological approaches (Smilie and Khan, 2010).

22.4.1 Physical Methods

Physical methods involved in the authentication of herbs and spices are macroscopic and microscopic structural evaluation and other parameters such as solubility, bulk density, texture, etc.

22.4.1.1 Macroscopic Analysis

Macroscopic analysis involves the morphological description of the plant part(s) that may be used in discriminating between plant species that are morphologically similar yet distinguishable and that could be used as a potential adulterant. It is based on parameters such as shape, size, color, texture, odor, surface characteristics etc. (Choudhary and Sekon, 2011) (Fig. 22.1). Traits considered for macroscopic analysis are stem features (woody or semiwoody/hard or soft/herbaceous/round or angular/fibrous or nonfibrous, smooth or rough texture, etc.); leaf shape, size, and morphology (eg, leaf margins: entire, undulate, dentate, serrate, lobed, pinnatifid); inflorescence characteristics, such as type of inflorescence (eg, spike, raceme, panicle, cyme, corymb, helicoid cyme, head); floral morphology (eg, epigynous/perigynous/hypogynous); stamen number and shape; number of carpels per ovary; number of seeds per carpel; root characteristics including surface texture, type (corm, bulb, rhizome); and tissue layering (banding patterns) (Smilie and Khan, 2010). Since these characteristics are judged subjectively and they closely resemble the genuine samples, the findings should be substantiated using microscopic methods.

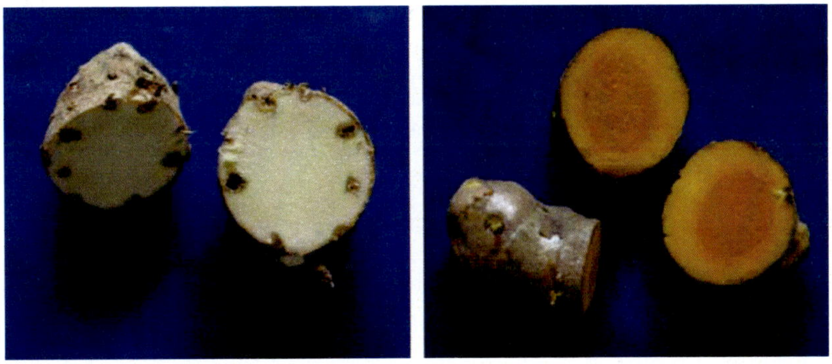

Figure 22.1 Rhizome color variation in *Curcuma aromatica* (left) and its counterfeit entity *Curcuma zedoaria* (right).

Some studies that incorporated macroscopic analysis as a tool for herb and spice authentication are listed in Table 22.2.

22.4.1.2 Microscopic Analysis

Microscopy, the observation of structural, cellular, and internal tissue features to differentiate between plant species (Revathy et al., 2012), is commonly employed in

Table 22.2 Authentication of Herbs and Spices Using Macroscopic Methods

Application	Traits Studied	References
Authentication of *Ephedra* species	Leaf and internode length	Joshi and Khan (2005)
Authentication of *Valeriana procera*	Sample diameter, rhizome color, taste, and odor	Joshi et al. (2005a)
Differentiating between two easily confused Chinese medicinal materials (willowleaf swallowwort rhizome and root from blackened swallowwort rhizome and root)	Rhizome characteristics	Zhao and Li (2007)
Authentication of *Jatropha curcas*	Leaf shape, size, margin, venation, apex, surface, color, and taste	Nayak and Patel (2010)
Authentication of *Cassia spectabilis* leaf	Leaf shape, size, and morphology	Torey et al. (2010)
Authentication of three "Snow Lotus herbs"	Capitula situation and arrangement	Chen et al. (2014)

case of powdered samples in which macroscopic characteristics are ineffective or indistinguishable. Microscopy techniques range from light to advanced electron microscopy techniques to analyze characteristics such as the presence or absence of hairs (trichomes), starch grains, oil glands, canals, particular cell types, seed or pollen morphology, and vascular traces (Smilie and Khan, 2010). Comparison of cell structure (anatomical features) with an authenticated specimen may reveal abnormal characteristics that may be attributed to the presence of foreign matter or species.

Selection of typical materials, preparation of slides, and observation of features are the three main steps involved in this procedure. Slides of transverse or longitudinal section, powder, and disintegrated tissues are prepared for microscopic investigation, and information is derived for species identification based on differences in the histological structure (Fig. 22.2).

Herb and spice authentication has been demonstrated using microscopic methods. Joshi and Khan (2005) and Joshi et al. (2005a) have illustrated the differentiation of *Ephedra* and *Valeriana* species in trade using microscopic analysis. The medicinal herb *Oldenlandia diffusa* could be completely distinguished from its confused species based on the fluorescence of its endodermal walls using fluorescence microscopy (Liang et al., 2006). Authentication of a Chinese herbal tea "Ku-Ding-Cha" was made based on the evaluation of its leaf blade, xylem cells, stone cells, and calcium oxalate crystals using light and polarized microscopy (Tam et al., 2006). Scanning electron microscopy (SEM) aided in the identification of *Illicium verum* (star anise), a medicinal herb and spice from its adulterant *Illicium anisatum* by displaying the differences in their epicarp morphologies (Fritz et al., 2008). Joshi et al. (2005b) has also successfully differentiated star anise from its adulterant using fluorescence microscopy. Cinnamon and cassia barks could also be distinguished using microscopy as

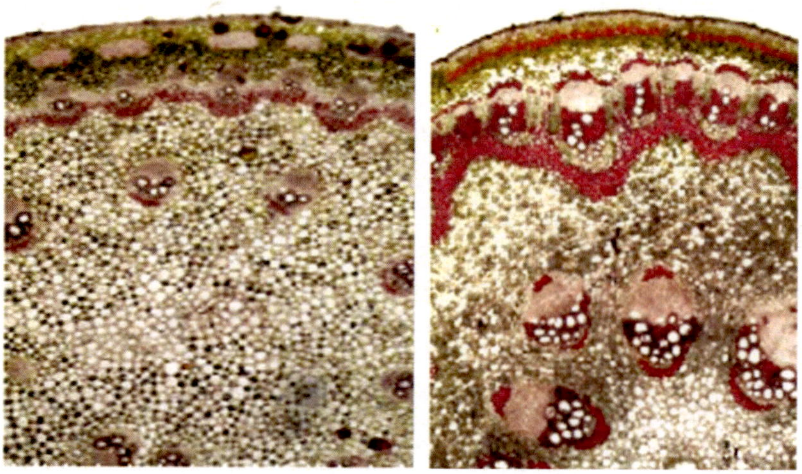

Figure 22.2 Stem anatomical variation in two species of *Piper. Piper colubrinum* (left) and *Piper nigrum* (right).

Table 22.3 Authentication of Herbs and Spices Using Microscopic Methods

Application	Technique	References
Detection of adulterants in black pepper powder	Microscopic analysis of spice powder	Tremlova (2001)
Authentication of Chinese patent medicine – Bo Ying compound	Light microscopy of the drug	Zhao et al. (2005)
Authentication of toxic and potent Chinese materia medica	Light microscopy of the drug	Xia et al. (2007)
Authentication of Asoka bark	Macroscopic and microscopic analysis of stem bark	Khatoon et al. (2009)
Authentication of *Ruta graveolens*	Light microscopy of root, stem, and leaves	Nazish et al. (2010)
Authentication of Neem (*Azadirachta indica*) from *Melia azedarach*	Scanning electron microscopy of pollens	Sulthana et al. (2011)
Comparative authentication of three "Snow Lotus herbs"	Light microscopy, polarized light microscopy and scanning electron microscopy of pollen grains, nonglandular hairs, and cells of inner surface of the microdiodange	Chen et al. (2014)
Identification of adulterants from powdered seasonings of chilli, black pepper, cumin, and mustard	Light microscopy of the spice powders	Zu and Zhao (2014)

cassia contained broader fibers, cork, and larger starch grains (Pruthi, 1998). Microscopic examination has revealed the presence of extraneous starch in some spices like coriander, cumin, chilli, and clove (FSSAI, 2012).

Some other examples in which microscopic analysis has aided in adulterant detection are itemized in Table 22.3.

Limitations of microscopy-based physical methods include the following:

- Difficulty in authentication of processed plant material
- Requires skilled expert
- Subjectivity
- Time consuming
- Difficulty in distinguishing two plant species that have similar morphology.
- Phenological variation
- Expressivity and penetrance
- Lack of diagnostic morphological characters.

22.4.2 Analytical Methods

Analytical techniques mainly use the chemical composition or organic components present in the plant for their identification and authentication. Depending on the basic principle, the techniques can be grouped into different types.

22.4.2.1 Chromatographic Techniques

TLC is the simplest, most versatile, and economic way of obtaining the chemical fingerprints of multiple herbal samples. The technique has been used to detect adulteration of herbs (Chau et al., 1998) and was proven to be the best approach in testing saffron purity (Mohammad et al., 2015). The presence of Sudan dye in chilli powder was detected using TLC by Darr et al. (2013).

In GC methods, the main components targeted are the volatile and semivolatile compounds present in the specimen, and the sensitivity of detection is high (Liang et al., 2004). Detection of adulteration of olive oil samples from sunflower seed oil was achieved using GC estimation of methyl esters of the oil components, steroids, and fatty acids. The technique could diagnose the contamination of olive oil by sunflower seed oil at least at 1% level with >95% certainty in bottling plants (Cercaci et al., 2003). Fatty acid as the purity indicator suggests the use of linolenic acid as the parameter for the detection of virgin olive oil with 5% of soybean oil (Gamazo-Vazquez et al., 2003).

HPLC can separate and identify amino acids, proteins, phenolic acids, etc. present in a compound. This is used in the detection of olive oil adulteration with other oils such as soybean oil, corn oil, and sunflower oil (Jabeur et al., 2014). Identification of black pepper powder adulterated with chilli (Parvathy et al., 2014), para red adulteration in red chilli powder, pickles, etc. (Riaz et al., 2009), could be done using HPLC. Detection of saffron components: crocins, picrocrocin, and safranal using HPLC has proved to be effective for determining the quality of the spice grown under different environmental and storage conditions (Lage and Cantrell, 2009). Sproll et al. (2008) developed a water HPLC system for analyzing the coumarin content of cinnamon, and the same was used for adulteration detection of true cinnamon with cassia cinnamon in Czech Republic retail markets. The high coumarin content in the market samples analyzed showed the adulteration of true cinnamon with cassia cinnamon (Blahov and Svobodov, 2012). The presence of Sudan dyes in hot chilli and spices could be detected using HPLC (Tateo and Bononi, 2004) with a detection limit of 3 mg/kg of the sample. Quantitative detection of adulteration of Notoginseng root extract with other *Panax* species was done by HPLC coupled with principal component analysis (PCA) (Wang et al., 2009).

Recent advances in the field of liquid chromatography such as micellar electrokinetic capillary chromatography (MECC), high-speed countercurrent chromatography (HSCCC), low-pressure size-exclusion chromatography (SEC), reversed-phase ion-pairing HPLC (RP-IPC-HPLC), and strong anion-exchange HPLC (SAX-HPLC) are reported to provide better separation of specific compounds found in herbal extracts (Kamboj, 2012). Using these techniques, levels of different components present in the spices/herbs can be detected, which denote the quality of the spices and herbs.

22.4.2.2 *Electrophoretic Methods*

Electrokinetic separation methods are used for capillary electrophoresis, an efficient way of documenting the purity and complexity of a compound depending on the presence of charged components. Capillary electrophoresis (CE) is a fast, precise, and sensitive analytical technique that employs narrow bore (20–200 μm) capillary tubes and facilitates the separation of both large and small molecules under the influence of high voltage (Xu, 1996). Separation is aided by differences in the electrophoretic and electro-osmotic movements of buffer solution and ions, induced as a result of the high voltage applied. Capillary electrophoretic methods include capillary zone electrophoresis, capillary gel electrophoresis, capillary isoelectric focusing, isotachophoresis, and micellar electrokinetic capillary chromatography.

Recently, the importance of capillary electrophoresis in the quality control of medicinal plants is being stressed (Ganzera, 2008). In the determination of active ingredients in herbal medicines, CE has proven to give accurate separation using only small quantities of samples (Liang et al., 2004). Wang et al. (2005) have generated a capillary electrophoretic fingerprint for the authentication of *Radix scutellariae*. The quality control of *Dendrobium candidum* was evaluated using a capillary electropherogram generated by electrophoresis through a fused silica capillary tube (Zha et al., 2009). Profiling and authentication of three species of *Scutellaria*, viz., *Scutellaria baicalensis, Scutellaria amoena*, and *Scutellaria lateriflora* were done by capillary electrophoresis (Reid, 2013). The potential of this technique in identifying possible synthetic adulterants ephedrine, norephedrine, caffeine, and furosemide in natural herbal medicines and dietary supplements for weight control was reported by Cianchino et al. (2007) using a fused silica capillary tube with sodium tetraborate buffer under a potential of 30 kV. Nonaqueous capillary electrophoresis using a fused silica capillary tube with sodium tetraborate methanolic solution as the background electrolyte was used to separate and quantify the crocin metabolites, the biologically active ingredients of saffron. The quality control of commercial saffron samples could be achieved by analyzing the electrophoretic data generated (Zougagh et al., 2005).

22.4.2.3 *Spectroscopic Analysis and Chemometrics*

Spectroscopy, the study of the interaction between electromagnetic radiation and matter, includes techniques like UV, visible, mid- or near infrared (MIR, NIR), Raman, fluorescence, and nuclear magnetic resonance (NMR) that allow nondestructive testing and the use of small samples to achieve identification (Meuren, 2010). Chemometrics is the discipline that uses mathematical, statistical, and other methods employing formal logic to select optimal measurement procedures and experiments and to provide maximum chemical information by analyzing chemical data (Massart et al., 1988). Analytical methods like spectroscopy generate multivariate data that is subjected to chemometric approaches like PCA, linear discriminant analysis, soft independent modeling of class analogy (SIMCA), artificial neural networks (ANNs), k-nearest neighbor analysis (KNN), etc. It has now developed into an indispensable tool for use in conjunction with chromatographic and spectroscopic analysis for quality control in fields such as medicine, environment, forensic analysis, etc. (Henrion and Henrion, 2001).

Spectroscopic analysis along with multivariate analysis using different chemometric approaches has paved the way for authentication of foodstuffs with special reference to spices and herbs. The artificial colorants added to saffron could be detected using UV—visible spectroscopy (Zalacain et al., 2015). UV—visible spectroscopy in conjunction with multivariate classification techniques like SIMCA, KNN, and partial least squares regression have aided in the detection of banned Sudan dyes and potent carcinogens in chilli samples purchased from retail markets (di Anibal, 2009). di Anibal (2014) has also reported the use of UV—visible spectroscopy and multivariate analysis as a screening tool for tracing Sudan I and a blend of Sudan I + IV dyes in culinary spices. Thyme, a medicinal herb, was authenticated using UV spectroscopy on a methanolic sample extract with chemometric tools like PCA, SIMCA, and a hierarchical clustering method (Gad et al., 2013).

Raman spectroscopy, MIR and NIR spectroscopy, along with multivariate analysis have proved their efficiency in authentication studies (Reid et al., 2006). Surface-enhanced Raman spectroscopy, an innovative methodology combined with multivariate classification analysis, was reported superior to Raman and FT Raman spectroscopy by di Anibal (2010), to differentiate culinary spices containing Sudan I dye, by comparing the fingerprint profiles generated. The efficiency of this method as a practical screening tool in samples adulterated with Sudan dye has been stressed.

NIR spectroscopy may be considered superior to the other methods owing to its high analytical speed, low cost, and reliability for qualitative and quantitative analysis. Absorption of light due to molecular vibrations in the NIR region (780—2500 nm) by components in the test sample coupled with chemometrics has helped in the authentication of herbal medicines (Wang and Yu, 2015) like *Paris* (Zhao et al., 2014), *Cortex phellodendri* (Chan et al., 2007), *Digitalis purpurea* (Kudo et al., 2000), *Radix puerariae* (Lau et al., 2009), *Dendrobium densiflorum* (Wang et al., 2009), *Ephedra* (Fan et al., 2010), *Rheum palmatum* (Wang et al., 2006), *Panax* (Chen et al., 2011), and spices like saffron (Zalacain et al., 2005). This technique was also successfully applied to authenticate herbal medicines and spices based on their geographical origin (Lai et al., 2011). NIR spectroscopy could clearly discriminate between Korean and Chinese *Angelicae gigantis* Radix with 100% accuracy on the basis of the unique 1625-nm band of decursin obtained in the Korean samples (Woo et al., 2005). Zalacain et al. (2005) also employed NIR spectroscopy coupled with discriminant analysis on 111 saffron samples from Spain, Greece, and Iran and observed that the Iranian saffron samples were most different while those from Spain and Greece were similar.

Fourier transform near infrared (FT-NIR) spectroscopy has evolved as a promising and sensitive tool for the analysis of herbs and spices (Schultz et al., 2003). Maree and Viljoen (2011) adopted FT-NIR and MIR spectroscopy for authentication of the commercially important *Pelargonium*. The absorption spectra of *Pelargonium sidoides* and its close relative *Pelargonium reniforme* were taken in the NIR and MIR regions. Analysis of the spectroscopic data by chemometric tools like PCA, orthogonal projection, and latent structures discriminant analysis revealed a phytochemical variation of 5.79% and 9.22%, respectively in the NIR and MIR regions. The data helped to identify seven absorption areas as putative biomarkers for differentiation between the two species. A rapid method based on FT-NIR combined with chemometric tools could discriminate *Salvia miltiorrhiza* var. *alba* according to their geographical origin with an accuracy of 100% (Duan et al., 2014).

NMR is an analytical tool with rapidity and reproducibility using minimal sample pretreatment. Site-specific natural isotope fractionation NMR and proton NMR (^{1}H NMR) are variants of NMR that are more specific and sophisticated techniques for food authentication (Reid et al., 2006). 1H NMR was used to discriminate authentic saffron from adulterated commercial material (Petrakis et al., 2015; Yilmaz et al., 2010). High-resolution ^{1}H NMR combined with chemometrics is used to develop a metabolic fingerprint capable of revealing the presence of Sudan dyes (I-IV) in commercial culinary spices (turmeric, curry, mild paprika, hot paprika; di Anibal., 2011). Metabolite fingerprinting by H1-NMR has also identified markers for the quality control of traded saffron (Ordoudi et al., 2015).

Mass spectrometry (MS) offers high sensitivity and chemical specificity enabling the accurate identification and quantification of analytes within complex food matrices (Ellis et al., 2015). Isotope ratios, trace elements, and molecular ions of ionic fragments serve as the chemical markers assessed by MS (Aceto, 2015). MS is often used in conjunction with liquid chromatography (LC) and GC in authentication studies. LC-MS has been used for the determination of illegal adulterants in herbal medicines and dietary supplements (Liang et al., 2006). Lau et al. (2003) reported the presence of synthetic adulterants in herbal medicine by LC-electron spray ionization MS. Ultra-fast liquid chromatography coupled with electron spray ionization tandem mass spectroscopy determined the presence of 18 adulterants in herbal medicines and health foods for male sexual potency (Ren et al., 2012). The presence of anabolic steroids in dietary supplements was established by high-throughput bioaffinity mass spectroscopy (Aqai et al., 2013). Variants of MS, like direct injection mass spectrometry and proton transfer reaction mass spectrometry, have found application in authentication of traded spices like black pepper, chilli paprika, nutmeg, vanilla, and saffron in conjunction with chemometric tools like PCA. Baseline fingerprints were generated for genuine spice and herb samples. Spectroscopic data subjected to PCA analysis indicated maximum variation between the selected variables, thereby distinguishing different spices and discriminating the genuine sample from the adulterated one (Silvis et al., 2015).

22.4.2.4 Hyphenated Techniques

Hyphenated techniques are developed from combining the chromatographic separation technique and spectroscopic detection technology to produce a single result. High-performance liquid chromatography—mass spectroscopy (HPLC-MS), gas chromatography—mass spectroscopy, capillary electrophoresis—mass spectroscopy, and liquid chromatography-NMR are some of the commonly used hybrid or hyphenated technologies deployed for adulteration detection in herbs and spices. The detection of Sudan red in chilli uses LC-MS (Rebane et al., 2010), and detection of banned dyes like Para Red, Sudan Orange G, Sudan I-IV, Sudan Red 7B, and Rhodamine B in spices uses HPLC-MS (Botek et al., 2007). Using high-performance liquid chromatography—electrochemical, blending as little as 5% marjoram or thyme into oregano herb could be detected (Zhang et al., 2013). Aflatoxin detection in spices by HPLC and other hyphenated techniques has proved to be effective in detecting aflatoxins in a range of 0.08—4.66 μg/kg (Romagnoli et al., 2007; Cho et al., 2008).

A review on the various hyphenated techniques in combination with chemometrics and statistical analysis used for the detection of synthetic adulterants in herbal samples and spices was done by Tzouros and Arvanitoyannis (2001) and Reinholds et al. (2015).

Some limitations of analytical methods do exist as follows:

- Variations in phytochemical profiles due to plant processing and the effect of environment conditions in which they grow;
- High cost of chemical standards;
- Overlapping of marker compounds in related but unwanted species;
- Absence of a marker compound for a particular botanical.

22.4.3 Biotechnological Methods

Biotechnological methods are classified into three main types: PCR-based, hybridization-based, and sequencing-based (Yip et al., 2007). The identity of an organism can be determined on the basis of its genetic content, the DNA, which is not affected by age, physiological condition, or environmental factors. Biotechnological approaches are much advanced in the field of authentication and discrimination and have the advantage of discriminating a species even if the morphological characteristics are changed such as in the case of powdered herbs and spices.

22.4.3.1 Non-PCR/Hybridization Based Methods

Hybridization methods work on the principle of generation of species-specific DNA profiles by hybridizing DNA digested with restriction enzymes and comparing it to labeled probes. It includes restriction fragment length polymorphism (RFLP), variable number tandem repeat (VNTR), microarray technique, etc. RFLP and VNTR are of limited application in adulteration detection while DNA microarray is more useful. It consists of many microscopic spots each of which contains identical single-stranded polymeric molecules of deoxyribonucleotides attached to a glass or polymer support (Marmirolli et al., 2010). In this method, the DNA extracted from the target of unknown origin is bound to the reporter probe in the microarray after which it is scanned to obtain a complete hybridization pattern generated by the release of fluorescent, chemiluminescent, calorimetric, or radioactive signals associated with the binding of the probe to the target DNA (Pereira et al., 2008). Array-based techniques include sequence-dependent (oligonucleotide microarray and gene probe microarray) and sequence-independent microarrays (diversity array technology, subtracted diversity technology, and suppression subtractive hybridization-based assay) (Niu et al., 2011).

Authentication using this chip-based method is a cheap, sensitive, and rapid tool for quality control of pharmaceuticals and nutraceuticals. Hybridization between the fluorescent targets and probes spotted on the microarray is utilized to identify the medicinal plants using DNA microarrays (Niu et al., 2011). However, problems related to reliability, reproducibility, sensitivity, and accuracy limit its application in quality control (Draghici et al., 2005).

22.4.3.2 PCR-Based Molecular Methods

PCR has a high potential in adulterant detection and authentication of commodities due to its simplicity, sensitivity, specificity, as well as rapid analysis time and low cost (Reid et al., 2006; Vidal et al., 2007; Mafra et al., 2008).

PCR-based molecular methods range from species-specific primer amplification (Sasaki et al., 2004), rDNA/18S rRNA gene (Cao et al., 2011), DNA fingerprinting methods that include random amplified polymorphic DNA (RAPD) (Williams et al., 1990), arbitrarily primed PCR (AP-PCR) (Welsh and McClelland, 1990), DNA amplification fingerprinting (DAF) (Anolles et al., 1991), intersimple sequence repeat (ISSR) (Zietkiewicz et al., 1994), directed amplification of minisatellite-region DNA (DAMD) (Heath et al., 1993), sequence characterized amplified regions (SCAR) (Paran and Michelmore, 1993), amplification refractory mutation system (ARMS) (Newton et al., 1989), simple sequence repeat (SSR) analysis (Litt and Lutty, 1989), single nucleotide polymorphism (SNP), among others.

RAPD and AP-PCR are most commonly used for the discrimination of closely related species as they involve the amplification of both coding and noncoding regions. The main advantage of RAPD is that no prior information regarding the gene is essential. ISSR markers are semiarbitrary markers amplified by PCR using primers that are much longer than RAPD primers. ISSR markers are reproducible and can be used as species-specific markers for authentication. RAPD is widely used for detecting adulterants in commercial plant materials due to its low operating cost and the ability to discriminate different botanical species. Though RAPD is a fast assay in which no sophisticated technology and no previous sequence information are needed, it is highly susceptible to variations in amplification conditions (Macpherson et al., 1993). However, if RAPD markers are converted to specific SCAR markers, they facilitate easy, sensitive, specific analysis, aiding in the large-scale screening of commercial samples for adulterants. SCAR markers are evolved from the specific RAPD primers or ISSR primers; they amplify characterized regions of a genome under stringent conditions and so are more reliable and reproducible (Paran and Michelmore, 1993).

SSRs/STRs mainly focus on the amplification of microsatellite regions in the genome, yielding a unique pattern for an individual, and are mostly used in authentication of plants showing inter-specific variation.

Quantitative competitive PCR (Zimmerman and Mannhalter, 1996) and real-time PCR (Lockley and Bardsley, 2000) approaches are used for quantitative estimation studies. They are probe-based quantitative estimations able to provide specific and sensitive detection of adulterants present in the sample. These different DNA-based techniques employed for adulteration detection in spices and herbs are summarized in Table 22.4.

DNA barcoding is a PCR-based technique that uses the sequence variation within a short standardized region, referred to as a "barcode," to distinguish between species (Hebert et al., 2003). In case of plants, barcoding genes vary depending on the species. The Consortium for the Barcode of Life suggests the use of *matK* (maturase K), *rbcL* (ribulose-1,5-bisphosphate carboxylase), internal transcribed spacer (*ITS*) or chloroplast spacer (*trnH-psbA*) as ideal loci for barcoding plants. Authentication using DNA barcodes has been performed for medicinal plants and herbs. SNPs specific to *Curcuma zedoaria*, an adulterant of *Curcuma longa*, were reported by Parvathy et al. (2015) on the basis of barcoding *ITS* locus (Table 22.5).

Phylogenetic analysis for taxonomic discrimination of Zingiberaceae species using DNA barcodes was reported by Selvaraj et al. (2008). Adulteration with starch and other fillers was detected in commercial turmeric samples using *psbA-trnH* and *rbcL* loci (Parvathy et al., 2015). Swetha et al. (2014), using the barcoding loci *rbcL,* could detect the presence of *Cinnamomum cassia* (source of coumarin, a hepatotoxin) in traded *Cinnamomum verum* samples. SNPs specific to *C. cassia* were identified by sequence analysis of the *rbcL* locus (Table 22.6). The first report on detection of adulteration of traded black pepper with chilli used the DNA barcoding method in which chilli specific amplicons of 600 bp clearly distinguished the adulterated black pepper powder from the genuine samples that produced 350 bp amplicons (Fig. 22.3) (Parvathy et al., 2014).

Adulteration detection in commercial samples of tea, olive oil, saffron, and medicinal plants has been successfully achieved using this DNA barcoding technique (Yuan et al., 2011; Stoeckle et al., 2011; Kumar et al., 2011; Vijayan and Tsou, 2010; Srirama et al., 2010; Gismondi et al., 2013).

Contamination of natural health products with animal constituents and other adulterant plant species was successfully detected using DNA barcoding (Wallace et al., 2012) proving the technique to be very efficient in discriminating both animal and plant constituents simultaneously. Newmaster et al. (2013) could successfully authenticate and detect substitution in 30 out of the 40 herbal products tested using DNA barcoding.

Next-generation sequencing (NGS) analysis provides us with a vast amount of data on the gene sequences, and these data can be used for the quantitative detection of admixtures in commercial samples. Meta-barcoding or meta-genetics uses high-throughput, next generation NGS strategies along with DNA barcoding. Meta-barcoding is also used in biodiversity analysis (Coissac et al., 2012; Christine et al., 2013). Cristescu (2014) in his paper on meta-barcoding reveals the vast number of global diversity studies using taxonomic and barcoding approaches together with NGS. High-throughput sequencing technologies are emerging for microbial and adulteration detection in food and spices (Galimberti et al., 2015).

Table 22.4 Adulterant or Contaminant Detection and Authenticity Assessment of Spices and Herbs Using DNA-Based Techniques

Application	Technique	Target Gene	References
Detection of cashew husk (*Anacardium occidentale* L.) adulteration in tea [*Camellia sinensis* (L.)] samples	Species-specific PCR	*ITS* of 5S rRNA	Dhiman and Singh (2003)
Differentiation of Arabica and Robusta coffee beans	PCR-Restriction Fragment Length Polymorphism (RFLP)	Chloroplast genome	Spaniolas et al. (2006)
Detection of allergenic celery (*Apium graveolens*) in food	Real-time PCR	Mannitol dehydrogenase	Hupfer et al. (2007), Mustorp et al. (2008)
Detection of allergenic celery in food	Species-specific PCR	Mannitol dehydrogenase	Dovicovicova et al. (2004)
Detection of allergenic mustard (*Sinapis alba*, *Brassica juncea*, *Brassica nigra*) in food	Real-time PCR	2S albumin	Mustorp et al. (2008)
Detection of allergenic sesame (*Sesamum indicum*) in food	Real-time PCR	*sinA*	Mustorp et al. (2008)
Detection of adulterants in traded turmeric powder	RAPD		Sasikumar et al. (2005)
	DNA barcoding	*rbcL*, *ITS*	Parvathy et al. (2015)
	SCAR		Dhanya et al. (2011a)
Detection of adulterant in traded chilli powder	RAPD		Dhanya et al. (2008)
	SCAR		Dhanya et al. (2011b)
Detection of adulterant in traded black pepper powder	SCAR		Dhanya et al. (2009)
	DNA barcoding	*psbA-trnH*, *rbcL*	Parvathy et al. (2014)

Continued

Table 22.4 Adulterant or Contaminant Detection and Authenticity Assessment of Spices and Herbs Using DNA-Based Techniques—cont'd

Application	Technique	Target Gene	References
Detection of adulterant in traded oregano	RAPD		Marieschi et al. (2009)
Discrimination of cinnamon (*Cinnamomum verum*) from its adulterants (*Cinnamomum cassia*, *Cinnamomum burmannii* and *Cinnamomum sieboldii*)	Sequencing; single strand conformation polymorphism (SSCP)	*trnL-trnF*	Kojoma et al. (2002)
	DNA barcoding	*rbcL*	Swetha et al. (2014)
Adulterant detection and authentication of medicinal *Panax* species	RAPD		Shaw et al. (1995), Shim et al. (2003), Wang et al. (2001), Ngan et al. (1999)
	RAPD		
	SCAR		
	PCR-RFLP	*ITS*1-5.8S-*ITS*2	
Identification of *Panax* species in herbal medicine preparations	RFLP, Gradient PCR		Shim et al. (2005)
Authentication of *Panax* species	Multiplex amplified refractory mutation system (MARMS)	*trn*K, 18S rRNA	Zhu et al. (2004)
Authentication of *Panax* species	Amplified fragment length polymorphism (AFLP), DAMD	–	Ha et al. (2002)
	AFLP-SCAR		Choi et al. (2008)
Discrimination of the Chinese drug "Ku-di-dan"(herba elephantopi) and "Pu gong ying" (herba taraxaci) from their adulterants	RAPD	–	Cao et al. (1996a,b)

Identification of the sources of medicinal Coptidis rhizoma (*Coptis* species) on the market	RAPD	–	Cheng et al. (1997)
Determination of components in herbal prescription	RAPD	–	Cheng et al. (1998a)
Discrimination of two very closely related medicinal plants *Anoectochilus formosanus* and *Anoectochilus koshunensis*	RAPD	–	Cheng et al. (1998b)
Discrimination of medicinal *Echinacea* species, viz., *E. angustifolia*, *E. pallida* and *E. purpurea*	RAPD SCAR	–	Nieri et al. (2003), Adinolfi et al. (2007)
Discrimination of medicinal *Melissa officinalis* at their subspecies level	RAPD	–	Wolf et al. (1999)
Discrimination of closely related dried *Scutellaria* plants, viz., *S. galericulata*, *S. lateriflora*, and *S. baicalensis*	RAPD	–	Hosokawa et al. (2000)
Discrimination of medicinal *Amomum villosum* samples from their adulterants	RAPD	–	Wang et al. (2000)
Discrimination of medicinal *Lycium* species from their closely related species	RAPD	–	Zhang et al. (2001)
Differentiation of *Lycium barbarum* from its common adulterant, Lycium *chinense* var. *potaninii*	SCAR	–	Sze et al. (2008)
Discrimination of *Saussurea lappa* from adulterants	Sequencing ITS	5S rRNA	Chen et al. (2008)
Authentication of *Alisma orientale*	PCR-RFLP, ARMS	*ITS*; nrDNA	Li et al. (2007)
Discrimination of the Chinese medicinal material *Gekko gecko* from its adulterants	Species-specific PCR	mitochondrial 12S rRNA	Liu et al. (2001)

Continued

Table 22.4 Adulterant or Contaminant Detection and Authenticity Assessment of Spices and Herbs Using DNA-Based Techniques—cont'd

Application	Technique	Target Gene	References
Authentication of *Pinellia ternata* and its related adulterants	PCR, PCR-SR	Mannose - binding lectin	Lin et al. (2006)
Discrimination of medicinal *Swertia mussotii* from related adulterants	Sequencing species-specific PCR	*ITS*	Xue et al. (2006)
Identification of *Ephedra sinica* dietary supplements such as plant mixtures and tablets or capsules	Sequencing	*psb*A-*trn*H	Techen et al. (2006)
Differentiation of medicinal plants *Euphorbia humifusa* and *E. maculata* from their adulterants	Real-time PCR	rDNA *ITS*1	Xue et al. (2008)
Identification of traded medicinal plant *Pueraria tuberosa* from its adulterants	SCAR	–	Devaiah and Venkatasubramanian (2008a)
Authentication of medicinal *Embelia ribes*	SCAR		Devaiah and Venkatasubramanian (2008b)
Identification of ginger (*Zingiber officinale*) from crude drugs and multicomponent formulations	SCAR	–	Chavan et al. (2008)
Discrimination of medicinal *Artemisia princeps* and *Artemisia argyi* from other *Artemisia* plants	SCAR	–	Lee et al. (2006)
Identification of true *Sinocalycanthus chinensis* in the seedling market	SCAR	–	Qian et al. (2006)
Detection of adulteration in traded *Phyllanthus* material in crude drug (dry leaf powder)	SCAR	–	Jain et al. (2008)

Identification of *Phyllanthus emblica* in commercial samples and a multicomponent Ayurvedic formulation	SCAR	–	Dhyaneshwar et al. (2006)
Determination of the components in an Ayurvedic herbal prescription, "Rasayana Churna"	RAPD	–	Shinde et al. (2007)
Authentication of five medicinal *Derris* species	RAPD	–	Sukrong et al. (2006)
Discrimination of *Aloe arborescens* from its adulterants	RAPD	–	Shioda et al. (2003)
Species identification in powdered plant materials of the genus *Cimicifuga* and *Trifolium*	RAPD	–	Xu et al. (2002)
Identification of *Atractylodes* plants in Chinese herbs and formulations	RAPD	–	Chen et al. (2001)
Discrimination of *Dryopteris crassirhizoma* and its adulterant species	Sequencing	cpDNA *rbcL*	Zhao et al. (2007)
Adulteration detection in *Crocus sativus*	SCAR	–	Marieschi et al. (2012)
Authentication of herbs and herbal drugs	SCAR	–	Kiran et al. (2010)
Identification of medicinal herb *Phyllanthus*	SCAR	–	Theerakulpisut et al. (2008)
Authentication of rhubarb	ISSR	–	Wang (2011)
Detecting the adulteration of *Dendrobium officinale*	Real-time PCR	–	Xu et al. (2012)
Identification of herbal drugs in tea mixtures	Real-time PCR, *ITS* sequencing	–	Slanc et al. (2006)

Modified from Dhanya, K., Sasikumar, B., 2010. Molecular marker based adulteration detection in traded food and agricultural commodities of plant origin with special reference to spices. Current Trends in Biotechnology and Pharmacy 4, 454–489.

Table 22.5 SNPs in *ITS* locus that Discriminate between *Curcuma longa* and *Curcuma zedoaria*

	Position of SNP and Nucleotide Substituted			
Species	**293**	**388**	**410**	**439**
C. longa	G	G	G	G
C. zedoaria	A	A	T	C

Parvathy, V.A., Swetha, V.P., Sheeja, T.E., Sasikumar, B., 2015. Detection of plant-based adulterants in turmeric powder using DNA barcoding. Pharmaceutical Biology 53, 1771–1779.

Table 22.6 SNPs Specific to *Cinnamomum cassia* in the *rbcL* Locus

	Position of SNP and Nucleotide Substituted		
Locus	**54**	**55**	**304**
C. verum	A	G	T
C. cassia	G	A	C

Swetha, V.P., Parvathy, V.A., Sheeja, T.E., Sasikumar, B., 2014 DNA Barcoding for discriminating the economically important *Cinnamomum verum* from its adulterants. Food Biotechnology 28, 183–194.

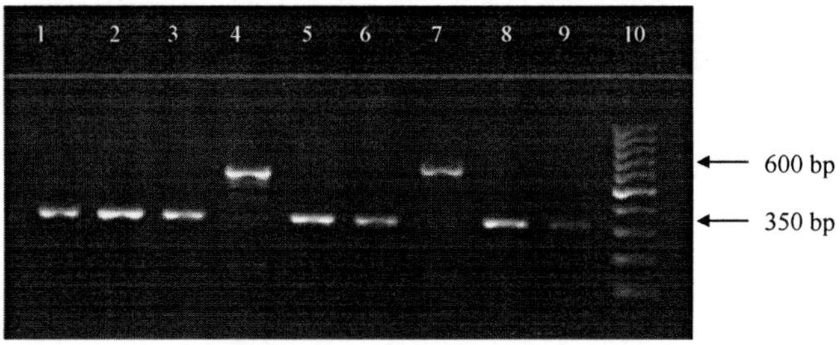

Figure 22.3 Amplification of *psbA-trnH* locus in traded black pepper powder (lane 1– *Piper nigrum*, lane 2– *Piper attenuatum*, lane 3– *Piper galeatum*, lane 4– *Capsicum annuum*, lane 5– Market sample 1, lane 6– Market sample 2, lane 7– Market sample 3, lane 8– Market sample 4, lane 9– Market sample 5, lane 10– 100 bp ladder).
Parvathy, V.A., Swetha, V.P., Sheeja, T.E., Leela, N.K., Chempakam, B., Sasikumar, B., 2014. DNA barcoding to detect chilli adulteration in traded black pepper powder. Food Biotechnology 28, 25–40.

22.4.3.3 High-Resolution Melting Analysis

Melting curve analysis is a fast and sensitive method for differentiating PCR products by fluorescence monitoring of the melting curve of double-stranded DNA that is intercalated by the dye SYBR green in a real-time PCR system (Ririe et al., 1997). It is a gel-free, quick, and inexpensive method that is widely used in pathogen identification, food authenticity, and biological diagnostics (Jiang et al., 2014).

The application of HRM in combination with DNA barcoding (Bar–HRM) has been reported in some authentication studies. Melting-curve analysis coupled with DNA barcoding using the *psbA-trnH* spacer was developed to detect adulterants like *Daucus carota, Carthamus tinctorius, Cinchona officinalis, Dendranthema morifolium, Nelumbo nucifera, Hemerocallis fulva*, and *Zea mays* in traded saffron, based on the differences in their melting point temperatures (Jiang et al., 2014). Authentication of the medicinal species *Sideritia* was successfully done using DNA barcode *ITS 2* coupled with HRM analysis (Kalivas et al., 2014). Bar-HRM using *rbcL* locus and the subsequent melting curve analysis could authenticate three medicinal *Acanthaceae* species (Osthanunkul et al., 2015). Singtonat et al. (2015) reported the application of this technique in detection of the toxic *Crotalaria spectabilis* in *Thunbergia laurifolia* herbal products in Thailand using the melting profiles of *matK, rbcL, rpoC1*, and *trnH*.

22.4.3.4 Immunological Methods

Immunological assays utilize antibodies that are produced in response to an antigen that shares a complementary structure to the antibody, and which, on binding, precipitates an antigen–antibody complex that thereby allows identification of the plant material (Rinaldi, 2007). Enzyme-linked immunosorbent assay (ELISA) is the most widely used immunoassay for the authentication of meat, dairy, and other products due to its specificity, simplicity, and sensitivity (Mackie, 1996). This technique involves an enzyme that detects the presence of an antigen or antibody in a sample. In the case of plants, antibodies are produced against a protein component of the plant. Two variants, indirect ELISA and sandwich ELISA, are employed for authentication purposes (Asensio et al., 2008). However, difficulty in distinguishing the components of a mixture limits its application.

Antibodies produced against ginsenoside Rg1 could discriminate different *Panax* species by the competitive ELISA method (Fukuda et al., 2000). Tanaka et al. (1999, 2005) have developed antibodies and monoclonal antibodies against ginsenoside Rb I that helped in the identification of different *Panax* species such as *Panax ginseng, Panax notoginseng, Panax quinquefolius*, and *Panax japonicas*. Xue et al. (2009) have employed an ELISA method to authenticate *Saussurea involucrate* in commercially prepared crude drugs.

22.4.3.5 Biosensors

Biosensors using nanotechnology are a robust invention for the detection of adulteration and authentication of herbs. The high sensitivity, selectivity, low cost, simplicity, miniaturization, portability, and integration in automated devices of biosensors make this a reliable technique for authentication and detection.

Electronic nose, a diagnostic instrument working on the basis of nanotechnology, was used in the adulteration detection of saffron (Heidarbeigi et al., 2015) and other spices and herbal products. Wilson (2013) describes the various applications of electronic nose in forestry and agriculture.

DNA/RNA aptamers in conjunction with nanotechnology have emerged as a new approach to adulteration detection. Aptamers are oligonucleotides, such as ribonucleic acid (RNA) and single-strand deoxyribonucleic acid (ssDNA), or peptide molecules that can bind to specific targets with high affinity and specificity due to their specific three-dimensional structures. The systematic evolution of ligands by exponential enrichment procedure through which a specific target aptamer (short oligonucleotides) is selected from a large amount of random oligonucleotide material provides the specificity and reproducibility for the technique. The aptamers, once conjugated to a nano chip, serve as a diagnostic kit. Baker et al. (2006) have developed an electronic, aptamer-based sensor for the detection of cocaine in biological fluids. Aptamer-based colorimetric detection of ochratoxins in 5 min was demonstrated by Yang et al. (2011) by using ochratoxin's aptamer as a recognition element and gold nanoparticle as indicator. Amaya-González et al. (2013) reported different aptamer-based techniques in the detection of pathogens and other substances in food. Immuno-based nanosensors form another group of diagnostic kits involving generation of monoclonal antibodies against specific targets and their detection (Bremer et al., 2009).

22.5 Future Perspectives and Conclusions

Spices and herbs assume special significance as they are high-value, export-oriented commodities extensively used for flavoring food and beverages, and in medicines, cosmetics, and perfumes. The worldwide spice and herbal market is worth US$9.4 million and 2.7 m tons were globally exported in 2014, showing a steady upward trend. Unlike the whole commodity, value-added items like powders are more amenable to adulteration as the foreign matter is more difficult to detect visually. The perceived biological activity of these commodities is linked to the quality of the items. Unfortunately, synthetic substances as well as natural products are increasingly finding their way into traded spices and herbs, adversely affecting their efficacy and public trust. Adulteration is also a major economic fraud involving public health. Reliable, easy, sensitive, and high-throughput traceability and authentication methods coupled with quality standards thus assume significance. Commercial adulteration diagnostic kits, if they can be developed, will be a very convenient way to ensure the quality of the traded herbs and spices.

References

Aceto, M., 2015. Food forensics. In: Pico, Y. (Ed.), Advanced Mass Spectrometry for Food Safety and Quality. Elsevier, Amsterdam, p. 460.

Adinolfi, B., Chicca, A., Martinotti, E., Breschi, M.C., Nieri, P., 2007. Sequence characterised amplified region (SCAR) analysis on DNA from the three medicinal *Echinacea* species. Fitoterapia 78, 43–45.

Al-Qurainy, F., Khan, S., Tarroum, M., Al-Hemaid, F.M., Ali, M.A., 2011. Molecular authentication of the medicinal herb *Ruta graveolens* (Rutaceae) and an adulterant using nuclear and chloroplast DNA markers. Genetics and Molecular Research 10, 2806–2816.

Amaya- González, S., Álvarez, N.S., Ordieres, A.J.M., Castañón, M.J.L., 2013. Aptamer-based analysis: a promising alternative for food safety control. Sensors 13, 16292–16311.

Anolles, G., Bassam, B.J., Gresshoff, P.M., 1991. DNA amplification fingerprinting using very short arbitrary oligonucleotide primers. Biotechnology 9, 553–557.

Aqai, P., Cevik, E., Gerssen, A., Haasnoot, W., Nielen, M.W.F., 2013. High throughput bio-affinity mass spectrometry for screening and identification of designer anabolic steroids in dietary supplements. Analytical Chemistry 85, 3255–3262.

Asensio, L., Gonzalez, I., Garcya, T., Martyn, R., 2008. Determination of food authenticity by enzyme linked immunosorbent assay (ELISA). Food Control 19, 1–8.

di Anibal, C.V., Odena, M., Ruisanchez, I., Callao, M.P., 2009. Determining the adulteration of spices with Sudan I-II-II-IV dyes by UV–visible spectroscopy and multivariate classification techniques. Talanta 79, 887–892.

di Anibal, C.V., 2010. Determination of Banned Sudan Dyes in Culinary Spices Through Spectroscopic Techniques and Multivariate Analysis (Doctoral thesis). Universitat Rovira I Virgili DL. T-1809–2011.

di Anibal, C.V., Ruisánchez, I., Callao, M.P., 2011. High resolution 1H Nuclear Magnetic Resonance spectrometry combined with chemometric treatment to identify adulteration of culinary spices with Sudan dyes. Food Chemistry 124, 1139–1145.

di Anibal, C.V., Rodriquez, S.M., Albertengo, L., 2014. UV-visible spectroscopy and multivariate classification as a screening tool to identify adulteration of culinary spices with Sudan I and blends of Sudan I + IV dyes. Food Analytical Methods 7, 1090–1096.

Baker, B.R., Lai, R.Y., Wood, M.S., Doctor, E.H., Heeger, A.J., Plaxco, K.W., 2006. An electronic, aptamer-based small-molecule sensor for the rapid, label-free detection of cocaine in adulterated samples and biological fluids. Journal of the American Chemical Society 128, 3138–3139.

Barbuto, M., Galimberti, A., Ferri, E., Labra, M., Malandra, R., Galli, P., et al., 2010. DNA barcoding reveals fraudulent substitutions in shark seafood products: the Italian case of "palombo" (*Mustelus* spp.). Food Research International 43, 376–381.

Blahova, J., Svobodova, Z., 2012. Assessment of coumarin levels in ground cinnamon available in the Czech retail market. Scientific World Journal 263851. http://dx.doi.org/10.1100/2012/263851.

Botek, P., Poustka, J., Hajšlová, J., 2007. Determination of banned dyes in spices by liquid chromatography–mass spectrometry. Czech Journal of Food Sciences 25, 17–24.

Bremer, M.G.E.G., Smits, N.G.E., Haasnoot, W., 2009. Biosensor immunoassay for traces of hazelnut protein in olive oil. Analytical and Bioanalytical Chemistry 395, 119–126.

Cao, H., But, P.P., Shaw, P.C., 1996a. Authentication of the Chinese drug "Ku-didan"(herba Elephantopi) and its substitutes using random-primed polymerase chain reaction (PCR). Acta Pharmaceutica Sinica 31, 543–553.

Cao, H., But, P.P., Shaw, P.C., 1996b. A molecular approach to identification of the Chinese drug 'Pu Gong Ying' (herba Taraxaci) and six adulterants by DNA fingerprinting using random primed polymerase chain reaction (PCR). Journal of Chinese Pharmaceutical Sciences 5, 186–194.

Cao, H., Sasaki, Y., Fushimi, H., Komatsu, K., 2011. Molecular analysis of medicinally used Chinese and Japanese *Curcuma* based on 18S rRNA gene and *trnK* gene sequences. Biological & Pharmaceutical Bulletin 24, 1389–1394.

Cercaci, L., Rodriguez-Estrada, M.T., Lercker, G., 2003. Solid phase extraction-thin-layer chromatography-gas chromatography method for the detection of hazelnut oil in olive oils by determination of esterified sterols. Journal of Chromatography A 985, 211–220.

Chan, C.O., Chu, C.C., Mok, D.K.W., Chau, F.T., 2007. Analysis of berberine and total alkaloid content in Cortex Phellodendri by near infrared spectroscopy (NIRS) compared with high-performance liquid chromatography coupled with ultra- visible spectrometric detection. Analytica Chimica Acta 592, 121–131.

Chau, F.T., Chan, T.P., Wang, J., 1998. A quantitative study of thin layer chromatography. Bioinformatics 14, 540–541.

Chavan, P., Warude, D., Joshi, K., Patwardhan, B., 2008. Development of SCAR (sequence-characterized amplified region) markers as a complementary tool for identification of ginger (*Zingiber officinale* Roscoe) from crude drugs and multicomponent formulations. Biotechnology and Applied Biochemistry 50, 61–69.

Chen, K.T., Su, Y.C., Lin, J.G., Hsin, L.H., Su, Y.P., Su, C.H., et al., 2001. Identification of Atractylodes plants in Chinese herbs and formulations by random amplified polymorphic DNA. Acta Pharmacologica Sinica 22, 493–497.

Chen, F., Chan, H.Y.E., Wong, K.L., Wang, J., Yu, M.T., But, P.P.H., et al., 2008. Authentication of *Saussurea lappa*, an endangered medicinal material, by ITS DNA and 5S rRNA sequencing. Planta Medica 74, 889–892.

Chen, Q., Yi, T., Tang, Y., Wong, L.L., Huang, X., Zhao, Z., et al., 2014. Comparative authentication of three "snow lotus herbs" by macroscopic and microscopic features. Microscopy Research and Technique 77, 631–641.

Chen, X., Wu, D., He, Y., Liu, S., 2011. Non destructive differentiation of *panax* species using visible and shortwave near-Infrared spectroscopy. Food and Bioprocess Technology 4, 753–761.

Cheng, K.T., Chang, H.C., Su, C.H., Hsu, F.L., 1997. Identification of dried rhizomes of *coptis* species using random amplified polymorphic DNA. Botanical Bulletin of Academia Sinica 38, 241–244.

Cheng, K.T., Tsay, H.S., Chen, C.F., Chou, T.W., 1998a. Determination of the components in a Chinese prescription, YuPing-Feng san, by RAPD analysis. Planta Medica 64, 563–565.

Cheng, K.T., Fu, L.C., Wang, C.S., Hsu, F.L., Tsay, H.S., 1998b. Identification of *Anoectochilus formosanus* and *Anoectochilus koshunensis* species with RAPD markers. Planta Medica 64, 46–49.

Cho, S.H., Lee, C.H., Son, Y.W., Lee, S.M., Choi, I.S., Kim, S.H., et al., 2008. Aflatoxins contamination in spices and processed spice products commercialized in Korea. Food Chemistry 107, 1283–1288.

Choi, Y.E., Ahn, C.H., Kim, B.B., Yoon, E.S., 2008. Development of species specific AFLP-derived SCAR marker for authentication of *Panax japonicus* C. A. MEYER. Biological and Pharmaceutical Bulletin 31, 135–138.

Choudhary, N., Sekon, B.S., 2011. An overview of advances in the standardization of herbal drugs. Journal of Pharmaceutical Education and Research. 2, 55–70.

Christine, E., Denise, L., Thomas, M., Richard, L.., Use of DNA metabarcoding to quantify the diversity of plant species utilized by a pollinator. In: Botany 2013 – Celebrating diversity, July 27–31, New Orleans, USA. Abstract ID – 734.

Cianchino, V., Acosta, G., Ortega, C., Martinez, L.D., Gomez, M.R., 2007. Food Chemistry 108, 1075–1081.

Coissac, E., Riaz, T., Puillandre, N., 2012. Bioinformatic challenges for DNA metabarcoding of plants and animals. Molecular Ecology 21, 1834–1847.

Cristescu, M.E., 2014. From barcoding single individuals to metabarcoding biological communities: towards an integrative approach to the study of global biodiversity. Trends in Ecology & Evolution 24, 566–571.

Darr, M.M., Idrees, W., Masoodi, F.A., 2013. Detection of Sudan dyes in red chilli powder by thin layer chromatography. Scientific Reports 2, 586.

Devaiah, K.M., Venkatasubramanian, P., 2008a. Development of SCAR marker for authentication of *Pueraria tuberose* (Roxb. ex. Willd.) DC. Current Science 94, 1306–1309.

Devaiah, K.M., Venkatasubramanian, P., 2008b. Genetic characterization and authentication of *Embelia ribes* using RAPD-PCR and SCAR marker. Planta Medica 74, 194–196.

Dhanya, K., Syamkumar, S., Jaleel, K., Sasikumar, B., 2008. Random amplified polymorphic DNA technique for the detection of plant based adulterants in chilli powder (*Capsicum annuum*). Journal of Spices and Aromatic Crops 17, 75–81.

Dhanya, K., Syamkumar, S., Sasikumar, B., 2009. Development and application of SCAR marker for the detection of papaya seed adulteration in traded black pepper powder. Food Biotechnology 23, 97–106.

Dhanya, K., Sasikumar, B., 2010. Molecular marker based adulteration detection in traded food and agricultural commodities of plant origin with special reference to spices. Current Trends in Biotechnology and Pharmacy 4, 454–489.

Dhanya, K., Syamkumar, S., Siju, S., Sasikumar, B., 2011a. SCAR markers for adulterant detection in ground chilli. British Food Journal 113, 656–658.

Dhanya, K., Syamkumar, S., Siju, S., Sasikumar, B., 2011b. Sequence characterized amplified region markers: a reliable tool for adulterant detection in turmeric powder. Food Research International 44, 2889–2895.

Dhiman, B., Singh, M., 2003. Molecular detection of cashew husk (*Anacardium occidentale*) adulteration in market samples of dry tea (*Camellia sinensis*). Planta Medica 69, 882–884.

Dhyaneshwar, W., Preeti, C., Kalpana, J., Bhushan, P., 2006. Development and application of RAPD-SCAR marker for identification of *Phyllanthus emblica* LINN. Biological and Pharmaceutical Bulletin 29, 2313–2316.

Dovicovicova, L., Olexova, L., Pangallo, D., Siekel, P., Kuchta, T., 2004. Polymerase chain reaction (PCR) for the detection of celery (*Apium graveolens*) in food. European Food Research and Technology 218, 493–495.

Draghici, S., Khatri, P., Eklung, A.C., Szallasi, Z., 2005. Reliability and reproducibility issues in DNA microarray measurements. Trends in Genetics 22, 101–109.

Duan, X., Zhang, D., Nie, L., Zhang, H., 2014. Rapid discrimination of geographical origin and evaluation of antioxidant activity of *Salvia miltiorrhiza* var. *alba* by Fourier transform near infra red spectroscopy. Spectrochimica Acta, Part A: Molecular and Biomolecular Spectroscopy 122, 751–757.

Ellis, H., Leandri, V., Hagfeldt, A., Boschloo, G., Bergquist, J., Shevchenko, D., 2015. Laser desorption/ionization mass spectrometry of dye sensitized solar cells: identification of the dye – electrolyte interaction. Journal of Mass Spectrometry 50, 734–739.

Fan, Q., Wang, Y., Sun, P., Liu, S., Li, Y., 2010. Discrimination of *Ephedra* plants with diffuse reflectance FT-NIRS and multivariate analysis. Talanta 80, 1245–1250.

Fritz, E., Olzant, S.M., Langer, R., 2008. *Ilicium verum* Hook. f. and *Ilicium anisatum* L.: anatomical characters and their value for differentiation. Scientia Pharmaceutica 76, 65–76.

FSSAI Manual of Methods for Analysis of Foods: Spices and Condiments, 2012. Food Safety and Standards Authority of India, Ministry of Health and Family Welfare, Government of India, p. 44.

Fukuda, N., Tanaka, H., Shoyama, Y., 2000. Formation of monoclonal antibody against a major ginseng component ginsenoside RgI and its characterisation: monoclonal antibody for a ginseng saponin. Cytotechnology 34, 197–204.

Gad, H.A., El-Ahmady, S.H., Abou-Shoer, M.I., Al-Azizi, M.M., 2013. A modern approach to the authentication and quality assessment of thyme using UV spectroscopy and chemometric analysis. Phytochemical Analysis 24, 520–526.

Galimberti, A., Bruno, A., Mezzasalma, V., Mattia, F., Bruni, I., Labra, M., 2015. Emerging DNA-based technologies to characterize food ecosystems. Food Research International 69, 424–433.

Gamazo-Vazquez, J., Garcia-Falcon, M.S., Simal-Gandara, J., 2003. Control of contamination of olive oil by sunflower seed oil in bottling plants by GC-MS of fatty acid methyl esters. Food Control 14, 463–467.

Ganzera, M., 2008. Quality control of herbal medicines by capillary electrophoresis: potential, requirements and applications. Elecrophoresis 29, 3489–3503.

Gismondi, A., Fanali, F., Labarga, J.M.M., Cailoa, M.G., Canini, A., 2013. *Crocus sativus* L. genomics and different DNA barcode applications. Plant Systematics and Evolution 299, 1859–1863.

Ha, W.Y., Shaw, P.C., Liu, J., Yau, F.C.F., Wang, J., 2002. *Panax ginseng* and *Panax quinquefolius* using amplified fragment length polymorphism (AFLP) and directed amplification of minisatellite region DNA (DAMD). Journal of Agricultural and Food Chemistry 50, 1871–1875.

Heath, D.D., Iwama, G.K., Devlin, R.H., 1993. PCR primed with VNTR core sequences yields species specific patterns and hypervariable probes. Nucleic Acids Research 21, 5782–6285.

Hebert, P.D.N., Cywinska, A., Ball, S.L., de Waard, J.R., 2003. Biological identification through DNA barcodes. Proceedings of the Royal Society of London 270, 313–321.

Heidarbeigi, K., Mohtasebi, S.S., Foroughirad, A., Varnamkhasti, M.G., Rafiee, S., Rezaei, K., 2015. Detection of adulteration in saffron samples using electronic nose. International Journal of Food Properties 18, 1391–1401.

Henrion, R., Henrion, G., 2001. Chemometrics. In: Gunzler, H., William, H. (Eds.), Handbook of Analytical Techniques. Wiley Publications, Germany, pp. 37–39.

Hosokawa, K., Minami, M., Kawahara, K., Nakamura, I., Shibata, T., 2000. Discrimination among three species of medicinal *Scutellaria* plants using RAPD markers. Planta Medica 66, 270–272.

Hupfer, C., Waiblinger, H.U., Busch, U., 2007. Development and validation of a real-time PCR detection method for celery in food. European Food Research and Technology 225, 329–335.

ISO (International Standards Organization), 1995. International Standard: Spices and Condiments- Nomenclature, First List, p. 676.

Jabeur, H., Zribi, A., Makni, J., Rebai, A., Abdelhedi, R., Bouaziz, M., 2014. Detection of Chemlali extra-virgin olive oil adulteration mixed with soybean oil, corn oil, and sunflower oil by using GC and HPLC. Journal of Agricultural and Food Chemistry 21, 4893–4904.

Jain, N., Shasany, A.K., Singh, S., Khanuja, S.P.S., Kumar, S., 2008. SCAR markers for correct identification of *Phyllanthus amarus, P. fraternus, P. debilis* and *P. urinaria* used in scientific investigations and dry leaf bulk herb trade. Planta Medica 74, 1–6.

Jiang, C., Liang, C., Yuan, Y., Chen, M., Jin, Y., Huang, L., 2014. Barcoding melting curve analysis for rapid, sensitive, and discriminating authentication of saffron (*Crocus sativus* L.) from its adulterants. BioMed Research International 2014, Article ID 809037. http://dx.doi.org/10.1155/2014/809037.

Joshi, V.C., Khan, I.A., 2005. Macroscopic and microscopic authentication of Chinese and North American species of *Ephedra*. Journal of AOAC International 88, 707–713.

Joshi, V.C., Navarrete, A., Khan, I.A., 2005a. Authentication of *Valeriana procera* Kunth and comparative account of five Valeriana species. Journal of AOAC International 88, 1621–1625.

Joshi, V.C., Pullala, V.S., Khan, I.A., 2005b. Rapid and easy identification of *Illicium verum* Hook. f. and its adulterant *Illicium anisatum* Linn. by fluorescent microscopy and gas chromatography. Journal of AOAC International 88, 703–706.

Kalivas, A., Ganopoulos, I., Xanthopoulou, A., Chatzopoulou, P., Tsaftaris, A., Mades, P., 2014. DNA barcode ITS2 coupled with high resolution melting (HRM) analysis for taxonomic identification of *Sideritis* species growing in Greece. Molecular Biology Reports 41, 5147–5155.

Kamboj, A., 2012. Analytical evaluation of herbal drugs. In: Vallisuta, O., Olimat, S.M. (Eds.), Drug Discovery Research in Pharmacognosy. Intech, Croatia, pp. 33–34.

Khatoon, S., Singh, N., Kumar, S., Srivastava, N., Rathi, A., Mehrotha, S., 2009. Authentication and quality evaluation of an important Ayurvedic drug – Asoka bark. Journal of Scientific and Industrial Research 68, 393–400.

Kiran, U., Khan, S., Mirza, K.J., Ram, M., Abdin, M.N., 2010. SCAR markers: a potential tool for authentication of herbal drugs. Fitoterapia 81, 969–976.

Kojoma, M., Kurihara, K., Yamada, K., Sekita, S., Satake, M., Iida, O., 2002. Genetic identification of cinnamon (*Cinnamomum* spp.) based on the *trnL-trnF* chloroplast DNA. Planta Medica 68, 94–96.

Kolhe, R., Acharya, R., Haricha, C.R., 2015. Application of random amplified polymorphic DNA markers for authentication of three different available source plant of a frequently used Ayurvedic drug Trivrut. European Journal of Biomedical and Pharmaceutical Sciences 2, 971–980.

Kudo, M., Watt, R.A., Moffat, A.C., 2000. Rapid identification of *Digitalis purpurea* using near-infrared reflectance spectroscopy. Journal of Pharmacy and Pharmacology 52, 1271–1277.

Kumar, S., Kahlon, T., Chaudhary, S., 2011. A rapid screening for adulterants in olive oil using DNA barcodes. Food Chemistry 127, 1335–1341.

Kumar, S.P., 2014. Adulteration and substitution in endangered ASU medicinal plants of India: a Review. International Journal of Medicinal and Aromatic Plants 4, 56–73.

Lage, M., Cantrell, C.L., 2009. Quantification of saffron (*Crocus sativus* L.) metabolites crocins, picrocrocin and safranal for quality determination of the spice grown under different environmental Moroccan conditions. Scientia Horticulture 121, 366–373.

Lai, Y., Ni, Y., Kokot, S., 2011. Discrimination of *Rhizoma corydalis* from two sources by near infrared spectroscopy supported by the wavelet transform and squares support vector machine methods. Vibrational Spectroscopy 56, 154–160.

Lau, A.J., Holmes, M.J., Woo, S.O., Koh, H.L., 2003. Analysis of adulterants in a traditional herbal medicinal product using liquid chromatography – mass spectrometry – mass spectrometry. Journal of Pharmaceutical and Biomedical Analysis 31, 401–406.

Lau, C.C., Chan, C.O., Chau, F.T., Mok, D.K., 2009. Rapid analysis of *Radix puerariae* by near-infrared spectroscopy. Journal of Chromatography A 1216, 2130–2135.

Lee, M.Y., Doh, E.J., Park, C.H., Kim, Y.H., Kim, E.S., Ko, B.S., et al., 2006. Development of SCAR marker for discrimination of *Artemisia princeps* and *A. argyi* from other *Artemisia* herbs. Biological & Pharmaceutical Bulletin 29, 629–633.

Li, X., Ding, X., Chu, B., Ding, G., Gu, S., Qian, L., et al., 2007. Molecular authentication of *Alisma orientale* by PCR-RFLP and ARMS. Planta Medica 73, 67–70.

Liang, Y.Z., Xie, P., Chan, K., 2004. Quality control of herbal medicines. Journal of Chromatography B 812, 53–70.

Liang, Q.L., Qu, J., Luo, G., Wang, Y., 2006a. Rapid and reliable determination of illegal adulterant in herbal medicines and dietary supplements by LC/MS/MS. Journal of Pharmaceutical and Biomedical Analysis 40, 305—311.

Liang, Z.T., Jiang, Z.H., Leung, K.S.Y., Peng, Y., Zhao, Z.Z., 2006b. Distinguishing the medicinal herb *Oldenlandia diffusa* from similar species of the same genus using fluorescence microscopy. Microscopy Research and Technique 69, 277—282.

Lin, J., Zhou, X., Gao, S., Wu, W., Liu, X., Sun, X., Tang, K., 2006. Authentication of *Pinellia ternata* and its adulterants based on PCR with specific primers. Planta Medica 72, 844—847.

Litt, M., Lutty, J.A., 1989. A hypervariable microsatellite revealed by in vitro amplification of a dinucleotide repeat within the cardiac muscle actin gene. American Journal of Human Genetics 44, 397—401.

Liu, Z., Wang, Y., Zhou, K., Han, D., Yang, X., Liu, X., 2001. Authentication of Chinese crude drug, Gecko, by allele- specific diagnostic PCR. Planta Medica 67, 385—387.

Lockley, A.K., Bardsley, R.G., 2000. DNA-based methods for food authentication. Trends in Food Science & Technology 11, 67—77.

Che Man, Y.B., Syahariza, Z.A., Mirghani, M.E.S., Jinap, S., Baker, J., 2005. Analysis of potential lard adulteration in chocolate and chocolate products using Fourier transform infrared spectroscopy. Food Chemistry 90, 815—819.

Mackie, M., 1996. Authentication of fish. In: Ashurt, P.R., Dennis, M.J. (Eds.), Food Authentication. Blackie Academic and Professional, London, pp. 140—170.

Macpherson, J.M., Eckstein, P.E., Scoles, G.J., Gajadhar, A.A., 1993. Variability of the random amplified polymorphic DNA assay among thermal cyclers, and effects of primer and DNA concentration. Molecular and Cellular Probes 7, 293—299.

Mafra, I., Ferreira, I.M.P.L.V.O., Oliveira, M.B.P.P., 2008. Food Authentication by PCR based methods. European Food Research and Technology 227, 649—655.

Marcus, D.M., Grollman, A.P., 2002. Botanical medicines-the need for new regulations. New England Journal of Medicine 347, 2073—2076.

Maree, J.E., Viljoen, A.M., 2011. Fourier transform near-and mid-infrared spectroscopy can distinguish between the commercially important *Pelargonium sidoides* and its close taxonomically *P. reniforme*. Vibrational Spectroscopy 55, 146—152.

Marieschi, M., Torelli, A., Poli, F., Sacchetti, G., Bruni, R., 2009. RAPD- based method for the quality control of Mediterranean oregano and its contribution to pharmacognostic techniques. Journal of Agricultural and Food Chemistry 57, 1835—1840.

Marieschi, M., Torelli, A., Bruni, R., 2012. Quality control of saffron (*Crocus sativus* L.): development of SCAR markers for the detection of plant adulterants used as bulking agents. Journal of Agricultural and Food Chemistry 60, 10998—11004.

Marmiroli, N., Peano, C., Maestri, E., 2010. Advanced PCR techniques in identifying food components. In: Lees, M. (Ed.), Food Authenticity and Traceability. Woodhead Publishing, Cambridge, p. 18.

Massart, D.L., Vandeginste, B.G.M., Deming, S.H., Michotte, Y., Kaufman, L. (Eds.), 1988. Chemometrics: A Textbook. Elsevier, Amsterdam.

Meuren, M., 2010. Spectrophotometric techniques. In: Lees, M. (Ed.), Food Authentication and Traceability. Wood head publishing, Cambridge, pp. 184—185.

Mohammad, I., Shukla, S.K., Shakeel, W., 2015. Rapid detection of adulteration in indigenous saffron of Kashmir valley, India. Research Journal of Forensic Sciences 3, 7—11.

Mustorp, S., Axelsson, C.E., Svensson, U., Holck, A., 2008. Detection of celery (*Apium graveolens*), mustard (*Sinapis alba, Brassica juncea, Brassica nigra*) and sesame (*Sesamum indicum*) in food by real-time PCR. European Food Research and Technology 226, 771—778.

Nayak, B.S., Patel, K.N., 2010. Pharmacognostic studies of *Jatropha curcas* leaves. International Journal PharmTech, Research 2, 140–143.

Nazish, I., Ali, M., Mir, R.S., Parvez, N., Yadav, S., Hwiva, N., et al., 2010. Application of Microscopy in authentication of Unani traditional plant *Ruta graveolens*. Pharma Science Monitor 1, 122–127.

Newmaster, S.G., Grguic, M., Shanmughanadhan, D., Ramalingam, S., 2013. DNA barcoding detects contamination and substitution in North American herbal products. BMC Medicine 11, 222–235.

Newton, C.R., Graham, A., Heptinstall, L.E., Powell, S.J., Summers, C., Kalsheker, N., et al., 1989. Analysis of any point mutation in DNA: the amplification refractory mutation system (ARMS). Nucleic Acids Research 17, 2503–2516.

Ngan, F., Shaw, P., But, P., Wang, J., 1999. Molecular authentication of *Panax* species. Phytochemistry 50, 787–791.

Nieri, P., Adinolfi, B., Morelli, I., Breschi, M.C., Simoni, G., Martinotti, E., 2003. Genetic characterization of the three medicinal *Echinacea* species using RAPD analysis. Planta Medica 69, 685–686.

Niu, L., Mantri, N., Li, C.G., Xue, C., Pang, E., 2011. Array based techniques for fingerprinting medicinal herbs. Chinese Medicine 6, 18–28.

Ordoudi, S.A., Cagliani, L.R., Lalou, S., Naziri, E., Tsimidou, M., Consonni, R., 2015. 1H NMR-based metabolomics of saffron reveals markers for its quality deterioration. Food Research International 70, 1–6.

Osthanunkal, M., Madesis, P., de Boer, H., 2015. Bar-HRM for authentication of plant based medicines: evaluation of three medicinal products derived from *Acanthaceae* species. PLoS One 10, e0128476.

Paran, I., Michelmore, R.W., 1993. Development of reliable PCR-based markers linked to downy mildew resistance genes in lettuce. Theoretical and Applied Genetics 85, 985–993.

Parvathy, V.A., Swetha, V.P., Sheeja, T.E., Leela, N.K., Chempakam, B., Sasikumar, B., 2014. DNA barcoding to detect chilli adulteration in traded black pepper powder. Food Biotechnology 28, 25–40.

Parvathy, V.A., Swetha, V.P., Sheeja, T.E., Sasikumar, B., 2015. Detection of plant-based adulterants in turmeric powder using DNA barcoding. Pharmacien Biologiste 53, 1771–1779.

Pereira, F., Carneiri, J., Amorim, A., 2008. Identification of species with DNA based technology: current progress and challenges. Recent Patents on DNA & Gene Sequence 2, 187–200.

Petrakis, E.A., Cagliani, L.R., Pollisiou, M.G., Consonni, R., 2015. Evaluation of saffron (*Crocus sativus* L.) adulteration with plant adulterants by (1) H NMR metabolite fingerprinting. Food Chemistry 173, 890–896.

Preethi, P.J., Padmini, K., Lohitha, M., Swetha, K., Priyanka, K., Rao, V.P., 2014. Adulterants and substitutes of foods and herbs: a review. International Journal of Analytical Chemistry 4, 213–217.

Pruthi, J.S., 1998. Quality Assurance in Spice and Spice Products: Modern Methods of Analysis. Allied Publishers, New Delhi.

Qian, Y.E., Ying-xiong, Q., Yan-qi, Q., Jianxin, C., Shu-zhen, Y., Ming-shui, Z., et al., 2006. Species–specific SCAR markers for authentication of *Sinocalycnthus chinensis*. Journal of Zhejiang University Science B 7, 868–872.

Rebane, R., Leito, I., Yurchenko, S., Herodes, K., 2010. A review of analytical techniques for determination of Sudan I–IV dyes in food matrixes. Journal of Chromatography A 1217, 2747–2757.

Reid, L.M., O'Donnell, C.M., Downey, G., 2006. Recent technological advances for the determination of food authenticity. Trends in Food Science & Technology 17, 344–353.

Reid, R.G., 2013. Capillary electrophoresis in the profiling and authentication of herbal medicines. In: Oral Presentation, International Conference and Exhibition on Traditional and Alternative Medicine, Radisson Blu Plaza Hotel, Hyderabad, 9 December 2013.

Reinholds, I., Esslinger, S., Bartkevics, V., Silvis, I.C.J., van Ruth, S.M., 2015. Analytical techniques combined with chemometrics for authentication and determination of contaminants in condiments: a review. Journal of Food Composition and Analysis 44, 56–72.

Ren, Y., Wu, C., Zhang, J., 2012. Simultaneous screening and determination of 18 illegal adulterants in herbal medicines and health foods for male sexual potency by ultra-fast liquid chromatography electrospray ionization tandem mass spectrometry. Journal of Separation Science 35, 2847–2857.

Revathy, S.S., Rathinamala, R., Murugeshan, M., 2012. Authentication methods for drugs used in Ayurvedha, Siddha and Unnani systems of medicine: an overview. International Journal of Pharmaceutical Sciences and Research 3, 2352–2361.

Riaz, N., Khan, R.A., Rahman, A., Ali, S., Yasmeen, S., Afza, N., 2009. Detection and determination of Para red in chillies and spices by HPLC. Journal of the Chemical Society of Pakistan 31, 151–155.

Rinaldi, C., 2007. Authentication of the *Panax* Genus Plants Used in Traditional Chinese Medicine (TCM) Using Random Amplified Polymorphic DNA (RAPD) Analysis (Doctoral thesis). The University of Western Australia.

Ririe, K.M., Rasmussen, R.P., Wittwer, C.T., 1997. Product differentiation by analysis of DNA melting curves during the polymerase chain reaction. Analytical Biochemistry 245, 154–160.

Romagnoli, B., Menna, V., Gruppioni, N., Bergamini, C., 2007. Aflatoxins in spices, aromatic herbs, herb-teas and medicinal plants marketed in Italy. Food Control 18, 687–701.

Sasaki, Y., Fushimi, H., Komatsu, K., 2004. Application of single-nucleotide polymorphism analysis of the *trnK* gene to the identification of *Curcuma* plants. Biological and Pharmaceutical Bulletin 27, 144–146.

Sasikumar, B., Syamkumar, S., Remya, R., John Zachariah, T., 2005. PCR based detection of adulteration in the market samples of turmeric powder. Food Biotechnology 18, 299–306.

Schulz, H., Schrader, B., Quilitzsch, R., Pfeffer, S., Kruger, H., 2003. Rapid classification of basil chemotypes by vibrational spectroscopy methods. Journal of Agricultural and Food Chemistry 51, 2475.

Selvaraj, D., Sarma, R.K., Sathishkumar, R., 2008. Phylogenetic analysis of chloroplast *mat* K gene from Zingiberaceae for plant DNA barcoding. Bioinformation 3, 24–27.

Sereena, K., Kumar, U.P., Remashree, B., 2011. Histochemical and phytochemical markers for the authentication of the Ayurvedic raw drug Hallakam (*Kaempferia rotunda*) and its marketed adulterant. International Journal of Pharmaceutical Sciences and Research 2, 2952–2958.

Shaw, P.C., But, P.P.H., 1995. Authentication of *Panax* species and their adulterants by random-primed polymerase chain reaction. Planta Medica 61, 466–469.

Shim, Y.H., Choi, J.H., Park, C.D., Lim, C.J., Cho, J.H., Kim, H.J., 2003. Molecular differentiation of *Panax* species by RAPD analysis. Archives of Pharmacal Research 26, 601–605.

Shim, Y.H., Park, C.D., Kim, D.H., Cho, J.H., Cho, M.H., Kim, H.J., 2005. Identification of *Panax* species in the herbal medicine preparations using gradient PCR method. Biological & Pharmaceutical Bulletin 28, 671–676.

Shinde, V.M., Dhalwal, K., Mahadik, K.R., Joshi, K.S., Patwardhan, B.K., 2007. RAPD Analysis for determination of components in herbal medicine. Evidence-Based Complementary and Alternative Medicine 4, 21–23.

Shioda, H., Satoh, K., Nagai, F., Okubo, T., Seto, T., Hamano, T., et al., 2003. Identification of *Aloe* species by random amplified polymorphic DNA (RAPD) analysis. Journal of the Food Hygienic Society of Japan 44, 203–207.

Silvis, I., Alewijn, M., van Ruth, S.M., 2015. Untargeted direct mass spectrometry for obtaining base-line fingerprints of authentic herbs and spices. Journal of Chromatography & Separation Techniques 6, 59.

Singhal, R.S., Kulkarni, P.R., Rege, D.V. (Eds.), 1997. Handbook of Indices of Food Quality and Authenticity. Woodhead Publishing Ltd, Cambridge.

Singtonat, S., Osthanunkul, M., 2015. Fast and reliable detection of toxic *Crotalaria spectabilis* Roth. in *Thunbergia laurifolia* Lindl. herbal products using DNA barcoding coupled with HRM analysis. BMC Complementary and Alternative Medicine 15, 162–170.

Slanc, P., Ravnikar, M., Štrukelj, B., Štrukelj, B., 2006. Identification of individual herbal drugs in tea mixtures using restriction analysis of ITS DNA and real-time PCR. Pharmazie 11, 912–915.

Smilie, T.J., Khan, I.A., 2010. A comprehensive approach to identifying and authenticating botanical products. Clinical Pharmacology & Therapeutics 87, 175–186.

Spaniolas, S., May, S.T., Bennett, M.J., Tucker, G.A., 2006. Authentication of coffee by means of PCR-RFLP analysis and lab-on-a-chip capillary electrophoresis. Journal of Agricultural and Food Chemistry 54, 7466–7470.

Sproll, C., Ruge, W., Andlauer, C., Godelmann, R., Lachenmeier, D.W., 2008. HPLC analysis and safety assessment of coumarin in foods. Food Chemistry 109, 462–469.

Srinivasan, K., 2000. Spices valued for more than taste and flavour of foods. In: De, A.K. (Ed.), Recent Trends in Spices and Medicinal Plants. Associated Publishing, New Delhi, pp. 31–34.

Srirama, R., Senthilkumar, U., Sreejayan, N., Ravikanth, G., Gurumurthy, B.R., Shivanna, M.B., et al., 2010. Assessing species admixtures in raw drug trade of *Phyllanthus*, a hepato-protective plant using molecular tools. Journal of Ethnopharmacology 130, 208–215.

Stoeckle, M.Y., Gamble, C.C., Kirpekar, R., Young, G., Ahmed, S., Damon, P., 2011. Commercial teas highlight plant DNA barcode identification successes and obstacles. Scientific Reports 1, 42.

Sukrong, S., Phadungcharoen, T., Ruangrungsi, N., 2006. DNA fingerprinting of medicinally used *Derris* species by RAPD molecular markers. Thai Journal of Pharmaceutical Sciences 29, 155–163.

Sulthana, S., Khan, M.A., Ahmad, M., Bano, A., Zafar, M., Shinwari, Z.K., 2011. Authentication of herbal medicine neem (*Azadirachta indica* A. Juss.) by using taxonomic and pharmacognostic techniques. Pakistan Journal of Botany 43, 141–150.

Swetha, V.P., Parvathy, V.A., Sheeja, T.E., Sasikumar, B., 2014. DNA Barcoding for discriminating the economically important *Cinnamomum verum* from its adulterants. Food Biotechnology 28, 183–194.

Sze, S.C., Song, J.X., Wong, R.N., Feng, Y.B., Ng, T.B., Tong, Y., et al., 2008. Application of SCAR (sequence characterized amplified region) analysis to authenticate *Lycium barbarum* (wolf berry) and its adulterants. Biotechnology and Applied Biochemistry 51, 15–21.

Tam, C.H., Peng, Y., Liang, Z.T., He, Z.D., Zhao, Z.Z., 2006. Application of microscopic techniques in authentication of herbal tea—Ku-Ding-Cha. Microscopy Research and Technique 69, 927–932.

Tanaka, H., Fukuda, N., Shoyama, Y., 1999. Formation of monoclonal antibody against a major ginseng component ginsenoside RbI and its characterisation. Cytotechnology 29, 115–120.

Tanaka, H., Fukuda, N., Yahara, S., Isoda, S., Yuan, C., Shoyama, Y., 2005. Isolation ofginsenoside RbI from *Kalopanax pictus* by eastern blotting using antiginsenoside RbI monoclonal antibody. Phytotherapy Research 106, 135–146.

Tateo, F., Bononi, M., 2004. Fast determination of Sudan I by HPLC/APCI-MS in hot chilli spices, and oven-baked foods. Journal of Agricultural and Food Chemistry 52, 655–658.

Techen, N., Khan, I.A., Pan, Z., Scheffler, B.E., 2006. The use of polymerase chain reaction (PCR) for the identification of *Ephedra* DNA in dietary supplements. Planta Medica 72, 241–247.

Theerakulpisut, P., Kanawapee, N., Maensiri, D., Bunnag, S., Chantaranothai, P., 2008. Development of species-specific SCAR markers for identification of three medicinal species of *Phyllanthus*. Journal of Systematic and Evolutionary Microbiology 46, 614–621.

Torey, A., Sasidharan, S., Yeng, C., Latha, L.Y., 2010. Standardization of *Cassia spectabilis* with respect to authenticity, assay and chemical constituent analysis. Molecules 15, 3411–3420.

Tremlova, B., 2001. Evidence of black pepper spice adulteration. Czech Journal of Food Sciences 19, 235–239.

Tzouros, N.E., Arvanitoyannis, I.S., 2001. Agricultural produces: synopsis of employed quality control methods for the authentication of foods and application of chemometrics for the classification of foods according to their variety or geographical origin. Critical Reviews in Food Science and Nutrition 41, 287–319.

Vidal, A.O., Schnerr, H., Rojmyr, M., Lysholm, F., Knight, A., 2007. Quantitative identification of plant genera in food products using PCR and pyrosequencing technology. Food Control 18, 921–927.

Vijayan, K., Tsou, C.H., 2010. DNA barcoding in plants: taxonomy in a new perspective. Current Science 99, 1530–1541.

Wallace, J.L., Boilard, S.M.A.L., Eagle, S.H.C., Spall, J.L., Shokralla, S., Hajibabaei, M., 2012. DNA barcodes for everyday life: routine authentication of Natural Health Products. Food Research International 49, 446–452.

Wang, P., Huang, F., Zhou, L., Cao, L., Liang, S., Xu, H., et al., 2000. Analysis of *Amomun villosum* species and some adulterants of Zingiberaceae by RAPD. Zhong Yao Cai 23, 71–74.

Wang, J., Ha, W.Y., Ngan, F.N., But, P.P.H., Shaw, P.C., 2001. Application of sequence characterized amplified region (SCAR) analysis to authenticate *panax* species and their adulterants. Planta Medica 67, 781–783.

Wang, C., Cao, Y.H., Xing, X.P., Ye, J.N., 2005. Fingerprint studies of *Radix scutellariae* by capillary electrophoresis and high performance liquid chromatography. Chromatographia 62, 283–288.

Wang, F., Zhang, Z., Cui, X., de Harrington, P.B., 2006. Identification of rhubarbs by using NIR spectrometry and temperature-constrained cascade correlation networks. Talanta 70, 1170–1176.

Wang, C., Xiang, B., Zhang, W., 2009. Application of two-dimensional near-infrared (2D-NIR) correlation spectroscopy to the discrimination of three species of Dendrobium. Journal of Chemometrics 23, 463–470.

Wang, C.Z., Ni, M., Sun, S., Li, X.L., He, H., Mehendale, S., 2009. Detection of adulteration of Notoginseng root extract with other *panax* species by quantitative HOLC coupled with PCA. Journal of Agricultural and Food Chemistry 57, 2363–2367.

Wang, X.M., 2011. Inter-simple sequence repeats (ISSR) molecular fingerprinting markers for authenticating the genuine species of rhubarb. Genome 5, 758–764.

Wang, P., Yu, Z., 2015. Species authentication and geographical origin discrimination of herbal medicines by near infrared spectroscopy: a review. Journal of Pharmaceutical and Biomedical Analysis 5, 277–284.

Welsh, J., McClelland, M., 1990. Fingerprinting genomes using PCR with arbitrary primers. Nucleic Acids Research 18, 7213–7218.

Wilhelmsen, E.C., 2004. Food adulteration. Food Science and Technology 138, 20131–22056.

Williams, J.G.K., Kubelik, A.R., Livak, K.J., Rafalski, J.A., Tingey, S.V., 1990. DNA polymorphisms amplified by arbitrary primers are useful as genetic markers. Nucleic Acids Research 18, 6531–6535.

Wilson, D.A., 2013. Diverse applications of electronic-nose technologies in agriculture and forestry. Sensors 13, 2295–2348.

Wolf, H.T., Berg, T., Czygan, F.C., Mosandl, A., Winckler, T., Zundorf, I., et al., 1999. Identification of *Melissa officinalis* subspecies by DNA fingerprinting. Planta Medica 65, 83–85.

Woo, Y.A., Kim, H.J., Kim, K., Ze, R., 2005. Near infrared (NIR) spectroscopy for the non – destructive and fast determination of geographical origin of *Angelica gigantis* Radix. Journal of Pharmaceutical and Biomedical Analysis 36, 955–959.

Xia, L., Bai, L.P., Yi, L., Liu, B.B., Chu, C., Liang, Z.T., et al., 2007. Authentication of the 31 species of toxic and potent Chinese Materia Medica (T/PCMM) by microscopic technique, part I: three kinds of toxic and potent animal CMM. Microscopy Research and Technique 70, 960–968.

Xu, Y., 1996. Tutorial: capillary electrophoresis. Chemical Educator 1, 1–14.

Xu, H., Fabricant, D.S., Piersen, C.E., Bolton, J.L., Pezzuto, J.M., Fong, H., et al., 2002. A preliminary RAPD-PCR analysis of *Cimicifuga* species and other botanicals used for women's health. Phytomedicine 9, 757–762.

Xu, H., Hou, B., Zhang, J., Tian, M., Yuan, Y., Niu, Z., Ding, X., 2012. Detecting adulteration of *Dendrobium officinale* by real-time PCR coupled with ARMS. International Journal of Food Science & Technology 47, 1695–1700.

Xue, C.Y., Li, D.Z., Lu, J.M., Yang, J.B., Liu, J.Q., 2006. Molecular authentication of the traditional Tibetan medicinal plant *Swertia mussotii*. Planta Medica 72, 1223–1226.

Xue, H.G., Wang, H., Li, D.Z., Xue, C.Y., Wang, Q.Z., 2008. Differentiation of the traditional Chinese medicinal plants *Euphorbia humifusa* and *E. maculate* from adulterants by TaqMan real-time polymerase chain reaction. Planta Medica 74, 302–304.

Xue, C.Y., Xuc, H.G., Li, D.Z., 2009. Authentication of the traditional Chinese medicinal plant *Saussurea involucrate* using enzyme – linked immunosorbent assay (ELISA). Planta Medica 75, 15. http://dx.doi.org/10.1055/s-0029-1234669.

Yang, C., Wang, Y., Marty, J.L., Yang, X.R., 2011. Aptamer based colorimetric biosensing of Ochratoxin A using unmodified gold nano particles indicator. Biosensors & Bioelectronics 26, 2724–2727.

Yilmaz, A., Nyberg, N.T., Mølgaard, P., Asili, J., Jaroszewski, J.W., 2010. 1H NMR metabolic fingerprinting of saffron extracts. Metabolismo 6, 511–517.

Yip, P.Y., Chau, C.F., Mak, C.Y., Kwan, H.S., 2007. DNA methods for identification of Chinese medicinal materials. Chinese Medicine 2, 9.

Yuan, M., Wei, M.F.U., Cheng, X.J., 2011. Identification of species within *Tetrastigma* (Miq.) Planch. (Vitaceae) based on DNA barcoding techniques. Journal of Systematic and Evolutionary Microbiology 49, 237–245.

Zalacain, A., Ordoudi, S.A., Diaz-Plaza, E.M., Carmona, M., Blazquez, I., Tsimidou, M.Z., 2005. Near infrared spectroscopy in saffron quality control: determination of chemical composition and geographical origin. Journal of Agricultural and Food Chemistry 53, 9337–9341.

Zalacain, A., Ordoudi, S.A., Blazquez, I., Diaz-Plaza, M., Carmona, M., Tsimidou, M.Z., Alonso, G.L., 2015. Screening method for the detection of artificial colors in saffron using derivative UV-vis spectrometry after precipitation of crocetin. Food Additives and Contaminants 22, 607–615.

Zha, X.Q., Luo, J.P., Wei, P., 2009. Identification and classification of *Dendrobium candidum* species by fingerprint technology with capillary electrophoresis. South African Journal of Botany 75, 276–282.

Zhang, K.Y.B., Leung, H.W., Yeung, H.W., Wong, R.N.S., 2001. Differentiation of *Lycium barbarum* from its related *Lycium* species using random amplified polymorphic DNA. Planta Medica 67, 379–381.

Zhang, Q., Thomas, D., Acworth, I., 2013. Evaluation of Herb and Fruit Juice Adulteration and Authenticity by Coulometric Array Detection and Pattern Recognition. Planta Medica 79, 125.

Zhao, Z., Hu, Y.N., Wong, Y.W., Gigi, W.W.C., Wu, K., Jiang, Z.H., Kang, T., 2005. Application of microscopy in authentication of Chinese patent medicine – Bo Ying compound. Microscopy Research and Technique 67, 305–311.

Zhao, Z., Hu, Y., Liang, Z., Yuan, J.P., Jiang, Z., Leung, K.S., 2006. Authentication is fundamental for standardization of Chinese medicines. Planta Medica 72, 865–874.

Zhao, Z.L., Leng, C.H., Wang, Z.T., 2007. Identification of *Dryopteris crassirhizoma* and the adulterant species based on cpDNA *rbcL* and translated amino acid sequences. Planta Medica 73, 1230–1233.

Zhao, Z.Z., Li, Y.S., 2007. Easily Confused Chinese Medicines in Hong Kong. Chinese Medicine Merchants Association Ltd., Hong Kong.

Zhao, Y., Zhang, J., Yuan, T., Shen, T., Li, W., Yang, S., et al., 2014. Discrimination of wild *Paris* based on near infrared spectroscopy and high performance liquid chromatography combined with multivariate analysis. PLoS One 9, e89100. http://dx.doi.org/10.1371/journal.pone.0089100.

Zhu, S., Fushimi, H., Cai, S., Komatsu, K., 2004. Species identification from ginseng drugs by multiplex amplification refractory mutation system (MARMS). Planta Medica 70, 189–192.

Zietkiewicz, E., Rafalski, A., Labuda, D., 1994. Genome fingerprinting by simple sequencerepeat (SSR)-anchored polymerase chain reaction amplification. Genomics 20, 176–183.

Zimmerman, K., Mannhalter, J.W., 1996. Technical aspects of quantitative competitive PCR. Biotechniques 21, 264–270.

Zougagh, M., Simonet, B.M., Rios, A., Valcarcel, M., 2005. Use of non aqueous capillary electrophoresis for the quality control of commercial saffron samples. Journal of Chromatography A 1085, 293–298.

Zu, H., Zhao, M., 2014. Study on the microscopic identification of adulterated plant origin powdered seasonings. Discourse Journal of Agriculture and Food Sciences 2, 264–269.

Tradition Meets High Tech for Authenticity Testing of Fruit Juices

23

P. Rinke
SGF International E.V., Nieder-Olm, Germany

Chapter Outline

23.1 Introduction

After scandals like the horse meat issue and the tragedy resulting from the addition of melamine to milk powder, food authenticity testing assumed more importance in general food analytics. However, fruit juices were already under intensive analytical authenticity control for decades. Adulteration is relatively easy to perform because of the chemical composition and the wide natural variation seen in juices. Addition of water and/or sugar, acidification, cheaper fruits, colorants, flavor, and vitamins are typical frauds that are performed with criminal intent and sometimes with a high level of sophistication to make the adulterated products as difficult as possible to detect (Fig. 23.1). Such economically driven frauds harm fair competition and enhance the risk of scandals and a bad public image for the industry. Both these facts were drivers for the early development of fruit juice authenticity testing.

Because of the scope of this chapter, there is unfortunately not enough room to give all of the technical details but it will try to give an overview of the most important control possibilities to assist the analyst or a laboratory's customer to select an appropriate analytical scope for specific problems.

Food safety considerations are not the main focus of this chapter but these typically include heavy metals, arsenic, pesticides, mycotoxins, and chemical residues, for example, from cleaning agents.

Furthermore, flavor analytics and vitamin analyses in fruit juices are also excluded here. These are large fields that can be embedded together with food safety analyses in a more general approach to foodstuff analysis.

DNA analyses can facilitate the differentiation of fruit species and varieties, neither of which are discussed in detail here. The application of this methodology to fruit

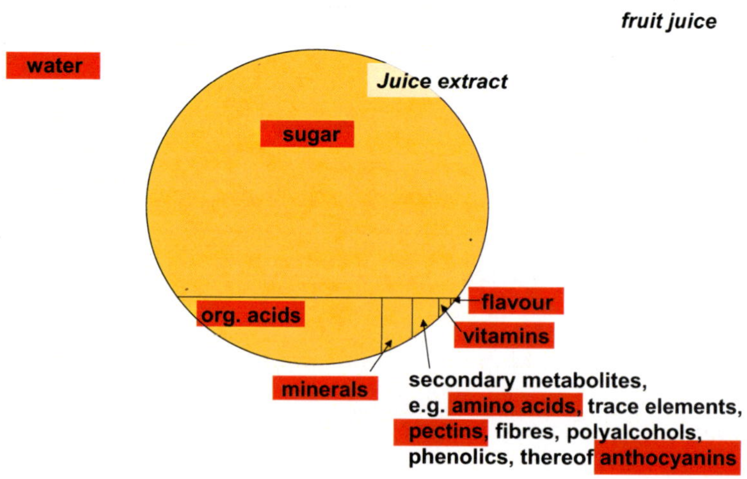

Figure 23.1 Schematic composition of a typical fruit juice. All compounds *highlighted in red* can be the subject of adulteration through addition.

juices is in a relatively early stage of development. Problems and limits are caused by degradation of the fruit DNA during processing, storage, and the product's low pH.

In this chapter, the term authenticity will include considerations of whether a product has been produced according to certain technological standards (Directive 2012/12/EC, 2012). Despite relatively good harmonization of legislation and industrial standards (CODEX STAN 247-2005), a product can be in conformity in one region but not in another. Some nonauthorized techniques can provide an illegal economic benefit or unfair sensory advantage. For example, it is not permitted in the European Union to coprocess *Citrus reticulata* varieties (mandarin and other hybrids) with *Citrus sinensis* (orange) (AIJN Code of Practice, 2015). However, in most other parts of the world, a certain percentage of the reticulata varieties are permitted in orange juice. The Codex Alimentarius is fixing a limit at a maximum of 10% of soluble solids from reticulata varieties for those countries where national legislation is permitting the blend (CODEX General Standard for Fruit Juices and Nectars, 2015). Other deviating national rules such as juice deacidification, enzyme use, water extraction of fruit pulp, addition of preservatives, and restoration of flavor must be taken into account when judging a product on a global market. Legal differences in the obligatory minimum Brix value or density for direct juices and juices reconstituted from concentrate probably have the biggest economic impact. These values relate to the juice extract and indirectly set limits for the amount of water present in a fruit juice. Therefore the relatively simple analysis for Brix (refractometric measurement expressed as percentage of dissolved sucrose) and/or density are two of the most important parameters in the fruit juice industry for authenticity control.

Authenticity control may include confirmation of a geographical origin of a fruit juice in cases where such a declaration for a product has been made. Besides this legal aspect, the analyst can use the analytical indication of an origin as supporting information for a refined interpretation of analytical figures. This will only be possible with experience and if regional specific reference materials and/or a suitable database is available.

The same is true for declared fruit varieties; these can have a large impact on sensory properties and raw material costs.

Fruit juice belongs to those food groups that are covered by very complex and extended analytics. For a successful interpretation, the analyst must know and consider a number of aspects, such as fruit juice species and varieties, process technology, geographical origin, seasonal deviations, types of possible frauds observed, and existing strategies to mask any adulteration. New supply areas, global warming, and progress in agriculture (providing new varieties) give an increasing dynamic to this already complex issue.

This may be the reason why there are only relatively few laboratories in the world that specialize in fruit juice analysis. Therefore progress in analytical techniques comes from a relatively small community of scientists and fruit juices are generally a minor focus for providers of modern analytical equipment. Together with the long history of fruit juice authenticity testing, this leads to the continued use of traditional methods together with sophisticated and modern developments (Hammond, 1995; Rossmann et al., 1990).

From today's view of analytics, one can consider that the transfer of stable isotopic measurements from the wine area to fruit juices in the early 1990s was the beginning of a broad introduction of modern analytics to the fruit juice field. Since then there has been a gradual evolution as a result of which traditional and more innovative and highly sophisticated techniques coexist. However, the combination of both these approaches should be considered the current state of the art for authenticity testing in fruit juices.

23.2 Overview of Methods Applied in Standard Control

For authenticity control of fruit juices a large number of aspects must be checked. The choice and combination of analyses chosen depends on the fruit type, product type, meta-data for the sample, and the availability of reference data.

In this chapter the analyses are classified as either conventional analyses or modern instrumental techniques. Chromatographic techniques, high-performance liquid chromatography (HPLC) and gas chromatography (GC), are grouped arbitrarily as conventional and traditional methods together with typical wet chemistry techniques even if this attribution may be incorrect in some cases. In most other cases, it is justified because the techniques have been using the same conditions for decades. For example, HPLC methods still deal with 30-cm columns and injection frequencies of up to 1 h or more. This is also because of the fact that fingerprinting methods play an important role and changes of methods would involve new database developments that may be time consuming and expensive to implement.

Conventional analyses are divided into quantitative determinations and fingerprinting methods. There are possible overlaps between both groups but it may help to structure the multitude of methods available in a typical fruit juice laboratory in this manner.

23.3 Conventional Methods

Table 23.1 lists a choice of quantitative parameters together with links to specific analytical questions and parameters typically used for this purpose. This matrix is indicative for the main fruit types but should be validated and adapted for every single case. Where applicable, the reference number of the respective method validated by the IFU (International Fruit and Vegetable Juice Association) is indicated (Website of International Fruit and Vegetable Juice Association).

Table 23.2 is a matrix linking some chromatographic methods with quality considerations. Even if most analyses deliver quantitative results, for the identified compounds the fingerprinting characters of these procedures are also important aspects in data interpretation.

Fingerprinting methods in fruit juice authentication have two main objectives, that is, the detection of marker substances for foreign fruits (Hofsommer, 1999; Goodner et al., 2001; Ooghe et al., 1994; Wilfried et al., 1997; Suarez Valles et al., 1994;

Table 23.1 Choice of Conventional Parameters and Their Use for Interpretation

Parameter	IFU Method (Website of International Fruit and Vegetable Juice Association)	Fruit Content	Sugar Addition	Organic Acid Addition	Foreign Fruit	Water Addition	Process Water Quality	Sulfitation	Technology (Citrus Juice)	Thermal Stress	Microbiological Indicator	Quality Processing Aids	Remaining Cleaning Agent
Brix/Density	1a, 8					x							
Total titratable acidity	3			x									
Potassium	33	x											
Formol number	30	x											
L-Malic acid	21	x		x									
D-Malic acid	64			x									
Magnesium	34	x											
Calcium	34	x							x				
Phosphorus	35	x											
D-Isocitric acid	54	x		x									
Proline	49	x			x								
Citric acid	22			x	x								x
Ratio citric/isocitric acid	22, 54			x									
pH	11			x									
Maltose/Isomaltose			x										
Chloride	37						x						
Sulfate	36						x	x					
Sulfur dioxide	7a							x					
Glucose	55		x										
Fructose	55		x										
Ratio glucose/fructose	55		x		x					x	x		

Continued

Table 23.1 **Choice of Conventional Parameters and Their Use for Interpretation—cont'd**

Parameter	IFU Method (Website of International Fruit and Vegetable Juice Association)	Fruit Content	Sugar Addition	Organic Acid Addition	Foreign Fruit	Water Addition	Process Water Quality	Sulfitation	Technology (Citrus Juice)	Thermal Stress	Microbiological Indicator	Quality Processing Aids	Remaining Cleaning Agent
Sucrose	56		x		x					x			
Total sugar (glucose, fructose, sucrose)	55, 56		x										
Share of sucrose versus total sugar	55, 56		x										
Lactic acid	19										x		
Ethanol	02										x		
5-Hydroxymethylfurfural	12									x			
Sodium	33						x					x	x
Nitrate	48						x						
Carotenoid profile (three fractions)	59				x								
Total carotenoids, β-carotene	44				x								
Sorbitol	32	x	x		x								
Water-soluble pectins	26								x				
Centrifugeable pulp	60								x				
Phlorin									x				
Ascorbic acid	17a			x						x			

Table 23.2 Chromatographic Methods With Fingerprint Character Used in Fruit Juice Authenticity Testing

	Sugar Addition	Foreign Fruit	Applicable in
Amino acid—HPLC or amino acid analyzer (IFU 57)		x	All fruits
Flavonoids—HPLC (IFU 58)		x	Citrus fruits
Anthocyanins—HPLC (IFU 71)		x	Red-colored fruits
Polymethoxylated flavanones—HPLC		x	Citrus fruits
Oligosaccharides—HPLC	x		Most fruits
Oligosaccharides—GC	x		Most fruits
Phenolic fingerprint—HPLC		x	All fruits
Carotenoid profile—HPLC		x	Yellow/orange-colored fruits
Organic acids—HPLC		x	All fruits

GC, Gas chromatography; *HPLC*, high-performance liquid chromatography.

Koswig et al., 1996; Hofsommer and Koswig, 2005; Hofsommer et al., 1989; Koswig and Hofsommer 1995; Koswig, 2006) and for sugar syrup (Low, 1995, 1996; Low et al., 1999; Swallow et al., 1991; Wudrich et al., 1993; Thavarajah and Low, 2006a; Swallow and Low, 1993; Low and Wudrich, 1993; Trotzer et al., 1994). With the exception of a gas chromatographic oligosaccharide analysis, all fingerprint analyses are performed by HPLC.

Some methods use direct injection or involve only simple sample preparation.

Flavonoids can be determined after dissolving a sample in ammonium oxalate solution with addition of dimethylformamide according to IFU method 58 (Website of International Fruit and Vegetable Juice Association).

Sample clean-up for the carotenoid fingerprint can be achieved by extraction after saponification (Rouseff et al., 1996).

The fingerprint of polymethoxylated flavanones is preceded by extraction and concentration.

To obtain a gas chromatographic fingerprint, the sample needs to be lyophilized prior to derivatization.

The most important authenticity aspects, including nonauthorized technologies, are discussed next.

23.3.1 Unauthorized or Undeclared Sugar Addition

Exogenous sugar can change the natural sugar profile that is typical for every individual fruit type. Reference is typically made to glucose, fructose, and sucrose and some important derived parameters such as the glucose-to-fructose ratio, sum of total sugars (glucose, fructose, and sucrose), and the share of sucrose in the total sugar. But for most adulteration, sugar types are involved to keep changes in the concentrations of these constituents inside the range of natural variation. Therefore traces of some typical marker substances for sugar syrups can give concrete hints about their addition. Starch-derived syrup can contain more maltose, maltotriose, isomaltose, or higher glucose oligosaccharides than are seen naturally in fruit juices. However, fruit types that naturally contain starch must be considered carefully.

If any product is adulterated by adding sugars from deionized juices of pome fruits (eg, apple or pear), the sugar alcohol sorbitol can be used as an important indicator for those fruit juices that have no native sorbitol content. Sorbitol is naturally present in pome fruits, stone fruits, and only a very few other fruit types like aronia berries Koswig and Hofsommer, 1999.

Furthermore, marker substances can be detected with a gas chromatographic fingerprinting method comprising silylation with *N*-trimethysilylimidazole and flame ionization detection developed by Prof. Nicholas Low (Low, 1995, 1996; Low et al., 1999; Swallow et al., 1991; Wudrich et al., 1993; Willems and Low, 2014) in a procedure often referred to as the "Low-GC method" and mentioned in Table 23.2 as "Oligosaccharides—GC." Typical side products in high-fructose corn syrup, invert sugar, and inulin hydrolyzate are detected by this approach. Maltose and isomaltose are indicators for starch-derived syrups. The marker substances for invert sugar are described as different combinations between glucose and fructose or two glucose molecules [*O*-α-D-glucopyranosyl-(1→3)-D-fructose, *O*-β-D-fructofuranosyl-(2→6)-D-glucose and *O*-α-D-glucopyranosyl-β-D-glucopyranoside] (Thavarajah and Low, 2006a).

A similar approach based on HPLC fingerprinting (Low and Wudrich, 1993; Trotzer et al., 1994) is less accurate and practically no longer in use. However, the detection of the typical glucose oligomer pattern, using HPLC, is still a valid method with which to characterize higher molecular weight degradation products from starch-based sugar syrups (mentioned in Table 23.2 as "Oligosaccharides—HPLC").

23.3.2 Unauthorized or Undeclared Addition of Organic Acids

A higher acidity level can be a sensory advantage and give a higher commercial value to certain types of fruit juice (eg, lemon, apple, cherry, blackcurrant). In a first step to detect addition of organic acids, the quantitative profile of the main organic acids in a juice sample must be checked against the natural relationship between the individual compounds. In particular, the ratio of citric acid/isocitric acid is an important characteristic for many fruit types of which citric acid is a major compound (Website of International Fruit and Vegetable Juice Association). Both acids are metabolites arising from the citrate cycle and have a more or less stable quantitative relationship in a defined fruit matrix. Isocitric acid has a chiral center and is naturally present as its D-isomer. A small amount of this acid may also appear as a cyclic lactone and therefore an alkaline hydrolysis is necessary to open the lactone and allow determination of the total D-isocitric acid content by an enzymic reaction procedure (Ref. IFU 53). If the hydrolysis step is omitted or other methods are applied, such as HPLC or capillary isotachophoresis, a deviation in absolute values will occur (Kvasnička et al., 2002), which can give significant differences in the citric-to-isocitrate ratio.

An interesting relationship in apple juices is the difference between the absolute concentration of malic acid and the titratable acidity with an endpoint at pH 7.0 and expressed as tartaric acid. The value for acidity is general slightly lower. Added malic acid disturbs the natural buffer system of the juice and leads to an increase of this difference, which is usually smaller than 1 g/L. This verification cannot be applied to juice with a naturally low acidity. Furthermore, it is not applicable for apple juices with a high content of galacturonic acid derived from pectin degradation when the extraction technology comprises an extremely strong use of pectinase activity (Will et al., 2000).

If commercial malic acid is added, depending on the quality of the additive, two marker substances can be detected. Fruits only contain the L-isomer of malic acid and the detection of D-malic acid indicates addition of a synthetic racemic mixture (D, L). An enzymic method for detection of D-malic acid exists (Website of International Fruit and Vegetable Juice Association). The other marker, fumaric acid (Website of AIJN Code of Practice; Website of International Fruit and Vegetable Juice Association), is a dehydration product of malic acid and is usually quantified by HPLC. However, today commercial malic acid, produced by fermentation processes, is available with only the L-malic isomer and is practically free of fumaric acid. In general, stable isotopic analyses are required to detect such adulteration now.

23.3.3 Water Addition/Overdilution

Adding water to fruit juices is a lucrative fraud and addition of small amounts of water can bring significant economic advantage to unscrupulous producers. Because of the large natural variation of fruit extracts (soluble solids content of a juice), the risk of failing to detect economically motivated adulteration by water addition to single strength products can be very high.

For products made from concentrates, the analyst can simply rely on a refractometric Brix determination or density measurement (Website of International Fruit and Vegetable Juice Association). For most fruit types a regulated minimum is fixed in the current EU fruit juice directive (Directive 2012/12/EC, 2012), Codex fruit juice standard (247, 2005), or the European Fruit Juice Association Code of Practice (AIJN CoP) (Website of AIJN Code of Practice).

Many authentic single strength products have a Brix or density higher than the minimum limit (Directive 2012/12/EC, 2012; Website of International Fruit and Vegetable Juice Association) because the standards take into account natural compositional variations. There is no other conventional method available to detect added water. In some cases, slightly increased sodium values can indicate possible water addition, for example, the maximum sodium level for orange juice is 30 mg/L

(Website of AIJN Code of Practice), which can reflect a typical, process-related contamination by sodium for juice concentrates. But a single strength juice with a sodium concentration of 20 mg/L is already suspicious. Unfortunately, standards do not differentiate between the maximum sodium value of single strength juices and juices made from concentrate. Therefore it is difficult to claim any sodium increase in single strength products which was caused by adulteration.

Suitable approaches for confirmation are described in the stable isotope section, discussed later.

23.3.4 Fruit Content

With the exception of authorized additives, a fruit juice must only contain authentic juice extracted by physical means from the fruit. Adulteration by addition of water or sugar syrup will decrease the fruit content. Checks are based on a number of selected analytical parameters (Table 23.1). Every parameter is compared individually with a typical average given in reference databases. Such a comparison allows a linear calculation of the theoretical fruit content for the selected parameters. Every parameter will result in a value for the fruit content. The consolidation of these values can be done by a simple average calculation or by taking into account the natural variability of each individual parameter. Parameters with low variation should have more impact on the final result.

$$\text{Example: FC(total)} = (f(i) * \text{FC}(i) + \ldots + f(n) * \text{FC}(n))/n$$

where, FC(total): predicted fruit content of the sample. $f(i)$: weighting factor for parameter i. n: number of parameters used.

Experience shows that at least five parameters should be used to verify a fruit content value. Different geographical origins and varieties of fruit can require separate evaluation.

Fruit content calculations are not standardized and often depend on in-house experience. Weighting factors and accepted tolerances in the case of observed deviations typically arise from the experience of the analyst. In many cases, reference datasets do not show a normal distribution, which limits the use of enhanced statistical methods.

23.3.5 Specific Marker Substances for Foreign Fruits

The mixing of pricey fruit juices with less expensive ones is a frequent economic fraud. There are certain substances that are characteristic of individual fruit species or groups of fruit. They can be used as marker compounds in other juice types (Hofsommer, 1999; Thavarajah and Low, 2006b; Koswig, 2006; Lee, 2015; Lehnert and Ara, 2014). Table 23.3 lists a selection of the most important markers used in juice analytics. The analyst should differentiate between unintended cross-contamination and intentional addition, a decision that may be assessed by evaluation of a number of different production batches. If all batches show evidence of mixtures, the admixture is highly unlikely to be unintentional.

Table 23.3 Typical Marker for Foreign Fruits in Fruit Juices

Adulterant	Marker Substance	Suitable for	Method
Pear	Arbutin	Most other juices	HPLC/UV phenolic compounds, proton-NMR
Apple	Phloridzin	Most other juices	HPLC/UV phenolic compounds
Pome and stone fruits	Sorbitol	Citrus, most berry fruits, tropicals	HPLC/EC, enzyme test
Lime	7-Methoxy- coumarin, further marker substances	Lemon juice	HPLC/UV(DAD) and/or MS
Lemon	Eriocitrin	Citrus juices	HPLC/UV flavonoid glycoside (IFU 58)
Grapefruit	Narangin	Citrus juices	HPLC/UV flavonoid glycoside (IFU 58)
Orange	Hesperidin	Passion fruit juice	HPLC/UV flavonoid glycoside (IFU 58)
Grape	Tartaric acid	Other juices	HPLC/UV (IFU 65)

HPLC/UV(DAD), high-performance liquid chromatography/ultraviolet (diode array detector); *HPLC/EC*, high-performance liquid chromatography/electrochemical; *MS*, mass spectrometry; *NMR*, nuclear magnetic resonance.

23.3.6 Indicators for Microbiological Damage

An authentic fruit juice is a product that is not fermented (CODEX STAN 247-2005; Directive 2012/12/EC, 2012). Lactic acid and ethanol are typical fermentation products Zhao et al, 2014 and are used as marker substances in the AIJN CoP (Website of AIJN Code of Practice). Depending on the fruit, different maximum values are fixed in the AIJN CoP. AIJN states a maximum of 500 mg/L of lactic acid for most fruits, whereas 200 mg/L is reported for citrus juices and up to 1000 mg/L in exceptional cases is allowed for elderberry products. Ethanol has a maximum limit of 3000 mg/L for all juices. These limits are references for authenticity assessment but in many cases they are much higher than tolerated by the industry to avoid negative sensorial effects.

In the case of vegetable juices, a lactic fermentation can be a voluntary process to lower the pH for stabilization purposes; however, any such fermentation must be stated on the product label.

Due to its volatility, ethanol plays a significant role in single strength products only and not in concentrates.

Glycerol and gluconic acid are typical metabolites in grape juice, which increase after microbiological activity (Malacrino et al., 2005; Biyela et al., 2009; Website of AIJN Code of Practice).

An increase in the level of volatile acids indicates that an aceto fermentation has taken place for all types of fruit juice (Website of AIJN Code of Practice). Volatile acids are recovered by steam distillation and quantified by titration (Website of International Fruit and Vegetable Juice Association). Alternatively, the amount of acetic acid can be measured by GC or by an enzymatic test. Acetic acid is generally the main volatile acid reported and is formed by fermentation of the sugars by *Acetobacterium*.

Furthermore, sorbitol has been mentioned as an indicator of microbiological problems in fruit types that naturally contain no sorbitol (Duvnjak et al., 1991).

23.3.7 Technology, Citrus Extraction

Citrus juices should only be extracted from the endocarp of the fruits. Coextraction of the peel leads to a product category other than "Fruit Juice," which is a legally defined denomination (CODEX STAN 247-2005; Directive 2012/12/EC, 2012). Furthermore, only water extraction of the excluded pulp for the production of juice concentrates is allowed by the European and Codex legislation (CODEX STAN 247-2005; Directive 2012/12/EC, 2012).

If these rules are not respected, products show increased values of water-soluble pectins, calcium, and phlorin (Website of AIJN Code of Practice; Louche et al., 1998; Scordino et al., 2004) and the ratio between the two flavonoids hesperidin and narirutin will be atypical. Determination of water-soluble pectins is part of a wet chemistry separation of three different pectin fractions with different solubilities and UV-spectrometric determination after a carbazole reaction with the galacturonic acid monomer (Website of International Fruit and Vegetable Juice Association). Phlorin can be determined by high-performance liquid chromatography/ultraviolet (HPLC/UV) or during proton-NMR (nuclear magnetic resonance) screening (Application note Bruker SGF Profiling) and enhanced levels of calcium can also be detected; these may be measured using either atomic absorption spectroscopy or inductively coupled plasma mass spectrometry (ICP-MS).

Products that contain high amounts of pulp [centrifugeable pulp $>10\%$ by IFU method 60 (Website of International Fruit and Vegetable Juice Association)] and some exceptional products with a particular process design can also show enhanced levels of water-soluble pectin. Again, product and process knowledge is essential for a correct interpretation of this elevated pectin level.

23.3.8 Cloud Stabilization

Pineapple juice often shows an unstable cloud and produces a solid precipitate that is not very attractive for consumers. Cloud stabilization by pectin addition is permitted by EU and Codex standards to counteract this effect. This additive must be labeled and its content should not exceed fixed maximum standards (Website of AIJN Code of Practice). Determination of water-soluble pectins by IFU method 26 (Website of International Fruit and Vegetable Juice Association) can be used for control of this parameter. Pectin addition to pineapple juice or juice concentrate, etc. may also be detected after its isolation by ^{13}C isotopic analysis (Hammond, 2006) as explained later.

23.3.9 Technology, Thermal Stress

5-Hydroxy-methyl-furfural (HMF) is a typical Maillard reaction product and an increased concentration indicates that a product was exposed either to an excessively high temperature during processing or unsuitable storage temperatures. Furthermore, the sugar profile of a product can change by acid-catalyzed inversion (hydrolysis) of sucrose. A decrease in sucrose concentration and an increase in glucose and fructose contents will be observed in such a case. This sugar profile change is a major alteration of the analytical composition but is generally only considered a quality matter.

Some fruit types like apple, mango, or pineapple are very sensitive to the formation of HMF, whereas other fruits, like citrus species, are less affected.

23.3.10 Technology, Sulfite Addition

Sulfur dioxide is permitted as a preservative in the European Union only in grape juice for sacramental use, lime, and lemon juice (Regulation (EC) No 1333/2008). However, bulk volumes of grape juice are often stored with sulfur dioxide for stabilization purposes. This product has to be desulfurized by vacuum distillation before packing as a consumer product. A correct desulfurization can be controlled by checking for sulfur dioxide remaining in the product—this has to be reduced to below 10 mg/L (Website of AIJN Code of Practice). This is one of the most difficult traditional methods used for control of fruit juices because of the potentially large interlaboratory reproducibility at the control concentration. It is based on a method initially developed for wine analytics where sulfur dioxide concentration above 100 mg/L are normal practice. The official IFU method 7a (Website of International Fruit and Vegetable Juice Association; Hofsommer, M. 2014) is based on a steam distillation and subsequent trapping of sulfurous acid, which can be quantified by titration. There is a strict requirement to follow the analytical procedure accurately and operators have to be sufficiently trained so that reproducible results are achieved. To date, more reproducible and faster methods such as HPLC biosensor-coupled approaches (Theisen, 2009; Patz et al., 1997) have not been established as standard procedures despite their better accuracy and lower limit of detection. Results are not always comparable between different methods; this is probably because sulfur dioxide is partially bound to the matrix and liberation rates are highly method dependent.

Sulfate is the oxidation product of sulfur dioxide and an increased sulfate value indicates in most cases a long storage time under sulfur dioxide.

23.3.11 Technology, Appropriate Process Water

Water used in any food plant for fruit washing, facility cleaning, and fruit processing should be of drinking water quality. At different steps of the juice process there is a risk of contamination as a result of compounds from the water entering the juice. Typical indicators for a possible contamination are elevated concentrations of sodium and nitrate ions. With some fruit types and regional specific exceptions, these components are usually present at trace concentrations only in pure juice. Elevated concentrations change the natural composition of a juice and can be considered as an authenticity issue. In addition, they can hint at possible further contamination. Theoretically, if a contamination is observed, there is an increased risk of finding other, maybe toxicologically relevant, contaminants.

A high sodium level can also arise from processing aids (eg, bentonite of insufficient quality which can release minerals) or from fruits growing under particular conditions (eg, in a salty soil). In this latter case, we cannot speak about a problem of authenticity.

23.3.12 Technology, Enzyme Treatment

Enzymes are used in industrial processes for juice production to break down cell walls, to influence the viscosity of the product and to increase juice extraction yield. In Europe, enzymatic liquefaction of fruit is not permitted and cellulases are only allowed as a minor side activity of other permitted enzymes. Cellobiose [glucopyranosyl-(1→4)-D-glucopyranose] is a breakdown product of cellulose and an increased concentration of this compound is an indicator for the use of a processing technology that is not permitted (Low and Hammond, 1996; Willems and Low, 2014).

Pectinases, which are allowed, form galacturonic acid and its oligomers. Excessive use of pectinases can be detected by measuring galacturonic acid levels. Juices containing elevated concentrations maybe legal but can be an indicator of poor quality.

23.4 Overview of Modern Techniques

23.4.1 Stable Isotope Analysis

Stable isotope analyses do not deal with the quantitative determination or quantitative fingerprint pattern of certain compounds but rather with a qualitative characterization of some elements in a substance contained in the juice. Analytical figures describe the relationship between nonradioactive heavier and lighter isotopes of the same element. The specific advantage of stable isotope analysis is its ability to differentiate between materials that are chemically identical (eg, sucrose from sugar beet and cane).

Stable isotope ratios of different compounds in fruit juices are mainly influenced by two factors:

- sources of hydrogen, oxygen, carbon, nitrogen, minerals, or other elements accumulated during the growing period of the fruit (Craig, 1961; Epstein and Mayeda, 1953; Friedman, 1953; Simpkins et al., 1999; Doner and Bills, 1981), and
- physical processes in the plant and biochemical pathways that selectively favor lighter or heavier isotopes and lead to characteristic isotopic fractionation (Bricout and Fontes, 1974; Farquhar et al., 2007; Bricout et al., 1972).

Different metabolic pathways to fix atmospheric carbon dioxide result in different levels of the heavy carbon isotope ^{13}C (Bender, 1971).

- C_3-plants use the Calvin cycle during photosynthesis and generally show the lowest accumulation of ^{13}C isotopes. Most fruit juices are derived from C_3-plants.
- C_4-plants use the Hatch—Slack pathway and have significantly higher rates of ^{13}C accumulation. No common fruit juices are produced from C_4-plants but sugar cane and corn are both C_4 plants and sugars from these are possible adulterants.
- Crassulacean acid metabolism (CAM) plants have rates of ^{13}C accumulation in between those of the C_3- and C_4-plants. The metabolism of CAM plants fixes carbon dioxide at night in a way similar to that of C_4-plants and it is stored as malate. At daylight, such plants use the carbon dioxide that was collected at night to perform photosynthesis following the Calvin cycle. Pineapple juice is the only commonly consumed fruit juice from this plant type; however, pitaya (dragon fruit) is also a CAM fruit that may be processed.

In water, the most important variations of naturally occurring deuterium and the oxygen ^{18}O isotope are caused by the water balance of a plant and its geographical origin. The evapotranspiration process of a plant plays an important role because the lighter isotopes have a slightly higher volatility (Farquhar et al., 2007) and so deuterium and ^{18}O are enriched in fruits and fruit juices. Both parameters can be used for water characterization but ^{18}O measurement dominates in commercial analysis.

Some trace minerals deliver a stable isotopic ratio that is characteristic for the age of the geological formation in which a plant has grown and from which it has extracted its nutrients. For instance, the strontium isotope ^{87}Sr enables, in a particular combination with isotope ratios of some lighter elements (H, C, N, S), the verification of a certain geographical origin (Rummel et al., 2010; Rossmann and Ara, 2013). In Africa the oldest soil strata on the surface of our planet can be found and these show extremely low values of the ^{87}Sr isotope.

Data for isotopic ratios are generally not expressed in absolute values but are quoted relative to a fixed standard, making the numbers easier to handle:

Carbon 13: Vienna Pee Dee Belemnite (vPDB)
Deuterium and Oxygen 18: Vienna Standard Mean Ocean Water (vSMOW) (Gonfiantini, 1978).

23.4.1.1 Principal Approaches in Stable Isotopic Measurement

For authenticity testing, an isotopic measurement can be performed on a whole juice, a separated fraction of the juice (eg, sugars, acids, pulp, etc.), isolated compounds (eg, sucrose, citric acid, etc.), or at site-specific atoms in a molecule (eg carbon atoms in the terminal position of malic acid).

Analysts speak about "internal referencing" when the relationship between two or more isotope ratios is obtained from different isolated parts of the same sample; these values are used for interpretation. Such an internal relationship shows much less natural variation of absolute values than is seen with the individual components. Thus internal referencing allows a more refined data interpretation to be made than is possible using a single analytical value for whole juices, fractions, or compounds. Site-specific internal correlation allows even more precise interpretation in some cases. Exogenous sugar, acid, or water can disturb easily the natural internal relationship of isotope ratios in a juice.

For different analytical approaches, different detection limits are published. Such data are generally indicative of a magnitude only. Natural variation in authentic juices and in the adulterant can lead to much better or poorer performance. As a rule of thumb, detection limits range from about 10% to 20% of added adulterant (eg, sugar, acids, water) with single parameter measurements. Approaches using internal referencing can reduce this by half or in some cases even more. In some cases, intramolecular site-specific ("positional") differentiation is the only effective method to detect an adulteration. Examples, such as the detection of added L-malic acid or the detection of C^4-derived sugars in juices from CAM plants, are described in later paragraphs.

Depending upon the analyte, sample preparation is more or less complex. For every sample clean-up step, such as precipitation, distillation, or chromatographic separation, care must be taken to ensure that no fractionation of the lighter and heavier isotopes results since any such change would cause a shift in the measured isotope ratio. As a general rule, more than 95% of the initial analyte amount must be recovered at each process step to ensure that there is no significant process fractionation.

Measurement of the isotope ratio is limited to a small number of techniques and isotope ratio mass spectrometry (IRMS) is the technique most commonly used. A sample to be measured is combusted internally to produce carbon dioxide, water, and other gases (N_2, SO_2). ^{13}C, ^{18}O, and D must be determined in separate measurements against standard substances with known isotope ratios. An advanced technique is the use of an elemental analyzer, which is coupled to a mass spectrometer via a GC column, thereby allowing the measurement of ^{13}C, D, ^{15}N, and ^{34}S in one run with good reproducibility.

Typical interlaboratory reproducibilities for ^{13}C measurements are usually around 0.5‰ PDB, even for complex sample preparations (Jamin et al., 2004). To obtain a relation to this figure note that the range for $\delta^{13}C$ defined as natural for sugar in orange juice by the AIJN CoP (Website of AIJN Code of Practice) is between −27‰ and −24‰ PDB and C_4-sugar has values from approximately −15‰ to −12‰ PDB. When mixing a fruit juice with an adulterant, values are changing in a linear way in relation to weight proportion of the analyte in both compounds of the blend.

An alternative instrument with which to measure D and ^{18}O in water is a cavity ring down spectrometer (CRDS) (Chesson et al., 2010; Beer et al., 2015); this technology determines absorption rates of light in the vapor phase of a sample. For lighter and heavier isotopes, separate spectral lines of a narrow bandwidth laser light can be registered to calculate the isotopic ratio. A disadvantage of this method is that other volatile organic compounds can lead to interferences. CRDS can also be used to measure ^{13}C ratios in carbon dioxide but for applications other than fruit juices (Becker et al., 2012; Maher et al., 2014). Some applications in environmental analytics are even carried out by portable devices. The method has the potential to implement isotopic measurements in more laboratories today because it is less expensive and easier to use. However, some improvement of reproducibility is still necessary and it is not yet clear if databases built up during the last few decades using IRMS are applicable to this technique.

Other elements in fruit juices can also be analyzed by isotopic techniques. These are lighter ones like nitrogen (^{15}N) and sulfur (^{35}S) or heavy metals like strontium (^{87}Sr) (Rummel et al., 2010; Rossmann and Ara, 2013).

Some sample preparation steps for site-specific measurements include the cleavage of specific molecules at certain sites and submission of these fractions to IRMS measurement (Jamin et al., 2000; Detection of added ascorbic acid). For other methods, the positional determination of D or ^{13}C is carried out via NMR measurement (Martin and Martin, 1995; Jamin et al., 2005).

When measuring any D/H ratio in organic molecules, it must be remembered that some protons and deuterium in certain molecules (eg, hydroxyl groups of sugars) can exchange easily with the surrounding medium. Derivatization techniques are able to remove these protons (Bricout and Koziet, 1987; Krueger, 1995; Dunbar and Schmidt, 1984; Doner et al., 1987) and these positions can be blocked in sugar molecules through nitrate ester formation. Selective oxidation to formate and precipitation as calcium salts is also possible. The derivatives can be measured via IRMS.

However, derivatization techniques are rarely used today. The controlled fermentation of sugars to ethanol, which allows a specific transfer of protons/deuterium to the ethanol molecule, is commonly applied. Details are given in the next paragraph, which deals with the method that is used for the detection of exogenous sugar in fruit juices.

23.4.1.2 Detection of Exogenous Sugar

Site-Specific Natural Isotope Fractionation-Nuclear Magnetic Resonance (SNIF-NMR) is an indirect analysis of the deuterium/hydrogen ratio in sugar contained in a fruit juice (Martin and Martin, 1995; Martin et al., 1994, 1996a,b; Gonzalez et al., 1998). Here the juice is fermented by a defined strain of *Saccharomyces cerevisiae* under controlled conditions and sugar is converted into ethanol. This ethanol is purified by distillation taking care to avoid isotopic fractionation. Therefore a practically complete collection of the ethanol is necessary but this can be achieved, for example, using high-performance distillation columns of the Cadiot type with a rotating band. The ethanol solution is submitted to a site-specific determination of the D/H ratios by NMR. Because the proton of the hydroxyl group is exchangeable with the medium (water), it cannot be used for the detection of any adulterant. The most important figure is the D/H ratio of the methyl group, called the $(D/H)_1$ value. The D/H ratio from the methylene group is called the $(D/H)_2$ value.

If sugar derived from certain C_3-plants, for example, from sugar beet or potato starch, is added to a juice, the measured deuterium concentration decreases. In general, the (D/H)1 value is sufficient for result interpretation but further refinement is possible in principle by data correction taking into account the $(D/H)_2$ value, derived from the methylene group, the relative distribution factor R ($R = 2\{(D/H)_2\}/(D/H)_1$) and the D/H valuc of the fermentation medium.

In parallel, the $^{13}C/^{12}C$ ratio for the ethanol obtained is determined by IRMS after combustion to carbon dioxide (Martin and Martin, 1995; Martin et al., 1996a). If sugars from a C_4-plant (eg, from sugar cane or corn starch) are added, the ^{13}C value

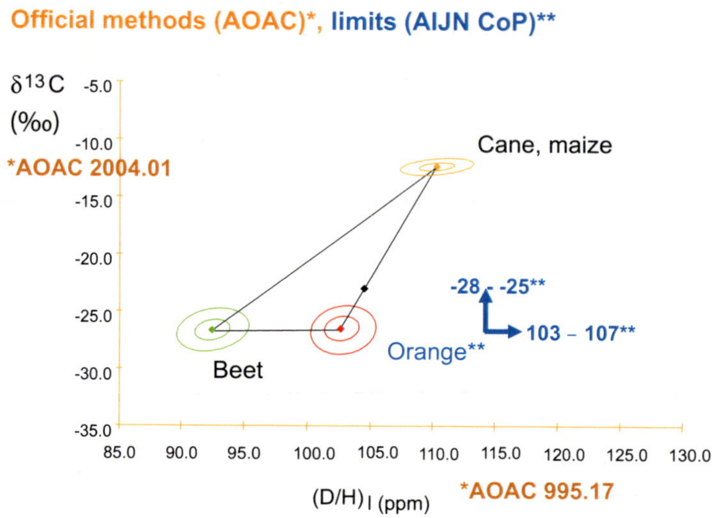

Figure 23.2 Differentiation between sugars from orange juice, beet or C4 sources using site-specific NMR in combination with IRMS (Thomas, 2009).

will increase. The combination of these results can be used to detect sugar addition for a large number of fruits derived from C_3-plants like orange juice, as shown in Fig. 23.2.

Because sugar syrups are very often of a C_4 origin (sugar cane, corn starch), ^{13}C measurement alone can detect a number of illegal sugar additions. Therefore the application of much faster methods than SNIF-nuclear magnetic resonance with less complex sample clean-up represents a valuable approach. The method with the least complex sample preparation involves determination of the ^{13}C level from the whole juice via IRMS after pyrolysis without any sample clean-up. As sugar is the main organic compound in most juices, the analytical result is a good indication of the isotopic characteristics of the sugar fraction (Doner and Phillips, 1981; Krueger et al., 1986; Doner and Bills, 1982; Doner et al., 1980).

Slightly better information can be obtained after purification of the sugar (Koziet et al., 1993). From a highly diluted juice, solid particles are separated by centrifugation and the organic acids fraction can be precipitated either using Carrez I and II solution or as their calcium salts using calcium hydroxide. The remaining clarified supernatant is freeze dried. This isolate is a mixture of different carbohydrates, mainly glucose, fructose, and sucrose, and can be used in IRMS measurements. In this way, interferences from other organic substances are avoided.

^{13}C values from ethanol ex sugar (obtained through fermentation of sugar) and from directly analyzed sugar or the whole juice are not comparable because carbon dioxide is lost in the fermentation process, which further depletes the sample, for example, the ^{13}C isotope ratio is ca. 1.5 per mil more negative. This means that a dedicated reference database must be used for each type of data.

Furthermore, the following difference measurements for internal referencing for ^{13}C values measured by IRMS are useful:

^{13}C sugar fraction—^{13}C acid fraction;	^{13}C sugar fraction—^{13}C pectin;
^{13}C sugar fraction—^{13}C of single organic acids;	^{13}C sugar fraction—^{13}C protein fraction;
^{13}C sugar fraction—^{13}C pulp;	^{13}C glucose—^{13}C fructose—^{13}C sucrose

^{13}C measurements of the acid fraction or of individual organic acids are also used for the detection of organic acids as explained later in this chapter. If the natural correlation between these values and the ^{13}C values for the sugar fraction are not as encountered in authentic material, the reason could be addition of sugar and/or acids. Any decision on which one is the adulterant must be taken on the basis of the absolute values and/or other internal isotope relationships or on conventional data for the sample.

Internal referencing using sugar pulp allows for a precise interpretation if it is known that the pulp in the product is from the same juice. In particular, in citrus juices, the addition of pulp or cells from other sources is quite frequent and legal. Isolation of pulp and the sugar fraction follows the European Standard method ENV 13070:1998. It is evident that this approach is limited to cloudy products and is not suitable for clarified juices.

Isolation of pectin can be performed after precipitation with ethanol and centrifugation according IFU method 26 (Website of International Fruit and Vegetable Juice Association) before freeze drying and measurement by IRMS. This type of approach can prove very useful in pineapple juices in which undeclared added pectin would typically be from a C_3 source (apple or citrus) (Hammond, 2006).

Protein can be isolated by bentonite precipitation (Jamin et al., 1996), allowing also the determination of the ^{15}N value. ^{15}N is, inter alia, under discussion as a parameter for the detection of wrongly declared organic juice qualities when applied fertilizer use does not conform to organic agricultural principles (Laursen et al., 2014; Rossmann and Ara, 2013; Rapisarda et al., 2010).

A further refinement of sugar detection could be the control of ^{13}C relationships between individual saccharides, for example, glucose, fructose, and sucrose. Isolation can be done by ion exchange purification of the juice to discard nonsugar compounds followed by preparative HPLC, which is critical in terms of isotope fractionation. Using this type of approach, the detection of added exogenous C_4 sugar can, in some cases, be improved significantly by a factor of two (González et al., 1999; Day et al., 1998).

Another approach applied to lemon and lime juices used an HPLC system online coupled to an IRMS. After separation, analytes are chemically oxidized to carbon dioxide, which is extracted online before being measured by IRMS to determine ^{13}C (Guyon et al., 2014). The HPLC separation runs with water only to avoid the presence of organic solvents during the oxidation step. Sucrose is completely hydrolyzed to fructose and glucose and the malic acid and citric acid are not separated but are measured as one peak. However, as this method uses minimal sample preparation, it is suitable for routine screening.

A particular case of illegal sugar addition is the addition of a C_4-plant-derived sugar to juice produced from CAM plants such as pineapple or pitaya (dragon fruit). As the difference in ^{13}C between C_4- and CAM plants is very small, even large amounts of such sugar addition are difficult to detect. To solve this problem, an approach was proposed based on positional quantitative ^{13}C-NMR of ethanol derived from the sugars (Thomas et al., 2010). Ethanol is formed through fermentation and distillation steps as mentioned previously for SNIF-NMR. The two CO_2 fixation routes lead to differences in the intramolecular distribution of the ^{13}C molecules in the sugars and this is transferred to the ethanol through specific biochemical reactions during fermentation. As a consequence, the difference between ^{13}C content in the methyl and the methylene groups of ethanol varies between CAM and C_4-plants and allows their discrimination. Sugars from CAM plants produce a higher content of ^{13}C in the methylene group than C_4-plants while sugar from C_4-plants has a higher ^{13}C content in the methyl group than their CAM counterparts. Differentiation is shown in Fig. 23.3.

23.4.1.3 Detection of Exogenous Organic Acids

Stable isotope analyses to detect addition of organic acids that are either not permitted, not declared, or both follow the same general principle as the detection of added sugar. For lemon or lime juice, in which citric acid is the main compound, ^{13}C analyses of the whole product can provide a first indication of whether large amounts of exogenous

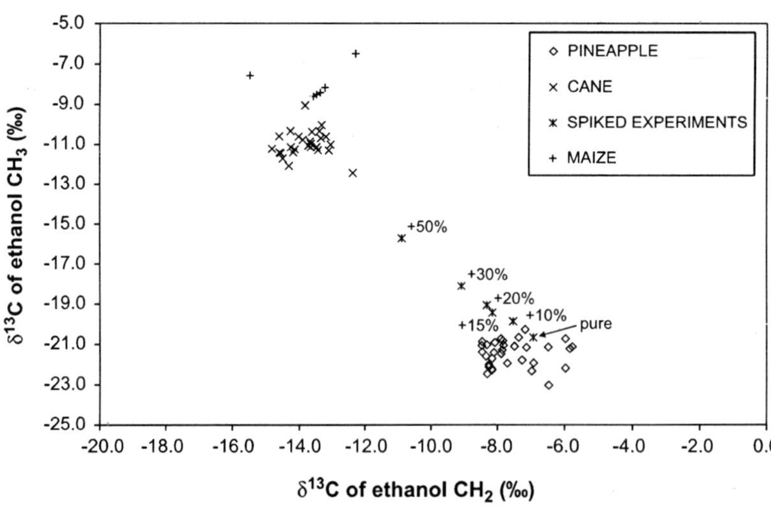

Figure 23.3 Differentiation of sugar derived from different biochemical pathways using positional ^{13}C-nuclear magnetic resonance measurement on ethanol ex. sugar.

acid derived from a C_4 plant or chemical syntheses from hydrocarbons have been added. However, the detection level is not sufficient for most observed adulterations and further purification steps are recommended (Doner, 1985).

Besides lemon and lime juice, other juice types may also be subject to illegal acid addition to improve sensory properties and the commercial value of a product. The acid fraction or the respective organic acid must be isolated for determination of the isotopic ratio. Again, internal referencing gives the best chance of fraud detection. Isolation of the organic acid fraction is part of the purification, described earlier, of the sugar fraction. Isolation of individual acids (citric acid and malic acid) can be achieved by preparative HPLC (Jamin et al., 1998) while isotopic ratios of the respective isolates are determined by IRMS.

Intramolecular referencing of ^{13}C was developed to improves the chance of detecting added commercial malic acid. Two approaches were followed: (1) enzymatic cleavage of the carbon at the 4th position and (2) chemical cleavage of the carbon at the 1st position (Jamin et al., 2000; Jamin, 2006). The ^{13}C value of the single carbon can be compared with the ^{13}C value for the whole malic acid molecule. Synthetic malic acids usually show quite a different internal relationship than that seen in malic acid extracted from apple juice or other authentic juices. Today, chemical cleavage of the C_1 carbon is mainly used because of the poor availability of the enzyme required to remove the carbon at the 4th position. A redox reaction with cerium(IV) sulfate leads to the liberation of carbon dioxide, which can be trapped and subjected to IRMS measurement.

A very similar technique can be applied to control the authenticity of ascorbic acid in a fruit juice, for example, in orange juice, blackcurrant, and acerola purée/juice containing products (Detection of added ascorbic acid; Jamin et al., 1998). Acerola fruits have high ascorbic acid contents and are used very often as a natural source for vitamin C in various recipes. Positional referencing of the carbon in position 1 produces good control results (Fig. 23.4). To avoid forming dehydroascorbic acid, sample preparation has to be carried out under reducing conditions using metabisulfite.

Another site-specific approach to detect smaller amounts of added citric acid is to simultaneously use ^{13}C and deuterium as indicators (Jamin et al., 2005). Purification of the organic acid with preparative HPLC allows the IRMS measurement of ^{13}C after pyrolysis. Before the deuterium determination can be carried out, the exchangeable protons have to be eliminated by precipitation as a calcium salt. Development of this method was based on former studies carried out by site-specific D/H measurement with NMR, which had shown the potential of deuterium as an indicator of fraud (Gonzalez et al., 1998). Because of the complex isolation steps required to collect sufficient citric acid for the NMR approach, it is hardly suitable for routine analysis.

A particular adulteration in grape juice can be the addition of tartaric acid from another botanical origin such as the tamarind fruit or from chemical synthesis. A method proposed for wine authenticity testing can be applied to this case. After isolation of the organic acid, a multivariate approach is applied using IRMS measurements of ^{13}C, ^{18}O, and deuterium to distinguish different sources of the analyte (Rojas et al., 2007).

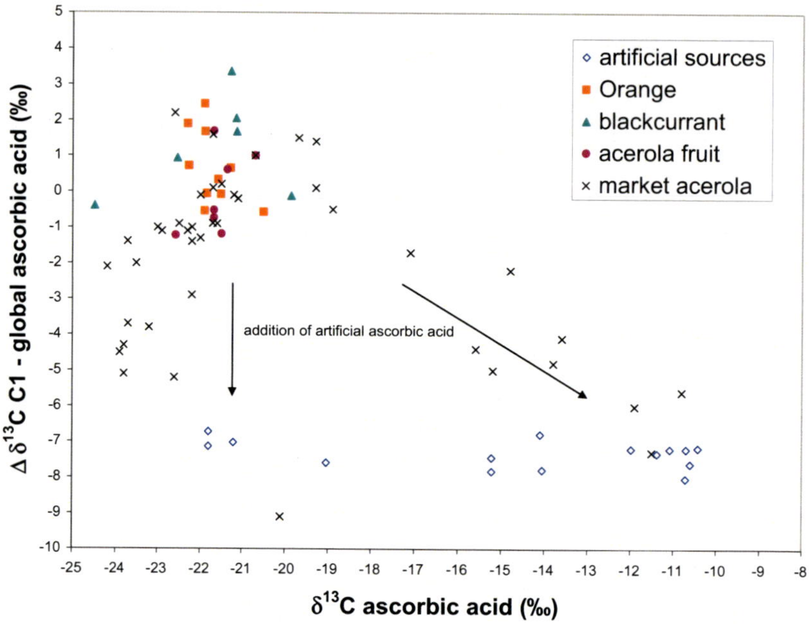

Figure 23.4 Bidimensional plot of results obtained for the global and positional analysis of ^{13}C deviations in (1) artificial ascorbic acid sources, (2) authentic fruit samples, and (3) market samples of acerola products (Jamin, 2009).

23.4.1.4 Detection of Exogenous Water Using ^{18}O Isotope

$^{18}O/^{16}O$ and D/H ratios are used as indicators of the presence of exogenous water (Website of AIJN Code of Practice; Kvasnička et al., 2002; Bricout et al., 1972; Dunbar and Wilson, 1983; Koziet et al., 1995). Water contained in a juice can be trapped during lyophilization of the sample and submitted to a mass spectrometric measurement. Through biochemical reactions and evapotranspiration of the plant, the heavier isotopes are enriched compared to rain, ground, or surface waters. By comparing the ^{18}O value with a minimum value as defined in the AIJN CoP (Website of AIJN Code of Practice) it is, in most cases, possible to distinguish between pure single strength juices and those made from concentrate, which contain mainly exogenous water. However, the addition of a small amount (c. 10%) of water to single strength juices can produce a significant, illegal economic advantage but still produce values inside the expected isotopic range and above the minimum Brix or density.

To lower the detection limit for added water, a method was successfully established by controlling the internal relationship between $^{18}O/^{16}O$ ratio present in the sugar and in the free water of the juice sample. The ^{18}O value for the sugar compounds is obtained indirectly by analysis of ethanol after sugar fermentation and distillation, in a manner similar to the SNIF-NMR method (Monsallier-Bitea et al., 2006; Thomas et al., 2013; Jamin et al., 2003). Because of its hygroscopic nature, sugar, isolated from juice by other means, would always contain low levels of retained water that

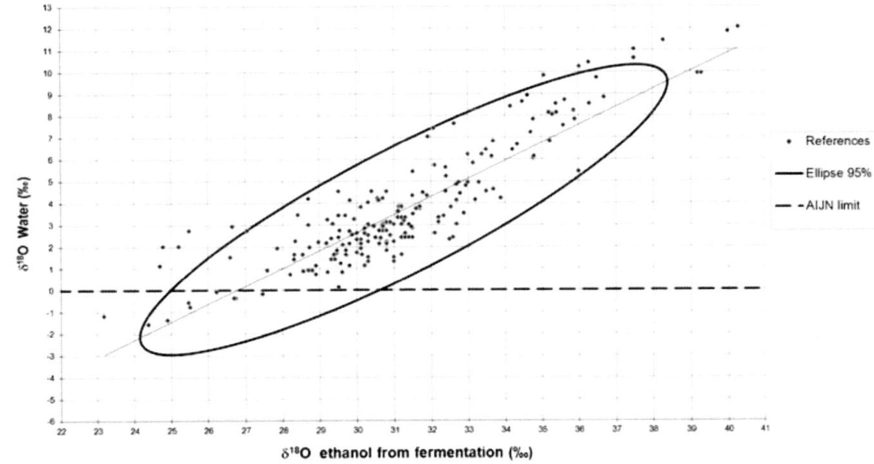

Figure 23.5 Correlation between ^{18}O ethanol and ^{18}O water in authentic orange juices from worldwide origins (Thomas et al., 2013).

can interfere with a direct ^{18}O measurement. During the growing period, water acts as the source of oxygen during sugar assimilation. Thus there must be a stable relation between the isotopic ratios of oxygen in the free water and in the sugar fraction. Fig. 23.5 demonstrates that this is true for authentic, laboratory pressed, juices. A risk remains that a particularly strong evaporation process, because of arid weather conditions or an excessive intake of water through irrigation or heavy rain shortly before harvest, can influence this interrelationship. Nevertheless, the method shows results that can be interpreted with a high level of confidence if a robust reference database is available for a given fruit type and the analytical procedure is followed exactly. If the measured internal relationship is not as expected, this could be because of water addition and/or sugar addition.

23.4.1.5 Confirmation of Origin

Confirmation of a declared or expected origin often requires a multivariate approach and can involve different types of analyses. Stable isotopes play an important role in this regard. Among a whole range of possible elements that may be used are the strontium isotopes ($^{87}Sr/^{86}Sr$), which can give relatively robust results if used as a single parameter. This minor atomic species, which is normally only present in minor quantities, is assimilated by the plant from the soil and every region has a typical $^{87}Sr/^{86}Sr$ ratio that is transferred to the fruit (Voerkelius et al., 2010; Trincherini et al., 2014; Rossmann and Rummel, 2006b). The method of choice for strontium isotope analysis is thermal ionization mass spectrometry and the specific substance to be analyzed is strontium nitrate (a solid sample). An alternative approach can be ICP-MS.

It had been observed that the $^{87}Sr/^{86}Sr$ ratio is more specific for a geographic origin than for a fruit type or production process. Thus an observation made for one fruit type can be applied in principle to other fruit types. In addition, there is, in general, a good correlation between the ratio of the liquid phase and the solid phase of a juice sample.

If both values deviate one from the other, this can be caused by a mixture of two products with different proportions between solids and the liquid phase, for example, by adding pulp or cells to any citrus juice from another production with deviating $^{87}Sr/^{86}Sr$ ratio, for example, from another origin.

Further multielement approaches are described that use a number of stable isotope ratios to define a typical pattern for one specific geographic origin. In this regard, data of D, ^{18}O, ^{13}C, ^{15}N, ^{34}S, and ^{87}Sr can be useful for chemometric data analyses (eg, principal component analysis, discriminant analyses) (Rummel et al., 2010; Rossmann and Ara, 2013; Ogrinc et al., 2009; Mimmo et al., 2015; Perez et al., 2006; Rossmann and Rummel, 2006a).

However, there are different studies that do not deal with isotope ratios but with quantitative patterns of different trace elements determined for different commodities and different origins (Perez et al., 2006; Bayer et al., 1980; Pellerano et al., 2008; Nikdel et al., 1985; Coetzee et al., 2005). ICP/MS techniques are generally applied for this type of analysis.

The confirmation or determination of any geographic origin is one of the most difficult challenges in fruit juice analysis. Experience shows that stable isotopes and/or extended trace element analyses can exclude a number of origins for a specific sample, which is precious information for many practical problems. But it demands large regional-specific databases for a large number of parameters. Further effort to complete reference data is still necessary. Chemometric models used for proton-NMR screening are a further powerful support as explained in the following chapter.

23.4.2 Proton-Nuclear Magnetic Resonance Screening—Spin Generated Fingerprint Profiling (SGF Profiling)

Proton-NMR screening is a fast and simple method delivering multiple information from one recorded spectrum. Targeted and untargeted results are collected by a combination of metabolomics and signal quantification (Rinke et al., 2007; Spraul et al., 2009a,b).

Other approaches using statistical evaluation of spectra which are based on infrared spectroscopy were presented (León et al., 2005; Gamal et al., 2011; Giusti et al., 2011). However lower signal resolution did not allow an exploitation with same extend of information, which maybe the reason that these technologies did not establish in fruit juice authenticity control until now.

Today SGF Profiling is the only described method of this kind for fruit juices. It uses a 400 MHz NMR instrument. Analysis time is only about 15 min per sample and the process can be automated to facilitate a large sample throughput.

Sample preparation consists of centrifugation and diluting a juice or a concentrate with buffer containing trisodium phosphate [sodium salt of 3-(trimethylsilyl)-propionate acid-d_4] as an internal standard and sodium azide for preservation. The pH of the buffer solution is 3.1 or 3.4 depending on fruit type. Use of these specific buffer solutions is essential to allow the required reproducibility to be achieved because of the pH sensitivity of the chemical shifts of some of the polar compounds (eg, organic acids).

A full proton-NMR spectrum is recorded at 300K. NOESYPRID pulse sequence with continuous wave presaturation of the water resonance is used. Baseline and phase corrections can be included in an automatic data treatment. The instrument configuration can be designed as a pushbutton system with a flow cell or individual tubes.

A standard routine includes J-resolved NMR spectroscopy (JRES), which allows better signal assignment to molecule structures, which show interferences by other compounds in the one-dimensional spectrum along the chemical shift axis (Rinke et al., 2007; Ludwig and Viant, 2010). JRES spectra are obtained by suppression J-coupling to separate chemical shift and J-coupling; both are projected on two different axes, which results in a two-dimensional spectrum.

The spectrum of a fruit juice sample is influenced by industrial processes along the whole production chain in the same way as they are by fruit type, variety, and growing conditions. An advantage of this method is that it can make statements about fruit juice process technology. One disadvantage is that only industrially produced reference samples are suitable for database production and means that laboratory-pressed juices are not suitable for this type of analysis.

The method delivers two types of results. If any signal of the NMR spectrum can be assigned to a juice compound and it can be integrated, quantification of the compound is possible. Depending on the number of protons present at a specific site of a molecule, signal intensities are registered. As every signal is caused by protons, the response factor is directly linear to the respective number of protons. Therefore no multiple calibration with individual standard substances is necessary. A further advantage is the possible reprocessing of previously recorded spectra. This means that in the future, if a new signal can be identified and it is suitable for integration, quantification of this "new compound" in already recorded spectra is possible. This enables the rapid development of quantitative databases from "old" spectra provided there have not been any modifications made to the method.

A number of compounds can be quantified from the NMR screening with automatic quantification routines. Depending on the matrix, a selection of parameters can be applied. Interferences and low concentration levels do not allow every parameter to be measured in every fruit (Application note Bruker SGF Profiling). The following list of compounds is indicative and subject to possible extension in the future. Many of the accessible parameters show identical results to those recorded using conventional and official methods so standard compositional databases, such as the AIJN CoP, can be used for interpretation.

Parameters that allow automatic quantification are:

4-Aminobutanoic acid	Chlorogenic acid	Gluconic acid	Proline
Acetaldehyde	Citramalic acid	Glucose	Pyruvic acid
Acetone	Citric acid	HMF	Quinic acid
Alanine	Ethanol	Isocitric acid	Shikimic acid
Arbutin	Formic acid	Lactic acid	Sorbic acid
Arginine	Fructose	Malic acid	Succinic acid
Benzaldehyde	Fumaric acid	Methanol	Sucrose
Benzoic acid	Galacturonic acid	Phlorin	Xylose

Calculated values:

Glucose/fructose	% Sucrose	Total sugar	Malic acid/quinic acid

Today, based on measurements of several hundred orange and apple juice samples with known conventional analytical figures, some analytical parameters can be determined with good accuracy by linear regression. In this context this means that obtained results are sufficiently close to values obtained by conventional analyses for a use in authenticity interpretation. Therefore no specific proton-generated signal is used for quantification—the whole spectrum is utilized. Values for total acidity, potassium, and magnesium are predictable for all test spectra that fit with statistical verification models. Deviating spectra are not suitable for determination by regression.

The full proton-NMR (^{1}H-NMR) spectrum permits another interpretation, which is based on a metabonomics approach, which has a strong untargeted character. Such chemometric approaches use different statistical models. Therefore the NMR spectrum is divided into different segments, or so-called buckets; the integral of one bucket corresponds to one data point. Performance of the method is linked to the selection and application of the statistical algorithm used. Depending on the data amount and its distribution, a large number of supervised or unsupervised methods (Adams, 1998) can be tested and validated, for example, by Monte Carlo cross-validation.

The same NMR experiment as for quantification can be used for all available models for any respective fruit type. Every model is designed to check a specific quality aspect. Thus a number of quality aspects can be checked from one spectrum. Targeted and untargeted results are generally obtained from the same database including a list of different models and quantification routines.

Statistical models to check authenticity need to be developed using a sufficient number of reference samples that are known to be authentic. This sample set must be representative for the population of possible samples from the respective product group. Depending on the complexity of the analytical problem and natural variation, the number of reference samples varies for each problem. As a general rule, 50–70 authentic samples are a minimum with which to build a qualified reference model. In addition, a regular update with normal product deviation (eg, new fruit varieties, new geographical origin, new process technologies, seasonal effects) is necessary.

Once the database has been built, no change in sample preparation or instrumental procedures can be made in future analysis as any such change could invalidate the models. Instrumental reproducibility is important when sharing one database between different NMR spectrometers and this can be an important restriction in the implementation of the method.

We can differentiate between two main types of statistical models, that is, classification and verification models.

Univariate verification models: These are used to check if an individual spectrum deviates from the reference group. Univariate analysis checks that every data point in a test sample falls within the range given by the reference spectra. Higher or lower signal intensities are indicated as a deviation and the cause must be checked. As NMR technology gives structural indication, the reason for any observed deviation can, in many cases, be explained directly by the ^{1}H-spectrum.

Multivariate verification models: These are more complex methods used to compare the spectrum of a test sample with corresponding spectra of reference materials. In this approach the overall pattern and relationship of signals to each other are more important than their absolute intensities.

Classification models: Such models differentiate between populations of samples (eg, samples of different origin or different product types). Mathematical PCA-based models can work in a multidimensional space, which is not conceivable by the human imagination.

However, experiences tend to show that the combination of individual models allows better class assignment. For every group of classes to be differentiated, a separate model is established and the sample spectrum is successively checked against each of these models. Based on group-specific signal characteristics for every model it can be stated that either the spectrum belongs to or does not belong to the group.

Some specific classification models involve combined approaches of pure chemometric models and knowledge of targeted marker compounds for one of the groups. An example is used for the detection of added peach products to apricot purée, a problem that is extremely difficult to solve with conventional analytics. Fig. 23.6 visualizes the principle and gives an idea about possible detection of peach in apricot purées. A combination of monitoring for peach marker signals from still unidentified compounds and a classification model gives a detection limit estimated at 10–20% based on soluble solids.

Some examples of possible classification are given in Table 23.4 (Application note Bruker SGF Profiling).

It should be pointed out that, as a general rule, all statistical models work within a defined probability. For example, a model with a limit of assignment fixed at 0.01 accepts that up to 1% of authentic samples will not be recognized as authentic. This is similar

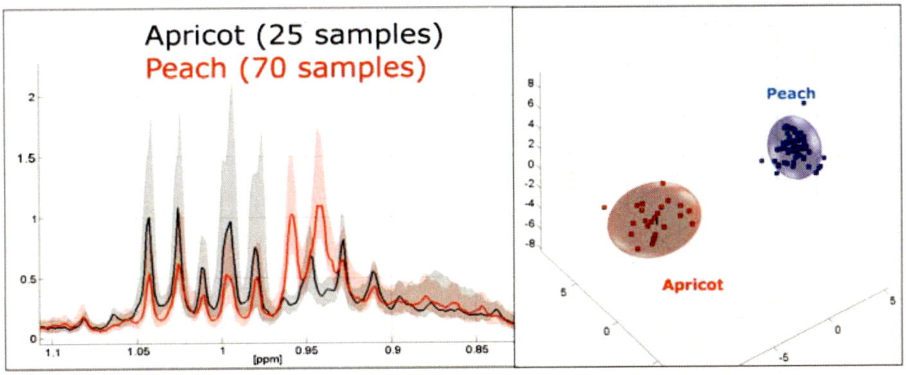

Figure 23.6 Extract of nuclear magnetic resonance spectra for reference samples of apricot purée (gray: range of distribution / black: average intensity) and peach purée (pink: range of distribution/red: average intensity) and a corresponding classification model (red: apricot / blue: peach).

Table 23.4 Overview About Existing Classification Models for Nuclear Magnetic Resonance Screening in Fruit Juice Analytics

Analytical Aspect	Classes to Differentiate
Origin apple juice	Poland/Germany
	Turkey
	China
	Hungary
	Spain/Italy
	Hungary
Origin orange juice	Brazil
	Spain
	Greece
	Belize/Costa Rica/Cuba
	Mexico
	United States
	Argentina/Paraguay/Uruguay
Origin lemon juice	Spain/Italy
	Argentina
Origin pineapple juice	Asia
	Middle America
	Brazil
Origin sour cherry juice	Poland
	Turkey
Origin mango purée	Mexico
	India
Product type apple juice	Direct juice
	Juice made from concentrate
Product type orange juice	Direct juice
	Juice made from concentrate
Product type lemon juice	Direct juice
	Juice made from concentrate
Product type pineapple juice	Direct juice
	Juice made from concentrate
Citrus type	Orange
	Blood orange
	Citrus reticulata

to databases for conventional parameters, which are also subject to misidentification of naturally occurring samples at extreme values of individual parameters.

Verification of fruit content: This is done principally in a way comparable to that described for fruit content calculation using conventional parameters but a much larger number of data points. Detected signals may also come from nonidentified compounds or accumulated interfering signals if reference samples show a low natural variance at a defined chemical shift. Multiple data points (integrals of buckets) can be selected for fruit content calculation. Thus masking a low fruit content by adding a mixture of defined chemicals, as is often done to confuse the conventional estimation, is nearly impossible as this/these addition/s would lead to deviations in other models too. One such model was the main way to show that a large proportion of raspberry products in the market were adulterated although this fact remained nearly undetected by other analytical means. Because of the cost and speed of proton-NMR screening, it allowed a large number of samples to be screened and suspicious samples were further analyzed using stable isotope techniques or quantitative compositional analyses, which confirmed the adulterations.

23.5 Case Study Combining Different Methods

A raspberry purée concentrate was first analyzed by SGF Profiling. The result stated a low fruit content. Fig. 23.7 shows a short part of the spectrum in comparison with the range of expectation for authentic raspberry products. The biological matrix of the

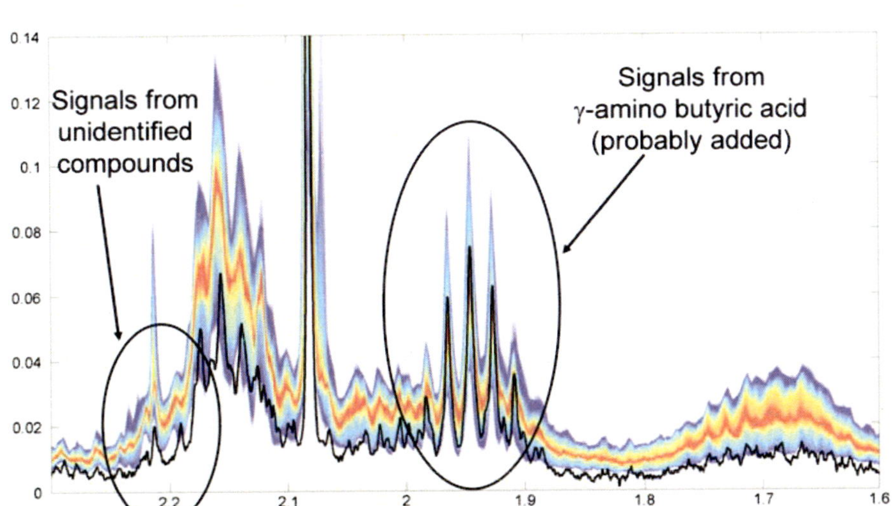

Figure 23.7 Extract from the proton-nuclear magnetic resonance spectrum of a raspberry purée concentrate market sample (*black line*) compared with the range of signal intensity from authentic reference samples (*colored ribbon*), all measured at half single strength concentration.

tested sample is clearly present in lower concentration than expected for authentic products.

To confirm the NMR result conventional analyses were carried out. As listed in Table 23.5 analyzed parameters were in accordance with AIJN CoP guide values. For a comparison the concentration factor calculated from the Brix value of the concentrate was used to convert values obtained for the concentrate to single strength.

Then the theoretical fruit content was calculated based on the internal database of SGF International e.V. The result with 105% should be considered as inside the expected range for authentic products.

Further investigations were carried out by analyzing isotopic parameters, summarized in Table 23.6. Every individual value was an absolute magnitude, which was

Table 23.5 Results of Conventional Analyses for a Sample of Raspberry Purée Concentrate, Expressed for a Brix of 8.5 degrees

Parameter	Result	AIJN CoP Guide Values
Potassium	2161 mg/kg	1300–2800 mg/kg
Total phosphorus	207 mg/kg	100–250 mg/kg
Magnesium	135 mg/kg	110–230 mg/kg
D-Isocitric acid	106 mg/kg	60–160 mg/kg
Formol number	18.9 (0.1 M NaOH mL/100 mL)	10–50 (0.1 M NaOH mL/100 mL)
Citric/isocitric ratio	151	80–240
Glucose/fructose ratio	0.82	0.6–0.95

Table 23.6 Results of Isotopic Analyses for a Sample of Raspberry Purée Concentrate

Parameter	Result	Result Evaluation
$\delta^{13}C$ sugar	−24.7‰ PDB	Pass (AIJN CoP: −24 to −27)
$\delta^{13}C$ acid fraction	−24.9‰ PDB	Pass
$\delta^{13}C$ pulp	−23.9‰ PDB	Pass
Difference $\delta^{13}C$ sugar-$\delta^{13}C$ acids	−0.2‰ PDB	Pass
Difference $\delta^{13}C$ sugar-$\delta^{13}C$	−0.85‰ PDB	Fail

AIJN CoP, European Fruit Juice Association Code of Practice; *PDB*, Pee Dee Belemnite.

not suspicious. Also the internal relation between ^{13}C of sugar and ^{13}C of acids was without giving any hint of adulteration. Only the relation between the ^{13}C value of the sugar fraction and the ^{13}C value of the pulp could clearly confirm the NMR result. A sugar addition of minimum 20% soluble solids was stated.

The ^{13}C value of the pulp is an analysis that is not chosen regularly by analysts and was performed in this case only because of the strong hint from NMR screening. Many products in the fruit juice industry are clarified and without any pulp. If, instead of a purée concentrate, the present case would have concerned a raspberry juice concentrate, which is usually a clarified product, the fraud was only detected by the SGF Profiling. A confirmation by any other currently applied method would have been hardly possible.

It must be supposed that the adulteration of adding sugar was carried out by an unserious producer having good knowledge of chemical composition and analytics. A cocktail of chemicals and/or other cheaper fruit products must have been added to adjust expected concentrations of compounds which are usually controlled by conventional targeted analyses. The NMR spectrum could even show that main amino acids where present in sufficient concentration to probably avoid that an amino acid analysis would easily indicate any problem with the product. Furthermore, a selection of sugar syrup and organic acids for the adulteration was performed to obtain unsuspicious isotopic data for absolute values and important internal relations. This example shows quite well that in some cases, as here, much criminal energy is applied and scientific knowledge is misused to counter quality control.

23.6 Importance of Databases and Documentation

Analytics are only useful if the data collected can be interpreted. Analytical accuracy is, in most cases, much higher than uncertainties in interpretation because of the natural variation seen in fruit juices, because we are dealing with natural and not formulated products. Only refined and robust databases combining a multitude of parameters can be used for effective control work. For the collection of reference samples, a particular effort is necessary to assure authenticity. These samples must constitute a representative collection from each production area of interest. In particular, for chemometric databases they must have undergone an industrial process so they "fit" with industrial products. However, this is equally applicable for some traditional analytical methods, for example, for water-soluble pectins. Every process may change the chemical composition of a fruit juice.

The quality of inferences arising from analytical testing increases with the quality of meta-data, which accompany any specific sample. Controlled and suitable traceability systems for products are important side aspects of fruit juice analysis to support data interpretation, which depends very often on origin, process data, varieties, seasonal particularities, or other meta-data.

Thus fruit juice authenticity testing has already become a multidisciplinary exercise in which the performance of analytical technology is no longer a standalone science. Modern food quality standards and traceability systems can provide useful and meaningful data to the analyst. For example, the European fruit juice industry has built up a global control system for semifinished goods (Website of SGF International e.V.) and European consumer products, which is unique in the food sector. This on-site control system is a good example of how to combine analytics and to assure reliable traceability through independent control audits and how to keep analytical databases up to date by sampling authentic and industrial reference material from all over the world. In fact, many of the innovations mentioned in this chapter have benefited from, and have only been possible because of, such sample collection.

23.7 Outlook

The number of fruit types, varieties, cultivation techniques, processing technologies, geographical origins, and seasonal particularities because of unusual weather conditions are increasing constantly. In parallel, unscrupulous producers are using more sophisticated means to try to mask any adulteration. Interpretation of analytical results will become much more complex in the future and authenticity testing will be more and more difficult. Reference materials must be collected and analyzed in greater numbers to keep databases suitable for pertinent controls.

In the opinion of the author, this can be achieved only by the combination of targeted and untargeted analytical techniques with a high degree of automation and throughput. Processing of large data volumes will be essential. NMR screening as described earlier is a first successful method in fruit juice analytics, which is strongly dependent on mathematical application and effective algorithm development. Including proton NMR screening in the analytical scope can lead to better profitability than using conventional analyses only. Despite a relatively expensive investment in NMR equipment this positive economic effect is caused by the fact that a number of quality aspects are checked simultaneously with one single experiment. This benefit will increase with the development of new and larger databases. Further, NMR applications, for example, with automated solid phase extraction, will lower detection limits in the future and provide much better molecular information via NMR in parallel with the untargeted information. Thus the return on investment for expensive equipment should improve in the near future.

The overlay in Fig. 23.8 shows the first results from studies tending to deliver a solution for a field of authenticity check, which still needs improvement for routine controls. This is the characterization of blends between citrus juices with weak differences in their chemical composition, like lemon and lime or orange and mandarin. The approach, followed in this study, is the combination of proton-NMR screening with an automatic sample clean-up using solid phase extraction. Upper spectra indicate clearly a number of specific marker compounds for lime juices, which are not detectable or have much less intensity in lemon juices. Typical lime patterns are registered. The lowest spectra in the graph result from standard SGF Profiling and are displayed with the same signal amplification to give an idea of increased sensitivity through sample clean-up. It must be pointed out that NMR has a large dynamic range and the standard spectra have much more information, as visible here. Furthermore, results look promising in terms of repeatability so that chemometric approaches should also be

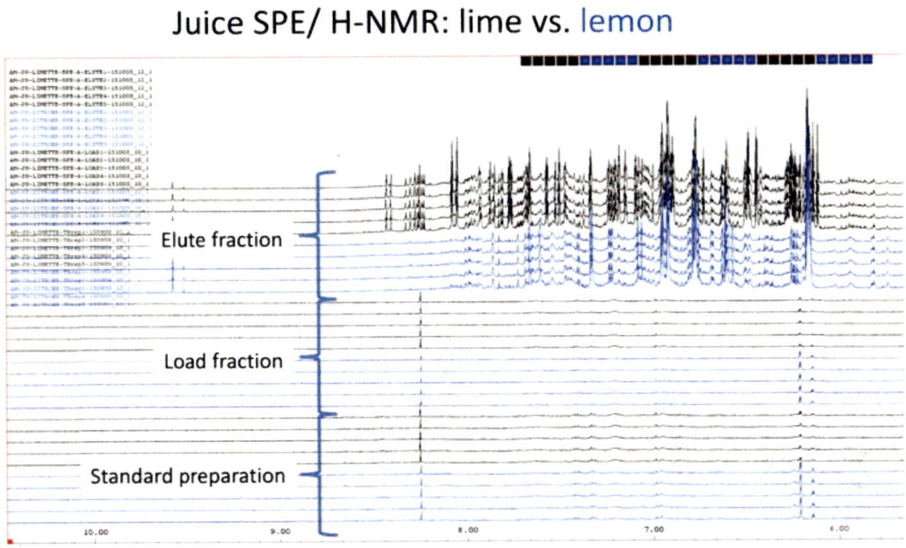

Figure 23.8 Comparison between standard spin generated fingerprint profiling and proton-nuclear magnetic resonance screening after solid phase extraction (SPE). The upper five spectra (in black) correspond to a lime juice sample after SPE, the following five (in blue) to a lemon juice. The lowest 10 spectra correspond to lime and lemon juice after standard procedure.

possible. Respective reference databases must be established after fixing optimal measurement conditions.

Furthermore, other techniques like chromatographic methods combined with high resolution mass spectroscopy (HRMS) will probably play an important role too. They will be used for authenticity testing and benefit also from the growing capacity to treat data today and in the future. These methods using precise molecular information in combination with untargeted metabonomic approaches are already under development (Dubin et al., 2014).

Both approaches, NMR and HRMS, are complementary and we see permanent progress in technology and data processing.

For economic reasons, synergies obtained by covering other quality aspects such as food safety are beneficial. Possible combinations of equipment to cover food safety risks and authenticity control in one analytical run are already realized. Major minerals like potassium, magnesium, calcium, and sodium can be analyzed by ICP-MS in parallel with toxic heavy metals. Chromatographic HRMS methods established for authenticity testing may be used for determination of pesticides, mycotoxins, and the verification of the pattern of secondary metabolites and other juice compounds in a single experiment.

Thus it is not an unrealistic vision that spectrometric techniques like NMR in combination with LC-HRMS, GC-HRMS, and ICP-MS could replace almost all other conventional methods in fruit juice authenticity testing. Stable isotope measurements will still play a role for specific analytical questions and provide confirmatory results in the case of suspicious findings. Greater use of isotopic techniques in laboratories will take place through the use of more economic technologies like the CRDS. Thus a typical fruit juice laboratory will work with a small number of sophisticated instruments and deal with mathematical treatment of large datasets. GC and HPLC instruments, enzymatic analyzers, and labor-intensive wet chemistry methods will gradually lose their importance.

However, it is difficult to imagine that some traditional basic parameters will disappear from specialized fruit juice laboratories. These are Brix, density, and total acidity measurement because they are used by the industry for a first characterization of the economic value of any fruit juice.

Acknowledgments

I thank David Hammond, Andreas Rossmann, and Wilhelm Rieth for the precious information and comments they have provided. Furthermore, I thank Eric Jamin, Freddy Thomas, and Markus Goedejohann for the authorization to use their graphs and figures.

References

Adams, M.J., 1998. The principles of multivariate analysis. In: Ashurst, Dennis (Eds.), Analytical Methods of Food Authentication, Chapter 12 309 − 336. Blackie, London.

Application note Bruker SGF Profiling, Release 3.0 Specifi cation Sheet © Bruker BioSpin 10/13 T132662. www.bruker.com/sgf.

Bayer, S., McHard, J.A., Winefordner, J.D., 1980. Determination of the geographical origins of frozen concentrated orange juice via pattern recognition. Journal of Agricultural and Food Chemistry 28 (6), 1306−1307.

Becker, M., Andersen, N., Fiedler, B., Fietzek, P., Körtzinger, A., Steinhoff, T., Friedrichs, G., 2012. Using cavity ringdown spectroscopy for continuous monitoring of $\delta^{13}C(CO_2)$ and fCO_2 in the surface ocean. Limnology Oceanography: Methods 10, 752−766.

Beer, C., Fiedler, Th., Hofsommer, M., November 3−6, 2015. Poster: using cavity ring-down spectroscopy for the detection of food fraud. In: 7th International Symposium on Recent Advances in Food Analysis. Prague.

Bender, M.M., 1971. Variations in the $^{13}C/^{12}C$ ratios of plants in relation to the pathway of photosynthetic carbon dioxide fixation. Phytochemistry 10, 1239−1244.

Biyela, B.N.E., du Toit, W.J., Divol, B., Malherhe, D.F., van Rensburg, P., 2009. The production of reduced-alcohol wines using Gluzyme Mono®10,000 BG-treated grape juice. South African Journal of Enology and Viticulture 30 (2).

Bricout, J., Fontes, J.C., 1974. Distinction analytique entre sucre de canne et sucre de betterave. Annales des Falsifications et de l'Expertise Chimique 716, 211−215.

Bricout, J., Koziet, J., 1987. Control of the authenticity of orange juice by isotopic analysis. Journal of Agricultural and Food Chemistry 35, 758−760.

Bricout, J., Fontes, J.-C., Merlivat, L., 1972. Sur la composition en isotopes stables de l'eau des jus d'oranges. Comptes Rendus de l'Académie des Sciences, Paris, Series D 274, 1803−1806.

Chesson, L.A., Bowen, G.J., Ehleringer, J.R., 2010. Analysis of the hydrogen and oxygen stable isotope ratios of beverage waters without prior water extraction using isotope ratio infrared spectroscopy (CRDS). Rapid Communications in Mass Spectrometry 24, 3205–3213.

Codex General Standard for Fruit Juices and Nectars (CODEX STAN 247-2005). http://www.codexalimentarius.org/standards/list-standards/en.

Coetzee, P.P., Steffens, F.E., Eiselen, R.J., Augustyn, O.P., Balcaen, L., Vanhaecke, F., 2005. Multi-element analysis of South African wines by ICP–MS and their classification according to geographical origin. Journal of Agricultural and Food Chemistry 53 (13), 5060–5066.

Craig, H., 1961. Isotopic variation in meteoritic water. Science 133, 1702–1703.

Day, M.P., Correia, P., Hammond, D.A., 1998. ^{13}C-IRIS – a refined method to detect the addition of cane/corn derived sugars to fruit juices and purees. Fruit Processing 8 (3), 86–90.

Detection of added ascorbic acid. Final Report of RTD Project Funded under the Fifth Framework Programme of the European Community within the Competitive and Sustainable Growth Programme, Measurement and Testing Activity. Contract N°: G6RD-CT-2002–00760. Coordination: SGF International e.V.

Directive 2012/12/EC, 2012. Council Directive Relating to Fruit Juices and Certain Similar Products Intended for Human Consumption of 19 April 2012.

Doner, L.W., Bills, D.D., 1981. Stable carbon isotope ratios in orange juice. Journal of Agricultural and Food Chemistry 29, 803–804.

Doner, L.W., Bills, D.D., 1982. Mass spectrometric ^{13}C/^{12}C determinations to detect high fructose corn syrup in orange juice. Collaborative study. Journal of the Association of Official Analytical Chemists 65, 608–610.

Doner, L.W., Phillips, J.C., 1981. Detection of high fructose corn syrup in apple juice by mass spectrometric ^{13}C/^{12}C analysis: collaborative study. Journal of the Association of Official Analytical Chemists 64, 85–90.

Doner, L.W., Krueger, H.W., Ressmann, R.H., 1980. Isotopic composition of carbon in apple juice. Journal of Agricultural and Food Chemistry 28, 362–364.

Doner, L.W., Ajie, H.O., Stenberg, L.S.L., Miburn, J.M., De Niro, M.J., Hicks, K.B., 1987. Detecting sugar beet syrups in orange juice by deuterium/hydrogen and oxygen-18/oxygen-16 analysis of sucrose. Journal of Agricultural and Food Chemistry 35, 610–612.

Doner, L.W., 1985. Carbon isotope ratios in natural and synthetic citric acid as indicators of lemon juice adulteration. Journal of Agricultural and Food Chemistry 33, 770–772.

Dubin, E., Dumas, A.-S., Lees, M., Jamin, E., Ginet, J., Rutledge, D.N., 2014. Are you sure that your blackcurrants are not aronia berries? In: Poster Presented at the 8ème Journées Scientifiques du Réseau Français de Métabolomique et de Fluxomique, Lyon.

Dunbar, J., Schmidt, J.L., 1984. Measurement of the ^{2}H(D)/^{1}H isotope ratios of the carbon bound hydrogen atoms of sugars. Fresenius' Journal of Analytical Chemistry 317, 853–857.

Dunbar, J., Wilson, A.T., July 1983. Oxygen and hydrogen isotopes in fruit and vegetable juices. Plant Physiology 72 (3), 725–727.

Duvnjak, Z., Turcotte, G., Duan, Z.D., 1991. Production of sorbitol and ethanol from Jerusalem artichokes by *Saccharomyces cerevisiae* ATCC 36859. Applied Microbiology and Biotechnology 35, 711–715.

Epstein, S., Mayeda, T., 1953. Variation of ^{18}O content of waters from natural sources. Geochimica et Cosmochimica Acta 4, 213–244.

Farquhar, G.D., Cernusak, L.A., Barnes, B., 2007. Heavy water fractionation during transpiration. Plant Physiology 143 (1), 11–18.

Friedman, I., 1953. Deuterium content of natural water and other substances. Geochimica et Cosmochimica Acta 4, 89–103.

Gamal, F.M., Mohamed, S.S., Safaa, K.H.K., Ahmed, M.S.H., Mohie, M.K., 2011. Application of FT-IR Spectroscopy for rapid and simultaneous quality determination of some fruit products. Nature and Science 9 (11).

Giusti, M.M., Atnip, A., Sweeney, C., Rodriguez-Saona, L.E., 2011. Rapid authentication of fruit juices by infrared spectroscopic techniques. In: Ebeler, S.E., Takeoka, G.R., Winterhalter, P. (Eds.), Progress in Authentication of Food and Wine, vol. 1081. American Chemical Society, pp. 275–299 (Chapter 20).

Gonfiantini, R., 1978. Standards for stable isotope measurements in natural compounds. Nature 271, 534–536.

Gonzalez, J., Jamin, E., Remaud, G., Martin, Y.-L., Martin, G.G., Martin, M.L., 1998. Authentication of lemon juices and concentrates by a combined multi-isotopc approach using SNIF-NMR$^{(R)}$ and IRMS. Journal of Agricultural and Food Chemistry 46 (6), 2200–2205.

González, J., Remaud, G., Jamin, E., Naulet, N., Martin, G.G., 1999. Specific natural isotope profile studied by isotope ratio mass spectrometry (SNIP-IRMS): (13)C/(12)C ratios of fructose, glucose, and sucrose for improved detection of sugar addition to pineapple juices and concentrates. Journal of Agricultural and Food Chemistry 47 (6), 2316–2321.

Goodner, K.L., Rouseff, R.L., Hofsommer, H.-J., 2001. Orange, mandarin and hybrid classification using multivariate statistics based on carotenoid profiles. Journal of Agricultural and Food Chemistry 49 (3), 1146–1150.

Guyon, F., Auberger, P., Gaillard, L., Loublanches, C., Viateau, M., Sabathié, N., Salagoïty, M.-H., Médina, B., 2014. $^{13}C/^{12}C$ isotope ratios of organic acids, glucose and fructose determined by HPLC-co-IRMS for lemon juices authenticity. Food Chemistry 146, 36–40.

Hammond, D.A., 1995. Authentication of fruit juices using traditional multi-component methods and a novel fingerprinting technique, pyrolysis-mass spectrometry. In: Nagy, S., Wade, R. (Eds.), Methods to Detect Adulteration of Fruit Juice Beverages, vol. 1. AgScience, pp. 84–111.

Hammond, D.A., March 2006. Detection of extracts from pineapple peels and cores in juice. In: Conference Proceedings of EU Funded Project "Pure Juice", G6RD – CT – 2002–00760, Darmstadt Germany. www.purejuice.org.

Hofsommer, H.-J., Koswig, S., 2005. Zum Nachweis von Aronia in schwarzer Johannisbeere. Flüssiges Obst 6, 289–293.

Hofsommer, H.-J., Klein, I., Grüning, J., Höpker, H.-R., 1989. Bestimmung von D-Aminosäuren in Fruchtsäften. Flüssiges Obst Jg. 56 (Heft. 10), 646–651.

Hofsommer, H.-J., 1999. New analytical techniques for judging the authenticity of fruit juices. Fruit Processing 12, 471–479.

Hofsommer, M., 2014. Zur Problematik der SO_2-Bestimmung in Traubensaft II. Flüssiges Obst 8, 345–346.

Jamin, E., Gonzalez, J., Bengoechea, I., Kerneur, G., Remaud, G., Itiondo, C., Martin, G.G., 1996. Proteins as intermoleuclar isotope reference for detection of adulteration of fruit juices. Journal of Agricultural and Food Chemistry 46, 5118–5123.

Jamin, E.R., Lees, M., Fuchs, G., Martin, G.G., 2000. Detection of added L- and D, L- malic acids in apple and cherry juices – site specific 13-IRMS method. Fruit Processing 11, 434–436.

Jamin, E., Guerin, R., Rétif, M., Lees, M., Martin, G.J., 2003. Improved detection of added water in orange juice by simultaneous determination of the oxygen-18/oxygen-16 isotope ratios of water and ethanol derived from sugars. Journal of Agricultural and Food Chemistry 51 (18), 5202–5206.

Jamin, E., Martin, F., Martin, G.G., May–June 2004. Determination of the $^{13}C/^{12}C$ ratio of ethanol derived from fruit juices and maple syrup by isotope ratio mass spectrometry: collaborative study. Journal of AOAC International 87 (3), 621–631.

Jamin, E.R., Lees, M., Thomas, F., 2005. Detection of exogenous citric acid in fruit juices by stable isotope ratio analysis. Journal of Agricultural and Food Chemistry 53, 5130–5133.

Jamin, E., Gonzalez, J., Bengoechea, I., Kerneur, G., Remaud, G., Naulet, N., et al., 1998. Measurements of $^{13}C/^{12}C$ ratios of sugars, malic acid, and citric acid as authenticity probes of citrus juices and concentrates. Journal of AOAC International 81, 604–609.

Jamin, E., March 2006. Detection of undeclared added organic acids. In: Conference Proceedings of EU Funded Project "Pure Juice", G6RD – CT – 2002–00760, Darmstadt Germany. www.purejuice.org.

Jamin, E., July/August 2009. Superfruits: Are they authentic? Fruit Processing 170–175.

Koswig, S., Hofsommer, H.-J., 1995. HPLC-Methode zur Untersuchung von Anthocyanen in Buntsäften und anderen gefärbten Lebensmitteln. Flüssiges Obst 62 (4), 125–130.

Koswig, S., Hofsommer, H.-J., 1999. Zur Analytik von Zuckeralkoholen in Fruchtsäften. In: Proceedings der 2. Fachtagung zur Ionenanalyse und Kapillarelektrophorese, Idstein, p. 183.

Koswig, S., Hofsommer, H.-J., Weiß, J., Jensen, D., 1996. Ionenchromatographische Untersuchung von Fruchtsäften. In: Proceedings der Fachtagung "Ionenanalyse mit Chromatographie und Kapillarelektrophores", München.

Koswig, S., 2006. Determination of foreign fruit types and fruit varieties – analyses, evaluation and practical problems. Fruit Processing 6, 401–407.

Koziet, J., Rossmann, A., Martin, G.J., Ashurst, P.R., 1993. Determination of carbon-13 content of sugars of fruit and vegetable juices. A European inter-laboratory comparison. Analytica Chimica Acta 271, 31–38.

Koziet, J., Rossmann, A., Martin, G.J., Johnson, P., 1995. Determination of oxygen-18 and deuterium content of fruit and vegetable juice-water – a European inter-laboratory comparison study. Analytica Chimica Acta 302, 29–37.

Krueger, D.A., Krueger, R.G., Krueger, H.W., 1986. Carbon isotope ratios of various fruits. Journal – Association of Official Analytical Chemists 63, 1181–1183.

Krueger, D.A., 1995. Detection of added sugar to fruit juices using carbon and hydrogen stable isotope ratio analysis. In: Nagy, S., Wade, R. (Eds.), Methods to Detect Adulteration of Fruit Beverage, vol. 1. AgScience, pp. 41–51.

Kvasnička, F., Voldřich, M., Pyš, P., Vinš, I., 2002. Determination of isocitric acid in citrus juice—a comparison of HPLC, enzyme set and capillary isotachophoresis methods. Journal of Food Composition and Analysis 15 (6), 685–691.

Laursen, K.H., Schjoerring, J.K., Kelly, S.D., Husted, S., 2014. Authentication of organically grown plants – advantages and limitations of atomic spectroscopy for multi-element and stable isotope analysis. Trends in Analytical Chemistry 59, 73–82.

Lee, J., 2015. Sorbitol, Rubus fruit, and misconception. Food Chemistry 166, 616–622.

Lehnert, N., Ara, V., 2014. Authenticity analysis of lemon juices concerning the adulteration with lime. Fruit Processing 10, 242.

León, L., Kelly, J.D., Downey, G., May 2005. Detection of apple juice adulteration using near-infrared transflectance spectroscopy. Journal of Applied Spectroscopy 59 (5), 593–599.

Louche, L.M.-M., Gaydou, E.M., Lesage, J.-C., 1998. Determination of phlorin as peel marker in orange (*Citrus sinensis*) fruits and juices. Journal of Agricultural and Food Chemistry 46 (10), 4193–4197.

Low, N.H., Hammond, D.A., 1996. Detection of inulin in apple juice by capillary gas chromatography. Fruit Processing 4, 135–139.

Low, N.H., Wudrich, G.G., 1993. Detection of inexpensive sweetener addition to grapefruit juice by HPLC-PAD. Journal of Agricultural and Food Chemistry 41 (6), 902–909.

Low, N.H., McLaughlin, M., Hofsommer, H.-J., Hammond, D.A., 1999. Capillary gas chromatographic detection of invert sugar in heated, adulterated, and adulterated and heated apple juice concentrates employing the equilibrium method. Journal of Agricultural and Food Chemistry 47 (10), 4261–4266.

Low, N.H., 1995. Apple and orange juice authenticity analysis by capillary gas chromatography with flame ionization detection. Fruit Processing 11, 362–367.

Low, N.H., 1996. Fruit juice authenticity analysis by capillary gas chromatography with flame ionization detection. Journal of AOAC International 79, 724–737.

Ludwig, C., Viant, M.R., January–February 2010. Two-dimensional J-resolved NMR spectroscopy: review of a key methodology in the metabolomics toolbox. Phytochemical Analysis 21 (1), 22–32. http://dx.doi.org/10.1002/pca.1186.

Maher, D.T., Santos, I.R., Tait, D.R., 2014. Mapping methane and carbon dioxide concentrations and $\delta^{13}C$ values in the atmosphere of two Australian coal seam gas fields. Water, Air & Soil Pollution 225, 2216.

Malacrino, P., Tosi, E., Caramia, G., Prisco, R., Zapparoli, G., 2005. The vinification of partially dried grapes: a comparative fermentation study of *Saccharomyces cerevisiae* strains under high sugar stress. Letters in Applied Microbiology 40 (6), 466–472.

Martin, G.J., Martin, G.G., 1995. NMR and MS stable isotope studies of fruit juice. In: Nagy, Wade (Eds.), Methods to Detect Fruit Beverage Adulteration. AgScience.

Martin, G., Guillou, C., Martin, Y.L., September 1994. SNIF-NMR® for detection of sugar additions in fruit juices. In: Proceedings of the IFU/SGF Symposium "Progress in Authenticity Assurance of Fruit Juices", Parma.

Martin, G.G., Hanote, V., Lees, M., Martin, Y.L., 1996a. Interpretation of combined ^{2}H SNIF-NMR® and ^{13}C SIRA MS analyses of fruit juices to detect added sugar. Journal of the Association of Official Analytical Chemists 79 (1), 62–72.

Martin, G.G., Wood, R., Martin, G.J., 1996b. Detection of added beet sugar in concentrated and single strength fruit juices by deuterium nuclear magnetic resonance (SNF-NMR® method): collaborative study. Journal of the Association of Official Analytical Chemists 79, 917–928.

Mimmo, T., Camin, F., Bontempo, L., Capici, C., Tagliavini, M., Cesco, S., Scampicchio, M., 11/2015. Traceability of different apple varieties by multivariate analysis of isotope ratio mass spectrometry data. Rapid Communications in Mass Spectrometry 29 (21), 1984–1990.

Monsallier-Bitea, C., Jamin, E., Lees, M., Zhang, B.L., Martin, G.J., 2006. Study of the influence of alcoholic fermentation and distillation on the oxygen-18/oxygen-16 isotope ratio of ethanol. Journal of Agricultural and Food Chemistry 54 (2), 279–284.

Nikdel, S., Nagy, S., Attaway, J.A., 1985. Trace metals: defining geographical origin and detecting adulteration of orange juice. In: Nagy, Attaway, Rhodes (Eds.), Adulteration of Fruit Juice Beverages. Marcel Dekker Inc, New York, pp. 81–105.

Ogrinc, N., Bat, K., Kosir, I.J., Golob, T., Kokkinofta, R., 2009. Characterization of commercial slovenian and cypriot fruit juices using stable isotopes. Journal of Agricultural and Food Chemistry 57 (15), 6764–6769.

Ooghe, W.C., Ooghe, S.J., Detavernier, C.M., Huyghebaert, A., 1994. Characterization of orange juice (*Citrus sinensis*) by flavanone glycosides. Journal of Agricultural and Food Chemistry 42, 2183–2190.

Patz, C.D., Galensa, R., Dietrich, H., 1997. Beitrag zur Bestimmung von Sulfit in Fruchtsäften mittels HPLC-Biosensor-Kopplung. Dsch Legensm Rundsch 93, 347–351.

Pellerano, R.G., Mazza, S.S., Marigliano, R.A., Marchevsky, E.J., 2008. Multielement analysis of Argentinean lemon juices by instrumental neutronic activation analysis and their classification according to geographical origin. Journal of Agricultural and Food Chemistry 56 (13), 5222–5225.

Perez, A.L., Smith, B.W., Anderson, K.W., 2006. Stable isotope and trace element profiling combined with classification models to differentiate geographical growing origin for 3 fruits (strawberry, blueberry and pear): effects of sub-region and variety. Journal of Agricultural and Food Chemistry 54 (13), 4506–4516.

Rapisarda, P., Camin, F., Fabroni, S., Perini, M., Torrisi, B., Intrigliolo, F., 2010. Influence of different organic fertilizers on quality parameters and the delta(15)N, delta(13)C, delta(2)H, delta(34)S, and delta(18)O values of orange fruit (*Citrus sinensis* L. Osbeck). Journal of Agricultural and Food Chemistry 58 (6), 3502–3506.

Regulation (EC) No 1333/2008 of the European Parliament and of the Council of 16 December 2008 on Food Additives, last amendment on October 12, 2015.

Rinke, P., Moitrier, S., Humpfer, E., Keller, S., Moertter, M., Godejohann, M., Hoffmann, G., Schaefer, H., Spraul, M., January/February 2007. An ^{1}H-NMR technique for high throughput screening in quality and authenticity control of fruit juice and fruit juice raw materials – SGF profiling. Fruit Processing 10–18.

Rojas, J.M.M., Cosofort, S., Reniero, F., Guillou, C., Serra, F., 2007. Control of oenological products: discrimination between different botanical sources of L-tartaric acid by isotope ratios mass spectrometry. Rapid Communication in Mass Spectrometry 21, 2447–2450.

Rossmann, A., Ara, V., September/October 2013. Multi element stable isotope analysis for fruit juice geographical origin and production control. Fruit Processing 192–196.

Rossmann, A., Rummel, S., March 9, 2006a. Geographical Origin Assignment EQCS Workshop Darmstadt. PURE JUICE. http://www.purejuice.org/WS_Presentations/ISOLAB_ppt.pdf.

Rossmann, A., Rummel, S., March 2006b. Geographical origin assignment. In: Conference Proceedings of EU Funded Project "Pure Juice", G6RD – CT – 2002–00760, Darmstadt Germany. www.purejuice.org.

Rossmann, A., Rieth, W., Schmidt, H.L., 1990. Möglichkeiten und Ergebnisse der Kombination von Messungen der Verhältnisse stabiler Wasserstoff und Kohlenstoff-Isotope mit Resultaten konventioneller Analysen (RSK Werte) zum Nachweis des Zuckerzusatzes zu Fruchtsäften. Zeitschrift für Lebensmittel-Untersuchung und -Forschung 191, 259–264.

Rouseff, R.L., Raley, L., Hofsommer, H.J., 1996. Application of DAD with a C_{30} RP column for the separation and identification of saponified orange juice carotenoids. Journal of Agricultural and Food Chemistry 44 (8), 2176–2181.

Rummel, S., Hoelzl, S., Horn, P., Rossmann, A., Schlicht, C., 2010. The combination of stable isotopic abundance ratios of H, C, N & S with ^{87}Sr/^{86}Sr for geographical origin assignment of orange juices. Food Chemistry 118, 890–900.

Scordino, M., Di Mauro, A., Passerini, A., Maccarone, E., December 15, 2004. Phloroglucinol from phlorin hydrolysis for testing quality of commercial orange juices and beverages. Journal of Agricultural and Food Chemistry 52 (25), 7469–7474.

Simpkins, W.A., Patel, G., Collins, P., Harrison, M., Goldberg, D., 1999. Oxygen isotope ratios of juice water in Australian oranges and concentrates. Journal of Agricultural and Food Chemistry 47 (7), 2606–2612.

Spraul, M., Schütz, B., Rinke, P., Koswig, S., Humpfer, E., Schäfer, H., Mörtter, M., Fang, F., Marx, U.C., Minoja, A., 2009a. NMR-based multi parametric quality control of fruit juices: SGF Profiling. Nutrients 1, 148–155.

Spraul, M., Schütz, B., Humpfer, E., Moertter, M., Schaefer, H., Koswig, S., Rinke, P., 2009b. Mixture analysis by NMR as applied to fruit juice quality control. Magnetic Resonance in Chemistry 47, S130–S137.

Suarez Valles, B., Santamaria Victorero, J., Mangas Alonso, J.J., Blanco Gomis, D., 1994. High-performance liquid chromatography of the neutral phenolic compounds of low molecular weight in apple juice. Journal of Agricultural and Food Chemistry 42 (12), 2732–2736.

Swallow, K.W., Low, N.H., 1993. Isolation and identification of oligosaccharide in a commercial beet medium invert syrup. Journal of Agricultural and Food Chemistry 41 (10), 1587–1592.

Swallow, K.W., Petrus, D., Low, N.H., 1991. Detection of orange juice adulteration with beet medium invert sugar using anion exchange liquid chromatography with pulsed amperometric detection. Journal – Association of Official Analytical Chemists 74, 341–345.

Thavarajah, P., Low, N.H., 2006a. Isolation and identification of select oligosaccharides from commercially produced total invert sugar with a proposed mechanism for their formation. Journal of Agricultural and Food Chemistry 54 (7), 2754–2760.

Thavarajah, P., Low, N.H., 2006b. Adulteration of apple with pear juice: emphasis on major carbohydrates, proline, and arbutin. Journal of agricultural and food chemistry 54 (13), 4861–4867.

Theisen, S., 2009. HPLC-IMER as a Fast and Sensitive Method for the Determination of Sulfur Dioxide in Foodstuffs Dissertation. Rheinische Friedrich-Wilhelms-Universität, Bonn.

Thomas, F., Randet, C., Gilbert, A., Silvestre, V., Jamin, E., Akoka, S., Remaud, G., Segebarth, N., Guillou, C., 2010. Improved characterization of the botanical origin of sugar by carbon-13 SNIF-NMR applied to ethanol. Journal of Agricultural and Food Chemistry 58, 11580–11585.

Thomas, F., Jamin, E., Hammond, D.A., 2013. ^{18}O internal referencing method to detect water addition in wines and fruit juices: collaborative study. Journal of the Association of Official Analytical Chemists 98 (3), 615–624.

Thomas, F., 2009. In: Presentation at: Customs 2013 Programme, Learning Days on Stable Isotopic Analyses. Czech Republic, Prague.

Trincherini, P.R., Baffi, C., Barbero, P., Pizzoglio, E., Spalla, S., 2014. Precise determination of strontium isotope ratios by TIMS to authenticate tomato geographical origin. Food Chemistry 145, 349–355 (2013).

Trotzer, A., Hofsommer, H.-J., Rubach, K., 1994. Kohlenhydratanalytik mit Anionenaustausch-Chromatographie und gepulster amperometrischer Detektion am Dionex DX-300 Chromatographie Modul. Flüssiges Obst 12, 581–589.

Voerkelius, S., Lorenz, G.D., Rummel, S., Quétel, C.R., Heiss, G., Baxter, M., Brach-Papa, C., Deters-Itzelsberger, P., Hoelzl, S., Hoogewerff, J., Ponzevera, E., Van Boacxstaele, M., Ueckermann, H., 2010. Strontium isotopic signatures of natural mineral waters, the reference to a simple geological map and its potential for authentication of food. Food Chemistry 118 (4), 933–940.

Website of AIJN Code of Practice. http://www.aijn.org/.

Website of International Fruit and Vegetable Juice Association. http://www.ifu-fruitjuice.com.

Website of SGF International e.V. www.sgf.org.

Wilfried, C., Ooghe, S.J., Christ'l, M., 1997. Detavernier detection of the addition of *Citrus reticulata* and hybrids to *Citrus sinensis* by flavonoids. Journal of Agricultural and Food Chemistry 45 (5), 1633–1637.

Will, F., Baukhage, K., Dietrich, H., 2000. Apple pomace liquefaction with pectinase and cellulase: analytical data of the corresponding juices. European Food Research and Technology 211, 291–297.

Willems, J.L., Low, N.H., 2014. Authenticity analysis of pear juice employing chromatographic fingerprinting. Journal of Agricultural and Food Chemistry 62 (48), 11737–11747.
Wudrich, G.G., McSheffrey, S., Low, N.H., 1993. Detection of the addition of variety of inexpensive sweeteners to pure orange juice (adulteration) by high performance liquid chromatography. Journal – Association of Official Analytical Chemists 76, 342–354.
Zhao, H., Zhou, F., Dziugan, P., Yao, Y., Zhang, J., Lv, Z., Zhang, B., 2014. Development of organic acids and volatile compounds in cider during malolactic fermentation. Czech Journal of Food Sciences 32 (1), 69–76.

Advances in Testing for Adulteration of Food Supplements

24

S.H. El-Ahmady, M.L. Ashour
Ain Shams University, Cairo, Egypt

Chapter Outline

24.1 Introduction

Food supplements are a fast growing, multibillion dollar market and therefore represent a major target of adulteration worldwide. Food supplements may be classified into three broad types: (1) substances that are essential nutrients such as vitamins, minerals, trace elements, essential fatty acids, and amino acids; (2) substances that are natural body metabolites and/or are naturally present in the diet and hence are not considered to be essential nutrients, but the additional intake of which may have health benefits or even the potential to alleviate disease; and (3) some supplements of plant or occasionally animal origin or their extracts that contain substances in the previous categories or other pharmacologically active substances and are claimed to have health-enhancing properties.

24.1.1 Forms of Food Supplements

Food supplements are generally sold over the counter and they are taken orally in specified doses in the form of pills, capsules, powders, or liquid preparations. They are not to be substituted for the normal diet but are intended to be additional to it. They are also not intended to be the only source of energy or fluid or a major contributor to energy or fluid intake. Usually, promotional material or brochures accompany the products carrying some health claims, while in other instances these indications may be present on the product label (Webb, 2006). The most common forms of supplements are described briefly in the following section (Jennings and Ottaway, 2008).

24.1.1.1 Tablets

This is the most common form of supplements in the market and they can take one of the following forms:

Swallowable tablets: The bulk of the supplement tablet market is in the form of film-coated tablets, made using directly compressible major ingredients.

Chewable tablets: These have become popular for the delivery of nutrients required in fairly large quantities (ie, hundreds of mg) and that have tastes acceptable or pleasant tastes.

Sustained-release tablets: These were developed to allow for the release of some micronutrients over a period of time rather than all at once in instances when this process is more effective. This is achieved by coating the particles of the nutrient with various thicknesses of a soluble coating.

Enteric-coated tablets: These tablets use coatings to delay the release of the active ingredient until an advanced stage of the digestive process and are favored for ingredients with a strong flavor such as garlic.
Multilayer tablets: These tablets are the state of the art in the pharmaceutical industry. Originally made to keep incompatible ingredients apart until they are digested by the consumer, they are now used because of their consumer appeal. The use of distinct layers to visually differentiate products (eg, vitamins and minerals) is visually attractive.

24.1.1.2 Capsules

These are a convenient method of carrying supplements in different forms, ie, powder, oil, oil-based suspension, or paste form. The main types include hard capsules and soft capsules as clarified following:

Hard capsules: A hard gelatin capsule shell has an advantage of masking the organoleptic properties of the active ingredients, which are generally filled with powders, granules, or specific oil-based suspensions. Minutes after swallowing, the shell disintegrates, releasing the active ingredients.
Soft capsules: Having the same advantages as hard capsules, soft capsules usually contain active ingredients in oil, oily suspension, or paste form, and thus are ideally suited for vitamins and other ingredients that naturally occur as oils.
Chewable capsules: These are a form of soft capsules that are made chewable by the addition of sweet additives.

24.1.1.3 Liquid Preparations

These preparations include syrups and water-based liquids, emulsions, and oil-based supplements. In general, syrups have been popular for many decades, mainly as vitamin products for children. Poor stability and microbial growth tend to be a problem in aqueous-based supplements, and rigorous stability tests are required in all new formulations. The less-common liquid forms are emulsions, which present a means of delivering a mixture of oil-soluble and water-soluble ingredients.

24.1.1.4 Powder Preparations

Most powdered supplements are intended to be mixed with water, milk, or fruit juice to make up a drink.

24.1.2 History of Use and Legislation

Legislation and establishment of certain criteria for the use of food supplements has been the subject of much debate over the past few years. In general, the main rule has been if a product claim is not substantiated with evidence that meets authority standards for efficacy in treating certain medical conditions, then it will not be licensed as a medicine and hence not allowed to be labeled with any medical claims.

Medicines law is not harmonized across the European Union (EU), and what may be freely sold in one EU member state as a food may be classified as medicinal in another EU member state. Recently, initial steps have been taken toward such harmonization but currently each state has its own regulations, which vary enormously from country to country. Prior to European harmonization, there are diverse regulations regarding the maximum permitted doses of vitamins and minerals that may be legally included in products available for over-the-counter sale as dietary supplements. The main aim for the European Commission (EC) will be to set maximum permitted levels of vitamins and minerals that can be present in products marketed as food supplements for general sale. An example for clarification involves vitamin C for which the EU recommended dietary allowance (RDA) is 60 mg, while it is legal to sell and buy such preparations containing 20 or more times this value in the United Kingdom (UK) and Sweden. On the contrary, in France, the general philosophy is that doses up to the RDA or a low multiple of it are regarded as foods but anything in excess of this is regarded as a medicine (Webb, 2006).

In the United Kingdom, the majority of food supplements are covered by food law, unless they have a medicinal effect or involve a medicinal claim including prevention, treatment, or curing any disease or medical condition. In such cases, they must be licensed under medicines legislation, which is the responsibility of the Medicines and Healthcare Products Regulatory Authority (MHRA). The EU Food Supplements Directive 2002/46 came into force on August 1, 2005, and is implemented in the United Kingdom by the Food Supplements (England) Regulations 2003 and equivalent regulations in Scotland, Wales, and Northern Ireland. The Regulations specify the vitamin and mineral substances permitted for use in food supplements and identify the units of measurement, labeling, presentation, and advertising allowed. It also defines food supplements as: "A concentrated source of a vitamin, mineral or other substance with a nutritional or physiological effect, alone, or in combination, sold in dose form." In the United Kingdom, responsibility for legislation on food supplements in England transferred from the Food Standards Agency to the Department of Health on October 1, 2010. With regard to herbal products, some herbal remedies are exempt from licensing if they consist solely of a dried or crushed part of the plant that is sold under its botanical name with no written recommendations for use on the packaging and provided they are made by a person who holds a special manufacturing license. Nowadays, they are regulated by the Traditional Herbal Medicines Directive, which is administered in the United Kingdom by the MHRA (Webb, 2006).

The regulation of dietary supplements in the United States is in many ways similar to that which existed in the United Kingdom prior to the influence of EU directives. Dietary supplements are regulated as foods rather than drugs by the US Food and Drug Administration (FDA). Unlike drugs, there is no requirement for manufacturers to show the efficacy of their product unless they make a specific health claim. The Dietary Supplement Health Education Act (DSHEA) of 1994 states that "Manufacturers and distributors of dietary supplements and dietary ingredients are prohibited from marketing products that are adulterated or misbranded. That means that these firms are responsible for evaluating the safety and labeling of their products before marketing to ensure that they meet all the requirements of DSHEA and FDA regulations.

FDA is responsible for taking action against any adulterated or misbranded dietary supplement product after it reaches the market." Consequently, it requires that manufacturers have evidence to support claims for nutritional support and the manufacturer may be required to include a disclaimer stating that the claim has not been evaluated by the FDA (Webb, 2006).

24.1.3 Production and Formulation

The quality of food supplements is not a trivial matter. Various concerns may arise in the preparation process such as absence of the active ingredients listed on the package or the precise amount and the identity of the active ingredients in the case of natural extracts. In the latter case, other doubts include the presence of potentially harmful contaminants and the bioavailability of the active ingredients. ConsumerLab.com is an independent testing organization in the United States, which has carried out very large numbers of product tests on dietary supplements for identity, strength, purity, and bioavailability. Further details of this testing together with sample results and some sample reports can be found on the ConsumerLab.com Website (Webb, 2006).

24.1.4 Health Benefits and Clinical Importance

The rationale behind the use of food supplements has always been to ensure adequacy of required nutritive essential elements and the prevention of deficiency diseases. In recent years, other purposes have evolved including the following: reduction of the risk of developing a chronic age-related disease such as cancer, heart disease, osteoporosis, or type 2 diabetes, boosting of the immune system, treating symptoms of clinical depression, boosting athletic and physical performance, or for general consumption during periods of pregnancy, illness, or old age. The following categories represent the main purposes for food supplement use:

24.1.4.1 Compensation for Diet Inadequacy

In general, nutrient deficiencies are uncommon in individuals who consume a variety of foods as well as enough food to satisfy their energy needs since different foods have different profiles of essential nutrients. A diverse diet also makes it less likely that any natural toxin or potentially toxic contaminants in some foods will be consumed in hazardous amounts. In some cases, individuals may have a perceived or potential inadequacy in their diet that leads to a specific nutrient deficiency as a result of a lower total amount of food eaten and/or the narrower range of foods selected. It is logical to assume that higher food consumption would lead to higher essential nutrient intake, although many individuals still suffer from inadequate intake of certain nutrients. Children, pregnant or lactating mothers, and the elderly tend to be at high risk of nutrient deficiency. Regarding nutrient requirements, the intake dose needed to prevent deficiency is quite modest and is generally safe.

24.1.4.2 Compensation for a Certain Nutrient

Some individuals may suffer from certain medical conditions that increase their need for certain nutrients. Examples include the following:

Pregnant women or women who are planning to conceive in the near future have been advised to take folic acid supplements to reduce the risk of neural tube defects in the baby appearing as spina bifida.

Pernicious anemia is an autoimmune disease that causes vitamin B12 deficiency due to a physiological defect that results in an inability to produce a gastric intrinsic factor necessary for its absorption. Regular injections of vitamin B12 are required to alleviate this condition.

Iron supplementation is commonly required in cases of substantial acute blood losses exemplified by heavy menstruation, internal bleeding, intestinal parasites, or even repeated pregnancies to reduce the risk of iron deficiency anemia.

Vitamin D supplement is required for elderly people and other individuals who are not regularly exposed to sunshine to reduce the risk of developing osteoporosis.

24.1.4.3 Treatment or Prevention of Nondeficiency Diseases

In this class of usage, there may be two apparent targets: (1) an acute benefit in cases when the supplement is used to alleviate certain symptoms, or (2) a long-term benefit. An example of the former includes women taking evening primrose oil to reduce the symptoms of premenstrual syndrome or reduce breast tenderness. An example of the alternative supplement usage that may take months or years to significantly make a difference is consumption of calcium supplements or eating foods with enhanced calcium levels when women are young to reduce the risk of osteoporosis fractures in old age.

24.1.4.4 Improvement of Athletic Performance

This subject is considered controversial since it may be acceptable to assume that heavy training may increase the requirement for nutrients and proteins, but on the other hand, if athletes are meeting their increased energy requirements for training, they should also be consuming more nutrients than the average, less active person. In turn, supplements are probably unnecessary and may sometimes even cause more problems than benefits.

24.1.5 Global Distribution, Value, and Pricing

In the United Kingdom, it was reported that, in the year 2000, just over one-third of UK men and nearly half of women said that they took dietary supplements and around three-quarters of these users said that they took them daily. In general, among all age groups, women are more prone to use supplements than men, and there is an increase in usage with age. Adverse publicity questioning supplements' efficacy or concerns about safety have always had a negative impact on sales. The estimated total UK market was worth around £355 million in 2000, about 8% less in real terms than the value of the market in 1996. UK sales dipped sharply in 1998 as a result of some negative publicity but seemed to recover gradually in 2001 (Webb, 2006).

National surveys of supplement use in the United States conclude that anywhere from 55% to 75% of the US population takes a vitamin or other dietary supplement. Americans spent $6.5 billion on dietary supplements in 1996, nearly doubling the 1990 total of $3.2 billion with a steady growth rate until 2004 (Hasler, 2005). The NBJ's Supplement Business Report of 2011 reported that the dietary supplement industry surpassed $30 billion in 2011; sales showed 7% annual growth representing $2 million in incremental sales in a year, indicating an increasing interest in supplementation amongst consumers as well as pharmaceutical buyers.

24.1.6 Impact on Society and Economy

Increased consumption of food supplements has been associated with many factors including the rise of health care costs and uncertainty in the health care system in some populations, which has led to a shift in consumer interest toward finding alternatives to solving health problems. Food supplements are perceived as safe, available, and effective in the long run and appear as attractive alternatives to the many classes of pharmaceuticals. However, the food supplement industry faces some challenges including new regulations and legislation imposed by national and international governing authorities to ensure good manufacturing practices and safety. These guidelines, as well as procedures for establishing concrete health claims in societies in which consumer awareness and availability of information is no longer an obstacle, may interfere with sales growth of these products. Another potential sales growth barrier is clinical substantiation especially when standard chemical fingerprints for the bioactive ingredients are absent as in the case of botanicals and multi-ingredient plant extracts. The vast range of supplements in the market usually leads to consumer inclination to cheaper brand products or buying from retail outlets and taking advantage of promotional offers or buying large packs, which consequently contributes to diminished sales growth. On the other hand, recent escalations of sales may be seen as a direct indication of positive consumer inclination toward supplementation.

24.2 Adulteration of Food Supplements

The purity and authenticity of food products and dietary supplements is regulated according to the Code of Federal Regulations under the regulatory authority of the FDA. According to federal regulations, an adulteration involves any component of a product whose identity is not as disclosed or whose quality is such that the material value of the product is compromised in any way in terms of quality, purity, or safety. A variety of adulteration methods are observed that reduce the value of the product and occur for different reasons. At the industrial level, good manufacturing practices (GMPs) in the production of dietary supplements are mandated by laws to help reduce the occurrence of adulteration, although this still remains a problem. Since the most common adulterations relate to the botanical types, the following section will mainly focus on herbal supplements and their adulteration (Upton et al., 2011).

24.2.1 Methods of Adulteration, Contamination, and Types of Adulterants

The many methods of adulteration of food supplements can be summarized as follows.

24.2.1.1 Botanical Substitution

This type of adulteration occurs mainly in the field as a result of poor identification by means of unskilled workers and collectors by which the intended plant may be substituted for another at the time of harvesting. Intentional substitution may include the admixture of other plants with no active constituents or even with exhausted plants. This type of adulteration may also include the addition of vegetable oil or mineral oil to oil-based supplements. The more expensive the product, the more it will be prone to substitution with less expensive substituents.

24.2.1.2 Incorporation of Impurities

The second most common form of adulteration is due to a variety of impurities ranging from dirt, mold, insects, and insect fragments through to the wrong plant part being mixed in with the desired portion. In general, natural products are not free of such foreign matter, but appropriate handling processes such as washing and garbling are implemented to minimize their presence. Specifications and limitations for most impurities are cited in pharmacopoeias.

24.2.1.3 Presence of Contaminants

In this case, natural products include additives ranging from yeasts, molds, and a variety of microbes to heavy metals as well as pesticide, herbicide, and fungicide residues. These contaminants not only represent another form of degradation but pose a health hazard as well.

24.2.1.4 Sophistication

Sophistication includes disguising products at suppliers level in various ways with the intention of making a large profit from cheap items. This may involve the use of dyes, forming different shapes of products using dough, or even spiking with cheap alternatives of ingredients to pass certain identification assays.

24.2.2 Examples of Reported Adulteration

A vast number of examples of adulteration of food supplements have been reported in the literature, mainly related to herbal products. An overview of recently reported examples is compiled in Tables 24.1–24.3 which present the matrix adulterated, the adulterant, and methods of detection.

Other examples, including reports that had a greater impact on society, are presented in this section. In 2003 dietary supplements labeled as ephedra free and sold in the San Francisco Bay area were found by the Food and Drug Laboratory of the

Table 24.1 Applications of Different Chromatographic Techniques in Food Supplement Authentication

Matrix	Adulterant	Method Utilized	References
Ixeris laevigata var. Oldhami	*Ixeris chinensis* and *Taraxacum formosanum*	HPLC-UV	Lu et al. (2000)
Soft drinks containing Cornus fruit extract (*Cornus mas*)	Phentolamine and sildenafil	TLC, LC-MS, HPLC-PDA	Mikami et al. (2002)
Dietary supplement capsule claimed to contain an extract of animal organs and traditional Chinese herbs and indicated for enhancing sexual activity	Sildenafil citrate	LC-MS/MS	Tseng and Lin (2002)
Ginkgo biloba	Colchicine	HPLC-UV/VIS	Petty et al. (2001)
	Rutin, quercetin	HPLC-PDA, LC-MS	Sloley et al. (2003), Harnly et al. (2012), Demirezer et al. (2014)
		HPLC-PDA, LC-MS, GCMS	van Beek and Montoro (2009)
Burdock root tea (*Arctium lappa*)	Atropine	GCMS	Rhoads et al. (1984)
Valerian, St. John's wort, Passion flower, Echinacea	Organochlorine pesticides	GC	Huggett et al. (2001)
Yohimbe extract	Caffeine, *Podophyllum hexandrum*	TLC, HPLC	De Smet and Smeets (1994)
Scutellaria lateriflora	*Teucrium canadense* and *T. chamaedrys*	LC-UV/MS, TLC	Gafner et al. (2003)

Continued

Table 24.1 Applications of Different Chromatographic Techniques in Food Supplement Authentication—cont'd

Matrix	Adulterant	Method Utilized	References
Traditional Indonesian herbal product Serbuk Jarem (Encok)	Phenylbutazone, caffeine, and oxyphenbutazone	LC-MS/MS	Lau et al. (2003)
Composition: *Myristicae semen, Blumeae folium, Kaemferiae rhizoma, Curcumae rhizoma, Retrofracti fructus*			
Dietary supplements used as weight reducers containing an extract of animal organs and traditional herbs	Thyroxine	LC-MS	Mikami et al. (2003)
Flos carthami	*Stigma croci*, and *Flos hemerocallis*	CE	Sun et al. (2003)
Achyranthes bidentata	*Cyathula officinalis* and *Strobilanthes forrestii*	HPLC	Ku et al. (2004)
Illicium verum	*Illicium anisatum*	GC	Joshi et al. (2005)
Chinese herbal capsules "Yong Gang"	Tadalafil, sildenafil	LC-MS/MS	Bogusz et al. (2006)
Chinese herbal capsules "Vigorous"	Sildenafil	LC-MS/MS	Bogusz et al. (2006)
Herbal capsules "Phyto Andro"	Sildenafil	LC-MS/MS	Bogusz et al. (2006)
Instant herbal powder "XKL"	Sildenafil	LC-MS/MS	Bogusz et al. (2006)
Herbal powder "Jamu Ragel" from Indonesia	Phenylbutazone, dipyrone	LC-MS/MS	Bogusz et al. (2006)
Chinese herbal drug for weight loss (LiDa Dai Dai Hua Jiao Nang)	Sibutramine	GCMS, HPLC-PDA	Jung et al. (2006)
Herbal product (Sensitex)	Tadalafil	LC-MS/MS	Zou et al. (2006a,b)

Dietary supplement named "Oyster plus"	Tadalafil	LC-MS/MS	Zou et al. (2006a,b)
Black cohosh	*Cimicifuga foetida, Cimicifuga heracleifolia, Cimicifuga dahurica, Cimicifuga americana*	HPTLC	Ankli et al. (2008)
		HPLC. LC/MS	Jiang et al. (2011), Masada-Atsumi et al. (2014)
Royal jelly	Yogurt, water, egg white, sweet condensed milk mixed with propolis, unripe banana, and corn starch slurry	HPLC-UV	Garcia-Amoedo and de Almeida-Muradian (2007)
Ginseng	Different cultivation age	GC/MS	Park et al. (2013), Yang et al. (2012)
Cassia bark (cortex *cinnamomi*) *Cinnamomum cassia*	*Cinnamomum wilsonii, Cinnamomum japonicum, Cinnamomum mairei* and *Cinnamomum burmanii*	HPLC	He et al. (2005)
Psoralea corylifolia	*P. corylifolia* from different localities	HPLC and LC-MS	Zhao et al. (2005)
Chamomile (*Matricaria chamomilla*)	*Anthemis nobilis, Matricaria aurea and Inula vestita*	TLC	Ahmad et al. (2009), Wang et al. (2004)
Scutellaria baicalensis	*Teucrium chamaedrys*	HPTLC	Hong et al. (2009)
Onosma hispida	*Geranium wallichianum*	TLC	Ahmad et al. (2010)
Gold Nine soft capsules composed of Chinese Caterpillar Fungus, Garter Snake, Monascus anka, Earthworm, Barbary Wolfberry fruit, common Yam Rhizome, Spina Date Seed, Dahurian Angelica root, Nutmeg, Tangerine Peel, Salad oil	Amlodipine, indapamide and valsartan	LC−HRMS and LC−MS−SPE/NMR	Kesting et al. (2010)

Continued

Table 24.1 Applications of Different Chromatographic Techniques in Food Supplement Authentication—cont'd

Matrix	Adulterant	Method Utilized	References
dietary supplements containing *Citrus aurantium* fruits	Synephrine, octopamine and tyramine	CE	Mercolini et al. (2010)
Dietary supplement MEGATON	A novel analogue of vardenafil	HPLC-PDA	Lee et al. (2011)
Red yeast rice products	Lovastatin	HPLC-PDA	Song et al. (2011)
Cod liver oil	Beef fat	GC-FID	Rohman and Man (2011)
Bupleurum chinense roots	*Aristolochia manshuriensis* roots	LC-MS, NMR	Rueda et al. (2012)
Isatis indigotica	*Baphicacanthis cusiae*	UPLC-PDA	Shi et al. (2012)
Dietary supplements composed of *Panax Ginseng, Tribulus terrestris, Rhodiola rosea, and Lepidium meyenii*	Sildenafil thio derivative	UPLC–TOF/MS and GC/MS	Damiano et al. (2014)
Gymnema sylvestre	Flavonoids rutin, quercetin, and kaempferol	HPLC-PDA and LC-MS/MS	Satheeshkumar et al. (2014)
Multivitamin supplement (Parabolon-S and Stanozolon-S)	Anabolic steroids Metandienone and stanozolol	GCMS, HPLC-PDA, LC-MS	Geyer et al. (2008)
Fish oil	Organochlorine pesticide	GCMS	Jacobs et al. (1998)

Table 24.2 Applications of Different Spectroscopic Techniques in Food Supplement Authentication

Matrix	Adulterant	Method Utilized	References
Echinacea purpurea	*Echinacea angustifolia, Echinacea pallida, or Parthenium integrifolium*	NIR	Laasonen et al. (2002)
Dietary supplements used as weight reducers containing an extract of animal organs and traditional herbs	Thyroxine	ELISA	Mikami et al. (2003)
Dietary supplement oil (olive oil)	Soya oil, sun flower oil, corn oil, walnut oil and hazelnut oil	FT-IR, NIR	Downey et al. (2002), Ozen et al. (2003), Christy et al. (2004)
Ginseng	Sawdust and *Platycodon grandiflorum*	IR	Yap et al. (2007)
	Other *Panax ginseng* species	2D-NMR	Kang et al. (2008)
	Panax quinquefolius	MALDI-MS	Lai et al. (2012)
	Different cultivation age	NMR	Park et al. (2013), Yang et al. (2012)
Herbal medicines and dietary supplements for weight loss	Sibutramine, phenolphthalein, synephrine	1H, 2D-NMR	Vaysse et al. (2010)

Continued

Table 24.2 Applications of Different Spectroscopic Techniques in Food Supplement Authentication—cont'd

Matrix	Adulterant	Method Utilized	References
Fish oil capsules	Trout, salmon, and cod oils	13C-NMR	Aursand et al. (2007)
Cod liver oil	Beef fat	FT-IR	Rohman and Man (2011)
Food supplements containing pure L-leucine	Discriminating between plant and animal sources	Elemental analyzer which was connected to an isotope ratio mass spectrometer	Huang et al. (2013)
Cynanchum stauntonii	*Cynanchum atrati, Cynanchum paniculati*	NIR	Dong et al. (2012)
Cortex Phellodendri	*Caulis mahoniae* and David poplar bark	SP-EE-F	Gu et al. (2012)
Thymus vulgaris	Other *Thymus*, *Satureja*, *Origanum*, *Plectranthus*, and *Eriocephalus* species	UV	Gad et al. (2013)
Angelicae Sinensis	*Levisticum officinale*	1H, COSY NMR	Li et al. (2015)

Table 24.3 Applications of Different DNA Profiling Techniques in Food Supplement Authentication

Matrix	Adulterant	Method Utilized	References
Tea (*Camellia sinensis*)	Cashew husk (*Anacardium occidentale*)	PCR	Dhiman and Singh (2003)
Stellaria media	*Myosoton aquaticum*	PCR	Huang et al. (2005)
Angelica decursiva (*Peucedanum decursivum*)	*Peucedanum praeruptorum* and *Anthricus sylvestris*	RAPD	Choo et al. (2009)
Cordyceps sinensis	*Cordyceps gunnii*	ITS	Chan et al. (2011)
Zingiber officinale	*Zingiber montanum and Zingiber zerumbet*	AFLP	Ghosh et al. (2011)
Tripterygium wilfordii	*Tripterygium regelii*	ITS	Law et al. (2011)
Clematis armandii, *Clematis montana*	Other species	RAPD and SCAR	Guo et al. (2010)
Cistanches herba (*Cistanche deserticola* and *Cistanche tubulosa*)	*Orobanche pycnostachya, Orobanche coerulescens, Boschniakia rossica, Cistanche salsa, Cistanche sinensis*, and *Cynomorium songaricum*	ITS	Sun et al. (2012)
Herba dendrobii	*Pholidota articulata and Flickingeria comate*	ITS	Wu et al. (2012)

Continued

Table 24.3 Applications of Different DNA Profiling Techniques in Food Supplement Authentication—cont'd

Matrix	Adulterant	Method Utilized	References
Ginseng	Other *Panax ginseng* species	RAPD, PCR-RFLP	Um et al. (2001), Diao et al. (2009)
	P. quinquefolius	DALP	Ha et al. (2001)
Boerhavia diffusa	*Trianthema portulacastrum* and *Trianthema monogyna*	PCR-RFLP	Biswas et al. (2013)
Gentiana scabra, *Gentiana manshurica*, *Gentiana triflora*, and *Gentiana rigescens*	*Podophyllum hexandrum* and *Gentiana rhodantha*	DNA barcodes using different spacers	Wong et al. (2013)
Stephania tetrandra	*Aristolochia fangchi*	DNA barcodes using matK, rbcL, trnH-psbA and trnL-trnF	Li et al. (2014)
Akebia quinata *Akebia trifoliata* *Akebia trifoliata* var. *australis*	*Aristolochia manshuriensis*	DNA barcodes using matK, rbcL, trnH-psbA and trnL-trnF multiplex-PCR	Li et al. (2014), Moon et al. (2015)
Aucklandia lappa	*Aristolochia debilis*	DNA barcodes using matK, rbcL, trnH-psbA and trnL-trnF	Li et al. (2014)

California Department of Health Services to contain significant concentrations of lead, arsenic, cadmium, and mercury.

Adulteration of Chinese herbal medicines (CHMs) poses a serious problem on many levels. The incorporation of synthetic drugs with known pharmacological activity, such as steroids, with the intention of increasing therapeutic efficacy, is one major problem and can lead to potentially serious adverse effects. An analysis of over 2609 Chinese herbal products prescribed in Taiwanese hospitals found that more than one-half contained between two and five synthetic drugs, while four samples contained at least six including NSAIDs, steroids, and analgesics (Huang et al., 1997). Other substances included phenylbutazone, phenytoin, glibenclamide, corticosteroids, chlorpropamide, fenfluramine, and indomethacin. To further underline the magnitude of this example, one reported case relates to a 56-year-old man from Indonesia who was admitted to an Australian hospital for hypoglycemia. Even though he insisted that his type 2 diabetes was controlled by diet only, it was discovered that he also took "Zhen Qi," a Traditional Chinese Medicine that was analyzed to reveal it contained glibenclamide (Huang et al., 1997). This type of adulteration has been the cause of many fatalities and life-threatening events. As recently as 2010, 336 out of 390 warnings for herbal products issued by regulatory authorities in the United Kingdom, the United States, Canada, Singapore, and Australia were directly due to a pharmaceutical contamination or adulteration (Roytas, 2015).

Substituting an effective ingredient with a much cheaper chemical component is another common practice. The requirements for *Ginkgo biloba* dietary supplements state that the commercial product must contain 24% Ginkgo flavonoids and 6% terpene lactones (ginkgolides and bilobalide). Since only total and not individual flavonoids were assessed, the addition of rutin and quercetin to the extract was a common adulteration procedure performed to ensure compliance with the relevant standard. In addition, organochlorine pesticide residues were detected in a number of Chinese herbal plants sold in Hong Kong (Fu and Xia, 2014).

24.3 Methods of Adulterant Detection

Food supplements represent a major target of adulteration of foods and pharmaceuticals worldwide. The absence of regulatory authorities, strict regulations and laws together with a scarcity of robust and reliable analytical methods to check compliance are the main causes for this problem (Vlietinck et al., 2009). Although many herbal products, nonessential fatty acids, and multivitamins are included as dietary supplements in many international pharmacopoeias and many plant monographs have been released, yet the majority of these food supplements have not been fully reported (Upton, 2011; Indian Pharmacopoeia Commission, 2010; British Pharmacopoeia Commission, 2009; Japanese Pharmacopoeia Commission, 2006; Pharmacopoeia of the People's Republic of China Commission 2005; European Pharmacopoeia Commission, 2004; Wagner and Ulrich-Merzenich, 2013; Wagner et al., 2011).

In most cases, profiling of dietary and food supplements is accomplished either by chromatographic or spectroscopic methods. However, when herbal supplements are included, microscopic examination and DNA barcoding may also be included. It is important to mention that the scope of this chapter is not to cite all the work done relating to concept validation or authentication of food supplements but rather to shed light on the most relevant work related to each technique. The main criteria used were the presence of the name of the dietary supplement and or its composition.

24.3.1 Chromatographic Techniques

Generally, the most widely used analytical approach involved in the analyses of food supplements is a combination of two chromatographic methods. Among these, thin-layer chromatography (TLC), high-performance liquid chromatography combined with ultraviolet (HPLC-UV) or photo diode array (PDA) or mass spectrometry (LC-MS), gas chromatography combined with mass spectrometry (GC-MS), or capillary electrophoresis (CE) are most commonly used (Jiang et al., 2010).

24.3.1.1 High-Performance Thin-Layer Chromatography

High-performance thin-layer chromatography (HPTLC) represents a more efficient form of normal TLC in which application of the samples, scanning and visualization of the spots are fully automated. Nevertheless, it is one of the simplest, low-cost, versatile, and specific methods that can be applied for the authentication of food supplements including herbal drugs (Srivastava, 2011; Upton, 2010). Generally, it is the method of choice when the mixture is not complicated and the components are of moderate to low polarity.

With HPTLC, Wagner et al. (2011) provided an in-depth analysis of over 100 Chinese plants that are not only used for their medicinal values but also as food supplements. Additionally, the American herbal Pharmacopoeia Association released about 25 monographs of many plants that are used as supplements. TLC was the principal method used in authentication of these valuable herbs (Upton, 1999a,b,c,d,e,f, 2000a,b,c,d, 2001a,b,c, 2002a,b, 2003a,b, 2004, 2007a,b, 2008, 2009, 2010a,b,c, 2012a,b; Romm and Upton, 2012). Inspired by early work, authentication of various species of famous food supplements such as Chamomile, Ginseng, Ginkgo, black Cohosh, and *Radix Puerariae* and *Scutellaria* as well as measurement of the consistency of their preparations became possible (van Beek and Montoro, 2009; Ankli et al., 2008; Ahmad et al., 2009; Wang et al., 2004; Hong et al., 2009; Xie et al., 2006; Chen et al., 2006).

Additionally, both TLC and HPTLC provide a useful tool with high sensitivity, better separation and reproducibility not only for the detection of adulteration with different species but also by other synthetic compounds. One of the most common adulterants is the use of the phosphodiesterase inhibitor sildenafil and its analogues in many food supplements including soft drinks containing the *Cornus* fruits extract or other dietary supplements marketed to address problems of sexual impotence. It is important to mention that the TLC technique was able to qualitatively detect the presence of these adulterants with similar accuracy as other more sophisticated techniques including LC/MS (Mikami et al., 2002; Cai et al., 2010). Adulteration of many slimming herbal supplements with sibutramine was also detected efficiently by this technique. However, the limited source of details on the product ingredients limits accurate analysis and justifiable detection results (Mathon et al., 2014; Phattanawasin et al., 2012; Chen et al., 2010).

24.3.1.2 Gas Chromatography–Coupled Techniques

The methods of choice for detection and quantitation of relatively low-molecular-weight organic compounds is GC and GC-MS for analysis of volatile constituents. This chromatographic technique exhibits a strong sensitivity, stability, and high efficiency for this class of secondary metabolites. Coupling with mass spectrometry reduces somewhat the analytical sensitivity compared to other GC detectors but still provides reliable data about the composition of mixtures (Wittkowski and Matissek, 1993; Carlin and Dean, 2013; Sparkman et al., 2011).

Among the most common application of the GC-MS technique, detection of organochloride pesticides in Valerian, Echinacea, and Passion flower represents a good illustration of this technique (Huggett et al., 2001) that was also employed for fish oil (Jacobs et al., 1998). Another good example is detection of beef fat adulteration of cod liver oil (Rohman and Man, 2011) or sibutramine in a Chinese herbal drug for weight loss (Jung et al., 2006).

Recently, many new efficient sample preparation methods have been developed. Among them, solid-phase microextraction (SPME), headspace microextraction (HME), headspace solid-phase microextraction (HS-SPME), and microextraction coupled with pressurized hot water extraction (PHWE) or microwave-assisted extraction (MAE) are the most known procedures (Jiang et al., 2010). These have permitted detection and characterization of many compounds in the picogram level even without the use of organic solvents. Additionally, derivatization of the relatively nonvolatile compounds in Gingko and Ginseng enable the determination of panaxoside and other Gingko flavonoids and determination of their cultivation age (van Beek and Montoro, 2009; Park et al., 2013).

24.3.1.3 High-Performance Liquid Chromatography–Coupled Techniques

This is the most common and reliable analytical tool used officially worldwide. With its wide range of applications and accuracy, it has become the easiest method in daily routine use for detection of adulteration of food supplements and herbal drugs (Wagner et al., 2011; Cai et al., 2012; Waksmundzka-Hajnos and Sherma, 2011; Ahuja and Rasmussen, 2007). Availability of a wide range of detectors capable of being coupled to HPLC allows for determination and quantitation of different food supplement components, and consequently it can be used in detection of possible adulterations.

For instance, analysis by HPLC-UV of flavonoid and coumarin content in *Ixeris laevigata*, a common folk medicine plant in Taiwan, allowed detection of adulteration by other species, ie, *Ixeris chinensis*, based on variation in content of four flavonoids, apigenin, apigenin-7-*O*-glucoside, luteolin, and luteolin-7-*O*-glucoside, and two coumarins, esculetin and esculin (Lu et al., 2000).

In the same context, many adulterants (mainly synthetic flavonoids) were detected in several Ginkgo and *Gymnema sylvestre* herbal preparations (Sloley et al., 2003; Demirezer et al., 2014; Satheeshkumar et al., 2014). In these cases, rutin and other synthetic flavonoids were detected at high levels indicating intentional addition.

However, application of HPLC was not limited to herbal products only. It was also used successfully to detect adulteration of Megaton (a food supplement) with a novel analogue of vardenafil (Lee et al., 2011), and the presence of the synthetic antihypercholesterolemia drug lovastatin in a red yeast rice product (Song et al., 2011).

Introduction of mass spectrometry as a hyphenated technique coupled with HPLC allowed better understanding of the nature of detected adulterants by obtaining information about their molecular weight and hence their chemical identity. This approach was used efficiently to detect anabolic steroids methandienone and stanozolol in multivitamin preparations (Geyer et al., 2008). Adulteration of the famous Chinese plant *Bupluerum* with the GABA(A) receptor modulator aristolactone from the nephrotoxic *Aristolochia manshuriensis* (Rueda et al., 2012) and detection of the PDA analogue tadalafil in a herbal product (Sensitex) and the dietary supplement "Oyster Plus" was also detected with this method (Zou et al., 2006a,b).

In the last decade, with the increasing demand for shortened analysis time, collection of more qualitative data on composition of the whole mixture, reduction of analytical running time, and minimization of the cost of solvent usage and disposal, a modified technique has emerged (Xu, 2013; Guillarme and Veuthey, 2012). Ultra-performance liquid chromatography (UPLC) provides an ultra-fast and precise tool that can be used to detect adulteration of sildenafil thio-derivatives in dietary supplements (Damiano et al., 2014).

As in GC-coupled techniques, sample preparation strategies have also developed considerably. In all cases, the main goal is to reduce sample size and improve reproducibility of the extraction method. Among the strategies developed, microwave-assisted extraction coupled with single-drop microextraction allows, eg, determination of trace synthetic estrogen adulterants in soybean isoflavone dietary supplements (Xiao et al., 2010).

24.3.1.4 Capillary Electrophoresis

Capillary electrophoresis is an effective analytical tool that can be used for rapid and efficient food supplement separation and authentication based on differences in electrophoretic progress as components migrate or move through narrow-bore capillary tubes. There are several variants of the CE procedure that differ in the driving force separating ions, but, due to the high cost, poor sensitivity, and the complexity of this procedure, there are no reports related to the detection of adulteration in food supplements.

Mercolini et al. (2010) were able to use a fast-CE analysis method to detect adrenergic amines in *Citrus aurantium* fruits and dietary supplements (Mercolini et al., 2010) while Sun and his coworkers recorded a fingerprint analysis of *Flos Carthami* by capillary electrophoresis to detect *Stigma Croci*, and *Flos Hemerocallis* (Sun et al., 2003).

It is worth mentioning that, as most food supplements are present as multicomponent mixtures, many tedious purification and fractionation steps to resolve these complex mixtures and allow their profiling are required. This might lead to the loss of certain key secondary metabolites, which may contribute in the overall bioactivity of these supplements. Therefore, most of these profiling methods are based on selection of certain markers to detect the presence of adulterants rather than characterization of the complex matrix. Additionally, the qualitative and quantitative analyses of food supplements containing this large number of components are a great challenge as compared to their synthetic counterparts because food supplements are mixtures of various components embedded in a natural matrix, and in most cases the compositions of these mixtures are either unknown or not clear. Consequently, sample preparation for analysis of these products will mostly require complex processing because the substances to be analyzed must be separated from a matrix, which is subject to natural variations. This requirement adds further sources of error and results in larger uncertainty in the methods than corresponding analyses of isolated active substances.

24.3.2 Spectroscopic Techniques

Spectroscopic techniques are not only coupled with other chromatographic techniques but could work as stand-alone tools for authentication of food supplements. There are many spectral methods used widely in the quality control of food supplements, such as Fourier-transform infrared spectroscopy (FT-IR), near-infrared (NIR), ultraviolet (UV), and nuclear magnetic resonance (NMR). Most of these techniques are simple, rapid, relatively cheap and require little or no prepreparation of the food samples. Jiang et al. (2010) summarized most of the relevant work carried out on the quality control of herbal drugs using spectroscopic techniques. Here we include most of the work done related to quality control of food supplements as well.

24.3.2.1 Fourier-Transform Infrared Spectroscopy

FT-IR mainly measures functional groups of the chemical constituents in a sample but it has been used widely for the identification, quality control, and supervision of the manufacturing process of food supplements and chemicals. Additionally, the fingerprint region of the IR spectrum may be used to detect adulteration of the main supplement. Using this technique, discrimination of plants from different habitats, manufacturers, and species has been reported as well as testing for adulteration of herbal medicines by inclusion of synthetic drugs.

Using this tool, it was possible to detect adulteration of Ginseng by sawdust and *Platycodon grandiflorum* via spectral differences and principal component analysis (PCA) of their infrared spectra (Yap et al., 2007); detection of adulteration of the dietary supplement olive oil with sunflower oil, soya oil, corn oil, walnut oil, and hazelnut oil has also been reported (Downey et al., 2002; Ozen et al., 2003). Additionally, adulteration of cod liver oil by beef fat was also detected (Rohman and Man, 2011).

24.3.2.2 Near-Infrared Spectroscopy

Compared to FT-IR, NIR spectroscopy has a higher precision and involves easier sample preparation. As a result, in recent years there has been an increasing trend toward the use of NIR for the qualitative and quantitative analysis of pharmaceutical products and raw materials (Workman and Weyer, 2008; Ciurczak and Drennen, 2002; Ozaki et al., 2007; Burns and Ciurczak, 2008). However, the limitation of NIR is that specific models for quantitation have to be established before analysis of test samples, and the time required for model development can be long.

By the NIR technique, Dong et al. (2012) were able to detect adulteration of *Cynanchum stauntonii* by both *Cynanchum atratum* and *Cynanchum paniculatum*, adulteration of olive oil by other vegetable oils (Downey et al., 2002), discriminate between different *Echinaceae* species (Laasonen et al., 2002), distinguish between different geographical varieties of *Paeonia lactiflora* (Lau et al., 2009), and to detect the adulteration of *Cortex Phellodendri* (Chan et al., 2007).

24.3.2.3 Nuclear Magnetic Resonance Spectroscopy

NMR represents perhaps one of the newest techniques applied to detect food authentication. The considerable cost of the instrumentation and consumables will undoubtedly limit their use to certain laboratories; this limitation is the main reason for the presence of only a few reports concerning the application of NMR to authentication of food supplements (Sun, 2008).

Among successful examples using NMR as an efficient tool in authentication of different *Ginseng* samples, Kang et al. were able to discriminate ginseng roots from various sources. Six different types of ginseng roots from China and Korea were analyzed by NMR-based metabolomics, and differentiation was based mainly on the large signals in the sugar region of the NMR spectrum. This approach was able to detect the adulteration of ginseng root powders and other herbal products from different origins (Kang et al., 2008). Recently, it was applied to determination of the origin not only of *Ginseng* samples but also to ago, the falsification of which represents a serious problem in the industry (Yang et al., 2012).

The same technique was used to analyze different types of *Danggui* (Li et al., 2015) while Chinese *Angelica* was found to contain higher levels of alanine, γ-aminobutyrate, adenosine, arginine, sucrose, α-glucose, β-glucose, tryptophan, and *cis*-Z,Z′-3a.7a′,7a.3a′-dihydroxyligustilide than European species.

Another good example of the application of high-resolution NMR spectroscopy pattern recognition in conjunction with multivariate analysis is in relation to commercial fish oil—related food products (Aursand et al., 2007). These tools have been used to provide a discrimination based on the nature, composition, refinement, and/or adulteration or authentication of the products. Based on this method, trout, salmon, and cod oils were completely and correctly classified.

24.3.2.4 Ultraviolet—Visible Spectroscopy

Ultraviolet—visible spectroscopy (UV—Vis) represents the oldest, and the simplest, method used in food authentication. However, in most cases it is coupled with other techniques such as HPLC, which were mentioned before (Section 24.3.1.3.). Nevertheless, rare reports about the application of UV–Vis technique as a rapid and cheap tool that can be used as daily routine work in authentication of herbal products or food supplements do exist.

Gad et al. (2013) used this technique alone to distinguish between different *Thymus* species and between thyme and many other common adulterants such as *Satureja*, *Origanum*, *Plectranthus*, and *Eriocephalus* species. The model was also able to classify closely related species in clusters using multivariate analysis of PCA and hierarchal cluster analysis (Gad et al., 2013).

If we were to draw some conclusions from this overview and point out significant factors that should be taken into consideration during the process of adulterant testing in food supplements, sample number is definitely an important aspect. In testing for adulteration in *Ginkgo biloba* supplements, the fingerprints of 18 commercially available supplements, 12 samples of raw *G. biloba* leaves and three *G. biloba* reference materials were analyzed in one study (Demirezer et al., 2014) and eight samples in a more recent one (van Beek and Montoro, 2009). The larger sample number accounts for more variability and produces more robust results from a statistical point of view. In another study developed for the detection of most common synthetic adulterants in herbal remedies using LC-ESI-MS-MS, 80 drugs belonging to various pharmacological classes were included in the study (Bogusz et al., 2006). In a highly acclaimed study conducted to establish levels of organochlorine residues in fish oils, 44 samples were collected from 15 countries between 1994 and 1995, including 38 purchased over the counter as dietary supplements (Jacobs et al., 1998). A study on the adulteration of olive oil reported the analysis of 138 oil samples comprising 46 pure extra virgin olive oils and the same oils adulterated with sunflower oil; these were analyzed by visible and NIR transflectance spectroscopy (Downey et al., 2002). Whether the testing is using chromatograms and areas of various peaks pertaining to different components or spectral data, multivariate analysis is a powerful technique and can be built on in future analyses.

The use of more than one chemical marker is also a valuable attribute to the analytical approach in testing for adulteration specifically in herbal products. In a study developed to distinguish black cohosh products from other similar species, the phytochemical fingerprints of 15 of these samples were established using HPLC-PDA and LC-MS techniques. Two marker compounds were used and were relevant to distinguish authentic black cohosh from most adulterants in commercially available black cohosh products (Jiang et al., 2011). In other studies, such as in case of Ginseng (Park et al., 2013), several biochemical metabolites were measured and used as statistical variables in multivariate models.

Another valid approach is to apply more than one method of testing—usually a chromatographic analysis together with one spectroscopic procedure or another fingerprinting technique such as genetic profiling. In case of herbal supplements, it is quite common to perform botanical authentication of the products in addition to a chemical investigation, which supports the procedure of adulteration testing. In a study performed to test and identify adulterants of black cohosh, metabolic profiling of 25 black cohosh products using LC-MS/MS followed genetic identification of the samples; adulterants were distinguished using three marker compounds

(Masada-Atsumi et al., 2014). In another study, the authentication of chamomile was performed using TLC, SEM, light microscopy, organoleptic procedures, UV, and IR analyses (Ahmad et al., 2010). In a study aimed to authenticate cod liver oil from beef fat by determining the level of the latter as a fat adulterant, gas chromatography with flame ionization detector (GC-FID) for fatty acid analysis, and FT-IR spectroscopy were exploited (Rohman and Man, 2011).

24.4 Global Agencies and Authorities Responsible for Drug and Food Supplement Safety

The Codex Alimentarius Commission was created in 1962 by two United Nations organizations, the Food and Agricultural Organization of the United Nations (FAO) and the World Health Organization (WHO), as an intergovernmental body to implement the Joint FAO/WHO Food Standards Program. Codex comprises more than 150 member countries and international organizations that meet and exchange information and ideas related to food safety and trade issues. Currently, Codex Alimentarius contains more than 200 standards, including topics such as labeling, additives, methods of analysis and sampling, food import and export inspection and certification, pesticides in foods, and contaminants. The code also deals with nutrition and foods for special dietary uses, which includes dietary supplements (Bagchi, 2014).

In the case of herbal supplements, standards of quality and identification are codified in national and international pharmacopoeias, which contain a list of medicinal drugs along with their uses, preparations, and dosages. Various herbal medicinal preparations are given the authority of law by governments of countries in which herbal products are used therapeutically and must be manufactured according to a very specific set of standards outlined by the national pharmacopoeia. For purity standards, assays and tests are provided and include a measure of foreign matter, ash content, loss of moisture upon drying, sometimes extractive matter, and occasionally other specifications. In the case of quality, the pharmacopoeias require a minimum amount of a specific constituent in the plant material that is associated with its biological activity.

The EC has passed few laws incorporating functional foods and drugs but not until recently has legislation been established to include most of the member states, which had their own regulations that varied from one country to another. The most recent legislation established in the area of food supplements passed by the EC was Directive 2002/46, which defines certain products and represents a first step in the harmonization process as it focuses only on vitamins and minerals.

In the United States, the FDA has substantial policing powers with respect to the regulation of dietary supplement products and their ingredients. In 1994 Congress passed the DSHEA, which governs most of the regulations pertaining to food supplements. The new law was a compromise not including all the restraints on FDA regulation of dietary supplements but imposed some significant new requirements for such products. However, all dietary ingredients in food supplements and ingredients that were not marketed prior to October 15, 1994, must be the subject of a notification to the FDA, documenting safety, to be submitted at least 75 days before marketing begins. On the other hand, FDA has the primary regulatory jurisdiction over the manufacture of botanical supplements and botanical drugs. GMPs mandated by law to be used in the manufacture of botanical dietary supplements override the issue of authenticity, purity, and quality to the extent of preventing any form of adulteration. In this context, manufacturers do not need to register their products with the FDA nor get FDA approval before producing or selling food supplements but must make sure that product label information is correct and not misleading. Postmarketing, the FDA is responsible for monitoring safety, eg, voluntary dietary supplement adverse event reporting and product information, such as labeling, claims, package inserts, and accompanying literature.

The International Alliance of Dietary Food Supplement Associations (IADSA) was created in 1998 and has developed into an alliance of more than 50 dietary supplement associations spread over six continents, which currently includes more than 9500 companies. IADSA works closely with international bodies such as Codex Alimentarius, WHO, and FAO to ensure that the views of the dietary supplement industry are taken into account in the development of relevant policies (Bagchi, 2014).

24.5 Future Perspectives

In an ongoing growing industry such as pharmaceuticals, in which some of the main concerns are quality control, efficacy, and safety, rigid and reliable bases for standardization are necessary. Scientific literature contains numerous references to the determination of various ingredients of food supplements such as vitamins, minerals, herbal products, and others, using different techniques. Many of these methods, either singly or coupled to other techniques, are of some concern due to a lack of selectivity or are recognized as complicated and tedious procedures requiring expensive instrumentation or hazardous reagents. Therefore, improvements in sensitivity and selectivity of these methods and combined techniques are still required. Another critical fact is the standardization of herbal supplements, especially multi-ingredient products, in which elucidation of reference markers for each ingredient remains a problem. With advances in multivariate analysis, scientists are now able to take into account different variables responsible for inconsistency in plant extracts allowing for better standardization procedures. It is hoped that these developing measures along with growing databases that include references on various plant bioactive markers will allow for improved and more accurate analyses, procedures and results.

References

Ahmad, M., Ajabkhan, M., Zafar, M., Hasan, A., Sultana, S., Shah, G.M., et al., 2009. Chemotaxonomic authentication of herbal drug chamomile. Asian Journal of Chemistry 21, 3395–3410.

Ahmad, M., Khan, M.A., Zafar, M., Arshad, M., Sultana, S., Abbasi, B.H., et al., 2010. Use of chemotaxonomic markers for misidentified medicinal plants used in traditional medicines. Journal of Medicinal Plants Research 4, 1244–1252.

Ahuja, S.H., Rasmussen, 2007. HPLC Method Development for Pharmaceuticals, first ed. In: Separation Science and Technology. Elsevier, Academic Press, Amsterdam, Boston.

Ankli, A., Reich, E., Steiner, M., 2008. Rapid high-performance thin-layer chromatographic method for detection of 5% adulteration of black cohosh with *Cimicifuga foetida*, *C. heracleifolia*, *C. dahurica*, or *C. americana*. Journal of AOAC International 91, 1257–1264.

Aursand, M., Standal, I.B., Axelson, D.E., 2007. High-resolution (13)C nuclear magnetic resonance spectroscopy pattern recognition of fish oil capsules. Journal of Agricultural and Food Chemistry 55, 38–47.

Bagchi, D., 2014. Nutraceutical and Functional Food Regulations in the United States and Around the World, second ed. Elsevier, AP, Amsterdam, Boston.

Biswas, K., Kapoor, A., Biswas, R., 2013. Authentication of herbal medicinal plant- *Boerhavia diffusa* L. using PCR-RFLP. Current Trends in Biotechnology and Pharmacy 7, 725–731.

Bogusz, M.J., Hassan, H., Al-Enazi, E., Ibrahim, Z., Al-Tufail, M., 2006. Application of LC-ESI-MS-MS for detection of synthetic adulterants in herbal remedies. Journal of Pharmaceutical and Biomedical Analysis 41, 554–564.

British Pharmacopoeia Commission, 2009. British Pharmacopoeia. Stationery Office, London.

Burns, D.A., Ciurczak, E.W., 2008. Handbook of Near-infrared Analysis, third ed. CRC Press, Boca Raton.

van Beek, T.A., Montoro, P., 2009. Chemical analysis and quality control of *Ginkgo biloba* leaves, extracts, and phytopharmaceuticals. Journal of Chromatography A 1216, 2002–2032.

Cai, Y., Cai, T.-G., Shi, Y., Cheng, X.-L., Ma, L.-Y., Ma, S.-C., et al., 2010. Simultaneous determination of eight PDE5-IS potentially adulterated in herbal dietary supplements with TLC and HPLC-PDA-MS methods. Journal of Liquid Chromatography & Related Technologies 33, 1287–1306.

Cai, B., Ong, S.P., Liu, X., 2012. High Performance Liquid Chromatography Fingerprinting Technology of the Commonly-used Traditional Chinese Medicine Herbs. World Scientific; Chemical Industry Press, Singapore; Hackensack, NJ, Beijing.

Carlin, M.G., Dean, J.R., 2013. Forensic Applications of Gas Chromatography, Analytical Concepts in Forensic Chemistry. CRC press, Boca Raton, London, New York.

Chan, C.O., Chu, C.C., Mok, D.K., Chau, F.T., 2007. Analysis of berberine and total alkaloid content in cortex phellodendri by near infrared spectroscopy (NIRS) compared with high-performance liquid chromatography coupled with ultra-visible spectrometric detection. Analytica Chimica Acta 592, 121–131.

Chan, W.-H., Ling, K.-H., Chiu, S.-W., Shaw, P.-C., But, P.P.-H., 2011. Molecular analyses of *Cordyceps gunnii* in China. Journal of Food and Drug Analysis 19, 18–25.

Chen, S.B., Liu, H.P., Tian, R.T., Yang, D.J., Chen, S.L., Xu, H.X., et al., 2006. High-performance thin-layer chromatographic fingerprints of isoflavonoids for distinguishing between *Radix Puerariae lobate* and *Radix Puerariae thomsonii*. Journal of Chromatography A 1121, 114–119.

Chen, S.P.L., Tang, M.H.Y., Ng, S.W., Poon, W.T., Chan, A.Y.W., Mak, T.W.L., 2010. Psychosis associated with usage of herbal slimming products adulterated with sibutramine: a case series. Clinical Toxicology 48, 832–838.

Choo, B.K., Moon, B.C., Ji, Y., Kim, B.B., Choi, G., Yoon, T., et al., 2009. Development of SCAR markers for the discrimination of three species of medicinal plants, *Angelica decursiva* (*Peucedanum decursivum*), *Peucedanum praeruptorum* and *Anthricus sylvestris*, based on the internal transcribed spacer (ITS) sequence and random amplified polymorphic DNA (RAPD). Biological & Pharmaceutical Bulletin 32, 24–30.

Christy, A.A., Kasemsumran, S., Du, Y., Ozaki, Y., 2004. The detection and quantification of adulteration in olive oil by near-infrared spectroscopy and chemometrics. Analytical Sciences 20, 935–940.

Ciurczak, E.W., Drennen, J.K., 2002. Pharmaceutical and Medical Applications of Near-infrared Spectroscopy. Marcel Dekker, New York.

Damiano, F., Silva, C., Vacondio, F., Mor, M., Gregori, A., Menozzi, M., et al., 2014. Analysis of illicit dietary supplements sold in the Italian market: identification of a sildenafil thioderivative as adulterant using UPLC-TOF/MS and GC/MS. Science & Justice 54, 228–237.

Demirezer, L.O., Buyukkaya, A., Ucakturk, E., Kuruuzum-Uz, A., Guvenalp, Z., Palaska, E., 2014. Adulteration determining of pharmaceutical forms of *Ginkgo biloba* extracts from different international manufacturers. Records of Natural Products 8, 394–400.

Dhiman, B., Singh, M., 2003. Molecular detection of cashew husk (*Anacardium occidentale*) adulteration in market samples of dry tea (*Camellia sinensis*). Planta Medica 69, 882–884.

Diao, Y., Lin, X.-M., Liao, C.-L., Tang, C.-Z., Chen, Z.-J., Hu, Z.-L., 2009. Authentication of *Panax ginseng* from its adulterants by PCR-RFLP and ARMS. Planta Medica 75, 557–560.

Dong, W.-J., Ni, Y.-N., Kokot, S., 2012. Quantitative analysis of two adulterants in *Cynanchum stauntonii* by near-infrared spectroscopy combined with multi-variate calibrations. Chemical Papers 66, 1083–1091.

Downey, G., McIntyre, P., Davies, A.N., 2002. Detecting and quantifying sunflower oil adulteration in extra virgin olive oils from the eastern mediterranean by visible and near-infrared spectroscopy. Journal of Agricultural and Food Chemistry 50, 5520–5525.

De Smet, P.A., Smeets, O.S., 1994. Potential risks of health food products containing yohimbe extracts. BMJ 309, 958.

European Pharmacopoeia Commission, European Pharmacopoeia, 2004. European Treaty Series. Council of Europe, Directorate for the Quality of Medicines, Strasbourg, fifth ed.

Fu, P.P., Xia, Q., 2014. Assessment of safety and quality assurance of herbal dietary supplements. In: Bagchi, D. (Ed.), Nutraceutical and Functional Food Regulations in the United States and Around the World. Elsevier Inc., Oxford, London.

Gad, H.A., El-Ahmady, S.H., Abou-Shoer, M.I., Al-Azizi, M.M., 2013. A modern approach to the authentication and quality assessment of thyme using UV spectroscopy and chemometric analysis. Phytochemical Analysis 24, 520–526.

Gafner, S., Bergeron, C., Batcha, L.L., Angerhofer, C.K., Sudberg, S., Sudberg, E.M., et al., 2003. Analysis of *Scutellaria lateriflora* and its adulterants *Teucrium canadense* and *Teucrium chamaedrys* by LC-UV/MS, TLC, and digital photomicroscopy. Journal of AOAC International 86, 453–460.

Garcia-Amoedo, L.H., de Almeida-Muradian, L.B., 2007. Physicochemical composition of pure and adulterated royal jelly. Quimica Nova 30, 257–259.

Geyer, H., Parr, M.K., Koehler, K., Mareck, U., Schaenzer, W., Thevis, M., 2008. Nutritional supplements cross-contaminated and faked with doping substances. Journal of Mass Spectrometry 43, 892–902.

Ghosh, S., Majumder, P.B., Sen Mandi, S., 2011. Species-specific AFLP markers for identification of *Zingiber officinale, Z. montanum* and *Z. zerumbet* (Zingiberaceae). Genetics and Molecular Research 10, 218–229.

Gu, Y., Ni, Y., Kokot, S., 2012. Solid phase excitation-emission fluorescence method for the classification of complex substances: cortex phellodendri and other traditional Chinese medicines as examples. Journal of Physical Chemistry A 116, 8949–8958.

Guillarme, D., Veuthey, J.-L., 2012. UHPLC in Life Sciences. Royal Society of Chemistry, Cambridge.

Guo, J.-L., Ren, Y., Chen, L., Pei, J., Wan, D.-G., 2010. Authentication of *Caulis clematidis armandii* ("Chuanmutong") and differentiation of its common adulterants using RAPD and SCAR markers. Journal of Medicinal Plants Research 4, 697–701.

Ha, W.Y., Yau, F.C., But, P.P., Wang, J., Shaw, P.C., 2001. Direct amplification of length polymorphism analysis differentiates *Panax ginseng* from *P. quinquefolius*. Planta Medica 67, 587–589.

Harnly, J.M., Luthria, D., Chen, P., 2012. Detection of adulterated *Ginkgo biloba* supplements using chromatographic and spectral fingerprints. Journal of AOAC International 95, 1579–1587.

Hasler, C.M., 2005. Regulation of Functional Foods and Nutraceuticals a Global Perspective. Blackwell Pub, Chicago, Iowa.

He, Z.D., Qiao, C.F., Han, Q.B., Cheng, C.L., Xu, H.X., Jiang, R.W., et al., 2005. Authentication and quantitative analysis on the chemical profile of Cassia bark (Cortex Cinnamomi) by high-pressure liquid chromatography. Journal of Agricultural and Food Chemistry 53, 2424–2428.

Hong, T., Jeong, M.L., Zahn, M., Fay, B.A., Lee, K., Hwangbo, H., et al., 2009. Detection of the potential adulterant *Teucrium chamaedrys* in *Scutellaria baicalensis* raw material and extract by high-performance thin-layer chromatography. Journal of AOAC International 92, 785–788.

Huang, W.F., Wen, K.C., Hsiao, M.L., 1997. Adulteration by synthetic therapeutic substances of traditional Chinese medicines in Taiwan. Journal of Clinical Pharmacology 37, 344–350.

Huang, W.-Z., Dong, T.-X., Qi, H.-Y., Lu, Z.-Q., Zhan, H.-Q., 2005. Identification of *Stellaria* media by PCR. Journal of Chinese Pharmaceutical Sciences 14, 144–148.

Huang, J., Nkrumah, P.N., Appiah-Sefah, G., Tang, S., 2013. Authentication of pure L-leucine products manufactured in China by discriminating between plant and animal sources using nitrogen stable isotope technique. Journal of Food Science 78, H490–H494.

Huggett, D.B., Khan, I.A., Allgood, J.C., Block, D.S., Schlenk, D., 2001. Organochlorine pesticides and metals in select botanical dietary supplements. Bulletin of Environmental Contamination and Toxicology 66, 150–155.

Indian Pharmacopoeia Commission, Indian Pharmacopoeia, 2010. Indian Pharmacopoeia Commission, Ghaziabad, 2010, sixth ed.

Jacobs, M.N., Santillo, D., Johnston, P.A., Wyatt, C.L., French, M.C., 1998. Organochlorine residues in fish oil dietary supplements: comparison with industrial grade oils. Chemosphere 37, 1709–1721.

Japanese Pharmacopoeia Commission, 2006. The Japanese Pharmacopoeia, fifteenth ed. Kosei Rodosho, Tokyo.

Jennings, S., Ottaway, P.B., 2008. Forms of food supplements. In: Ottaway, P.B. (Ed.), Food Fortification and Supplementation: Technological, Safety and Regulatory Aspects. Woodhead Publishing Limited and CRC Press LLC, USA.

Jiang, Y., David, B., Tu, P., Barbin, Y., 2010. Recent analytical approaches in quality control of traditional Chinese medicines—a review. Analytica Chimica Acta 657, 9–18.

Jiang, B., Ma, C., Motley, T., Kronenberg, F., Kennelly, E.J., 2011. Phytochemical fingerprinting to thwart black cohosh adulteration: a 15 *Actaea* species analysis. Phytochemical Analysis 22, 339–351.

Joshi, V.C., Srinivas, P.V., Khan, I.A., 2005. Rapid and easy identification of *Illicium verum* Hook. f. and its adulterant *Illicium anisatum* Linn. by fluorescent microscopy and gas chromatography. Journal of AOAC International 88, 703–706.

Jung, J., Hermanns-Clausen, M., Weinmann, W., 2006. Anorectic sibutramine detected in a Chinese herbal drug for weight loss. Forensic Science International 161, 221–222.

Kang, J., Lee, S., Kang, S., Kwon, H.N., Park, J.H., Kwon, S.W., et al., 2008. NMR-based metabolomics approach for the differentiation of ginseng (*Panax ginseng*) roots from different origins. Archives of Pharmacal Research 31, 330–336.

Kesting, J.R., Huang, J., Sorensen, D., 2010. Identification of adulterants in a Chinese herbal medicine by LC-HRMS and LC-MS-SPE/NMR and comparative in vivo study with standards in a hypertensive rat model. Journal of Pharmaceutical and Biomedical Analysis 51, 705–711.

Ku, Y.-R., Ho, Y.-L., Chen, C.-Y., Ho, L.-K., Chang, Y.-S., 2004. Analysis of N-cis- and N-trans-Feruloyl 3-Methyldopamine in Achyranthes bidentata by HPLC. Journal of Liquid Chromatography & Related Technologies 27, 727–736.

Laasonen, M., Harmia-Pulkkinen, T., Simard, C.L., Michiels, E., Raesaenen, M., Vuorela, H., 2002. Fast identification of *Echinacea purpurea* dried roots using near-infrared spectroscopy. Analytical Chemistry 74, 2493–2499.

Lai, Y.-H., So, P.-K., Lo, S.C.-L., Ng, E.W.Y., Poon, T.C.W., Yao, Z.-P., 2012. Rapid differentiation of *Panax ginseng* and *Panax quinquefolius* by matrix-assisted laser desorption/ionization mass spectrometry. Analytica Chimica Acta 753, 73–81.

Lau, A.-J., Holmes, M.J., Woo, S.-O., Koh, H.-L., 2003. Analysis of adulterants in a traditional herbal medicinal product using liquid chromatography-mass spectrometry-mass spectrometry. Journal of Pharmaceutical and Biomedical Analysis 31, 401–406.

Lau, C.C., Chan, C.O., Chau, F.T., Mok, D.K., 2009. Rapid analysis of *Radix Puerariae* by near-infrared spectroscopy. Journal of Chromatography A 1216, 2130–2135.

Law, S.K.-Y., Simmons, M.P., Techen, N., Khan, I.A., He, M.-F., Shaw, P.-C., et al., 2011. Molecular analyses of the Chinese herb Leigongteng (*Tripterygium wilfordii* Hook.f.). Phytochemistry 72, 21–26.

Lee, H.-M., Kim, C.S., Jang, Y.M., Kwon, S.W., Lee, B.-J., 2011. Separation and structural elucidation of a novel analogue of vardenafil included as an adulterant in a dietary supplement by liquid chromatography-electrospray ionization mass spectrometry, infrared spectroscopy and nuclear magnetic resonance spectroscopy. Journal of Pharmaceutical and Biomedical Analysis 54, 491–496.

Li, M., Au, K.-Y., Lam, H., Cheng, L., But, P.P.-H., Shaw, P.-C., 2014. Molecular identification and cytotoxicity study of herbal medicinal materials that are confused by *Aristolochia* herbs. Food Chemistry 147, 332–339.

Li, Z.-Y., Zhang, Z.-Z., Du, G.-H., Qin, X.-M., 2015. Comparative analysis of *Danggui* and European *Danggui* using nuclear magnetic resonance-based metabolic fingerprinting. Journal of Pharmaceutical and Biomedical Analysis 103, 44–51.

Lu, K.-L., Ku, Y.-R., Wen, K.-C., Ho, L.-K., Chang, Y.-S., 2000. Analysis of flavonoids and coumarins in *Ixeris laevigata* var. *Oldhami* by HPLC. Journal of Liquid Chromatography & Related Technologies 23, 2573–2583.

Masada-Atsumi, S., Kumeta, Y., Takahashi, Y., Hakamatsuka, T., Goda, Y., 2014. Evaluation of the botanical origin of black cohosh products by genetic and chemical analyses. Biological & Pharmaceutical Bulletin 37, 454–460.

Mathon, C., Ankli, A., Reich, E., Bieri, S., Christen, P., 2014. Screening and determination of sibutramine in adulterated herbal slimming supplements by HPTLC-UV densitometry. Food Additives & Contaminants: Part A 31, 15–20.

Mercolini, L., Mandrioli, R., Trere, T., Bugamelli, F., Ferranti, A., Raggi, M.A., 2010. Fast CE analysis of adrenergic amines in different parts of *Citrus aurantium* fruit and dietary supplements. Journal of Separation Science 33, 2520–2527.

Mikami, E., Ohno, T., Matsumoto, H., 2002. Simultaneous identification/determination system for phentolamine and sildenafil as adulterants in soft drinks advertising roborant nutrition. Forensic Science International 130, 140–146.

Mikami, E., Ohno, T., Matsumoto, H., Sekita, S., 2003. Detection of thyroxine in dietary supplements using an enzyme-linked immunosorbent assay. Journal of Health Sciences 49, 547–550.

Moon, B.C., Ji, Y., Lee, Y.M., Kang, Y.M., Kim, H.K., 2015. Authentication of *Akebia quinata* DECNE. from its common adulterant medicinal plant species based on the RAPD-derived SCAR markers and multiplex-PCR. Genes Genomics 37, 23–32.

Ozaki, Y., McClure, W.F., Christy, A.A., 2007. Near-infrared Spectroscopy in Food Science and Technology. Wiley-Interscience, Hoboken, New Jersey.

Ozen, B.F., Weiss, I., Mauer, L.J., 2003. Dietary supplement oil classification and detection of adulteration using Fourier transform infrared spectroscopy. Journal of Agricultural and Food Chemistry 51, 5871–5876.

Park, H.E., Lee, S.-Y., Hyun, S.-H., Kim, D.Y., Marriott, P.J., Choi, H.-K., 2013. Gas chromatography/mass spectrometry-based metabolic profiling and differentiation of ginseng roots according to cultivation age using variable selection. Journal of AOAC International 96, 1266–1272.

Petty, H.R., Fernando, M., Kindzelskii, A.L., Zarewych, B.N., Ksebati, M.B., Hryhorczuk, L.M., et al., 2001. Identification of colchicine in placental blood from patients using herbal medicines. Chemical Research in Toxicology 14, 1254–1258.

Pharmacopoeia of the People's Republic of China Commission, 2005. Pharmacopoeia of the People's Republic of China, English ed. Chemical Industry Press, Beijing, China.

Phattanawasin, P., Sotanaphun, U., Sukwattanasinit, T., Akkarawaranthorn, J., Kitchaiya, S., 2012. Quantitative determination of sibutramine in adulterated herbal slimming formulations by TLC-image analysis method. Forensic Science International 219, 96–100.

Rhoads, P.M., Tong, T.G., Banner Jr., W., Anderson, R., 1984. Anticholinergic poisonings associated with commercial burdock root tea. Journal of Toxicology Clinical Toxicology 22, 581–584.

Rohman, A.Y., Man, B., 2011. Authentication analysis of cod liver oil from beef fat using fatty acid composition and FTIR spectra. Food Additives & Contaminants: Part A, Chemistry, Analysis, Control, Exposure & Risk Assessment 28, 1469–1474.

Romm, A.J., Upton, R., 2012. Blue Cohosh Root and Rhizome: *Caulophyllum Thalictroides* (L.) Michx., *C. Giganteum* (Farw.) Loconte & W.H. Blackw.: Standards of Analysis, Quality Control, and Therapeutics. American Herbal Pharmacopoeia, Scotts Valley, CA.

Roytas, D., 2015. Clinical outcomes, safety, and efficacy of chinese herbal medicines. In: Ghosh, D., Bagchi, D., Konishi, T. (Eds.), Clinical Aspects of Functional Foods and Nutraceuticals. CRC Press/Taylor & Francis Group, Florida, USA.

Rueda, D.C., Zaugg, J., Quitschau, M., Reich, E., Hering, S., Hamburger, M., 2012. Discovery of GABA(A) receptor modulator aristolactone in a commercial sample of the Chinese herbal drug "Chaihu" (Bupleurum chinense roots) unravels adulteration by nephrotoxic *Aristolochia manshuriensis* roots. Planta Medica 78, 207–210.

Satheeshkumar, N., Shantikumar, S., Komali, M., 2014. Identification and quantification of aldose reductase inhibitory flavonoids in herbal formulation and extract of *Gymnema sylvestre* using HPLC-PDA and LC-MS/MS. Chromatography Research International 1–8, 518175.

Shi, Y.-H., Xie, Z.-Y., Wang, R., Huang, S.-J., Li, Y.-M., Wang, Z.-T., 2012. Quantitative and chemical fingerprint analysis for the quality evaluation of *Isatis indigotica* based on ultra-performance liquid chromatography with photodiode array detector combined with chemometric methods. International Journal of Molecular Sciences 13, 9035–9050.

Sloley, B.D., Tawfik, S.R., Scherban, K.A., Tam, Y.K., 2003. Quality control analyses for Ginkgo extracts require analysis of intact flavonol glycosides. Journal of Food and Drug Analysis 11, 102–107.

Song, F., El-Demerdash, A., Lee, S.-J.S.H., Smith, R.E., 2011. Fast screening of lovastatin in red yeast rice products by flow injection tandem mass spectrometry. Journal of Pharmaceutical and Biomedical Analysis 57, 76–81.

Sparkman, O.D., Penton, Z., Kitson, F.G., 2011. Gas Chromatography and Mass Spectrometry: A Practical Guide, second ed. Academic Press, Burlington.

Srivastava, M., 2011. High-performance Thin-layer Chromatography (HPTLC). Springer, Heidelberg, New York.

Sun, Y., Guo, T., Yin, S., Li, F., 2003. Fingerprint analysis of Flos Carthami by capillary electrophoresis. Journal of Chromatography B: Analytical Technologies in the Biomedical and Life Sciences 792, 147–152.

Sun, Z., Song, J., Yao, H., Han, J., 2012. Molecular identification of *Cistanches Herba* and its adulterants based on nrITS2 sequence. Journal of Medicinal Plants Research 6, 1041–1045.

Sun, D.-W., 2008. Modern Techniques for Food Authentication. Elsevier/Academic Press, Amsterdam; Boston.

Tseng, M.-C., Lin, J.-H., 2002. Determination of sildenafil citrate adulterated in a dietary supplement capsule by LC/MS/MS. Journal of Food and Drug Analysis 10, 112–119.

Um, J.Y., Chung, H.S., Kim, M.S., Na, H.J., Kwon, H.J., Kim, J.J., et al., 2001. Molecular authentication of *Panax ginseng* species by RAPD analysis and PCR-RFLP. Biological & Pharmaceutical Bulletin 24, 872–875.

R. Upton, et al. (Eds.), 2011. To Be or Not To Be? A Focus on Botanical Adulteration in American Herbal Pharmacopoeia®. CRC Taylor & Francis Group Florida, USA.

Upton, R., 1999a. Hawthorn Leaf With Flower : *Crataegus* Spp.: Analytical, Quality Control, and Therapeutic Monograph. American Herbal Pharmacopoeia, Santa Cruz, CA.

Upton, R., 1999b. Valerian Root: *Valeriana officinalis*: Analytical, Quality Control, and Therapeutic Monograph. American Herbal Pharmacopoeia, Santa Cruz, CA.

Upton, R., 1999c. Hawthorn Berry: *Crataegus* Spp.: Analytical, Quality Control, and Therapeutic Monograph. American Herbal Pharmacopoeia, Santa Cruz, CA.

Upton, R., 1999d. Astragalus root: *Astragalus membranaceus* & *Astragalus membranaceus* Var. *mongholicus*: Analytical, Quality Control, and Therapeutic Monograph. American Herbal Pharmacopoeia, Santa Cruz, CA.

Upton, R., 1999e. Schisandra Berry: *Schisandra chinensis*: Analytical, Quality Control and Therapeutic Monograph. American Herbal Pharmacopoeia, Santa Cruz, CA.

Upton, R., 1999f. Willow Bark: *Salix* Spp.: Analytical, Quality Control, and Therapeutic Monograph. American Herbal Pharmacopoeia, Santa Cruz, CA.

Upton, R., 2000a. Cramp Bark: *Viburnum opulus*: Analytical, Quality Control, and Therapeutic Monograph. American Herbal Pharmacopoeia, Santa Cruz, CA.

Upton, R., 2000b. Ashwagandha Root: *Withania somnifera*: Analytical, Quality Control, and Therapeutic Monograph. American Herbal Pharmacopoeia, Santa Cruz, CA.

Upton, R., 2000c. Black Haw Bark: *Viburnum prunifolium*: Analytical, Quality Control, and Therapeutic Monograph. American Herbal Pharmacopoeia, Santa Cruz, CA.

Upton, R., 2000d. Reishi Mushroom: *Ganoderma lucidum*: Standards of Analysis, Quality Control, and Therapeutics. American Herbal Pharmacopoeia, Santa Cruz, CA.

Upton, R., 2001a. Goldenseal Root: *Hydrastis canadensis*: Standards of Analysis, Quality Control, and Therapeutics. American Herbal Pharmacopoeia, Santa Cruz, CA.

Upton, R., 2001b. Chaste Tree Fruit: *Vitex Agnus-castus*: Standards of Analysis, Quality Control, and Therapeutics. American Herbal Pharmacopoeia, Santa Cruz, CA.

Upton, R., 2001c. Bilberry Fruit: *Vaccinium myrtillus* L.: Standards of Analysis, Quality Control, and Therapeutics. American Herbal Pharmacopoeia, Santa Cruz, CA.

Upton, R., 2002a. Black Cohosh Rhizome: *Actaea racemosa* L., Syn. *Cimicifuga racemosa* (L.) Nutt.: Standards of Analysis, Quality Control, and Therapeutics. American Herbal Pharmacopoeia, Santa Cruz, CA.

Upton, R., 2002b. Cranberry fruit: *Vaccinium macrocarpon* aiton: Standards of Analysis, Quality Control, and Therapeutics. American Herbal Pharmacopoeia, Santa Cruz, CA.

Upton, R., 2003a. Dang Gui Root: *Angelica sinensis* (Oliv.) Diels: Standards of Analysis, Quality Control, and Therapeutics. American Herbal Pharmacopoeia, Santa Cruz, CA.

Upton, R., 2003b. Ginkgo Leaf, Ginkgo Leaf Dry Extract: *Ginkgo biloba* L.: Standards of Analysis, Quality Control, and Therapeutics. American Herbal Pharmacopoeia, Scotts Valley, CA.

Upton, R., 2004. Echinacea Purpurea Root: *Echinacea purpurea* (L.) Moench: Standards of Analysis, Quality Control, and Therapeutics. American Herbal Pharmacopoeia, Scotts Valley, CA.

Upton, R., 2007a. Echinacea Purpurea Aerial Parts: *Echinacea purpurea* (L.) Moench: Standards of Analysis, Quality Control, and Therapeutics. American Herbal Pharmacopoeia, Scotts Valley, CA.

Upton, R., 2007b. American Herbal Pharmacopoeia., Feverfew Aerial Parts: *Tanacetum parthenium* (L.) Schultz Bip: Standards of Analysis, Quality Control, and Therapeutics. American Herbal Pharmacopoeia and Therapeutic Compendium. American Herbal Pharmacopoeia, Scotts Valley, CA.

Upton, R., 2008. Uva Ursi Leaf: *Arctostaphylos uva-ursi* (L.) Spreng: Standards of Analysis, Quality Control, and Therapeutics. American Herbal Pharmacopoeia, Scotts Valley, CA.

Upton, R., 2009. Stinging Nettle Herb: *Urtica dioica* L., *Urtica urens* L.: Standards of Analysis, Quality Control and Therapeutics. American Herbal Pharmacopoeia, Scotts Valley, CA.

Upton, R.T., 2010d. Use of high-performance thin layer chromatography by the American herbal pharmacopoeia. Journal of AOAC International 93, 1349–1354.

Upton, R., 2010a. Stinging Nettle Root: *Urtica dioica* L.: Standards of Analysis, Quality Control, and Therapeutics. American Herbal Pharmacopoeia, Scotts Valley, CA.

Upton, R., 2010b. Echinacea Angustifolia Root: *Echinacea augustifolia* DC: Standards of Analysis, Quality Control and Therapeutics Therapeutics. American Herbal Pharmacopoeia, Scotts Valley, CA.

Upton, R., 2010c. Echinacea Pallida Root: *Echinacea pallida* (Nutt.) Nutt.: Standards of Analysis, Quality Control, and Therapeutics. American Herbal Pharmacopoeia, Scotts Valley, CA.

Upton, R., 2011. American Herbal Pharmacopoeia: Botanical Pharmacognosy–microscopic Characterization of Botanical Medicines. American Herbal Pharmacopoeia/CRC Press, Boca Raton, Florida.

Upton, R., 2012a. American Ginseng Root: *Panax quinquefolius* L.: Standards of Analysis, Quality Control, and Therapeutics. American Herbal Pharmacopoeia, Scotts Valley, CA.

Upton, R., 2012b. Aloe Vera Leaf, Aloe Vera Leaf Juice, Aloe Vera Inner Leaf Juice, *Aloe vera* (L.) Burm. F.: Standards of Identity, Analysis, and Quality Control. American Herbal Pharmacopoeia, Scotts Valley, CA.

Vaysse, J., Balayssac, S., Gilard, V., Desoubdzanne, D., Malet-Martino, M., Martino, R., 2010. Analysis of adulterated herbal medicines and dietary supplements marketed for weight loss by DOSY 1H-NMR. Food Additives & Contaminants: Part A 27, 903–916.

Vlietinck, A., Pieters, L., Apers, S., 2009. Legal requirements for the quality of herbal substances and herbal preparations for the manufacturing of herbal medicinal products in the European Union. Planta Medica 75, 683–688.

Wagner, H., Ulrich-Merzenich, G., 2013. Evidence and Rational Based Research on Chinese Drugs. Springer, Vienna; New York.

Wagner, H., Bauer, R., Melchart, D., Staudinger, A., Xiao, P., 2011. Chromatographic Fingerprint Analysis of Herbal Medicines Thin-layer and High Performance Liquid Chromatography of Chinese Drugs. Springer, New York.

Waksmundzka-Hajnos, M., Sherma, J., 2011. High Performance Liquid Chromatography in Phytochemical Analysis. CRC Press, Boca Raton, Florida.

Wang, Y., Tang, H., Nicholson, J.K., Hylands, P.J., Sampson, J., Whitcombe, I., et al., 2004. Metabolomic strategy for the classification and quality control of phytomedicine: a case study of chamomile flower (*Matricaria recutita* L.). Planta Medica 70, 250–255.

Webb, G.P., 2006. Dietary Supplements and Functional Foods. Blackwell Pub., Oxford, Ames, Iowa.

Wittkowski, R., Matissek, R., 1993. Capillary Gas Chromatography in Food Control and Research. Technomic Publishing Co., Inc., Lancaster.

Wong, K.-L., But, P.P.-H., Shaw, P.-C., 2013. Evaluation of seven DNA barcodes for differentiating closely related medicinal *Gentiana* species and their adulterants. Chinese Medicine 8, 16/1–12.

Workman, J.L., Weyer, 2008. Practical Guide to Interpretive Near-infrared Spectroscopy. CRC Press, Boca Raton.

Wu, C.-T., Gupta, S.K., Wang, A.Z.-M., Lo, S.-F., Kuo, C.-L., Ko, Y.-J., et al., 2012. Internal transcribed spacer sequence based identification and phylogenic relationship of *Herba Dendrobii*. Journal of Food and Drug Analysis 20, 143–151.

Xiao, X., Yin, Y., Hu, Y., Li, G., 2010. Microwave-assisted extraction coupled with single drop microextraction and high-performance column liquid chromatography for the determination of trace estrogen adulterants in soybean isoflavone dietary supplements. Journal of AOAC International 93, 849–854.

Xie, P., Chen, S., Liang, Y.Z., Wang, X., Tian, R., Upton, R., 2006. Chromatographic fingerprint analysis—a rational approach for quality assessment of traditional Chinese herbal medicine. Journal of Chromatography A 1112, 171–180.

Xu, Q.A., 2013. Ultra-high Performance Liquid Chromatography and Its Applications. Wiley, Hoboken, New Jersey.

Yang, S.-O., Shin, Y.-S., Hyun, S.-H., Cho, S., Bang, K.-H., Lee, D., et al., 2012. NMR-based metabolic profiling and differentiation of ginseng roots according to cultivation ages. Journal of Pharmaceutical and Biomedical Analysis 58, 19–26.

Yap, K.Y.-L., Chan, S.Y., Lim, C.S., 2007. Authentication of traditional Chinese medicine using infrared spectroscopy: distinguishing between ginseng and its morphological fakes. Journal of Biomedical Science 14, 265–273.

Zhao, L., Huang, C., Shan, Z., Xiang, B., Mei, L., 2005. Fingerprint analysis of *Psoralea corylifolia* L. by HPLC and LC-MS. Journal of Chromatography B: Analytical Technologies in the Biomedical and Life Sciences 821, 67–74.

Zou, P., Hou, P., Low, M.-Y., Koh, H.-L., 2006a. Structural elucidation of a tadalafil analogue found as an adulterant of a herbal product. Food Additives and Contaminants 23, 446–451.

Zou, P., Hou, P., Oh, S.S.-Y., Low, M.-Y., Koh, H.-L., 2006b. Electrospray tandem mass spectrometric investigations of tadalafil and its analogue. Rapid Communications in Mass Spectrometry 20, 3488–3490.

Chemometrics for Food Authenticity Applications

25

P. Oliveri, R. Simonetti
University of Genova, Genova, Italy

Chapter Outline

25.1 Introduction

The necessity of verifying authenticity of food products is a very ancient issue, required to detect many types of commercial frauds. In many cases, frauds involve the addition of ingredients of low value to expensive products for financial reasons. Other common adulterations have the purpose of camouflaging the bad appearance and taste of rotten food (Bush, 2002). In the past, such deceptions were rudimentary and, therefore, often easily discovered by a careful visual examination or by the use of basic instruments (balances, magnifying glasses, or microscopes) (Hart, 1952).

Through the ages, adulteration practices became more refined in order to overcome advances in analytical controls. In recent decades, a particular type of fraud has concerned claims around food geographical provenance. The reason for this may be found in the increased emphasis on food origin that is widespread in contemporary culture due to several reasons including confidence in locally produced products, specific sensory properties, and even perceived health values (Luykx and Van Ruth, 2008). Frauds concerning food provenance represent a financial loss for the consumer who often pays a considerable price premium when a food is labeled with a declaration of production within a specific region.

Verification of food authenticity claims is a complex analytical task, and the evaluation of a single parameter is rarely sufficient. Numerous analytical techniques are currently applied in the investigation of food authenticity. These include chromatographic techniques, mass spectrometry (MS), spectroscopic (ultraviolet–visible, near infrared, mid-infrared, Raman, fluorescence and nuclear magnetic resonance) methods, DNA-based approaches, enzymatic procedures and -omics approaches (Lees, 2003; Sun, 2008).

The best way to get useful information from such data is to process them by multivariate pattern recognition methods, which facilitate consideration of intercorrelations between measured variables, providing what is called an analytical fingerprint. Indeed, multivariate pattern recognition emulates mathematically the learning mechanisms typical of the human brain and, therefore, tends to exploit the information available as efficiently as possible. Actually, the scientific literature shows that multivariate pattern recognition approaches are able to provide effective models to verify the authenticity of foods while the univariate approach often fails.

Pattern recognition methods can be used for different purposes such as data exploration and the development of predictive models. The output of these models can be qualitative or quantitative, depending on the particular purpose. A proper validation of predictive models is always required to provide reliable predictions.

In this chapter, the principal chemometric methods, both unsupervised and supervised, which are currently applied for food authenticity assessment, are presented. In particular, the most important preprocessing transformations are described, with a focus on their application potential and limits. Data visualization and exploration techniques are discussed with a real example concerning food authentication. Supervised methods for qualitative and quantitative modeling are described together with the related evaluation parameters and the most common validation strategies.

25.2 Multivariate Data Analysis

25.2.1 Preprocessing

25.2.1.1 Row Preprocessing

Digital signals, which are commonly provided by current analytical instruments, usually require suitable pretreatment(s) prior to chemometric analysis. One of the major aims of signal pretreatment is to improve the quality of signals by removal of unwanted information (ie, information not related to the chemical characterization of the system under investigation), the origin of which may be related either to electric interferences or with surrounding effects. Such spurious signal variations may be random or systematic. Random noise is generally due to sporadic interferences or is associated with random phenomena (eg, Brownian motions of particles and thermal motion of electrons—the so-called Johnson–Nyquist noise), which usually follow a standard normal or a Poisson probability distribution. It is usually characterized by a higher frequency than the useful signal. On the contrary, systematic unwanted variations are commonly due to instrumental trends or to external influences. They may affect the signal with baseline shifts and/or drifts, which can be considered as a low-frequency contribution, or with global intensity variations. A further problem in the collection of a series of analytical signals may involve horizontal shifts—a typical situation for chromatographic data and, in some cases, for spectral data. In order to fix this problem, several methods for peak alignment have been proposed, the most important of which are based on the correlation between a selected reference profile and the signals to be aligned (Nielsen et al., 1998; Jellema, 2009; Savorani et al., 2010).

When digital signals are assembled into a data matrix following the chemometric convention, each signal corresponds to a row and each instrumental variable corresponds to a column. For this reason, signal preprocessing is also known as row preprocessing. The mathematical row transforms usually operate independently on each signal.

Classical techniques for reduction of random noise include the moving average—or boxcar—filters, Savitzky–Golay smoothing (Savitzky and Golay, 1964) and Fourier transform (FT)-based filters (Reis et al., 2009).

For the elimination, or minimization, of systematic interferences or effects, a number of mathematical methods are commonly employed, the most common of which are derivatives and the standard normal variate (SNV) transform. These can be applied either singularly or in combination.

Derivatives

Numerical derivatives applied to digital signals typically correct for baseline shifts and/or drifts. Furthermore, derivatives enhance apparent resolution of overlapping peaks and may accentuate small structural differences between very similar signal features (Taavitsainen, 2009).

In more detail, the first derivative of a signal $y = \mathrm{f}(x)$, defined as the rate of change of y with x (ie, $y' = dy/dx$), provides a correction for baseline shifts.

The second derivative, which can be considered as a further derivation of the first derivative ($y'' = d^2y/dx^2$), provides a correction for both baseline shifts and drifts.

For digital signals affected by random noise, characterized by high-frequency slope variations, derivation usually causes an amplification of noise. A common way to overcome this drawback is signal smoothing. A typical example of a smoothing-derivation algorithm is that proposed by Savitzky and Golay (1964).

Standard Normal Variate Transform

The SNV transform, or row autoscaling, is a pretreatment particularly used for spectral data, which allows correction for both baseline shifts and global intensity variations (Barnes et al., 1989). Each signal (x_i) is row centered by subtracting its mean ($\overline{x}_i$) from each single value ($x_{i,v}$), and then scaled by dividing by the signal standard deviation (s_i):

$$x^*_{i,v} = \frac{x_{i,v} - \overline{x}_i}{s_i} \tag{25.1}$$

After transformation, each signal presents a mean equal to 0 and standard deviation equal to 1.

SNV has the peculiarity of possibly shifting informative regions along the signal range, so that the interpretation of the results by reference to the original signals should be performed with caution (Fearn, 2009).

25.2.1.2 Column Preprocessing

Column preprocessing corrects for systematic differences between variables, acting on each variable individually.

Column Centering

Each measured value of a variable is corrected by subtracting the corresponding column mean value ($\overline{y}_v$):

$$y^*_{i,v} = y_{i,v} - \overline{y}_v \tag{25.2}$$

This transformation corrects for systematic location differences among variables—the mean value of each column after transformation becomes null.

Column Autoscaling

Column autoscaling is the pretreatment most appropriate in the case of variables of different nature. It corrects for systematic location and dispersion differences by dividing each value of a column-centered variable by the standard deviation of the corresponding column (s_v). This transformation makes variables dimensionless and gives all of them the same a priori importance (mean values equal to 0 and standard deviations equal to 1).

$$y_{i,v}^{*} = \frac{y_{i,v} - \bar{y}_v}{s_v} \quad (25.3)$$

25.2.2 Exploratory Methods

25.2.2.1 Principal Component Analysis

Principal component analysis (PCA) is one of the basic and most useful tools in the branch of multivariate analysis. Such an exploratory method, originating in the work of K. Pearson (1901), always offers an overview of the problem studied, may be employed for feature and noise reduction purposes, and may constitute the basis for more complex pattern recognition techniques (eg, SIMCA or PCR, which will be described in subsequent paragraphs).

Based on the assumption that a high variability (ie, a high-variance value) is synonymous with a high amount of information, PCA algorithms search for the maximum variance direction in the multidimensional space of the original data, preferably passing through the data centroid. In order to perform a centered rotation, data has to be mean-centered column-wise. The maximum variance direction represents the first principal component (PC). The second PC is defined as the direction that keeps the maximum variance among all directions orthogonal to the first PC, and so on. It follows that PCs are not intercorrelated (Jolliffe, 2002).

Since the variance value of each variable depends on its scale, it becomes difficult to compare and impossible to combine information from variables of different nature, unless properly normalized; column autoscaling (see Eq. (25.3)) is the pretreatment most commonly applied for this purpose.

The PCs are expressible as linear combinations of the original variables—the coefficients that multiply each variable represent the cosine values (director cosines) of the angles between the PCs and the original variables. These values, called loadings, may vary between -1 and $+1$; the larger their absolute value, the larger the contribution of the original variable to the PC. In fact, high absolute values of the cosines indicate that the two directions are close.

The rotation from the space of the original variables to the PC space is expressible, in terms of matrix algebra, by means of the following product:

$$\mathbf{D} = \mathbf{S} * \mathbf{L}^{\mathrm{T}} + \mathbf{E} \quad (25.4)$$

where **D** is the original data matrix, constituted by m samples (rows) described by n variables (columns), **L** is the loading orthogonal matrix, and **S** is the so-called score matrix (Fig. 25.1).

The score values can be used as coordinates to project samples in the Cartesian space defined by the new variables (PCs); such graphs are called score plots.

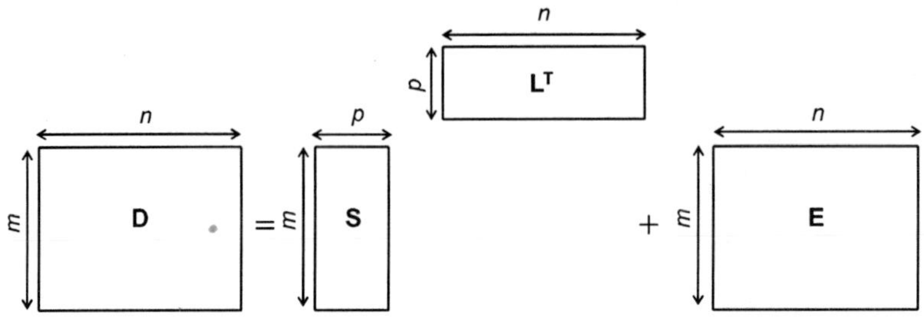

Figure 25.1 General scheme of a principal component analysis decomposition.

The loading values, showing the contributions of the original variables to the PCs, can be represented in scatter or profile graphs called loading plots.

Scatter representations of both samples (scores) and variables (loadings) are called biplots (Geladi et al., 2003; Kjeldahl and Bro, 2010). Since PCs are not intercorrelated, no duplicate information is shown in PC plots.

Fig. 25.2 represents an example of a typical PCA output, which is derived from a PCA performed on the table olive NIR data set (Oliveri et al., 2013). The data set contains FT-NIR spectra (recorded over the spectral range 9000–4200 cm^{-1}, at 4 cm^{-1} resolution) on ground table olives belonging to three different cultivars (*Taggiasca*, *Leccino*, and *Coquillo*). Spectral data have been previously submitted to SNV transform and column autoscaled in order to eliminate unwanted signal variations. The two Cartesian axes correspond to the first (lower-order) two PCs, which together show more than 85% of the information (defined as explained variance) enclosed in the original multidimensional data space.

The subplots clearly show the structures existing among samples, and the interrelations existing among variables and between samples and variables.

In more detail, from Fig. 25.2A (score plot) it is possible to notice groupings among samples, which correspond to the three olive categories: *Taggiasca* (red squares), *Leccino* (blue squares), and *Coquillo* (green squares). Information about the dispersion of samples within each class can also be deduced.

In particular, it appears that PC1—which accounts for about 70% of the total variance, ie, information—is the direction effective in distinguishing between *Leccino* and the other two cultivars. Similarly, PC2 (explaining about 15% of total variance) is useful to differentiate mainly *Coquillo* samples from the other two groups.

To estimate the importance of the spectral variables measured to characterize the different cultivars, the loading plots have to be examined. Fig. 25.2B is a typical loading scatter plot, from which it is usually possible to identify the variables most important to define the two PCs considered, ie, the points located at the extremes of the plot.

Nevertheless, in the case of spectral data, interpretation of such plots is not very straightforward, due to the high number of points—corresponding to the spectral variables—present within the plot.

In such cases, representation of loading profiles, like those in Fig. 25.2C, may aid in understanding in a more direct and simple way the importance of individual or groups

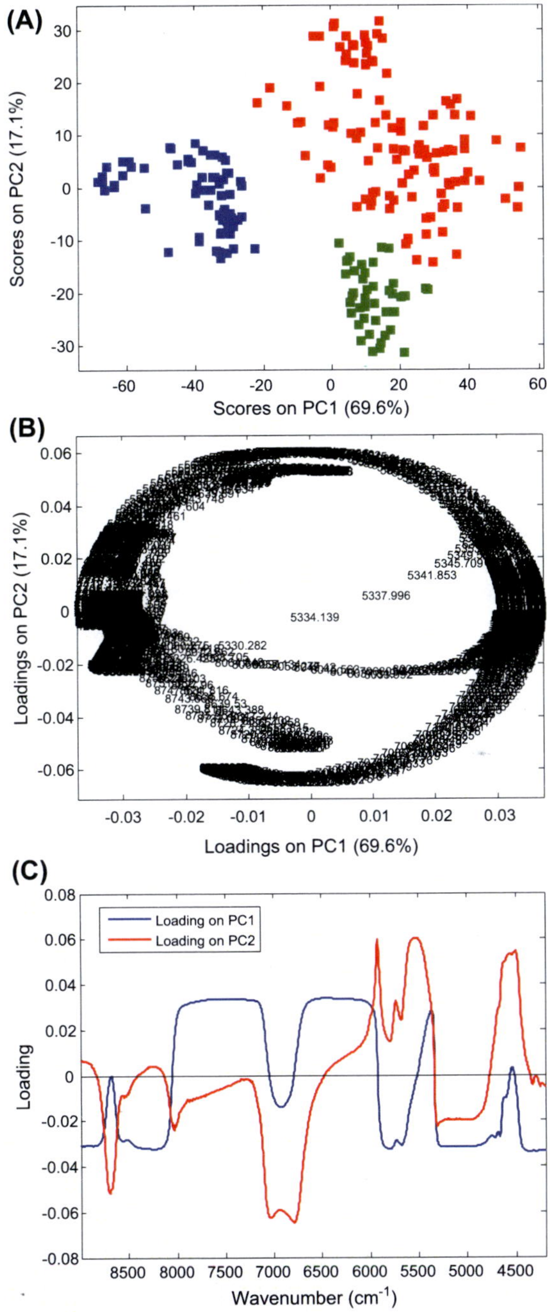

Figure 25.2 Example of PCA score plot (A), loading scatter plot (B), and loading profiles on PC1 and PC2 (C) for the autoscaled and SNV transformed olive data. The scores (*colored squares*) correspond to the olive samples of cultivars Coquillo (green), Taggiasca (red), and Leccino (blue), respectively.

of variables. In fact, this plot can be directly compared with the original spectral profiles, possibly allowing a chemical interpretation of important bands.

For instance, Fig. 25.2C suggests that NIR bands around 6700 cm^{-1} are the most important in defining PC1 and, consequently, in differentiating *Leccino* olives from *Taggiasca* and *Coquillo*. Conversely, bands around 8700, 7050, 6800, 5900, 5550, and 4550 cm^{-1}, respectively, exhibit the highest absolute value of loading on PC2. This means that such spectral regions are the most important in characterizing *Coquillo* olives with respect to the other two cultivars.

Further considerations may be drawn by looking at the distribution of samples inside each class. For instance, it can be easily seen that *Coquillo* olives are characterized by the lowest within-class variability while the *Taggiasca* cultivar is characterized by the highest dispersion. This type of information may also be extremely important for characterization purposes.

25.2.2.2 Multiway Data Analysis

The conceptual evolution of exploratory analysis for datasets organized in three (or more) dimensions—such as *N* samples described by *V* variables measured at *T* times, or *N* samples evaluated for *V* attributes evaluated by *M* panelists—is represented by multiway methods. The multiway methods most commonly applied in chemometrics are parallel factor analysis (PARAFAC) and Tucker (Bro, 2006).

25.2.2.3 Multivariate Curve Resolution

Multivariate curve resolution (MCR) (Tauler, 1995, 2001; Tauler et al., 1995) is a family of chemometric methods used for the deconvolution of complex analytical responses arising from unresolved multicomponent mixtures.

Any multicomponent system that gives as a result data matrices that can be described by a bilinear model can be analyzed by MCR methods.

The goal of MCR is the bilinear decomposition (Eq. (25.5)) of the data matrix **D** into the "true" pure response profiles associated with the variation of each contribution in the row and the column directions (matrices **C** and $\mathbf{S}^T$, respectively), which are responsible for the observed data variance.

$$\mathbf{D} = \mathbf{C} * \mathbf{S}^T + \mathbf{E} \tag{25.5}$$

Multivariate curve resolution—alternating least squares (MCR-ALS) is the most common MCR method used in chemometrics. It solves Eq. (25.5) iteratively by an alternating least squares algorithm, which calculates concentration **C** and pure spectra $\mathbf{S}^T$ matrices by optimally fitting the data matrix **D** (Fig. 25.3).

This optimization is performed for a proposed number of components and using initial estimates of **C** and $\mathbf{S}^T$ that can be obtained, for instance, in the case that they are unknown, by applying evolving factor analysis (EFA) (Maeder, 1987) or SIMPLe-to-use Interactive Self-modeling Mixture Analysis (SIMPLISMA) (Windig and Guilment, 1991) methods.

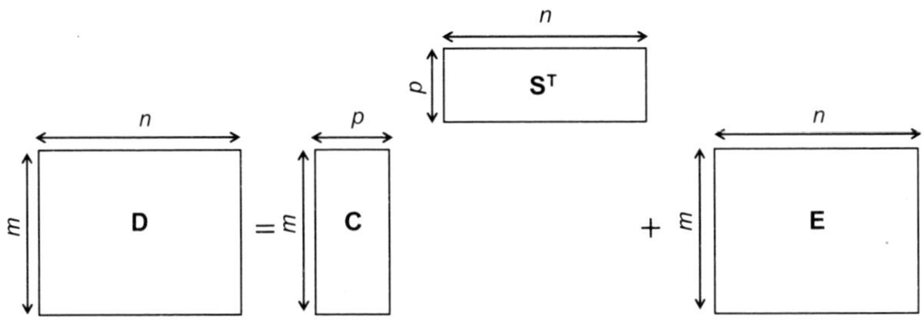

Figure 25.3 General scheme of an MCR decomposition.

The choice of the optimal component number can be based on the knowledge of the system studied or by evaluating PCA outcomes.

During optimization, several constraints, such as nonnegativity, unimodality, closure, trilinearity, selectivity, or/and other shape or hard-modeling constraints can be applied in order to properly model the shape of the **C** and $\mathbf{S}^T$ profiles, taking into account chemical or physical knowledge.

When in two consecutive iterative cycles, relative differences in standard deviation of the residuals between experimental and ALS calculated data values are less than a previously selected value, convergence is achieved.

The difference (**E**) between the original data **D** and the data reproduced from the $\mathbf{C} * \mathbf{S}^T$ product obtained by MCR-ALS is defined lack of fit and represents one of evaluation parameters for the optimization procedure.

25.2.2.4 Cluster Analysis

Cluster exploratory analysis includes a family of methods able to identify groupings among samples and/or variables by means of a similarity measurement (Vandeginste et al., 1998). Similarity among samples is defined as an inverse function of the distance between them. Similarity among variables can be estimated, for instance, by means of the correlation coefficient.

Frequently, similarity is normalized by the maximum value encountered within the data set. It follows that S values may vary between 0 (samples or variables more dissimilar) and 1 (samples or variables coincident).

Cluster analysis can be performed using two main approaches: hierarchical and nonhierarchical. Hierarchical methods can in turn be agglomerative or divisive. The first ones start considering as many clusters as objects; then objects are joined in consecutive steps, on the basis of similarity, until a final situation is reached in which all of the objects are included in a unique cluster. Divisive methods follow exactly the opposite procedure (see Fig. 25.4). In both cases, the number of meaningful clusters is finally defined by the operator evaluating the outcomes, often by looking at a dendrogram. A dendrogram is a plot in which the similarities corresponding to each fusion/ partition step are represented. In more detail, one of the two axes corresponds to similarity, while the second one identifies the objects in an arbitrary order without any physical implication.

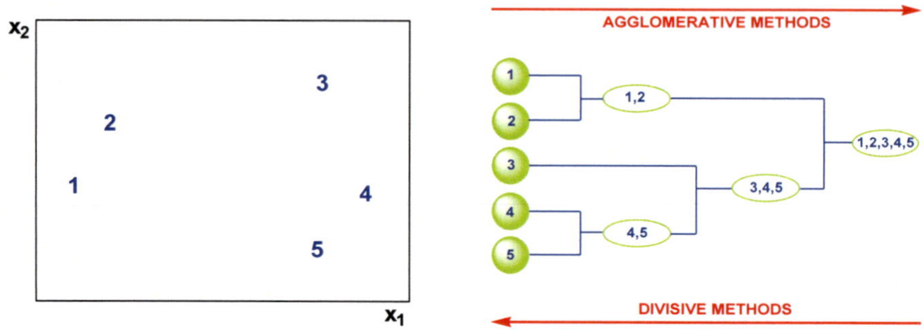

Figure 25.4 Example outline of agglomerative and divisive clustering approaches illustrated with a simulated data set containing five samples described by two variables.

25.2.3 Supervised Qualitative Modeling: Classification and Class Modeling

Analytical controls on food adulterations and, more generally, verification of food authenticity claims usually require qualitative answers.

Chemometric tools that provide qualitative rules and models useful to characterize a sample concerning a given qualitative property are typically represented by discriminant classification and class-modeling techniques. Such qualitative properties define classes that samples belong to. In more detail, classes (or categories) can be defined as groups of samples having in common the same values of discrete variables or proximate values of continuous variables. Frequently, these variables are qualitative factors that cannot be determined experimentally. For this reason, mathematical models able to predict their values—and, therefore, the class to which they belong—from some experimentally measurable predictors are often required.

Discriminant classification techniques require a number of predefined classes (at least two) to be meaningfully defined. They operate by defining a mathematical delimiter between each couple of classes and, consequently, dividing the space of experimental data in as many subspaces as there are classes. On this basis, each new sample will be unambiguously assigned to the class to which it more probably belongs, even in the case of objects that are not pertinent to any class studied.

Conversely, class-modeling techniques characterize a single class of interest by defining an enclosed region in the domain of experimental data—the so-called class space. If a new sample falls within this space, it is considered compatible with the characteristics of the class of interest, otherwise it is considered as anomalous or nongenuine. This is essentially the question to be answered in most food authentication studies (Forina et al., 2008; Oliveri and Downey, 2012).

25.2.3.1 Evaluation Parameters

The outcomes of discriminant classification can be summarized in the so-called confusion matrix, the rows of which represent the actual classes to which samples belong and the columns of which represent the classes to which samples have been assigned by the classification rule.

The success rate is usually evaluated by the classification (or prediction) rate, ie, the percentage of samples correctly classified (or predicted). The term "classification" usually refers to the training sample set, while "prediction" usually indicates estimations on test samples.

A class model is characterized by two parameters: sensitivity and specificity. Sensitivity is the percentage of samples belonging to the modeled class that are correctly recognized as compliant by the model. Specificity is the percentage of samples extraneous to the modeled class that are correctly recognized as noncompliant by the model.

Efficiency of a given class model is defined as the mean (preferably, the geometric mean) of its sensitivity and specificity.

Usually, factors that provide an increment of sensitivity determine a specificity decrease, and vice versa. Depending on the particular problem under study, it may be preferable to maximize one of the two parameters. Not uncommonly, models commissioned by producer consortia for authentication of a food product are required to have 100% sensitivity in order to endorse each of the affiliated and approved producers as genuine.

When specificity is used for optimizing a class model, it should be considered that the choice of the optimal model will be partially influenced by information from classes extraneous to the modeled one.

Classification and class-modeling techniques can be grouped into three main categories:

- distance-based techniques
- probability-based techniques
- experience-based techniques.

25.2.3.2 Distance-Based Techniques

K-nearest Neighbors

K-nearest neighbors (*k*-NN) represents a very intuitive approach for performing discriminant classification on the basis of distances between samples (Vandeginste et al., 1998).

The number of *k* neighbor samples to be considered has to be fixed. Then, for a given sample to be classified, the algorithm identifies the *k* nearest samples of known class membership, in the multivariate space of the measured variables.

Usually, nearness between two samples *i* and *j* is evaluated as an inverse function of the multivariate Euclidean distance $D_{i,j}$:

$$D_{i,j} = \sqrt{(\mathbf{x}_i - \mathbf{x}_j)^{\mathrm{T}}(\mathbf{x}_i - \mathbf{x}_j)} \tag{25.6}$$

where $\mathbf{x}_i$ and $\mathbf{x}_j$ are the sample data vectors, $x_{i,v}$ is the value of variable v for sample i, and $x_{j,v}$ is the value of variable v for sample j.

To perform classification, generally, a majority vote is employed, meaning that the test sample is classified into the class to which the majority of the *k* selected objects belong. Even k values permit ambiguous classifications and for this reason, odd values of k are generally preferred.

Despite its simple mathematical basis, k-NN provides complex nonlinear delimiters—generally expressible as piecewise linear functions—between pairs of classes (see Fig. 25.5). The delimiter usually becomes more complex for small values of k, while it tends to a linear function with increasing k.

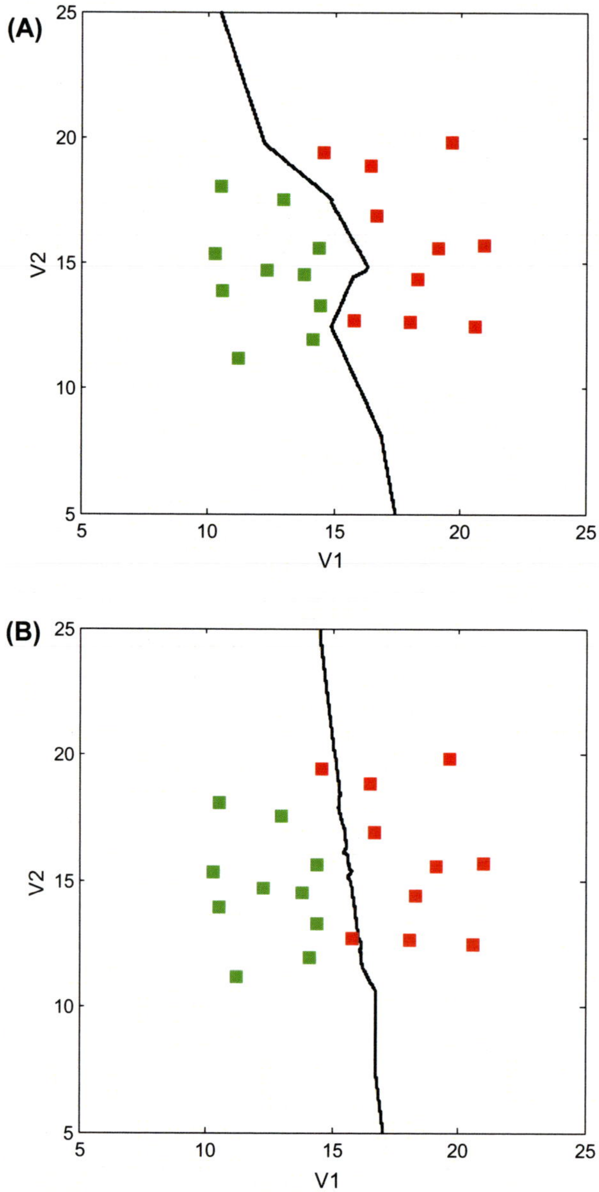

Figure 25.5 Example (*simulated data*) of k-NN class delimiters for $k = 1$ (A) and $k = 9$ (B).

Being a nonprobabilistic method, *k*-NN is free from statistical assumptions—such as normality of variable distributions—and requirements around limitations on the number of variables. This assures a wide applicability (Vandeginste et al., 1998; Dudoit et al., 2002). On the other hand, being a distance-based method, it is particularly sensitive to scaling and transforms applied to the data.

Soft Independent Modeling of Class Analogy

Class-modeling was introduced into chemometrics by Svante Wold (Wold and Sjöström, 1977), with the soft independent modeling of class analogy (SIMCA) method. This method performs PCA on the samples of the class to be modeled, generally after within-class autoscaling or centering. Then, a number of low-order PCs—ideally the significant ones—is identified. They define the so-called inner space, which is the space containing the useful information. The SIMCA model is defined by the range of the sample scores on the PCs of the inner space and it has, therefore, the shape of a segment (one PC, as in Fig. 25.6), a rectangle (two PCs), a parallelepiped (three PCs), or a hyper-parallelepiped (more than three PCs). The score range can be enlarged or reduced, mainly depending on the number of samples, to avoid the possibility of under- or overestimation of the true variability (Forina and Lanteri, 1984). The higher-order principal components not used to describe the model define the space of uninformative variability, called the outer space. The standard deviation of the

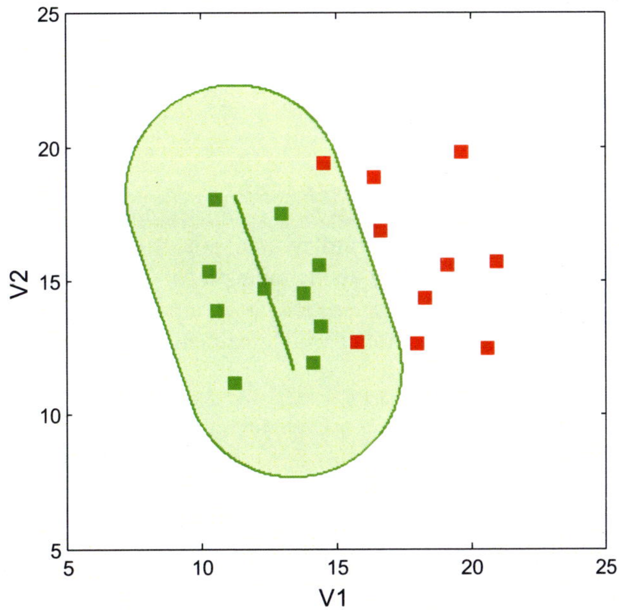

Figure 25.6 SIMCA normal-range model (*green segment*) with monodimensional inner space and the corresponding class space at 95% confidence level (*shaded region enclosed by the green line*) for the class of interest (*simulated data*).

distance of training samples from the model, in the outer space, corresponds to the class standard deviation. A critical distance is obtained by means of the Fisher *F* statistics, at a given confidence level, and it is used to define the boundaries of the SIMCA class space around the model. The SIMCA distance can be defined in several ways corresponding to the different versions of SIMCA proposed by different authors (Durante et al., 2011).

25.2.3.3 Probability-Based Techniques

Linear Discriminant Analysis

Linear discriminant analysis (LDA) is a probability-based discriminant classification method developed by Fisher (1936). The algorithm estimates multivariate probability density functions for each class, starting from location and dispersion parameters estimated by the experimental data; therefore, it is considered a parametric probabilistic technique.

LDA assumes that the probability density distributions within each class are multivariate normal, with the same dispersion for all the classes. For this reason, the same variance-covariance matrix is used to describe all of the probability distributions and it is computed as a pooled variance-covariance matrix. In the bivariate case, the probability density function is bell shaped—its elliptic sections correspond to equal probability density points and are characterized by the same Mahalanobis distance from the centroid.

Mahalanobis distance can be considered as a Euclidean distance (see Eq. (25.6)) modified to take into account the dispersion and the correlation of all the variables:

$$D_{i,j} = \sqrt{(\mathbf{x}_i - \mathbf{x}_j)^{\mathrm{T}} \mathbf{P}^{-1} (\mathbf{x}_i - \mathbf{x}_j)} \tag{25.7}$$

where **P** is the pooled variance-covariance matrix.

Using the same **P** for different classes, the ellipses obtained from the individual class distributions present equal eccentricity and axis orientation; they only differ in their location. Ellipses corresponding to the same probability density for a pair of classes intersect at two points. These intersection points are connectable by a straight line, which defines the linear delimiter (after which the method is named) between couples of classes (see Fig. 25.7).

Quadratic Discriminant Analysis

Quadratic discriminant analysis (QDA) is a probability-based parametric classification technique that can be considered as an evolution of LDA for nonlinear class separations. QDA also assumes that probability density distributions are multivariate normal but it admits different dispersions for the different classes. Consequently, the probability distribution of each class is described by its own variance-covariance matrix and the ellipses of different classes differ for eccentricity and axis orientation (Geisser, 1964). The intersection points of each pair of corresponding ellipses (at the same probability

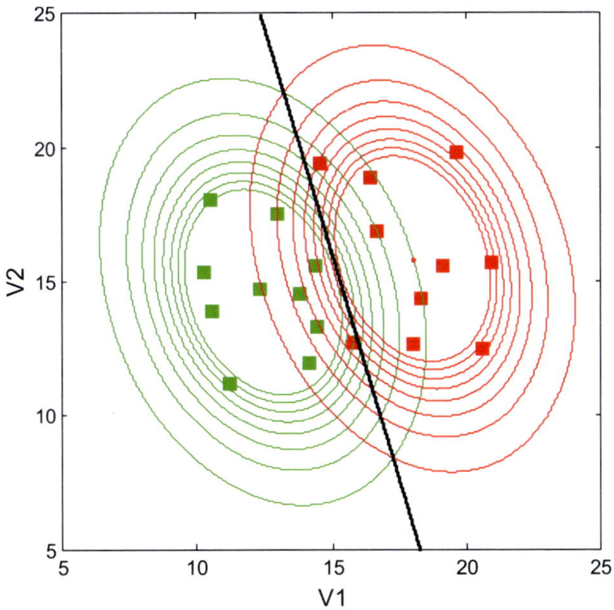

Figure 25.7 Linear class delimiter and associated isoprobability ellipses for LDA hypotheses (*simulated data*).

density level) can be connected, obtaining a quadratic delimiter between the classes (black line in Fig. 25.8).

Unequal Class Models

Unequal class models (UNEQ) is a probability-based class-modeling technique introduced by Derde and Massart (1986) as an evolution of the work on multivariate quality control by Hotelling (1947).

The method can also be considered as a modeling version of QDA; it is also based on the hypothesis of a multivariate normal distribution in the class to be modeled. The critical Mahalanobis distance that defines the width of the class space is determined by application of the Hotelling's T^2 statistics at a selected confidence level (see Fig. 25.9). The class space has the shape of an ellipse (bivariate case), an ellipsoid (trivariate case), or a hyper-ellipsoid (multivariate case) the eccentricity and orientation of which depend on the correlation between the variables and on their dispersion.

These probabilistic techniques present some restrictions on the number of samples, in relation to the number of variables, for a given data set. From a strictly mathematical point of view, samples have to be one more than the number of measured variables. Nevertheless, in order to obtain reliable results, these techniques should be applied in cases when the ratio between the number of objects in a given category and the number of variables is at least three. Furthermore, the number of objects in each class

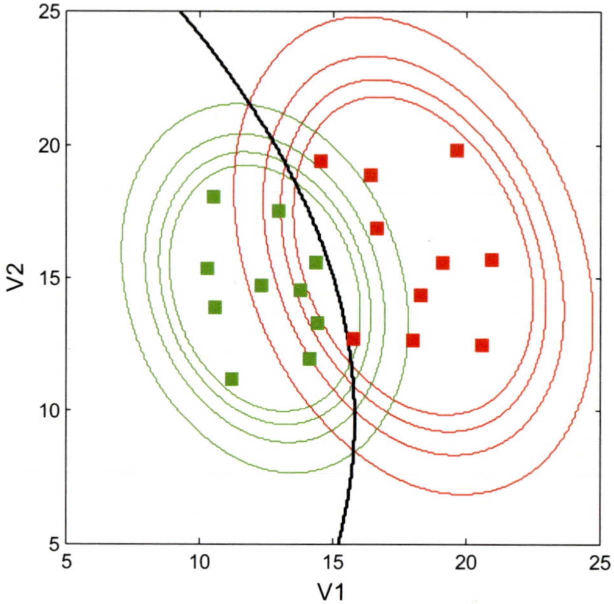

Figure 25.8 Quadratic class delimiter and associated isoprobability ellipses for QDA hypotheses (*simulated data*).

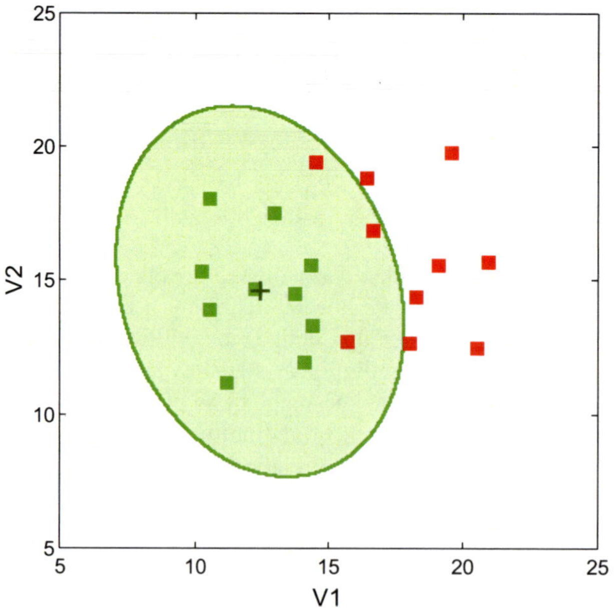

Figure 25.9 UNEQ class model (*green cross*) and the corresponding ellipsoidal class space at 95% confidence level (*shaded region enclosed by the green line*) for the class of interest (*simulated data*).

should be nearly balanced; it is not advisable to work with these methods when ratios between the number of samples in different categories are greater than three (Derde and Massart, 1989).

In cases involving many variables, it is possible to apply LDA, QDA, and UNEQ following a preliminary reduction in the number of variables, which can be achieved, for instance, by a PCA-based compression.

Potential Functions Methods

Potential functions were applied for the first time as probability-based modeling methods by Coomans and Broeckaert (1986). The probability density distribution of the class to be modeled is estimated as the sum of individual contributions of training samples. A variety of functions can be used to define such contributions, the most common of which are Gaussian-like functions. A smoothing coefficient, formally analogous to the standard deviation of the Gaussian probability function, determines the shape of the function. Such a coefficient can be the same for all the samples of a given class (fixed potential) or it can be determined locally as a function of sample density; the latter strategy, known as normal variable potential, is useful when the underlying multivariate distribution is very irregular and characterized by nonuniform density regions (Forina et al., 1991).

The resulting overall probability distribution can assume very irregular shapes, capable of effectively describing complex situations (see the example in Fig. 25.10).

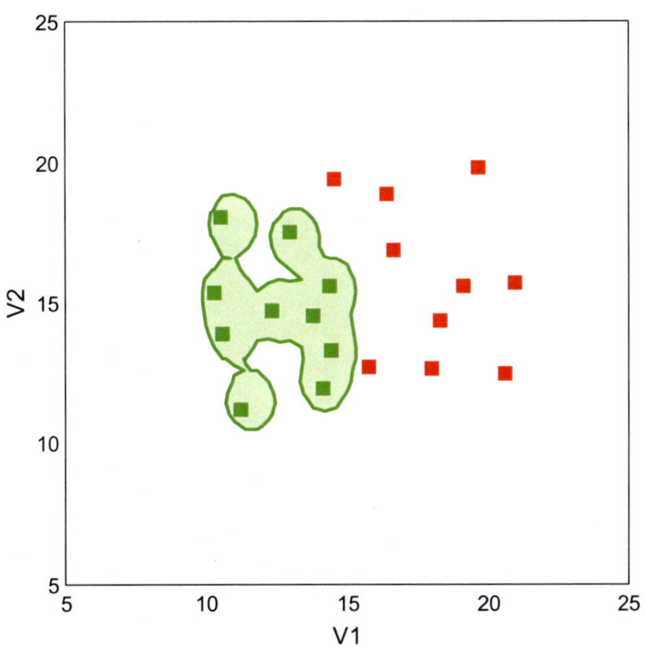

Figure 25.10 Potential function class space at 95% confidence level (*shaded region enclosed by the green line*) for the class of interest (*simulated data*).

The critical value of the probability density distribution, which determines the boundary of the class space, at a selected confidence level is obtained from the critical value of the chi-squared distribution with the so-called equivalent determinant method or with analogue alternative strategies (Forina et al., 1991).

25.2.4 Supervised Quantitative Modeling: Regression

Quantitative models are used to quantify properties of interest on samples using a number of measured variables, called predictors.

Regression models can be univariate or multivariate, depending on the number of predictors and, eventually, of response variables involved. From the point of view of the order of the modeled relationship, models can be linear or nonlinear.

25.2.4.1 Ordinary Least Squares

The ordinary least squares (OLS) method looks for the combination of parameters of the linear model (intercept and slope) that provides the minimum value for the squared residuals (ie, the squared differences between the values estimated by the model and the corresponding true values). The confidence interval for each predicted value can be easily computed.

OLS can be applied as well to multivariate data, namely when the predictors are two or more. In such cases, the method is also referred to as multivariate linear regression (MLR) (Draper and Smith, 1981).

The mathematical model can be expressed in the matrix notation as:

$$\widehat{\mathbf{y}} = \mathbf{X}^{\mathrm{T}}\mathbf{b} \tag{25.8}$$

where $\hat{\mathbf{y}}$ is the vector of the predicted values, $\mathbf{X}$ is the matrix of the predictors augmented with a column of 1, necessary for the estimation of the intercept values, and $\mathbf{b}$ is the column vector of the regression coefficients. The regression coefficients are estimated by:

$$\mathbf{b} = \left(\mathbf{X}^{\mathrm{T}}\mathbf{X}\right)^{-1}\mathbf{X}^{\mathrm{T}}\mathbf{y} \tag{25.9}$$

The elements of the vector $\mathbf{y}$ are the values of the response variable measured for a set of training samples and used for building the model.

The uncertainty of the estimation of coefficients varies inversely with the determinant of the information matrix ($\mathbf{X}^{\mathrm{T}}\mathbf{X}$), which, in the univariate case, corresponds to the variance of the predictor. In the multivariate case, the determinant value depends on the variance of the predictors and on their intercorrelation; high intercorrelations provide a small determinant of the information matrix, which means a large uncertainty of the coefficients and, consequently, unreliable results.

This is a common hurdle when instrumental signals (such as spectra) are used as predictors. In fact, in such cases, contiguous variables are considerably intercorrelated, with correlation coefficient near to 1. In such cases, the determinant of the information matrix would be very small and OLS prediction unreliable.

25.2.4.2 Principal Component Regression

Principal component regression (PCR) performs principal component analysis on the matrix of predictors **X** and uses the scores of samples on a reduced number of significant principal components as new predictors to perform OLS regression. Since the PCs are orthogonal and, therefore, uncorrelated by definition (Jolliffe, 1982), the information matrix derived is not affected by problems related to the determinant.

PCR is very efficient in many cases, but it is not always the case that the significant, lowest-order PCs (which, by definition, explain the highest amount of variance) are the most correlated with the response variable. Therefore, there is a risk of discarding (in the highest-order PCs, not used as predictors) information that would be useful for the prediction.

25.2.4.3 Partial Least Squares Regression

Partial least squares (PLS) regression, also referred to as projections on latent structures, conceptually represents a supervised evolution of PCR (Wold et al., 2001). The latent structures, more frequently called latent variables (LVs) or PLS components, are directions in the space of the predictors characterized by the maximum covariance with the selected response variable. The optimal complexity of the PLS model, ie, the most appropriate number of LVs, is determined by studying the trend of the error as a function of the number of LVs. The error is usually evaluated by computing the standard deviation of the error of calibration (SDEC), estimated with the training samples, and the standard deviation of the error of prediction (SDEP), estimated with test objects:

$$\text{SDEC or SDEP} = \sqrt{\frac{\sum_{i=1}^{N} \left(y_i - \hat{y}_i\right)^2}{N}} \tag{28.10}$$

where y_i is the actual value of the response variable y for sample i, $\hat{y}_i$ is the corresponding value computed or predicted by the model, and N is the number of samples.

The calibration error usually decreases when increasing the LV number because data fitting increases (leading eventually toward overfitting). Conversely, the profile of the prediction error usually presents a minimum at a certain number of LVs and then rises again (see Fig. 25.11); this indicates that the subsequent LVs introduce noise into the model. A simple and practical criterion to identify optimal model complexity is the choice of the number of LVs corresponding to the absolute minimum of SDEP or, better, to its first local minimum. In the example of Fig. 25.11, the optimal complexity could be identified between three and five LVs.

PLS variants have been proposed for developing nonlinear models and for simultaneously predicting two or more response variables (PLS-2) (Wold et al., 2001).

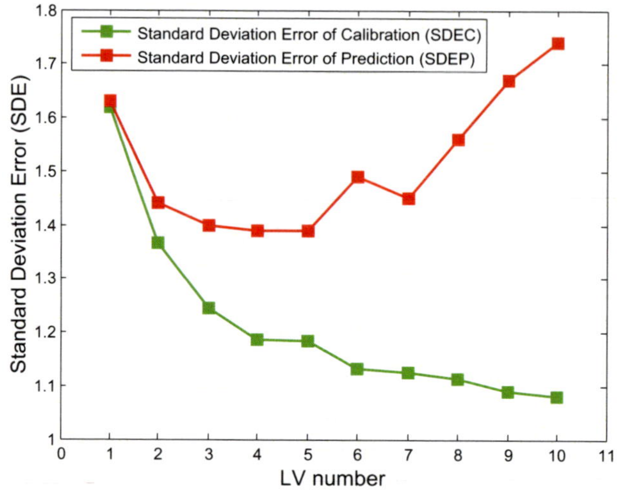

Figure 25.11 Typical trends for calibration and prediction errors as a function of LV number (PLS model complexity).

Furthermore, if class indices are taken as dummy response variables, PLS may work as a classification method, which is usually referred to as discriminant PLS (D-PLS) or PLS discriminant analysis (PLS-DA) (Barker and Rayens, 2003).

25.2.5 Artificial Neural Networks

Artificial neural networks (ANNs) are a family of versatile nonparametric tools that can be employed for several different purposes, from exploratory data analysis to qualitative and quantitative predictive modeling. ANN models are nonlinear and are generally well suited to complex problems. A typical scheme of a multilayer feed-forward artificial neural network (MLF-ANN), which represents one of the most widespread implementations, is shown in Fig. 25.12.

MLF-ANN comprises a number of computational elements, called neurons, generally organized in three layers (Zupan, 1994). In the first one, the input layer, there are usually N neurons that correspond to the original predictors. The predictors are scaled (generally range scaled).

The first layer transmits the value of the predictors to the second—internal—layer. All of the neurons of the input layer are connected to the J neurons of the second layer by means of weight coefficients, meaning that the J elements of the hidden layer receive, as information, a weighted sum Y of the values from the input layer. They transform the information received (Y) by means of a suitable transfer function, frequently a sigmoid.

These neurons transmit information to the third—output—layer, as a weighted combination (K) of their values. The neurons in the output layer correspond to the

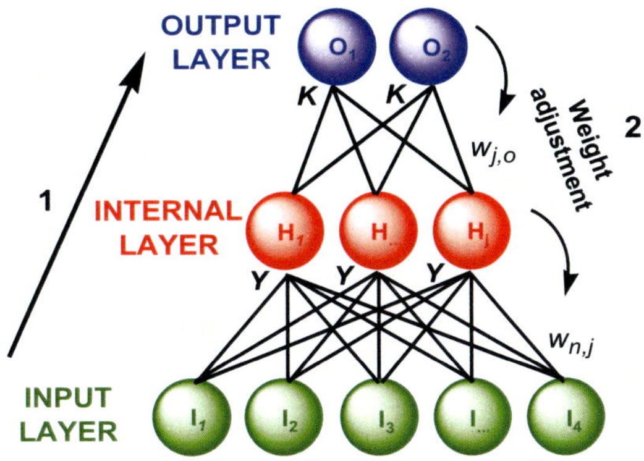

Figure 25.12 Typical scheme of initialization, evolution, adjustment, and prediction mechanisms for a multilayer feed-forward artificial neural network (MLF-ANN).

response variables, which, in the case of classification, are the coded class indices. The output neurons transform the information K, from the hidden layer, by means of a further sigmoid or semilinear function.

After a first random initialization of the values, a learning procedure modifies the weights $w_{n,j}$ and $w_{j,o}$ during several optimization cycles in order to improve the performances of the net. The correction of the weights at each step is proportional to the prediction error of the previous cycle. This optimization of many parameters and the large number of learning cycles considerably increase the risk of overfitting and, for this reason, a thorough validation is required, with a consistent number of objects. In conclusion, ANN use should be limited only to the cases in which other simpler techniques fail and, primarily, when a great number of samples is available.

Another type of widely employed ANN is represented by the Kohonen's self-organizing maps (SOMs), used for unsupervised exploratory analysis, and by the counterpropagation (CP) neural networks, used for nonlinear regression and classification (Kohonen, 2001). Also these tools require a considerable number of objects to build reliable models together with a rigorous validation.

25.2.6 Model Validation

Supervised chemometric methods usually develop models with the purpose of predicting a qualitative or quantitative property of interest. The estimation of the actual predictive ability on new samples is a fundamental issue for providing reliable predictions and it is achieved through model validation. The most common validation strategies divide the available samples into two subsets: a training (or calibration) set used for developing the model and an evaluation (or test) set used to assess its prediction capability. Samples in the evaluation set should be completely extraneous to the model, meaning that no information from them should be used neither for model building nor in the preprocessing stages. This helps to avoid overestimations of the prediction ability.

In many methods, some parameters can be tuned and optimized in the search for a setting that provides the maximum predictive ability for a given sample set. In such cases, the correct approach would involve three sample subsets: a training set, an optimization set, and an evaluation set—the optimization set being used to find the best modeling settings and the evaluation set being used to estimate the actual reliability of the final model.

Evaluation of the predictive ability of a model can be performed in a unique step or many times with different evaluation sets, depending on the strategy adopted.

Evaluation of the predictive ability of a model is an experimental procedure and is therefore affected by an error. For this reason, prediction rate results should be presented together with their confidence interval, which can be estimated by applying appropriate statistical distributions as a function of the number of samples used for validation (Forina et al., 2001, 2007).

25.2.6.1 Single Evaluation Set

The single evaluation set is the simplest scheme for model validation: a fraction—usually between 10% and 50%—of the available samples is excluded from the training set and constitutes the evaluation set. The subdivision may be arbitrary, random, or performed by way of uniform sampling designs, such as the Kennard and Stone and the duplex algorithm (Kennard and Stone, 1969; Snee, 1977), which provide two subsets that are uniformly distributed and representative of the total sample variability.

25.2.6.2 Cross-Validation

The cross-validation (CV) approach is probably the most common validation procedure. Available samples (N) are divided into G cancellation groups following a systematic scheme (eg, Venetian blinds or contiguous blocks). The model is computed G times; each time, one of the cancellation groups is used as the evaluation set while the remaining groups jointly constitute the training set. At the end of the procedure, each sample has been used $G-1$ times for building a model and once for evaluation. The number of cancellation groups is arbitrary and usually ranges from three to N. CV with N cancellation groups is generally known as a leave-one-out procedure (LOO). LOO has the advantage of being independent of the order of samples while, when $G < N$, different orders of the samples may supply different outcomes. However, especially in the case for numerous sample sets, predictions made on single samples, although repeated many times, may produce overoptimistic results. An extensive validation strategy would consist in performing CV many times with different numbers of cancellation groups, from three up to N. Another possibility is to repeat CV, for a given number $G < N$ of cancellation groups, each time permuting the order of the samples and thus obtaining a different group composition each time.

25.2.6.3 Repeated Evaluation Set

The repeated evaluation set procedure, often referred to as Monte Carlo validation, is based on the computation of many models (hundreds or thousands), each time selecting a different evaluation set by random selection. Thus, samples may fall many times, or even no times at all, in the evaluation set. This strategy requires a longer computational time but one that is generally still practical on modern computers.

25.2.7 Future Trends

Analytical instrumentation is continuously evolving and the amount of data recorded is often considerable. As an example, spectroscopic techniques operating at high-resolution levels may produce thousands of data for a single spectrum. Consequently, high-performance algorithms and computational tools, able to manage and process megavariate data, are more and more often required. Furthermore, many analytical techniques produce data structured as three-dimensional arrays; this is the typical case for hyperspectral imaging methods (Gowen et al., 2014) and for bidimensional spectroscopic and chromatographic methods (Lenhardt et al., 2015; Tranchida et al., 2016). Also in these cases, appropriate chemometric approaches are required, and this is one of the most important current research fields (Burger and Gowen, 2011).

25.2.8 An Overview on Chemometric Software

In recent decades, the number of available software tools for chemometric data processing has considerably increased. An overview of a selection of software packages for chemometric analysis and their main features is contained in Table 25.1. Software tools for multivariate analysis can be divided into three main categories on the basis of their scope and application field. The first type (represented, eg, by Minitab and XLStat) is software for multivariate statistical analysis in general. Such programs usually include the most common techniques for data exploration and modeling, but no specific tools for the processing of analytical data. The second type is represented by dedicated chemometric packages; in this case, specific techniques for analysis of chemical/physical data, such as signal transformations and/or curve resolution methods, are implemented. The third category (not included in the overview reported in Table 25.1), which includes software provided together with specific analytical instrumentation, is the one that usually contains tools that are more strictly aligned to the processing of the particular type of data measured by the instrument.

Further possible classifications concern the distinction between free and commercial software, or between open-source and closed-source programs. Finally, a number of tools are provided as stand-alone packages that just need to be installed and executed; others are implemented as extensions of well-established platforms (eg, Excel, Matlab, and R).

Table 25.1 Comparison of a Selection of Software Tools for Multivariate Analysis

Software	Company	Stand-Alone/ Environment-Specific	Signal Preprocessing	PCA	Multi-way	MCR	Cluster Analysis	Classification	Class-Modeling	Regression	Variable Selection	DoE
The Unscrambler X	CAMO	Stand-alone	SNV, smoothing, Detrending, MSC, EMSC, OSC, derivatives (Savitzki-Golay, Norris Gap, Gap-segment), COW	Yes, with test set projection	No	Yes	No	LDA, SVM-DA	SIMCA	PCR, PLS, MLR	MUT	Factorial design, mixture design, Plackett-Burman design, D-optimal design, Central Composite design
PLS-toolbox/ Solo	Eigenvector Research Inc.	Matlab-dependent/ stand-alone	SNV, row profiles, smoothing, Detrending, OSC, MSC, EMSC, derivatives (Savitzki-Golay), WLS, COW	Yes, with test set projection	MPCA, PARAFAC, multiway PLS (N-PLS)	Yes	Hierarchical agglomerative and k-means	k-NN, LDA, QDA, PLS-DA, SVM-DA (SVM-C)	SIMCA	MLR, CLS, PCR, PLS, LWR, SVM-R	GA, I-PLS	No
Pirouette	InfoMetrix Inc.	Stand-alone	SNV, smoothing, MSC, derivatives	Yes, with test set projection	No	Yes	Hierarchical	k-NN, PLS-DA	SIMCA	PCR, PLS, CLS, LWR, ALS	No	No
Minitab17	Minitab Inc.	Stand-alone	No	Yes	No	No	Hierarchical and non-hierarchical	LDA, QDA	No	OLS, PLS, nonlinear regression, Poisson regression	Stepwise	Factorial design, response surface design, mixture design, Taguchi design, Plackett-Burman design, D-optimal design

XLStat	Addinsoft SARL/ Microsoft Corporation	MS-Excel-dependent	No	Yes	No	No	Hierarchical agglomerative and k-means	LDA, QDA, PLS-DA, k-NN, CART	No	OLS, PLS, PCR, CART, nonlinear methods,	No	Screening design, Surface response design, mixture design
SIMCA	Umetrics	Stand-alone	SNV, derivatives, OSC, MSC, wavelet	Yes	No	No	Hierarchical, PLS-Trees	PLS-DA, OPLS-DA, O2PLS-DA	SIMCA	PLS, OPLS, O2PLS	No	No
R-based chemometric software	Italian chemometrics group	R-dependent	SNV, derivatives, row profiles	Yes, with test set projection	Tucker3	No	No	LDA, QDA	No	PCR, PLS-1, PLS-2, MLR	No	D-optimal design
PARVUS	Prof. Michele Forina - University of Genova	Stand-alone	SNV, row profiles, smoothing, Detrending, MSC, EMSC, derivatives (Savitzki-Golay), Consensus	Yes, with test set projection	No	No	Hierarchical and non-hierarchical, ANN (Kohonen maps)	k-NN, LDA, QDA, PLS-DA, ANN	UNEQ, SIMCA, PFM, MRM, CAMM	OLS, PCR, PLS-1, PLS-2, ACE, ANN	ISE, IPW, IPOW, UVE, I-PLS, GOLPE, GA, select	No

The following table is not intended to provide a complete and too detailed review of the available chemometric software nor to supply a comparison for commercial purposes. For more information and details about the reviewed software, the reader is referred to the individual developers or sellers. *SNV*, standard normal variate; *MSC*, multiplicative scatter correction; *EMSC*, extended multiplicative scatter correction; *OSC*, orthogonal signal correction; *COW*, correlation optimized warping; *WLS*, weighted least squares; *PCA*, principal component analysis; *MPCA*, multiway (unfold) principal components analysis; *PARAFAC*, PARAllel FACtor analysis; *PLS*, partial least squares; *ANN*, artificial neural networks; *MCR*, multivariate curve resolution; *LDA*, linear discriminant analysis; *SVM-DA*, support vector machines discriminant analysis; *k-NN*, k-nearest neighbors; *PLS-DA*, partial least squares discriminant analysis; *SVM-C*, support vector machines classification; *QDA*, quadratic discriminant analysis; *CART*, classification and regression trees; *O(2)PLS-DA*, orthogonal (2) partial least squares discriminant analysis; *SIMCA*, soft independent modeling of class analogy; *UNEQ*, UNEQual class models; *PFM*, potential function methods; *MRM*, multivariate range modeling; *CAMM*, caiman analogue modeling methods; *PCR*, principal component regression; *MLR*, multivariate linear regression; *CLS*, classical least squares; *LWR*, locally weighted regression; *ALS*, alternating least squares; *OLS*, ordinary least squares; *ACE*, alternating conditional expectations; *MUT*, martens uncertainty test; *GA*, genetic algorithms; *I-PLS*, interval partial least squares; *ISE*, iterative stepwise elimination; *IPW*, iterative predictor weighting; *IPOW*, iterative predictors and objects weighting; *UVE*, uninformative variable elimination; *GOLPE*, generating optimal linear PLS estimations.

Acknowledgment

Financial support by the Italian Ministry of Education, Universities and Research (MIUR) is acknowledged – Research Project SIR 2014 "Advanced strategies in near infrared spectroscopy and multivariate data analysis for food safety and authentication," RBSI14CJHJ (CUP: D32I15000150008).

References

Barker, M., Rayens, W., 2003. Partial least squares for discrimination. Journal of Chemometrics 17, 166–173.

Barnes, R.J., Dhanoa, M.S., Lister, S.J., 1989. Standard normal variate transformation and de-trending of near-infrared diffuse reflectance spectra. Applied Spectroscopy 43 (5), 772–777.

Bro, R., 2006. Review on multiway analysis in chemistry – 2000–2005. Critical Reviews in Analytical Chemistry 36, 279–293.

Burger, J., Gowen, A., 2011. Data handling in hyperspectral image analysis. Chemometrics and Intelligent Laboratory Systems 108, 13–22.

Bush, J.E., 2002. "By Hercules! the more common the wine, the more wholesome!": science and the adulteration of food and other natural products in ancient Rome. Food and Drug Law Journal 57, 573–602.

Coomans, D., Broeckaert, I., 1986. Potential Pattern Recognition in Chemical and Medical Decision Making. Research Studies Press, England. Letchworth.

Derde, M.P., Massart, D.L., 1986. UNEQ: a disjoint modelling technique for pattern recognition based on normal distribution. Analytica Chimica Acta 184, 33–51.

Derde, M.P., Massart, D.L., 1989. Evaluation of the required sample size in some supervised pattern recognition techniques. Analytica Chimica Acta 223, 19–44.

Draper, N.R., Smith, H., 1981. Applied Regression Analysis, second ed. Wiley, New York.

Dudoit, S., Fridly, J., Speed, P., 2002. Comparison of discrimination methods for the classification of tumors using gene expression data. Journal of the American Statistical Association 97, 77–87.

Durante, C., Bro, R., Cocchi, M., 2011. A classification tool for N-way array based on SIMCA methodology. Chemometrics and Intelligent Laboratory Systems 106, 73–85.

Fearn, T., 2009. The effect of spectral pre-treatments on interpretation. NIR News 20, 16–17.

Fisher, R.A., 1936. The use of multiple measurements in taxonomic problems. Annals of Eugenics 7, 179–188.

Forina, M., Lanteri, S., 1984. Chemometrics: mathematics and statistics in chemistry. In: Kowalski, B.R. (Ed.), NATO ASI Series, Ser. C, vol. 138. Reidel Publishing Co., Dordrecht, pp. 439–466.

Forina, M., Armanino, C., Leardi, R., Drava, G., 1991. A class-modelling technique based on potential functions. Journal of Chemometrics 5, 435–453.

Forina, M., Lanteri, S., Rosso, S., 2001. Confidence intervals of the prediction ability and performance scores of classifications methods. Chemometrics and Intelligent Laboratory Systems 57, 121–132.

Forina, M., Lanteri, S., Casale, M., 2007. Multivariate calibration. Journal of Chromatography A 1158, 61–93.

Forina, M., Oliveri, P., Lanteri, S., Casale, M., 2008. Class-modeling techniques, classic and new, for old and new problems. Chemometrics and Intelligent Laboratory Systems 93, 132–148.

Geisser, S., 1964. Posterior odds for multivariate normal distributions. Journal of the Royal Statistical Society: Series B Methodological 26, 69–76.

Geladi, P., Manley, M., Lestander, T., 2003. Scatter plotting in multivariate data analysis. Journal of Chemometrics 17, 503–511.

Gowen, A., Burger, J., Esquerre, C., Downey, G., O'Donnell, C., 2014. Near infrared hyperspectral image regression: on the use of prediction maps as a tool for detecting model overfitting. Journal of Near Infrared Spectroscopy 22, 261–270.

Hart, F.L., 1952. A history of the adulteration of food before 1906. Food Drug Cosmetic Law Journal 7, 5–22.

Hotelling, H., 1947. Multivariate quality control. In: Eisenhart, C., Hastay, M.W., Wallis, W.A. (Eds.), Techniques of Statistical Analysis. McGraw-Hill, New York, pp. 111–184.

Jellema, R.H., 2009. Variable shift and alignment. In: Brown, S.D., Tauler, R., Walczak, B. (Eds.), Comprehensive Chemometrics, vol. 2. Elsevier, Amsterdam, pp. 85–108.

Jolliffe, I.T., 1982. A note on the use of principal components in regression. Journal of the Royal Statistical Society: Series C (Applied Statistics) 31 (3), 300–303.

Jolliffe, I.T., 2002. Principal Component Analysis, second ed. Springer, New York, pp. 201–207.

Kennard, R.W., Stone, L.A., 1969. Computer aided design of experiments. Technometrics 11, 137–148.

Kjeldahl, K., Bro, R., 2010. Some common misunderstandings in chemometrics. Journal of Chemometrics 24, 558–564.

Kohonen, T., 2001. Self Organizing Maps, third ed. Springer, New York.

Lees, M., 2003. Food Authenticity and Traceability. Woodhead Publishing Ltd, Cambridge, UK.

Lenhardt, L., Bro, R., Zeković, I., Dramićanin, T., Dramićanin, M.D., 2015. Fluorescence spectroscopy coupled with PARAFAC and PLS DA for characterization and classification of honey. Food Chemistry 175, 284–291.

Luykx, D.M.A.M., Van Ruth, S.M., 2008. An overview of analytical methods for determining the geographical origin of food products. Food Chemistry 107, 897–911.

Maeder, M., 1987. Evolving factor analysis for the resolution of overlapping chromatographic peaks. Analytical Chemistry 59, 527–530.

Nielsen, N.-P.V., Carstensen, J.M., Smedsgaard, J., 1998. Aligning of single and multiple wavelength chromatographic profiles for chemometric data analysis using correlation optimised warping. Journal of Chromatography A 805, 17–35.

Oliveri, P., Downey, G., 2012. Multivariate class modeling for the verification of food-authenticity claims. TRAC Trends in Analytical Chemistry 35, 74–86.

Oliveri, P., Casolino, M.C., Casale, M., Medini, L., Mare, F., Lanteri, S., 2013. A spectral transfer procedure for application of a single class-model to spectra recorded by different NIR spectrometers for authentication of olives in brine. Analytica Chimica Acta 761, 46–52.

Pearson, K., 1901. On lines and planes of closest fit to systems of points in space. Philosophical Magazine 2 (6), 559–572.

Reis, M.S., Saraiva, P.M., Bakshi, B.R., 2009. Denoising and signal-to-noise ratio enhancement: Wavelet transform and Fourier transform. In: Brown, S.D., Tauler, R., Walczak, B. (Eds.), Comprehensive Chemometrics, vol. 2. Elsevier, Amsterdam, pp. 25–55.

Savitzky, A., Golay, M.J.E., 1964. Smoothing and differentiation of data by simplified least squares procedure. Analytical Chemistry 36, 1627–1639.

Savorani, F., Tomasi, G., Engelsen, S.B., 2010. Icoshift: a versatile tool for the rapid alignment of 1D NMR spectra. Journal of Magnetic Resonance 202, 190–202.

Snee, R., 1977. Validation of regression models: methods and examples. Technometrics 19, 415–428.

Sun, D.W., 2008. Modern Techniques for Food Authentication. Academic Press/Elsevier, London, UK.

Taavitsainen, V.M., 2009. Denoising and signal-to-noise ratio enhancement: derivatives. In: Brown, S.D., Tauler, R., Walczak, B. (Eds.), Comprehensive Chemometrics, vol. 2. Elsevier, Amsterdam, pp. 57–66.

Tauler, R., Smilde, A.K., Kowalsky, B.J., 1995. Selectivity, local rank, three-way data analysis and ambiguity in multivariate curve resolution. Journal of Chemometrics 9, 31–58.

Tauler, R., 1995. Multivariate curve resolution applied to second order data. Chemometrics and Intelligent Laboratory Systems 30, 133–146.

Tauler, R., 2001. Calculation of maximum and minimum band boundaries of feasible solutions for species profiles obtained by multivariate curve resolution. Journal of Chemometrics 15, 627–646.

Tranchida, P.Q., Franchina, F.A., Dugo, P., Mondello, L., 2016. Comprehensive two-dimensional gas chromatography-mass spectrometry: recent evolution and current trends. Mass Spectrometry Reviews 35, 524–534. http://dx.doi.org/10.1002/mas.21443.

Vandeginste, B.G.M., Massart, D.L., Buydens, L.M.C., De Jong, S., Lewi, P.J., Smeyers-Verbeke, J., 1998. Handbook of Chemometrics and Qualimetrics, vol. 20B. Elsevier, Amsterdam.

Windig, W., Guilment, J., 1991. Interactive self-modeling mixture analysis. Analytical Chemistry 63, 1425–1432.

Wold, S., Sjöström, M., 1977. SIMCA: a method for analysing chemical data in terms of similarity and analogy. In: Kowalski, B.R. (Ed.), Chemometrics: Theory and Applications, ACS Symposium Series, vol. 52. American Chemical Society, Washington, pp. 243–282.

Wold, S., Sjöström, M., Eriksson, L., 2001. PLS-regression: a basic tool of chemometrics. Chemometrics and Intelligent Laboratory Systems 58, 109–130.

Zupan, J., 1994. Introduction to artificial neural network (ANN) methods: what they are and how to use them. Acta Chimica Slovenica 41, 327–352.

Advances in Testing for Adulteration in Honey

26

F. Ulberth
European Commission, Geel, Belgium

Chapter Outline

26.1 Introduction

Honey is a natural product that has been valued for its sweetening properties since ancient times and has a long history of medicinal use. To comply with internationally accepted standards, honey can only be minimally processed by centrifugation, mild heating, and, if necessary to avoid foreign matter, filtered. Additives must not be added. The FAO/WHO Codex Alimentarius standard for honey (CODEX STAN 12-1981) describes the product as:

> *Honey is the natural sweet substance produced by honey bees from the nectar of plants or from secretions of living parts of plants or excretions of plant sucking insects on the living parts of plants, which the bees collect, transform by combining with specific substances of their own, deposit, dehydrate, store and leave in the honey comb to ripen and mature.*

The Codex standard also requires that no other food ingredient or additive shall be added, no pollen or other constituent removed except where this is unavoidable in the removal of foreign inorganic or organic matter, and that honey shall not be heated or processed to such an extent that its essential composition is changed and/or its quality impaired. Furthermore, the standard lays down compositional requirements and quality provisions such as the content of moisture, glucose, fructose, sucrose, hydroxymethylfurfural (HMF), free acidity, diastase activity, and electrical conductivity.

Provisions of the Codex standard are intended to facilitate international trade but also to protect the well-being of consumers (therefore the standard contains certain provisions on contaminants and residues).

A number of jurisdictions have transposed CODEX STAN 12-1981 into national law, sometimes in slightly amended and extended form. For example, Council Directive 2001/110/EC builds on the Codex standard and lays down further provisions related to labeling and to the mode of production and/or presentation. This Directive allows labeling the floral or vegetable origin of honey if the product comes wholly or mainly from the indicated source and possesses the organoleptic, physicochemical, and microscopic characteristics of the botanical source, and the regional, territorial, or topographical origin if the product comes entirely from the indicated source. Honeys with an indicated origin command higher prices on the market as consumers appreciate and value their unique sensory properties and sometimes also their medicinal effects such as in the case of Manuka (*Leptospermum scoparium*) and Kanuka (*Kunzea ericoides*) honeys.

The worldwide demand for honey has risen over the past decades, whereas production in most countries has remained constant, except in the case of China where production more than doubled in the period 1993 to 2013 (Fig. 26.1). China is also the largest supplier of honey to the European market, with imports amounting to more than 83,000 tons (FAOSTAT, 2015). Prices for Chinese honey tend to be lower than European Union domestic products due to cheaper labor costs.

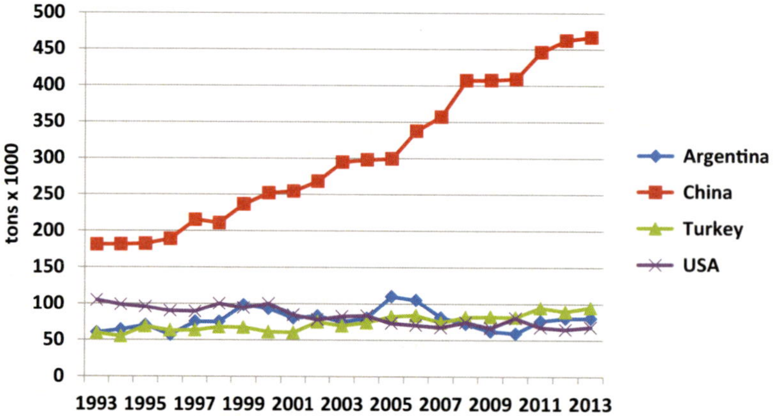

[AU2] **Figure 26.1** Honey production by the top-five producing nations (FAOSTAT, 2015).

Whenever demand for a certain product is high and supply is short, an incentive exists for unscrupulous operators in the supply chain to engage in fraudulent manipulations to improve profits. In the case of honey, the two basic fraud situations with which control authorities are confronted are:

- Extension of honey by sugar syrups of various origins
- Misdescription of botanical and/or geographic origin of honey

Other aspects of honey authenticity relate to undeclared filtration to remove pollen, undeclared pasteurization, and removal of water from unripe "green" honey (Bogdanov and Martin, 2002).

The International Honey Commission (IHC) has published a compendium of harmonized methods (http://www.ihc-platform.net/ihcmethods2009.pdf), which is of great use in the verification of the provisions of the Codex standards as well as national legislation related to honey quality. They are widely used to control whether honey conforms to marketing standards laid down by international guidelines and national legislation but are not always effective enough to detect fraudulent manipulations.

In the quest to find markers of honey authenticity, numerous approaches have been tried with varying success. Honey is a natural product and its composition is influenced by a wide range of factors that are difficult to control. Its basic composition is fairly constant, with a water content generally less than 20 g/100 g, 37–39 g/100 g fructose, 30–32 g/100 g glucose (fructose-to-glucose ratio usually 1.2:1.0), 0.5–2 g sucrose and 0.2 g/100 g ash. However, the amount of minor and trace components such as oligosaccharides, amino acids, volatiles, phenolic substances. and trace elements varies to a great extent depending on the composition of the floral nectar bees forage on. This latter is influenced by the plant species, soil, climate, latitude and altitude, and environmental pollution of the foraging area; in addition, during processing and storage of honey, certain compositional changes occur. This multifaceted mechanism makes it difficult to identify a set of markers that allow a robust classification of honeys of unknown provenance. However, when sugar syrups are deliberately added to honey for extension of the product, certain substances that do not naturally occur in honey may be introduced; such substances may well serve as markers of adulteration.

Sensory analysis by a trained panel may effectively serve to identify unifloral honey based on sensory attributes such as color, taste and aroma. The International Honey Commission developed harmonized terminology and a description of European unifloral honey (Piana et al., 2004). A glossary of terms used in sensory description of unifloral honey was agreed and arranged as an "aroma and odor wheel of honey." The aim of the method, which is based on a number of ISO standards related to sensory analysis (ISO 4121, ISO 6658, ISO 6564), is to detect sensory defects and to assess the conformity of the aroma profile with certain, agreed upon standard descriptions for unifloral honey.

Combining sensory analysis with conventional physicochemical tests (conductivity, pH, free acidity, etc.) has been reported to be of help in characterizing and differentiating unifloral honeys from various geographical origins (Bertoncelj et al., 2011; Rodríguez et al., 2015).

26.2 Processes Used in Identification of Adulteration in Honey

As in any other food forensics work, targeted or untargeted methods can be used to detect adulterated or misdescribed honey (Fig. 26.2). Adulteration of honey by addition of sugar syrups is usually targeted by the analysis of specific markers, while for detection of wrongly described geographical and botanical honey origin, both targeted and untargeted profiling methods are employed. The botanical and the geographical origin of a honey influence at the same time certain characteristic properties (traces of organic and inorganic substances), and, therefore, profiling methods can serve both purposes. However, the analyst needs to know beforehand either the geographical or the botanical origin to judge whether the other has been declared correctly.

Numerous reports exist reviewing many aspects of honey composition, authenticity, and traceability (Anklam, 1998; Arvanitoyannis et al., 2005; Kaškonienė and Venskutonis, 2010; Wang and Li, 2011; Zábrodská and Vorlová, 2014; Missio da Silva et al., 2016).

26.2.1 Detection and Quantification of Sugar Syrup Addition to Honey

Since genuine honey is an extensive commodity and similar products of lower economic value exist, fraudsters are tempted to extend honey by adding sugar syrups for economic gain. Chemically speaking, honey is a concentrated solution of a few

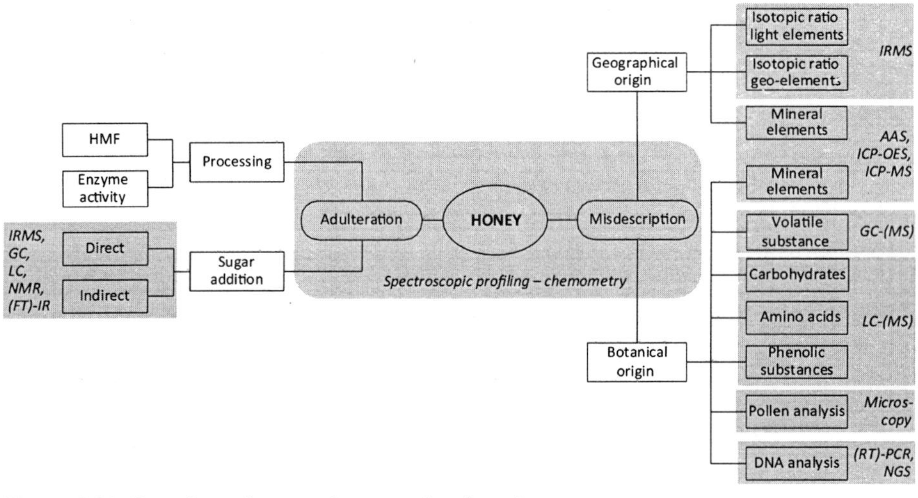

Figure 26.2 Overview of approaches to authenticate honey.

sugars (fructose, glucose, and sucrose) and certain other disaccharides and oligosaccharides occurring at low concentrations. Usually the fructose-to-glucose ratio is around 1.2:1.0 although quite a degree of variation exists depending on honey floral origin (Escudero et al., 2014). Crystallization behavior of honey is primarily influenced by its glucose content; those samples with a concentration lower than 30%[1] usually take longer to crystallize, eg, honeydew, chestnut, eucalyptus, while sunflower, rape and lime honeys with a higher glucose content will granulate more rapidly (Manikis and Thrasivoulou, 2001). For this reason, the simple addition of pure glucose syrup would not only be easy to detect but, more importantly, exert negative effects on the crystallization behavior of honey. Addition of sucrose would also be easy to detect by one of the sugar methods harmonized and validated by the International Honey Commission (Table 26.1), although the naturally present

Table 26.1 Conventional Parameters for Estimating Honey Quality and Authenticity

Parameter	Method Principle	Type of Adulteration/Misdescription Detected
Moisture	Refractometry	Water addition
Electrical conductivity	Electrochemistry	Botanical origin (unifloral honeys)
Ash	Gravimetry	Botanical origin
Acidity	Titrimetry	Deterioration (fermentation)
		Botanical origin
Hydroxymethyl-furfural (HMF)	Colorimetry Chromatography	Sugar syrups produced by acid hydrolysis Heat treatment Freshness
Diastase	Colorimetry	Heat treatment
Invertase		Freshness
Sugars Fructose Glucose Sucrose Maltose	Chromatography GLC-FID LC-RID LC-PAD	Sugar syrup addition Botanical origin
Proline	Colorimetry	Honey maturity

Harmonized and validated methods of analysis for those parameters were made available by the International Honey Commission (http://www.ihc-platform.net/ihcmethods2009.pdf).

[1] Percentages in this chapter relate to mass/mass.

enzyme invertase can partially convert sucrose to a mixture of fructose and glucose. Inverted sugar syrup (IS), which is a mixture of glucose and fructose and therefore much closer in composition to honey, can be detected by its elevated content of HMF if acid is used for the sucrose hydrolysis (Anklam, 1998). More modern processes for producing invert syrup use enzymes and avoid the formation of HMF.

High-fructose corn syrup (HFSC) is most commonly used for the fraudulent extension of honey because of its ready availability at comparatively low cost. HFSC 55 is fairly similar to honey; it contains approximately 55% fructose, 41% glucose, and 4% other (oligo)saccharides (White, 2008), and addition of up to 50% will not push the sugar composition outside of the Codex specifications. Of course, larger amounts of added sugar syrups will dilute the levels of other minor components of genuine honey such as certain di- and oligosaccharides (turanose, trehalose, erlose, melezitose, etc.), minerals, phenolic and volatile compounds, N-containing substances, etc.; however, the wide natural variation of these substances lessens their value as authenticity indicators. More appropriate is the use of marker substances that are exogenous to honey and that are introduced by the extension with sugar syrups.

26.2.1.1 Chromatography

Although HFCS material is chromatographically refined, samples contain a measureable quantity of oligosaccharides that are not converted to glucose and fructose; consequently, these are good markers for the detection of HFCS addition to honey. High-performance anion-exchange chromatography coupled with pulsed amperometric detection (HPAEC-PAD) is a suitable technique for the determination of oligosaccharides. Morales et al. (2006, 2008) applied this technique to detect admixture of corn syrup (CS) and HFCS to genuine honey samples after separation of the oligosaccharides from the bulk of other sugars through the use of charcoal. High-molecular-weight oligosaccharides with a degree of polymerization (DP) of DP3 to DP16 were present in CS and HFCS samples. Admixture of 5% CS to honey was clearly detectable but the sensitivity of the method for detecting HFCS was lower. Multivariate statistical methods such as linear discriminant analysis (LDA) and partial least-squares (PLS) regression analysis were applied to chromatographic data of honey and honey/sugar syrup mixtures obtained by HPAEC-PAD (Cordella et al., 2005). Preprocessing of the chromatographic data was necessary before applying the statistical routines. Correct classification rates (>95%) were obtained for authentic and adulterated samples (96.5% overall correct classification) using LDA followed by canonical analysis. HPAEC-PAD was used after sample preparation by solid phase extraction (SPE) on Envi-ChromP (styrene/divinyl benzene copolymer resin) to enrich oligosaccharides in bee-feeding sugar syrup (10% fructose, 45% glucose, 30% maltose, 13% maltotriose, and 2% higher oligosaccharides). Oligo-/polysaccharides up to DP 18 were detected in the syrup. Addition of this type of syrup at the 1% level in all three floral types of honey (acacia, mountain polyfloral, and polyfloral) tested was readily detected (Megherbi et al., 2009).

A different liquid chromatographic approach using an ultra-performance column and detection by evaporative light scattering (UPLC—ELSD) allowed determination of maltooligosaccharides originating from syrups at limits of quantification (LOQ) ranging from 0.30 to 0.60 mg/g honey. In one report, 290 honey samples taken from the Chinese market were analyzed and it was concluded that honey samples should be regarded as imitation or adulterated product if the contents of maltose, maltotriose, maltotetraose, maltopentaose, maltohexaose, and maltoheptaose are greater than or equal to 5.0, 148.0, 13.0, 5.0, 2.0, and 4.0 mg/g, respectively (Zhou et al., 2014).

Wang et al. (2015) claimed to have found a marker in high fructose syrups (HFS) obtained from different plant sources (corn, rice, cassava) that elutes from a Carbomix Ca-NP5, 8% cross-linkage column at a certain retention time. This marker was absent in the pure honeys surveyed (only a small hump in the baseline was seen for some honeys, which would theoretically correspond to 1% HFS addition). The marker was tentatively identified as a mixture of oligosaccharides with DP4 (maltopentaose, maltohexaose, and maltoheptaose) by retention time matching to authentic standards. A limit of detection of 1% rice HFS in honey was reported. The ease of sample preparation (dilution of honey) and simplicity of instrumentation (isocratic HPLC with refractive index detection) and use of pure water as eluent makes this method attractive for routine application, although the chromatographic run time is rather long (30 min).

A marker for the presence of rice syrup in honey was developed by another Chinese group (Xue, 2013); this is of great relevance because the addition of rice syrup is difficult to detect even by analysis of carbon isotopes. The marker compound was identified as 2-acetylfuran-3-glucopyranoside (AFGP) by mass spectrometry (MS) and nuclear magnetic resonance (NMR) spectroscopy. It absorbs at 280 nm, which allows detection by a UV or diode array detector (DAD) after HPLC separation. AFPG was found to be absent in genuine honey ($n = 186$) but was present in rice syrups at a concentration of 92 ± 60 mg/kg, which allows to detect addition of 10% rice syrup to honey.

Difructose anhydrides (DFAs) are nonfermentable, pseudodisaccharides that consist of two fructose residues and present different structural varieties according to their linkage type. They do not occur in honey but in fructose-rich syrups (Ruiz-Matute et al., 2007). Before being determined by GLC-FID or GLC-MS, the majority of honey sugars need to be removed by fermentation with *Saccharomyces cerevisiae*. Detection as low as 5% addition of fructose-rich syrups (HFCS or IS) in honey was feasible by this approach. The same approach has been used to detect addition of high-fructose inulin syrup (HFIS) to honey. Besides DFA, inulotriose proved to be a good marker for the presence of HFIS in honey (Ruiz-Matute, 2010). Inulotriose was an even better marker for HFIS as it occurred at substantially higher levels, which rendered the fermentation step to enrich DFAs unnecessary, does not occur in honey, and is specific for HFIS. Addition of HFIS down to 1% can be detected by this approach.

Du et al. (2015) generated a comprehensive system for testing honey extension using different syrups by UPLC-quadrupole/time-of-flight mass spectrometry targeting AFGP, DFA and polysaccharides (DP 12-19) in a single chromatographic run. An Acquity UPLC BEH Amide column (2.1 mm × 100 mm, 1.7 μm) was used to separate the markers within 15 min, and they were detected by high-resolution accurate mass spectrometry. This method has the advantage of allowing simultaneous detection of a variety of syrups (rice, corn, inverted beet, and cane) added to honey at levels down to 10%.

26.2.1.2 Mass Spectrometry

Stable carbon isotope ratio analysis (SCIRA) by isotopic ratio mass spectrometry (IRMS) is a widely used tool to discriminate material originating from plants. Plant tissue contains a lower ratio of $^{13}C/^{12}C$ in comparison to atmospheric CO_2 and this depletion ($\delta^{13}C$) is more pronounced in plants that use the Calvin–Benson cycle for carbon fixation (C3 plants) than in C4 plants, which use the Hatch-Slack pathway. Flowering plants and blossoms of trees that bees usually visit belong to the C3 plant group while sugar cane and corn are C4 plants. $\delta^{13}C$ values for C3 plants range from -23 to $-28‰$ while for C4 species it is -9 to $-15‰$, when using the Vienna Pee Dee Belemnite as a reference; honey's average $\delta^{13}C$ value is $-25.4‰$ and that of HFCS is $-9.7‰$ (Elflein and Raezke, 2008). Consequently, SCIRA is an excellent tool to detect sugar cane or corn-based syrup addition to honey; honeys with $\delta^{13}C$ values less negative than $-23.5‰$ are considered adulterated (White and Winters, 1989). For the IRMS analysis, honey is combusted first in an elemental analyzer (EA) and the different masses of the formed gases separated by a magnetic field before being detected by a Faraday cup detector array. In the AOAC 998.12 standardized method, which is widely applied for checking authenticity of honey, the $\delta^{13}C$ value of the isolated protein fraction of honey serves as an internal standard (AOAC International, 1998). The difference between the $\delta^{13}C$ values of a honey and the protein fraction isolated from it should not exceed 1‰. AOAC 998.12 allows detection of the addition of sugar syrups obtained from C4 plants down to a level of 7%; sugars from C3 plants can, however, not be reliably detected. The principles of AOAC 998.12 have been widely applied and its utility has been confirmed by numerous authors (Cotte et al., 2007; Schellenberg et al., 2010; Çinar et al., 2014). Even indirect sugar addition by feeding C4 syrups to bees could be detected by SCIRA (Guler et al., 2014). Certain irregularities, eg, with Manuka honey, have been reported (Rogers et al., 2010); these authors initially identified pollen as the reason why authentic Manuka honeys failed the C4 sugar test by SCIRA. They proposed removal of pollen and other insoluble material by filtration so that only the pure protein is isolated and used in the AOAC 998.12 method. Further studies did not confirm that the presence of pollen was the source of the irregularities but indicated that ripened Manuka honeys high in antibacterial nonperoxide activity have unusually high negative $\delta^{13}C$ protein values while their $\delta^{13}C$ honey value is within the normal range; this results in an apparent C4 sugar content above 7% (Rogers et al., 2014). Therefore, an amendment of AOAC 998.12 has been proposed; this would read: *Pure honey (free of corn or cane sugars) yields a value of "apparent" C-4 sugars of* $\leq 7\%$. *New Zealand's Manuka honey may exceed this value, but will have honey* $\delta^{13}C$ *values which are in the normal range (more negative than* $-24.7‰$*) and an apparent C-4 sugar content no greater than 13.0%.*

To lower the detection limit for C4 sugars and also allow detection of C3 sugars, Cabañero et al. (2006) introduced a combination of liquid chromatography using a ligand exchange column and IRMS (LC-IRMS) for SCIRA of the individual main sugars in honey. Differences (Δ) in the $\delta^{13}C$ values of sucrose, fructose, and glucose were of diagnostic value for identifying adulteration by C4 as well as C3 sugars. In genuine honey Δ $\delta^{13}C$ between fructose and glucose was 0.0 ± 0.3‰, between fructose and sucrose 1.2 ± 0.4‰, and between glucose and sucrose 1.3 ± 0.4‰. A difference in the $\delta^{13}C$ [fru-glu] lower than −0.6 and/or values of $\delta^{13}C$ [gluc-suc] higher than 2 indicates the addition of sugar syrups. Addition of C3 sugars can be detected at levels of between 5% and 10%, while sensitivity for C4 sugars is even better (around 1%). Elflein and Raezke (2008) suggested to make not only use of the LC-IRMS data for the disaccharides (sucrose), fructose, and glucose, but also to include the honey trisaccharides and the protein fraction. Their decision rule for genuine honey requires Δ δ13C [fru-glu] to be ±1.0 and all differences between [fructose and disaccharides/trisaccharides/protein], [glucose and disaccharides/trisaccharides/protein], [disaccharides and trisaccharides/protein] and [trisaccharides and protein] to be within a range of ±2.1. Similar results were reported by a Chinese research group (Fei et al., 2011).

26.2.1.3 *Optical Spectroscopy*

Spectroscopy in the near infrared (NIR, c. 14000–4000 cm^{-1}) and the mid-infrared (MIR, c. 4000–400 cm^{-1}) wavelength ranges are widely used techniques for quality control of food and feed, including authenticity issues. Recorded absorption spectra contain information about the chemical makeup of the sample analyzed and can be used in combination with multivariate statistics for quantifying targeted substances or classification of samples (eg, genuine/adulterated) based on partial or complete spectral profiles.

Numerous reports exist describing the successful application of vibrational spectroscopy either for the detection of sugar syrups or the quantification of individual syrups added to honey. The former is mostly used in combination with multivariate classification methods while, for the latter purpose, regression models are employed. Before multivariate data analysis, spectra may be pretreated using various transformations (normalization, derivatives, Savitsky–Golay smoothing, etc.).

Application of IR techniques for quality control of honey has been reviewed recently (Cozzolino et al., 2011).

Detection of addition of inverted beet syrup to honey using Fourier transform IR (FT-IR) spectroscopy and an attenuated total reflectance (ATR) sampling accessory was reported by Sivakesava and Irudayaraj (2001). PLS regression allowed accurate prediction of the amount of added syrup in the case of three different honey types. Classification of the adulterants involved (fructose, glucose, sucrose, inverted beet, and cane sugar syrups) was also possible using LDA (Sivakesava and Irudayaraj, 2002). A similar approach was applied by Kelly et al. (2004) to detect honey adulteration by sugar solutions; the study was later extended to discriminate between genuine Irish honey and honey adulterated with inverted beet syrup and HFSC syrup (Kelly et al., 2006a). Soft independent modeling of class analogy (SIMCA) and PLS classification were employed to classify correctly 96.2%, 97.5%, 95.8%, and 91.7% of samples of authentic honey and honey adulterated by beet sucrose, dextrose syrups, and partial invert corn syrup, respectively. In a separate study, the standard error of prediction, a metric that indicates the accuracy of a regression model, varied between 1.5% and 2.1% for corn syrup, 2.1% and 3.0% for HFCS syrup and 1.4% and 2.5% for inverted sugar using a PLS calibration model and FT-IR data (Gallardo-Velazquez et al., 2009). Similar values for predicting the amount of corn, invert, and cane sugar syrups by PLS regression were found by Rios-Corripio et al. (2012).

NIR is another technique that has been successfully used to detect honey adulterated by sugar syrups. The main absorption bands that are useful for discriminating adulterated samples are in the range of 6000–10,000 cm^{-1}. Downey et al. (2004) used this technique for the detection of fructose and glucose solutions (individual and in combination) in honey. Later, Kelly et al. (2006b) first applied SIMCA for classification and then PLS regression for quantification of the level of adulteration by beet invert syrup and HFCS. Chen et al. (2011) used a fiber-optic diffuse reflectance probe immersed into honey to collect NIR spectra that were, after preprocessing, treated by PLS discriminant analysis (PLS-DA) to identify addition of HFCS. An interesting phenomenon was described by Bazar et al. (2016), who demonstrated by using aquaphotomics-based evaluations that addition of HFCS triggered a disturbance in water molecular structures in honey. This aided the interpretation of the PLS and principal component regression (PCR) models used for estimating the HFCS addition level. The usefulness of several algorithms for sample classification (least-squares support vector machine, support vector machine, back propagation artificial neural network, LDA, and *k*-nearest neighbors) for the detection of sugar syrups by NIR were compared (Zhu et al., 2010). Best classification models were achieved with least-squares support vector machine together with the use of wavelet transformation for compressing spectral data (total accuracy >95% correct classification).

Raman spectroscopy is a related technique offering advantages similar to MIR and NIR for detection of adulterants in honey. Using PLS-DA, HFCS, and maltose syrup additions to honey were detected with high rates of correct classification, with a total accuracy of 91.1% (authentic honey vs adulterated honey with HFCS), 97.8% (authentic honey vs adulterated honey with maltose syrup), and 75.6% (authentic honey vs adulterated honey with HFCS and maltose syrup) (Li et al., 2012).

Recently, fluorescence spectroscopy has attracted attention as a powerful technique for characterizing food (Christensen et al., 2006). Three-dimensional fluorescence spectra were used to build PLS calibration models (after spectral preprocessing to remove Rayleigh and Raman scattering) for quantification of rice syrup in honey by either PLS or back propagation neural network routines; the latter proved to be superior (Chen et al., 2014a). Unfortunately, the number of different honeys and syrup samples studied in this report was rather low.

26.2.1.4 Nuclear Magnetic Resonance Spectroscopy

NMR-based profiling of food has found wide application in controlling food quality, authenticity, and traceability. The majority of publications explain the use of NMR spectroscopy for authentication of botanical and/or geographical origin of honey. Bertelli et al. (2010) used one-dimensional (1D) and two-dimensional (2D) NMR to detect sugar syrups added to 63 authentic honey samples (robinia, eucalyptus, citrus, chestnut, and multifloral). Preprocessed NMR spectra were used for factor analysis and general discriminant analysis (GDA) to classify authentic and adulterated samples. The cross-validated model developed using 1D spectra correctly classified 95% of the authentic and adulterated honeys. All of the authentic honeys were assigned to the correct class; only adulterated honeys ($n = 6$) were misclassified. More than 800 globally sourced honey samples have been profiled by NMR in an attempt to build a universally applicable honey screening procedure (Spiteri et al., 2015). Using a statistical technique called independent components analysis, NMR spectra of authentic honeys were compared to commercial honey samples and two signals identified that were indicative of sugar addition to honey. Those markers were validated by adding commercial sugar syrups to honey, although no strict linear relationship between signal strength and level of addition was observed. Nevertheless, sugar syrup addition was in most instances detectable at levels of 10% or higher. Another way of detecting sugar addition was via the dilution effect on minor sugars of honey, although in this case the addition was only recognized at levels greater than 20%.

An economically interesting application for detecting HFCS addition by using low-field proton NMR has been described (Ribeiro et al., 2014). Two water populations were observed by fitting measured relaxation times to a multiexponential curve, with addition of HFCS to blossom honey leading to an observed increase in relaxation times. Unfortunately, only a few samples were included in this study.

26.2.1.5 Other Techniques

Several sensing approaches based on the measurement of physical properties have been proposed as well. Sensors based on dielectric properties to detect addition of sucrose syrup (Guo et al., 2011), on cyclic voltammetry to detect rice syrup in *Angelica* honey (Cai et al., 2013), and on an electronic tongue to detect rice and corn syrup in honey (Bougrini et al., 2016) have been described.

The fructose/glucose ratio in honey is a factor determining the crystallization rate of honey, which in turn governs the rheological properties of honey. Syrup addition decreased viscosity (η), storage (G'), and loss modulus (G'') values of the control honey samples, which suggested that the use of steady, dynamic, and creep analysis would be a novel tool to detect honey adulteration by fructose and sucrose syrups (Yilmaz et al., 2014).

26.2.2 Geographical and Botanical Origin

Minor component composition of honey is determined by the chemical makeup of the nectar produced by the plant species visited by bees and the pedioclimatic environment the plants grow in. For this reason, the composition of unifloral honey obtained from different geographical regions may be expected to differ to a certain extent (Kropf et al., 2010).

26.2.2.1 Analysis of Pollen (Melissopalynology)

Melissopalynology is regarded as the "gold standard" for determining botanical as well as geographical origin of honey. To be of use for the latter, the characteristic flora of the region the honey comes from has to be known. An experienced operator is needed to recognize and classify the pollen grains present in honey and a large library of pollen grains is necessary for comparative purposes. Usually, the proportion of the pollen grains typical for the floral source is estimated, although in some situations the absolute amount of the denominating pollen grains might be more useful. Unifloral honey practically does not exist; to be denominated an unifloral honey, the relative frequency of the pollen of the denominating *taxon* shall exceed 45%. A harmonized procedure for microscopic pollen evaluation has been described (Von der Ohe et al., 2004). Although pollen of certain *taxa* can be under- or overrepresented, eg, *Citrus* pollen could be represented at <10% of all constituent pollen in authentic *Citrus* honey.

Developments in molecular biology have opened new alternatives to the microscopic evaluation of pollen. TaqMan™ assays were developed for the detection of acacia, broom, citrus, clover, heather, eucalyptus, lavender, linden, oak, olive, rape, rockrose, rosemary, sunflower, and sweet chestnut with the aim of identifying the geographical origin of honey (Laube et al., 2010). This approach proved to be successful in authentication of Corsican honey (Miel de Corse), but it requires a priori knowledge of the plant species likely to be found.

DNA (meta)barcoding was applied by Valentini et al. (2010), Hawkins et al. (2015), Richardson et al. (2015), Bruni et al. (2015), and Galimberti et al. (2015) to characterize the *taxa* of pollen collected either from beehives or isolated from honey. A multiplex next-generation sequencing approach was also described (Keller et al., 2015). Those new approaches will certainly find more application in the future and more data are needed to evaluate their potential for honey authentication.

26.2.2.2 Phytochemical Markers

As pollen analysis requires a considerable level of expertise that is not always available, development of chemical markers for authenticity has received considerable attention. As unifloral honeys mostly have a particular taste and aroma, substances responsible for the sensory properties of honey have been proposed to serve as markers of botanical origin. This subject has been recently reviewed by Kaskonienė and Venskutonis (2010) and Manyi-Loh et al. (2011).

Flavor is perhaps the most distinctive characteristic of unifloral honey as the responsible volatile components are transferred from the floral source to honey. Nevertheless, during the processing of nectar to honey, volatiles can be added by bees and processing (heating) and storage can also lead to changes in the pattern of volatiles. In addition, the way the volatile fraction is isolated can also change its patterns. For example, techniques involving heating (distillation) can lead to the de novo formation of volatiles via Maillard reactions. In addition, even for the same botanical source, nectar composition can vary due to climatic and geological influences at a given geographical location.

Several hundred volatile compounds have been isolated from honey and attempts have been made to identify individual substances characteristic for a given floral source. Recently, methods avoiding excessive heat such as head-space sampling, either static or dynamic or using solid-phase microextraction (SPME) fibers, have been favored over methods involving distillation (Manyi-Loh et al., 2011). For example, using SPME as an isolation technique, methyl anthranilate was reported as a marker of citrus honey, p-methyl acetophenone, carvacrol, and 8-*p*-menthen-1,2-diol for lime tree; ethenyl phenyl acetate for thyme; phenyl acetonitrile for dandelion; aminoacetophenone for chestnut; and nonanoic and acetoin for Italian eucalyptus honey (Piasenzotto et al., 2003). Kaskonienė and Venskutonis (2010) and Manyi-Loh et al. (2011) present an overview of volatiles found in unifloral honey. Even if specific volatile marker compounds can play an important role in characterizing the botanical origin of honeys, it is more the profile—in qualitative as well as quantitative terms—of several compounds that is responsible for the typical aroma of a specific honey variety. Spanish honeys were chemometrically classified based on their volatile composition and sensory descriptive analysis by a panel (Castro-Vazquez et al., 2009). Seisonen at al. (2015) combined SPME and gas chromatographic (GC) separation of honey volatiles with olfactometry, a technique in which trained persons sniff and describe the sensory attributes of substances separated by GC. Substances making up the isolated volatiles were quite similar for four botanical origins, but, using hierarchical cluster analysis and correspondence analysis, it was possible to separate heather honey, whose aroma was described as containing "sweet" and "candy-like" notes, raspberry honeys involving "green" notes, and alder buckthorn with "honey" and "floral" notes.

A wide array of phenolic compounds are synthesized by plants and, therefore, are also present in nectar. They are responsible for the antioxidant capacity of honey (Gheldof et al., 2002) but they were also suggested to be a class of phytochemicals that could be used as botanical markers (Tomas-Barberan et al., 2001). Using HPLC coupled to a DAD, hesperetin was identified as a good marker for citrus honey, kaempferol for rosemary honey, and quercetin for sunflower honey. Abscisic acid, which had been reported to be a possible marker for heather honey, was also detected in rapeseed, lime tree, and acacia honeys. Ellagic acid in heather honey and the hydroxycinnamates caffeic, *p*-coumaric, and ferulic acids in chestnut, sunflower, lavender and acacia honeys were also detected. Other detection systems including an electrochemical detector (Zhao et al., 2016), electrospray ionization tandem mass spectrometry (Mattonai et al., 2016) or high-resolution accurate mass spectrometry (Keckes et al., 2013a) have been studied; all groups used PCA as a chemometric tool for the identification of unifloral honey clustering on the based on their phenolic profile. However, in a study encompassing 119 unifloral honey samples from pine, thyme, fir, and orange blossom obtained from 14 different regions of Greece, traditional physicochemical parameters in combination with LDA provided classification results that were as accurate as those developed using phenolic profiles (Karabagias et al., 2014). This should not be seen as a disadvantage of the profiling method; it simply shows the potential of traditional analysis in combination with chemometric data evaluation. Three-dimensional synchronous fluorescence spectroscopy (3D-SFS) was applied to phenolic compounds isolated by SPE to generate signatures (contour plots), which allowed a straightforward discrimination of honeys coming from acacia, buckwheat, heather, linden, and multifloral sources (Sergiel et al., 2014). Another application of 3D-fluorescence spectroscopy was described by Karoui et al. (2007), who directly scanned 62 honey samples of different botanical origins from Switzerland using a front-face accessory, and the obtained data were treated by PCA and factorial discriminant analysis. Correct classification rates of 100% and 90% were obtained for calibration and validation samples, respectively.

Free amino acid profiles have been used as an indicator of honey origin. Amino acid composition depends on the floral origin and the influence of production area. In addition, bees add amino acids during honey production, notably proline, which traditionally serves as a maturity indicator. The profile of free amino acids in honey can be determined either by HPLC or GC and, in combination with chemometric data analysis, has been used for creating classification models to discriminate honeydew and floral honey (Iglesias et al., 2004) and botanical sources (Gonzalez-Paramas et al., 2007; Rebane and Herodes, 2008; Keckes et al., 2013b; Kivrak, 2015).

26.2.2.3 Mineral Elements

Honey mineral content is determined by environmental, geographical, and botanical factors, and the interplay between them needs to be considered when the information content of the mineral profile is intended to be used for authentication purposes (Bogdanov et al., 2007). On top of these factors, pollution of the environment, in particular with Cd, Pb, and Hg, needs to be taken into consideration. Honey mineral content varies between 0.1% and 0.2%, and potassium occurs in the highest proportions (Solayman et al., 2016). Electrical conductivity correlates well with mineral content and is, therefore, also a useful indicator for botanical origin authenticity.

Numerous reports exist in which the use of mineral elements in combination with pattern recognition methods have been used to classify botanical and/or geographical origin. Table 26.2 provides an overview of more recent publications.

26.2.2.4 Spectroscopic Profiling

Information produced by spectral analysis of honey is not only used for detection of the addition of sugar syrups but also for classification according to botanical and geographical origin. Several different strategies have been described using either enriched honey fractions before NMR analysis or honey per se; in the latter case, targeted analysis of certain marker compounds or untargeted profiling can be used (Ohmenhaeuser et al., 2013).

Proton NMR spectra of chloroform extracts of 353 Italian honey samples (acacia, chestnut, linden, orange, eucalyptus, honeydew, multifloral) were acquired using a 600 MHz instrument (Schievano et al., 2012). Multivariate data treatment involved PCA, orthogonal projection to latent structures-discriminant analysis (O2PLS-DA), naïve Bayes classifiers, and support vector machines. In the next step, specific biomarkers for floral origin were identified: chrysin and pinocembrin for acacia, γ-lactam

[AU1] **Table 26.2 Mineral Analysis as a Tool for Discriminating Geographical and Botanical Origin of Honey (Yücel and Sultanoglu, 2013)**

	Analytical Technique	Statistical Technique	Samples	Origin	Botanical Source
Terrab et al. (2004)	ICP-OES	PCA	24	Spain	Thyme
Chudzinska and Baralkiewicz (2011)	ICP-MS	CA, PCA, LDA, C&RT	140	Poland	Honeydew, buckwheat, rape
De Alda-Garcilope et al. (2012)	AAS	CA, ANOVA	Unknown	Spain "Miel de Granada"	Chestnut, rosemary, thyme, avocado, orange blossom, mountain range, multifloral
Di Bella et al. (2015)	ICP-OES, ICP-MS	PCA, CDA	39	Italy	Orange blossom, lemon blossom, chestnut, eucalyptus, acacia, sulla, wildflower
Ursulin-Trstenjak (2015)	ICP-MS	PCA, ANOVA	200	Croatia	Black locust
Czipa et al. (2015)	ICP,OES, ICP-MS	LDA	34	Hungary	Acacia, rape, sunflower, multifloral
Chen et al. (2014b)	ICP-MS	PCA, PLS-DA, BP-ANN	163	China	Linden, vitex, rape, acacia
Yücel and Sultanoglu (2013)	ICP-OES	CA, PCA	45	Turkey	Citrus, eucalyptus, petroselinum, calluna, multifloral
Necemer et al. (2009)	TXRF	PCA, RDA	264	Slovenia	Acacia, lime, chestnut, spruce, fir, blossom, forest
Dos Santos et al. (2008)	AAS	CA, PCA	52	Brazil	Unknown

ICP-OES, inductively coupled plasma-optical emission spectroscopy; *ICP-MS*, inductively coupled plasma-mass spectroscopy; *AAS*, atomic absorption spectroscopy; *TXRF*, total-reflection X-ray fluorescence; *CA*, cluster analysis; *PCA*, principal component analysis; *ANOVA*, analysis of variance; *C&RT*, calibration and regression tree analysis; *CDA*, canonical discriminant analysis; *BP-ANN*, back-propagation artificial neural network; *RDA*, regularized discriminant analysis.

ester of 3-(2′-pyrrolidinyl)-kynurenic acid for chestnut, 8-hydroxylinalool and caffeine for orange, dehydrovomifoliol for eucalyptus, a diacylglycerylether for honeydew, and 4-(1-hydroxy-1-methylethyl)cyclohexa-1,3-diene-carboxylic and 4-(1-methylethenyl) cyclohexa-1,3-diene-carboxylic acid for linden. Those markers were further characterized by chromatographic purification of honey extracts, NMR, and MS (Schievano et al., 2013). SPE followed by NMR and chemometric data analysis was also used to classify Italian unifloral honeys (Beretta et al., 2008).

Using whole ^{1}H-NMR spectra in combination with PCA was not successful in separating multifloral honey samples according to geographical origin, but a hierarchical approach better preserved the information content of very-low-intensity NMR signals, which would otherwise be influenced by the main sugar signals. Hierarchical PLS-DA succeeded in separating multifloral honeys according to geographical origin (Consonni and Cagliani, 2008). By contrast, ^{1}H-NMR coupled with multivariate statistics was shown to be an efficient tool for classification of honey samples of different botanical origins. Two-dimensional NMR (^{1}H—^{13}C heteronuclear multiple bond correlation spectroscopy) was used next to ^{1}H-NMR to generate spectra that were then evaluated by PCA and GDA for grouping samples according to their botanical origin (multifloral, eucalyptus, chestnut, citrus); 2D-NMR was more effective for clustering (Lolli et al., 2008).

Saccharides in 86 Italian honeys were studied by ^{1}H and ^{1}H—^{13}C NMR spectroscopy allowing the identification of 19 sugars; PCA and OPLS-DA of the saccharide data together with some unidentified compounds allowed grouping of honey samples according to floral origin (Consonni et al., 2012). This same research group also demonstrated the use of NMR profiling for discriminating honeys according to geographical origin (Consonni et al., 2013). The anomeric sugar region between 4.400 ppm and 5.700 ppm was the most informative part of the ^{1}H-NMR spectrum for saccharide resonance assignment. OPLS-DA separated Chinese, Hungarian, Italian, and South American multifloral honey samples. Although less sensitive, ^{13}C-NMR was used to quantitate 14 mono-, di-, and trisaccharides in Greek honey; the data can be used for authenticating floral origin (Kazalaki et al., 2015).

Site-specific natural isotopic fractionation measured by NMR was also investigated for characterization of honey geographic origin. Honey sugars are converted into alcohol by fermentation, which is then distilled off and analyzed by NMR using a deuterium probe to determine the (D/H) ratio in the three isotopomers of ethanol: CH_2DCH_2OH(I), CH_3CHDOH(II), and CH_3CH_2OD(III). Usually the $(D/H)_I$ ratio is the most useful parameter. In this way it was possible to characterize acacia honey but the $(D/H)_I$ isotopic ratios of chestnut and lavender honey were equivalent (Cotte et al., 2007).

The mid-IR spectrum of a large number of honey samples from Switzerland and Germany ($n = 1206$, collected over several years) together with multivariate data treatment allowed an accurate classification of rape, lime tree, false acacia, heather, cornflower, clover, sunflower, and honeydew honeys (Etzold and Lichtenberg-Kraag, 2008). FT-IR with an ATR device was used to verify the origin of honey samples ($n = 150$) from Europe and South America. Recorded spectra were transformed by first- and second-derivative and standard normal variate (SNV) and analyzed using

PLS regression, factorial discriminant analysis (FDA), and SIMCA. The latter technique produced correct classifications of up to 100% but models describing some classes had very high false-positive rates. Overall correct classification of 93.3% was obtained for honeys by PLS discriminant analysis, while FDA techniques correctly classified 94.7% of honey samples (Hennessy et al., 2008). Ruoff et al. (2006) used the same instrumental technique and PCA and LDA of the recorded spectra to authenticate 11 unifloral honey types. Classification error rates ranged from <0.1% (polyfloral, heather, honeydew, metcalfa, oak, fir honey) to 8.3% (alpine rose honey). Similar results were reported using the same technique to classify 506 unifloral Croatian honeys by PLS-DA (Hennessy et al., 2010). The fingerprint spectral region (1800−700 cm^{-1}) was preprocessed by a particular Savitzky−Golay filtering algorithm. Receiver operating curve analysis was conducted to find an optimal cut-off (threshold) value for the PLS-DA models developed to ensure minimal misclassification (Svecnjak et al., 2015). FT-Raman spectroscopy (Corvucci et al., 2015) as well as front-face synchronous fluorescence spectroscopy and multivariate data evaluation (Lenhardt et al., 2014) were also effective in classifying floral origin, while NIR has been reported to be a useful tool for tracing the geographical origin (Woodcock et al., 2009).

26.3 Outlook

Untargeted and targeted profiling techniques based on various spectroscopy platforms have been successfully used to discriminate honey and other agro-food commodities on the basis of their geographical and botanical origin. Reliable and complete databanks are the cornerstone of such methods to unleash the full power of metabolomics approaches. Data collections containing spectra, compositional data, and metadata, which have to be generated using a large number of authentic samples covering as much as possible compositional variation due to geology, geography, plant species etc., have to be generated. Access to such samples is the key to success. Even more important is the sharing of this information with the scientific community, perhaps by using cloud computing. Such initiatives are underway and should continue. Otherwise, research groups have to rebuild databanks in isolation thereby wasting scarce resources. Another aspect that needs special consideration is the validation of statistical models in order to obtain robust classifications, which can be used to resolve disputes among trading partners or for official control purposes.

References

Anklam, E., 1998. A review of the analytical methods to determine the geographical and botanical origin of honey. Food Chemistry 63 (4), 549−562.

AOAC Official Method 998.12 C-4 Plant Sugars in Honey Internal Standard Stable Carbon Isotope Ratio Method, 2013. AOAC International, Rockville, MD, USA.

Arvanitoyannis, I.S., Chalhoub, C., Gotsiou, P., Lydakis-Simantiris, N., Kefalas, P., 2005. Novel quality control methods in conjunction with chemometrics (multivariate analysis) for detecting honey authenticity. Critical Reviews in Food Science and Nutrition 45 (3), 193–203.

Bazar, G., Romvari, R., Szabo, A., Somogyi, T., Éles, V., Tsenkova, R., 2016. NIR detection of honey adulteration reveals differences in water spectral pattern. Food Chemistry 194, 873–880.

Beretta, G., Caneva, E., Regazzoni, L., Bakhtyari, N.G., Maffei Facino, R., 2008. A solid-phase extraction procedure coupled to 1H NMR, with chemometric analysis, to seek reliable markers of the botanical origin of honey. Analytica Chimica Acta 620 (1–2), 176–182.

Bertelli, D., Lolli, M., Papotti, G., Bortolotti, L., Serra, G., Plessi, M., 2010. Detection of honey adulteration by sugar syrups using one-dimensional and two-dimensional high-resolution nuclear magnetic resonance. Journal of Agricultural and Food Chemistry 58 (15), 8495–8501.

Bertoncelj, J., Golob, T., Kropf, U., Korosec, M., 2011. Characterisation of Slovenian honeys on the basis of sensory and physicochemical analysis with a chemometric approach. International Journal of Food Science & Technology 46 (8), 1661–1671.

Bogdanov, S., Martin, P., 2002. Honey authenticity: a review. Mitteilungen aus Lebensmitteluntersuchung und Hygiene 93, 232–254.

Bogdanov, S., Haldimann, M., Luginbühl, W., Gallmann, P., 2007. Minerals in honey: environmental, geographical and botanical aspects. Journal of Apicultural Research 46 (4), 269–275.

Bougrini, M., Tahri, K., Saidi, T., El Alami El Hassani, N., Bouchikhi, B., El Bari, N., 2016. Classification of honey according to geographical and botanical origins and detection of its adulteration using voltammetric electronic tongue. Food Analytical Methods. http://dx.doi.org/10.1007/s12161-015-0393-2.

Bruni, I., Galimberti, A., Caridi, L., Scaccabarozzi, D., De Mattia, F., Casiraghi, M., Labra, M., 2015. A DNA barcoding approach to identify plant species in multiflower honey. Food Chemistry 170, 308–315.

Cabañero, A.I., Recio, J.L., Rupérez, M., 2006. Liquid chromatography coupled to isotope ratio mass spectrometry: a new perspective on honey adulteration detection. Journal of Agricultural and Food Chemistry 54, 9719–9727.

Cai, J., Wu, X., Yuan, L., Zhou, L., Zhou, A., 2013. Determination of Chinese Angelica honey adulterated with rice syrup by an electrochemical sensor and Chemometrics. Analytical Methods 5 (9), 2324–2328.

Castro-Vazquez, L., Díaz-Maroto, M.C., Gonzalez-Viñasa, M.A., Pérez-Coelloa, M.S., 2009. Differentiation of monofloral citrus, rosemary, eucalyptus, lavender, thyme and heather honeys based on volatile composition and sensory descriptive analysis. Food Chemistry 112 (4).

Chen, L., Xue, X., Ye, Z., Zhou, J., Chen, F., Zhao, J., 2011. Determination of Chinese honey adulterated with high fructose corn syrup by near infrared spectroscopy. Food Chemistry 128 (4), 1110–1114.

Chen, Q., Qi, S., Li, H., Han, X., Ouyang, Q., Zhao, J., 2014a. Determination of rice syrup adulterant concentration in honey using three-dimensional fluorescence spectra and multivariate calibrations. Spectrochim. Acta Part A: Molecular and Biomolecular Spectroscopy 131, 177–182.

Chen, H., Fan, C., Chang, Q., Pang, G., Hu, X., Lu, M., Wang, W., 2014b. Chemometric determination of the botanical origin for Chinese honeys on the basis of mineral elements determined by ICP-MS. Journal of Agricultural and Food Chemistry 62 (11), 2443–2448.

Christensen, J., Nørgaard, L., Bro, R., Engelsen, S.B., 2006. Multivariate autofluorescence of intact food systems. Chemical Reviews 106 (6), 1979–1994.

Chudzinska, M., Baralkiewicz, D., 2011. Estimation of honey authenticity by multielements characteristics using inductively coupled plasma-mass spectrometry (ICP-MS) combined with chemometrics. Food and Chemical Toxicology 49 (11), 284–290.

Çinar, S.B., Ekşi, A., Coşkun, I., 2014. Carbon isotope ratio (13C/12C) of pine honey and detection of HFCS adulteration. Food Chemistry 157, 10–13.

Consonni, R., Cagliani, L.R., 2008. Geographical characterization of polyfloral and acacia honeys by nuclear magnetic resonance and chemometrics. Journal of Agricultural and Food Chemistry 56 (16), 6873–6880.

Consonni, R., Cagliani, L.R., Cogliati, C., 2012. NMR characterization of saccharides in italian honeys of different floral sources. Journal of Agricultural and Food Chemistry 60 (18), 4526–4534.

Consonni, R., Cagliani, L.R., Cogliati, C., 2013. Geographical discrimination of honeys by saccharides analysis. Food Control 32, 543–548.

Cordella, C., Militão, J.S.L.T., Clément, M.-C., Drajnudel, P., Cabrol-Bassc, D., 2005. Detection and quantification of honey adulteration via direct incorporation of sugar syrups or bee-feeding: preliminary study using high-performance anion exchange chromatography with pulsed amperometric detection (HPAEC-PAD) and Chemometrics. Analytica Chimica Acta 531 (2), 239–248.

Corvucci, F., Nobili, L., Melucci, D., Grillenzoni, F.-V., 2015. The discrimination of honey origin using melissopalynology and Raman spectroscopy techniques coupled with multivariate analysis. Food Chemistry 169, 297–304.

Cotte, J.F., Casabianca, H., Lhéritier, J., Perrucchietti, C., Sanglar, C., Waton, H., Grenier-Loustalot, M.F., 2007. Study and validity of 13C stable carbon isotopic ratio analysis by mass spectrometry and 2H site-specific natural isotopic fractionation by nuclear magnetic resonance isotopic measurements to characterize and control the authenticity of honey. Analytica Chimica Acta 582 (1), 125–136.

Cozzolino, D., Corbella, E., Smyth, H.E., 2011. Quality control of honey using infrared spectroscopy: a review. Applied Spectroscopy Reviews 46 (7), 523–538.

Czipa, N., Andrási, D., Kovács, B., 2015. Determination of essential and toxic elements in Hungarian honeys. Food Chemistry 175, 536–542.

De Alda-Garcilope, C., Gallego-Picó, A., Bravo-Yagüe, J.C., Garcinuño-Martínez, R.M., Fernández-Hernando, P., 2012. Characterization of Spanish honeys with protected designation of origin "miel de Granada" according to their mineral content. Food Chemistry 135 (3), 1785–1788.

Di Bella, G., Lo Turco, V., Potortì, A.G., Bua, G.D., Fede, M.R., Dugo, G., 2015. Geographical discrimination of Italian honey by multi-element analysis with a chemometric approach. Journal of Food Composition and Analysis 44, 25–35.

Dos Santos, J.S., Dos Santos, N.S., Dos Santos, M.L.P., Dos Santos, S.N., Lacerda, J.J.D.J., 2008. Honey classification from semi-arid, Atlantic and transitional forest zones in Bahia, Brazil. Journal of the Brazilian Chemical Society 19 (2), 502–508.

Downey, G., Fouratier, V., Kelly, J.D., 2004. Detection of honey adulteration by addition of fructose and glucose using near infrared transflectance spectroscopy. Journal of Near Infrared Spectroscopy 11 (6), 447–456.

Du, B., Wu, L., Xue, X., Chen, L., Li, Y., Zhao, J., Cao, W., 2015. Rapid screening of multiclass syrup adulterants in honey by ultrahigh-performance liquid chromatography/quadrupole time of flight mass spectrometry. Journal of Agricultural and Food Chemistry 63, 6614–6623.

Elflein, L., Raezke, K.-P., 2008. Improved detection of honey adulteration by measuring differences between 13C/12C stable carbon isotope ratios of protein and sugar compounds with a combination of elemental analyser - isotope ratio mass spectrometry and liquid chromatography - isotope ratio mass spectrometry (δ13C-EA/LC-IRMS). Apidologie 39 (5), 574–587.

Escuredo, O., Dobre, I., Fernandez-Gonzalez, M., Seijo, M.C., 2014. Contribution of botanical origin and sugar composition of honeys on the crystallization phenomenon. Food Chemistry 149, 84–90.

Etzold, E., Lichtenberg-Kraag, B., 2008. Determination of the botanical origin of honey by Fourier-transformed infrared spectroscopy: an approach for routine analysis. European Food Research and Technology 227, 579–586.

Fei, X., Wu, B., Sehn, C., Ding, T., Li, L., Lu, Y., 2011. Honey adulteration detection using liquid chromatography/elemental analysis-isotope ratio mass spectrometry. Chinese Journal of Chromatography 29, 15–19.

Food and Agriculture Organization of the United Nations, Statistics Division, 2015. http://faostat3.fao.org/.

Galimberti, A., De Mattia, F., Bruni, I., Scaccabarozzi, D., Sandionigi, A., Barbuto, M., Casiraghi, M., Labra, M., 2015. A DNA barcoding approach to characterize pollen collected by honeybees. PLoS One. http://dx.doi.org/10.1371/journal.pone.0109363.

Gallardo-Velazquez, T., Osorio-Revilla, G., Zuñiga-de Loa, M., Rivera-Espinoza, Y., 2009. Application of FTIR-HATR spectroscopy and multivariate analysis to the quantification of adulterants in Mexican honeys. Food Research International 42, 313–318.

Gheldof, N., Wang, X.-H., Engeseth, N.J., 2002. Identification and quantification of antioxidant components of honeys from various floral sources. Journal of Agricultural and Food Chemistry 50 (21), 5870–5877.

Gonzalez-Paramas, A.M., García-Villanova, R.J., Gomez Barez, J.A., Sanchez Sanchez, J., Ardanuy Albajar, R., 2007. Botanical origin of monovarietal dark honeys (from heather, holm oak, pyrenean oak and sweet chestnut) based on their chromatic characters and amino acid profiles. European Food Research and Technology 226 (1–2), 87–92.

Guler, A., Kocaokutgen, H., Garipoglu, A.V., Onder, H., Ekinci, D., Biyik, S., 2014. Detection of adulterated honey produced by honeybee (*Apis mellifera* L.) colonies fed with different levels of commercial industrial sugar (C3 and C4 plants) syrups by the carbon isotope ratio analysis. Food Chemistry 155, 155–160.

Guo, W., Liu, Y., Zhu, X., Wang, S., 2011. Dielectric properties of honey adulterated with sucrose syrup. Journal of Food Engineering 107 (1), 1–7.

Hawkins, J., de Vere, N., Griffith, A., Ford, C.R., Allainguillaume, J., Hegarty, M.J., Baillie, L., Adams-Groom, B., 2015. Using DNA metabarcoding to identify the floral composition of honey: a new tool for investigating honey bee foraging preferences. PLoS One. http://dx.doi.org/10.1371/journal.pone.0134735.

Hennessy, S., Downey, G., O'Donnell, C., 2008. Multivariate analysis of attenuated total reflection-Fourier transform infrared spectroscopic data to confirm the origin of honeys. Applied Spectroscopy 62 (10), 1115–1123.

Hennessy, S., Downey, G., O'Donnell, C.P., 2010. Attempted confirmation of the provenance of Corsican PDO honey using FT-IR spectroscopy and multivariate data analysis. Journal of Agricultural and Food Chemistry 58 (17), 9401–9406.

Iglesias, M.T., De Lorenzo, C., Polo, M.D.C., Martín-Álvarez, P.J., Pueyo, E., 2004. Usefulness of amino acid composition to discriminate between honeydew and floral honeys. Application to honeys from a small geographic area. Journal of Agricultural and Food Chemistry 52 (1), 84–89.

ISO 4121, 2003. Sensory Analysis – Guidelines for the Use of Quantitative Response Scales. International Organization for Standardization, Geneva.

ISO 6564, 1985. Sensory Analysis – Methodology – Flavour Profile Methods. International Organization for Standardization, Geneva.

ISO 6658, 2005. Sensory Analysis – Methodology – General Guidance. International Organization for Standardization, Geneva.

Karabagias, I.K., Vavoura, M., Nikolaou, C., Badeka, A.V., Kontakos, S., Kontominas, M.G., 2014. Floral authentication of Greek unifloral honeys based on the combination of phenolic compounds, physicochemical parameters and chemometrics. Food Research International 62, 753–760.

Karoui, R., Dufour, E., Bosset, J.-O., De Baerdemaeker, J., 2007. The use of front face fluorescence spectroscopy to classify the botanical origin of honey samples produced in Switzerland. Food Chemistry 101, 314–323.

Kaškonienė, V., Venskutonis, P.R., 2010. Floral markers in honey of various botanical and geographic origins: a review. Comprehensive Reviews in Food Science and Food Safety 9, 620–634.

Kazalaki, A., Misiak, M., Spyros, A., Dais, P., 2015. Identification and quantitative determination of carbohydrate molecules in Greek honey by employing ^{13}C NMR spectroscopy. Analytical Methods 7 (14), 5962–5972.

Kečkeš, S., Gašić, U., Veličković, T.Ć., Milojković-Opsenica, D., Natić, M., Tešić, Ž., 2013a. The determination of phenolic profiles of Serbian unifloral honeys using ultra-high-performance liquid chromatography/high resolution accurate mass spectrometry. Food Chemistry 138 (1), 32–40.

Kečkeš, J., Trifković, J., Andrić, F., Tešić, Z., Milojković-Opsenica, D., 2013b. Amino acids profile of Serbian unifloral honeys. Journal of the Science of Food and Agriculture 93 (13), 3368–3376.

Keller, A., Danner, N., Grimmer, G., Ankenbrand, M., von der Ohe, K., von der Ohe, W., Rost, S., Härtel, S., Steffan-Dewenter, I., 2015. Evaluating multiplexed next-generation sequencing as a method in palynology for mixed pollen samples. Plant Biology 17, 558–566.

Kelly, J.D., Downey, G., Fouratier, V., 2004. Initial study of honey adulteration by sugar solutions using mid-infrared (MIR) spectroscopy and chemometrics. Journal of Agricultural and Food Chemistry 52 (1), 33–39.

Kelly, J.D., Petisco, C., Downey, G., 2006a. Application of Fourier transform mid-infrared spectroscopy to the discrimination between Irish artisanal honey and such honey adulterated with various sugar syrups. Journal of Agricultural and Food Chemistry 54, 6166–6171.

Kelly, J.D., Petisco, C., Downey, G., 2006b. Potential of near infrared transflectance spectroscopy to detect adulteration of Irish honey by beet invert syrup and high fructose corn syrup. Journal of Near Infrared Spectroscopy 14, 139–146.

Kivrak, I., 2015. Free amino acid profiles of 17 Turkish unifloral honeys. Journal of Liquid Chromatography & Related Technologies 38 (8), 855–862.

Kropf, U., Golob, T., Nečemer, M., Kump, P., Korošec, M., Bertoncelj, J., Ogrinc, N., 2010. Carbon and nitrogen natural stable isotopes in Slovene honey: adulteration and botanical and geographical aspects. Journal of Agricultural and Food Chemistry 58, 12794–12803.

Laube, I., Hird, H., Brodmann, P., Ullmann, S., Schöne-Michling, M., Chisholm, J., Broll, H., 2010. Development of primer and probe sets for the detection of plant species in honey. Food Chemistry 118, 979–986.

Lenhardt, L., Zekovica, I., Dramicanin, T., Dramicanin, M.D., Bro, R., 2014. Determination of the botanical origin of honey by front-face synchronous fluorescence spectroscopy. Applied Spectroscopy 68 (5), 557–563.

Li, S., Shan, Y., Zhu, X., Zhang, X., Ling, G., 2012. Detection of honey adulteration by high fructose corn syrup and maltose syrup using Raman spectroscopy. Journal of Food Composition and Analysis 28, 69–74.

Lolli, M., Bertelli, D., Plessi, M., Sabatini, A.G., Restani, C., 2008. Classification of Italian honeys by 2D HR-NMR. Journal of Agricultural and Food Chemistry 56 (4), 1298–1304.

Manikis, I., Thrasivoulou, A., 2001. La relacion entre las características fisicoquímicas de la miel y los parametros de sensibilidad a la cristalizacion. Apiacta 36 (2), 106–112.

Manyi-Loh, C.E., Ndip, R., Clarke, A.M., 2011. Volatile compounds in honey: a review on their involvement in aroma, botanical origin determination and potential biomedical activities. International Journal of Molecular Sciences 12, 9514–9532.

Mattonai, M., Parri, E., Querci, D., Degano, I., Ribechini, E., 2016. Development and validation of an HPLC-DAD and HPLC/ESI-MS2 method for the determination of polyphenols in monofloral honeys from Tuscany (Italy). Microchemical Journal 126, 220–229.

Megherbi, M., Herbreteau, B., Faure, R., Salvador, A., 2009. Polysaccharides as a marker for detection of corn sugar syrup addition in honey. Journal of Agricultural and Food Chemistry 57 (6), 2105–2111.

Missio da Silva, P., Gauche, C., Valdemiro Gonzaga, L., Costa, C.O.A., Fett, R., 2016. Honey: chemical composition, stability and authenticity. Food Chemistry 196, 309–323.

Morales, V., Sanz, M.L., Olano, A., Corzo, N., 2006. Rapid separation on activated charcoal of high oligosaccharides in honey. Chromatographia 64 (3/4), 233–238.

Morales, V., Corzo, N., Sanz, M.L., 2008. HPAEC-PAD oligosaccharide analysis to detect adulterations of honey with sugar syrups. Food Chemistry 107 (2), 922–928.

Necemer, M., Kosir, I.J., Kump, P., Kropf, U., Jamnik, M., Bertoncelj, J., Ogrinc, N., Golob, T., 2009. Application of total reflection X-ray spectrometry in combination with chemometric methods for determination of the botanical origin of Slovenian honey. Journal of Agricultural and Food Chemistry 57 (10), 4409–4414.

Ohmenhaeuser, M., Monakhova, Y.B., Kuballa, T., Lachenmeier, D.W., 2013. Qualitative and quantitative control of honeys using NMR spectroscopy and chemometrics. ISRN Analytical Chemistry. http://dx.doi.org/10.1155/2013/825318.

Piana, M.L., Persano Oddo, L., Bentabol, A., Bruneau, E., Bogdanov, S., Guyot Declerck, C., 2004. Sensory analysis applied to honey: state of the art. Apidologie 35, S26–S37.

Piasenzotto, L., Gracco, L., Conte, L., 2003. Solid phase micro extraction (SPME) applied to honey quality control. Journal of the Science of Food and Agriculture 83, 1037–1044.

Rebane, R., Herodes, K., 2008. Evaluation of the botanical origin of Estonian uni- and polyfloral honeys by amino acid content. Journal of Agricultural and Food Chemistry 56 (22), 10716–10720.

Ribeiro, R.D.O.R., Marsico, E.T., Carneiro, C.D.S., Guerra Monteiro, M.L., Junior, C.C., Jesus, E.F.O.D., 2014. Detection of honey adulteration of high fructose corn syrup by low field nuclear magnetic resonance (LF 1H NMR). Journal of Food Engineering 135, 39–43.

Richardson, R.T., Lin, C.-H., Sponsler, D.B., Quijia, J.O., Goodell, K., Johnson, R.M., 2015. Application of ITS2 metabarcoding to determine the provenance of pollen collected by honey bees in an agroecosystem. Applications in Plant Sciences. http://dx.doi.org/10.3732/apps.1400066.

Rios-Corripio, M.A., Rojas-López, M., Delgado-Macuil, R., 2012. Analysis of adulteration in honey with standard sugar solutions and syrups using attenuated total reflectance-Fourier transform infrared spectroscopy and multivariate methods. CyTA — Journal of Food 10 (2), 119—122.

Rodríguez, I., Serrano, S., Galán-Soldevilla, H., Piva, G., Ubera, J.L., 2015. Sensory analysis integrated by palynological and physicochemical determinations plays a key role in differentiating unifloral honeys of similar botanical origins (Myrtaceae honeys from southern Spain). International Journal of Food Science & Technology 50 (7), 1545—1551.

Rogers, K.M., Somerton, K., Rogers, P., Cox, J., 2010. Eliminating false positive C4 sugar tests on New Zealand Manuka honey. Rapid Communications in Mass Spectrometry 24, 2370—2374.

Rogers, K.M., Sim, M., Stewart, S., Phillips, A., Cooper, J., Douance, C., Pyne, R., Rogers, P., 2014. Investigating C-4 sugar contamination of manuka honey and other New Zealand honey varieties using carbon isotopes. Journal of Agricultural and Food Chemistry 62, 2605—2614.

Ruiz-Matute, A.I., Soria, A.C., Martínez-Castro, I., Sanz, M.L., 2007. A new methodology based on GC-MS to detect honey adulteration with commercial syrups. Journal of Agricultural and Food Chemistry 55, 7264—7269.

Ruiz-Matute, A.I., Rodríguez-Sánchez, S., Sanz, M.L., Martínez-Castro, I., 2010. Detection of adulterations of honey with high fructose syrups from inulin by GC analysis. Journal of Food Composition and Analysis 23, 273—276.

Ruoff, K., Luginbühl, W., Künzli, R., Iglesias, M.T., Bogdanov, S., Bosset, J.O., von der Ohe, K., von der Ohe, W., Amadò, R., 2006. Authentication of the botanical and geographical origin of honey by mid infrared spectroscopy. Journal of Agricultural and Food Chemistry 54 (18), 6873—6880.

Schellenberg, A., Chmielus, S., Schlicht, C., Camin, F., Perini, M., Bontempo, L., Heinrich, K., Kelly, S.D., Rossmann, A., Thomas, F., Jamin, E., Horacek, M., 2010. Multielement stable isotope ratios (H, C, N, S) of honey from different European regions. Food Chemistry 121 (3), 770—777.

Schievano, E., Stocchero, M., Morelato, E., Facchin, C., Mammi, S., 2012. An NMR-based metabolomic approach to identify the botanical origin of honey. Metabolomics 8 (4), 679—690.

Schievano, E., Morelato, E., Facchin, C., Mammi, S., 2013. Characterization of markers of botanical origin and other compounds extracted from unifloral honeys. Journal of Agricultural and Food Chemistry 61, 1747—1755.

Seisonen, S., Kivima, E., Vene, K., 2015. Characterisation of the aroma profiles of different honeys and corresponding flowers using solid-phase microextraction and gas chromatography—mass spectrometry/olfactometry. Food Chemistry 169.

Sergiel, I., Pohl, P., Biesaga, M., Mironczyk, A., 2014. Suitability of three-dimensional synchronous fluorescence spectroscopy for fingerprint analysis of honey samples with reference to their phenolic profiles. Food Chemistry 145, 319—326.

Sivakesava, S., Irudayaraj, J., 2001. Detection of inverted beet sugar adulteration of honey by FTIR spectroscopy. Journal of the Science of Food and Agriculture 81 (8), 683—690.

Sivakesava, S., Irudayaraj, J., 2002. Classification of simple and complex sugar adulterants in honey by mid-infrared spectroscopy. International Journal of Food Science & Technology 37 (4), 351—360.

Solayman, M., Islam, M.A., Paul, S., Ali, Y., Khalil, I., Alam, N., Gan, S.H., 2016. Physicochemical properties, minerals, trace elements, and heavy metals in honey of different origins: a comprehensive review. Comprehensive Reviews in Food Science and Food Safety 15 (1), 219–233.

Spiteri, M., Jamin, E., Thomas, F., Rebours, A., Lees, M., Rogers, K.M., Rutledge, D.N., 2015. Fast and global authenticity screening of honey using ^{1}H-NMR profiling. Food Chemistry 189, 60–66.

Svečnjak, L., Bubalo, D., Baranović, G., Novosel, H., 2015. Optimization of FTIR-ATR spectroscopy for botanical authentication of unifloral honey types and melissopalynological data prediction. European Food Research and Technology 24 (6), 1101–1115.

Terrab, A., Hernanz, D., Heredia, F.J., 2004. Inductively coupled plasma optical emission spectrometric determination of minerals in thyme honeys and their determination of geographical discrimination. Journal of Agricultural and Food Chemistry 52 (11), 3441–3445.

Tomás-Barberán, F.A., Martos, I., Ferreres, F., Radovic, B.S., Anklam, E., 2001. HPLC flavonoid profiles as markers for the botanical origin of European unifloral honeys. Journal of the Science of Food and Agriculture 81 (5), 485–496.

Uršulin-Trstenjak, N., Levanić, D., Primorac, L., Bošnir, J., Vahčić, N., Šarić, G., 2015. Mineral profile of Croatian honey and differences due to its geographical origin. Czech Journal of Food Sciences 33 (2), 156–164.

Valentini, A., Miquel, C., Taberlet, P., 2010. DNA barcoding for honey biodiversity. Diversity 2 (4), 610–617.

Von der Ohe, W., Persano Oddo, L., Piana, M.L., Morlot, M., Martin, P., 2004. Harmonized methods of melissopalynology. Apidologie 35, S18–S25.

Wang, J., Li, Q.X., 2011. Honey chemical composition, characterization, and differentiation. Advances in Food and Nutrition Research 62, 89–137.

Wang, S., Guo, Q., Wang, L., Lin, L., Shi, H., Cao, H., Cao, B., 2015. Detection of honey adulteration with starch syrup by high performance liquid chromatography. Food Chemistry 172, 669–674.

White, J.W., Winters, K., 1989. Honey protein as internal standard for stable carbon isotope ratio detection of adulteration honey. Journal of the Association of Official Analytical Chemists 72, 907–911.

White, J.S., 2008. Straight talk about high-fructose corn syrup: what it is and what it ain't. American Journal of Clinical Nutrition 88 (6), 1716S–1721S.

Woodcock, T., Downey, G., O'Donnell, C., 2009. Near infrared spectral fingerprinting for confirmation of claimed PDO provenance of honey. Food Chemistry 114 (2), 742–746.

Xue, X., Wang, Q., Li, Y., Wu, L., Chen, L., Zhao, J., Liu, F., 2013. 2-Acetylfuran-3-Glucopyranoside as a novel marker for the detection of honey adulterated with rice syrup. Journal of Agricultural and Food Chemistry 61, 7488–7493.

Yilmaz, M.T., Tatlisu, N.B., Toker, O.S., Karaman, S., Dertli, E., Sagdic, O., Arici, M., 2014. Steady, dynamic and creep rheological analysis as a novel approach to detect honey adulteration by fructose and saccharose syrups: correlations with HPLC-RID results. Food Research International 64, 634–646.

Yücel, Y., Sultanoğlu, P., 2013. Characterization of Hatay honeys according to their multi-element analysis using ICP-OES combined with chemometrics. Food Chemistry 140 (1–2), 231–237.

Zábrodská, B., Vorlová, L., 2014. Adulteration of honey and available methods for detection – a review. Acta Veterinaria Brno 83, S85–S102.

Zhao, J., Du, X., Cheng, N., Chen, L., Zue, X., Ahzo, J., Wu, L., Cao, W., 2016. Identification of monofloral honeys using HPLC-ECD and chemometrics. Food Chemistry 194, 167–174.

Zhou, J., Qid, Y., Ritho, J., Duan, L., Wu, L., Diao, Q., Li, Y., Zhao, J., 2014. Analysis of maltooligosaccharides in honey samples by ultra-performance liquid chromatography coupled with evaporative light scattering detection. Food Research International 56, 260–265.

Zhu, X., Li, S., Shan, Y., Zhang, Z., Li, G., Su, D., Liu, F., 2010. Detection of adulterants such as sweeteners materials in honey using near-infrared spectroscopy and chemometrics. Journal of Food Engineering 101 (1), 92–97.

Index

'*Note:* Page numbers followed by "f" indicate figures and "t" indicate tables.'

E

H

J

K

O

P

Q

S